Trail Guide to the Body

Seventh Edition

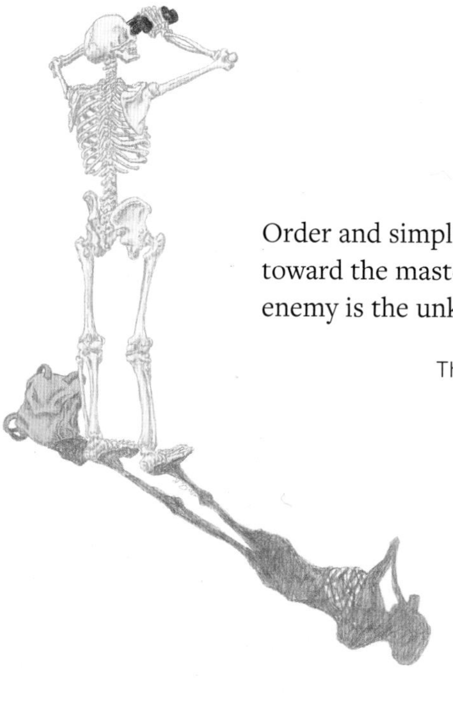

Order and simplification are the first steps toward the mastery of a subject—the actual enemy is the unknown.

Thomas Mann, *The Magic Mountain*

Since 1997, the mission of Books of Discovery has been to bring health care providers around the world the very best learning tools for anatomy, palpation, kinesiology, physiology, and pathology. It is always gratifying to know that a high school athlete in Florida, a first-time mother in Vancouver, or a journeyman bricklayer in Liverpool has received quality care from a practitioner who has benefited from our products.

We believe clear and practical information about the human body should be available to everyone—student, practitioner, patient, and layperson. It is, after all, where we live, and a better understanding can only strengthen how we move, think, and feel. This belief inspires us to serve individuals and schools all across the globe each and every day. Best wishes and happy trails.

Andrew Biel, Founder
Books of Discovery

Books of Discovery's products are manufactured with soy-based ink, and we strive to produce books in an environmentally friendly and socially responsible manner. Since 1997 we have donated more than $100,000 to reforestation and conservation projects.

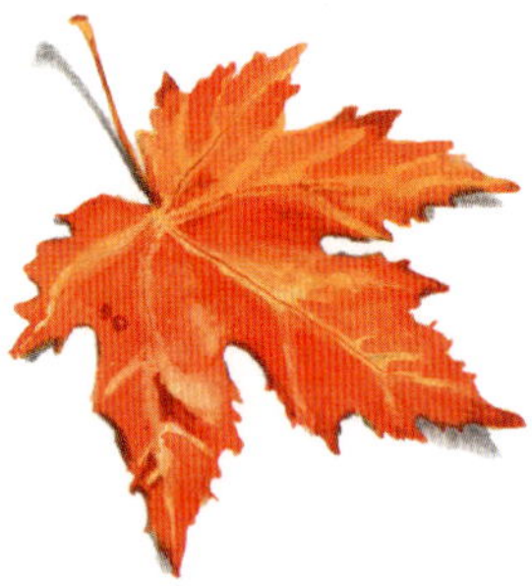

Trail Guide to the Body

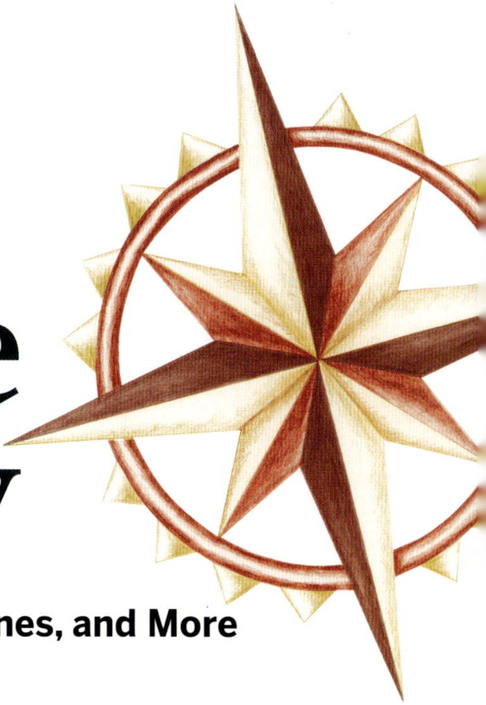

A Hands-On Guide to Locating Muscles, Bones, and More

Seventh Edition

Andrew Biel

Illustrations by Robin Dorn

Seventh Edition

Books of Discovery
Boulder, Colorado USA
booksofdiscovery.com
800.775.9227

Printed in China

ISBN: 978-0-9987850-7-3

10 9 8 7 6 5 4 3 2 1

Grateful acknowledgment is made to reprint an excerpt from:
The Magic Mountain by Thomas Mann
Copyright 1927. Used by permission of Random House, Inc., Alfred Knopf, Inc., Publisher

Excerpt from “Little Gidding” in *Four Quartets*, copyright 1942 by T.S. Eliot and renewed 1970 by Esme Valerie Eliot, reprinted by permission of Houghton Mifflin Harcourt Publishing Company

Author photo by Ross Pruden

Design and composition: Jessica Xavier, Planet X Design
Colorist: Dana Ecklund

Contents

3 Forearm & Hand 105

4 Spine & Thorax 167

5 Head, Neck & Face 225

7 Leg & Foot 347

Acknowledgments

The long and winding path of creation is often strewn with boulders and lacking in signposts. Luckily my path was cleared by the sharp machetes of many expert field guides and hiking partners.

It is always a pleasure to work with an artist as committed and talented as Robin Dorn. A heartfelt nod of gratitude to Lyn Gregory for her encouragement, patience, and suggestions.

I was blessed to have a wonderful support team for the seventh edition: Many thanks to Jessica Xavier for her design concept and Dana Ecklund for his persistence and eye for detail. I don't know where I'd be without Books of Discovery's dynamic duo of Rhoni Hirst and Tim Herbert. Many thanks to the incredible BOD team of Linda Lee, Louisa McGarty, Tracy McDermott, Eva Sissener, Danielle Schroeder Kraft, Renee Malis, Michael Diehl, and Julia Hellerman.

Special thanks to Brenda Hadenfeldt for editing the text and to Alan Bernhard, our managing editor, for helping us keep on track.

Much gratitude to Adrienne Asta, Katherine Brady, Gabe Byars, Debra Curties, Lisa Dubroff, Ruth Ford, David Freker, Eric Fuchs, Margo Greicar, Reed Handerly, Susanne Higgins, Chad Howland, Amelia Iams, Andrew Jurdan, Mari Knettle, Jeff Leatherman, Vic Liberi, Whitney Lowe, Kelly Lumpkin, Arlene Moskowitz, Maj Lis Nash, Lisa Nelson, Sunny Nilchavee, Marnie Vanden Noven, Nora St. John, Katherine Schofield, Nate Short, Bob Stow, Tracy Sullivan, Joey Swearingen, Donna Sweeney, Teresa Tetting, Jordan Tucker, and Colin Wallace.

The modeling and photography could not have happened without the patience of Bob "Obo" Baker, Charlie Chilson, Jason Glunt, Alex Gregory, Kennedy Hirst, Johanna Kasten, Nathan Musselman, Matt Samet, and Jennifer Spinelli.

Continued thanks to Paul and Aileen Biel, Jennifer Booksh, Kate Bromley, Clint Chandler, Robert Karman, Chris Maisto, Jackie Phillips, Marty Ryan, Anthony Sayre, and Diana Thompson.

I am very grateful to the following people for their expertise, research, and encouragement: Leon Chaitow, Sandy Fritz, John White, Sharon Babcock, Cynthia Christy, Ann Ekes, Daniel Gebo, Jim Holland, George C. Kent, Don Kelley, Lee Haines, Mary Marzke, Susan Parke, and John Zurhourek. Special thanks to Lurana Bain and Dr. Tawny Chamberlain for helping to develop the chapter openers.

Thank you also to Adam Bailey, Jessica Basamanowicz, Nancy Benerofe, Alexis Brereton, Deb Brockman, Mary Bryan, Patrick Bufi, Sylvia Burns, Kendra Busby, Kirk Butler, Sean Castor, Thomas Crown, Kathryn Dean, Kathy Eike, Jessica Elliott, Jean Marie Fay, Vicky Fosie, Dawn Fosse, Joanne Fowler, Gaye Franklin, Joanna Gardner, Christina Goehrig, Steve Goldstein, Laura Goularte, Alyce Green-Davis, Leslie Grounds, Joanne Guidici, Petra Guyer, Nicholas Hammersley, Debra Harrison, Anne Hartshorn, Meghan Heath, Carrie Henderson, Ian Hubner, Melissa Iverson, Mary Lynn Jackson, Leslie Jowett, Alison Kim, Erica King, Kimberly Kiriaki, Elinore Knutson, Beth Langston, Dave Lawrence, Kate McConnell, Becky Masters, Audra Meador, Chris Meier, Sandy Merrell, Steve Miller, Elizabeth Milliken, Debra Nelli, Eric Newberg, Rama Newton, Sally Nurney, Dave Oder, Jillian Orton, Anita Quinton, Dee Reeder, Coleen Renee, Obie Roe, Penny Rosen, Thea Satrom, Janice Schwartz, Sare Selko, Gerald Sexton, Joy Shaw, Penelope Thompson, Jaime Tousignant, Danny Tseng, Zdenka Vargas, Brian Weyand, Damon Williams, Ashley Wilson, Cynthia Wold, and Pantelis Zafiriou.

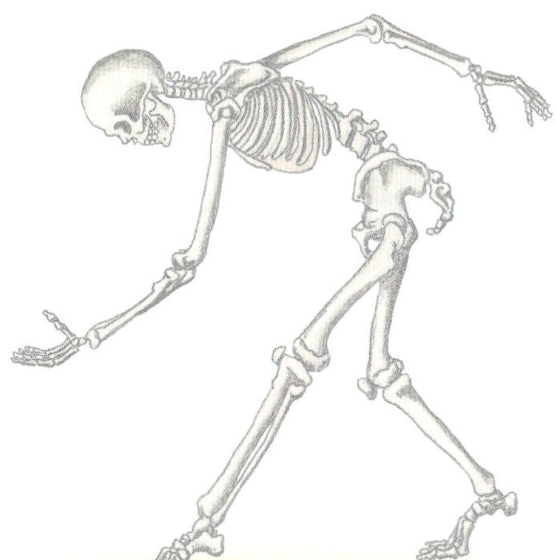

Preface

We shall not cease from exploration
And the end of all our exploring
Will be to arrive where we started
And know the place for the first time.

T. S. Eliot, *Four Quartets*

Many years ago, as a skinny ten-year-old, I remember pinching the flesh under my armpit only to accidentally locate a muscle. When I moved my arm in a certain way, the flesh would harden and slip into my fingers. "Wow," I said to myself. "I didn't think I *had* any muscles!"

I told my parents about my discovery, and they suggested that I check the encyclopedia (this was long before Google) to see which muscle I had found. The Latin names I encountered only confused me, but for months I showed everyone I met my one and only muscle.

I continued to be fascinated with the parts and pieces of the body and with how these all seemed to work together to produce movement, breath, even life itself. During my training as a bodyworker, I learned that the mysterious muscle of my armpit was the latissimus dorsi. Soon I learned how to palpate other muscles as well as the various tendons, bones, and tissues located throughout the body. I also realized the importance of palpation for tissue assessment and for performing safe and effective manual therapy techniques.

Later, as an instructor of bodywork and palpatory anatomy, I became familiar with many books describing and illustrating the anatomy of the body. I found few, however, that demonstrated how to locate and explore the body's structures manually. *Trail Guide to the Body* is designed to do just that: to teach you to map, navigate, and "gain your bearings" on the human body.

In preparation for any journey, it helps if you know the lay of the land you will be traveling. For every health care provider, a thorough understanding of the location and interrelationship of the body's structures is essential. The "hands-on" practitioner, however, cannot merely take a guided bus tour of the body, viewing it from afar and only hearing of its amazing qualities. She must undertake instead the actual/physical exploration through a geography that is never exactly the same on any two individuals. Rolling up her sleeves, she must rely on her hands and her senses to learn about the most challenging and fascinating of all terrains—the human body.

So, welcome! You are about to embark on the journey of a lifetime with this book as your trusty guide.

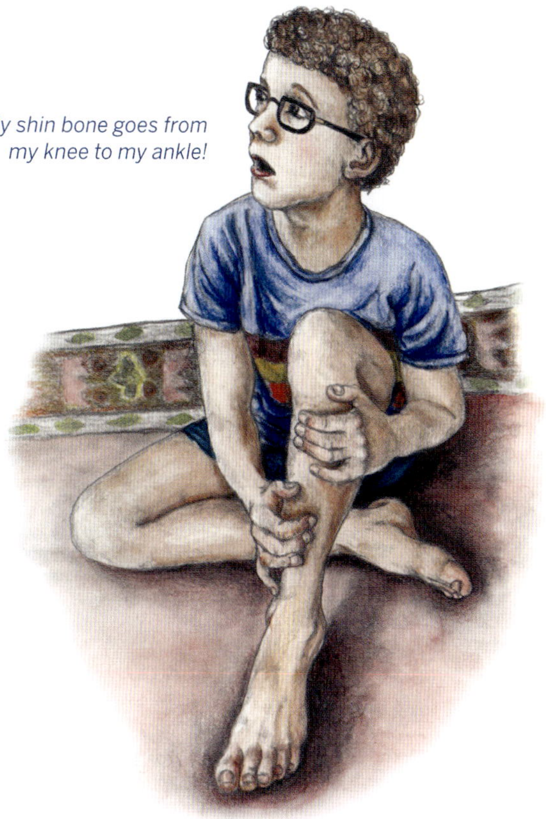

How to Use This Book

***Trail Guide to the Body* has seven chapters,** six of which focus on different regions of the body. In each of these six chapters, the topographical contours that can be seen on the surface of the skin and exercises to explore the skin and fascia are outlined first (**a**).

These are followed by the bones and bony landmarks (the bone's hills, dips, and ridges) (**b**).

Then the muscles of the region are presented (**c**).

Finally, other structures, such as ligaments, nerves, arteries, and lymph nodes, are accessed (**d**).

a

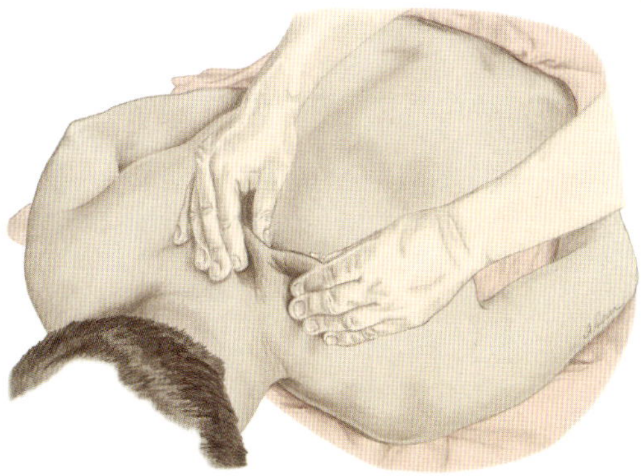

2.4 Partner prone, as you lift and twist the tissue of the upper back

b

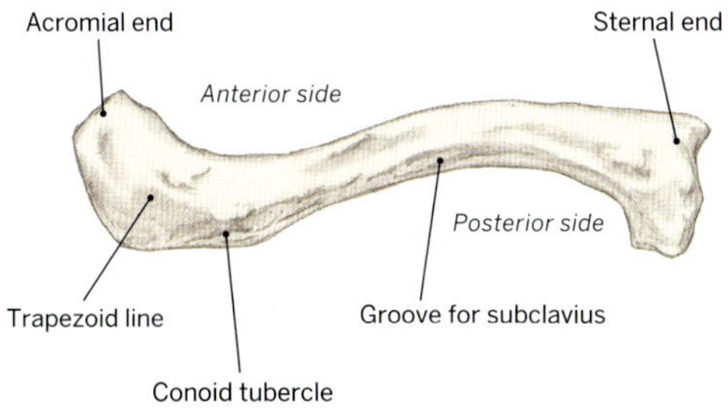

2.13 Inferior view of right clavicle

c

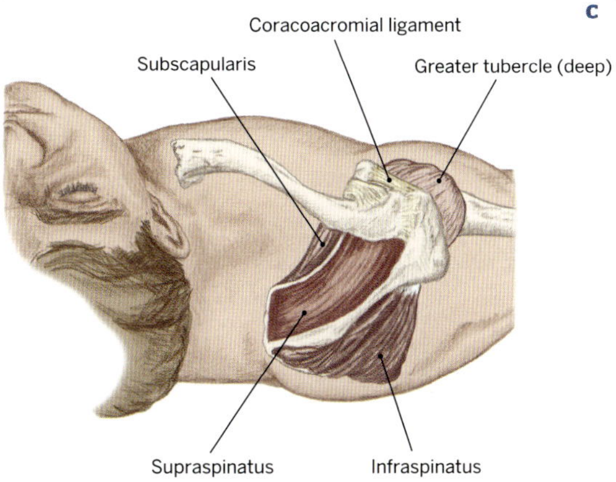

2.78 Superior view of right shoulder, showing rotator cuff muscles

d

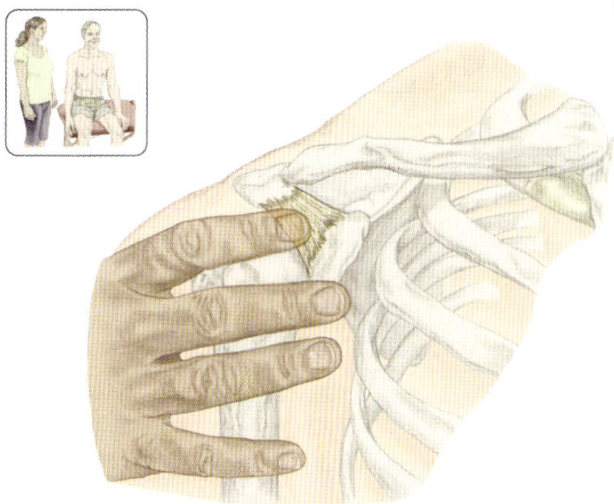

2.139 Anterior view of right shoulder, as you palpate the coracoacromial ligament

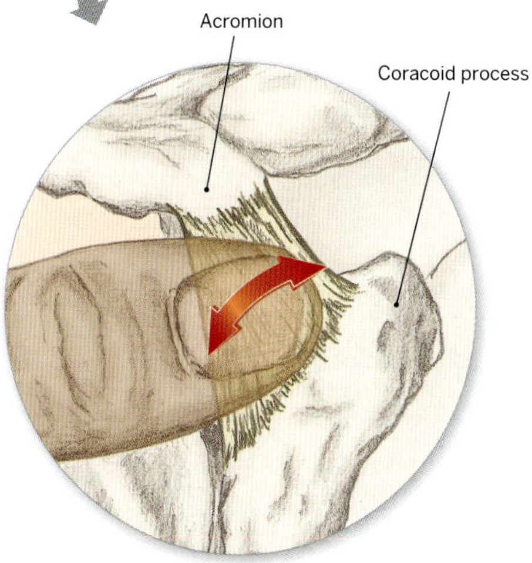

Palpation Framework

The textbook is designed around the following scenario: You follow along with the text and palpate on a partner (friend or classmate) who is on a bodywork table or seated in a chair. Step-by-step instructions walk you through the palpation process for each structure (**e**).

The bony landmarks highlighted in the text can be thought of as "trail markers." They are used as stepping-off points to locate muscles and tendons. Wherever possible, a region's bony landmarks have been strung together to form a trail (**f**).

These trails are designed to help you understand the connections between structures. Without a path to follow, you, the traveler, would be lost in a jungle of flesh and bones with no idea of your trail's location. You and your travel partner will find the journey more enjoyable and valuable if you have a trail to lead you to your destination point.

View the techniques described as helpful tour guides. When first palpating, it is best to follow the specific instructions. After you have located a structure, it is recommended that you adapt and explore other methods to find the approach that works best for you. Wherever possible, an optional method for locating a structure has been included (**g**).

e

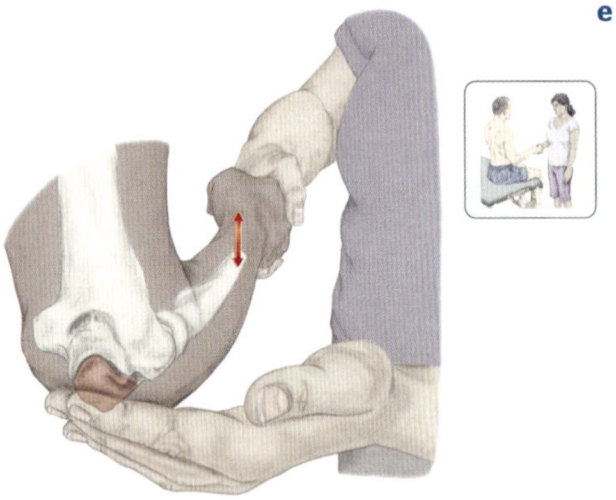

3.14 Posterior view of right elbow, as you palpate the olecranon process

Olecranon process

1. Partner seated. Shake hands with your partner and explore the large, superficial knob at the elbow. Palpate and explore its angular surface and sides.
2. Passively flex and extend the elbow, noticing how the olecranon process feels in various positions (**3.14**).

f

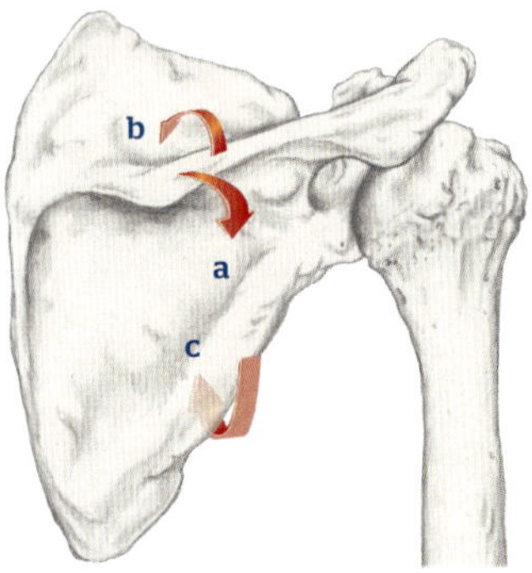

Trail 2 In the Trenches leaps off the spine of the scapula and sinks into the three basins of the scapula.

a Infraspinous fossa
b Supraspinous fossa
c Subscapular fossa

g

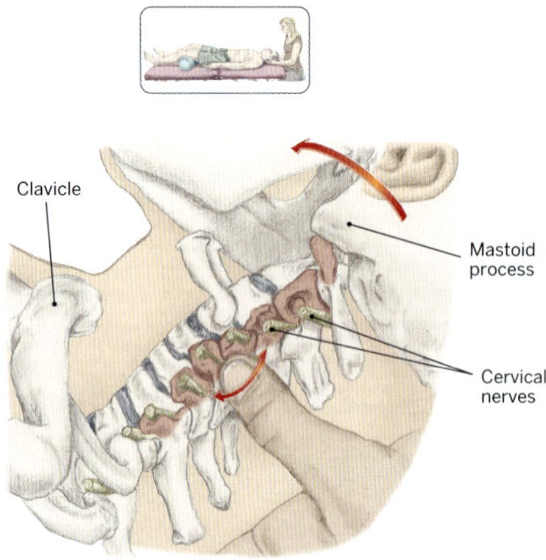

4.35 Partner supine, lateral view of neck with head *rotated away* from the side you are palpating

TVPs of cervicals

1. Partner supine. Place your fingers on the side of the neck below the earlobes.
2. Using your flat thumbpads, slide anteriorly and posteriorly to feel the ridge of TVPs. Explore the length of the neck (**4.34**).
3. You might not feel the tips of individual processes, but the ridge formed by the TVPs beneath the overlying tissue instead.

Are you palpating inferior to the earlobe? Do you feel a subtle ridge running down the side of the neck? If you passively flex, laterally flex, or rotate the neck, can you feel the TVPs move individually?

1. Partner supine. Rotate the head 45° to the right. With the head in this position, the TVPs form a line from the left mastoid process to the center of the shaft of the clavicle (**4.35**).
2. Draw an imaginary line from these two landmarks and visualize and palpate the TVPs along the path.

h

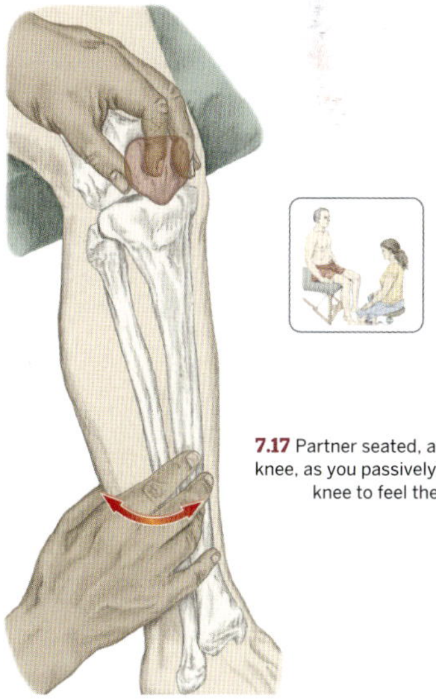

7.17 Partner seated, anterior view of right knee, as you passively flex and extend the knee to feel the patella shift

If you are a student, you are advised to proceed step by step, repeat certain methods when necessary, and explore the body along the way. If you are a more experienced practitioner, you may want to pick and choose your destinations. As with any worthwhile journey, veering off course to explore other areas often leads to wonderful discoveries. Please feel free to veer.

The procedures outlined are gentle and rarely uncomfortable, yet it is best to practice on an individual with no serious health conditions. Your partner may either wear loose, thin clothing or be undressed and draped with a sheet to enable you to palpate more easily.

Sometimes your partner will be asked to lie or sit passively on the table (**h**). At other times, she may be asked to move a limb, bend a joint, or contract a group of muscles. These movements should be done smoothly and according to the specific instructions of the text to enable you to explore the region thoroughly.

Talk to your partner before palpating so she will understand her role. Also, clarify beforehand which areas of the body you would like to palpate and explore so she will know what to expect.

Learning Objectives

Following this user's guide section, you will find the section of Learning Objectives. Use these as your goals for building skills and developing knowledge as you explore each chapter.

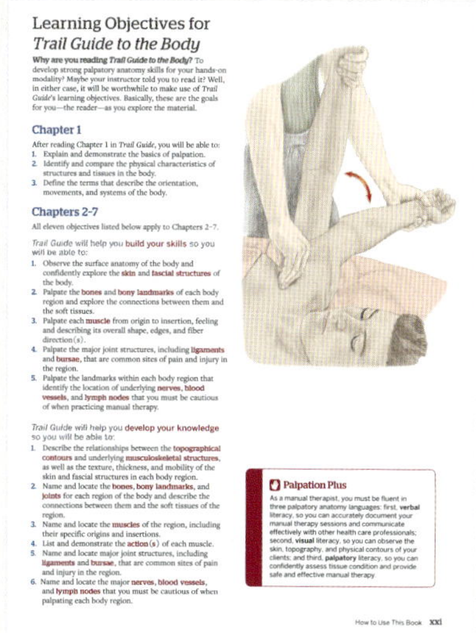

Learning Objectives for *Trail Guide to the Body*

Why are you reading *Trail Guide to the Body*? To develop strong palpatory anatomy skills for your hands-on modality? Maybe your instructor told you to read it? Well, in either case, it will be worthwhile to make use of *Trail Guide*'s learning objectives. Basically, these are the goals for you—the reader—as you explore the material.

Chapter 1

After reading Chapter 1 in *Trail Guide*, you will be able to:

1. Explain and demonstrate the basics of palpation.
2. Identify and compare the physical characteristics of structures and tissues in the body.
3. Define the terms that describe the orientation, movements, and systems of the body.

Chapters 2-7

All eleven objectives listed below apply to Chapters 2-7.

Trail Guide will help you **build your skills** so you will be able to:

1. Observe the surface anatomy of the body and confidently explore the **skin** and **fascial structures** of the body.
2. Palpate the **bones** and **bony landmarks** of each body region and explore the connections between them and the soft tissues.
3. Palpate each **muscle** from origin to insertion, feeling and describing its overall shape, edges, and fiber direction(s).
4. Palpate the major joint structures, including **ligaments** and **bursae**, that are common sites of pain and injury in the region.
5. Palpate the landmarks within each body region that identify the location of underlying **nerves, blood vessels**, and **lymph nodes** that you must be cautious of when practicing manual therapy.

Trail Guide will help you **develop your knowledge** so you will be able to:

1. Describe the relationships between the **topographical contours** and underlying **musculoskeletal structures**, as well as the texture, thickness, and mobility of the skin and fascial structures in each body region.
2. Name and locate the **bones, bony landmarks**, and **joints** for each region of the body and describe the connections between them and the soft tissues of the region.
3. Name and locate the **muscles** of the region, including their specific origins and insertions.
4. List and demonstrate the **action**(s) of each muscle.
5. Name and locate major joint structures, including **ligaments** and **bursae**, that are common sites of pain and injury in the region.
6. Name and locate the major **nerves, blood vessels**, and **lymph nodes** that you must be cautious of when palpating each body region.

Palpation Plus

As a manual therapist, you must be fluent in three palpatory anatomy languages: first, **verbal** literacy, so you can accurately document your manual therapy sessions and communicate effectively with other health care professionals; second, **visual** literacy, so you can observe the skin, topography, and physical contours of your clients; and third, **palpatory** literacy, so you can confidently assess tissue condition and provide safe and effective manual therapy.

How to Use This Book xxi

Chapter-Opening Features

Each chapter begins with a dynamic illustration of the body in motion, with select muscles of the body region highlighted. An opening story introduces the chapter and includes "See for yourself" activities to try out, and a chapter table of contents is provided for easy reference.

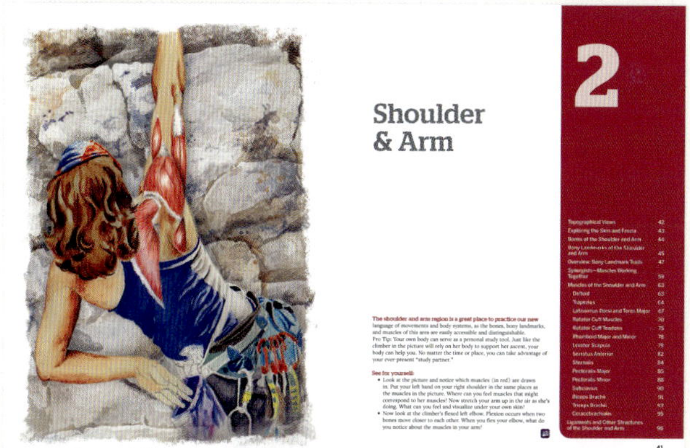

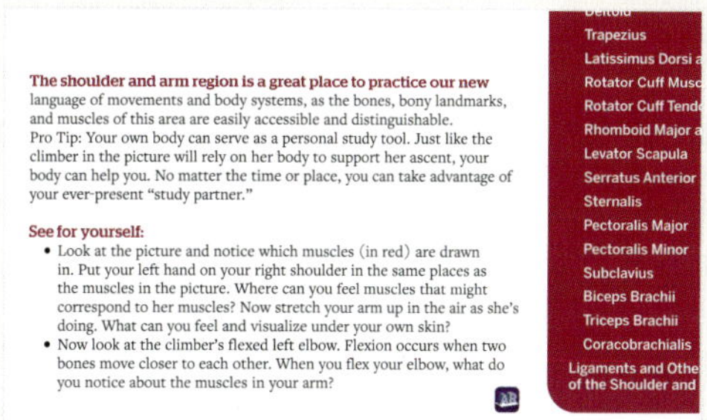

The shoulder and arm region is a great place to practice our new language of movements and body systems, as the bones, bony landmarks, and muscles of this area are easily accessible and distinguishable.
Pro Tip: Your own body can serve as a personal study tool. Just like the climber in the picture will rely on her body to support her ascent, your body can help you. No matter the time or place, you can take advantage of your ever-present "study partner."

See for yourself:

- Look at the picture and notice which muscles (in red) are drawn in. Put your left hand on your right shoulder in the same places as the muscles in the picture. Where can you feel muscles that might correspond to her muscles? Now stretch your arm up in the air as she's doing. What can you feel and visualize under your own skin?
- Now look at the climber's flexed left elbow. Flexion occurs when two bones move closer to each other. When you flex your elbow, what do you notice about the muscles in your arm?

Key

Name of structure

▶ indicates that a video clip is included in the "For Students" section of our website, booksofdiscovery.com

Introduction describing a structure's function, depth, and relationship to other structures

A table of the **A**ction, **O**rigin, **I**nsertion, and **N**erve innervation of the muscle. The primary action is listed first. The predominant spinal nerve levels are in **bold**.

O and **I** Illustration showing the **Origin** and **Insertion**

Activities when this muscle is activated or recruited

Muscles of the Forearm and Hand

Forearm & Hand

Brachialis ▶

The brachialis is a strong elbow flexor that lies deep to the biceps brachii (p. 91) on the anterior arm (**3.70**, **3.71**). It has a flat yet thick belly. Ironically, however, the brachialis's girth only helps the biceps to bulge further from the arm, making brachialis the biceps's best friend.

Although it lies underneath the biceps, portions of the brachialis are accessible. Its lateral edge, sandwiched between the biceps and triceps brachii, is superficial and palpable. The distal aspect of the brachialis is also accessible as it passes along either side of the biceps tendon.

BRACHIALIS	
A	**Flex** the elbow (humeroulnar joint)
O	Distal half of anterior surface of humerus
I	Tuberosity and coronoid process of ulna
N	Musculocutaneous, small branch from radial C**5**, **6**

When Do You Use Your Brachialis?

- Bringing food from the plate to your mouth
- Picking up a load of anatomy books
- Carrying a baby's car seat

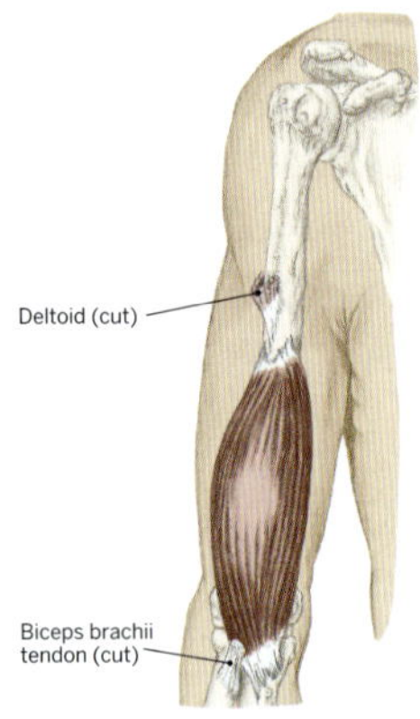

3.70 Anterior view of right arm, showing brachialis

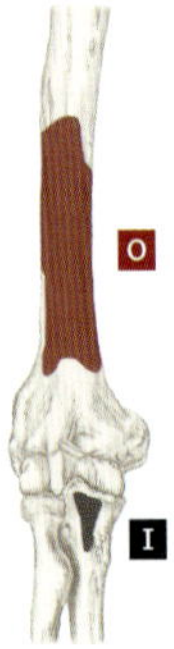

3.71 Anterior view of right arm, showing origin and insertion of brachialis

Step-by-step instructions on how to **palpate** a structure

"Check It" questions will confirm your location. They may ask you about your location in relation to a nearby structure or ask you or your partner to create a movement. Unless otherwise indicated, the answer to each question should be "Yes!"

Alternative palpatory routes

Pronunciation and **etymology** of anatomical terms

Look for **Mr. Bones** sharing cautionary advice or other helpful hints.

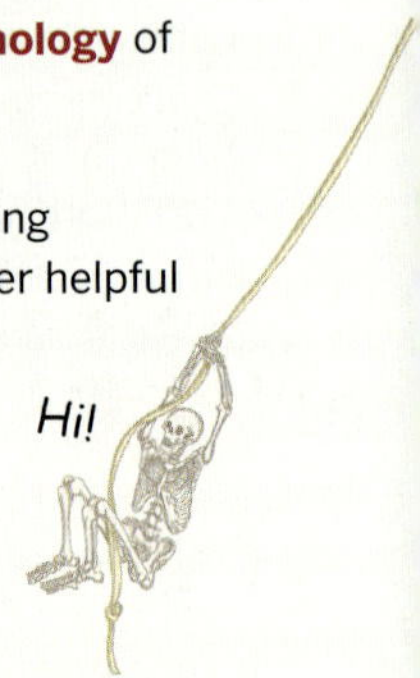

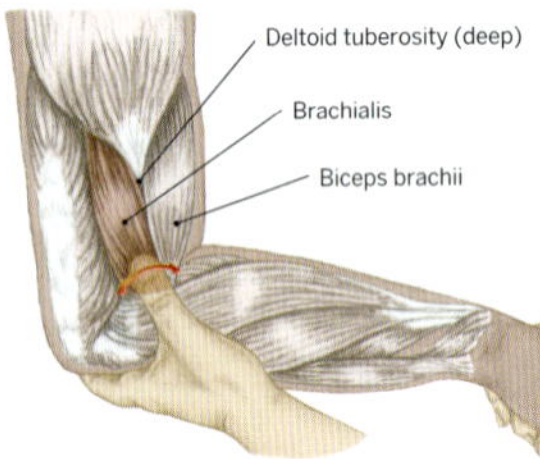

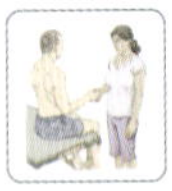

3.72 Lateral view of right forearm, as you strum across the edge of brachialis

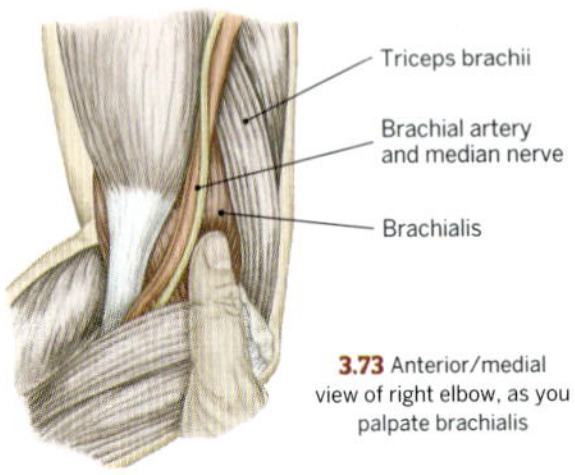

3.73 Anterior/medial view of right elbow, as you palpate brachialis

Brachialis

1. Shake hands with your partner and flex the elbow to 90°. Distinguishing the muscle tissue of the biceps brachii from that of the brachialis is important. Ask your partner to flex her elbow against your resistance and isolate the edges of the round biceps brachii belly.
2. With the arm relaxed, slide laterally half an inch off the distal biceps. The edge of the brachialis can be detected by rolling your fingers across its surface. As you strum across its solid edge, you will feel a pronounced "thump" (**3.72**).
3. Continuing to strum across its edge, follow it distally to where it disappears into the elbow.
4. Locate the distal biceps tendon. Palpate along either side of the tendon for portions of the deeper brachialis (**3.73**).

Can you roll across a distinct wad of muscle on the lateral side of the arm? Can you follow it distally toward the inner elbow? Locate the triceps and biceps brachii. Are the brachialis fibers between them on the lateral arm?

Locate the deltoid tuberosity. Slide distally straight down the lateral side of the arm and explore for the edge of the brachialis.

brachial	*bray-key-al*	L. relating to the arm
brachialis	*bray-key-al-is*	

130 Trail Guide to the Body

Look for insets that accompany many of the figures. These show either a zoomed-out view of where an illustrated structure is located in the body or the positions of you and your partner.

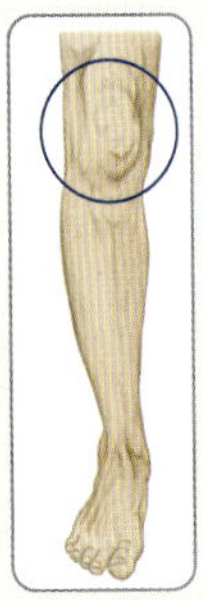

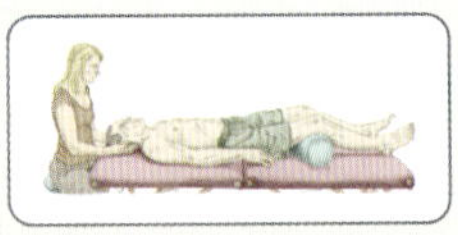

AOIN Tables and OI Illustrations

The AOIN tables are quick guides to the **A**ction, **O**rigin, **I**nsertion, and **N**erve innervation of a muscle. The primary action is listed first, and the predominant spinal nerve levels are highlighted in **bold**. Also included are examples of activities and movements in which the body uses the muscle. Accompanying illustrations show the **Origin** and **Insertion** attachment sites.

	TERES MAJOR
A	**Extend** the shoulder (glenohumeral joint) **Adduct** the shoulder (G/H joint) **Medially rotate** the shoulder (G/H joint)
O	Inferior angle and lower one-third of lateral border of the scapula
I	Crest of the lesser tubercle of the humerus
N	Lower subscapular C5, **6**, 7

When Do You Use Your Teres Major?

- Unzipping the back of your dress
- Walking with crutches
- Climbing up a rope when storming a castle

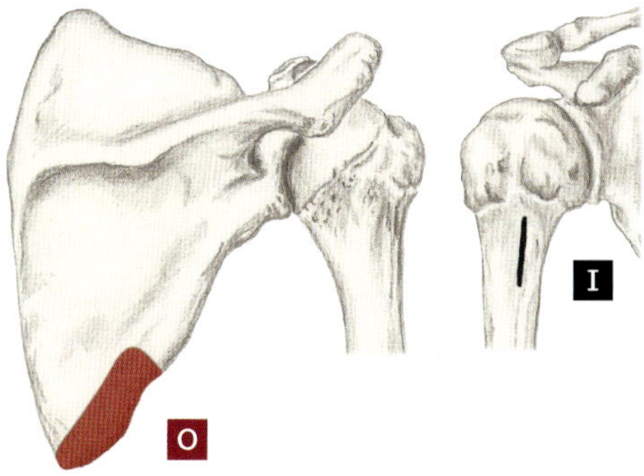

2.68 Posterior view (left) and anterior view (right) of right shoulder, showing origin and insertion of teres major

Palpation Plus

Palpation Plus features offer a variety of palpation tips and information, such as how to locate additional structures, how to differentiate muscles that are close together, and how to ensure a comfortable palpation experience for both you and your partner.

> **Palpation Plus**
>
> When the neck is flexed, the spinous process of C-7 shifts superiorly. T-1, however, is buckled in by the first ribs and does not move. With your partner seated, place a finger on the spinous processes of C-7 and T-1. Have your partner slowly flex his neck and observe both processes. Does C-7 tilt superiorly while T-1 is stationary?

Discover More

For historical notes, interesting facts, and supplemental information, check out the Discover More features. Who discovered that blood circulates throughout the body? How many miles of arteries, veins, and capillaries does a human have? What is the most frequently used joint in the body? Discover More will tell you!

> **Discover More**
>
> C-6 has a large anterior tubercle called the carotid tubercle. Its name corresponds to the carotid artery (p. 271) that passes immediately lateral to it. Although you would not want to, you can occlude the carotid artery by placing your finger lateral to the cricoid cartilage and pressing in a posterior direction against the carotid tubercle. Long ago this dramatic maneuver was used in emergency rooms as a last-ditch effort to stem hemorrhaging inside the skull.

Comparative Anatomy

Learn how the anatomy of humans and other living creatures are similar or different in the Comparative Anatomy features. From ants, bees, and reptiles to dogs, cats, horses, and giraffes, many different critters are highlighted, along with interesting evolutionary developments.

> **Comparative Anatomy**
>
> The pisiform is much larger on quadrupeds such as dogs (right), on whom it protrudes posteriorly above the heel of the front paw. This arrangement allows the flexor carpi ulnaris muscle that attaches to the pisiform greater leverage and power to flex the wrist when running on all fours. A human's pisiform is only a pea-sized knob. It is, nevertheless, still useful for kneading bread dough.

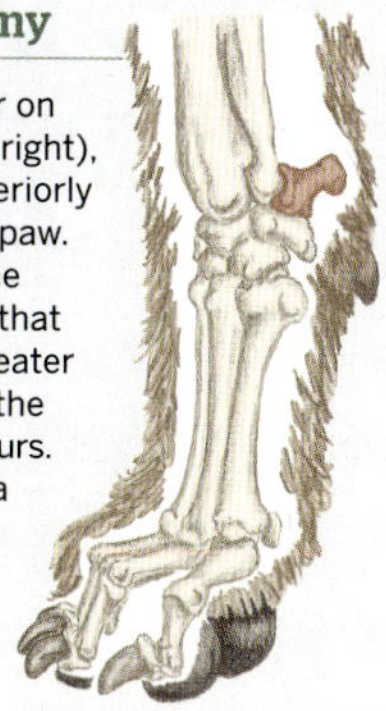

Synergists—Muscles Working Together

Each body region chapter includes sections of Synergists—Muscles Working Together to show how muscles work together to create movements, such as flexion, extension, abduction, adduction, pronation, supination, and rotation. Complete lists of synergists are also found in Appendix C.

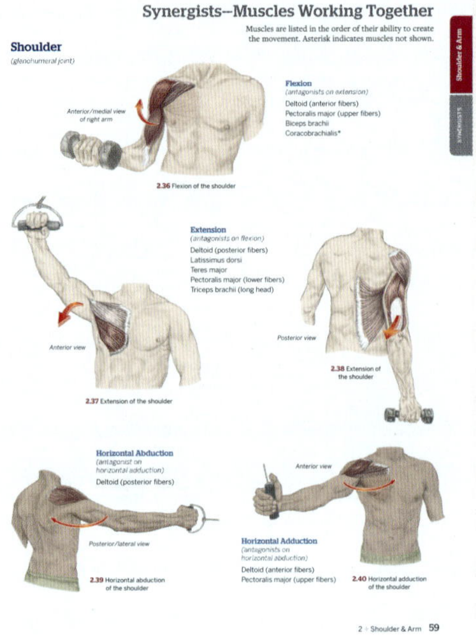

Appendixes

A Day in the Life of Your Nervous System

New to this edition is a detailed and fully illustrated appendix that explores the nervous system. Interweaving a story of how a body makes use of the nervous system throughout a typical day, this section covers the organization of the system, its components and distribution, dermatomes and myotomes, and proprioception and muscle function.

Muscles of Facial Expression Attachment Sites

This concise table summarizes the actions, origins, and insertions for muscles innervated by the facial nerve.

Synergists—Muscles Working Together

This section provides complete lists of synergists to summarize and expand on the Synergists sections within the chapters.

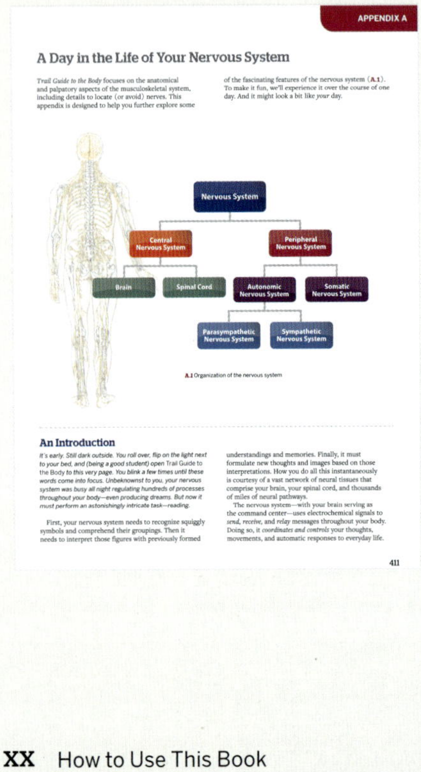

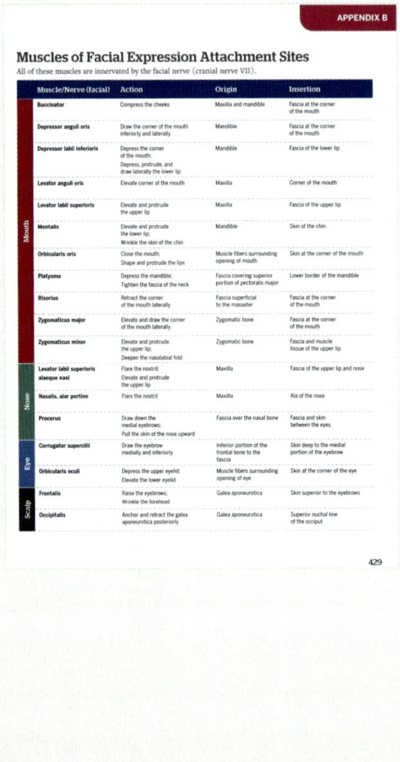

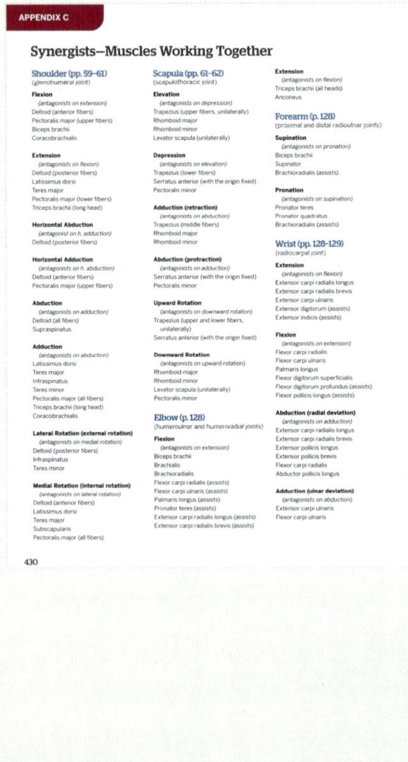

Learning Objectives for *Trail Guide to the Body*

Why are you reading *Trail Guide to the Body*? To develop strong palpatory anatomy skills for your hands-on modality? Maybe your instructor told you to read it? Well, in either case, it will be worthwhile to make use of *Trail Guide*'s learning objectives. Basically, these are the goals for you—the reader—as you explore the material.

Chapter 1

After reading Chapter 1 in *Trail Guide*, you will be able to:
1. Explain and demonstrate the basics of palpation.
2. Identify and compare the physical characteristics of structures and tissues in the body.
3. Define the terms that describe the orientation, movements, and systems of the body.

Chapters 2-7

All eleven objectives listed below apply to Chapters 2–7.

Trail Guide will help you **build your skills** so you will be able to:
1. Observe the surface anatomy of the body and confidently explore the **skin** and **fascial structures** of the body.
2. Palpate the **bones** and **bony landmarks** of each body region and explore the connections between them and the soft tissues.
3. Palpate each **muscle** from origin to insertion, feeling and describing its overall shape, edges, and fiber direction(s).
4. Palpate the major joint structures, including **ligaments** and **bursae**, that are common sites of pain and injury in the region.
5. Palpate the landmarks within each body region that identify the location of underlying **nerves**, **blood vessels**, and **lymph nodes** that you must be cautious of when practicing manual therapy.

Trail Guide will help you **develop your knowledge** so you will be able to:
1. Describe the relationships between the **topographical contours** and underlying **musculoskeletal structures**, as well as the texture, thickness, and mobility of the skin and fascial structures in each body region.
2. Name and locate the **bones**, **bony landmarks**, and **joints** for each region of the body and describe the connections between them and the soft tissues of the region.
3. Name and locate the **muscles** of the region, including their specific origins and insertions.
4. List and demonstrate the **action(s)** of each muscle.
5. Name and locate major joint structures, including **ligaments** and **bursae**, that are common sites of pain and injury in the region.
6. Name and locate the major **nerves**, **blood vessels**, and **lymph nodes** that you must be cautious of when palpating each body region.

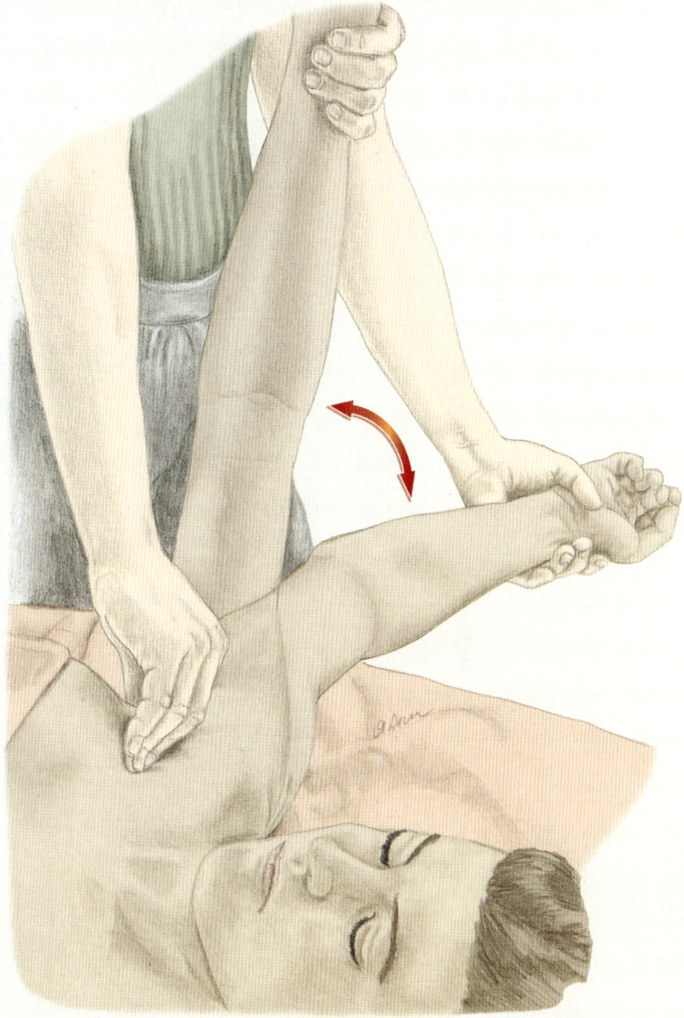

Palpation Plus

As a manual therapist, you must be fluent in three palpatory anatomy languages: first, **verbal** literacy, so you can accurately document your manual therapy sessions and communicate effectively with other health care professionals; second, **visual** literacy, so you can observe the skin, topography, and physical contours of your clients; and third, **palpatory** literacy, so you can confidently assess tissue condition and provide safe and effective manual therapy.

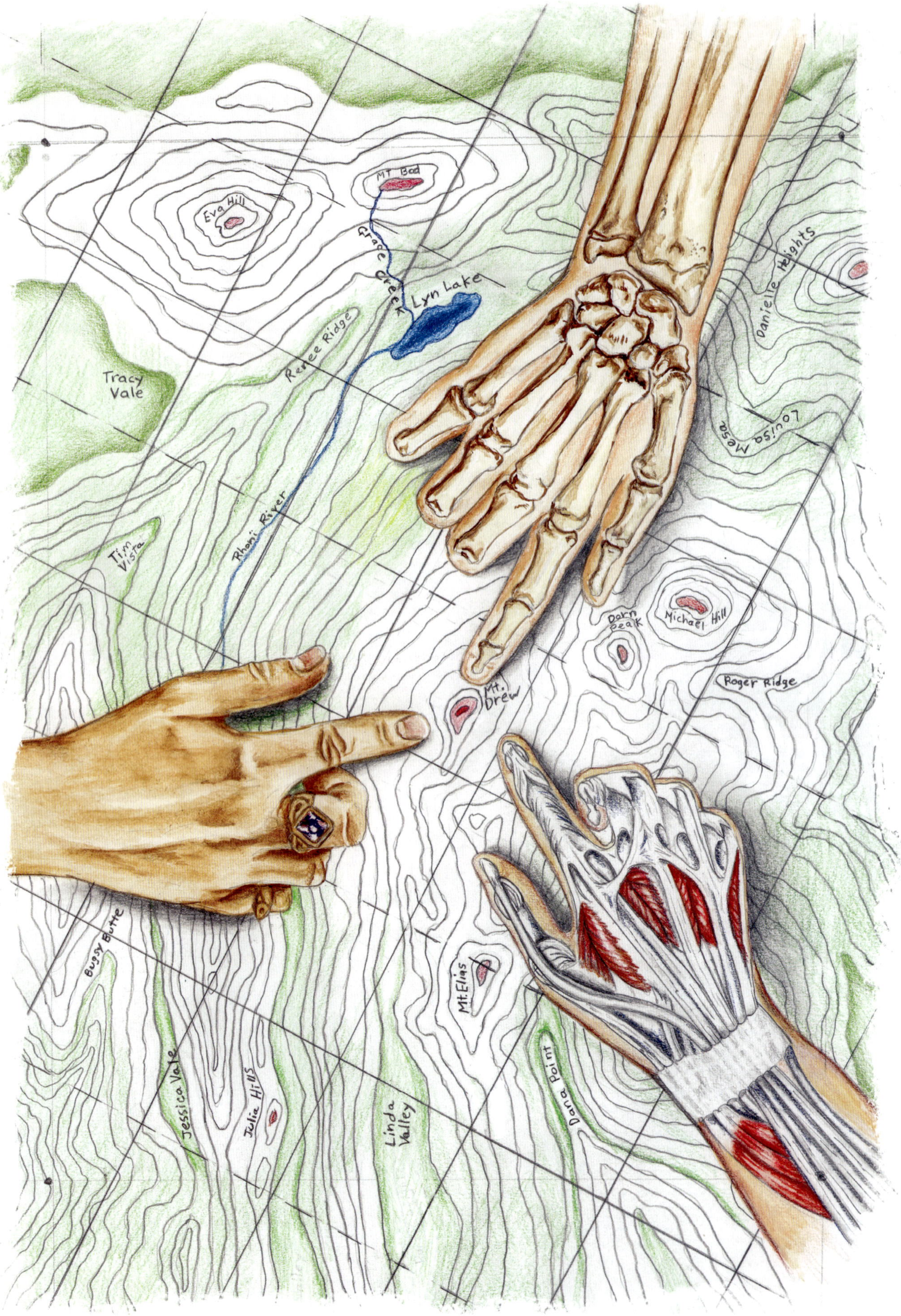
MT Bod
Eva Hill
Grace Creek
Lyn Lake
Renee Ridge
Tracy Vale
Danielle Heights
Louisa Mesa
Rhoni River
Tim Vista
Dorn Peak
Michael Hill
Mt. Drew
Roger Ridge
Bugsy Butte
Mt. Elias
Jessica Vale
Julia Hills
Linda Valley
Dana Point

1

Navigating the Body

Like a map-based app on your cell phone that helps you arrive at your destination, this book is your guide to navigating the human body. Instead of roads and intersections, you'll find hard surfaces (bones), meaty portions (muscles), and knobby areas (joints), along with general shapes and textures.

We'll begin by learning the basics of palpation and different types of textures. Then we'll introduce some new words—terms that describe body regions, movements, and systems. Finally, we'll use palpation skills to explore those areas and the structures that produce movement of the body. Speaking of which, how well do you know your own body? It helps you carry a backpack, ride a bike, and brush your teeth. But have you considered all its different parts and how they work together? When we're very familiar with something, we say, "I know it like the back of my hand!" Let's see.

See for yourself:

- Look at your hand. Where is the skin the thickest? Thinnest? Why do you think the palm feels different from the back of your hand?
- Continue exploring your hand. Where can you see dark lines (veins) below the surface? How about structures that look like ropes (tendons) or hard knobs of bone that make up the joints?
- Look at your arm. As you bend and straighten your elbow, where can you see structures moving beneath the skin?

Palpation Basics ▶

Palpation means to examine or explore by touching (an organ or area of the body), usually as a diagnostic aid. It is an art and a skill that involves **(1) locating** a structure, **(2) becoming aware** of its characteristics, and **(3) assessing** its quality or condition so you can deter-mine how to treat it.

The first two aspects of palpation—locating and being attentive to the body's structures—require a thorough knowledge of functional anatomy and experience through mindful, hands-on practice. This is the focus of *Trail Guide to the Body*. Assessment—the third aspect of palpation—is a vast subject requiring a book of its own.

Because bodies come in a variety of sizes and shapes, it might seem unrealistic that one trail guide could apply to all of them. If the terrain is never the same, what is the use of a map? Even though the topography, shape, and proportion of each person are unique, the body's composition and structures are virtually identical on all individuals. The differences are simply qualitative: it is easy to find many structures on a person with a slender build and more challenging on a physique with bulky muscles or a large amount of adipose (fatty) tissue (**1.1**).

As an experience involving all the senses, **palpation requires receptive hands and fingers, open eyes, listening ears, calm breath, and a quiet mind.** As you explore the terrain and texture of the body, be sure to bring along all of your sensing tools.

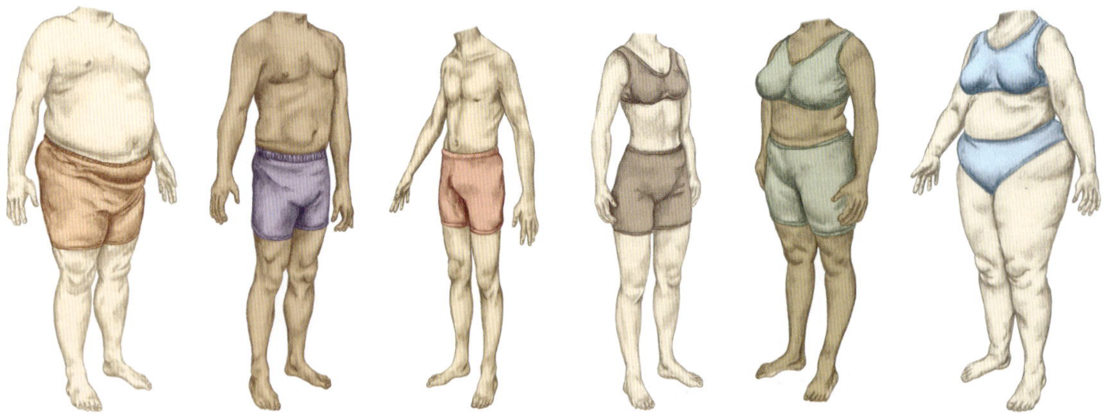

1.1 Each of us has a different body type; yet, even though our bodies are shaped differently, we all have the muscles, bones, and other tissues described in *Trail Guide to the Body.*

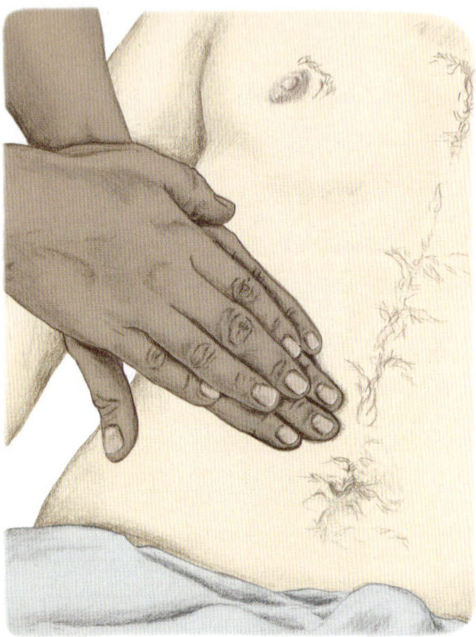

1.2 Using a firm top hand and a soft bottom hand

Making Contact

Let your hands and fingers be **responsive** and **sensitive**. Relaxed, patient hands will allow the body's contours, temperature, and structures to come more easily into your awareness.

For greater sensitivity and stability, **try laying one hand upon the other**, using the top hand to create the necessary pressure while the bottom hand remains relaxed (**1.2**). This will allow the bottom hand to stay receptive as the top hand directs movement and depth.

Smaller structures can be located by using one or two fingertips (**1.3**). **Larger structures** are best palpated with your whole hand. By sculpting out all of the sides and edges, full-hand contact helps to define the complete shape of a region or structure and also allows for a greater understanding of the interrelationships of structures (**1.4**). When palpating, you may want to **close your eyes** (**1.5**) periodically to enhance your awareness.

▶ indicates that a video clip is included in the "For Students" section of our website, booksofdiscovery.com

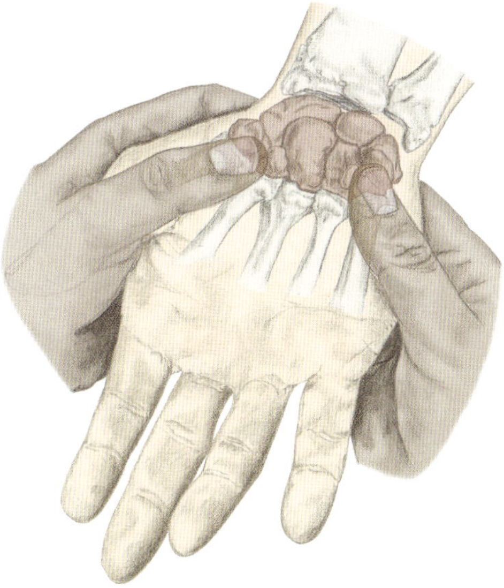

1.3 Using your thumbpads to explore the small carpal bones in the wrist

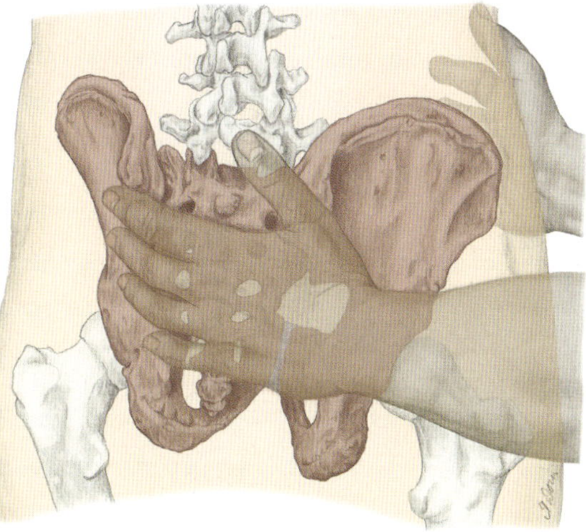

1.4 Using your entire hand to palpate the pelvis and sacrum

Working Hard vs. Working Smart

Often in the excitement of trying to locate something (whether it be a muscle or a set of car keys), you search so earnestly that your mental and physical awareness begins to diminish. Frustration arises, your breath stalls, and your hands ultimately become insensitive. You begin to work hard. Instead of working hard, you can work smart by reading the information about the structure before you palpate. Also, as you palpate, visualize what you are trying to access and verbalize to your partner what you are feeling.

Work smart by first locating the structure you wish to palpate on your own body before palpating it on your partner's. Self-palpation will improve your kinesthetic understanding of what you are looking for on your partner. Also, read the information aloud. Hearing the language as you are reading the text will improve your understanding and retention of the information.

Lastly, be patient with your learning process. Allow yourself to "make a wrong turn and get lost" on the body. Chances are you are close to what you are seeking. By letting your senses recognize the body's trail signs, you will get to where you want to be.

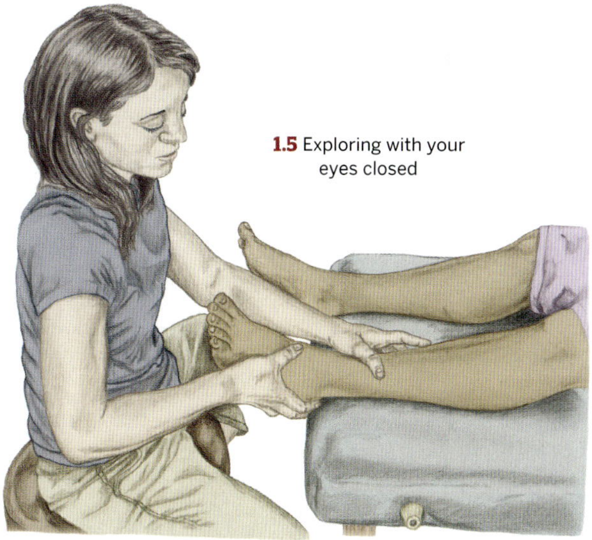

1.5 Exploring with your eyes closed

Less Is More

As you begin exploring the body, you might not be able to access things as readily as you wish. A common reaction is to press harder and deeper with your hands and fingers. However, instead of pushing into the muscles and other tissues, try to invite the tissues into your hands. Gentle contact will allow your hands to be sensitive, whereas excessive pushing only numbs the fingers, making for an uncomfortable experience for your partner (**1.6**).

Even deep structures are best accessed with mild pressure. Paradoxically, the deeper you move into the body, the slower and softer your touch needs to be. Ultimately, palpation at different levels of the body is not a question of pressure, but of intention. Having a clear intention as you seek out various structures will make for an easier, smoother journey.

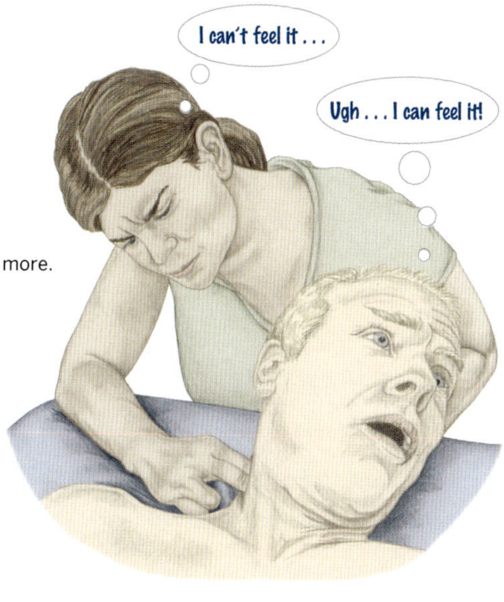

1.6 Less is more.

Rolling and Strumming

When outlining the shape or edge of a bone, try rolling your fingers or thumb **across**, rather than **along**, its surface. This is similar to checking the sharpness of a knife by sliding your finger across the blade. Do the same with the ropy fibers of muscle tissue. Like strumming the strings of a guitar, this method will help you ascertain the muscle's fiber direction and tensile state (**1.7**).

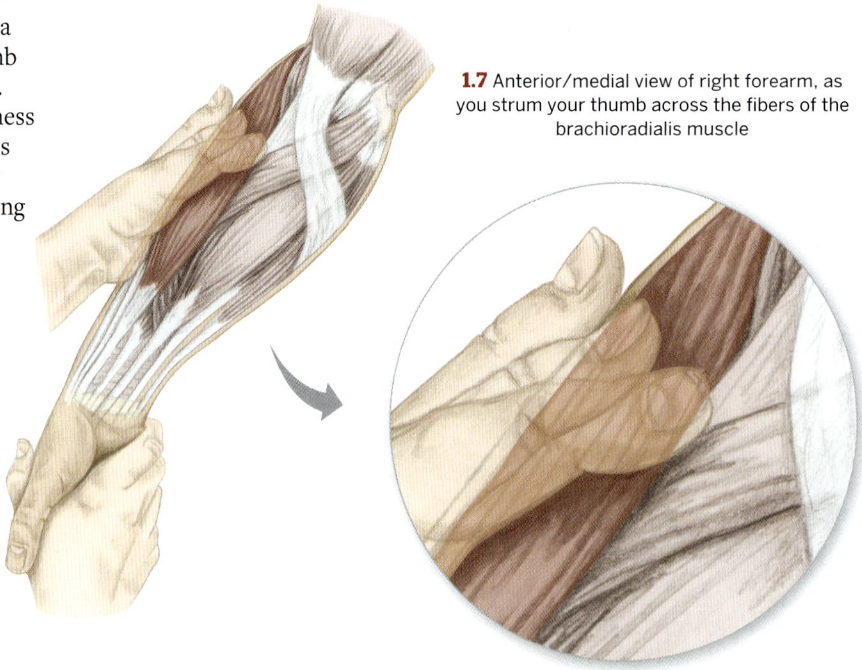

1.7 Anterior/medial view of right forearm, as you strum your thumb across the fibers of the brachioradialis muscle

Palpation Plus

Here is a simple exercise to increase your tactile sensitivity and palpatory skills. You will need this textbook and a human hair. Lay the hair beneath a single page. Close your eyes and palpate through the page, trying to locate the hair.

When you find the hair, reposition it and add another page. Continue to add pages until you can no longer locate the hair. How many pages can you palpate through?

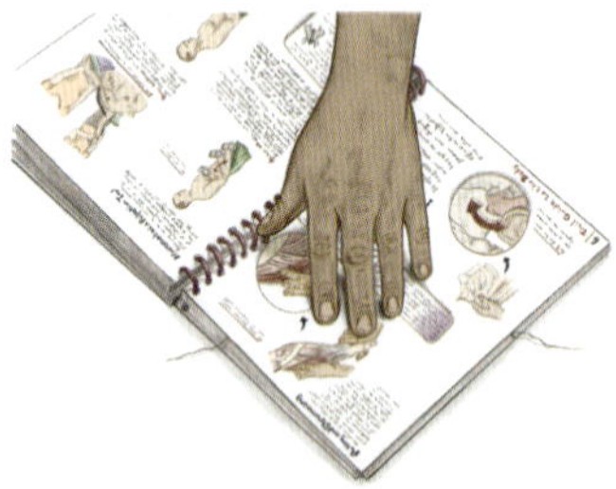

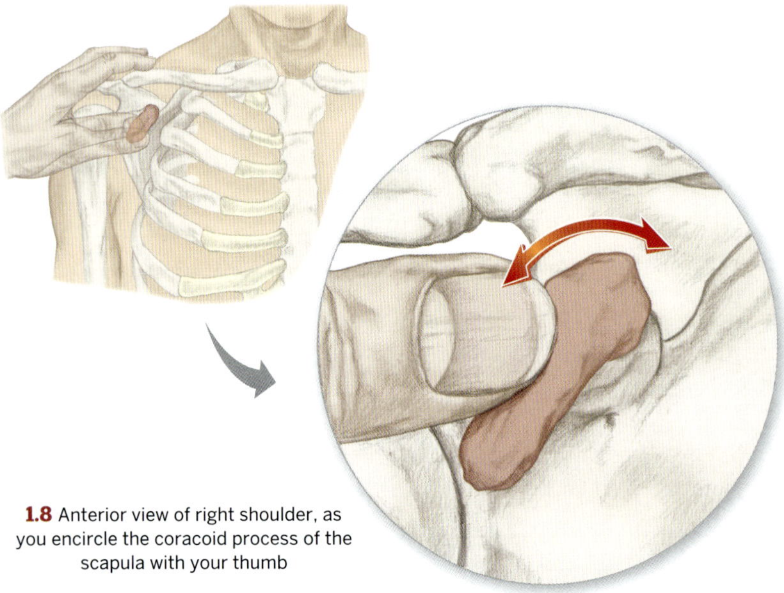

1.8 Anterior view of right shoulder, as you encircle the coracoid process of the scapula with your thumb

Movement and Stillness

If you were to compare the texture of newspaper with rough sandpaper, you would naturally want to rub your fingers across their surfaces. In contrast, when you lay your hand on an expectant mother's abdomen, hoping to feel the fetus move, you naturally keep your hand still and quiet. Similarly, when you want to determine the fiber direction of a muscle or sculpt the shape of a bone, **move your hands along its surface** (**1.8**). However, when you want to feel a muscle contract or a bone move, **keep your hands still** and follow the movement. Put simply, if the structure you are palpating is stationary, **move** your hands across it; if it is moving, **stay still**.

Movement as a Palpation Tool

Throughout the text, you will be asked to create specific movement on a partner's body with or without that person's help. These movements will help to verify the location of structures as well as any changes occurring in the tissues as a result.

Active movement is performed by your partner. He actively moves his body while you palpate or observe the movement. For example, the text may say, "Ask your partner to slowly flex his elbow while you palpate his biceps brachii muscle." All active movements performed by your partner should be slow and smooth—as changes in tissue are difficult to follow during fast, jerky motions (**1.9**).

Sometimes you might be instructed to ask your partner to contract and relax a muscle. For example, "To feel the forearm flexors, lay your hand on your partner's forearm and ask him to alternately flex and relax his wrist." The on-and-off aspect of this technique will not only help you locate muscles and tendons but will also give you the opportunity to feel the difference between contracted and relaxed tissue.

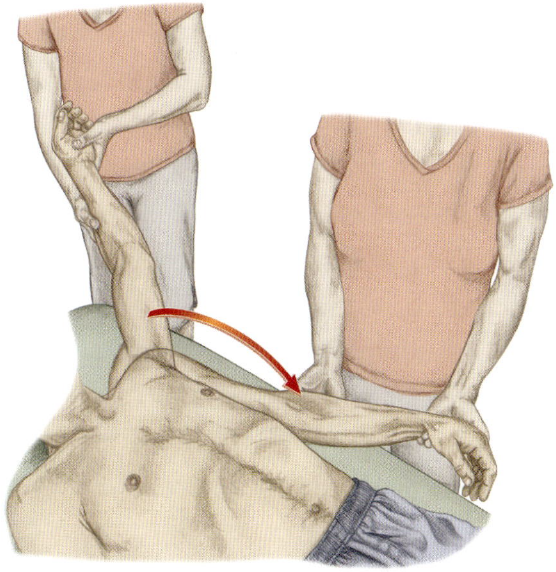
1.10 Passive flexion and extension of the shoulder

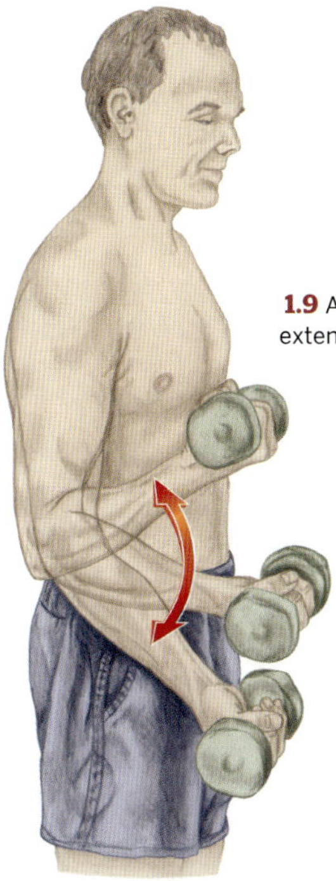
1.9 Active flexion and extension of the elbow

Passive movement is the opposite of active movement: Your partner relaxes while you move his body. For example, when the text says, "Passively flex and extend the shoulder," you will move the arm while your partner remains passive and allows the action to occur (**1.10**).

Resisted movement requires both of you to act: Your partner attempts to perform an action against your gentle resistance. For example, "To feel the elbow flexors contract, ask your partner to flex his elbow against your resistance" (**1.11**). As he meets the gentle resistance of your hand, no movement will occur at your partner's elbow. In this text, resisted movements are used to distinguish and compare the lengths, shapes, and edges of different muscle bellies and tendons.

Comparative Anatomy

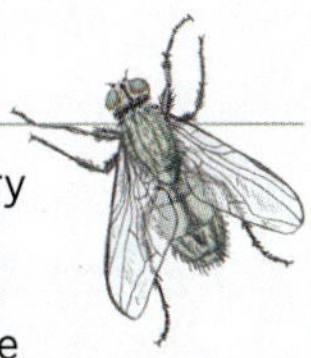

An adult has over 600,000 sensory receptors in the skin—more nerve endings than any other part of the body. The fingertips are among the most sensitive areas, with up to 50,000 nerve endings every square inch. The fingertips are so sensitive that a single touch sensor can respond to a pressure of less than 1/1,400 of an ounce—the weight of an average housefly.

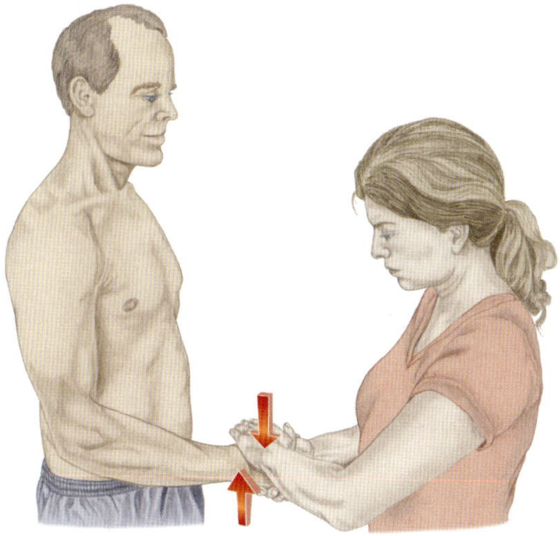
1.11 Resisted flexion of the elbow

Discover More

Leonardo da Vinci (1452–1519), who dissected bodies secretly at night, was the first to depict his anatomical findings. His anatomical illustration, laid out in more than 750 drawings, not only is detailed and accurate but also reveals many of the structural variations that can be seen when comparing bodies.

The anomalies shown in the drawings were not a case of Leonardo the artist dominating Leonardo the scientist; as he was a true Renaissance man, there can be little question that he drew exactly what he saw in the cadavers.

The structures of the human body do not always conform to the standard anatomical model. Structural differences have been recorded in almost every muscle, bone, major blood vessel, and organ in the body. Recognizing that the guidebook may not always coincide exactly with the geography of a particular body will help to prevent confusion and possible frustration.

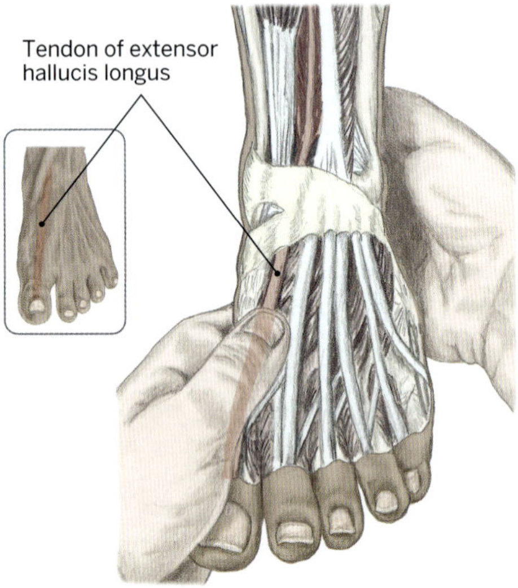

1.12 Dorsal view of left foot, as you explore a skinny tendon on the surface

When in Doubt, Ask the Body

While palpating, you may be confused or have questions about the body's structures and their whereabouts. **When in doubt, ask the body you are palpating.** For example, you may wonder, "What skinny tendon is this I see running along the top of the foot?" (**1.12**). The best advice would be to follow it in both directions and see where it leads you. If it runs from the big toe to the ankle and becomes taut when the toe is extended, it is the tendon of extensor hallucis longus (p. 382). **Always remember, you are never alone; the body is waiting to help you.**

All of the structures outlined in *Trail Guide to the Body*, with their Latin or Greek names, unique shapes, and buried positions, are inside you, your partner, and your patients. These structures have been there for years, waiting for you to discover them. Have faith and you will be able to locate them.

Palpation Plus

Three Principles of Palpation

1. Move slowly. Haste only interferes with sensation.
2. Avoid using excessive pressure. Less is truly more.
3. Focus your awareness on what it is you are feeling. In other words, be present.

Also, you can practice your palpation skills on yourself at any time. Daily routines such as waiting in line or riding the bus are wonderful opportunities to explore the malleable skin, tiny bones, and sinewy muscles of your forearms and hands.

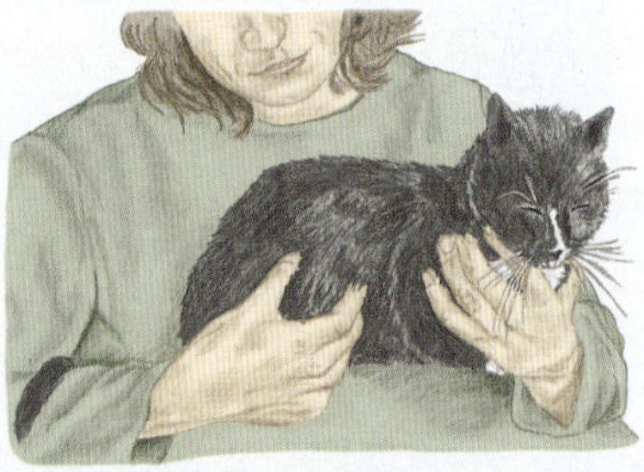

Comparative Anatomy

Dogs, cats, horses, and other animals offer a wonderful opportunity to compare musculoskeletal anatomy through palpation. For example, the next time you are petting your neighbor's cat, take a moment to locate its scapula. Compare the scapula's shape, location, and surrounding tissues to those of a human's or dog's. The anatomical differences may surprise you, but the similarities will amaze you.

Creating Your Palpatory Journal ▸

Do you remember the first movie you ever saw? How about that initial bite of (what would soon become) your favorite food? Chances are that these encounters created lasting impressions. You might recall details of later films or subsequent helpings of that scrumptious dish, but over time your senses and memory of those secondary encounters probably diminished.

Learning to palpate is no different. Our initial hands-on experiences can cast long shadows over future encounters. For example, exploring the shape, density, and fibers of the deltoid muscle for the first time can be formative. But as you become more familiar and less surprised by the muscle, later encounters will leave less of an impact.

The repetitive practice involved with learning a new skill, such as the martial arts, dance, or palpation, requires constant presence of the mind and body. It's a difficult journey—but an invaluable one that can be enhanced by creating a palpatory journal (**1.13**). Like a personal diary, your journal is a chronicle of your hands-on experiences. You could store your palpatory stories in your head, but it's certainly more effective to record them in a small notebook or on your computer.

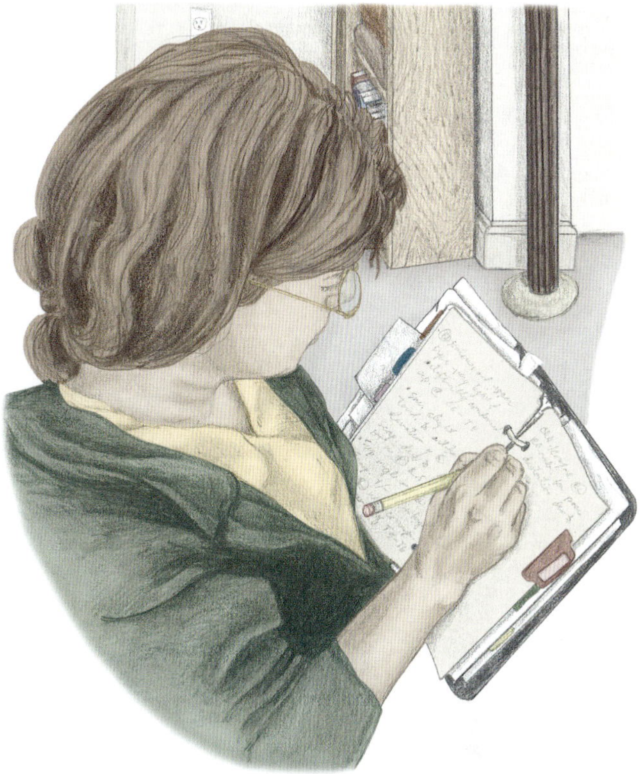

1.13 Taking time to chronicle your palpation experiences will provide an enduring resource that you can revisit during your learning journey.

- Initially, your journal remarks may be broad and undefined. "The deltoid was tight." "The hamstrings felt ropy." As your palpatory instinct develops greater awareness of the body's nuances, so will your ability to articulate your findings. "I was able to shift the fascia of the upper chest caudally but not laterally." "Left iliotibial tract was inseparable from vastus lateralis. Hypertonicity was an eight on a scale from one to ten."
- Your notebook can also include impressions, ideas, questions, and correlations. For example, "This week I palpated several different gastrocnemius muscles and noticed that four were particularly tender and had limited range of motion. Is this common or just coincidence?" Or "67-year-old male: The superficial fascia surrounding his hamstrings felt like bubble wrap. I've noticed this with two other seniors."
- Of course, journaling is a "head-based" activity and palpation is strongest when it is connected to the hands, heart, and gut. You may want to abandon words altogether and, instead, use colored pens to draw your experiences, or speak your findings into a small audio recorder. The best part is that there are no right or wrong answers.

Over time, whether you have explored the tissues of twenty or two hundred individuals, your journal will begin to fill with your thoughts and findings. Your palpatory journal will have evolved into something else—a memoir that you can read through and use to reflect on all of your adventures.

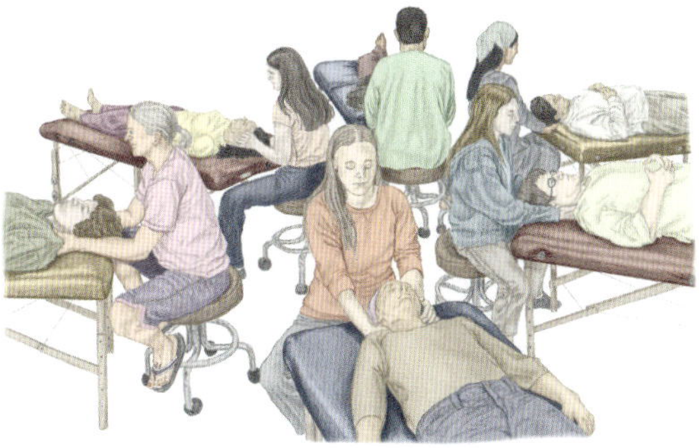

Palpation Plus

Palpating a variety of bodies in succession can create an unparalleled hands-on experience. This can be easily accomplished with a "round robin," where you rotate with others to palpate a series of people. Classroom settings (above), study sessions with friends, or even social gatherings offer opportunities for a round robin. The key to a productive round robin is maintaining awareness of the similarities and differences you are feeling from one person to the next.

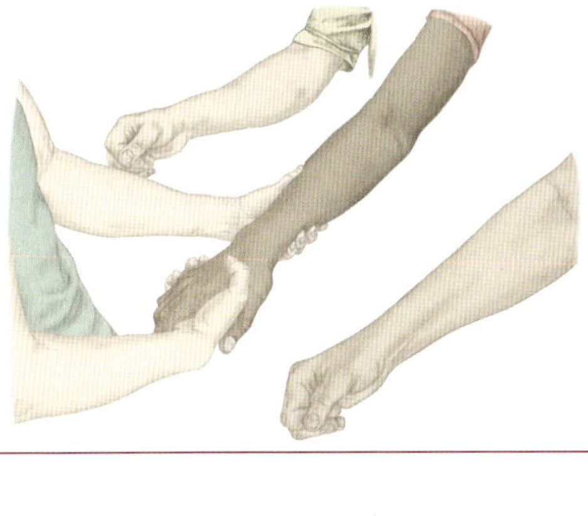

Exploring the Textural Differences of Structures ▸

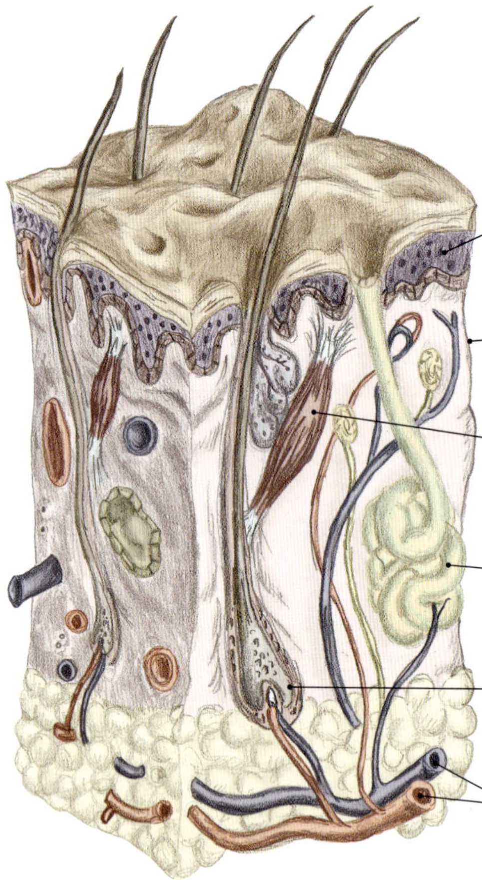

1.14 Cross section of the skin

This section is designed to help you identify and compare the physical characteristics of the various structures and tissues in the body. Understanding the textural differences between structures will help you to determine which techniques to apply on a particular body part in your hands-on practice.

Following are descriptions of various structures in their "normal," healthy condition. The tissue's basic structural design will be identical on everyone, but, of course, the particular quality or feel of a tissue will be as unique as the individual you are palpating. For example, a long-distance runner may have lean, sinewy bands of muscle tissue while an individual leading a sedentary lifestyle may have a very different quality to his muscles. Although the feel of the muscle tissue is different, its design and composition are the same.

Skin

Although often regarded as merely the body's covering, the skin is, in fact, the largest organ of the body (**1.14**). On an adult male, the skin can cover a surface area of 19 square feet and weigh nearly 10% of the total body weight. The skin averages about 1/20 of an inch in thickness, with the eyelids having the thinnest skin—less than 1/500 of an inch. The skin is intimately connected with the superficial fascia and deeper tissues, and its texture, thickness, and flexibility vary throughout the body.

Skin

For example, palpate the skin on the back of your hand. Note its thin, delicate, and pliable quality. Then turn your hand over and explore the palmar surface. Here the skin has a thicker, tougher layering.

Discover More

Most anatomy classrooms are haunted by a human skeleton. Hanging from a hook or set on a stand, it is most likely plastic, since real skeletons are difficult to dig up these days (which is how they were often acquired in anatomy's scandalous past). Close examination of a skeleton, real or not, with your eyes and hands is an opportunity not to be missed. Why? Because palpation, to a large degree, is about visualization. So, whenever you get a chance to spend some quality time with Mr. Bones, take it. After inspecting its pelvis and other features, you might discover that Mr. Bones is actually ***Ms.*** Bones!

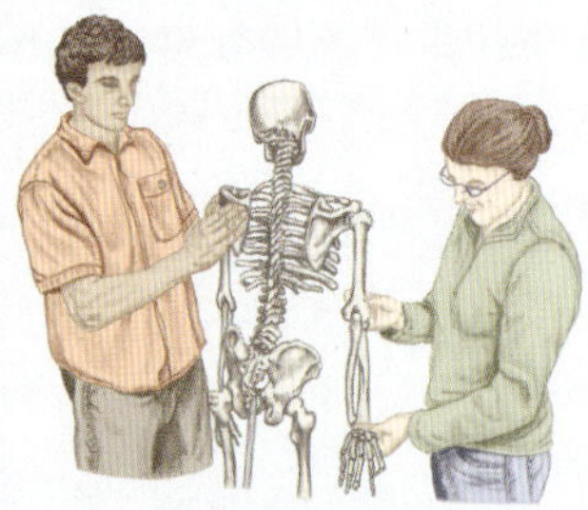

Bone

Bones and bony landmarks (the hills, valleys, and bumps on the surface of bones) are easy to distinguish from other tissues because they have a solid feel. Of course, the bones shift along with their surrounding structures during movement.

Sometimes other structures can feel like bone; for example, when a muscle contracts against resistance, its belly and tendons become very hard. Ligaments also can have a particularly solid quality. The shape and rigidity of bones and bony landmarks are constant, unlike muscles, which can transform from a soft to a hard state and back again.

Muscle

Skeletal muscle, the voluntary contractile tissue that moves the skeleton, is composed of muscle cells (fibers), layers of connective tissue (fascia), and numerous nerves and blood vessels.

A muscle's infrastructure is similar to that of an orange: a broad sheet of fascia encases the whole fruit, deeper layers of fascia separate the orange into "wedges" (the portions you eat after peeling), and finally, a thin coating of tissue surrounds each individual, tiny "bud" of fruit (**1.15**).

If we then apply this analogy to a muscle, a layer of fascia (epimysium) encases the muscle "belly," a deeper layer (perimysium) wraps the long muscle fibers into bundles, and finally, each microscopic muscle fiber is bound in fascia (endomysium) (**1.16**). Unlike an orange, however, a muscle's layers of connective tissue merge at either end of the muscle to form a strong tendon. The tendon attaches the muscle to a bone.

Muscle tissue has three specific physical characteristics that help to distinguish it from other tissues. First, **muscle tissue has a striated texture**—similar to a plank of unsanded wood. This is different from tendons, which have a smoother feel. The fibrous quality of a muscle belly is caused by bundles of muscle fibers running in a particular direction.

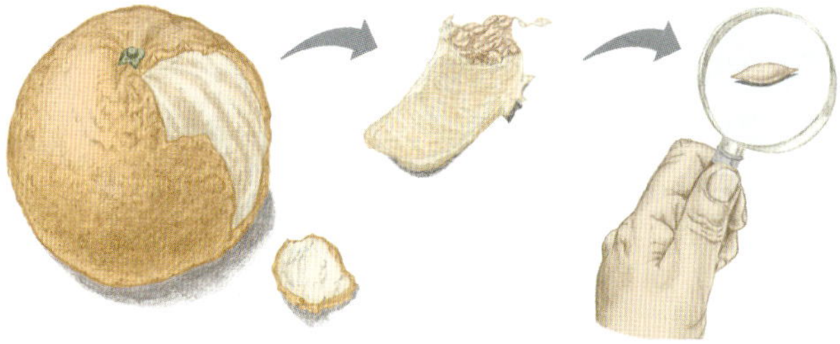

1.15 Peeling an orange. Fascial layering is highlighted.

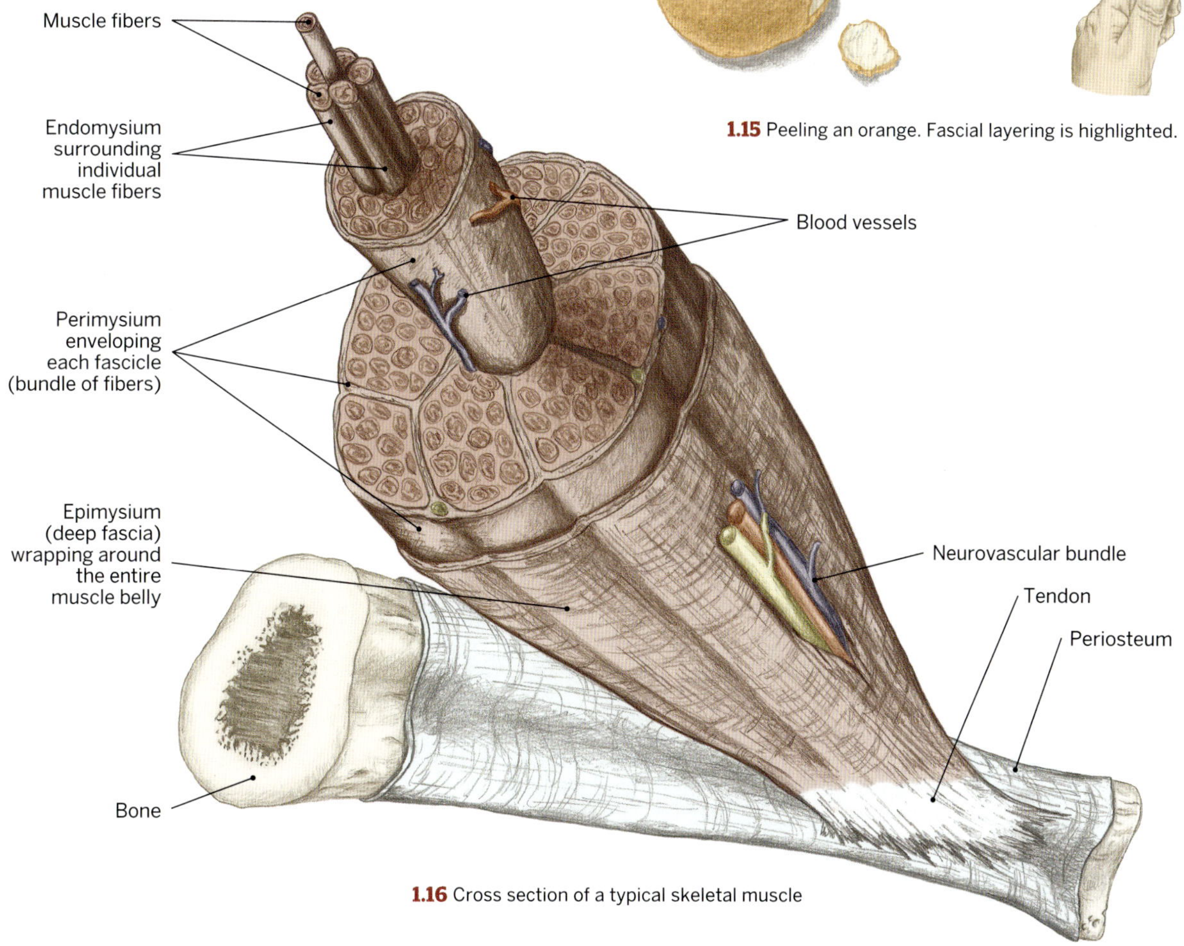

1.16 Cross section of a typical skeletal muscle

Discover More

In order for a specific movement to occur, muscles have to play particular roles. A muscle (or group of muscles) that carries out an action is called the **agonist**. A muscle that supports the agonist is called a **synergist**. A muscle that performs an action opposite of the agonist is called an **antagonist**. So when you ***dorsiflex*** your ankle (p. 27), the agonist is the tibialis anterior. It is supported in this movement by two synergists, the extensor digitorum longus and extensor hallucis longus (p. 382). Playing the role of antagonists to the tibialis anterior are the gastrocnemius and soleus (p. 375). Conversely, when you ***plantar flex*** your ankle (p. 27), the roles reverse: now the agonists are the gastrocnemius and soleus, the synergists are the other plantar flexors of the ankle, and the antagonists are the tibialis anterior, extensor digitorum longus, and extensor hallucis longus.

Second, **the direction of the muscle fibers** can be used to determine the specific muscle you are palpating. Depending on the shape and design of a muscle (see box below), the direction of its fibers may be parallel, convergent, or diagonal. For example, the erector spinae muscles (p. 196) have vertical fibers that run parallel to the spine. Identifying their fiber direction can help you distinguish the erector spinae from the oblique and horizontal fibers of the other back muscles.

Lastly, **muscle tissue is unique because it can be in a contracted or relaxed state**. When a muscle is relaxed, it often has a soft, malleable feel; when contracted, it has a firm, solid quality. As the tension in muscle tissue changes, surrounding tissues like tendons and fascia also change, becoming taut or loose.

How can you palpate a muscle that is deep to a superficial, overlying muscle? In some areas, the overlying muscle can be shifted to the side. At other times, you can slowly compress your fingerpads beyond the superficial muscle into the deeper tissues, using the different textures and fiber directions as guides. This is similar to palpating through your sweater, shirt, and skin to access a muscle in your arm.

Muscle

Discover the three distinguishing features of muscle tissue by palpating your biceps brachii—the muscle on the front of the arm (**1.17**). Keep your arm relaxed and feel for the biceps's ropy fibers. Note how its fiber direction runs distally (down the arm). Then contract and relax the biceps and sense how it tightens into a solid mass and relaxes into a soft wad.

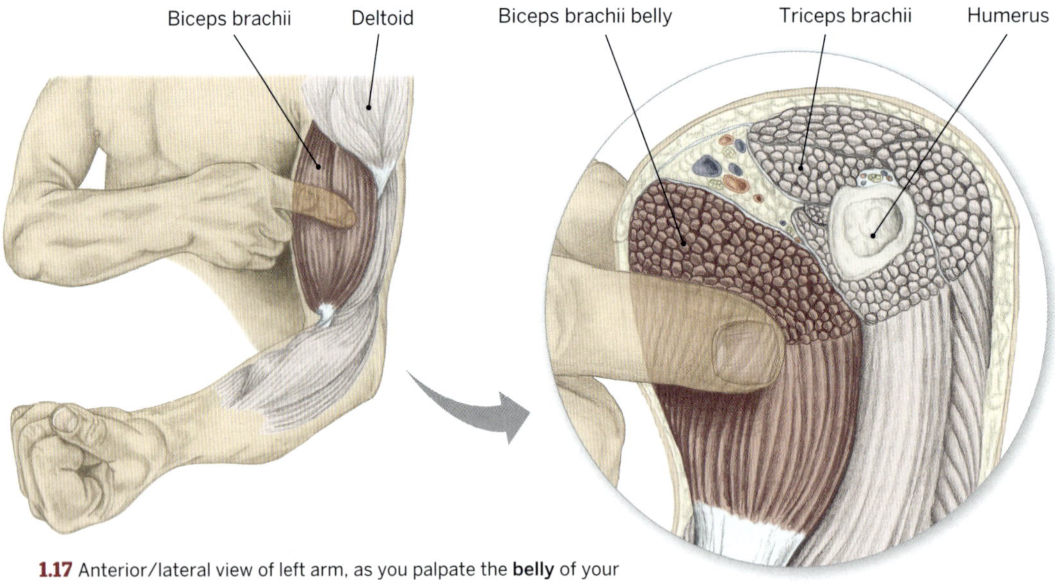

1.17 Anterior/lateral view of left arm, as you palpate the **belly** of your biceps brachii muscle. A cross section close-up is shown at right.

Muscle bellies have a variety of designs and shapes. *Parallel* muscles, as their name suggests, have long muscle fibers that run parallel to the length of the muscle. *Pennate* muscles have shorter fibers that run obliquely to their tendons.

See "Shapes and Arrangements of Muscles" in the Muscles–Part 2 chapter in *Trail Guide to Movement* for a full list of muscles' designs.

Five types of parallel muscles

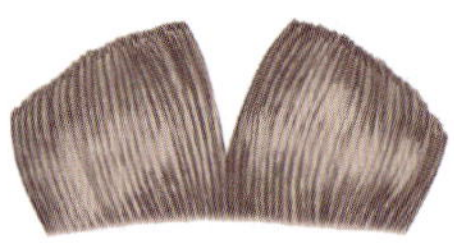

Flat
(frontalis, p. 258)

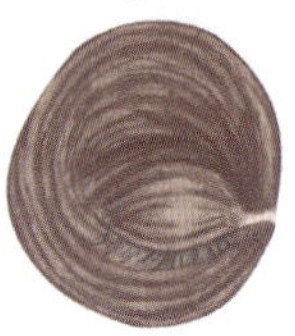

Sphincter
(orbicularis oculi, p. 268)

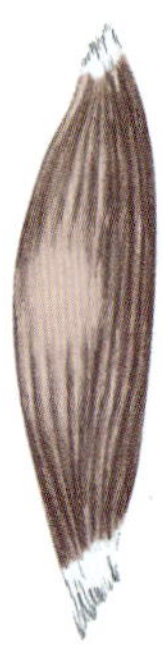

Fusiform
(brachialis, p. 130)

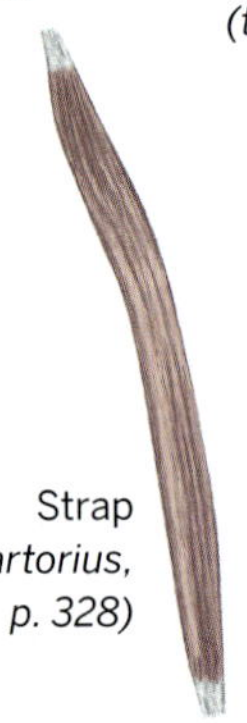

Strap
(sartorius, p. 328)

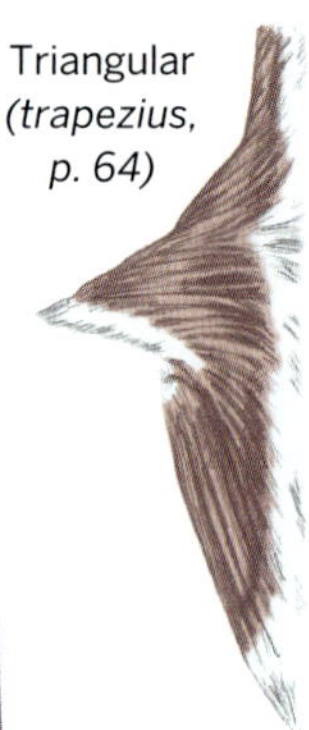

Triangular
(trapezius, p. 64)

Three types of pennate muscles

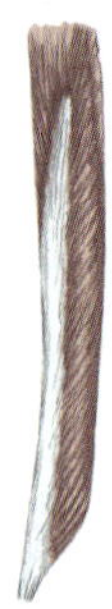

Unipennate
(tibialis posterior, p. 385)

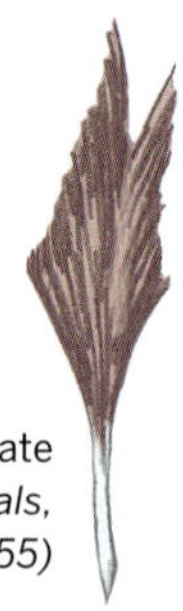

Bipennate
(lumbricals, p. 155)

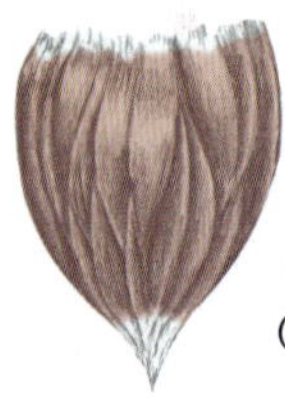

Multipennate
(deltoid, p. 63)

Tendon

Tendons attach muscle to bone. More accurately, they connect muscles to the periosteum—the connective tissue that surrounds the bone (p. 9). Tendons are composed of dense connective tissue shaped into bundles of parallel collagen fibers. Each end of a muscle has one or more tendons.

Tendons come in a variety of shapes and sizes. Some are short and wide like those of the gluteus maximus at the buttocks. Others are long and thin, such as the tendinous cables of your wrist. A broad, flat tendon is called an *aponeurosis*. An example is the galea aponeurotica (p. 262) that extends across the top of your cranium. All tendons have a smooth, tough, almost resilient feel to them, regardless of their shapes.

Tendon

Locate the distal tendon of the biceps brachii by holding your elbow in a flexed position (**1.18**). First, locate the biceps's muscle belly and follow it distally toward your inner elbow. As you progress, the muscle belly will become more slender and, at the crease of the inner elbow, it will become a smooth, thin tendon. It may feel like a taut strand of cable. Explore around either side of this tendon.

Ligament

Ligaments connect bones together at a joint. Their task is to strengthen and stabilize joints. Like tendons, ligaments are made of dense connective tissue. But unlike a tendon's parallel fiber arrangement, a ligament's fibers have a more uneven configuration.

The design and length of ligaments vary. Many simply cross a joint and blend in with the deeper joint capsule, like the ankle's deltoid ligament (**1.19**). Others span a distance between several bones, like the supraspinous ligament of the back (p. 219).

Ligaments often have a dense, taut feel and sometimes their fiber directions are palpable. If you want to distinguish a tendon from a ligament, explore its attachments and variable tension. A *tendon* connects a muscle belly to a bone, while a *ligament* attaches a bone to another bone. A *tendon* will become taut or slack depending on whether it is shortened or lengthened or if its muscle belly is contracted. A *ligament* will remain taut throughout all movements or states of contraction.

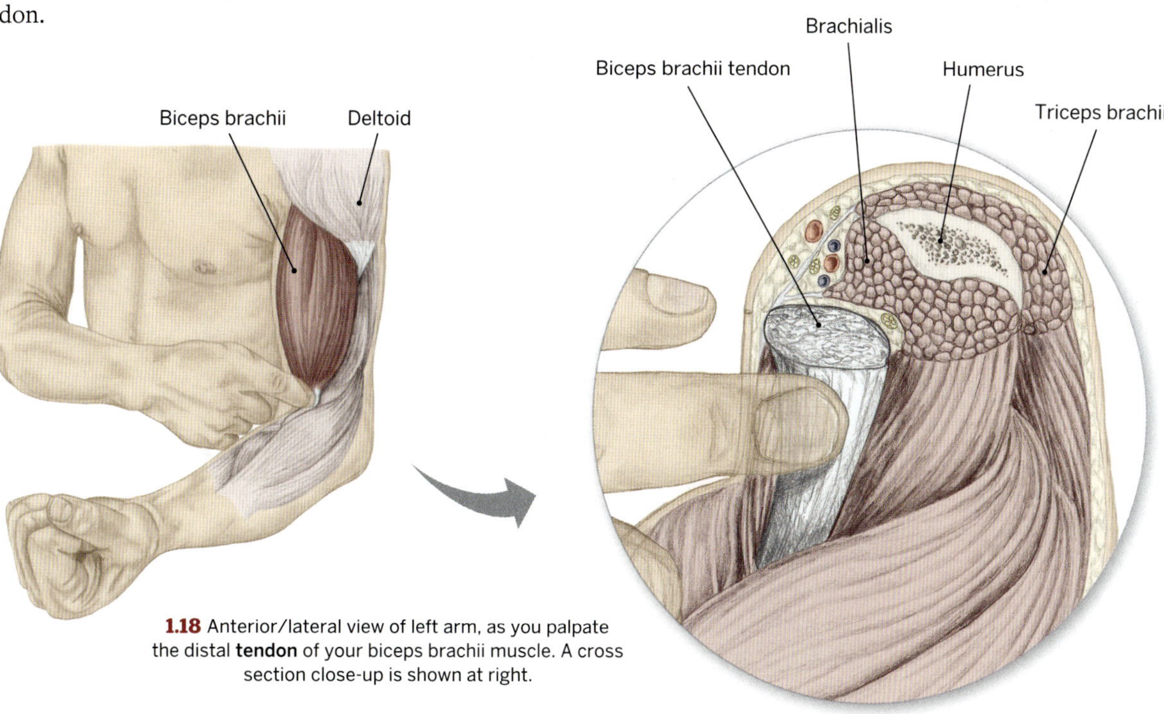

1.18 Anterior/lateral view of left arm, as you palpate the distal **tendon** of your biceps brachii muscle. A cross section close-up is shown at right.

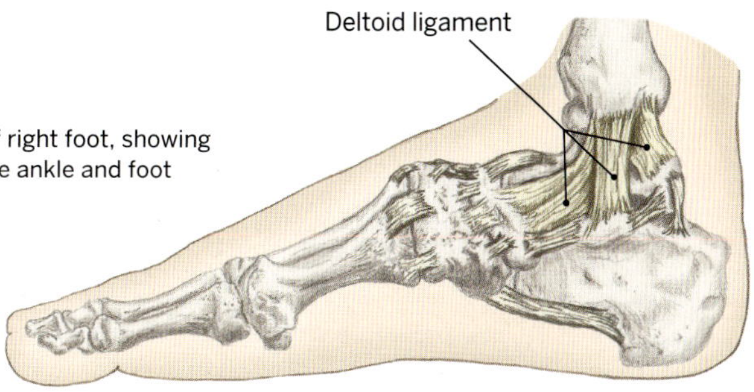

1.19 Medial view of right foot, showing ligaments of the ankle and foot

aponeurosis	*ap*-o-nu-*ro*-sis	Grk. *apo*, from + *neuron*, nerve or tendon
ligament	*lig*-a-ment	L. a band

Fascia

Like tendons and ligaments, fascia is a form of dense connective tissue. It is a continuous sheet of fibrous membrane located beneath the skin and around muscles and organs. This fascial system forms a three-dimensional matrix of connective tissue extending throughout the body from head to toe.

There are two types of fascia: superficial and deep. **Superficial fascia** is located immediately deep to the skin and covers the entire body. Often perceived as a thin sheet, superficial fascia is actually a spacial layering filled with adipose tissue, nerves, blood and lymph vessels, and connective tissue (**1.20**). The density of the superficial fascia varies from very thin (on the back of the hand) to quite thick (the sole of the foot).

Deep fascia has a more complex design. It surrounds muscle bellies, holding them together and separating them into functional groups. It also fills in the spaces between muscles and, like superficial fascia, carries blood vessels and nerves. Portions of the deep fascia penetrate into the muscle belly and encase each tiny muscle fiber.

Because of its ubiquitous quality, the fascial system requires an experienced, sensitive touch for precise palpation. On the next page are three simple exercises that can help you get a basic feel of the fascia and its relationship to other structures.

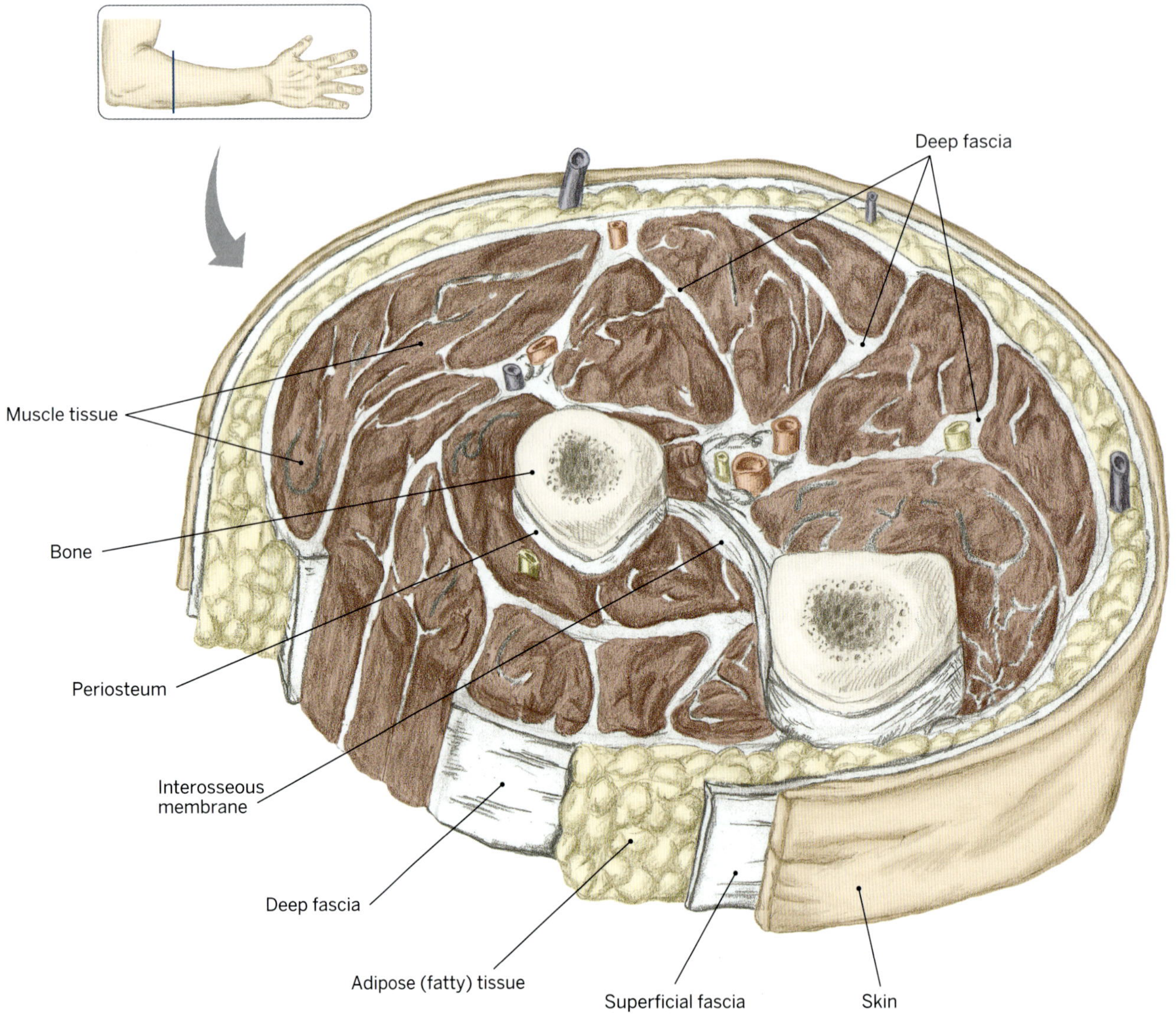

1.20 Cross section of the forearm, showing the arrangement of bone, muscle, and fascia

Explore your fascia

Pull up the skin on the back of your hand (**1.21**). Notice how the skin does not pull up entirely (as when you pull a baggy shirt away from your body). This is because the fascia is holding the skin down. Try this on your knee and various other parts of your body and notice how it is easier to lift the skin and fascia in some areas and more difficult in others (**1.22**).

Here is an exercise to demonstrate the omnipresent, yet phantomlike, nature of fascia. Put a latex glove on your partner's hand, followed by a thick winter glove. If you explore your partner's hand, you will immediately detect the texture and thickness of the winter glove and the general shape of the hands and fingers. The latex glove (representing the fascia), however, may be more challenging to detect.

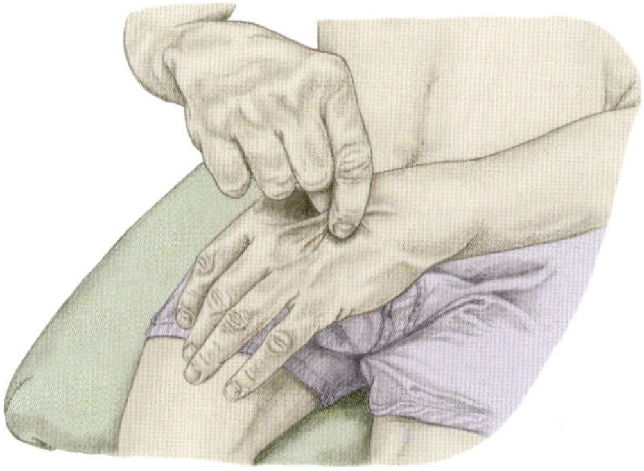

1.21 Exploring the fascia of the back of your left hand

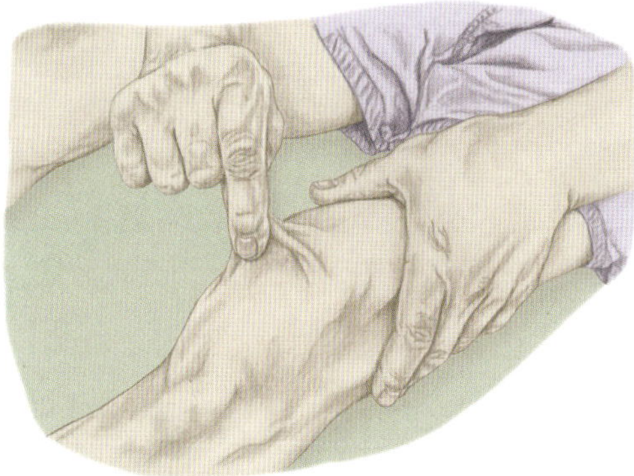

1.22 Exploring the fascia on your left knee

Continuity of the fascial sheet

This exercise is designed to give you a sense of the continuity of the fascial sheet throughout the body and of how pulling on one portion of this sheet can affect another. Draw a small *X* on your forearm. Place your fingerpads approximately two inches away from the *X*. Using the gentle pressure of your fingerpads, slowly move the skin of your arm in various directions away from the mark (**1.23**).

Notice how the *X* stretches and responds easily when you pull in a certain direction, yet may not move as easily when pulled in another direction. As you continue, reposition your fingers farther away from the *X* so, eventually, you are pulling across the skin of the hand.

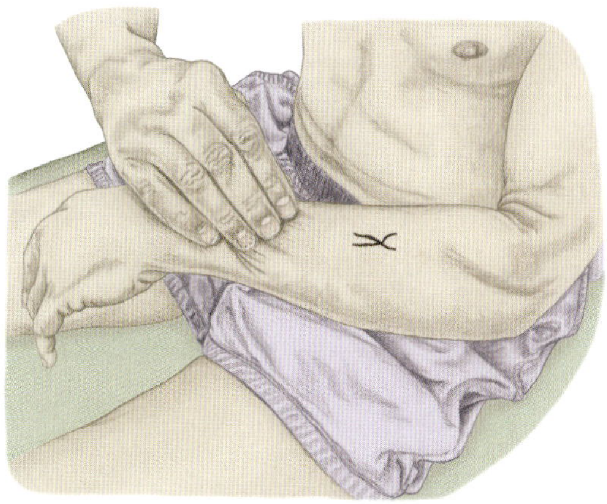

1.23 Exploring your superficial fascia near an *X* drawn on your left forearm

Retinaculum

A retinaculum is a structure that holds an organ or tissue in place. In relation to muscular connective tissue, a retinaculum is a transverse thickening of the deep fascia that straps tendons down in a particular location or position. For example, the retinacula of the ankle stabilize the tendons that traverse the sharp curve of the ankle (**1.24**).

Most retinacula are superficial and accessible. A retinaculum can be distinguished from its deeper tendons by its different fiber direction. A retinaculum will have transverse fibers that run perpendicular to the deeper tendons.

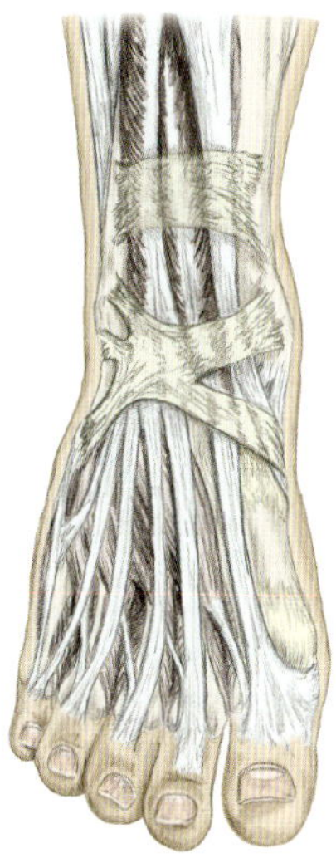

1.24 Dorsal view of right foot, showing retinacula of the ankle

retinaculum	*ret*-i-*nak*-u-lum	L. halter, band, rope
retinacula	*ret*-i-*nak*-u-la	plural for retinaculum

Artery and Vein

Arteries and veins have distinct features that you can palpate. For example, the pulse of the heart can be felt when pressing on an artery but not on a vein. Arteries are often situated on the protected side of an appendage and buried deep to the musculature. Some veins can be palpated superficially and are easily seen on the dorsal surfaces of the hands and feet.

Locating an artery is not only necessary for determining the pulse, but also important when palpating other structures. For example, when palpating the sternocleidomastoid muscle in the neck, it is crucial for you to be aware of the location of the carotid artery (p. 271), the chief blood vessel supplying the head and neck, so you avoid pressing on it. If an artery is occluded for a sustained period of time during palpation, the distal portion of the appendage will begin to tingle or become numb.

Vein

Let your arm hang at your side for a minute, allowing the blood to fill the superficial veins of your hand and forearm. The veins will swell with the increased pressure and become visible. For more dramatic results, gently squeeze your forearm with your opposite hand or apply a tourniquet (**1.25**).

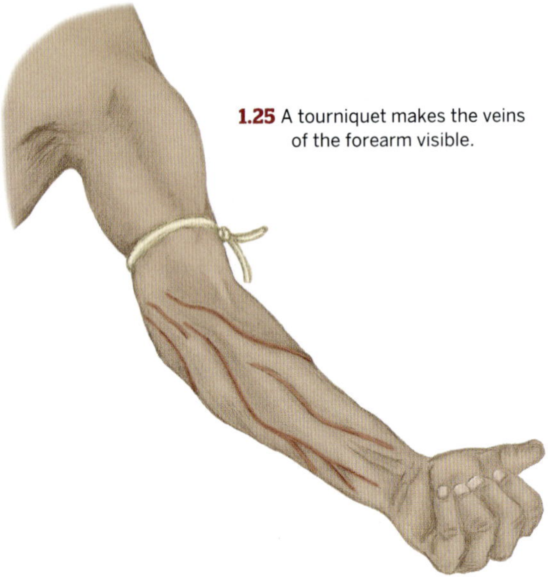

1.25 A tourniquet makes the veins of the forearm visible.

Bursa

A bursa is a small, fluid-filled sack that reduces friction between two structures (**1.26**). Situated primarily around joints, most of the body's six hundred bursae cushion skin, tendons, ligaments, muscles, or organs from the hard surfaces of bones. They are also located between two muscles, two tendons, a tendon and a ligament, or a muscle and a ligament.

Bursitis, inflammation of a bursa, is a common disorder accompanied by tenderness in the area and crepitation (cracking and clicking sounds) of the joint. When inflamed, superficial bursae are easily palpable and sometimes visible. In their normal state, however, bursae are generally not palpable.

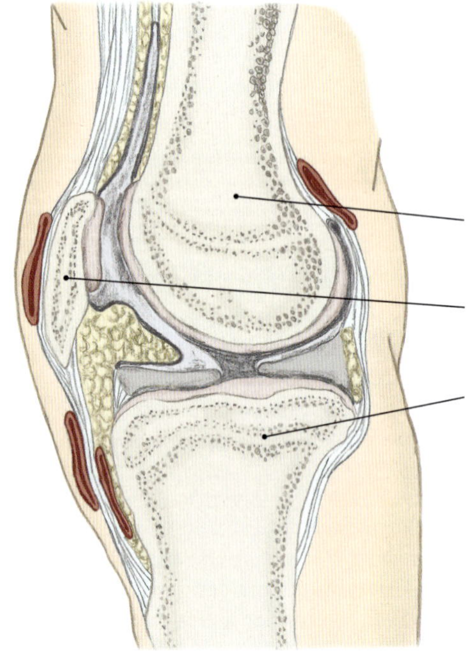

1.26 Cross-section view of knee. Some of the bursae of the knee are highlighted in red.

Discover More

William Harvey (1578–1657), often regarded as the first experimental scientist, discovered that blood circulates throughout the body. Along with describing the cardiovascular system, he explained how veins are equipped with valves that prevent blood from flowing backward between heartbeats. To prove his theory, Harvey tied a tourniquet around an

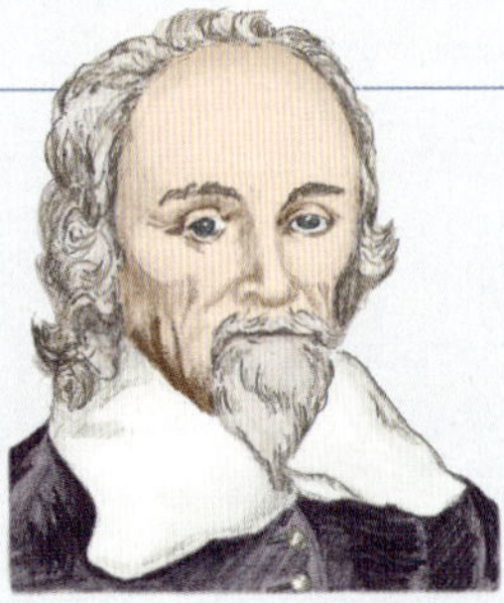

assistant's arm and allowed the blood to pool in the distal veins. He observed small swellings along the paths of veins, which he thought were valves. Harvey pressed on a valve and pushed the blood out of the vein to the next valve. As he held his finger on the distal valve, the proximal valve prevented blood from flowing backward and the vein remained empty.

bursa *bur*-sah L. a purse

Nerve

Nerve vessels are tube-shaped, mobile, and tender when compressed (**1.27**). Although sections of nerves and plexuses (bundles of nerves) can be accessed throughout the body, they are best avoided. Compression or impingement of a nerve may create a sharp, shooting sensation locally or down the corresponding appendage.

Lymph Node

Lymph nodes collect lymphatic fluid from lymphatic vessels. They are bean-shaped and may range in size from a tiny pea to an almond. Lymph nodes are located throughout the body, with palpable groups of nodes found in the body's creases, such as the groin, axilla, and neck (**1.28**). Healthy lymph nodes are roundish, slightly movable, and nontender. They differ from other glands, which are usually larger and have irregular, lumpy surfaces.

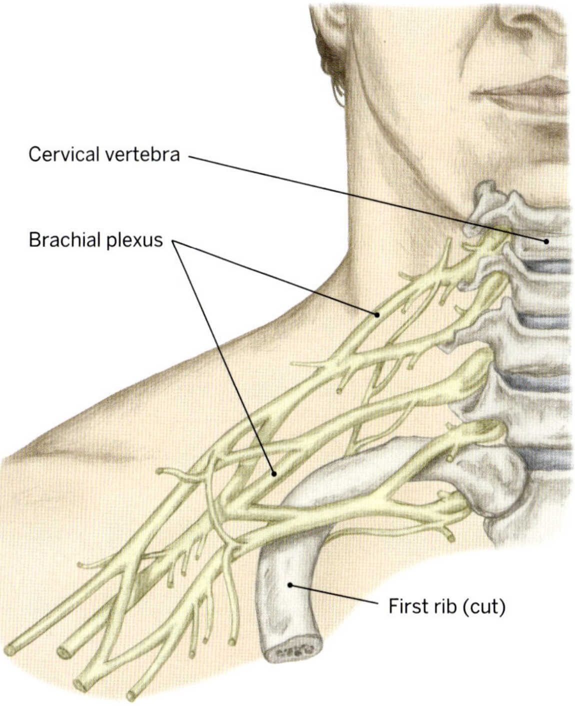

1.27 Anterior view of neck and right shoulder, showing the brachial plexus

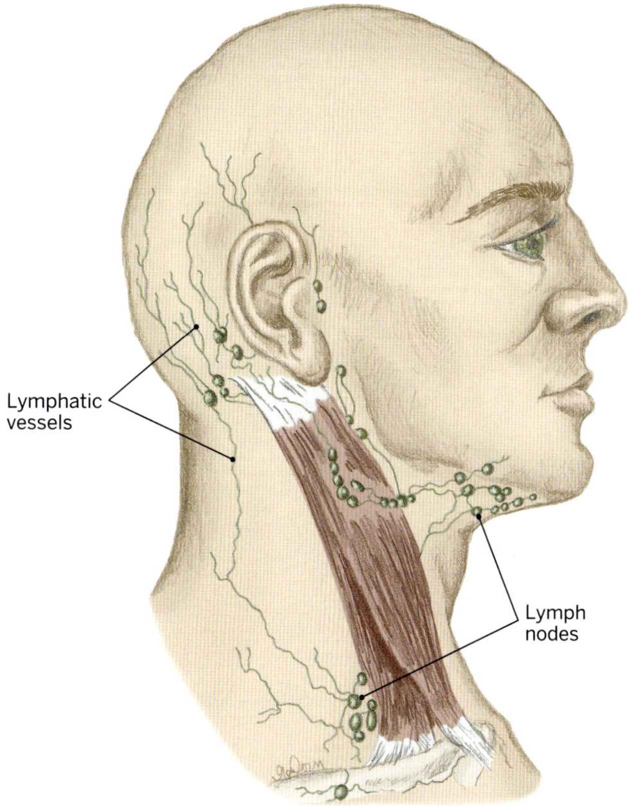

1.28 Lateral view of head and neck, showing cervical lymph nodes

Discover More

Adipose (fatty) tissue is a form of loose connective tissue. It is deposited at many levels throughout the body, including the marrow of long bones, around the kidneys, the padding around joints, and behind the eyeballs. Needless to say, some of these areas are outside the reach of this text. The most palpable location for adipose tissue is in the subcutaneous layer of tissue between the skin and superficial fascia. This layer of adipose varies in thickness throughout the body and may have different consistencies. Adipose usually has a gelatinous (jellylike) consistency, making it easy to sink the fingers into and detect deeper structures.

Stand up and squeeze the flesh of your own buttocks to feel adipose tissue. Yes, you might feel silly, but note the superficial layer of adipose. Then tighten the muscles of your buttocks and feel the textural difference between the adipose and the deeper muscles.

adipose	*a*-di-*pose*	L. fat, copious
gland		L. acorn
plexus	*plek*-sus	L. interwoven

Orientation of the Body

Regions of the Body

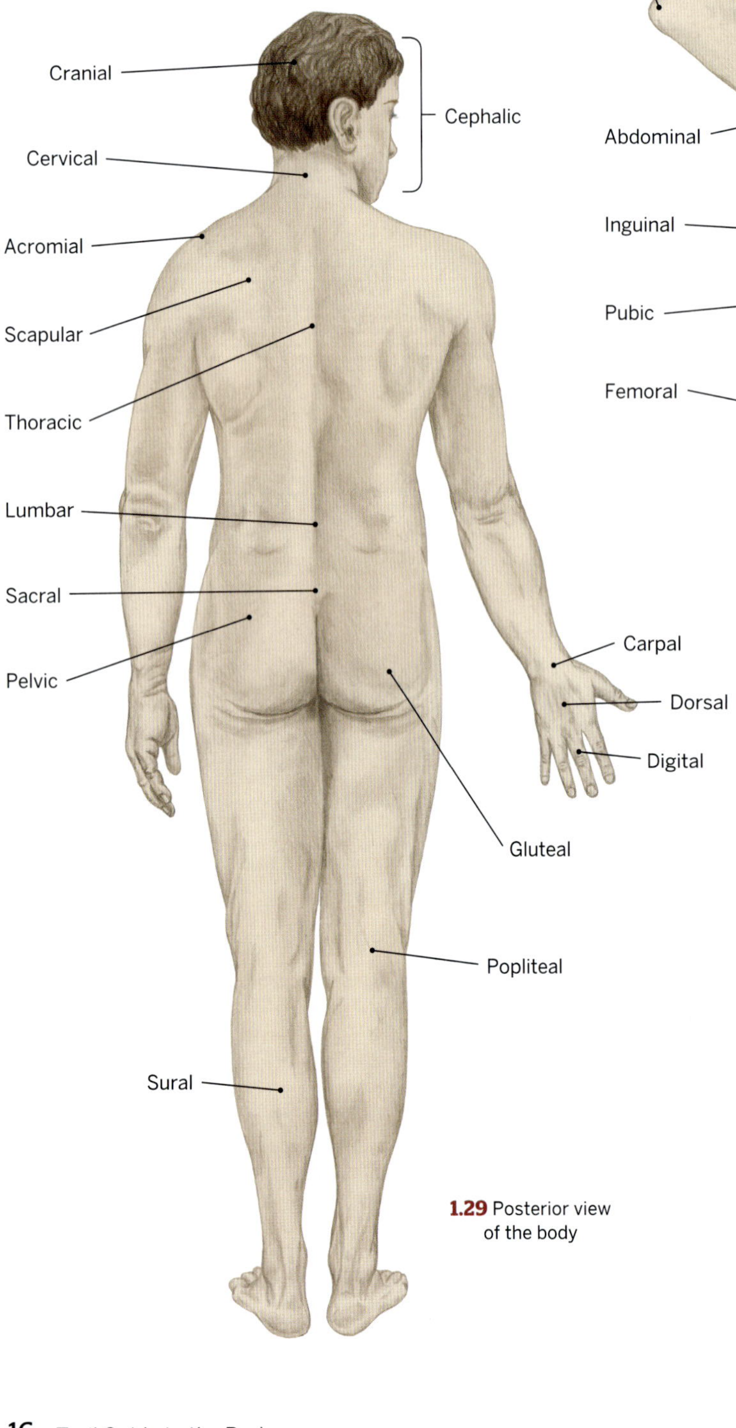

1.29 Posterior view of the body

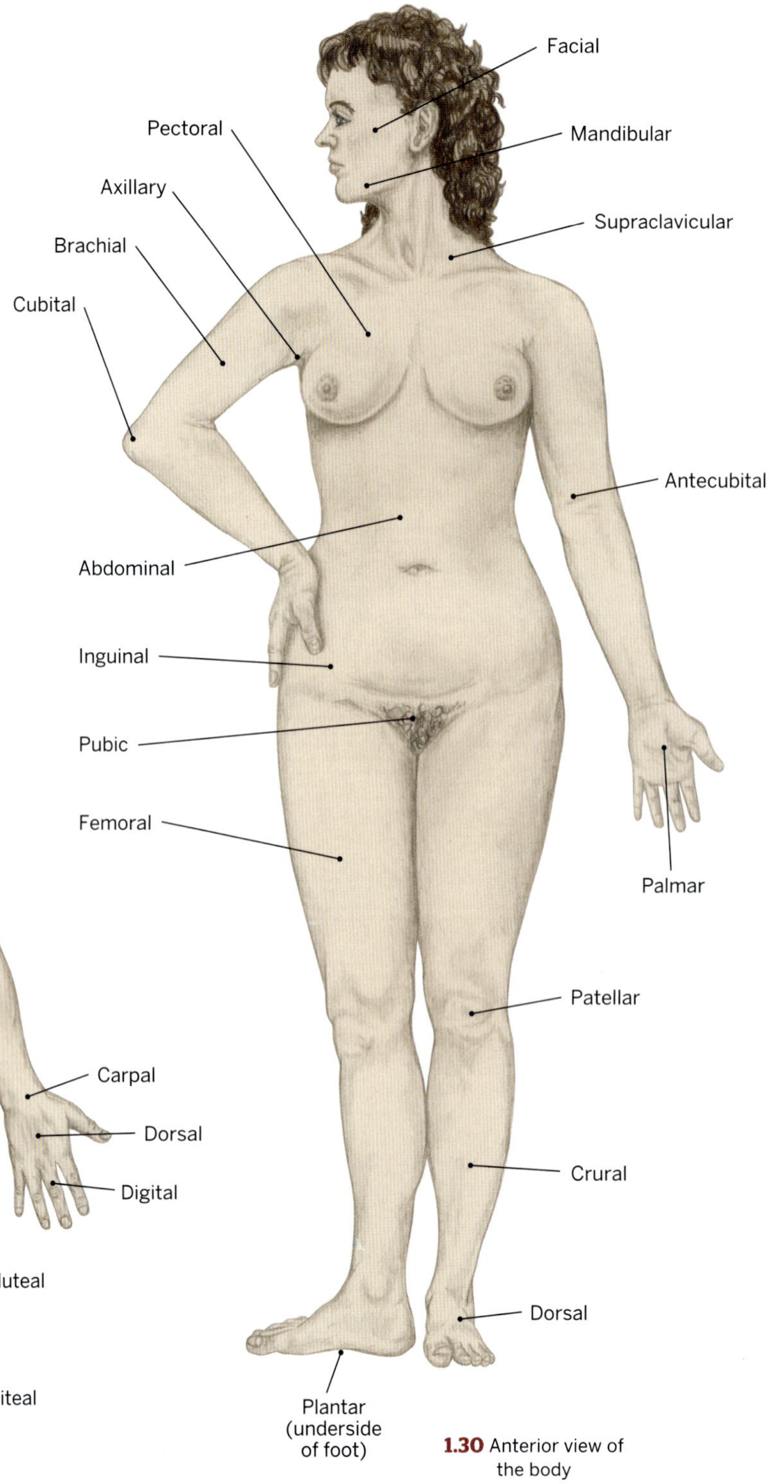

1.30 Anterior view of the body

Planes of Movement

When the body is in the standard anatomical position, standing erect with the palms facing forward (**1.31**), it can be divided into three imaginary planes (**1.32**). These planes help clarify and specify movements.

The **sagittal plane** divides the body into left and right halves. The descriptive terms medial and lateral correlate to the sagittal plane; the actions of flexion and extension occur along this plane. The midline (or midsagittal plane) runs down the center of the body, dividing the sagittal plane into symmetrical halves.

The **frontal (or coronal) plane** divides the body into front and back portions. The terms anterior and posterior relate to the frontal plane; the actions of adduction and abduction happen along this plane.

Dividing the body into upper and lower parts is the **transverse plane**. The terms superior and inferior refer to the transverse plane; rotation happens within this plane.

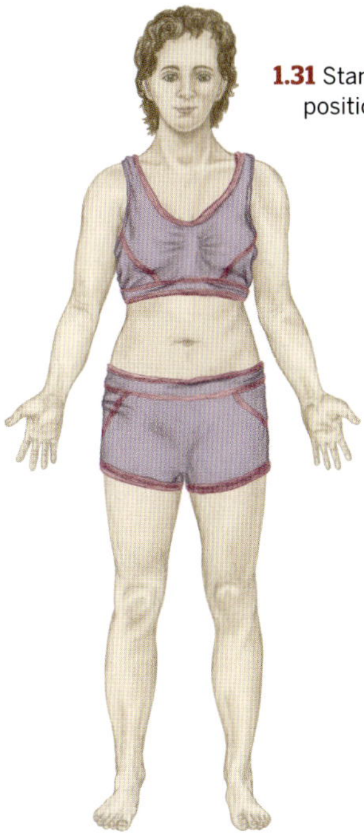

1.31 Standard anatomical position of the body

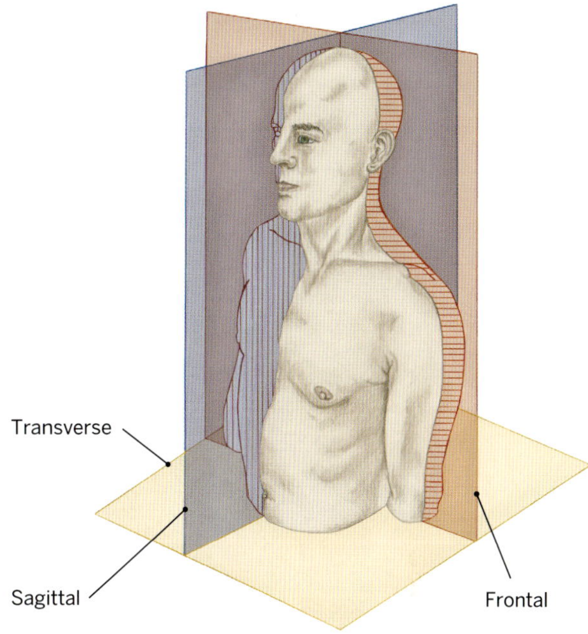

1.32 Planes of the body

Directions and Positions

Specific terms are used to help communicate location, direction, and position of body structures. These terms replace more general references like "up there" or "north of here," which are less precise and can be confusing. Each direction is paired up with its complementary direction.

Superior refers to a structure closer to the head. **Inferior** means closer to the feet (**1.33**). "The shoulders are *superior* to the knees." "The knees are *inferior* to the shoulders."

The terms **cranial** (closer to the head) and **caudal** (closer to the buttocks) are used when referring to structures on the trunk (**1.34**). For example, "The umbilicus is *caudal* to the clavicles." "The clavicles are *cranial* to the umbilicus."

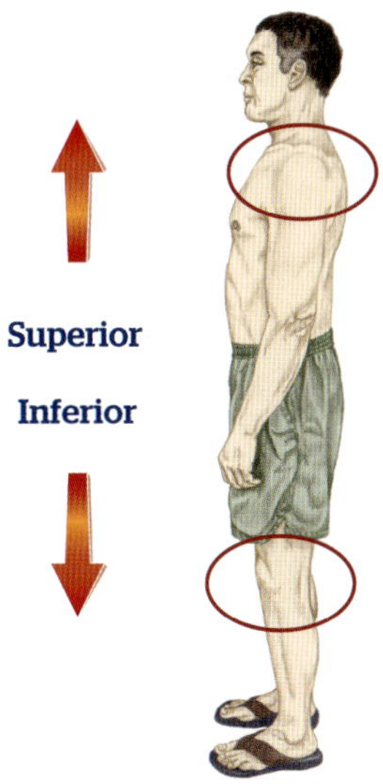

1.33 Superior and inferior directions

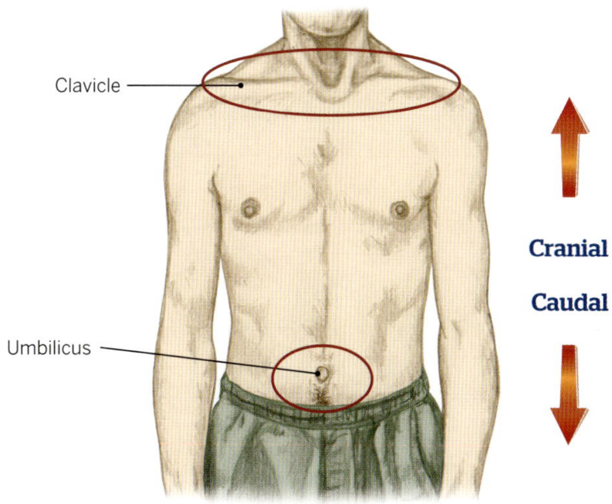

1.34 Cranial and caudal directions

sagittal	*saj*-i-tal	L. arrowlike
coronal	ko-*ro*-nal	L. crownlike
transverse	*trans*-verse	L. across, turned across

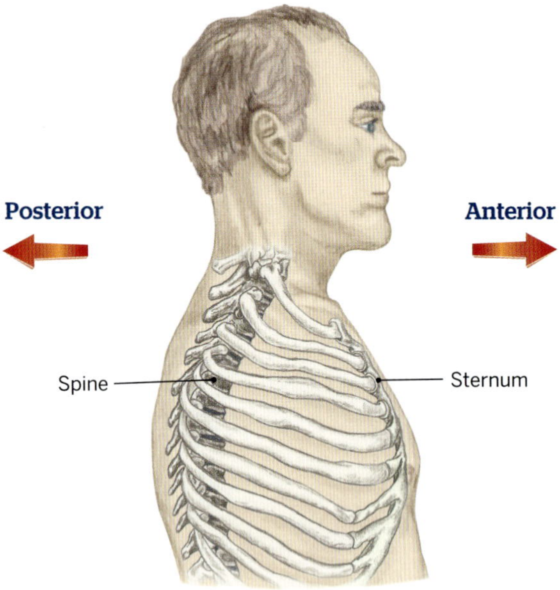

1.35 Posterior and anterior directions

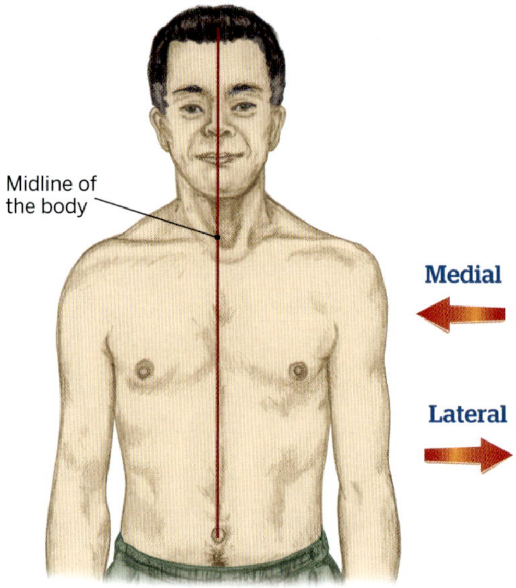

1.36 Medial and lateral directions

Posterior pertains to a structure further toward the back of the body than another structure. **Anterior** refers to a structure further in front. "The sternum is *anterior* to the spine" (**1.35**). These directions are also referred to as dorsal (posterior) and ventral (anterior).

Medial pertains to a structure closer to the midline (or center) of the body. **Lateral** refers to a structure further away from the midline. "The nose is *medial* to the ears." "The ears are *lateral* to the nose" (**1.36**).

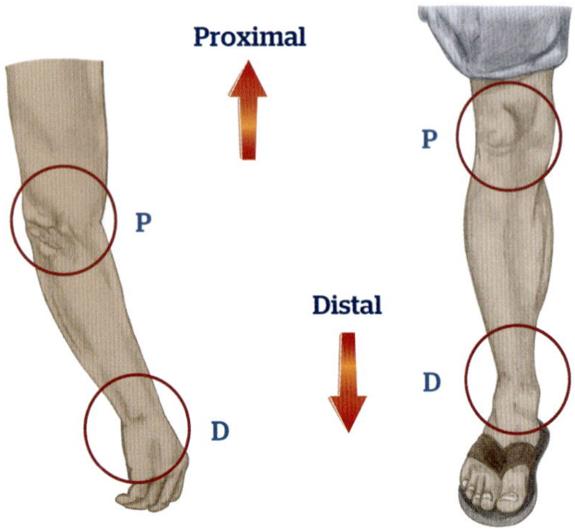

1.37 Proximal and distal directions

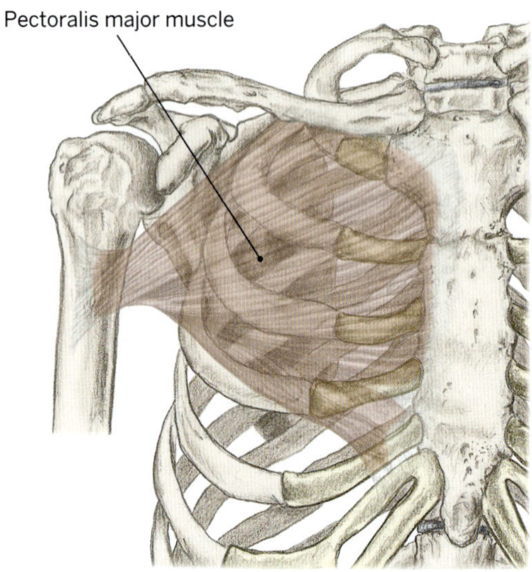

1.38 Pectoralis major is superficial to the ribs; the ribs are deep to pectoralis major.

Distal means a structure further away from the trunk or the body's midline. **Proximal** designates a structure closer to the trunk. These directions are used only when referring to the arms and legs. "The elbow is *proximal* to the wrist." "The ankle is *distal* to the knee" (**1.37**).

Superficial describes a structure closer to the body's surface. **Deep** refers to a structure deeper in the body. "The pectoralis major muscle is *superficial* to the ribs." "The ribs are *deep* to the pectoralis major" (**1.38**).

Movement Terminology

Movement of the body occurs at the joints, where bones articulate (or connect). Although movement affects the placement of bones, the terminology of movement always refers to joints. Bending your knee is called "flexion of the knee." "Flexion of the leg" would require an ambulance. See pages 22–27 for descriptions of movement at specific joints.

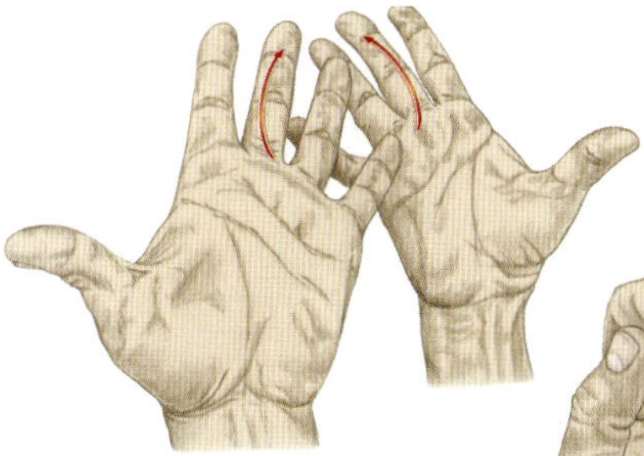

1.39 Extension of the fingers

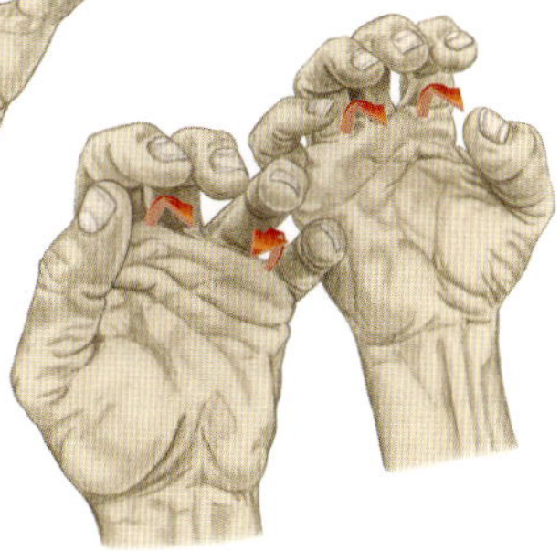

1.40 Flexion of the fingers

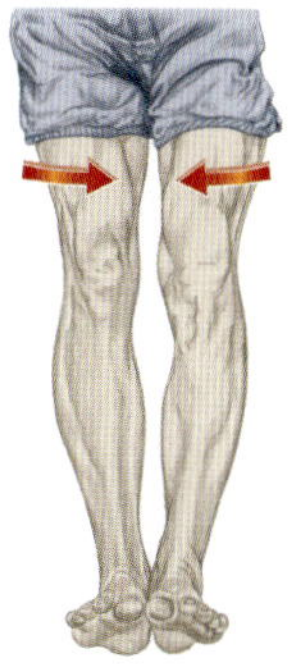

1.42 Adduction of the hips

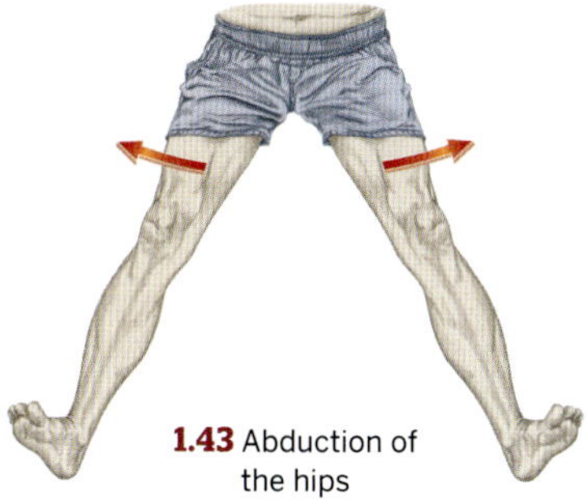

1.43 Abduction of the hips

Extension (**1.39**) is movement that straightens or opens a joint. In anatomical position, most joints are extended. When a joint can extend beyond its normal range of motion, it is called hyperextension. **Flexion** (**1.40**) is movement that bends a joint or brings the bones closer together. In a fetal position, most joints are in a flexed position (**1.41**). Both flexion and extension take place along the sagittal plane.

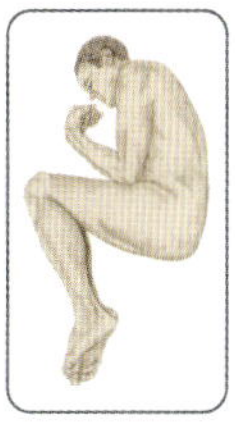

1.41 In the fetal position, most joints are flexed.

Adduction (**1.42**) of a joint brings a limb medially toward the body's midline ("adding to the body"). **Abduction** (**1.43**) moves a limb laterally away from the midline ("abduct or carry away"). These actions happen along the frontal plane and pertain only to the appendages. To adduct the fingers or toes is to bring them together; to abduct is to spread them apart.

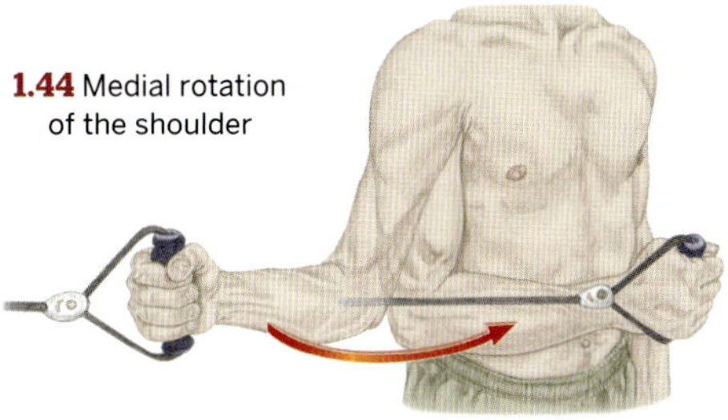

1.44 Medial rotation of the shoulder

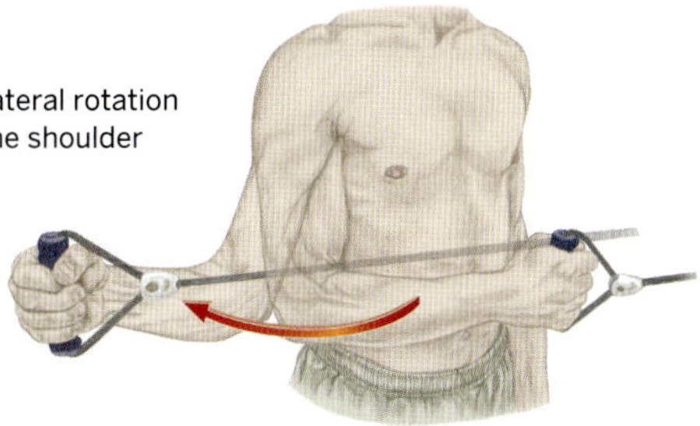

1.45 Lateral rotation of the shoulder

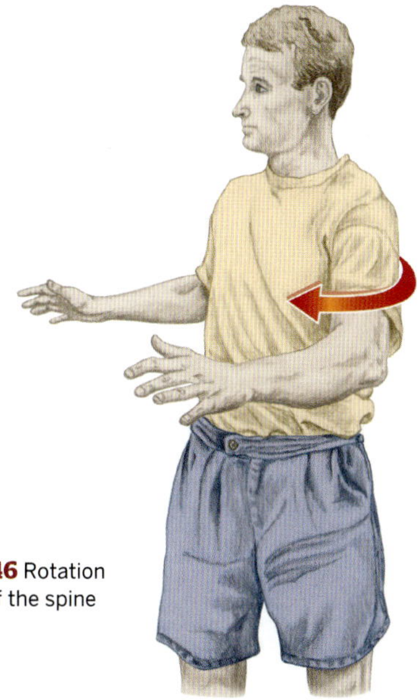

1.46 Rotation of the spine

Medial rotation (**1.44**) and **lateral rotation** (**1.45**) (sometimes referred to as internal and external rotation) occur at the shoulder and hip joints. When the joint medially rotates, the limb turns in toward the midline. Lateral rotation swings the limb away from the midline.

Rotation (**1.46**) pertains only to the axial skeleton (p. 28), specifically the head and vertebral column. Rotation of the head and neck occurs as a driver turns to check whether a car is coming from behind in the next lane. These movements happen along the transverse plane.

ab- (as in *abduct*) L. away from
ad- (as in *adduct*) L. toward

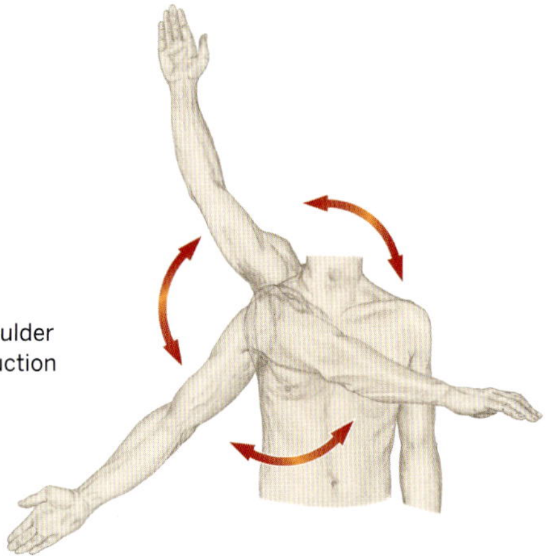

1.47 Shoulder circumduction

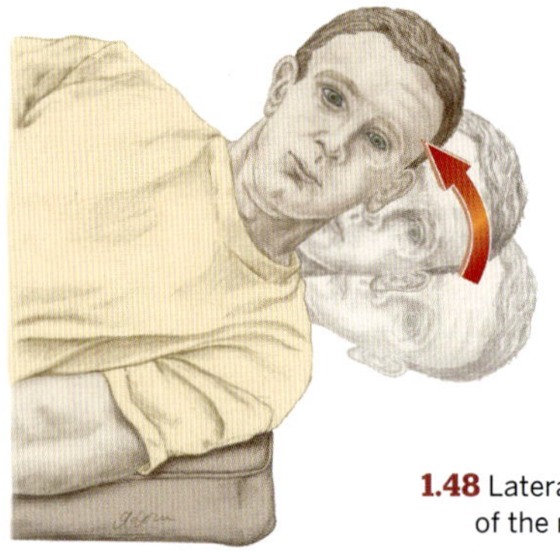

1.48 Lateral flexion of the neck

Circumduction (**1.47**) is possible only at the shoulder and hip joints. It involves a combination of flexion, extension, adduction, and abduction; together these actions create a cone-shaped movement. Swimming the backstroke requires circumduction at the shoulder joint.

Lateral flexion (**1.48**) occurs only at the axial skeleton—for example, when the neck or vertebral column bends laterally to the side.

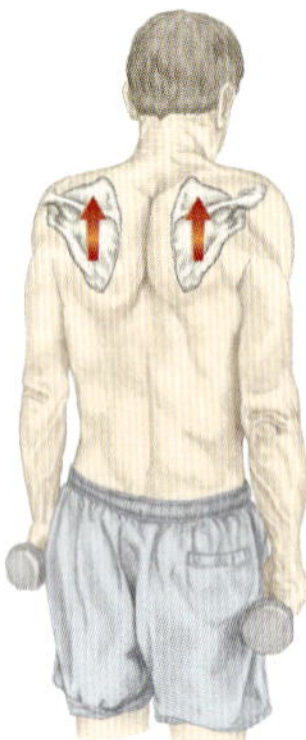

1.49 Elevation of the scapula

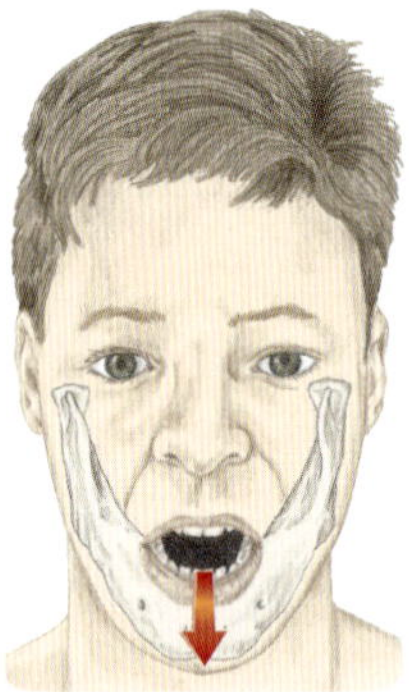

1.50 Depression of the jaw (mandible)

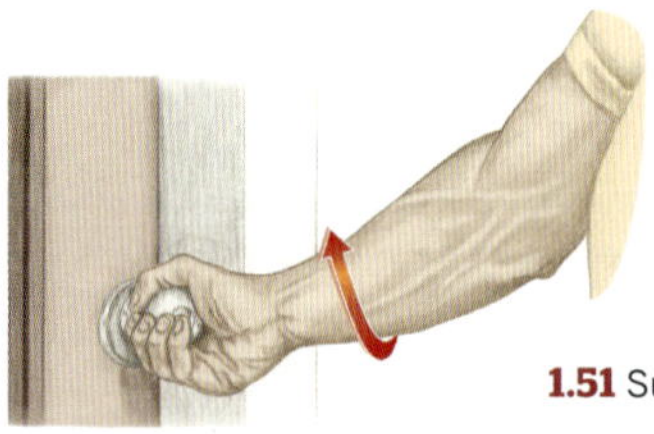

1.51 Supination of the forearm

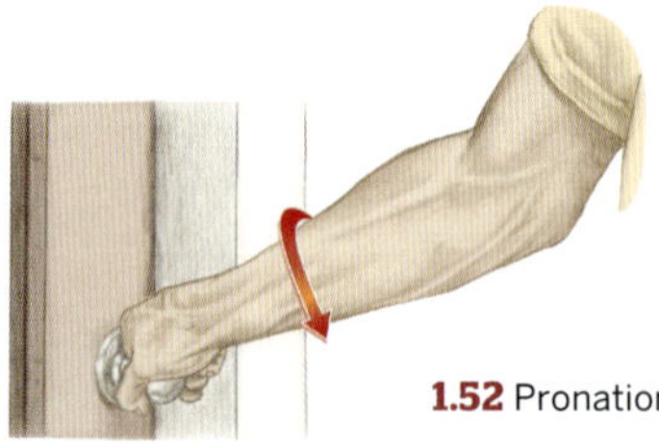

1.52 Pronation of the forearm

Elevation (**1.49**) and **depression** (**1.50**) refer to the movement of the scapula and jaw. Elevation is movement superiorly. Depression is movement inferiorly.

Supination (**1.51**) and **pronation** (**1.52**) describe the pivoting action of the forearm. Supination ("carrying a bowl of soup") occurs when the radius and ulna lie parallel to one another. Pronation ("prone to spill it") takes place when the radius crosses over the ulna, turning the palm down. Supination and pronation also occur at the feet.

Discover More

The names of many bones, bony landmarks, and muscles may initially look and sound foreign. They are—most anatomical terms are Latin or Greek. However, the source or story behind the terms can help to clarify their meaning. Take the phrase "infraspinous fossa of the scapula." The **scapula** is a flat bone of the shoulder. In Latin, scapula means "shoulder blade"—its common name.

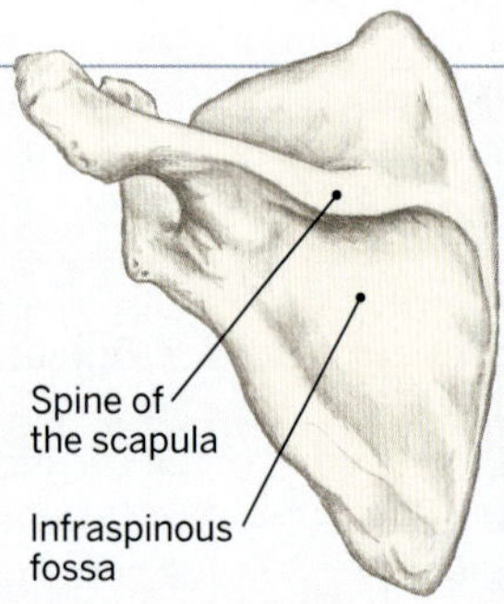

Fossa translates as "shallow depression." **Infraspinous** is a directional term (like north or southwest). It means inferior (infra-) to the spine of the scapula (-spinous). Put this all together and the "infraspinous fossa of the scapula" translates as "the shallow depression located below the spine of the shoulder blade." Keep an eye peeled for translations and phonetic descriptions at the bottom of pages.

supinate	***su***-pi-nate	L. bent backward
pronate	***pro***-nate	L. bent forward

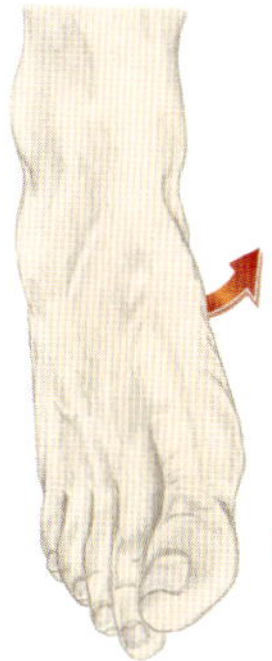

1.53 Inversion of the foot

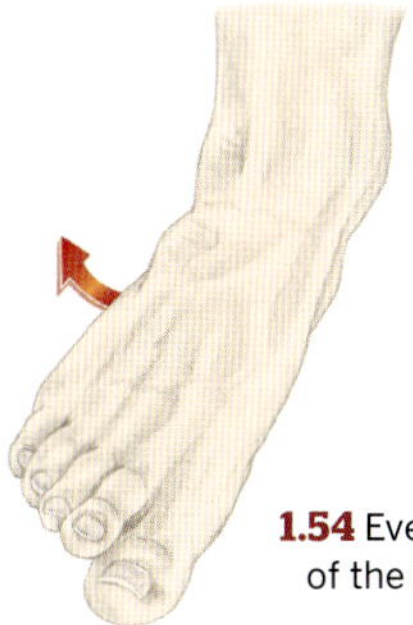

1.54 Eversion of the foot

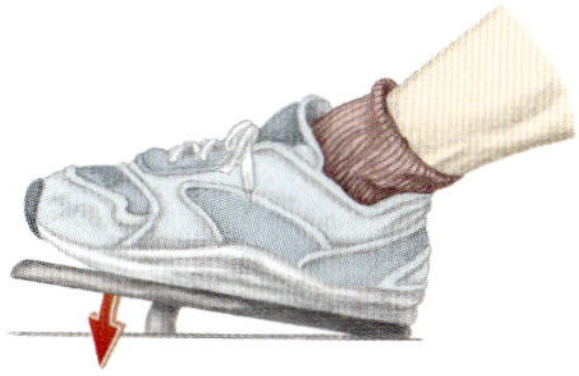

1.55 Plantar flexion at the ankle

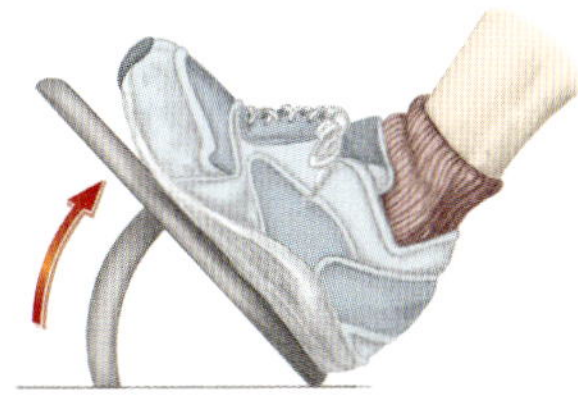

1.56 Dorsiflexion at the ankle

Inversion (**1.53**) and **eversion** (**1.54**) occur as a combination of movements of several joints of the feet. Inversion ("turn in") elevates the foot's medial side and brings the sole of the foot medially. Eversion ("turn out") elevates the foot's lateral side and moves the sole laterally.

Plantar flexion (**1.55**) and **dorsiflexion** (**1.56**) refer only to movement at the ankle. Plantar flexion is performed by moving the ankle to point your foot into the earth or stepping on a car's gas pedal. Dorsiflexion is the opposite movement, such as moving the ankle to let off the gas pedal.

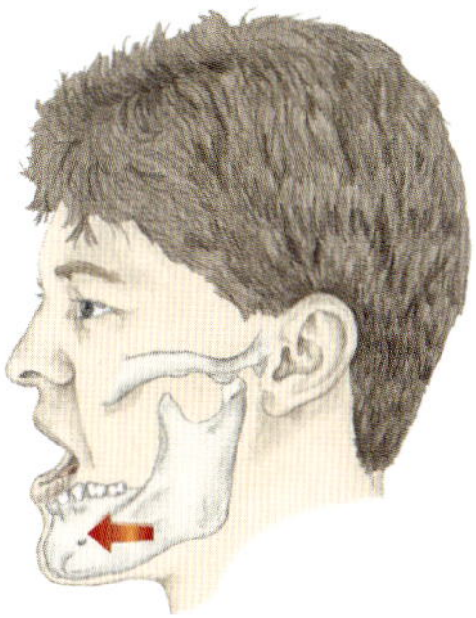

1.57 Protraction of the jaw (mandible)

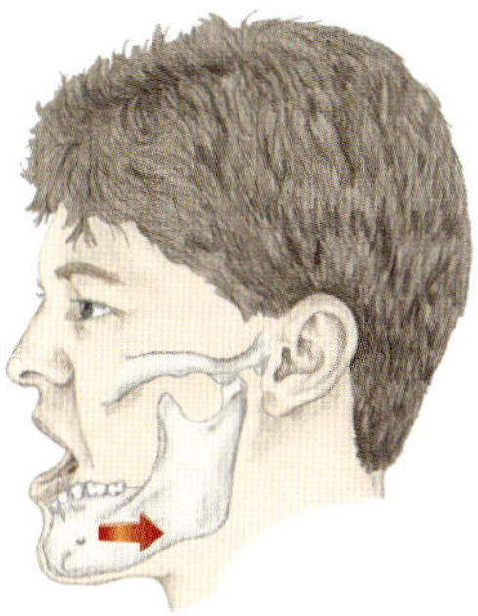

1.58 Retraction of the jaw (mandible)

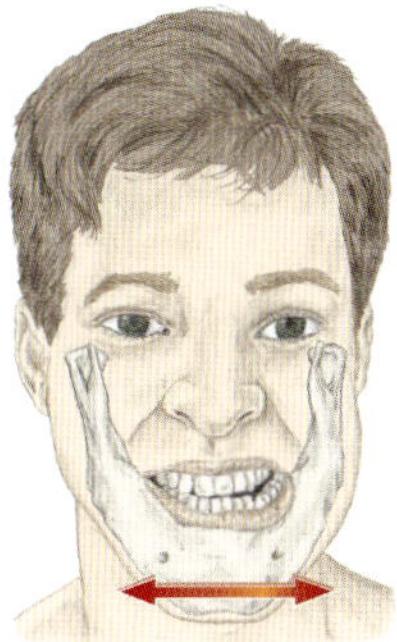

1.59 Lateral deviation of the jaw (mandible)

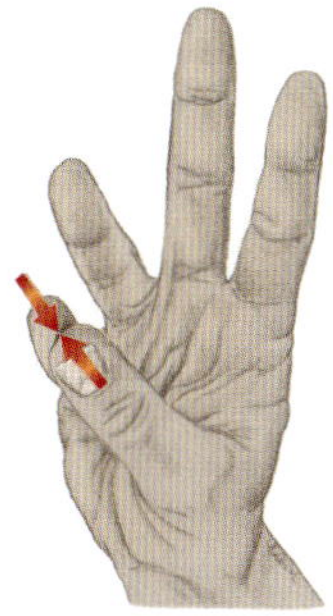

1.60 Opposition of the thumb

Protraction (**1.57**) and **retraction** (**1.58**) pertain to the scapula, clavicle, head, and jaw. Protraction ("protrude") occurs when one of these structures moves anteriorly. Retraction ("retreat") is movement posteriorly.

Deviation (**1.59**) means to wander from the usual course. Lateral deviation occurs at the mandible during talking or chewing.

Opposition (**1.60**) happens only at the carpometacarpal joint of the thumb. It occurs when the thumbpad crosses the palm toward the last (pinkie) finger.

Palpation Plus

Depending on the structure being palpated, ***Trail Guide*** will ask you to position your partner in a few different ways.

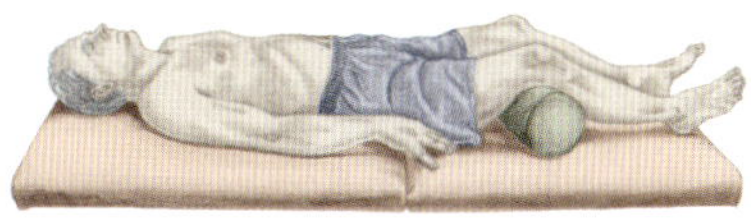

Supine *("on your spine") is to lie face up. A bolster behind the knees might be nice for your partner.*

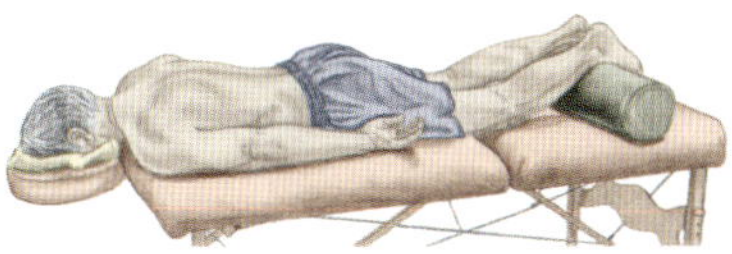

Prone *is to lie on the table face down. A bolster under the ankles is nice for this position.*

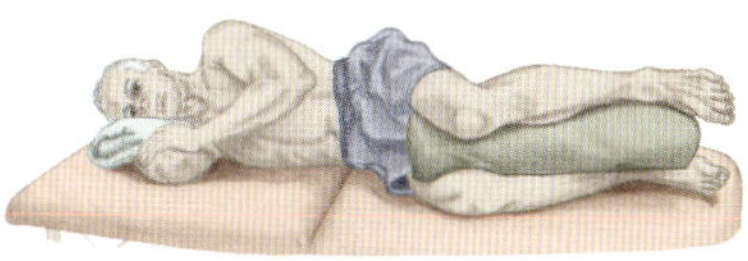

For ***side lying****, consider a bolster between the knees and a pillow under the head.*

dorsi	***dor***-si	L. of the back
plantar	***plan***-tar	L. the sole of the foot

Movements of the Body

Spine and Thorax

(vertebral column)

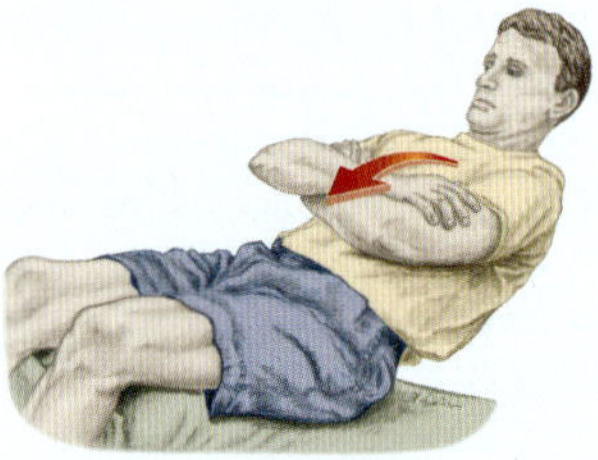

1.61 Flexion of the vertebral column

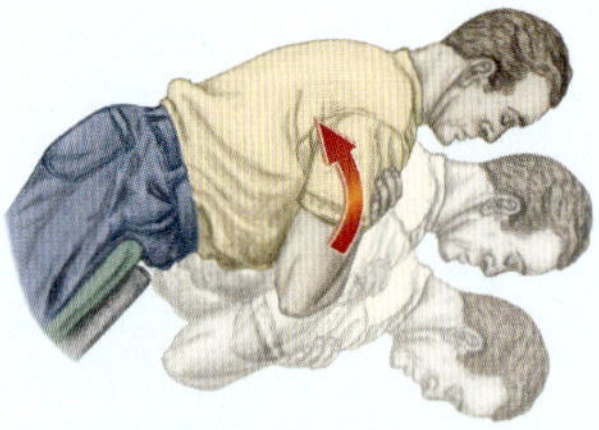

1.62 Extension of the vertebral column

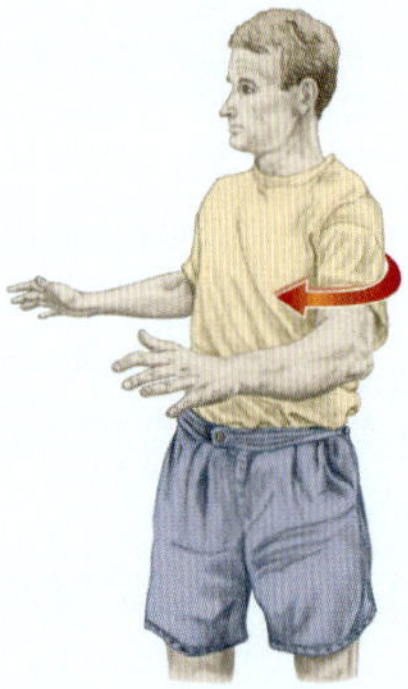

1.63 Rotation of the vertebral column

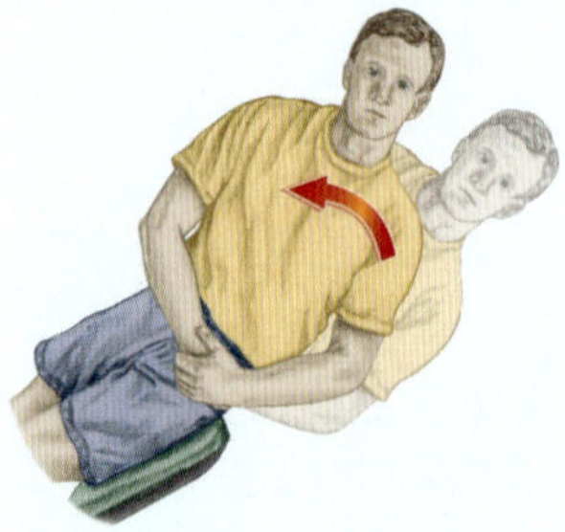

1.64 Lateral flexion of the vertebral column

Neck

(cervical spine)

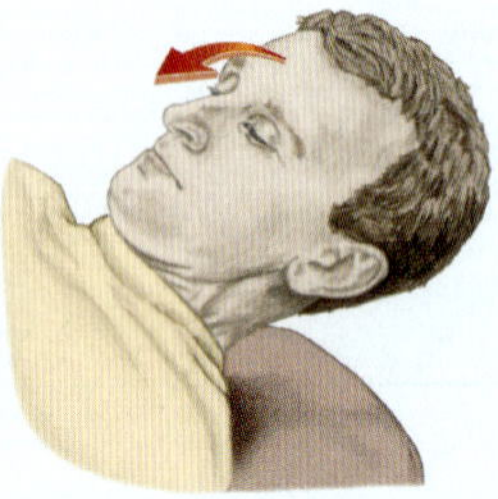

1.65 Flexion of the neck

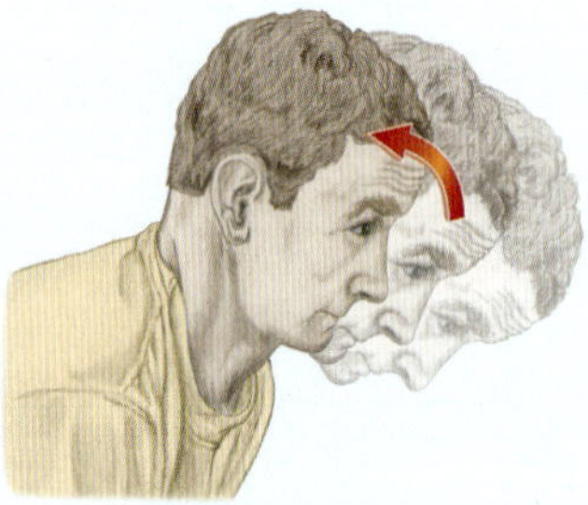

1.66 Extension of the neck

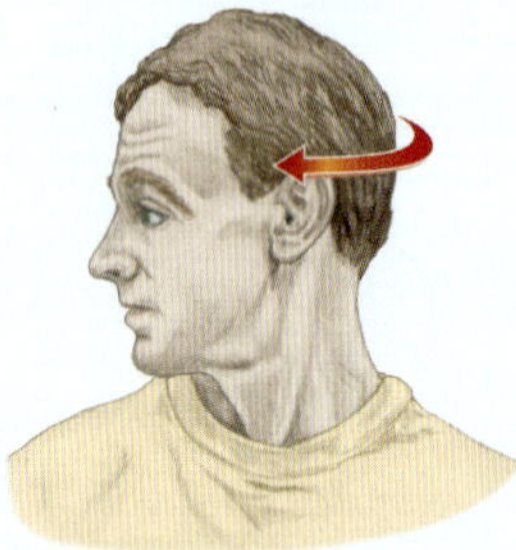

1.67 Rotation of the neck

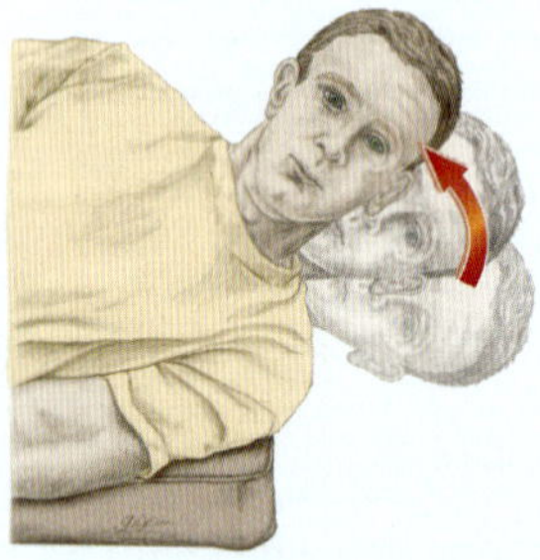

1.68 Lateral flexion of the neck

Ribs/Thorax

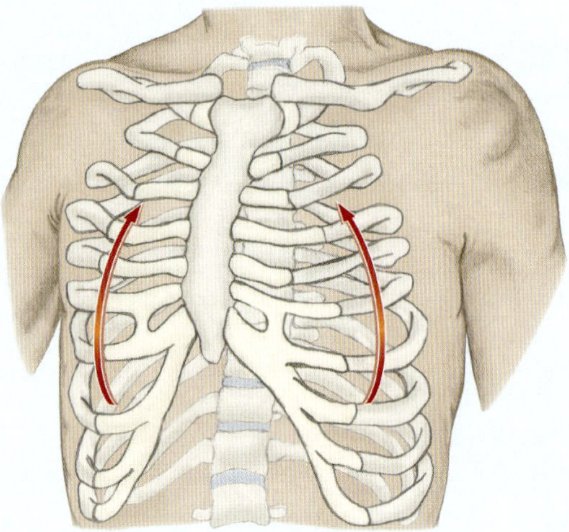

1.69 Elevation/expansion of the ribs/thorax *(inhalation)*

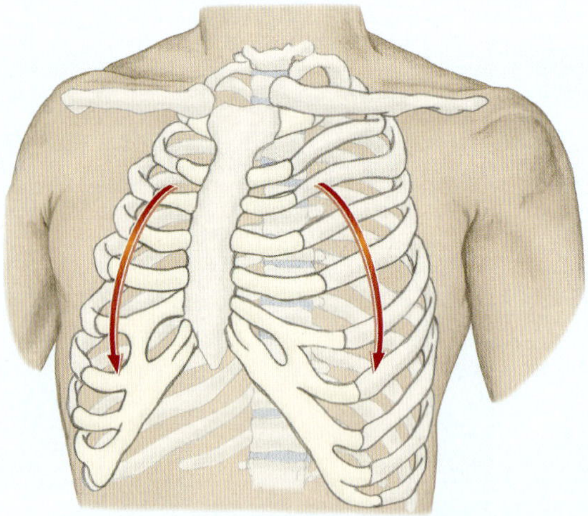

1.70 Depression/collapse of the ribs/thorax *(exhalation)*

Scapula

(scapulothoracic joint)

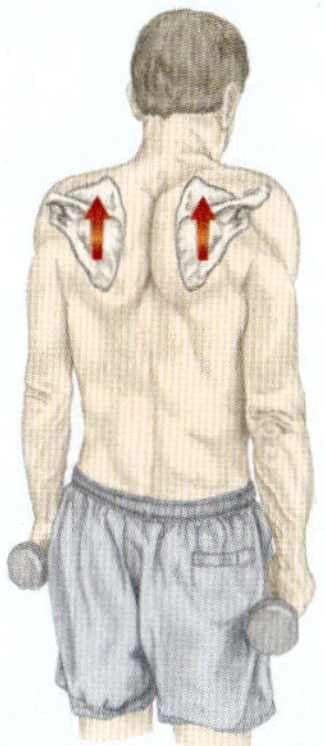

1.71 Elevation of the scapula

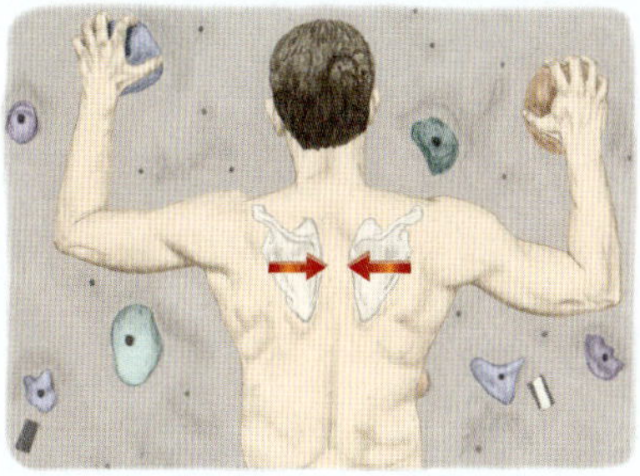

1.72 Adduction of the scapula (*retraction*)

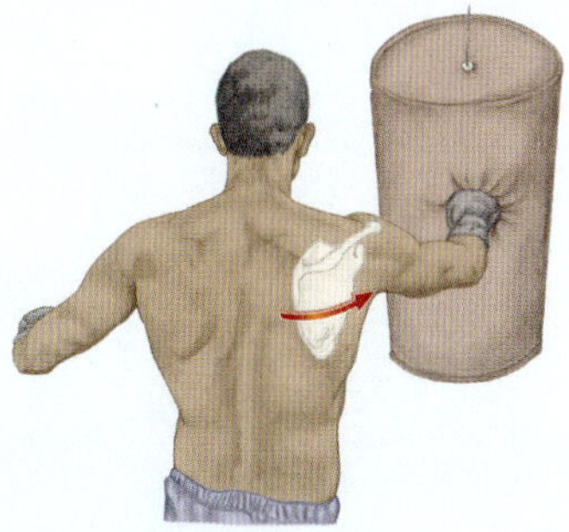

1.75 Abduction of the scapula *(protraction)*

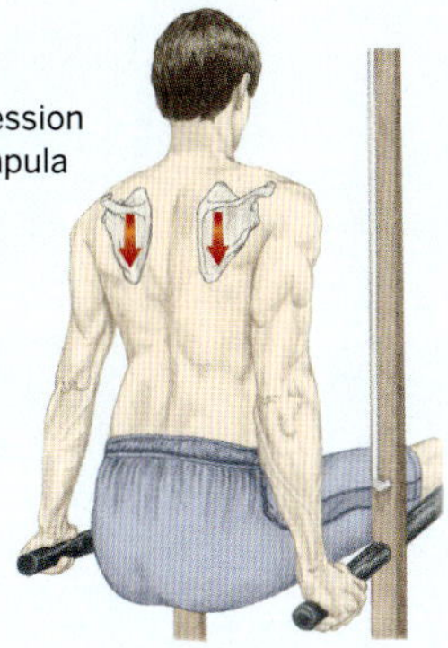

1.73 Depression of the scapula

Upward rotation of left scapula

Downward rotation of right scapula

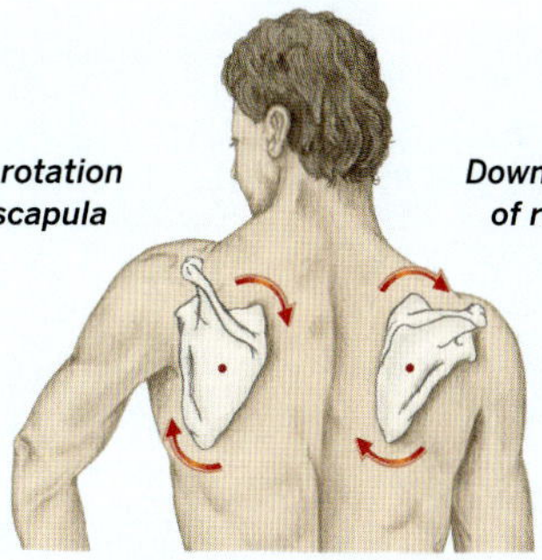

1.74 Upward and downward rotation of the scapula

The scapula can also tilt anteriorly or posteriorly. For **anterior tilt**, the coracoid process shifts anteriorly while the inferior angle moves posteriorly. During **posterior tilt**, the opposite movements occur.

Shoulder

(glenohumeral joint)

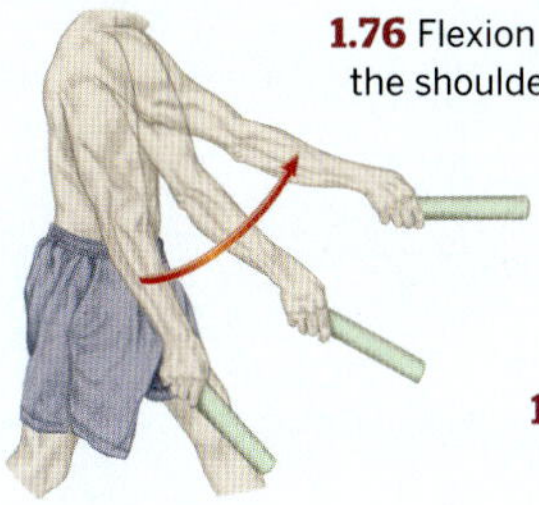

1.76 Flexion of the shoulder

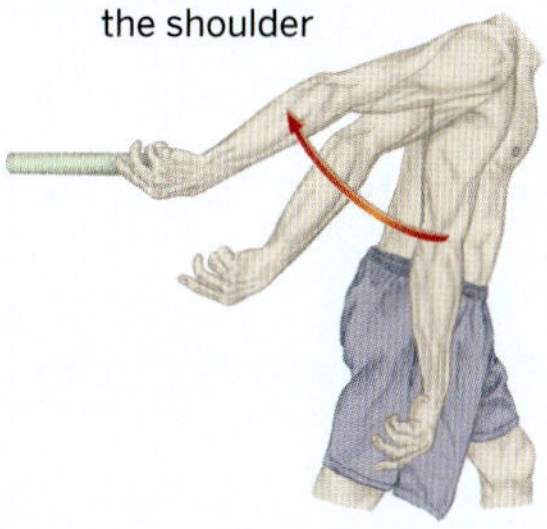

1.77 Extension of the shoulder

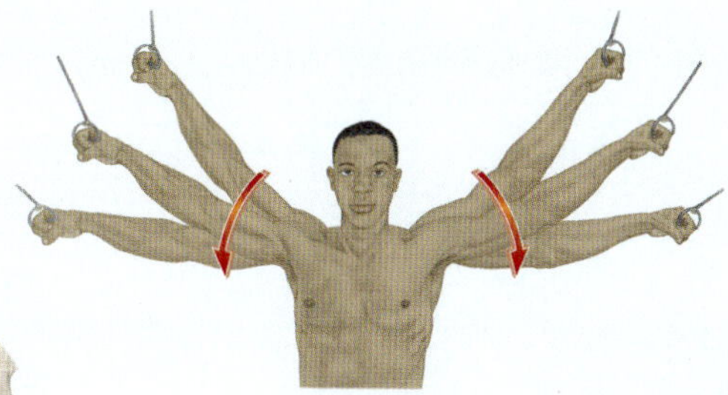

1.78 Adduction of the shoulder

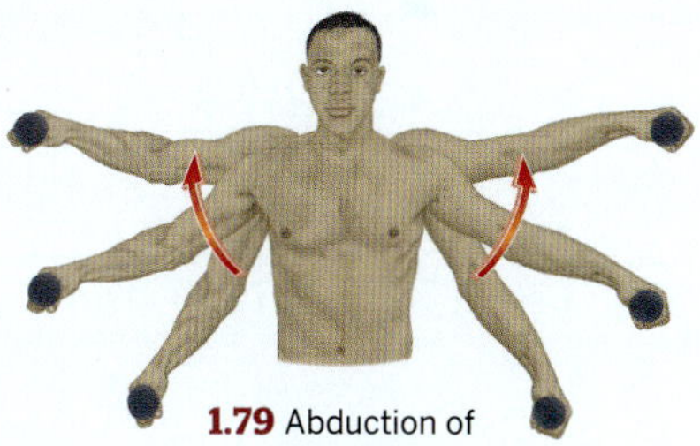

1.79 Abduction of the shoulder

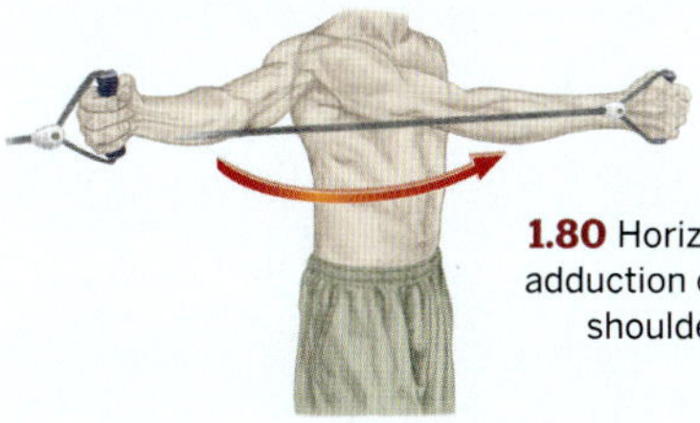

1.80 Horizontal adduction of the shoulder

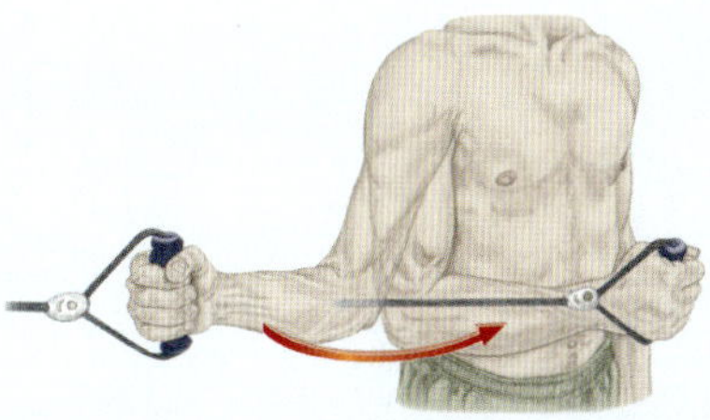

1.82 Medial rotation of the shoulder *(internal rotation)*

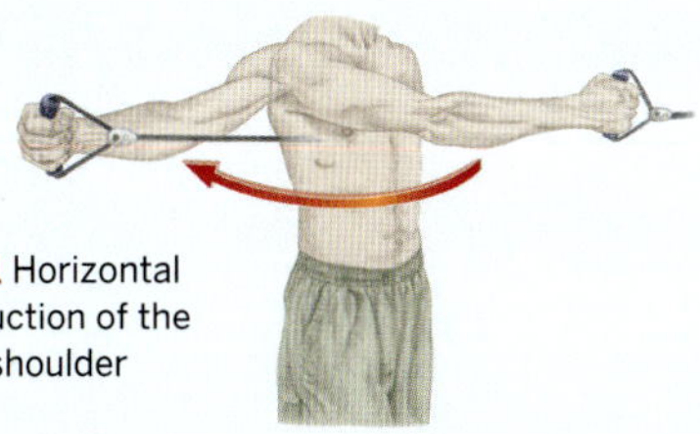

1.81 Horizontal abduction of the shoulder

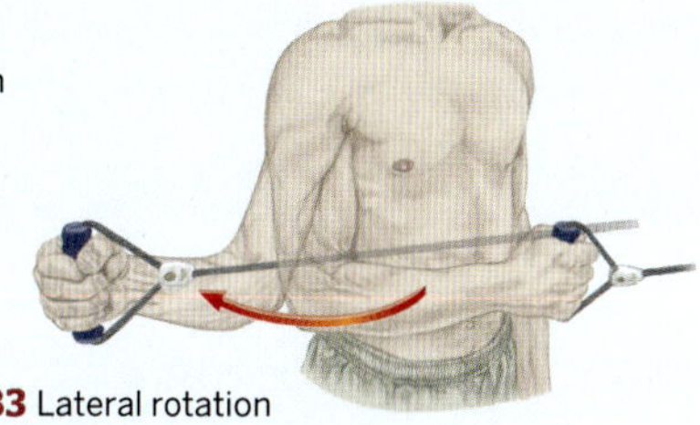

1.83 Lateral rotation of the shoulder *(external rotation)*

Elbow and Forearm

(humeroulnar and humeroradial joints at the elbow, proximal and distal radioulnar joints at the forearm)

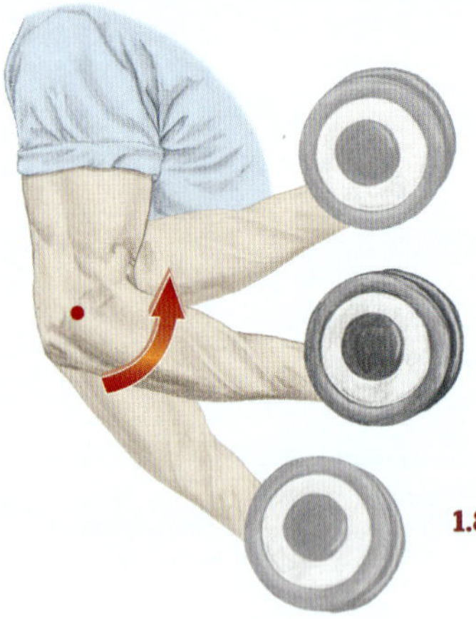

1.84 Flexion of the elbow

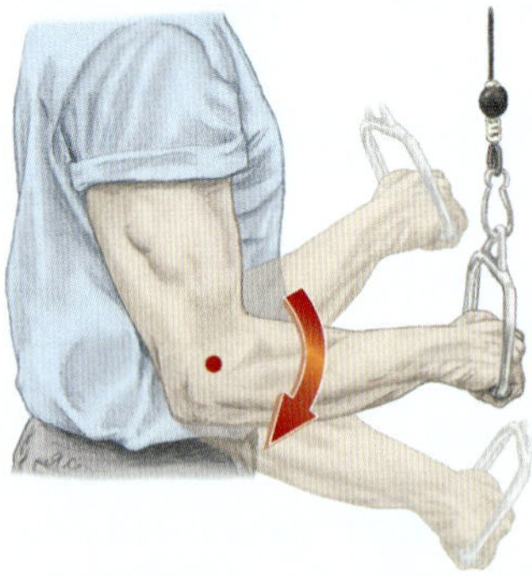

1.85 Extension of the elbow

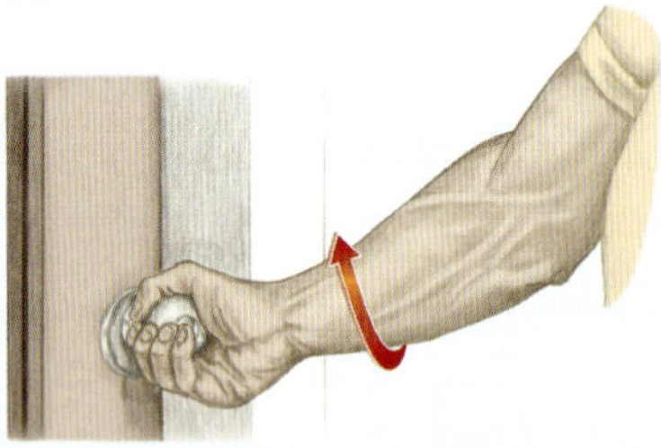

1.86 Supination of the forearm

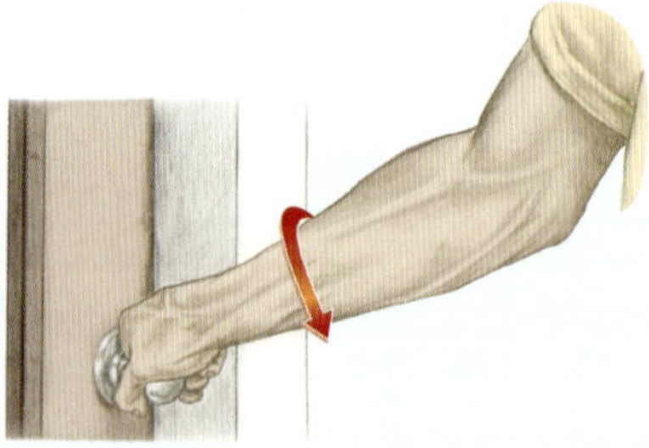

1.87 Pronation of the forearm

Wrist

(radiocarpal joint)

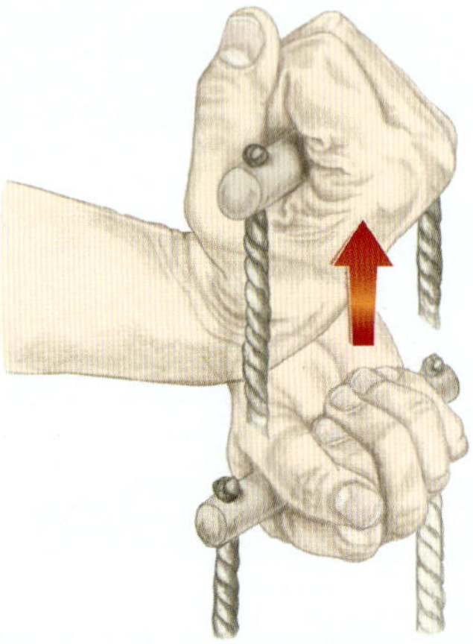

1.88 Flexion of the wrist

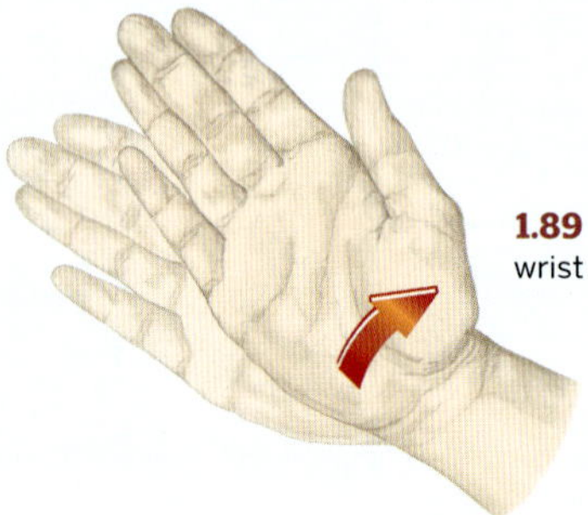

1.89 Abduction of the wrist (*radial deviation*)

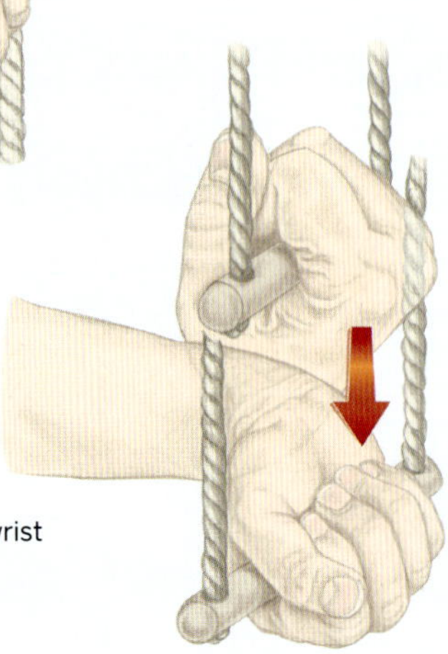

1.90 Extension of the wrist

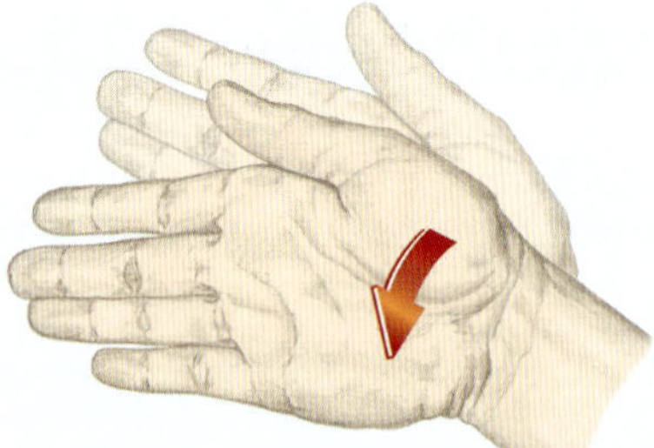

1.91 Adduction of the wrist (*ulnar deviation*)

Thumb

(first carpometacarpal and metacarpophalangeal joints)

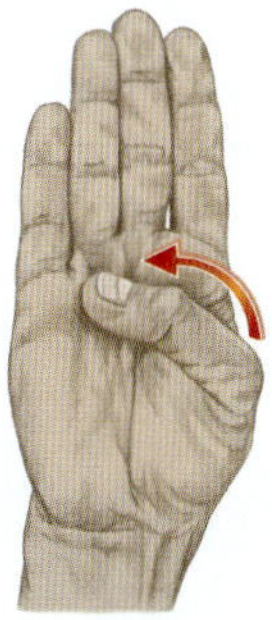

1.92 Flexion of the thumb

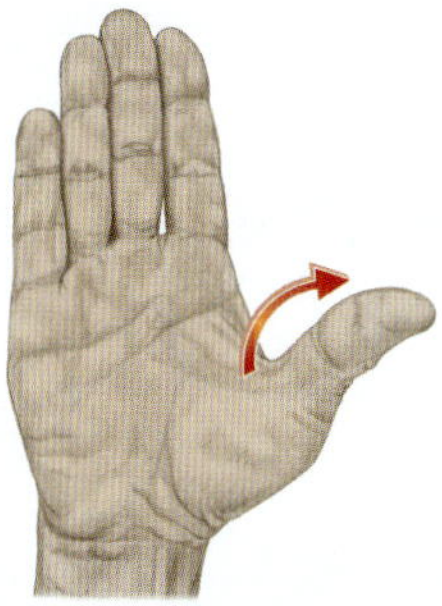

1.93 Extension of the thumb

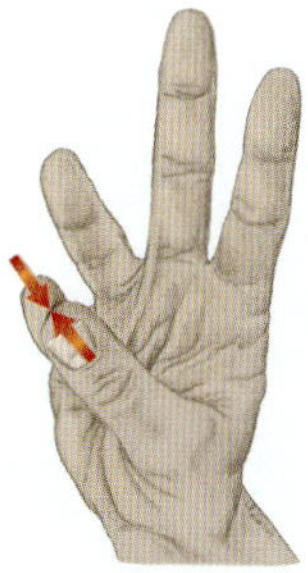

1.94 Opposition of the thumb

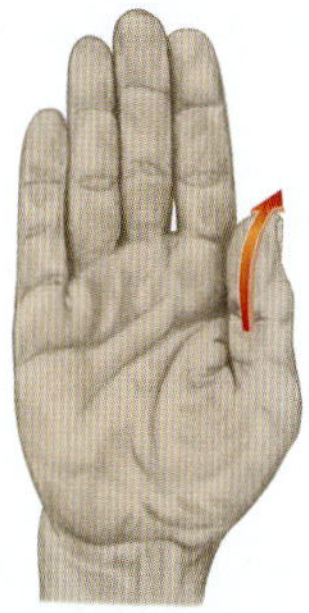

1.95 Adduction of the thumb

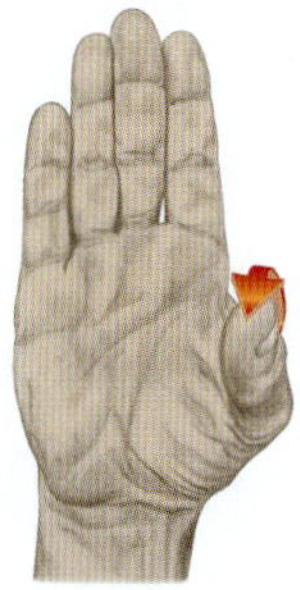

1.96 Abduction of the thumb

Fingers

(metacarpophalangeal, proximal and distal interphalangeal joints)

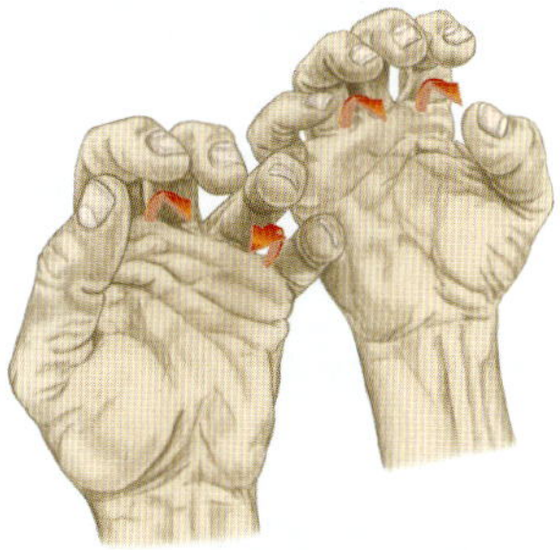

1.97 Flexion of the fingers

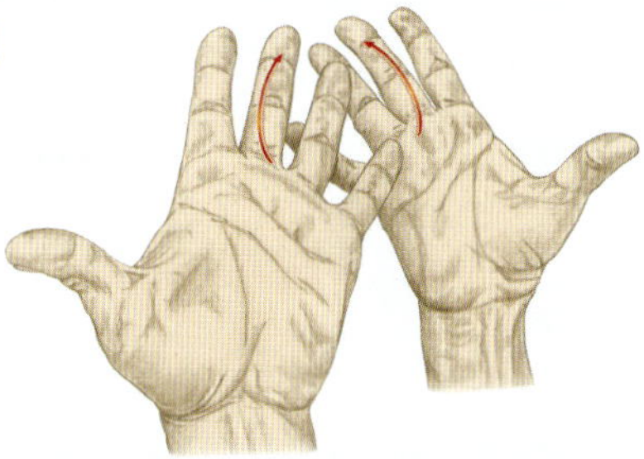

1.98 Extension of the fingers

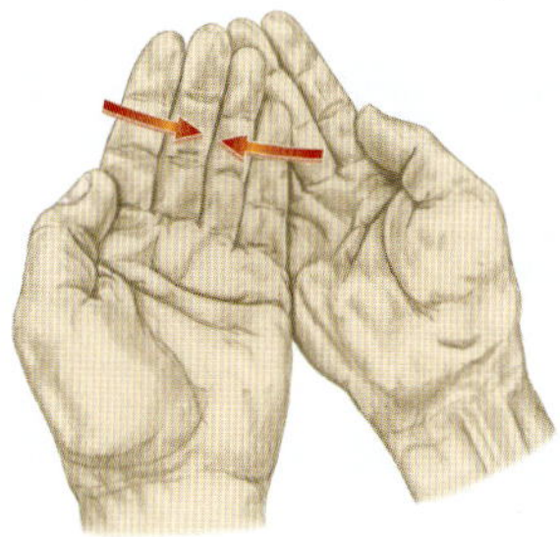

1.99 Adduction of the fingers

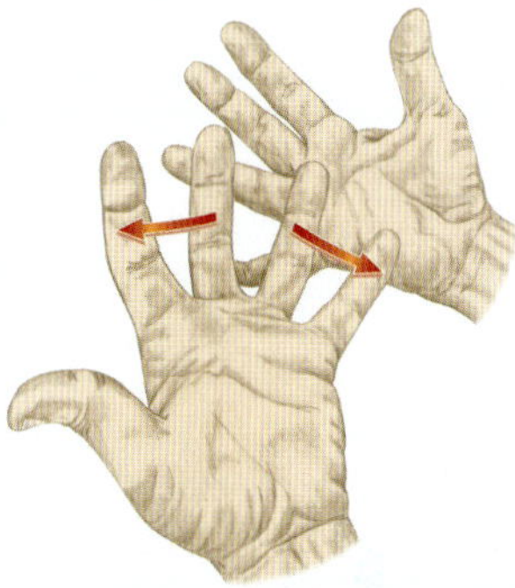

1.100 Abduction of the fingers

Mandible

(temporomandibular joint)

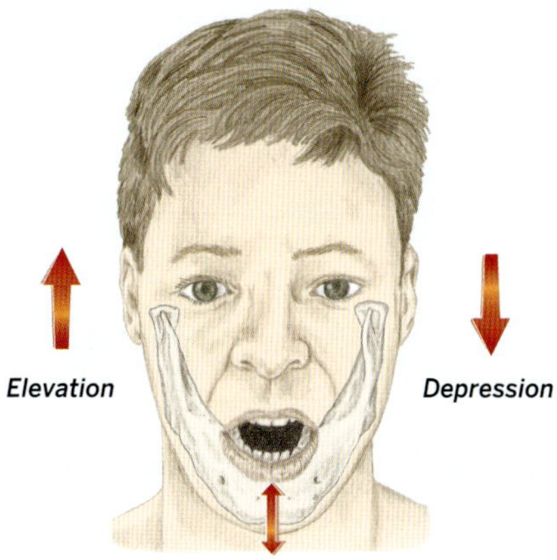

1.101 Elevation and depression of the mandible

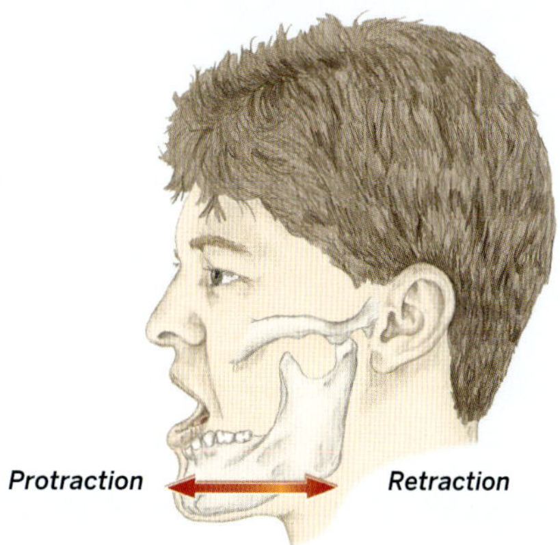

1.102 Protraction and retraction of the mandible

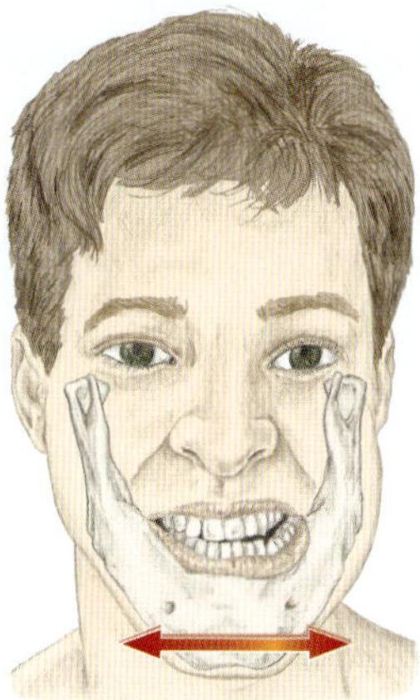

1.103 Lateral deviation of the mandible

Pelvis

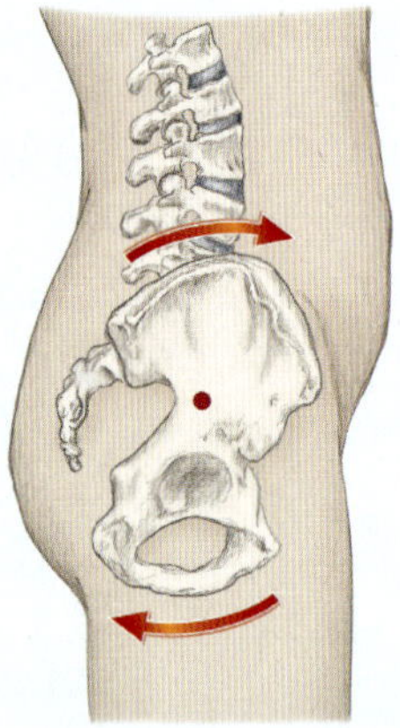

1.104 Anterior tilt of pelvis (*downward rotation*)

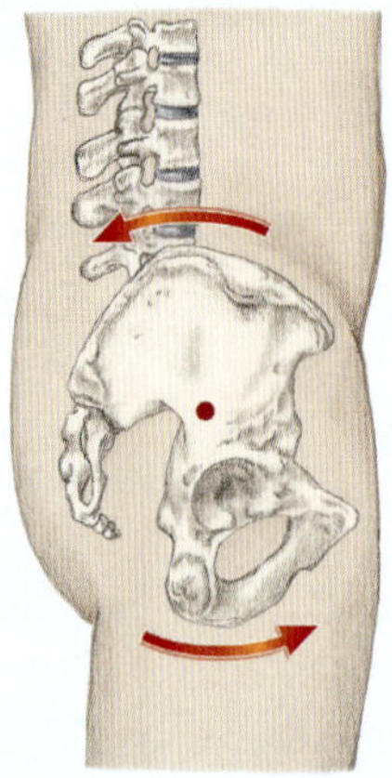

1.105 Posterior tilt of pelvis (*upward rotation*)

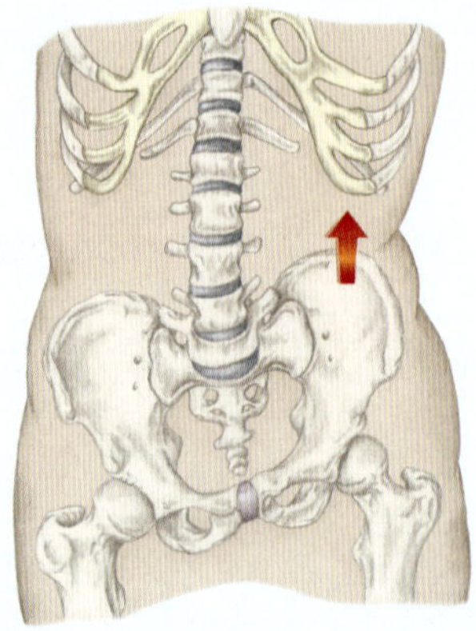

1.106 Lateral tilt of pelvis (*elevation*)

Hip

(*coxal joint*)

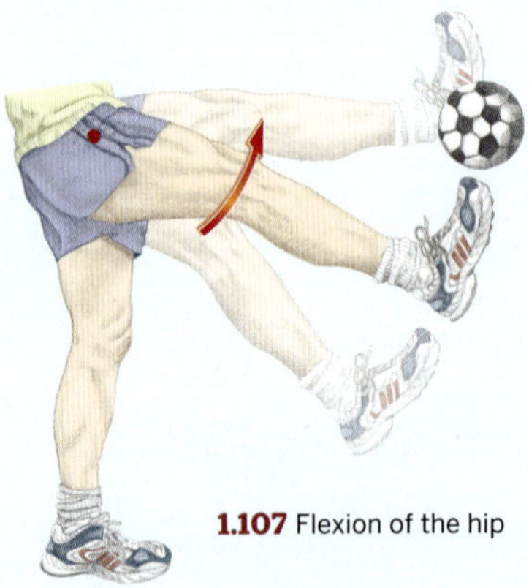

1.107 Flexion of the hip

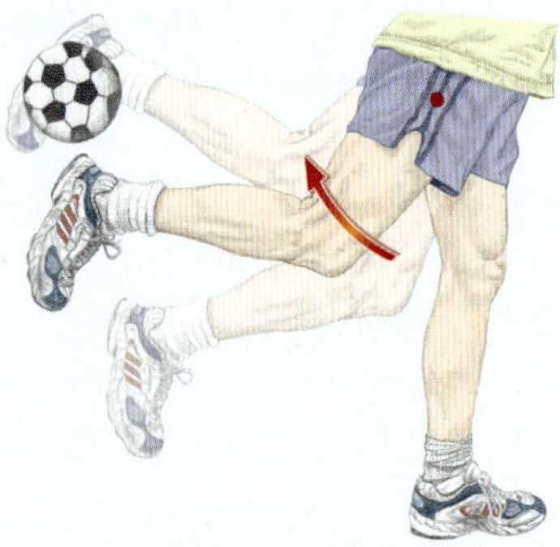

1.108 Extension of the hip

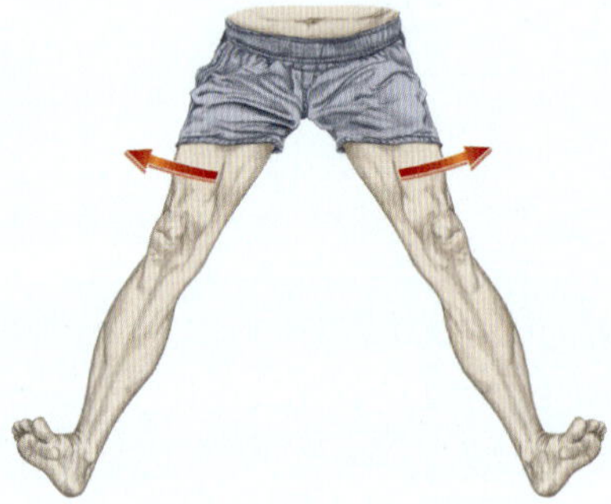

1.109 Abduction of the hip

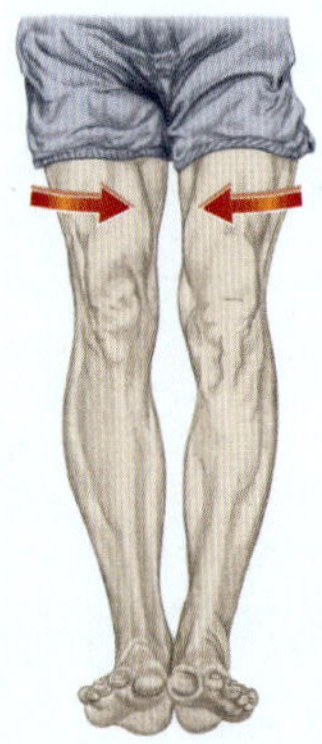

1.110 Adduction of the hip

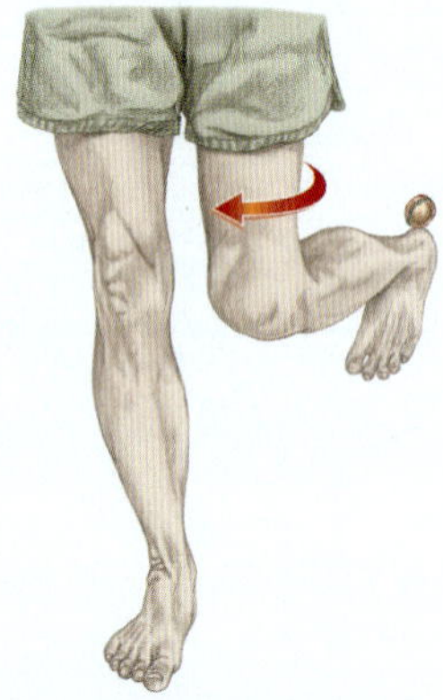

1.111 Medial rotation of the hip (*internal rotation*)

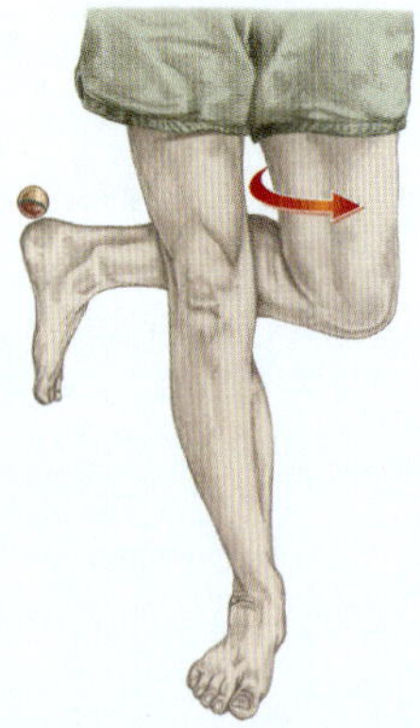

1.112 Lateral rotation of the hip (*external rotation*)

Knee

(tibiofemoral joint)

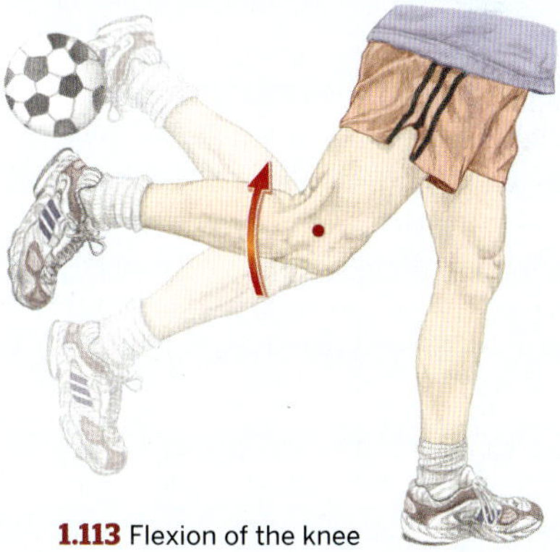

1.113 Flexion of the knee

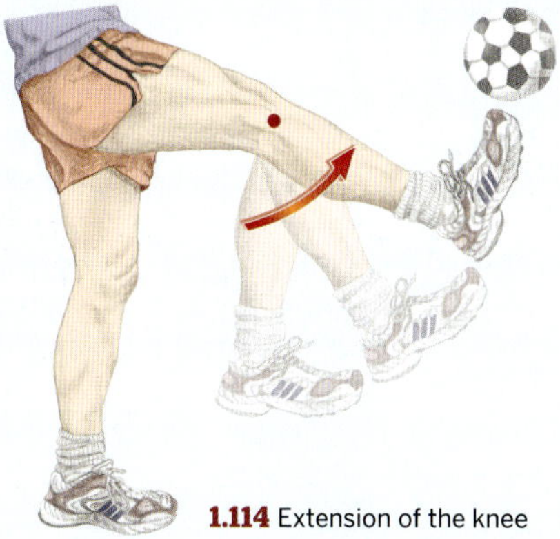

1.114 Extension of the knee

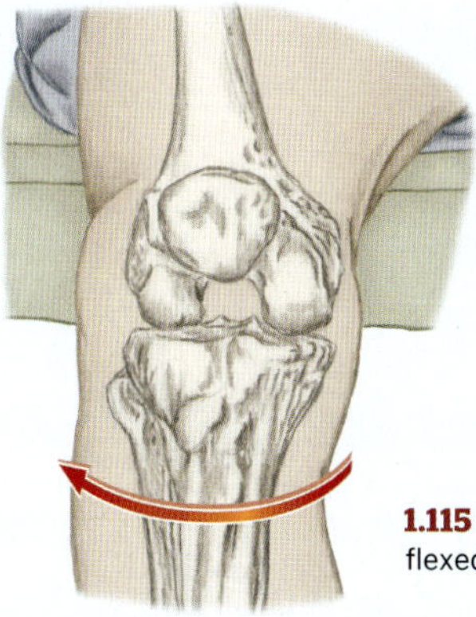

1.115 Lateral rotation of flexed knee (*right knee*)

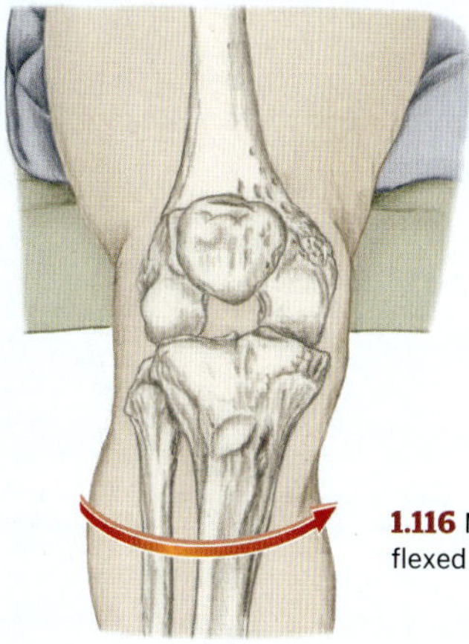

1.116 Medial rotation of flexed knee (*right knee*)

Ankle, Foot, and Toes

(talocrural, talotarsal, tarsometatarsal, midtarsal, metatarsophalangeal, and interphalangeal joints)

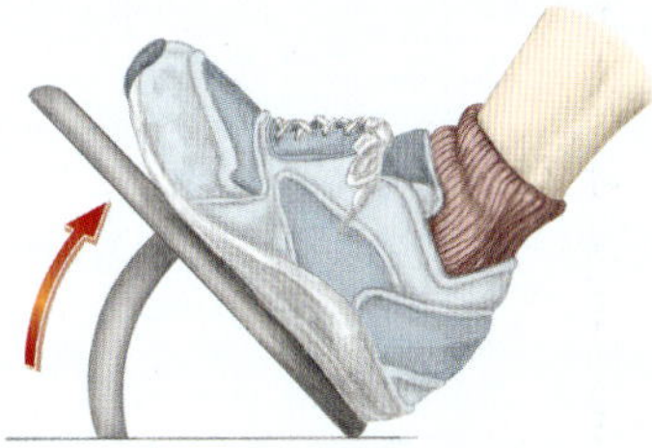

1.117 Dorsiflexion of ankle

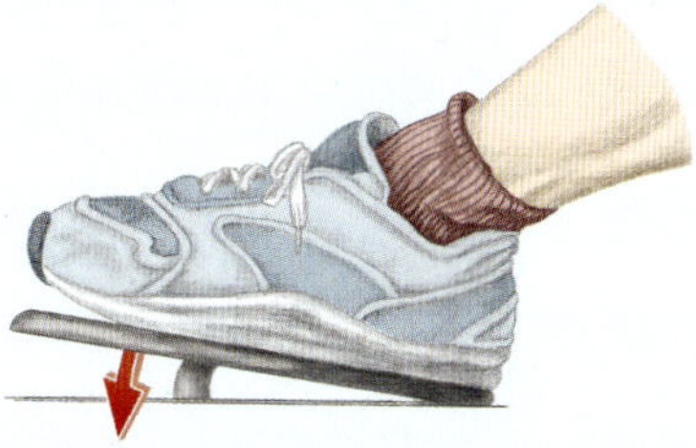

1.118 Plantar flexion of ankle

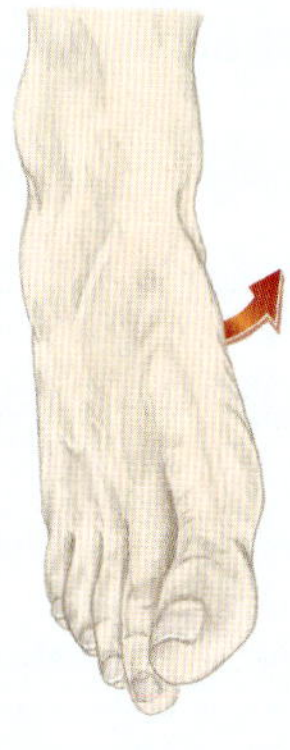

1.119 Inversion of foot

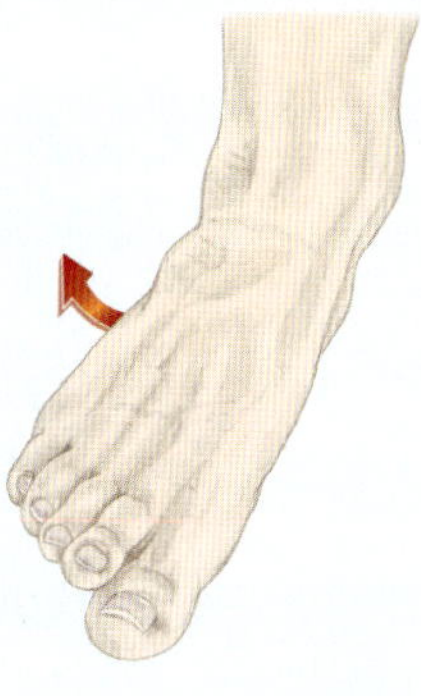

1.120 Eversion of foot

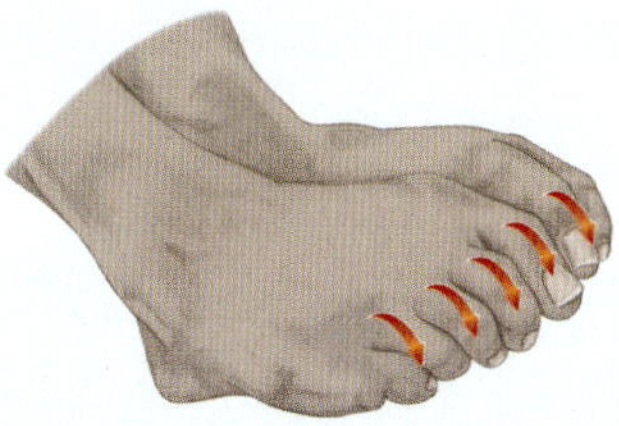

1.121 Flexion of toes

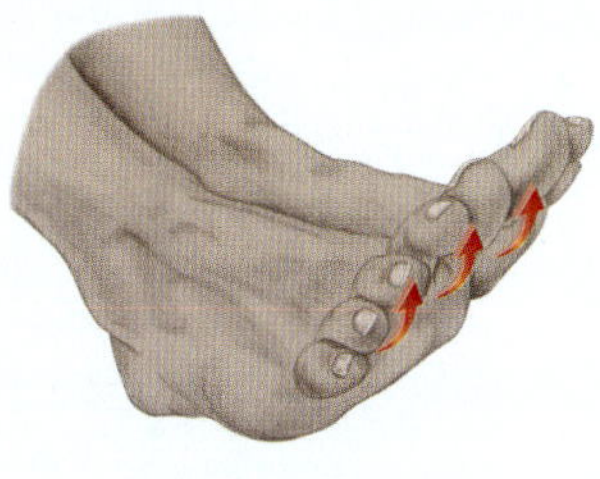

1.122 Extension of toes

Systems of the Body

The Skeletal System

The bones are linked together to form the skeleton. The skeleton is divided into two sections: the axial and the appendicular skeletons. The **axial** skeleton is the skeleton's center (**1.123**). It includes the cranium, vertebral column, ribs, sternum, and hyoid bone. The **appendicular** ("appendages") skeleton (**1.124**) is composed of the arms and legs, including the pectoral girdle (scapula and clavicle) and pelvic girdle (hips).

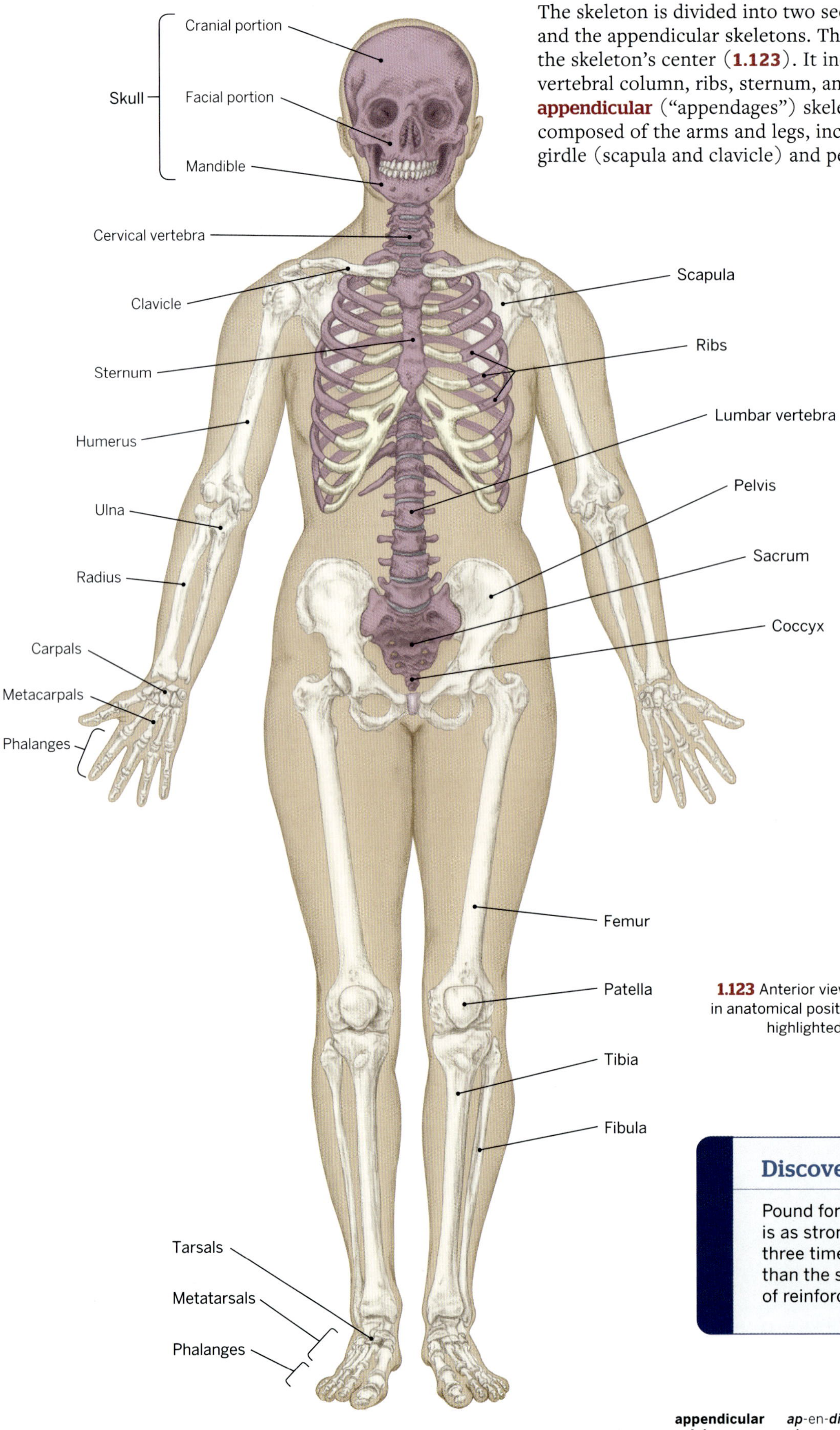

1.123 Anterior view of the skeleton in anatomical position, axial skeleton highlighted in purple

Discover More

Pound for pound, bone is as strong as steel and three times stronger than the same quantity of reinforced concrete.

appendicular	*ap*-en-*dik*-u-lar	L. to hang to
axial	*ak*-see-al	L. axle
skeleton	*skel*-et-on	Grk. dried up

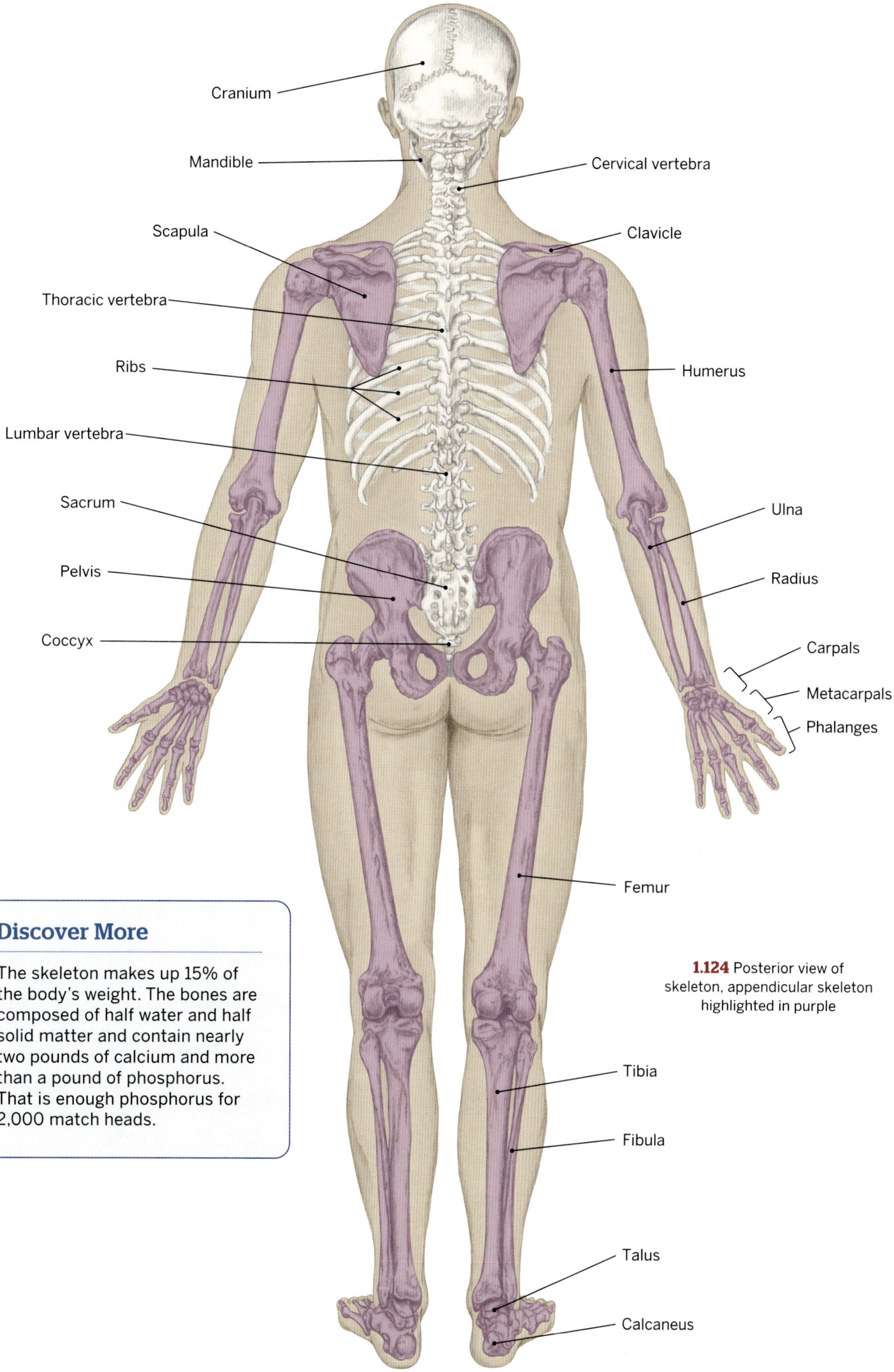

1.124 Posterior view of skeleton, appendicular skeleton highlighted in purple

Discover More

The skeleton makes up 15% of the body's weight. The bones are composed of half water and half solid matter and contain nearly two pounds of calcium and more than a pound of phosphorus. That is enough phosphorus for 2,000 match heads.

Types of Joints

A joint, or articulation, is the point of contact between bones. A joint's **structure determines its function**. All articulations have a fibrous, cartilaginous, or synovial structure. Because of their design, fibrous and cartilaginous joints have little or no movement capability. **Synovial joints**, however, **contain a joint cavity** (absent in fibrous and cartilaginous joints). This space allows for movement at the synovial joint. Although synovial joints all have the same basic structural components, they have different movement capabilities. There are six types of synovial joints: ball-and-socket, ellipsoid, hinge, saddle, gliding, and pivot.

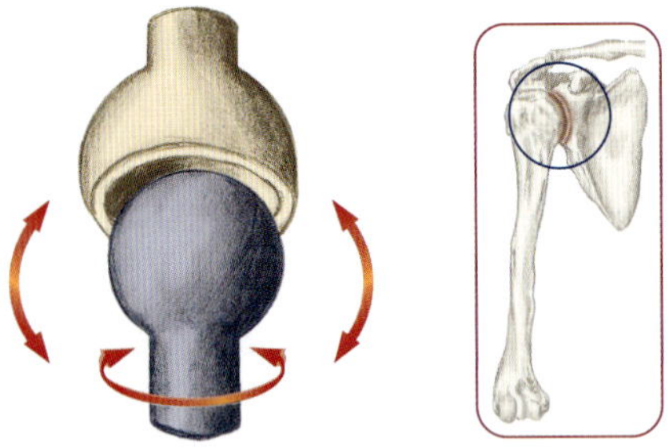

1.125 Ball-and-socket joint (left); anterior view of right shoulder joint (right)

A **ball-and-socket joint** is self-explanatory: A spherical surface of one bone fits into the dish-shaped depression of another bone. Such a joint is capable of movement in every plane. The shoulder (or glenohumeral joint) is an example of a joint capable of circumduction (**1.125**).

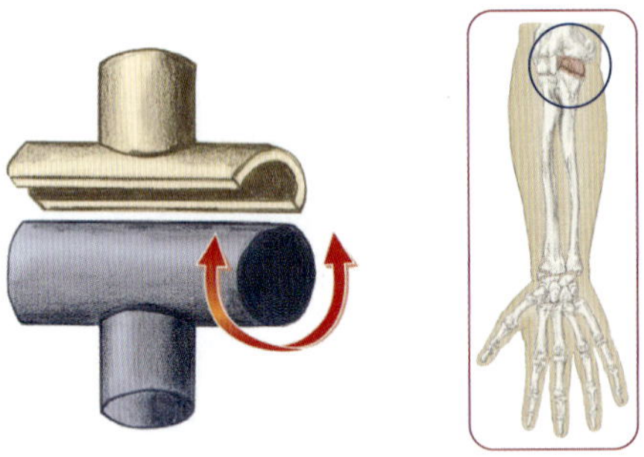

1.127 Hinge joint (left); anterior view of right elbow joint (right)

A **hinge joint** allows only flexion and extension, similar to the movements of a door hinge. An example of a hinge joint is the elbow (humeroulnar) joint (**1.127**).

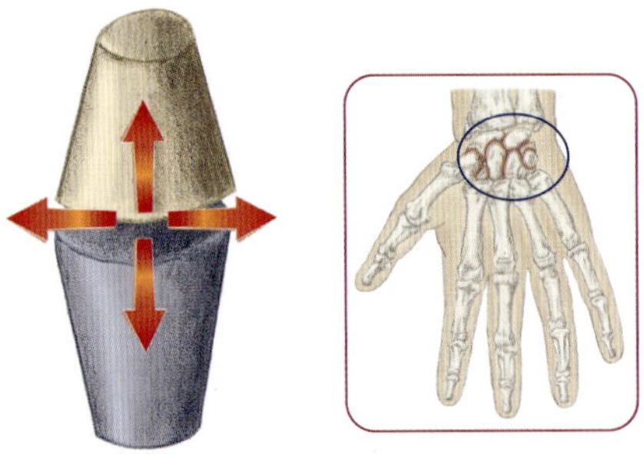

1.129 Gliding joint (left); anterior view of right wrist (right)

A **gliding joint** is usually between two flat surfaces and allows the least movement of all synovial joints. Only small shifting movements are possible at these articulations, such as those between the carpal bones in the wrist or tarsal bones in the foot (**1.129**).

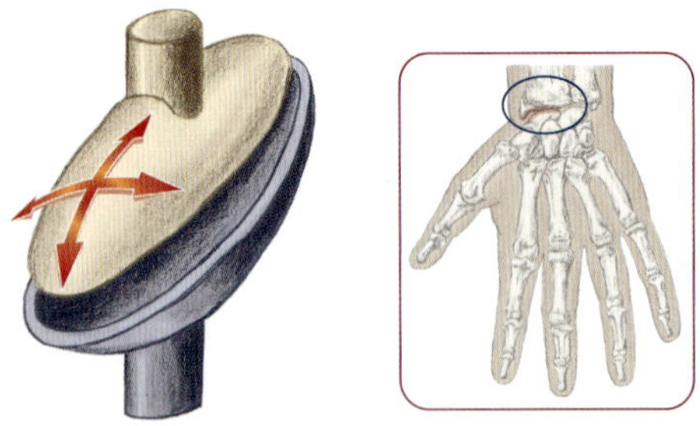

1.126 Ellipsoid joint (left); anterior view of right wrist joint (right)

An **ellipsoid joint** consists of the oval-shaped end of one bone articulating with the elliptical basin of another bone. It permits flexion/extension and abduction/adduction as seen at the wrist (radiocarpal) joint (**1.126**).

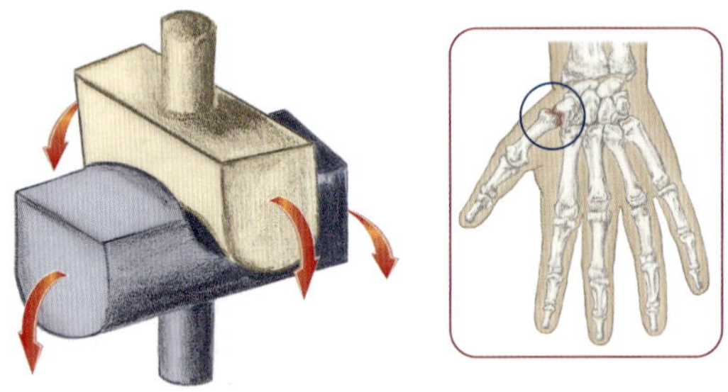

1.128 Saddle joint (left); anterior view of right thumb (right)

A **saddle joint** is a modified ellipsoid joint composed of convex and concave articulating surfaces—like two saddles. The joint between the trapezium (one of the small carpal bones in the wrist) and the first metacarpal bones is an example of a saddle joint (**1.128**).

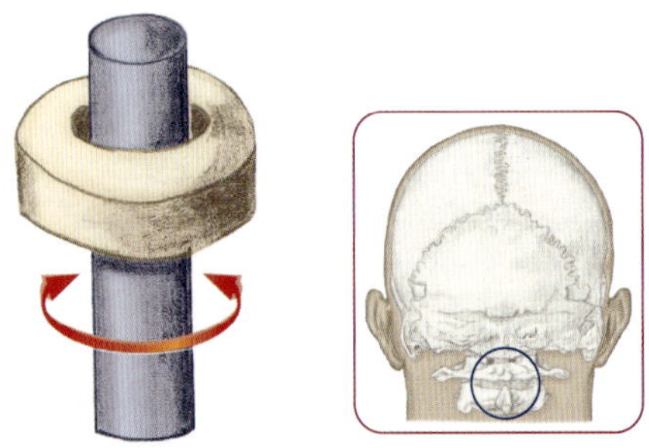

1.130 Pivot joint (left); posterior view of atlantoaxial joint (right)

A **pivot joint** is designed to allow one bone to rotate around the surface of another bone. For example, rotation of the head occurs because of the pivot joint between the first and second cervical vertebrae (the atlantoaxial joint) (**1.130**).

joint		L. to join
synovial	sin-**o**-ve-al	L. *synovia*, joint fluid

The Muscular System

A muscle's name can give you clues to its specific features. The name reflects either a muscle's shape (rhomboid), location (temporalis), fiber direction (external oblique), action (adductors), or attachment sites (coracobrachialis).

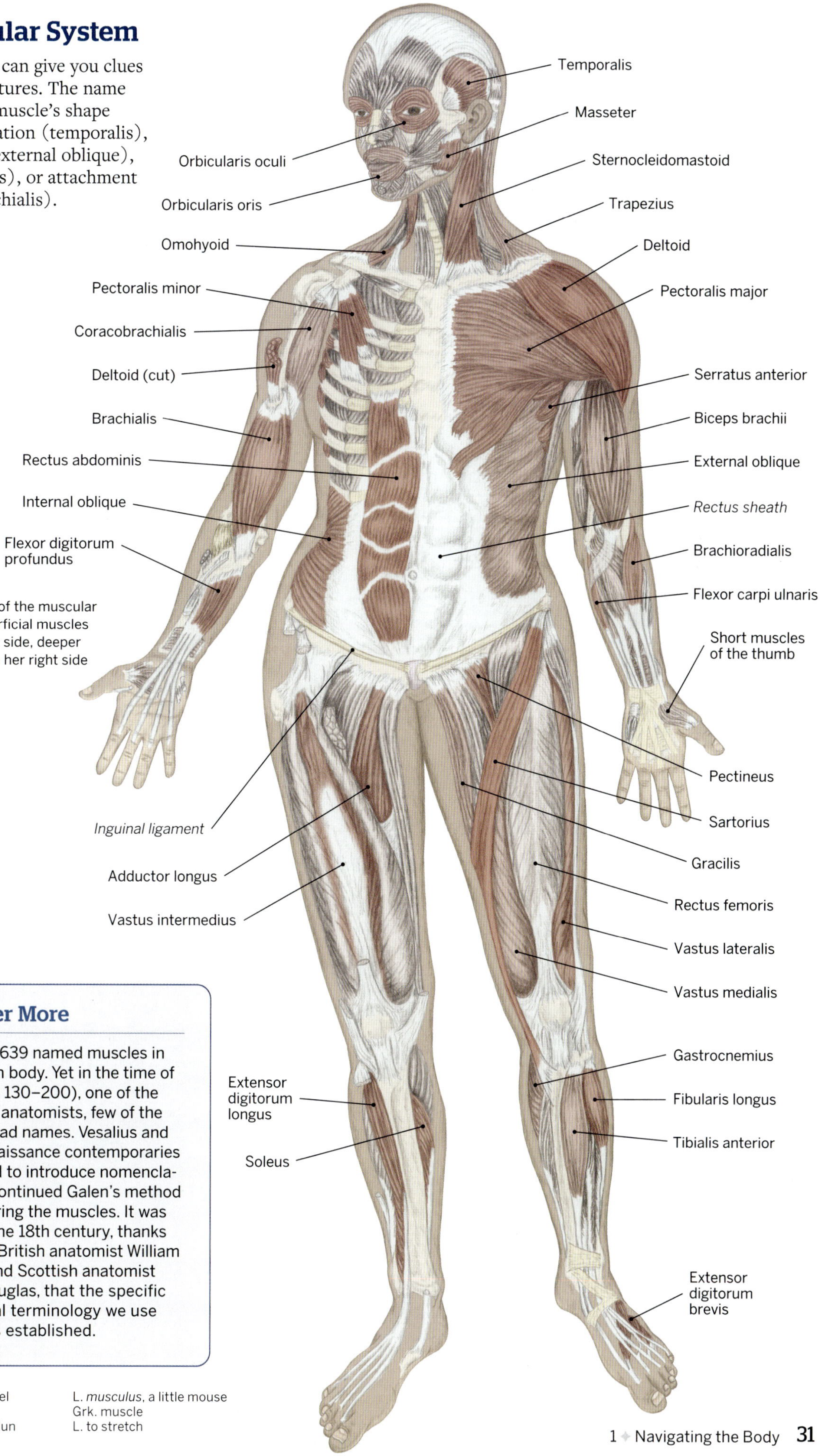

1.131 Anterior view of the muscular system, with superficial muscles shown on her left side, deeper muscles shown on her right side

Discover More

There are 639 named muscles in the human body. Yet in the time of Galen (AD 130–200), one of the first great anatomists, few of the muscles had names. Vesalius and other Renaissance contemporaries attempted to introduce nomenclature, yet continued Galen's method of numbering the muscles. It was not until the 18th century, thanks largely to British anatomist William Cowper and Scottish anatomist James Douglas, that the specific myological terminology we use today was established.

muscle	*mus*-el	L. *musculus*, a little mouse
myo-		Grk. muscle
tendon	*ten*-dun	L. to stretch

At either end of the muscle is a tendon, which attaches the muscle to a bone. Each muscle has an origin and an insertion. The origin is the attachment to the more stationary bone and the insertion is the connection to the more mobile bone.

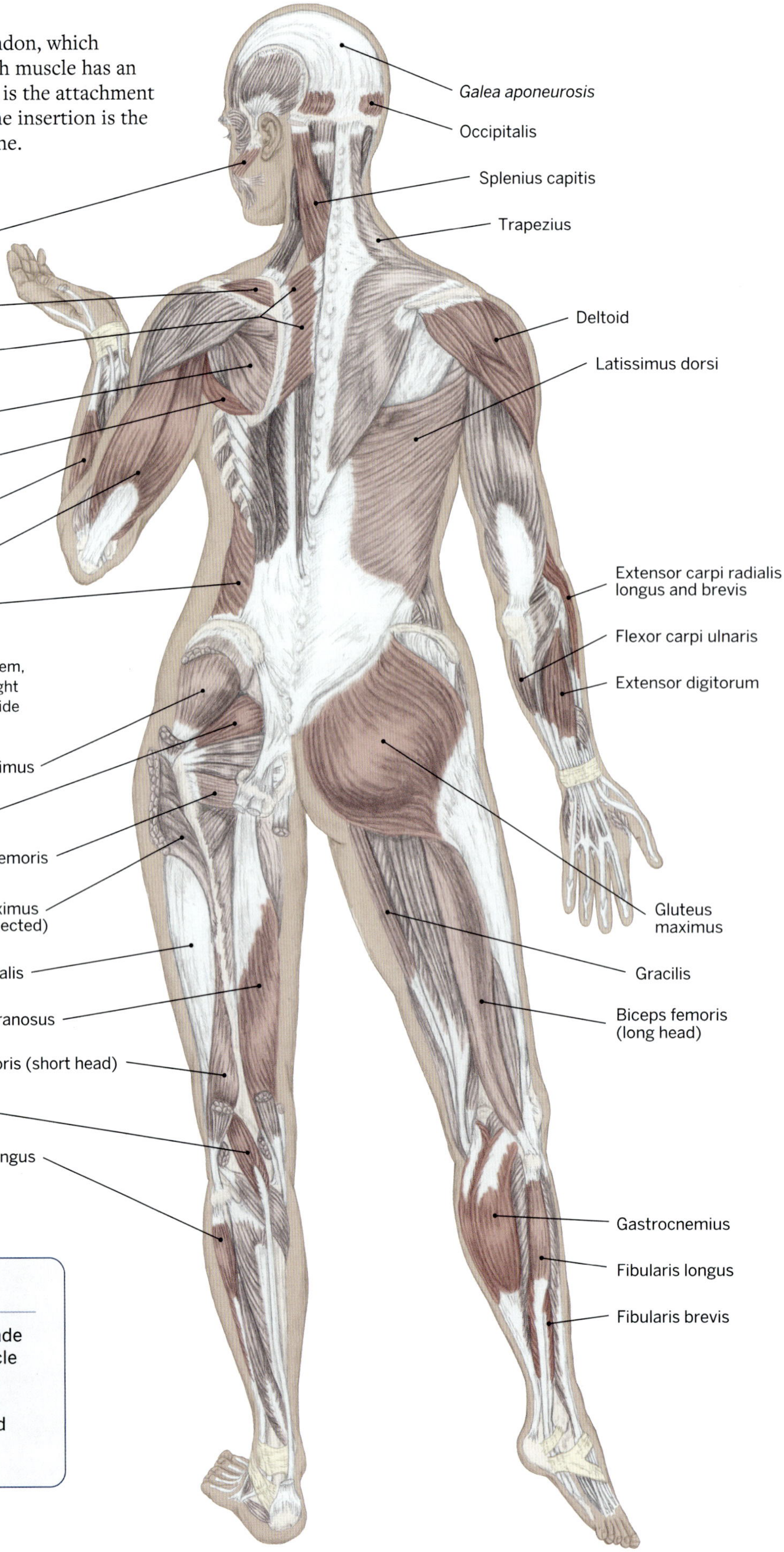

1.132 Posterior view of the muscular system, with superficial muscles shown on her right side, deeper muscles shown on her left side

Discover More

The muscular system is made up of some six trillion muscle fibers. Each fiber is thinner than a human hair but can support up to one thousand times its own weight.

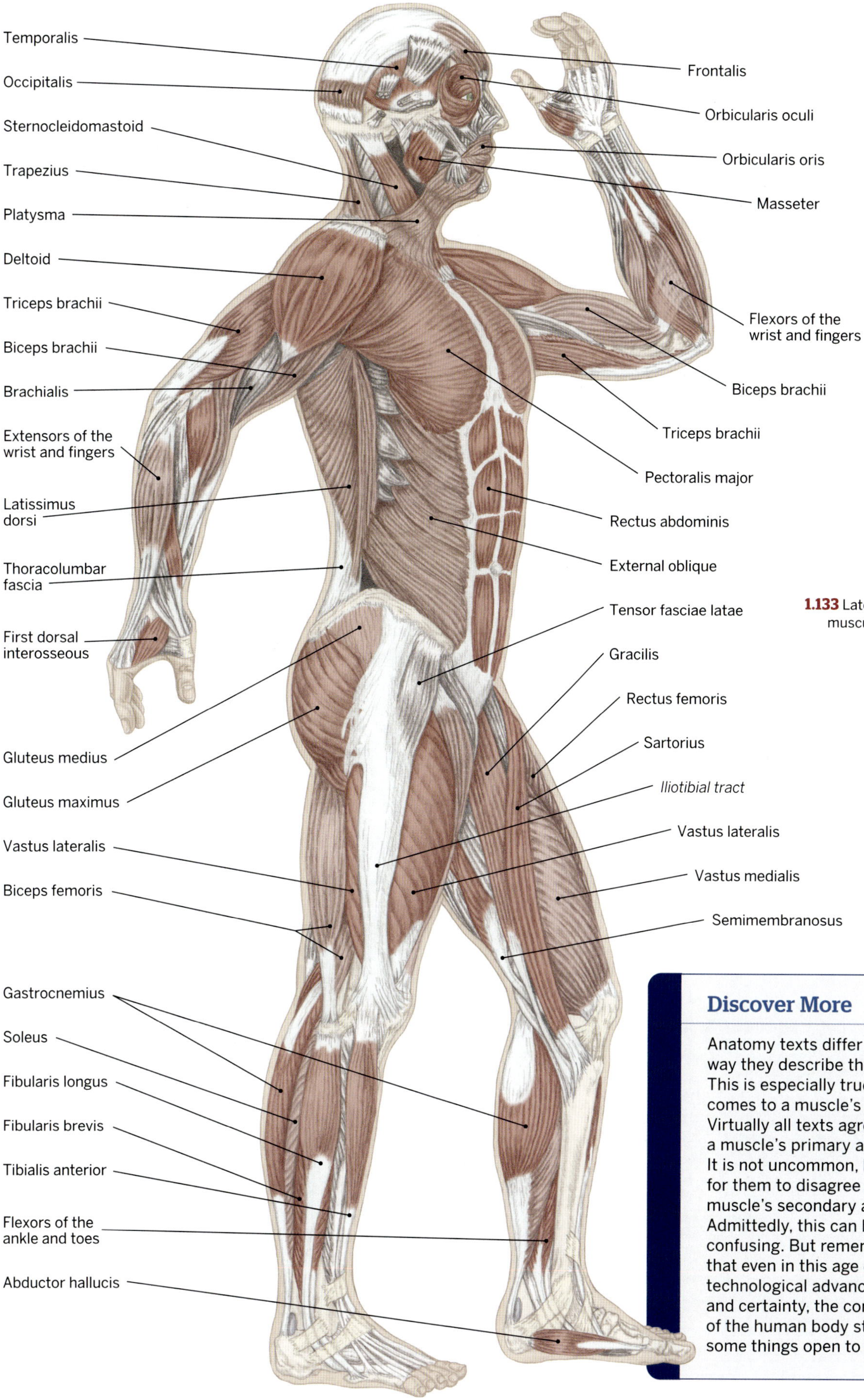

1.133 Lateral view of the muscular system

Discover More

Anatomy texts differ in the way they describe the body. This is especially true when it comes to a muscle's actions. Virtually all texts agree upon a muscle's primary action(s). It is not uncommon, however, for them to disagree about a muscle's secondary actions. Admittedly, this can be confusing. But remember that even in this age of great technological advancement and certainty, the complexity of the human body still leaves some things open to debate.

The Fascial System

The following illustrations show aspects of the fascia from both topographical and cross-section viewpoints.

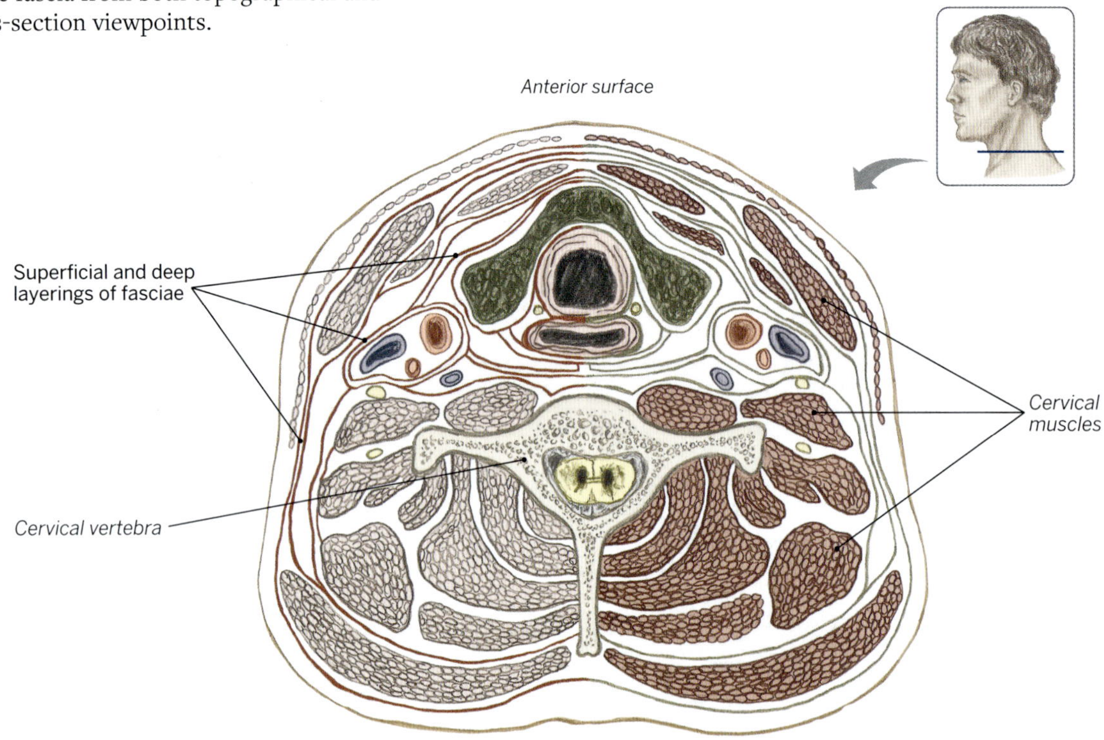

1.134 Cross section of the neck highlighting layers of fasciae (left) and cervical muscles (right)

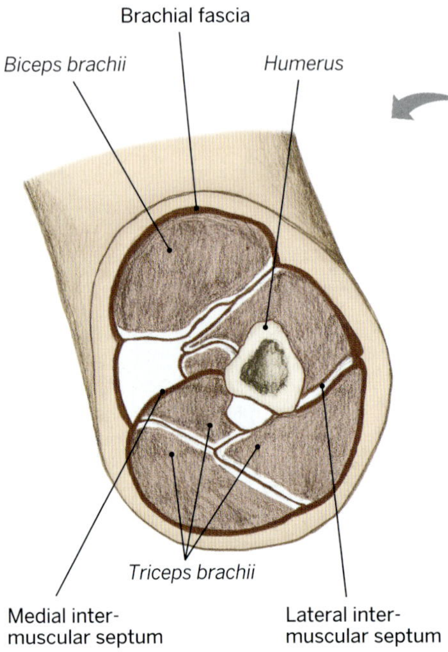

1.135 Cross section of left arm

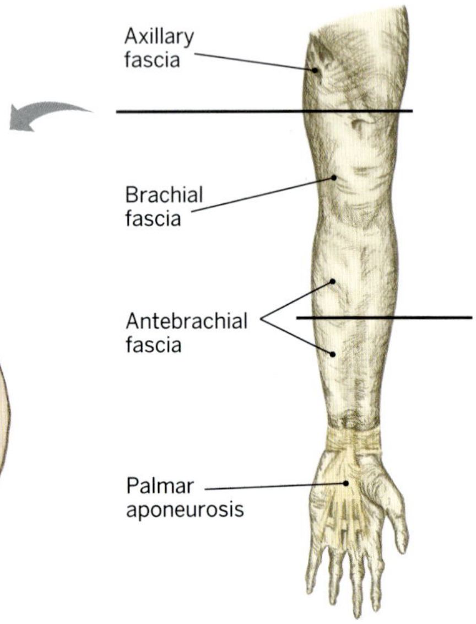

1.136 Anterior view of left arm, forearm, and hand, skin removed

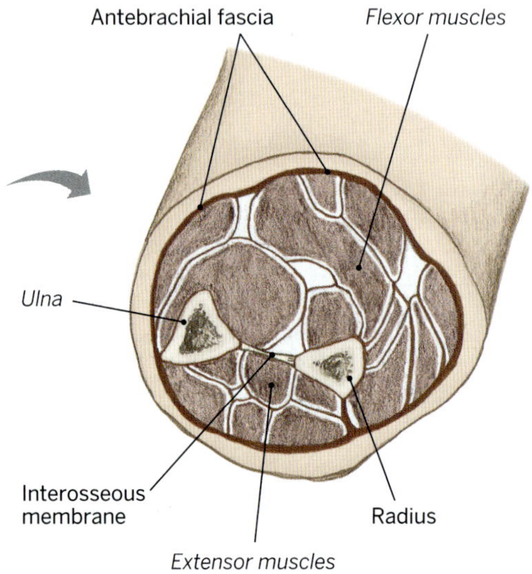

1.137 Cross section of left forearm

fascia	***fash***-ah	L. a band, bandage
retinaculum	***ret***-i-***nak***-u-lum	L. halter, band, rope
septum	***sep***-tum	L. enclosure

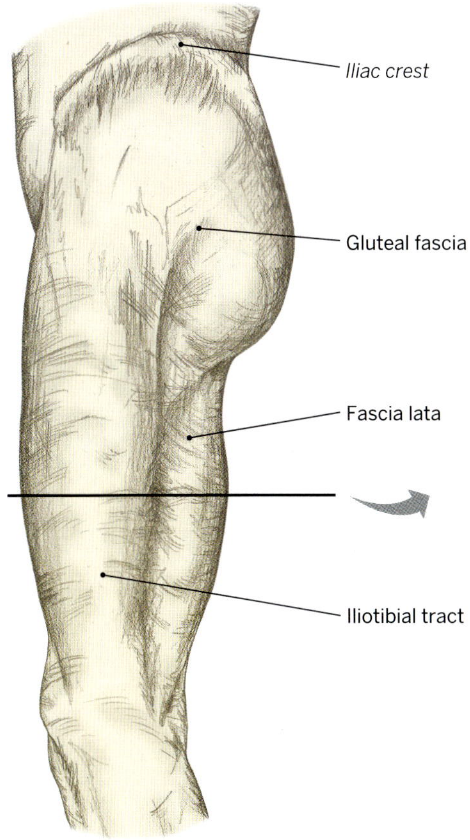

1.138 Fascia of the lateral left thigh and pelvis, skin removed

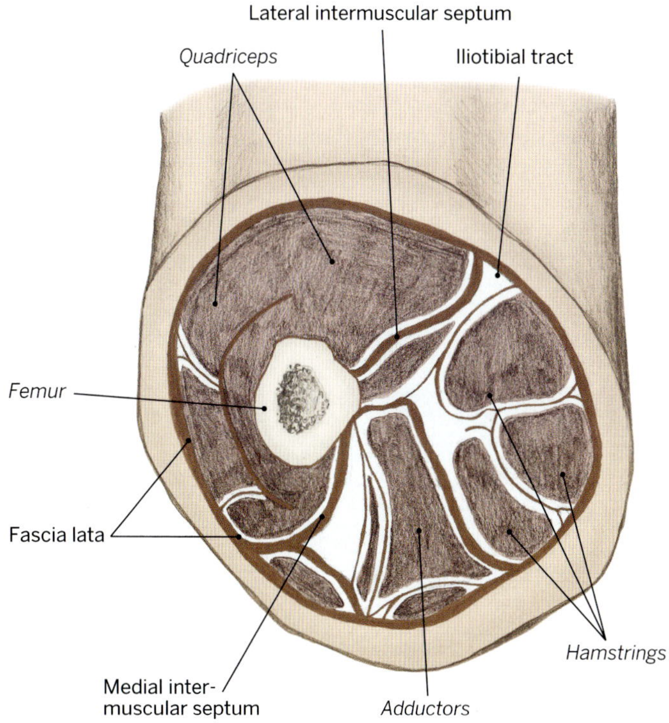

1.139 Cross section of left thigh

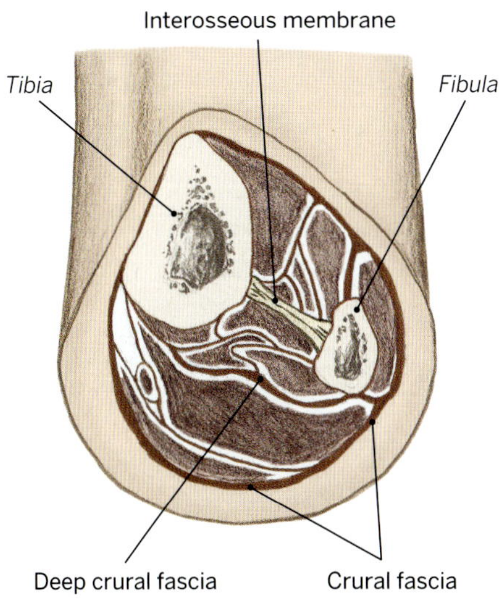

1.140 Cross section of left leg

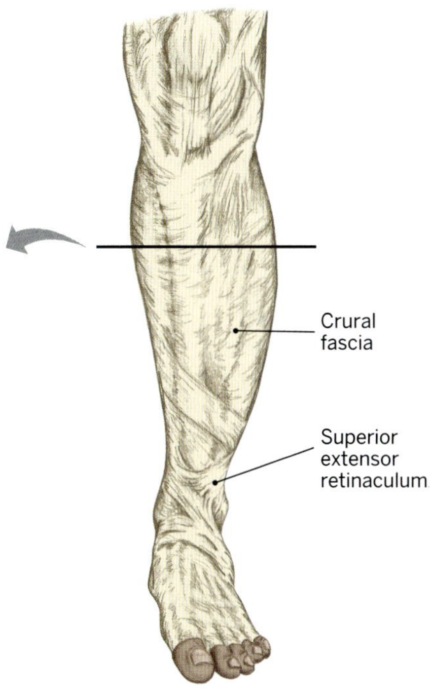

1.141 Anterior view of left leg and foot, skin removed

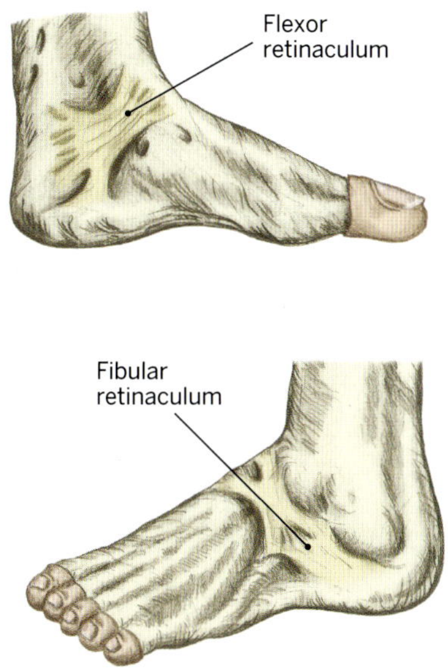

1.142 Medial view (top) and lateral view (bottom) of left foot, skin removed

aponeurosis	***ap***-o-nu-***ro***-sis	Grk. *apo*, from + *neuron*, nerve or tendon
septa	***sep***-ta	plural for septum

The Cardiovascular System

Arteries and veins are the blood vessels of the cardiovascular system (**1.143, 1.144**). They form an amazing network that transports blood from the heart, brings it to the body's tissues, and then carries it back to the heart.

Arteries carry blood away from the heart. As an artery moves away from the heart, it divides into smaller branches. Arterioles, the smallest branches, divide into millions of microscopic vessels called capillaries. The walls of the capillaries serve as nutrient and waste exchange sites between the body's tissues and the blood. The capillaries then merge back together, creating small veins or venules that then unite to form the larger veins that carry the blood back to the heart.

Arteries

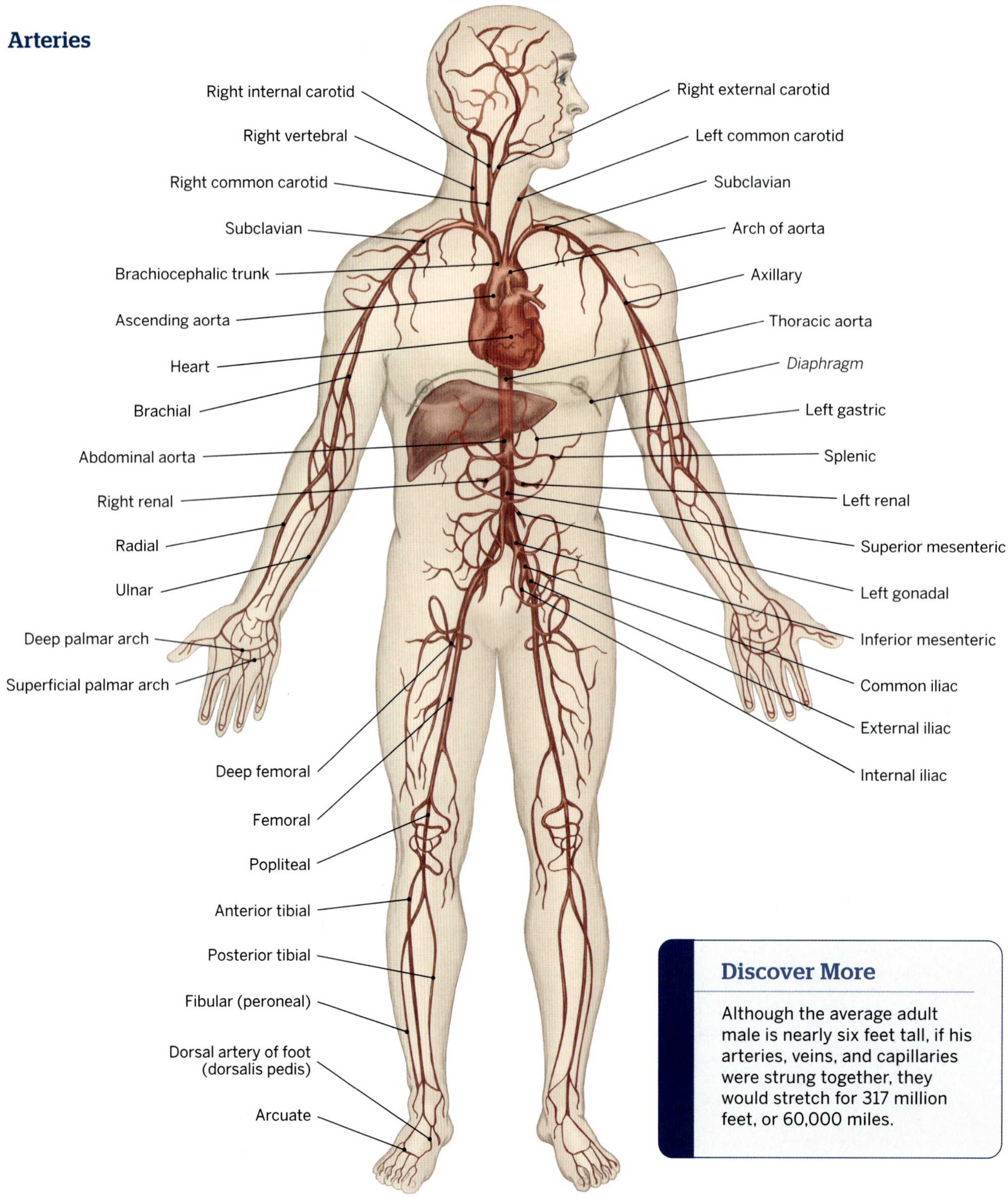

1.143 Anterior view of major arteries of the body

Discover More

Although the average adult male is nearly six feet tall, if his arteries, veins, and capillaries were strung together, they would stretch for 317 million feet, or 60,000 miles.

artery	***ar***-ter-ee	Grk. windpipe
capillary	***kap***-i-***lar***-ee	L. hairlike
vein		L. vessel

Veins

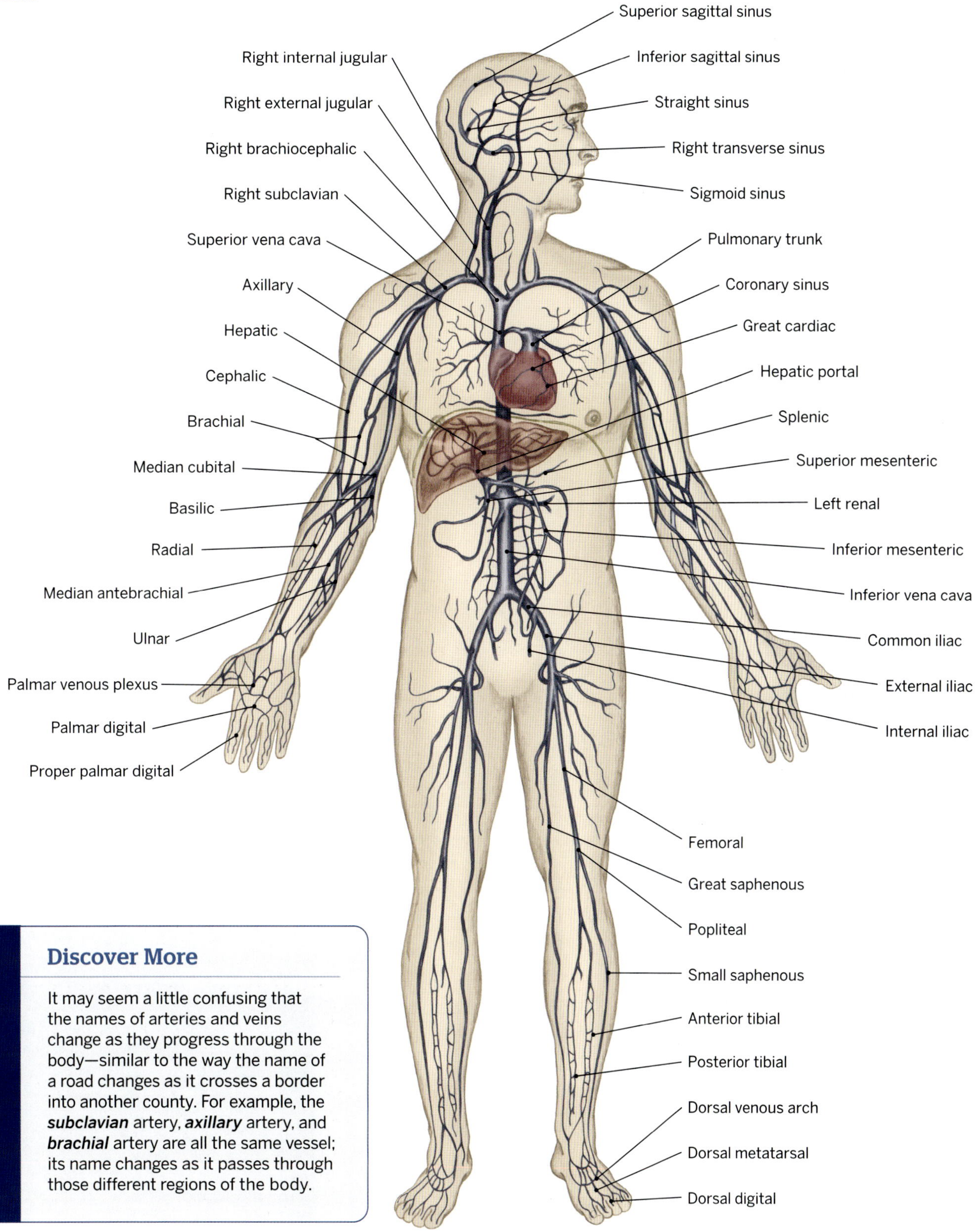

1.144 Anterior view of major veins of the body

Discover More

It may seem a little confusing that the names of arteries and veins change as they progress through the body—similar to the way the name of a road changes as it crosses a border into another county. For example, the ***subclavian*** artery, ***axillary*** artery, and ***brachial*** artery are all the same vessel; its name changes as it passes through those different regions of the body.

The Nervous System

The nervous system is the body's functional headquarters. It senses, interprets, and responds to the body's needs in order to maintain homeostasis, or equilibrium. The brain and spinal cord make up the central nervous system, while the remaining aspects form the peripheral nervous system (**1.145**). Many nerves branch off the spinal cord and exit through the sides of the vertebrae. Some of these nerves regroup to form a plexus. The main plexuses are the cervical, brachial, lumbar, and sacral. The individual branches of a nerve plexus split off and have names that correspond to the regions they innervate.

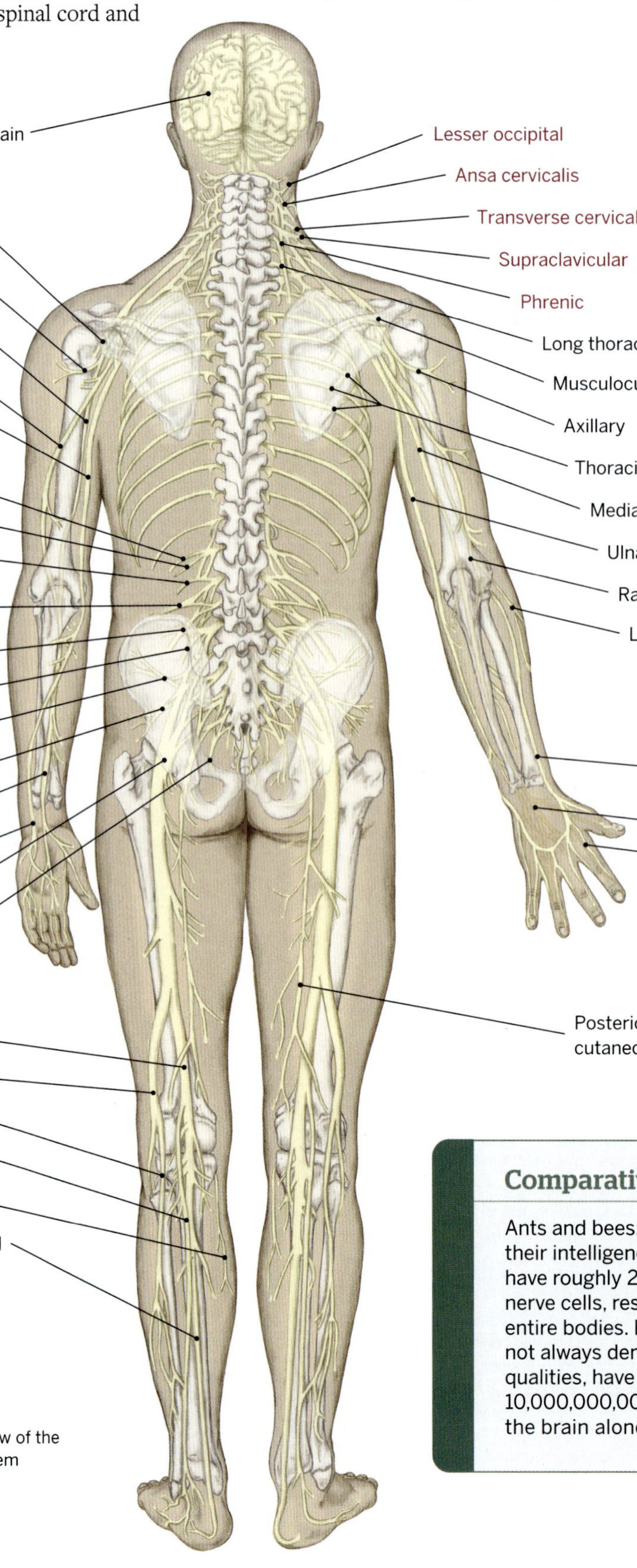

1.145 Posterior view of the nervous system

Comparative Anatomy

Ants and bees, both revered for their intelligence and diligence, have roughly 250 and 900 nerve cells, respectively, in their entire bodies. Humans, who do not always demonstrate such qualities, have an estimated 10,000,000,000 nerve cells in the brain alone.

The Lymphatic System

The lymphatic system is composed of several organs, yellow fluid called lymph, small microscopic vessels called lymphatics, and lymph nodes (**1.146**). These structures perform many functions throughout the body, such as draining the interstitial fluid that escapes from capillaries and transporting it back to the heart. Lymphatic vessels carry fats from the intestines to the blood. Lymphatic tissue also helps the body's immune system defend against foreign cells, microbes, and cancer cells.

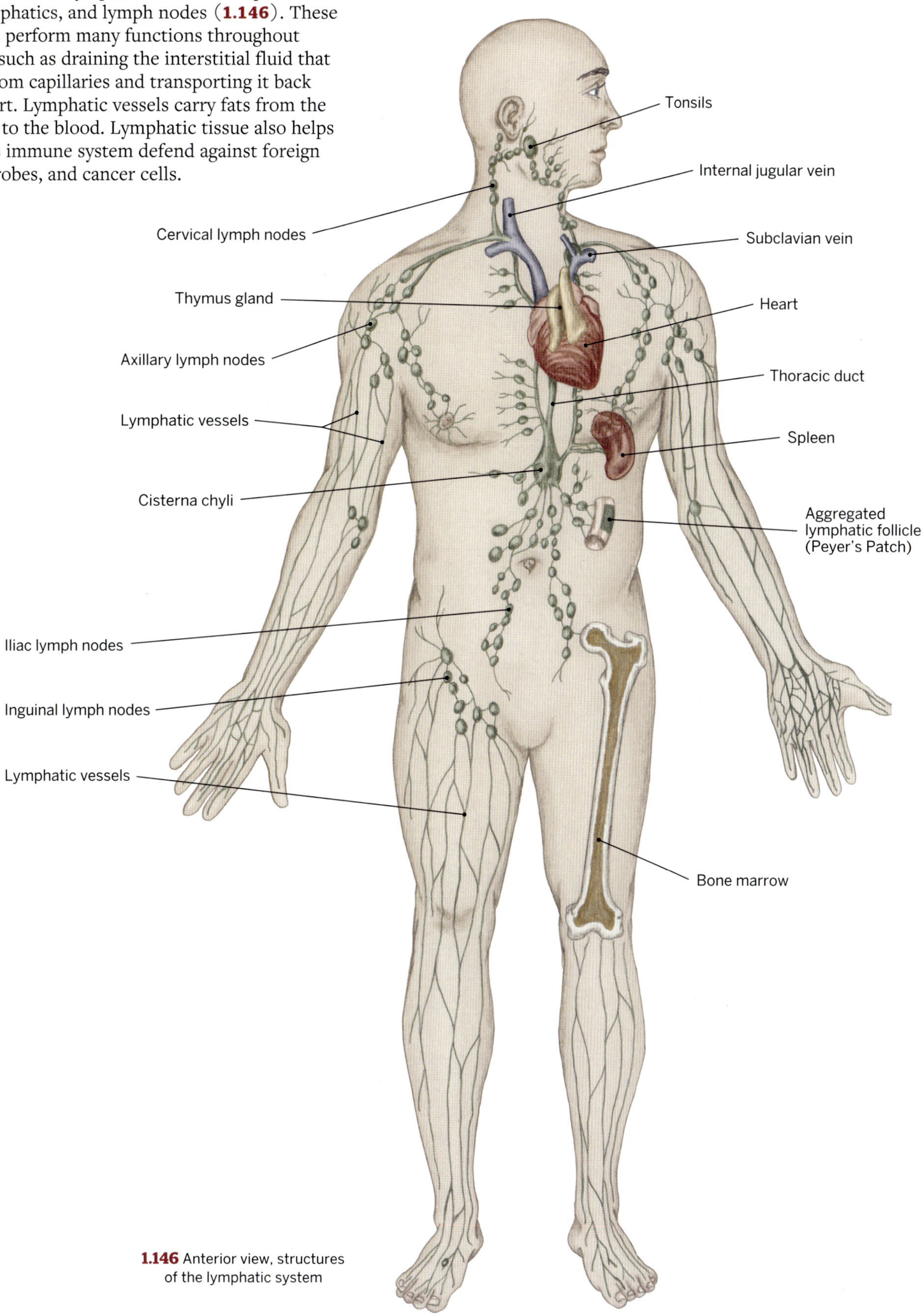

1.146 Anterior view, structures of the lymphatic system

interstitial	*in*-ter-*stish*-al	L. placed between
lymph	limf	L. pure spring water
cisterna chyli	sis-*turn*-a *ki*-lee	L. reservoir + Grk. juice

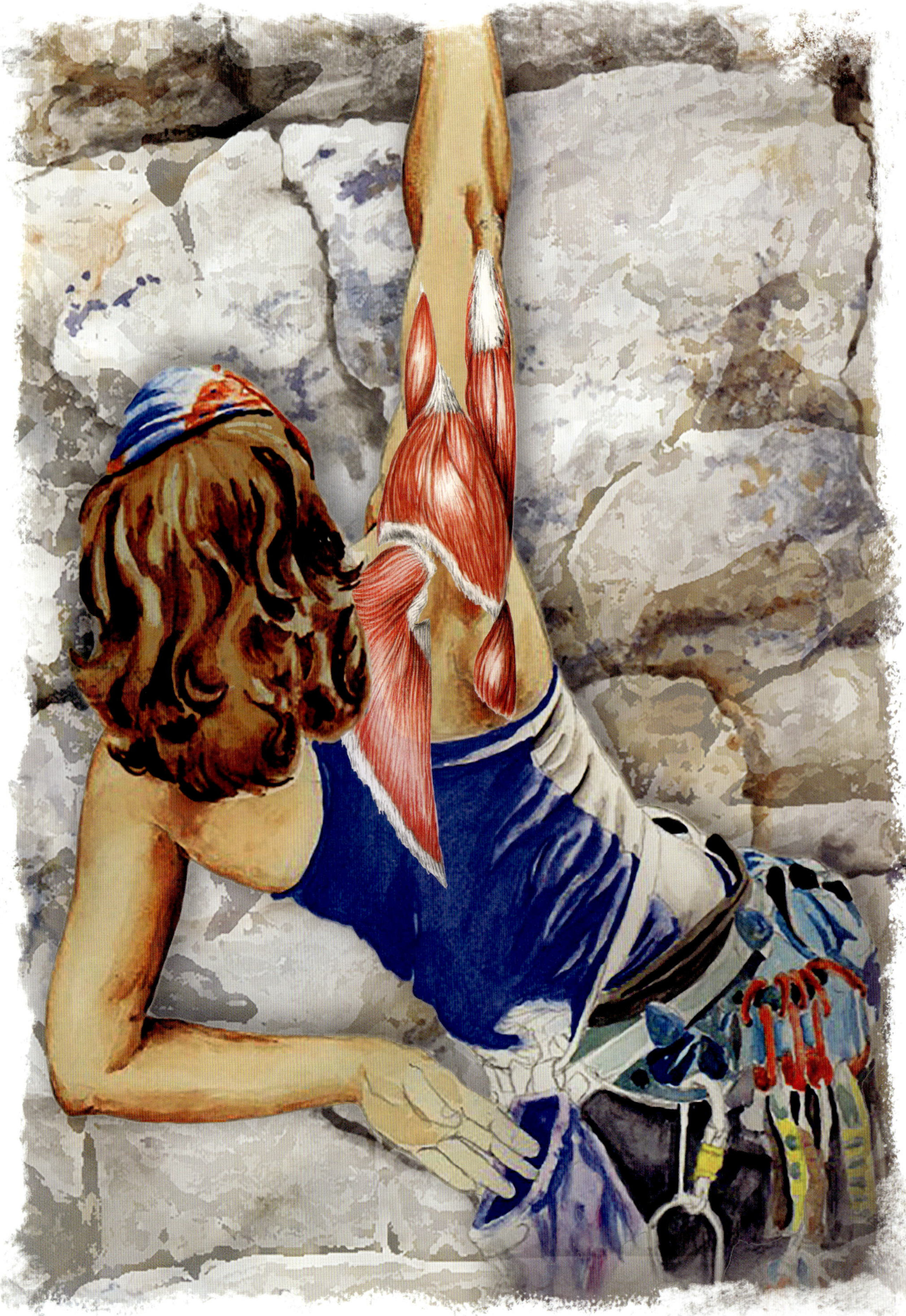

2

Shoulder & Arm

The shoulder and arm region is a great place to practice our new language of movements and body systems, as the bones, bony landmarks, and muscles of this area are easily accessible and distinguishable.
Pro Tip: Your own body can serve as a personal study tool. Just like the climber in the picture will rely on her body to support her ascent, your body can help you. No matter the time or place, you can take advantage of your ever-present "study partner."

See for yourself:

- Look at the picture and notice which muscles (in red) are drawn in. Put your left hand on your right shoulder in the same places as the muscles in the picture. Where can you feel muscles that might correspond to her muscles? Now stretch your arm up in the air as she's doing. What can you feel and visualize under your own skin?
- Now look at the climber's flexed left elbow. Flexion occurs when two bones move closer to each other. When you flex your elbow, what do you notice about the muscles in your arm?

Topographical Views

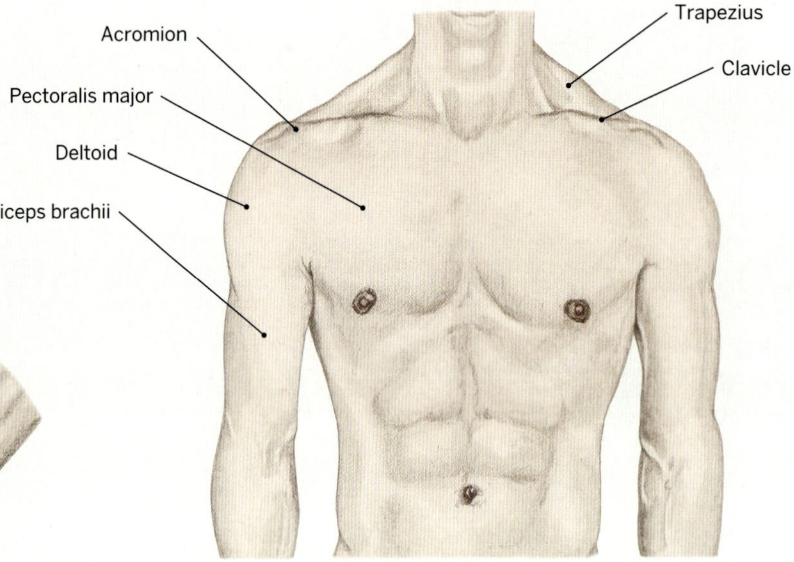

2.1 Anterior view of upper body

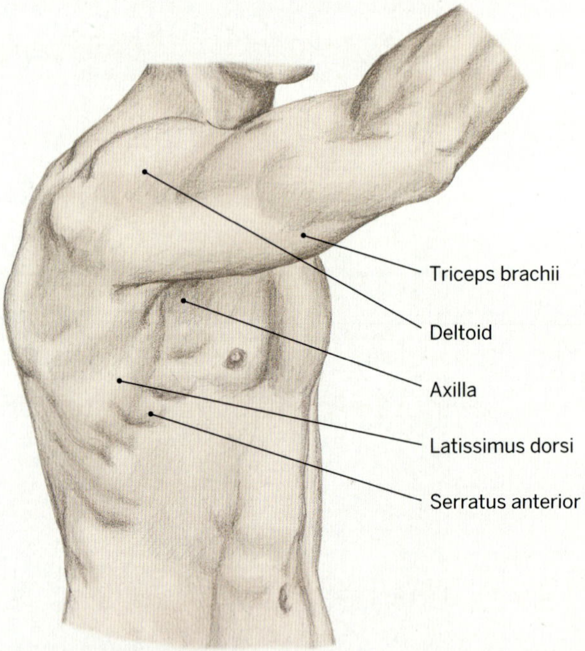

2.2 Anterior/lateral view of upper body

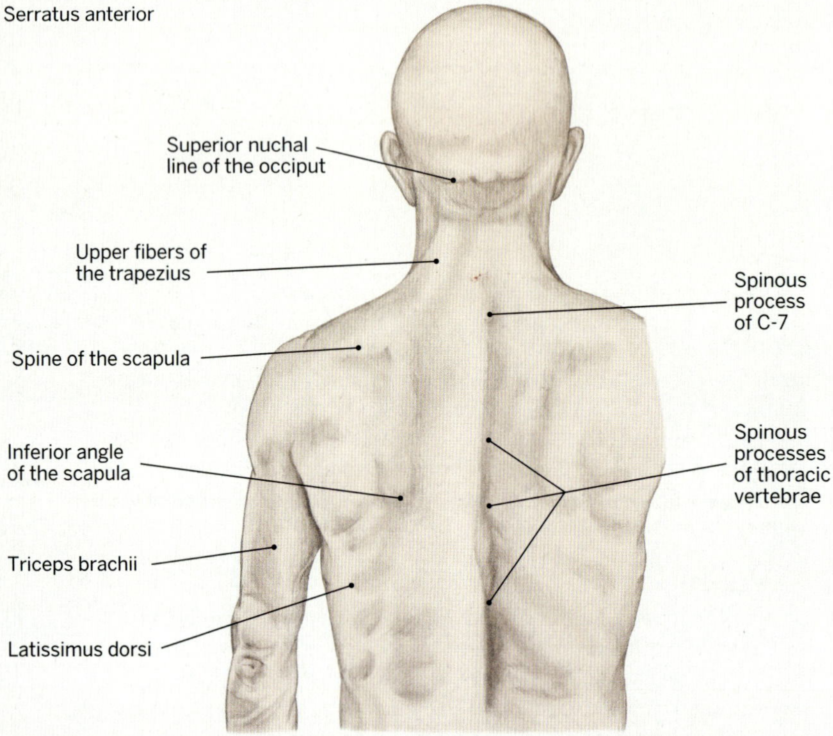

2.3 Posterior view of upper body

Exploring the Skin and Fascia

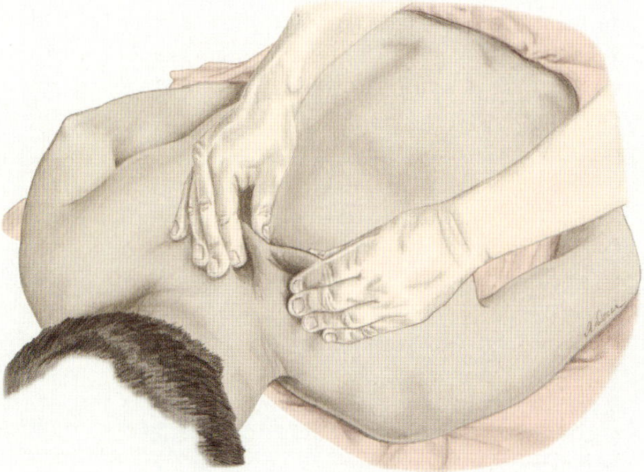

2.4 Partner prone, as you lift and twist the tissue of the upper back

Back

1. Partner prone. Begin by gently lifting the skin and fascia of the upper back. As you raise it away from the thicker, deeper musculature, twist the tissue from side to side (**2.4**). Compare the changes in tissue as you explore the top of the shoulders, arms, and upper chest.
2. Take particular note of the tissue's changes in thickness and elasticity. For example, the skin and fascia superficial to the spine of the scapula may be dense and matted, whereas the tissue at the top of the shoulder, only a few inches away, may be thin and mobile.

Chest

1. Partner supine. Slowly sink your fingers into the skin of the upper chest. Then gently shift the tissue from side to side (**2.5**). Try moving it in all directions, sensing its mobility, resistance, and temperature.
2. Compare this tissue with other areas of the shoulder and arm, including the axilla (armpit) and the area near the clavicle.

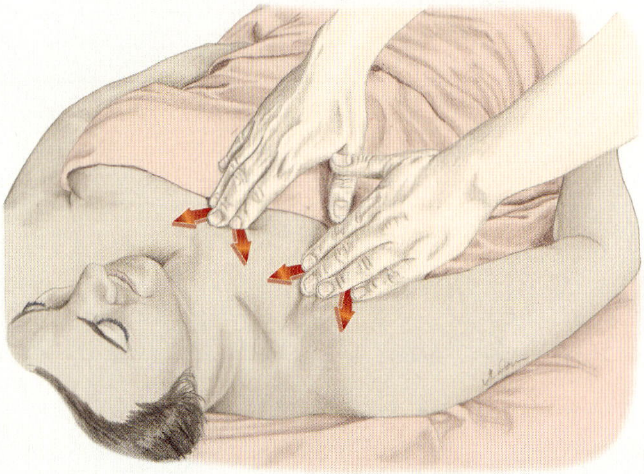

2.5 Partner supine, as you sink your fingers into the upper chest

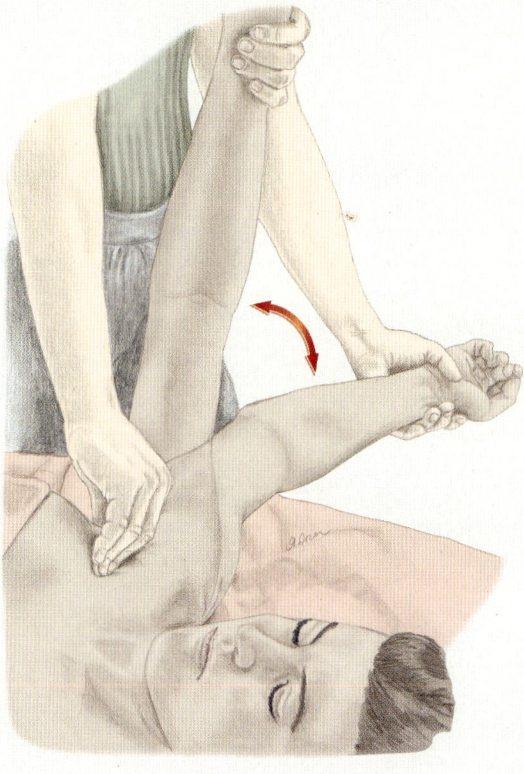

2.6 Partner supine, as you feel shifts in the skin during movement

Chest in movement

1. Partner supine. Here is an opportunity to feel the skin and fascia shorten or stretch. Holding your partner's arm at the wrist, gently grasp the tissue of the upper chest.
2. Encourage your partner to relax her arm as you passively move it up and down (horizontal abduction and adduction) (**2.6**). Note the changes you feel in the tissues.
3. Try this same action while grasping the tissue near the clavicle, sternum, or latissimus dorsi. Explore different movements at the shoulder, feeling how virtually all the skin of the upper chest, shoulder, and arm shifts to accommodate even a simple action.

Bones of the Shoulder and Arm

The shoulder complex is made up of three bones: the clavicle, scapula, and humerus (**2.7**). The **clavicle**, or collarbone, is superficial and runs horizontally along the top of the chest at the base of the neck. It articulates laterally with the acromion of the scapula (acromioclavicular joint) and medially with the sternum (sternoclavicular joint). Both joints are synovial joints. The sternoclavicular joint is the single attachment site between the upper appendicular and axial skeletons.

The **scapula** is the triangular-shaped bone of the upper back. Along with the clavicle, the scapula plays a vital role in stabilization and movement of the arm. The scapula has several fossae, corners, and ridges that serve as attachment sites for seventeen muscles.* The scapula glides across the posterior surface of the thorax to form the scapulothoracic joint. However, because this articulation does not have any of the usual joint components, it is considered a false joint.

The **humerus** is the bone of the arm. The proximal humerus articulates with the glenoid fossa of the scapula to form the glenohumeral joint. The glenohumeral joint is a synovial, ball-and-socket joint with a wide range of movement. The deltoid muscle and numerous tendons surround the proximal humerus and the glenohumeral joint.

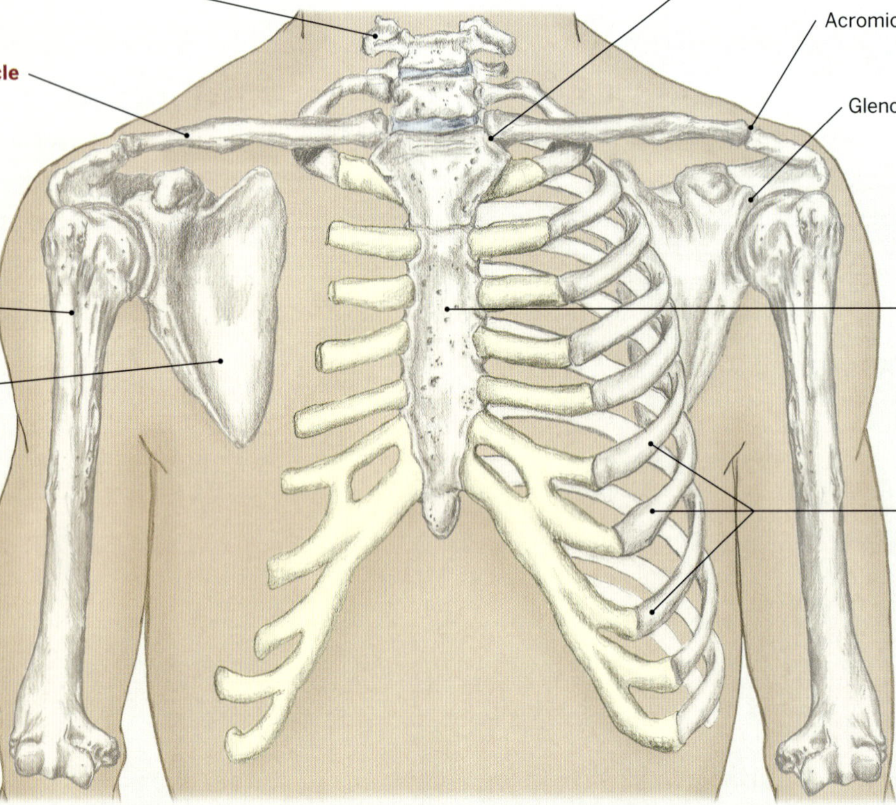

2.7 Anterior view of bones of the shoulder complex, with ribs removed on his right side

Comparative Anatomy

The clavicle is the first bone to start ossifying (hardening) in a human fetus; paradoxically, it is the last to completely develop—often not until the late teens or early twenties. This fact, along with its superficial location, may explain why the clavicle is one of the most frequently broken bones in the body.

A quadruped, such as a dog or cat, however, is not concerned with breaking its clavicle. Since a quadruped's scapula is positioned on the lateral side of the trunk (as opposed to a human's, which lies on the posterior side of the trunk), its clavicle is not as essential to the movement of the shoulder complex. Actually, cats have a thin sliver for a clavicle, and dogs have just a small piece of cartilage.

A bird's clavicles are joined to form a furcula. The single unit of the furcula acts as a strut, offering greater stability to the large pectoral muscles during flight. The furcula is what we split apart when vying for the long end of the "wishbone."

*The 17th muscle is the omohyoid, p. 255.

clavicle	*klav*-i-k'l	L. little key
furcula	*fur*-ku-la	L. a little fork
humerus	*hu*-mer-us	L. upper arm

Bony Landmarks of the Shoulder and Arm

The Scapula

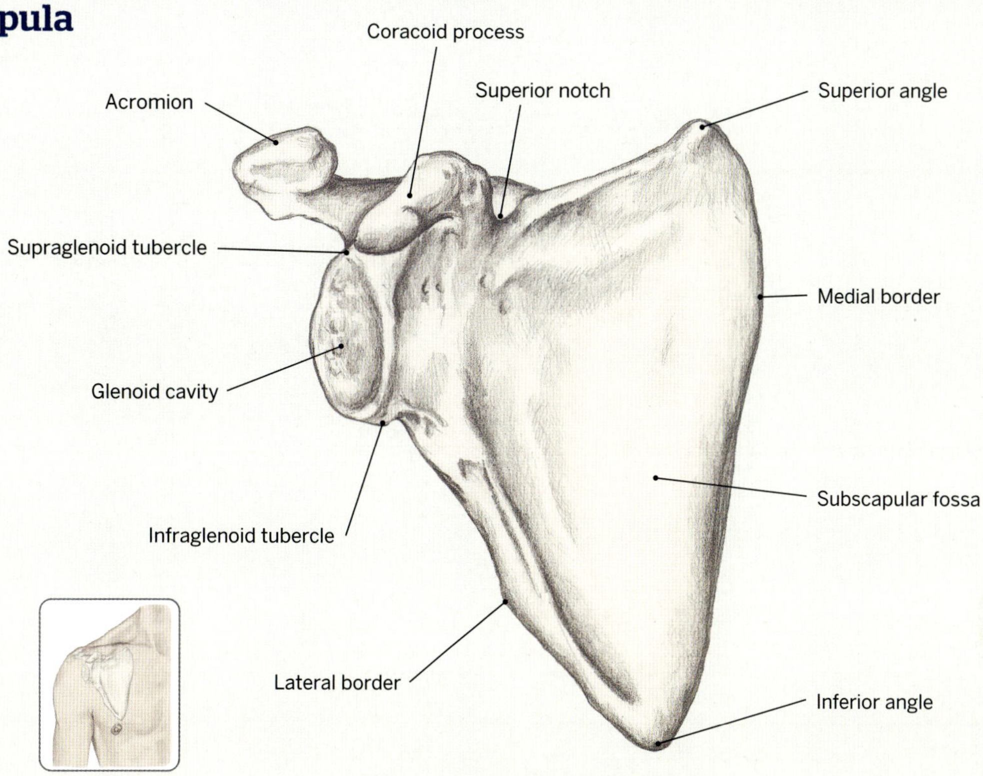

2.8 Anterior view of right scapula

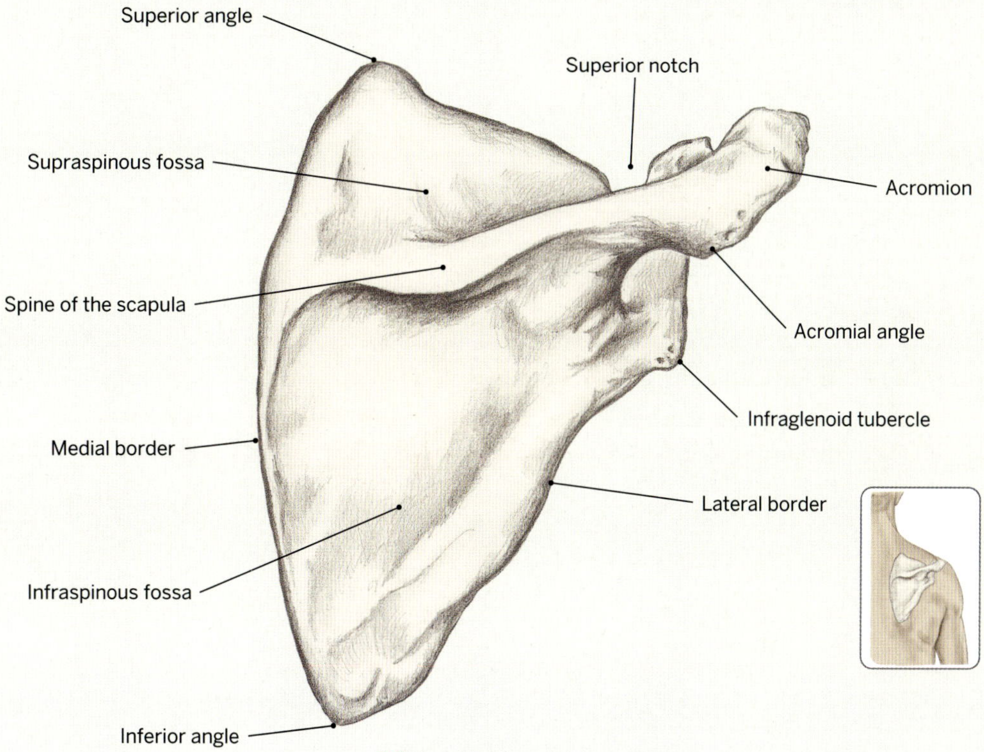

2.9 Posterior view of right scapula

process	***pros***-es	L. going forth
scapula	***skap***-u-la	L. shoulder blade
scapulae	***skap***-u-lay	plural for scapula

The Humerus and Clavicle

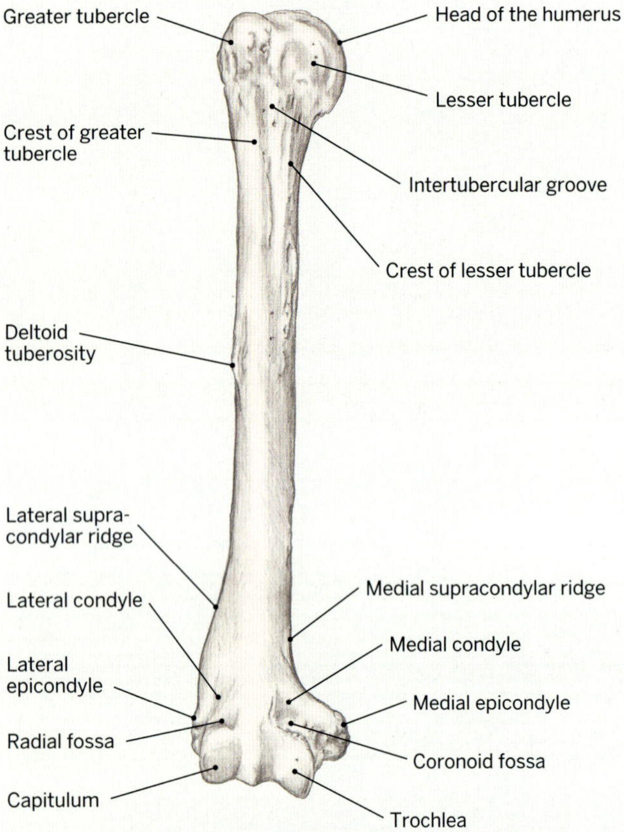

2.10 Anterior view of right humerus

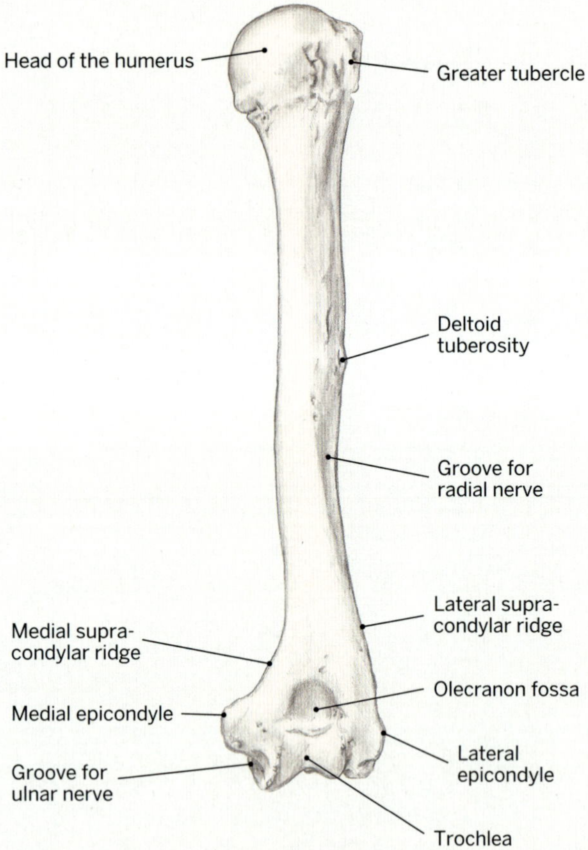

2.11 Posterior view of right humerus

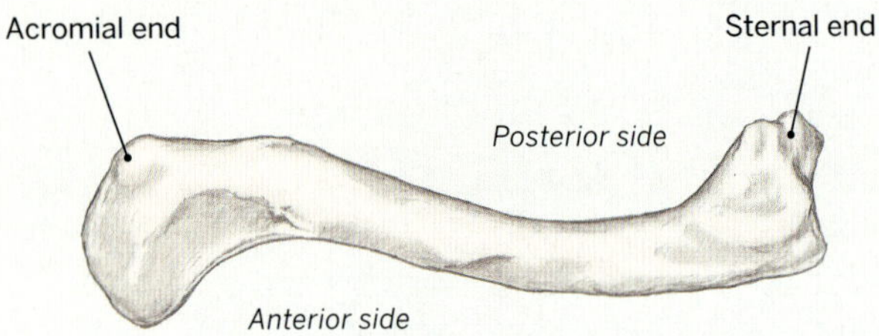

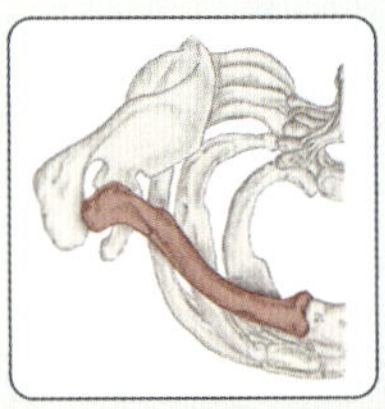

2.12 Superior view of right clavicle

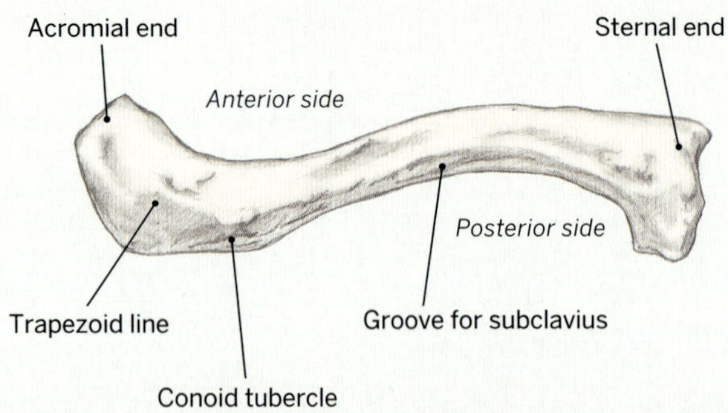

2.13 Inferior view of right clavicle

Overview: **Bony Landmark Trails**

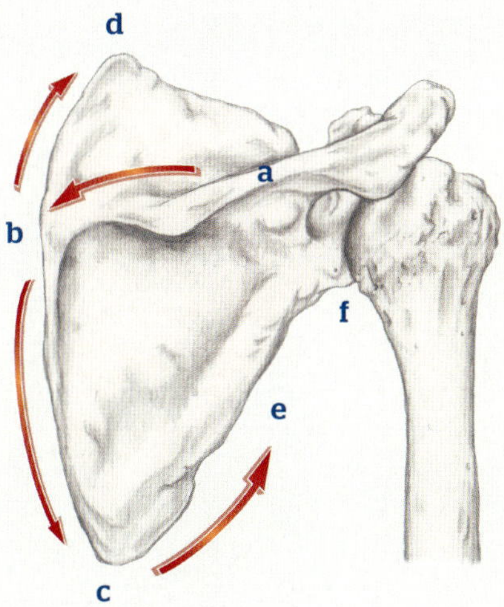

Trail 1 Along the Edges explores the sides and corners of the posterior scapula.

a Spine of the scapula
b Medial border
c Inferior angle
d Superior angle
e Lateral border
f Infraglenoid tubercle

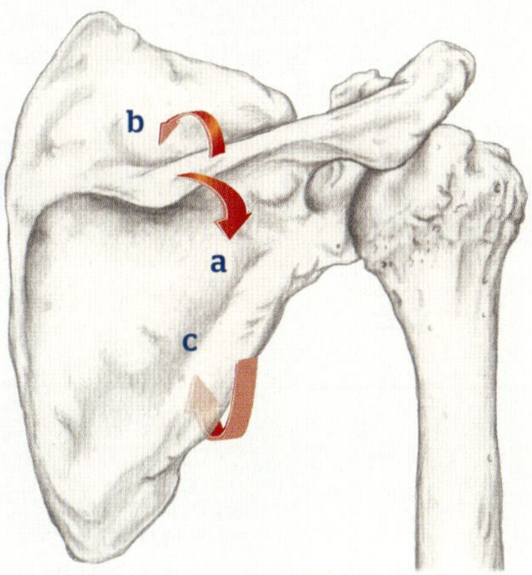

Trail 2 In the Trenches leaps off the spine of the scapula and sinks into the three basins of the scapula.

a Infraspinous fossa
b Supraspinous fossa
c Subscapular fossa

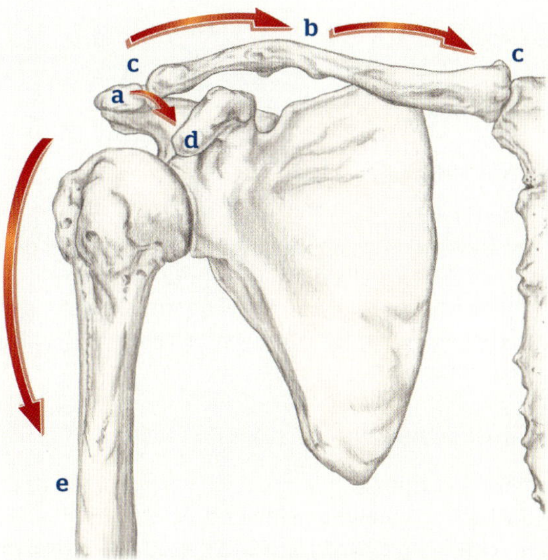

Trail 3 Springboard Ledge leads around to the anterior shoulder, using the scapula's acromion as a jumping-off point.

a Acromion
b Clavicle
c Acromioclavicular and sternoclavicular joints
d Coracoid process
e Deltoid tuberosity

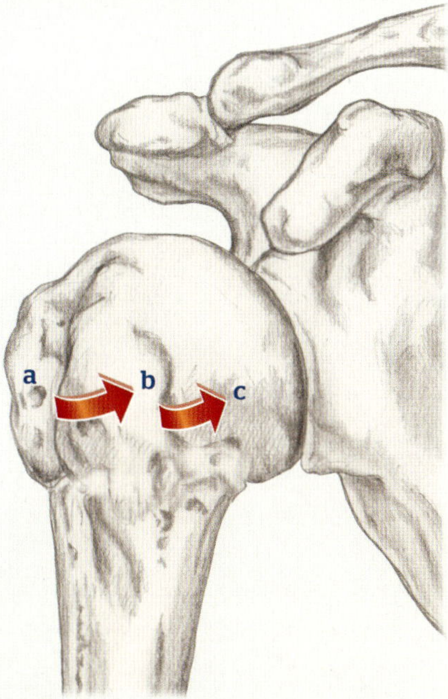

Trail 4 Two Hills and a Valley focuses on the three landmarks located along the anterior, proximal humerus.

a Greater tubercle
b Intertubercular groove
c Lesser tubercle

Trail 1 Along the Edges ▸

Spine of the Scapula

The spine of the scapula is a superficial ridge located just off the top of the shoulder. It runs at an oblique angle to the body, spanning from the acromion to the medial border. It is an attachment site for the posterior deltoid (p. 63) and middle and lower fibers of the trapezius (p. 64).

Scapula - spine

1. Partner prone. Lay your hand across the upper back and slide your fingertips inferiorly until they roll over the superficial spine (**2.14**).
2. Strum your fingers vertically, palpating its width and edges. Also explore its entire length by palpating laterally toward the acromion and medially toward the vertebral column.

As you strum your fingers over the spine, do you feel a ditch of soft tissue above and below it? If your partner slowly elevates his scapula, does the spine elevate as well?

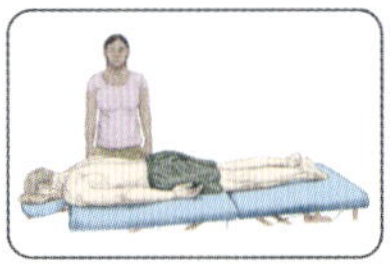

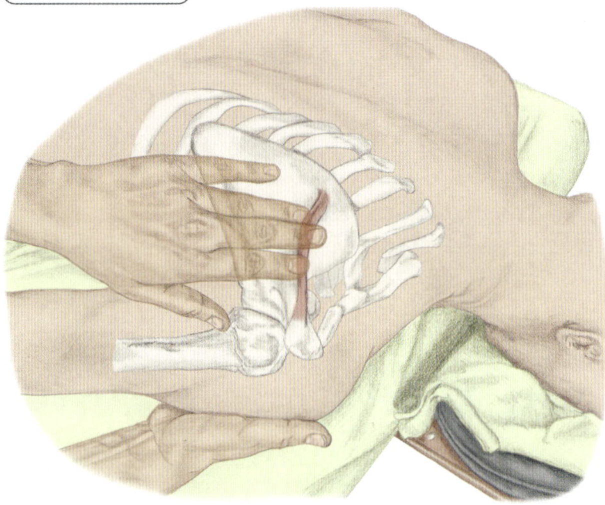

2.14 Partner prone, as you locate the spine of the scapula

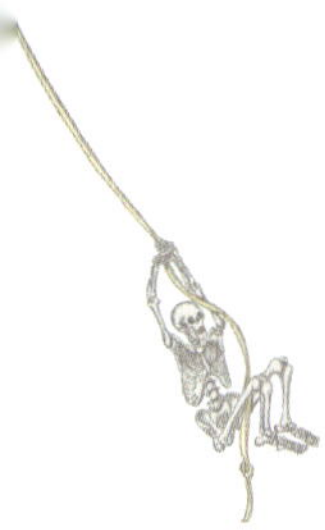

Because of its central location, the spine of the scapula makes a great base camp for locating other landmarks. If you become lost or confused while palpating the scapula, return to its spine.

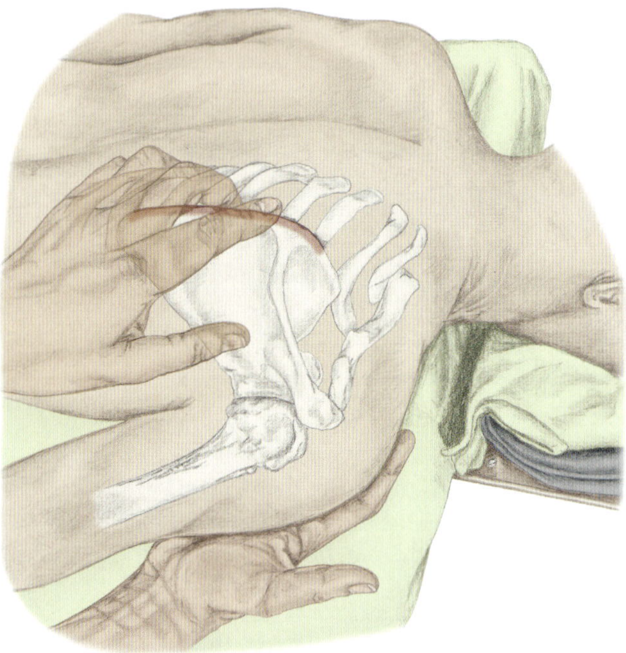

2.15 Partner prone, as you sculpt out the medial border

Medial Border

The medial border is the long edge of the scapula that runs parallel to the vertebral column. It can measure five to seven inches in length, depending on body type. The medial border is an attachment site for the rhomboids (p. 78) and serratus anterior (p. 82) and is deep to the trapezius.

Scapula - medial border

1. Partner prone. Place your partner's hand in the small of his back to raise the medial border off the ribs. For more exposure, scoop and raise the shoulder with one hand.
2. Locate the spine of the scapula and glide your fingertips medially until they slide off the spine onto the medial border (**2.15**).
3. Follow the medial border inferiorly and superiorly; note that it extends further inferiorly from the spine of the scapula than superiorly.

Does the edge you feel run vertically?

Inferior Angle

There are two angles of the scapula, one on either end of the medial border. The inferior angle is superficial and located at the medial border's lower end.

Scapula - inferior angle

1. Partner prone. Place your partner's hand in the small of his back. Glide your fingers inferiorly along the medial border.
2. At the end of the medial border, the edge of the scapula will turn a corner and start to rise superiorly and laterally. This corner is the inferior angle (**2.16**).

Can you sculpt around the inferior angle and pinch it with your fingertip and thumb?

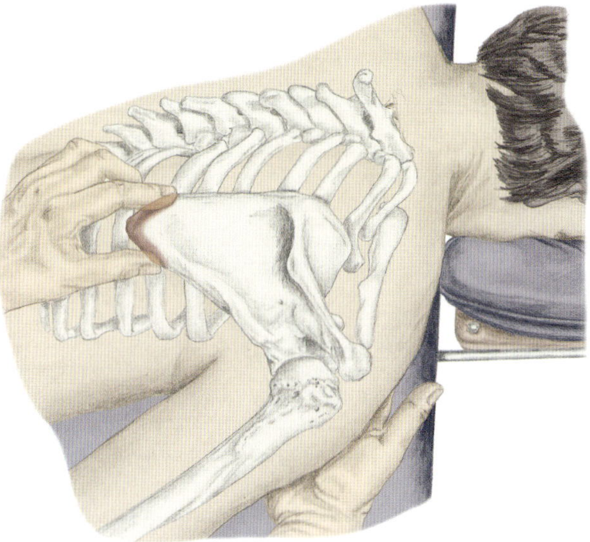

2.16 Partner prone, as you pinch the inferior angle

Discover More

The term "winged scapula" refers to a postural condition in which the medial border falls away from the rib cage and visibly protrudes posteriorly. Often indicating a weak serratus anterior muscle, a winged scapula may also involve the muscles that pull the shoulder girdle anteriorly, such as the pectoralis major and minor.

Actually, a degree of scapular winging normally occurs with scapular abduction. For example, when a boxer throws a punch (and fully abducts the scapula), the glenoid fossa is facing anteriorly. In order for this to happen, the medial border must shift posteriorly away from the rib cage. If this winging of the scapula did not occur, the glenoid fossa would not move anteriorly and the boxer would be flat on the canvas in the first round.

Superior Angle

The superior angle is located at the superior end of the medial border. It serves as an attachment site for the levator scapula muscle (p. 79). Because the angle is located deep to the trapezius muscles (p. 64), it may not be as easy to isolate as the inferior angle.

Scapula - superior angle

1. Partner prone. Scoop the shoulder with your hand to raise it off the table. This will soften the overlying muscles.
2. Locate the medial border. Slide your fingertips superiorly along the border to find the superior angle (**2.17**).
3. You may need to move an inch superior to the spine of the scapula to reach the superior angle.

Sculpt out the superior angle and note if it is continuous with the medial border. Locate both the inferior angle and the superior angle. Note the distance between them and gently slide the scapula superiorly and inferiorly.

With your partner side lying, elevate the scapula toward the ear. As the scapula falls away from the rib cage, the superior angle will be quite palpable.

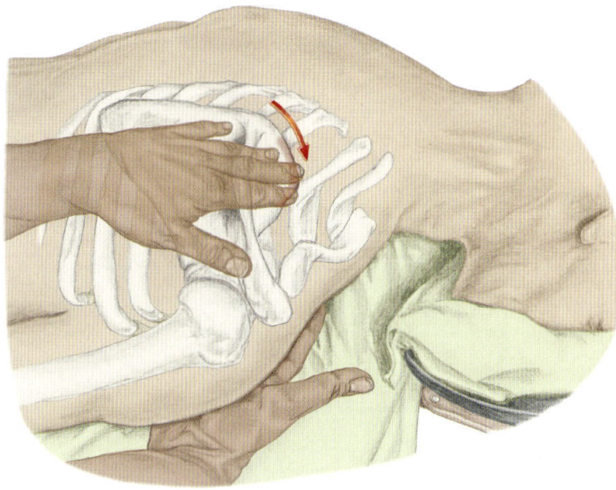

2.17 Partner prone, as you isolate the superior angle

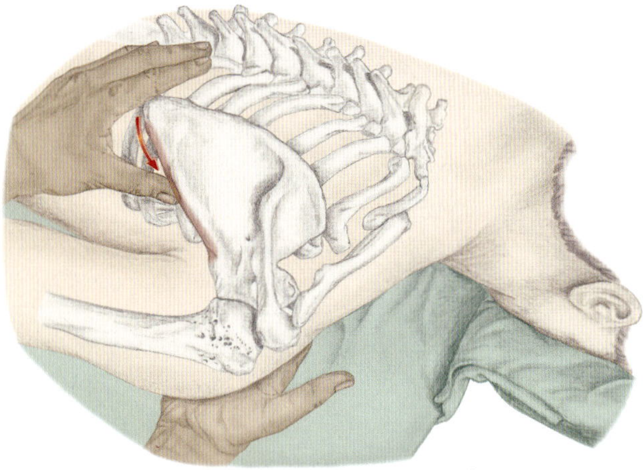

2.18 Partner prone, as you palpate the lateral border

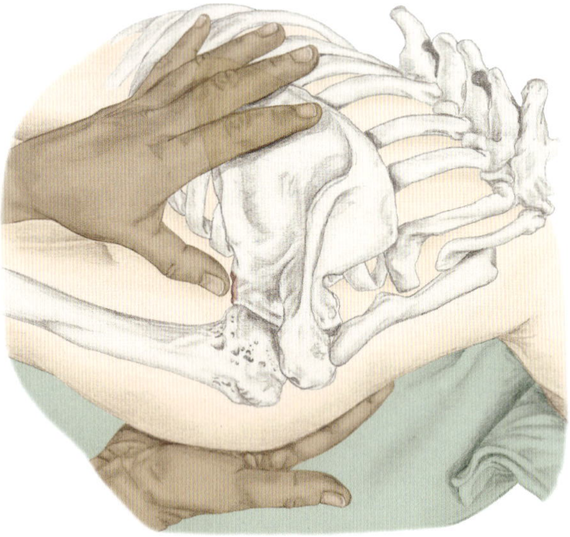

2.19 Partner prone, as you access the infraglenoid tubercle

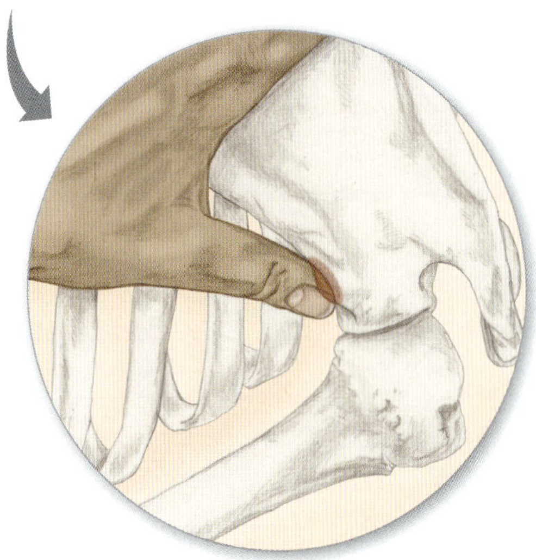

Lateral Border

The lateral border extends superiorly and laterally from the inferior angle toward the axilla, or "armpit." It is an attachment site for the teres major and teres minor muscles (pp. 67, 70) and, due to the thickness of these tissues, might not be as clearly defined as the medial border.

Scapula - lateral border

1. Partner prone. Drape the arm off the side of the table. Slide your thumb from the inferior angle superiorly along the lateral border.
2. Follow the border in the direction of the axilla. If the musculature is too thick to palpate through, try curling your thumb underneath the tissue (**2.18**). This is most effective when locating the infraglenoid tubercle (see below).

Is the edge of bone you are palpating continuous with the inferior angle? As you follow it superiorly, does it lead you in the direction of the axilla?

Try the above method with your partner's hand in the small of his back.

Infraglenoid Tubercle

The infraglenoid tubercle is located at the most superior aspect of the lateral border. The tubercle is not a distinguishable point, but a small spot that serves as an attachment site for the long head of the triceps brachii (p. 93). It lies deep to the teres minor and deltoid muscles.

Exploring the infraglenoid tubercle often elicits tenderness in the surrounding tissues. By using your broad thumbpad, you will be able to palpate more precisely without causing pain.

Scapula - infraglenoid tubercle

1. Partner prone. Locate the lateral border.
2. Slide along the lateral border to its most superior portion (**2.19**). To access the landmark directly, you can either compress through the overlying muscles or curl underneath them.

Are you along the edge of the lateral border? Are you on the posterior side of the axilla?

tubercle *tu*-ber-kl L. a little swelling

Infraspinous Fossa

The scapula contains three fossae, or depressions: the infraspinous, supraspinous, and subscapular. Each fossa is designed to accommodate a muscle belly and its tendinous attachments. The infraspinous fossa is the triangular area inferior to the spine of the scapula; it is filled with the infraspinatus muscle (p. 70).

Scapula - infraspinous fossa

1. Partner prone. Palpate the spine of the scapula, its medial border, and its lateral border to isolate the infraspinous fossa.
2. Cradle the inferior angle in the webbing between your index finger and thumb. Your index finger will rest along the medial border, your thumb along the lateral border (**2.20**).
3. Place a finger of the opposite hand along the length of the spine of the scapula. The triangular-shaped area you isolate is the infraspinous fossa.

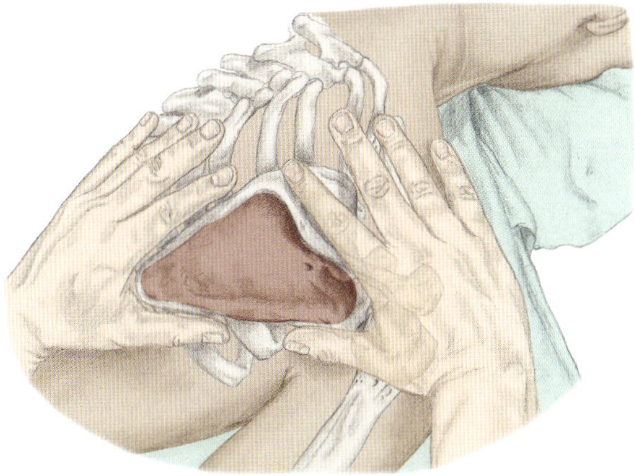

2.20 Partner prone, as you isolate the infraspinous fossa

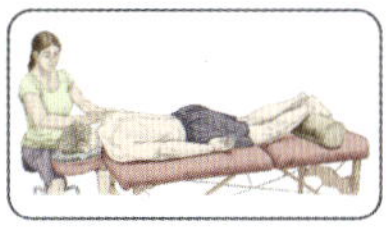

Supraspinous Fossa

The supraspinous fossa is located superior to the spine of the scapula. It is small in size, yet quite deep. Because the supraspinatus muscle (p. 70) attaches to and lies in this basin, the supraspinous fossa is difficult to access directly.

Scapula - supraspinous fossa

1. Partner prone. Drop your thumbpad inferiorly and laterally from the superior angle into the fossa, or lay your thumb along the spine of the scapula and raise it superiorly into the fossa.
2. Although the fossa is covered by the trapezius and supraspinatus muscles, explore as much as you can of its size and shape (**2.21**).
3. Slide your thumbs laterally, noting how the fossa becomes thinner and finally ends at the junction of the acromion and clavicle. Actually, the fossa continues underneath the acromion, although it is inaccessible.

Are you superior to the spine of the scapula? If you strum your thumbs vertically, can you palpate the supraspinatus fibers running horizontally toward the acromion?

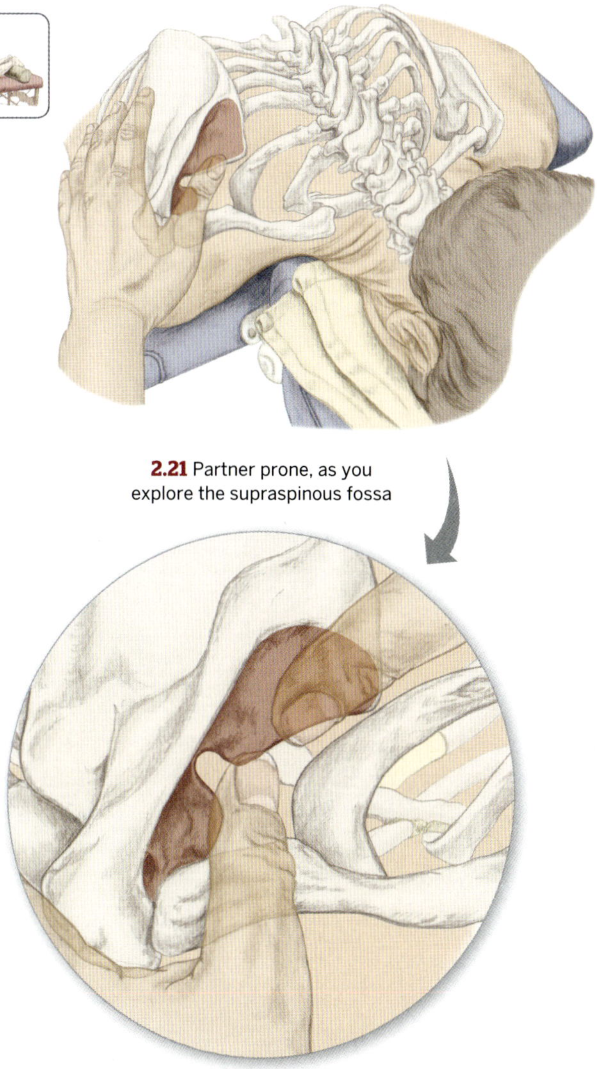

2.21 Partner prone, as you explore the supraspinous fossa

fossa *fos*-a L. a shallow depression

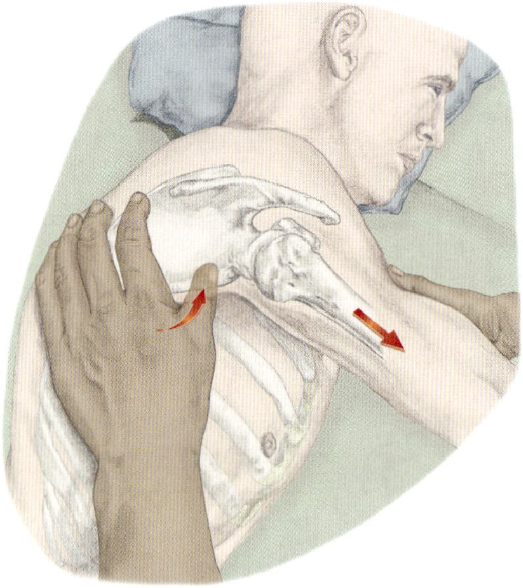

2.22 Partner side lying, as you access the lateral side of the subscapular fossa. This fossa can be tender when palpated, so move slowly and check in with your partner.

Subscapular Fossa

The subscapular fossa is located on the scapula's anterior (or underside) surface, next to the rib cage. It is the attachment site for the subscapularis (p. 70) and the location of the serratus anterior muscle (p. 82).

The fossa can be challenging to access, due to the scapula's close proximity to the rib cage and the numerous muscle bellies surrounding it.

Scapula - subscapular fossa

1. Partner side lying. This position allows the scapula to slide away from the rib cage for easier access (**2.22**).
2. Place your thumb at the middle of the lateral border. Be sure to position your thumb anterior to the large mass of muscles along the lateral border.
3. Slowly sink and curl your thumbpad onto the surface of the fossa. Use your other hand to maneuver the arm and scapula for a position that best allows your thumb to sink into the tissue. You may only be able to sink an inch into the fossa.

*Can you feel the rib cage and anterior surface of the scapula on either side of your thumb? Try this same approach with your partner prone (**2.23**).*

Here is a method for palpating the medial portion of the subscapular fossa. The fossa may or may not be accessible, depending on the tissue's flexibility.

1. Partner side lying. Flex your partner's shoulder and lay your fingertips along the medial border. With the other hand, move the scapula posteriorly (bringing the medial border off the ribs) (**2.24**).
2. Slowly curl your fingers through the rhomboid and trapezius muscles, under the scapula and onto the fossa.

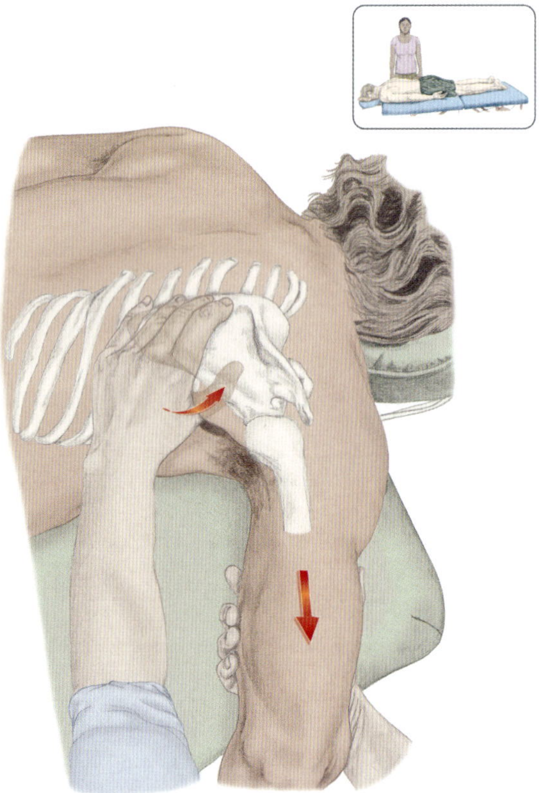

2.23 Partner prone, as you palpate the lateral side of the subscapular fossa

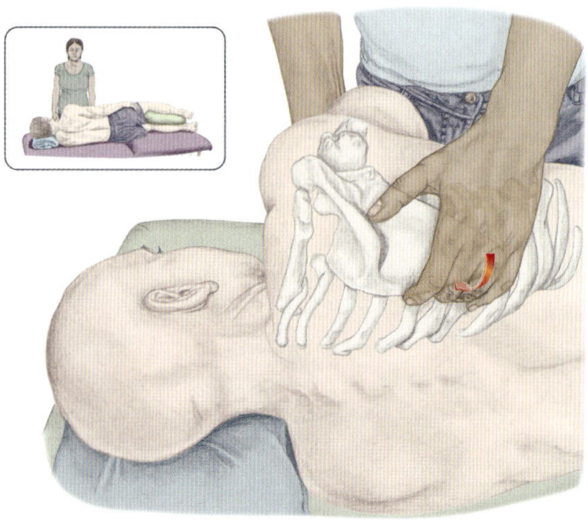

2.24 Partner side lying, as you access the medial side of the subscapular fossa

Acromion

The acromion is the lateral aspect of the spine of the scapula and is located at the top of the shoulder. It has a flat surface and articulates with the clavicle's lateral end. The acromion serves as an attachment site for the deltoid (p. 63) and trapezius (p. 64) muscles.

The acromial angle is the small corner that can be felt along the acromion's lateral/posterior aspect (see p. 45).

Acromion

1. Partner seated or supine. Locate the spine of the scapula.
2. Follow the spine as it rises superiorly and laterally to the top of the shoulder. Use your fingerpads to explore the acromion's flat surface (**2.25**).
3. Explore and sculpt around all sides of the acromion and its attachment to the clavicle.

Is the bone you are palpating superficial and directly on the top of the shoulder? Can you feel the small point of the acromial angle on the posterior edge of the acromion?

Clavicle

The superficial clavicle lies horizontally across the upper chest and has a gentle S shape. It is an attachment site for a number of muscles. Both ends of the clavicle are superficial and accessible. The lateral end is relatively flat and often rises slightly higher than the acromion. The medial end is round and articulates with the sternum.

Clavicle

1. Partner seated. Locate the acromion and walk your fingers medially onto the shaft of the clavicle.
2. Grasp the clavicle's cylindrical body between your finger and thumb and explore its length from the acromion to the sternum. Observe how its acromial end rises superiorly while its sternal end curves inferiorly (**2.26**).

Have your partner move his shoulder anteriorly, and the shaft of the clavicle will protrude visibly. Can you locate the medial and lateral ends of the clavicle simultaneously?

With your fingers at either end of the clavicle, ask your partner to elevate and depress, then adduct and abduct his scapula. As the scapula moves, notice how the ends of the clavicle shift their positions.

acromion a-*cro*-me-on Grk. *akron*, top + *omos*, shoulder

Trail 3 Springboard Ledge ▸

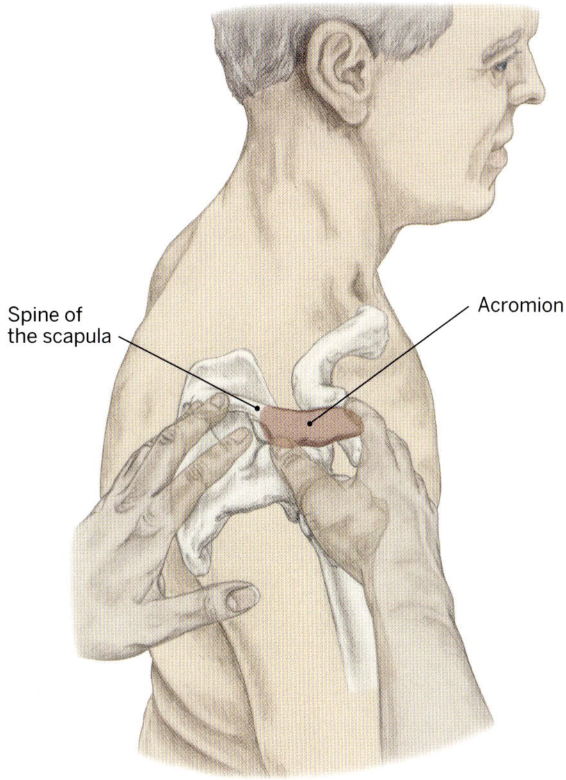

2.25 Partner seated, as you explore the acromion's flat surface

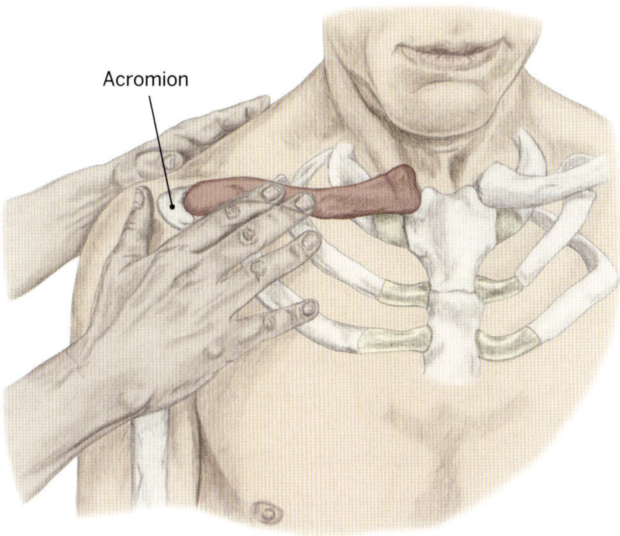

2.26 Partner seated, as you explore the clavicle (highlighted in red)

Acromioclavicular and Sternoclavicular Joints

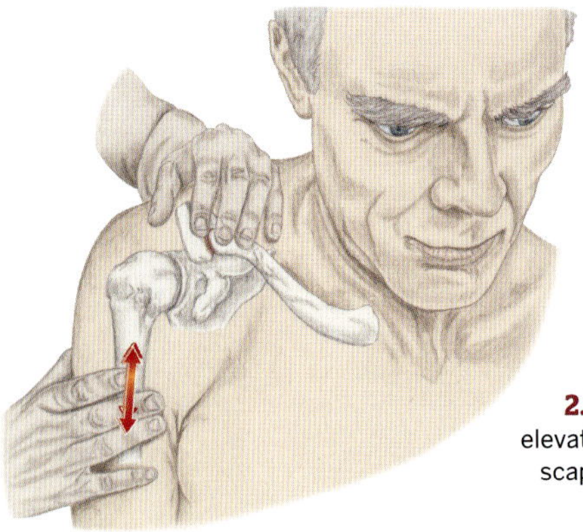

2.27 Partner seated, elevating and depressing his scapula while you access the A/C joint

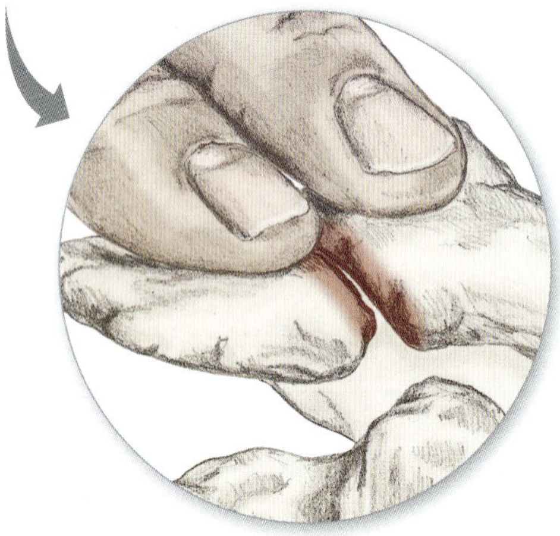

The **acromioclavicular (A/C) joint** is the small articulation between the acromion of the scapula and the acromial end of the clavicle. The anterior and superior surfaces of this thin crevice can be palpated directly.

The **sternoclavicular (S/C) joint** is the articulation between the sternal end of the clavicle and the sternum. Unlike the slender, smooth A/C joint, the S/C joint is wedge-shaped and contains a small, impalpable fibrous disc. At rest, only the inferior portion of the sternal end makes contact with the sternum. When the clavicle is elevated, the sternal end pivots on the sternum.

A/C joint

1. Partner seated or supine. Locate the acromion.
2. Glide medially toward the clavicle. Your finger will feel a small "step" as you rise up onto the surface of the clavicle.
3. Backtrack slightly. Just lateral to the step will be the A/C joint's slender ditch.

*Does the acromial end of the clavicle lie slightly higher than the acromion? Place a finger where you believe the A/C joint to be and ask your partner to slowly elevate and depress his scapula (**2.27**). As the scapula rises, do you feel the joint space widen slightly? As it depresses, does the joint space diminish?*

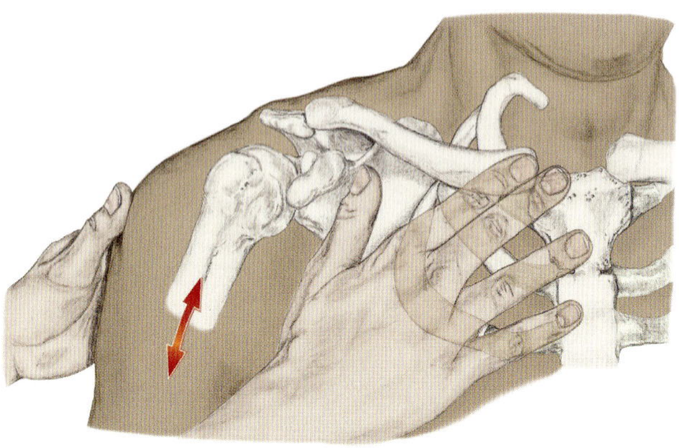

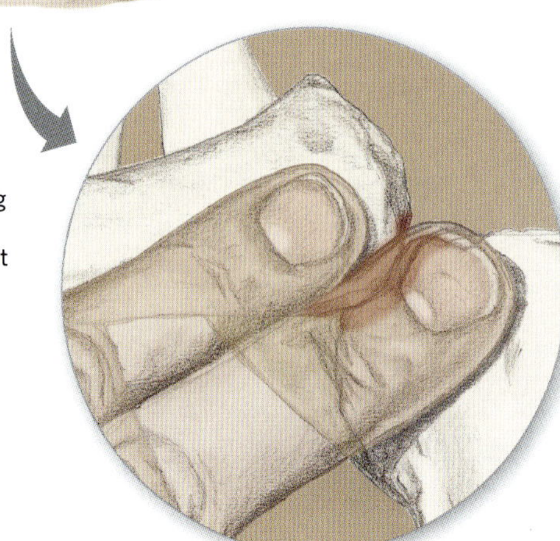

2.28 Partner seated, elevating and depressing his scapula while you palpate the S/C joint

S/C joint

1. Partner seated or supine. Slide your fingers medially along the shaft of the clavicle.
2. Just lateral to the body's centerline, the shaft will broaden to become the bulbous sternal end.
3. Locate the S/C joint by sliding your finger medially off the sternal end. Passively elevate, depress, and abduct the scapula. Then explore the changes occurring at the S/C joint.

*Place a finger where you believe the S/C joint to be and ask your partner to slowly elevate and depress his scapula (**2.28**). Can you feel the joint space widen and diminish?*

acromioclavicular	a-***kro***-me-o-kla-***vik***-u-lar
sternoclavicular	***ster***-no-kla-***vik***-u-lar

Coracoid Process

The coracoid process of the scapula is the beak-like projection found inferior to the shaft of the clavicle. Depending on the position of the scapula, it is often found in the deltopectoral groove (p. 58) between the deltoid and pectoralis major fibers. The coracoid process can be tender when palpated, so proceed carefully.

Coracoid process

1. Partner seated or supine. Lay your thumb along the lateral shaft of the clavicle.
2. Slide inferiorly off the clavicle no more than an inch and a half. Locate the tip of the coracoid process by compressing your fingerpads into the tissue (**2.29**).
3. As the coracoid becomes more apparent, get a better understanding of its shape and size by sculpting a circle around its edges.

✓ *Are you inferior to the shaft of the clavicle? Passively move the scapula with your other hand and feel the coracoid follow your movements.*

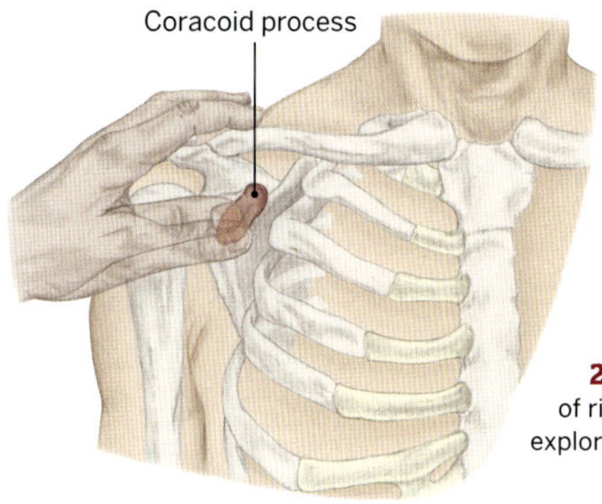

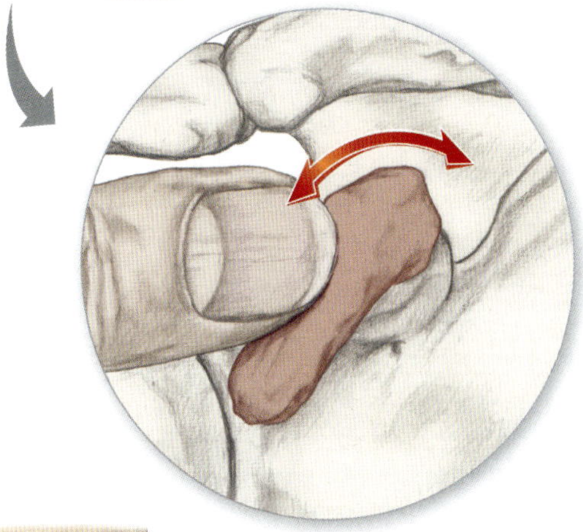

2.29 Anterior view of right shoulder, as you explore the coracoid process

Deltoid Tuberosity

The deltoid tuberosity is located on the lateral side of the mid-humeral shaft. It is a small, low bump that serves as an attachment site for the converging fibers of the deltoid muscle (p. 63).

Deltoid tuberosity

1. Partner seated or supine. Locate the acromion.
2. Slide off the acromion and down the lateral aspect of the arm (**2.30**).
3. When you reach the halfway point between the shoulder and elbow, there will be a small mound on the lateral side of the arm.

✓ *If your partner abducts his shoulder, do the deltoid fibers converge where you are palpating?*

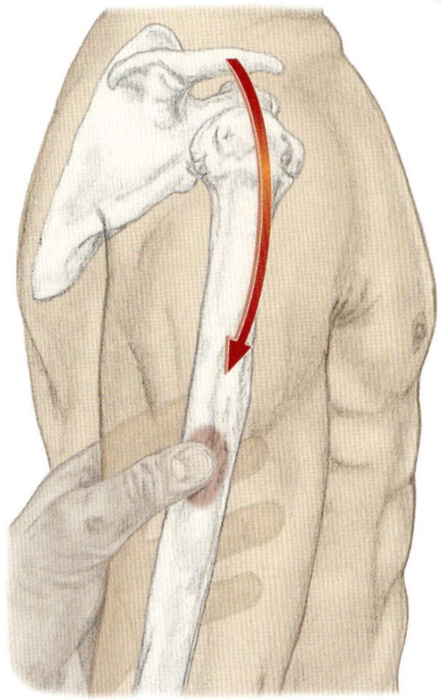

2.30 Lateral view of right shoulder, as you access the deltoid tuberosity

Discover More

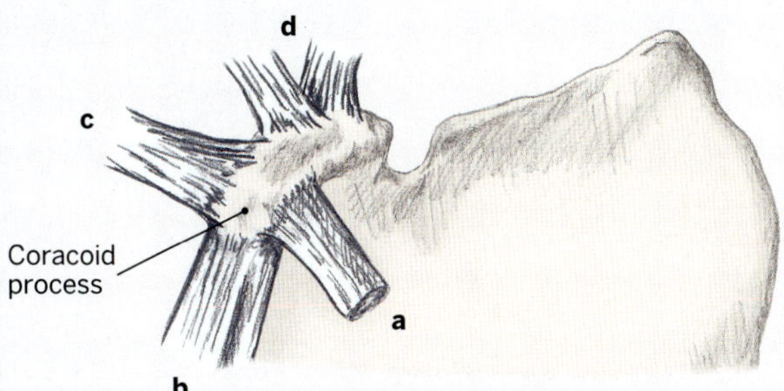

Anterior view of right scapula

The coracoid process is an attachment site for several tendons and ligaments. The arrangement of these structures can be illustrated in a clockwise fashion. On the right scapula, the pectoralis minor tendon (**a**) connects at four o'clock, while the coracobrachialis and biceps brachii tendons (**b**) lie at seven o'clock. The coracoacromial ligament (**c**) attaches at ten o'clock and the coracoclavicular ligaments (**d**) attach further posteriorly on the coracoid process at eleven o'clock and midnight.

coracoid	*kor*-a-koyd	Grk. raven's beak
tuberosity	*tu*-ber-*os*-i-tee	L. a swelling

Trail 4 Two Hills and a Valley ▸

Greater and Lesser Tubercles, Intertubercular Groove

These three landmarks are located on the proximal humerus deep to the deltoid muscle. The **greater tubercle** is located inferior and lateral to the acromion. It is shaped more like a low mound than a pointy hill. The greater tubercle is an attachment site for three of the four rotator cuff muscles—supraspinatus, infraspinatus, and teres minor (p. 70).

The **lesser tubercle** is smaller than the greater tubercle and is an attachment site for the fourth rotator cuff muscle—subscapularis (p. 70). The **intertubercular groove** is situated between the greater and lesser tubercles and is roughly a pencil's width in diameter. Within the groove lies the tendon of the long head of the biceps brachii, which can be tender; you should palpate gently in this region.

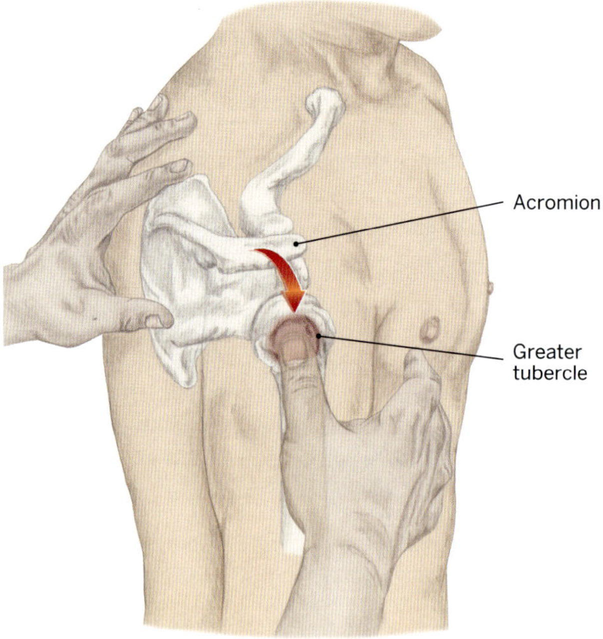

2.31 Lateral view of right shoulder, as you slide off the acromion to the greater tubercle

Greater tubercle

1. Partner seated or supine. Shaking hands with your partner, locate the acromion.
2. Slide off the acromion inferiorly and laterally approximately one inch (**2.31**).
3. The solid surface located deep to the deltoid fibers will be the greater tubercle. You may feel a small dip between the acromion and the tubercle.

Intertubercular groove and lesser tubercle

1. Partner seated or supine. Place your thumb on the greater tubercle (**2.32**, **a**).
2. Begin to rotate the arm laterally. As the humerus rotates, the greater tubercle (**a**) will move out from under your thumb and be replaced by the slender ditch of the intertubercular groove (**b**).
3. As you continue to laterally rotate the arm, your thumb will rise out of the groove onto the lesser tubercle (**c**).

✔ *Place your thumb at the greater tubercle and passively rotate the arm medially and laterally. Do you feel the "bump-ditch-bump" sequence as the three landmarks pass beneath your thumb? Are you horizontal to the level of the coracoid process?*

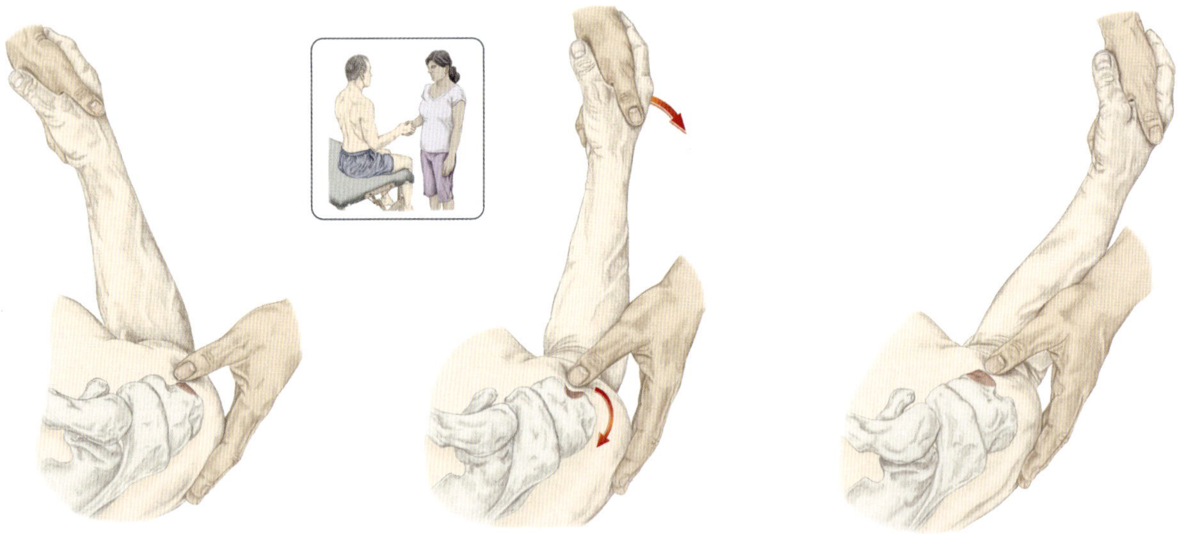

a Greater tubercle **b** Intertubercular groove **c** Lesser tubercle

2.32 Superior views of rotating the right humerus, as you palpate the tubercles and intertubercular groove

intertubercular **in**-tur-tu-**ber**-ku-lar

Overview: **Muscles of the Shoulder and Arm**

The muscles of the shoulder and arm are an amazingly diverse group. Some of them span across the back and rib cage, some attach at the cranium, and others extend down to the elbow. All of the muscles create movement at the shoulder complex (formed by the scapula, clavicle, and humerus). Some also elevate the ribs, extend the head and cervical vertebrae, or bend the elbow (**2.33-2.35**).

The superficial muscles of the shoulder and back are presented first, followed by the deeper muscles of the back and, lastly, the muscles of the arm. Some muscles are presented together to better understand how they function as a group.

Although the instructions for each muscle or muscle group specify the position in which to place your partner (prone, supine, or seated), exploration in all positions is encouraged for a better understanding of the muscle(s) and the surrounding structures.

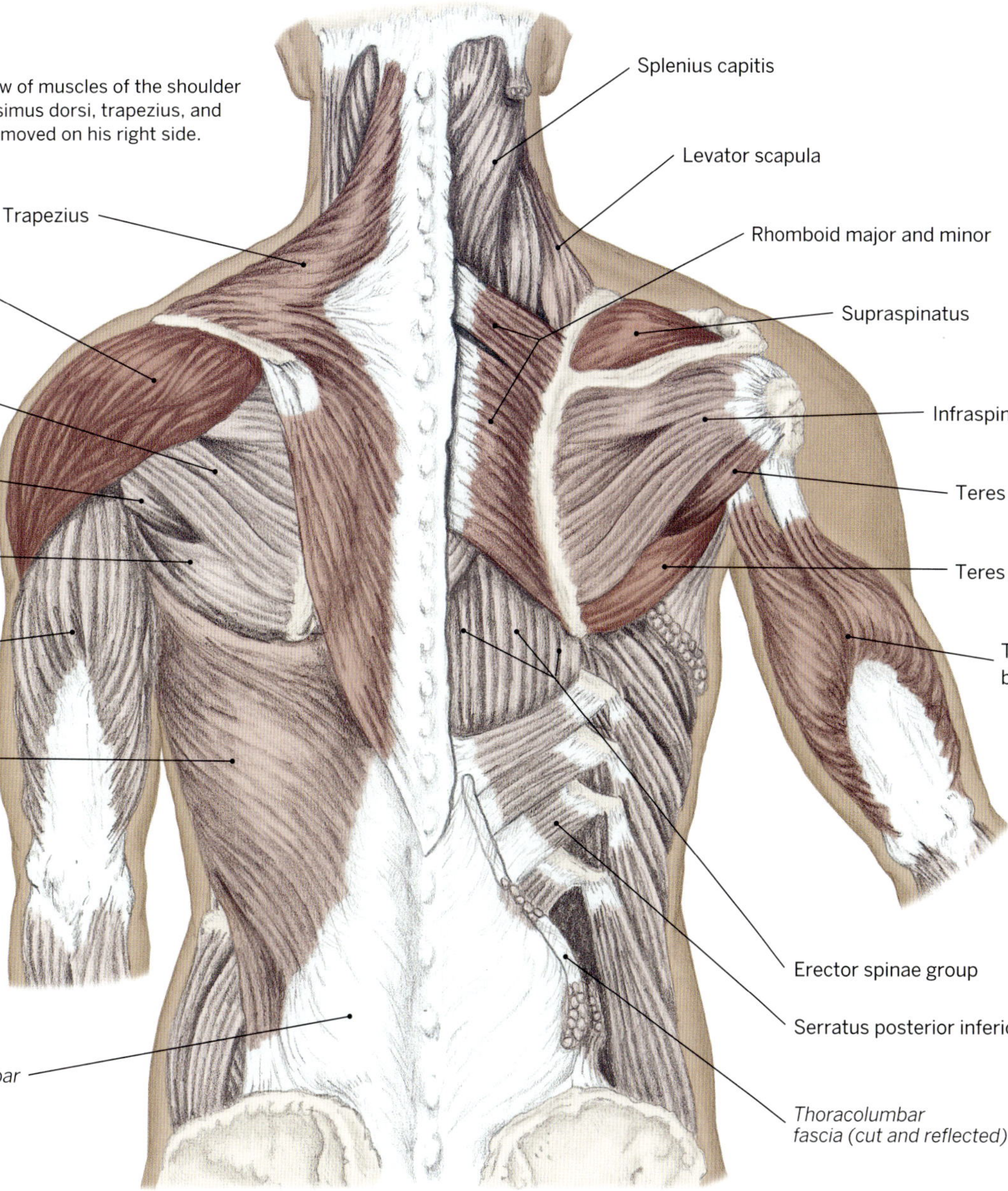

2.33 Posterior view of muscles of the shoulder and back. Latissimus dorsi, trapezius, and deltoid are removed on his right side.

Discover More

The trapezius received its present name from the British anatomist William Cowper (c. 1700). Previously, it was called the musculus cucullaris (L. muscle hood) because the two trapezius muscles together resemble a monk's hood.

Overview: **Muscles of the Shoulder and Arm,** *continued*

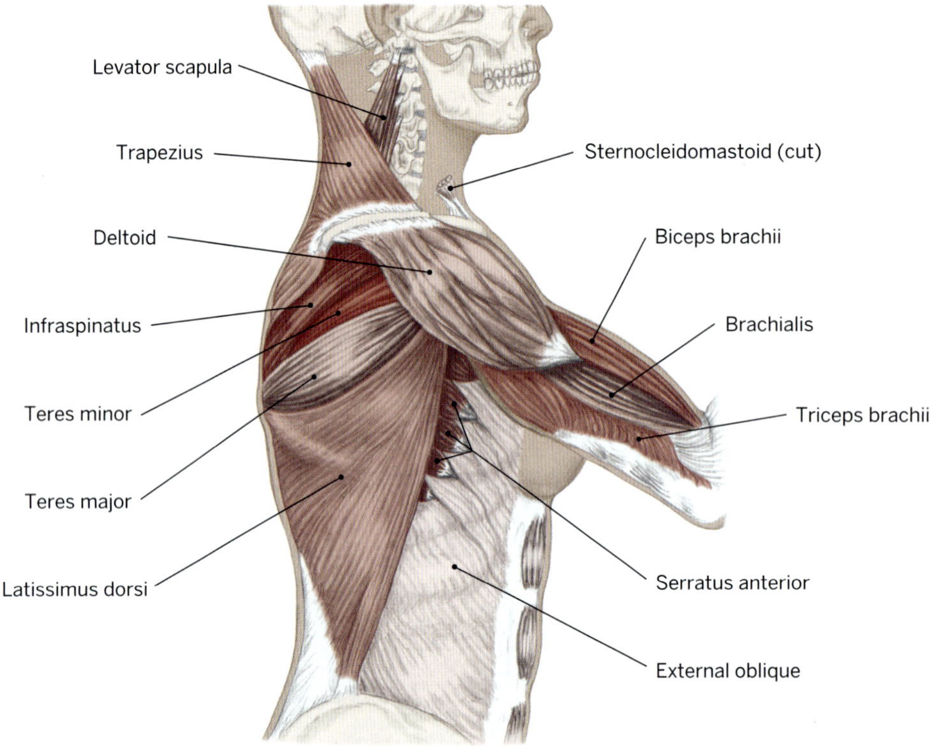

2.34 Lateral view of muscles of the torso, shoulder, and arm

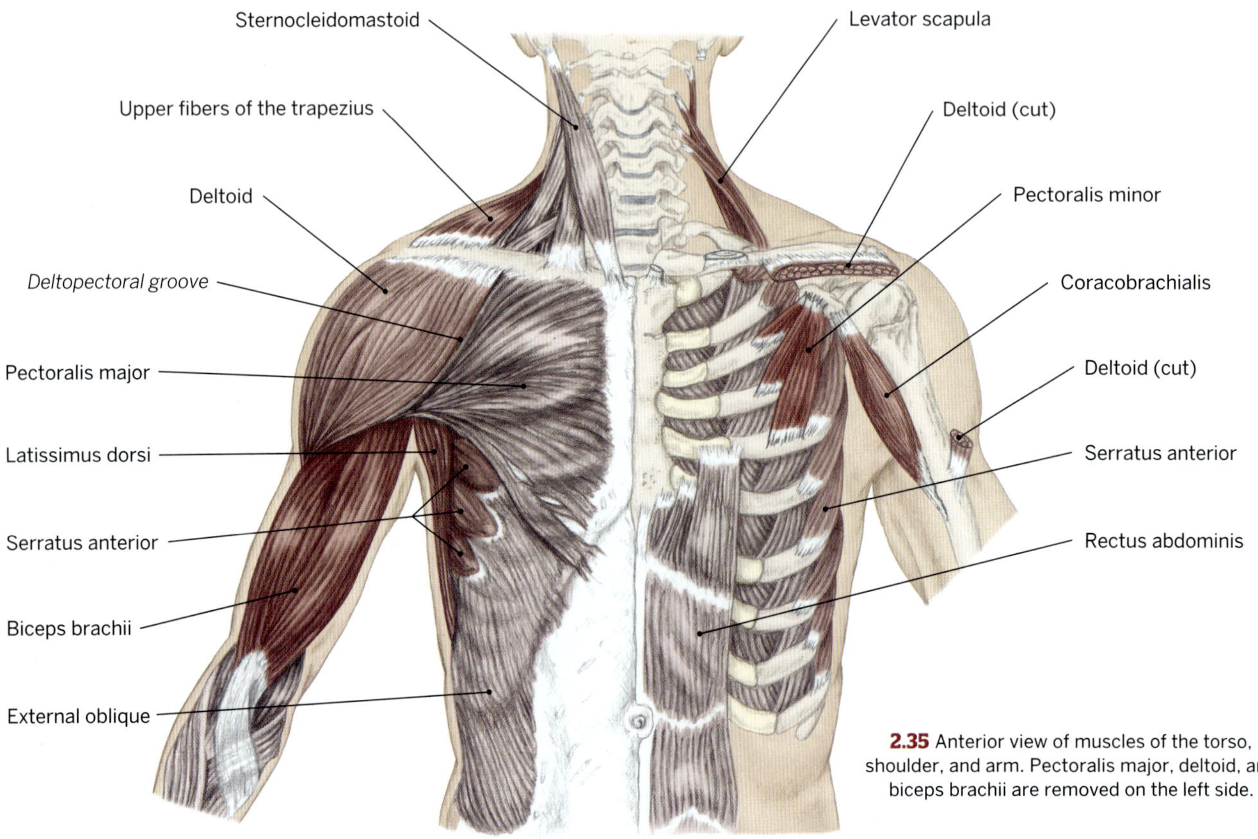

2.35 Anterior view of muscles of the torso, shoulder, and arm. Pectoralis major, deltoid, and biceps brachii are removed on the left side.

Synergists—Muscles Working Together

Muscles are listed in the order of their ability to create the movement. Asterisk indicates muscles not shown.

Shoulder

(glenohumeral joint)

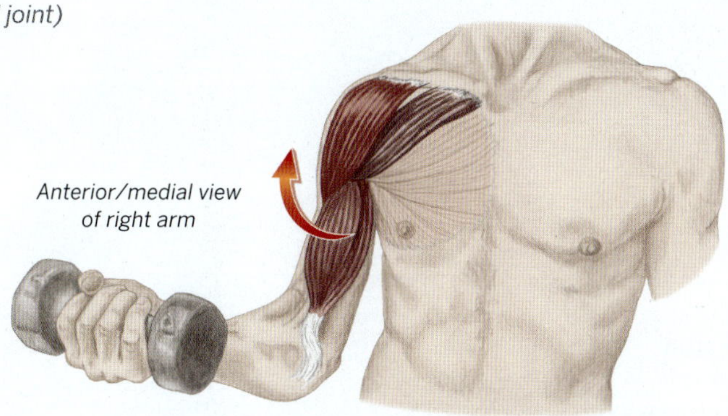

2.36 Flexion of the shoulder

Flexion

(antagonists on extension)

Deltoid (anterior fibers)
Pectoralis major (upper fibers)
Biceps brachii
Coracobrachialis*

Extension

(antagonists on flexion)

Deltoid (posterior fibers)
Latissimus dorsi
Teres major
Pectoralis major (lower fibers)
Triceps brachii (long head)

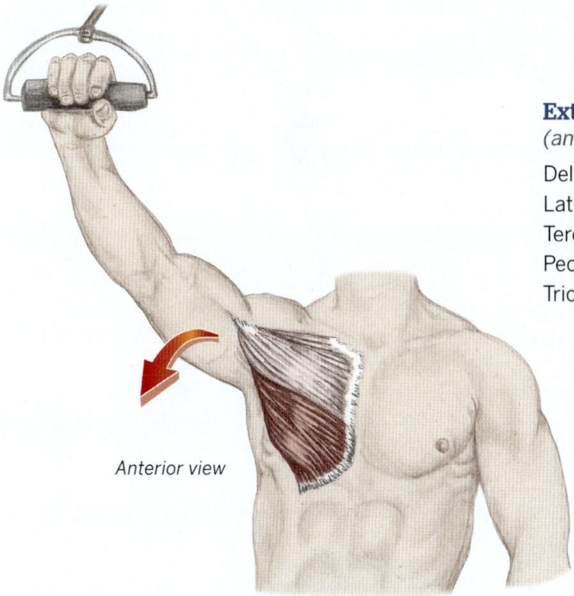

2.37 Extension of the shoulder

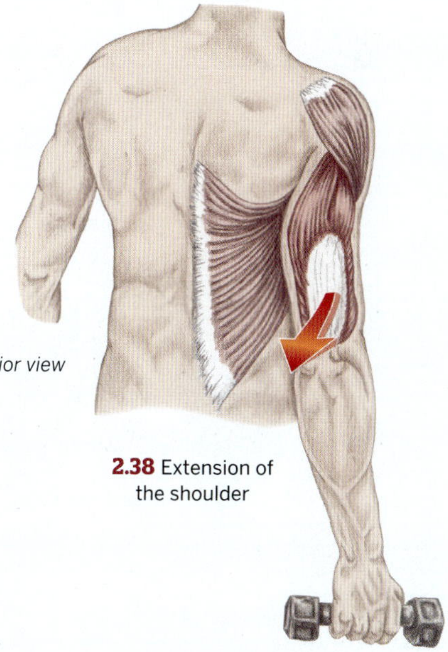

2.38 Extension of the shoulder

Horizontal Abduction

(antagonist on horizontal adduction)

Deltoid (posterior fibers)

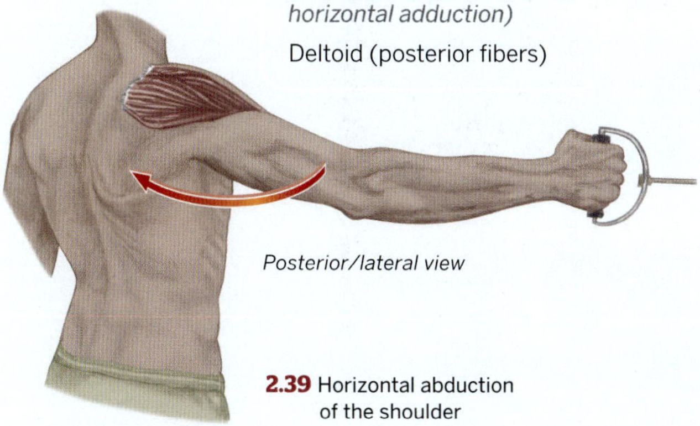

2.39 Horizontal abduction of the shoulder

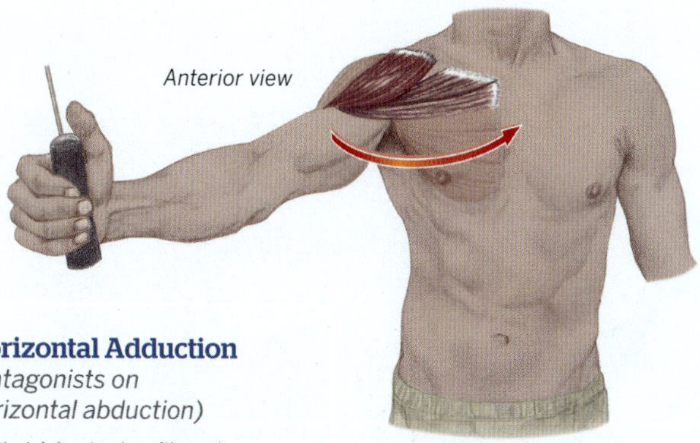

Horizontal Adduction

(antagonists on horizontal abduction)

Deltoid (anterior fibers)
Pectoralis major (upper fibers)

2.40 Horizontal adduction of the shoulder

Shoulder

(glenohumeral joint)

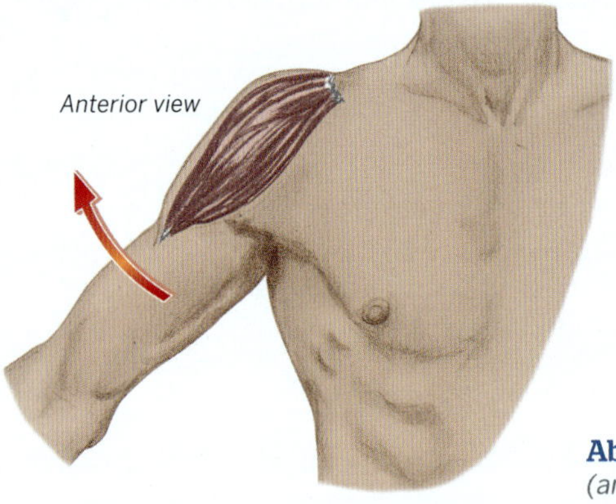

2.41 Abduction of the shoulder

Abduction

(antagonists on adduction)

Deltoid (all fibers)
Supraspinatus

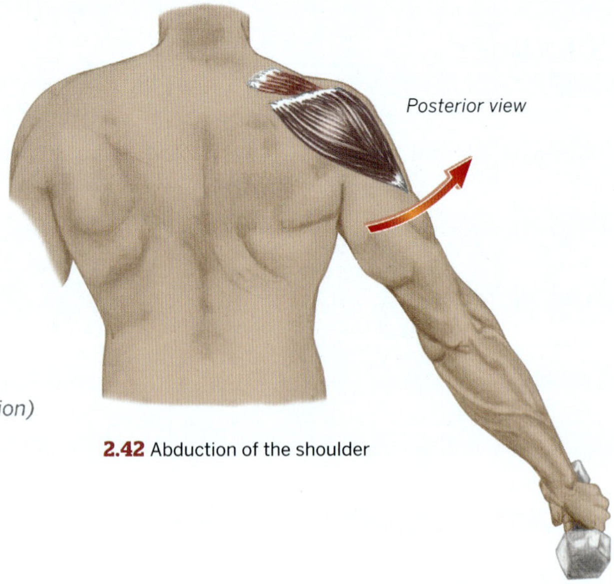

2.42 Abduction of the shoulder

Adduction

(antagonists on abduction)

Latissimus dorsi
Teres major
Infraspinatus
Teres minor
Pectoralis major (all fibers)
Triceps brachii (long head)
Coracobrachialis

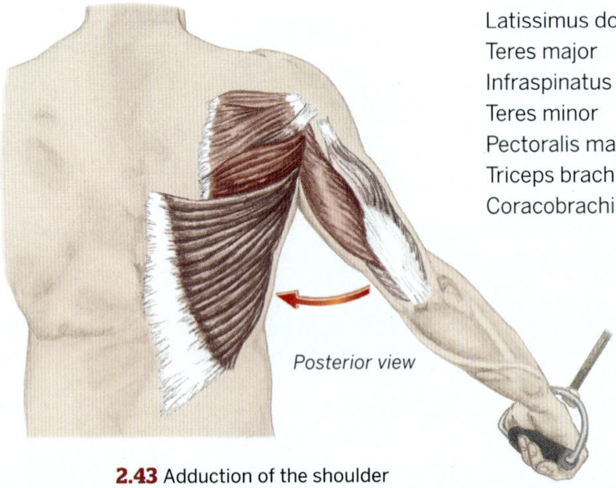

2.43 Adduction of the shoulder

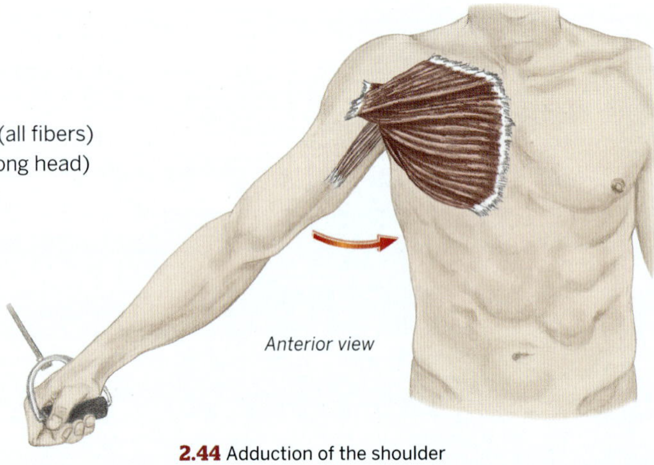

2.44 Adduction of the shoulder

Lateral Rotation (external rotation)

(antagonists on medial rotation)

Deltoid (posterior fibers)
Infraspinatus
Teres minor

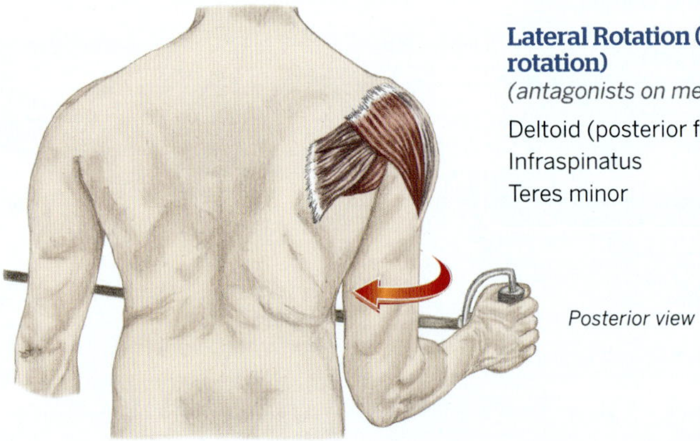

2.45 Lateral rotation (external rotation) of the shoulder

Shoulder

(glenohumeral joint)

Medial Rotation (internal rotation)

(antagonists on lateral rotation)

Deltoid (anterior fibers)
Latissimus dorsi
Teres major
Subscapularis
Pectoralis major (all fibers)

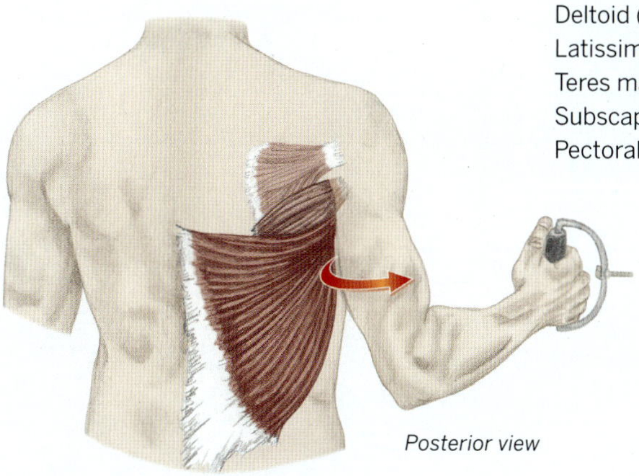

2.46 Medial rotation (internal rotation) of the shoulder

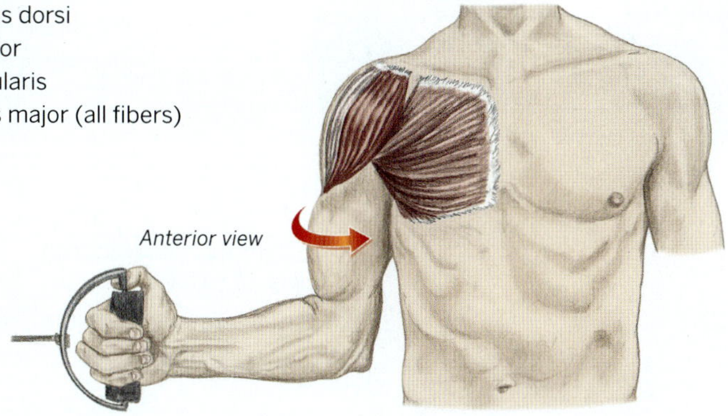

2.47 Medial rotation (internal rotation) of the shoulder

Scapula

(scapulothoracic joint)

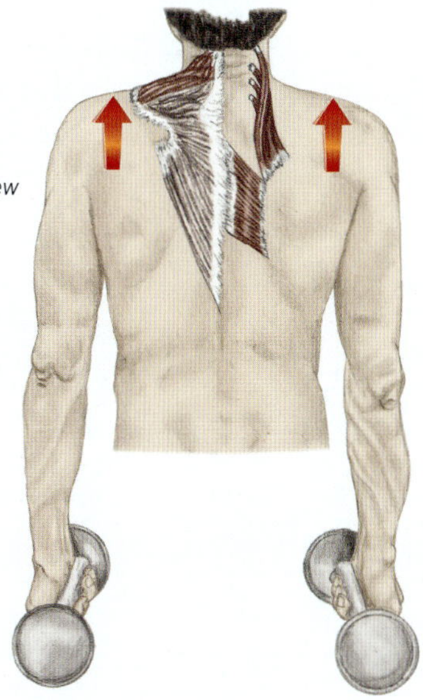

Elevation

(antagonists on depression)

Trapezius (upper fibers, unilaterally)
Rhomboid major
Rhomboid minor
Levator scapula (unilaterally)

2.48 Elevation of the scapula

Depression

(antagonists on elevation)

Trapezius (lower fibers)
Serratus anterior (with the origin fixed)
Pectoralis minor

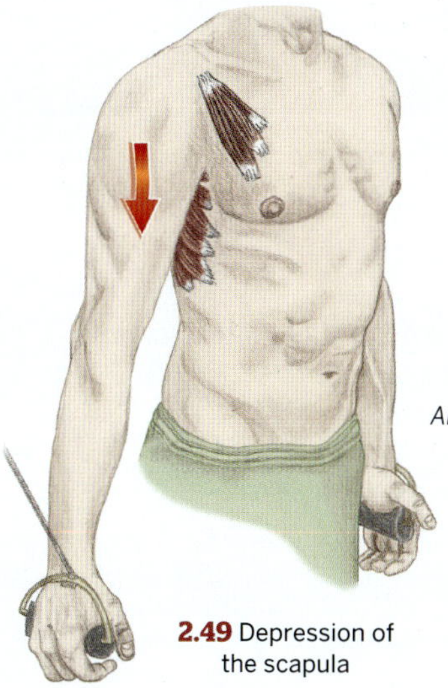

2.49 Depression of the scapula

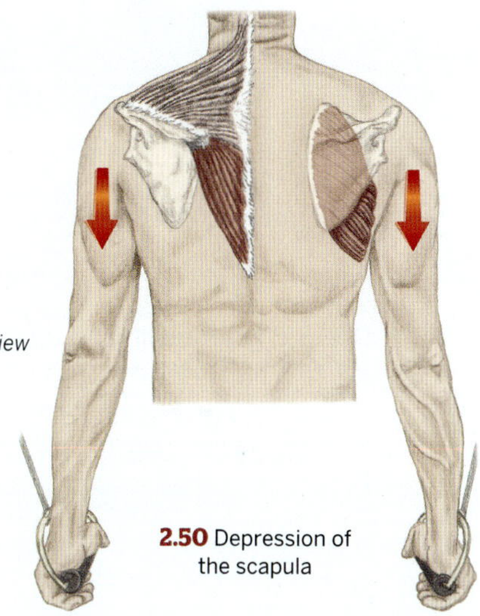

2.50 Depression of the scapula

Scapula

(scapulothoracic joint)

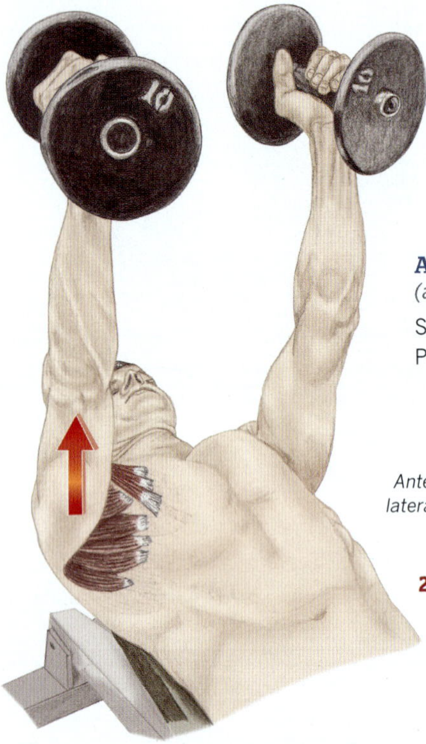

Abduction (protraction)

(antagonists on adduction)

Serratus anterior (with the origin fixed)
Pectoralis minor

2.51 Abduction (protraction) of the scapula

Adduction (retraction)

(antagonists on abduction)

Trapezius (middle fibers)
Rhomboid major
Rhomboid minor

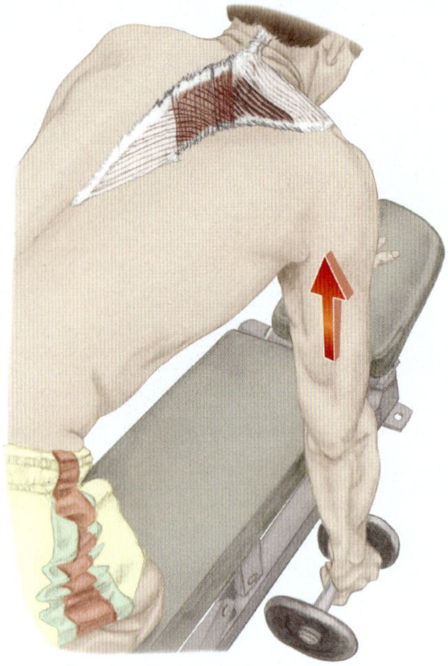

2.52 Adduction (retraction) of the scapula

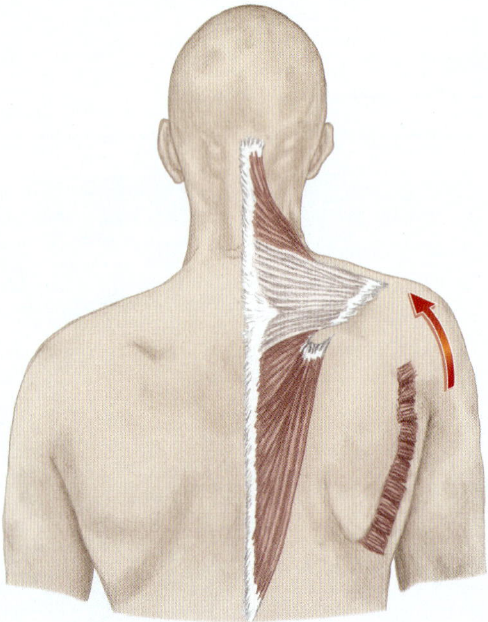

Upward Rotation of the Scapula

(antagonists on downward rotation)

Trapezius (upper and lower fibers)
Serratus anterior (with the origin fixed)

2.53 Upward rotation of the scapula

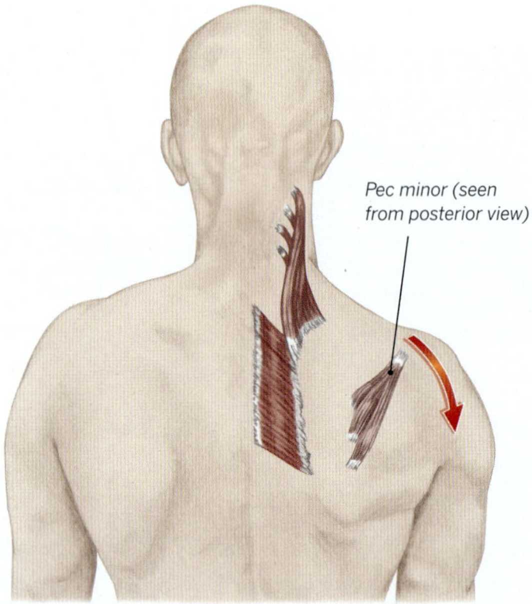

Downward Rotation of the Scapula

(antagonists on upward rotation)

Rhomboid major
Rhomboid minor
Levator scapula
Pectoralis minor

2.54 Downward rotation of the scapula

Muscles of the Shoulder and Arm

Deltoid ▶

The triangle-shaped deltoid is located on the cap of the shoulder. The origin of the deltoid (which is, interestingly enough, identical to the insertion of the trapezius) curves around the spine of the scapula and clavicle, forming a V shape. From this broad origin, the fibers converge down the arm to attach at the deltoid tuberosity (**2.55**, **2.56**).

The deltoid fibers can be divided into three segments: the anterior, middle, and posterior fibers. All three groups abduct the humerus, but the anterior and posterior fibers are antagonists in both flexion/extension and medial/lateral rotation.

	DELTOID
A	*All fibers:* **Abduct** the shoulder (glenohumeral joint) *Anterior fibers:* **Flex** the shoulder (G/H joint) **Medially rotate** the shoulder (G/H joint) **Horizontally adduct** the shoulder (G/H joint) *Posterior fibers:* **Extend** the shoulder (G/H joint) **Laterally rotate** the shoulder (G/H joint) **Horizontally abduct** the shoulder (G/H joint)
O	Lateral one-third of clavicle, acromion, and spine of scapula
I	Deltoid tuberosity
N	Axillary C**5**, **6**

When Do You Use Your Deltoid?

- Virtually all movements that involve the shoulder
- Slipping your arms into a jacket
- Raking, shoveling, sawing

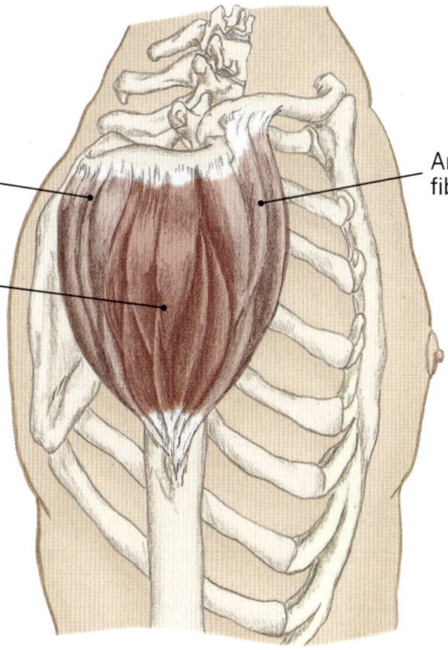

2.55 Lateral view of right shoulder, showing the three segments of the deltoid

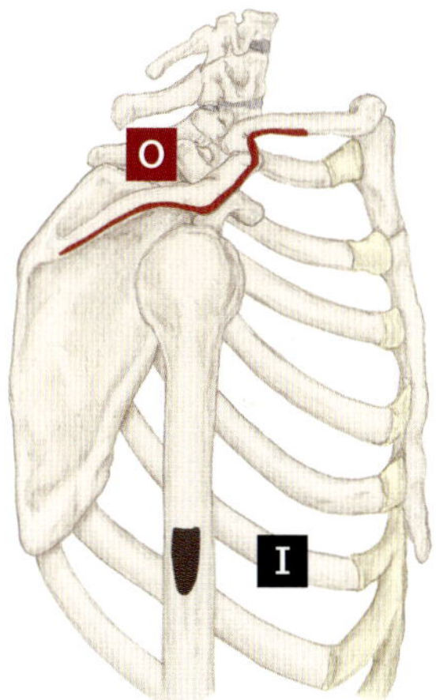

2.56 Lateral view of right shoulder, showing origin and insertion of deltoid

Belly of the deltoid

1. Partner seated. Locate the spine of the scapula, the acromion, and the lateral one-third of the clavicle. Note the V shape these landmarks form.
2. Locate the deltoid tuberosity.
3. Palpate between these landmarks to isolate the superficial, convergent fibers of the deltoid. Be sure to explore the deltoid's most anterior and posterior aspects.

*Are the fibers you feel superficial and do they converge toward the deltoid tuberosity? If your partner alternately abducts and releases, do you feel the fibers contract and relax (**2.57**)?*

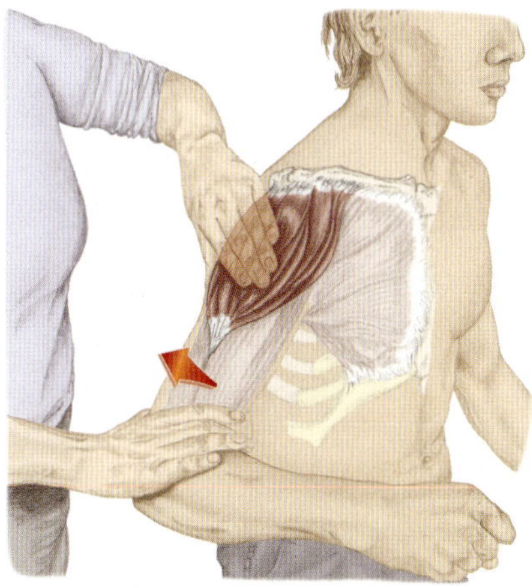

2.57 Partner seated, alternately abducting and releasing while you palpate the deltoid

▶ indicates that a video clip is included in the "For Students" section of our website, booksofdiscovery.com

deltoid *del*-toid Grk. *delta*, capital letter *D* (Δ) in the Greek alphabet

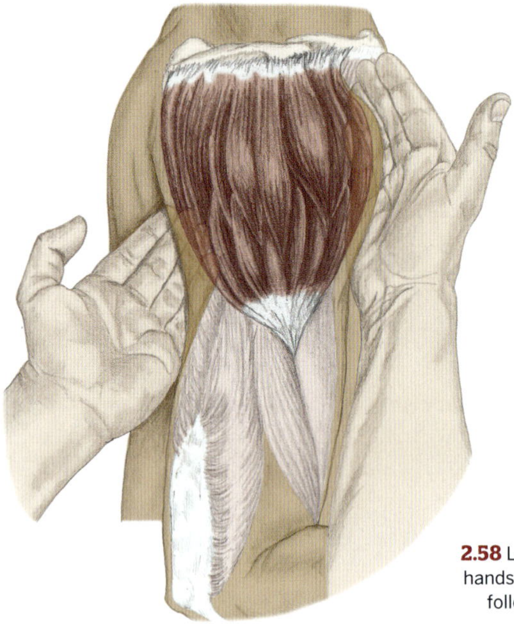

2.58 Lateral view of right shoulder. Use both hands to sculpt out the edges of the deltoid, following them down to the tuberosity.

Palpation Plus

Deltoid as antagonist to itself

To feel the antagonistic abilities of the deltoid's anterior and posterior fibers:

1. Shaking hands with your partner, place your other hand on the deltoid.
2. Keeping his elbow next to his side, ask your partner to medially and laterally rotate his arm against your resistance. Can you sense the anterior fibers contracting upon medial rotation and relaxing upon lateral rotation, and vice versa for the posterior fibers?

Trapezius ▶

The trapezius lies superficially along the upper back and neck. Its broad, thin fibers blanket the shoulders, attaching to the occiput (the bone at the base of the head, p. 231), lateral clavicle, scapula, and spinous processes of the thoracic vertebrae (**2.59–2.61**).

The trapezius fibers can be divided into three groups: upper (descending) fibers, middle fibers, and lower (ascending) fibers. The upper and lower fibers are antagonists in elevation and depression of the scapula, respectively. All fibers of the trapezius are easy to palpate.

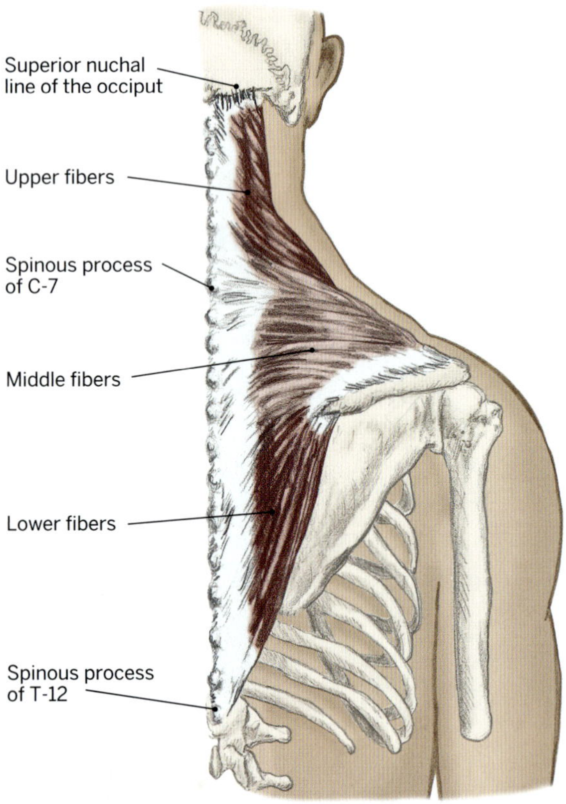

2.59 Posterior view of right shoulder and neck, showing trapezius

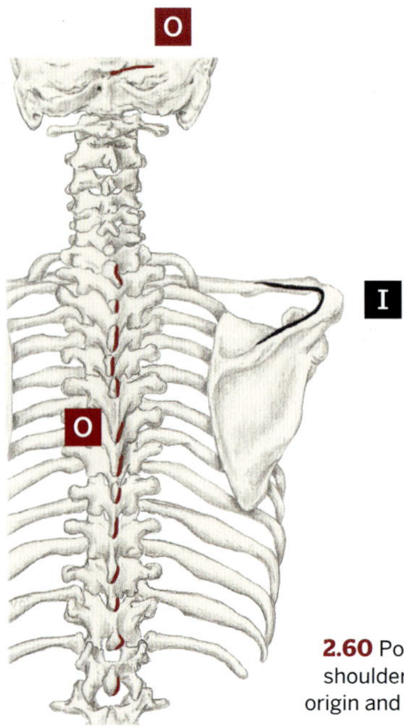

2.60 Posterior view of right shoulder and neck, showing origin and insertion of trapezius

TRAPEZIUS

A

Upper fibers:

Bilaterally:

Extend the head and neck

Unilaterally:

Laterally flex the head and neck to the same side

Rotate the head and neck to the opposite side

Elevate the scapula (scapulothoracic joint)

Upwardly rotate the scapula (S/T joint)

Middle fibers:

Adduct the scapula (S/T joint)

Stabilize the scapula (S/T joint)

Lower fibers:

Depress the scapula (S/T joint)

Upwardly rotate the scapula (S/T joint)

O External occipital protuberance, medial portion of superior nuchal line of the occiput, ligamentum nuchae, and spinous processes of C-7 through T-12

I Lateral one-third of clavicle, acromion, and spine of the scapula

N Spinal portion of cranial nerve XI (accessory) and ventral ramus C2, **3**, **4**

When Do You Use Your Trapezius?

- Holding a smartphone between your shoulder and ear
- Carrying articles strapped across the shoulder (backpack, purse)
- Carrying boxes or furniture with both hands

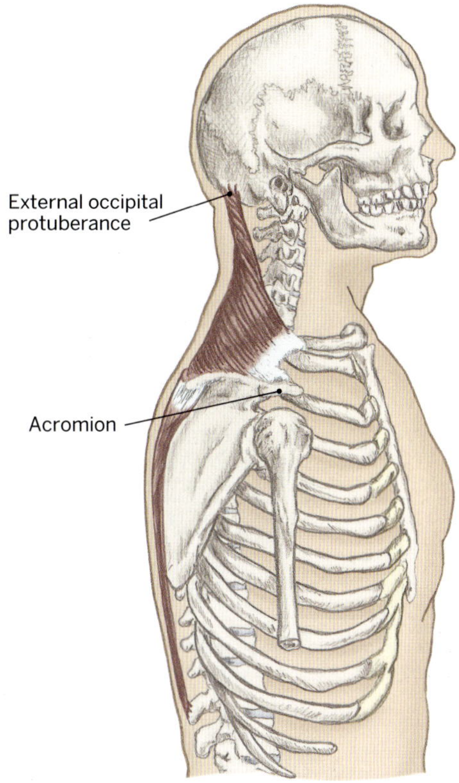

2.61 Lateral view of right shoulder and neck, showing trapezius

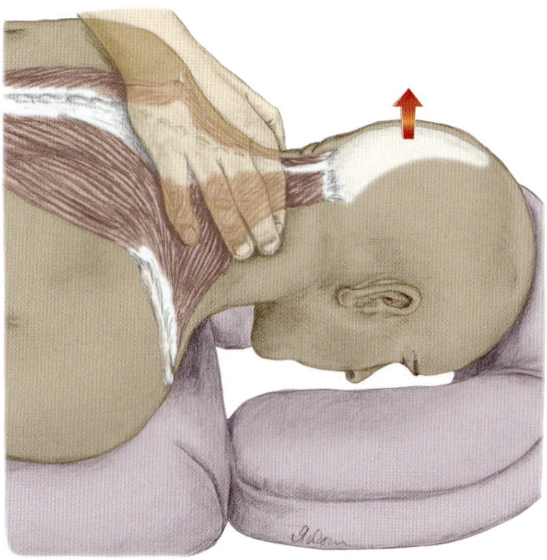

2.62 Partner prone, as you palpate the upper fibers of the trapezius

Upper fibers of the trapezius

1. Partner prone. These fibers form the easily accessible flap of muscle lying across the top of the shoulder. Along the posterior neck they are surprisingly skinny, each being only an inch wide.
2. Grasp the superficial tissue on the top of the shoulder and feel the upper trapezius fibers. Take note of their slender quality (**2.62**).
3. Follow the fibers superiorly toward the base of the head at the occiput. To feel the fibers along the posterior neck contract, stand at the side of the table and ask your partner to extend his head "a quarter inch off the face cradle." Then follow the fibers inferiorly to the lateral clavicle.

Is the muscle you are grasping thin and superficial? Grasp the fibers along the top of the shoulder and have your partner elevate his scapula gently toward his ear. Do the muscle fibers become taut?

trapezius	tra-***pee***-ze-us	Grk. a little table or trapezoid shape
nuchae	***nu***-kay	L. nape of neck
occiput	***ok***-si-put	L. the back of the skull

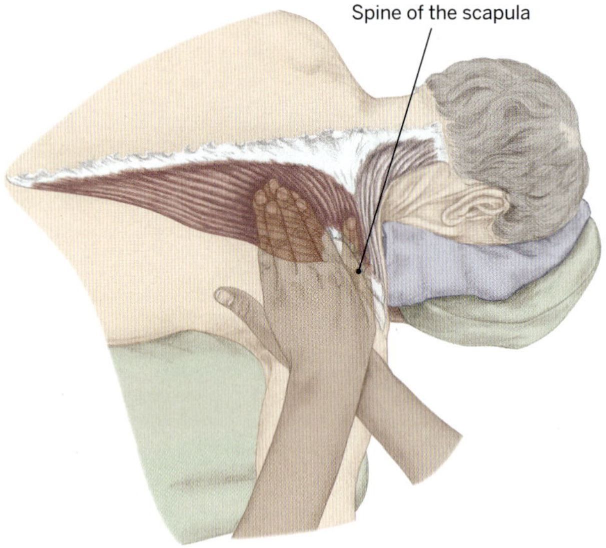

2.63 Partner prone, as you access the middle and lower fibers of the trapezius

Middle fibers of the trapezius

1. Partner prone. Locate the spine of the scapula.
2. Slide medially from the spine of the scapula onto the trapezius and move your fingers across its fibers (**2.63**). The trapezius fibers are superficial and thin, so explore at a superficial level and not deeper into the rhomboids or erector spinae muscles.

Palpate the middle fibers and ask your partner to adduct his scapula. "Bring your shoulder up off the table." Can you feel any contraction in the fibers?

Discover More

As your partner extends his head, you will likely see two parallel "speed bumps" running along the posterior neck. These bulges are formed primarily by the deeper semispinalis capitis muscle (p. 200), with the trapezius muscles draped on top.

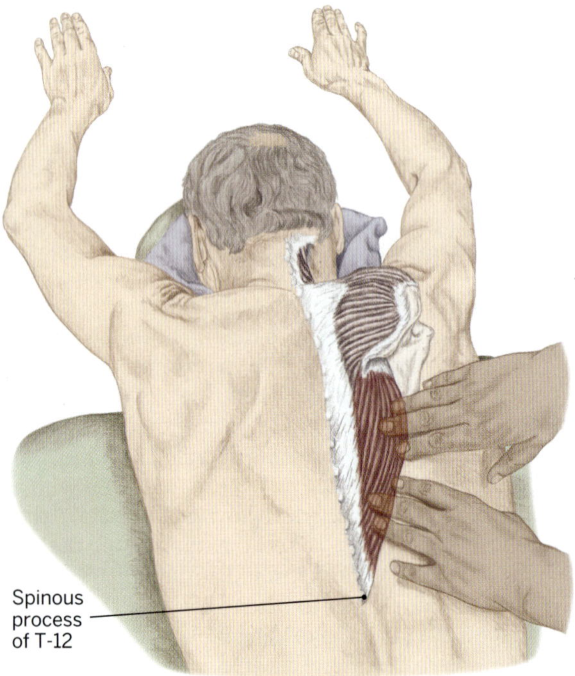

2.64 Partner prone, with arms reaching out in front of him, as you palpate the superficial fibers of the trapezius

Lower fibers of the trapezius

1. Partner prone. Locate the edge of the lower fibers by drawing a line from the spine of the scapula to the spinous process of T-12 (p. 177).
2. Palpate along this line and push your fingers into the edge of the lower fibers. Ask your partner to hold his arms out in front of him (like Superman) and feel for the superficial fibers of the trapezius (**2.64**).
3. Attempt to lift the lower fibers between your fingers, raising them off the underlying musculature.

Another way to feel the lower fibers contract is to ask your partner to depress his shoulder. Do the lower fibers run at a gentle angle toward the scapula (rather than parallel with the vertebral column like the erector spinae muscles)?

Latissimus Dorsi and Teres Major ▶

The **latissimus dorsi** is the broadest muscle of the back. Its thin, superficial fibers originate at the low back, ascend the side of the trunk, and merge into a thick bundle at the axilla (**2.65**, **2.67**). Both ends of the latissimus dorsi are difficult to isolate; however, its middle portion next to the lateral border of the scapula is easy to grasp.

The **teres major** is called "lat's little helper" because it is a complete synergist with the latissimus dorsi (**2.66**, **2.68**). It is superficial and located along the scapula's lateral border between the latissimus dorsi and teres minor. Although they share names, the teres major and teres minor rotate the arm in opposite directions—the major medially, the minor laterally.

The latissimus dorsi and teres major are sometimes called the "handcuff muscles" because their actions collectively bring the arms into the "arresting" position!

LATISSIMUS DORSI

A	**Extend** the shoulder (glenohumeral joint) **Adduct** the shoulder (G/H joint) **Medially rotate** the shoulder (G/H joint)
O	Inferior angle of scapula, spinous processes of last six thoracic vertebrae, last three or four ribs, thoracolumbar fascia, and posterior iliac crest
I	Intertubercular groove of the humerus
N	Thoracodorsal C**6**, **7**, **8**

When Do You Use Your Latissimus Dorsi?

- Steering a kayak with a paddle
- Unzipping the back of your dress
- Walking with crutches

TERES MAJOR

A	**Extend** the shoulder (glenohumeral joint) **Adduct** the shoulder (G/H joint) **Medially rotate** the shoulder (G/H joint)
O	Inferior angle and lower one-third of lateral border of the scapula
I	Crest of the lesser tubercle of the humerus
N	Lower subscapular C5, **6**, 7

When Do You Use Your Teres Major?

- Unzipping the back of your dress
- Walking with crutches
- Climbing up a rope when storming a castle

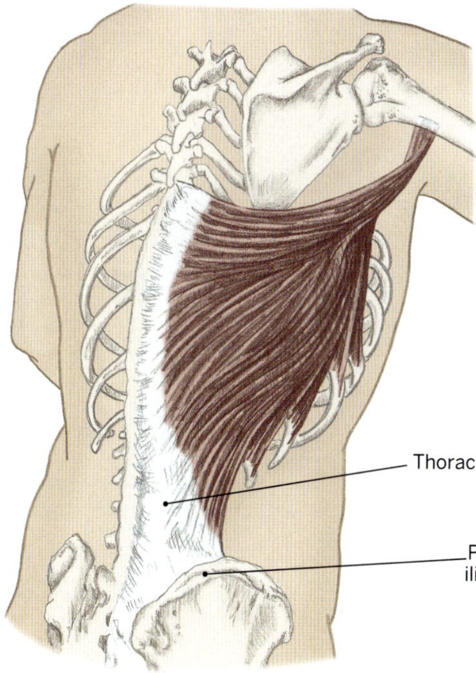

2.65 Lateral/posterior view of right shoulder and torso, showing latissimus dorsi

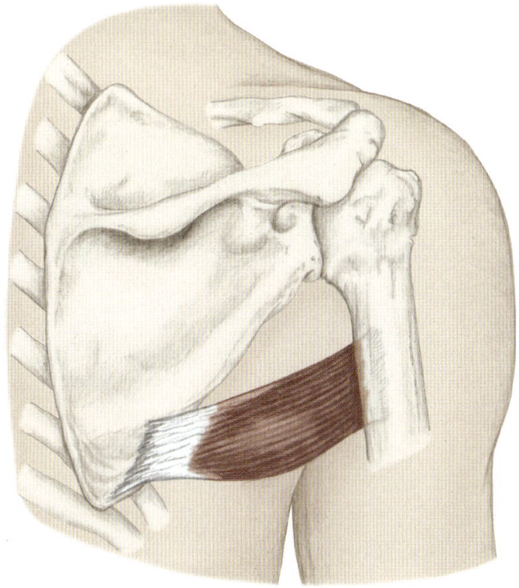

2.66 Posterior view of right shoulder, showing teres major

Discover More

The latissimus dorsi not only moves the arm but, because of its broad origin, can also affect the trunk and spine. Contraction of the left latissimus dorsi assists in lateral flexion of the trunk to the left. If the arm is fixed, as when hanging from a bar, the latissimus will assist in extension of the spine and tilting of the pelvis anteriorly and laterally.

latissimus dorsi	la-*tis*-i-mus *dor*-si	L. widest of the back
teres	*teh*-reez	L. rounded, finely shaped

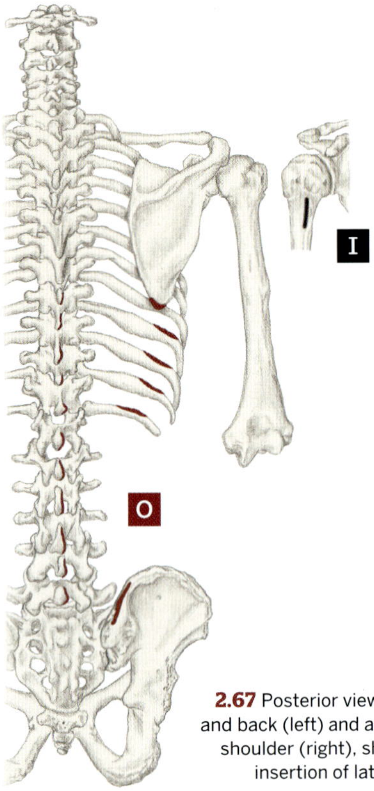

2.67 Posterior view of right shoulder and back (left) and anterior view of right shoulder (right), showing origin and insertion of latissimus dorsi

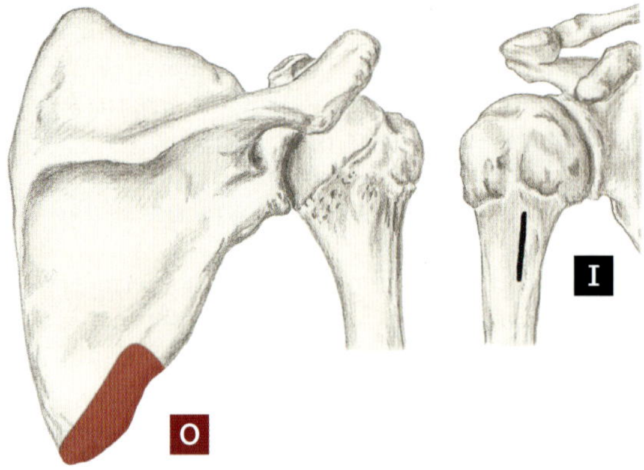

2.68 Posterior view (left) and anterior view (right) of right shoulder, showing origin and insertion of teres major

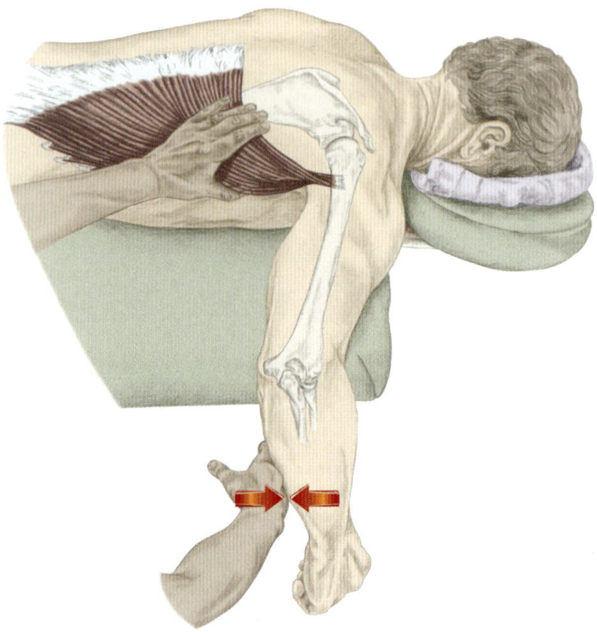

2.69 Partner prone, medially rotating his shoulder against your resistance while you palpate the latissimus fibers

Latissimus dorsi

1. Partner prone with the arm off the side of the table. Locate the scapula's lateral border.

2. Using your fingers and thumb, grasp the thick wad of muscle tissue lateral to the lateral border. This is the latissimus dorsi (and perhaps some of teres major). Note how this muscle tissue flares off the side of the trunk.
3. Feel the latissimus fibers contract by asking your partner to medially rotate his shoulder against your resistance. "Swing your hand up toward your hip" (**2.69**). As this occurs, follow the latissimus fibers superiorly into the axilla and inferiorly on the ribs.

To ensure you are not just lifting the skin, grasp the tissue and let it slowly slip out between your fingers. Do you feel the muscle's fibrous texture or just the skin's jellylike quality?

Latissimus dorsi

1. With your partner supine, cradle the arm in a flexed position. Then grasp the tissue of the latissimus located beside the lateral border.
2. Ask your partner to extend his shoulder against your resistance. "Press your elbow toward your hip." This will force the latissimus to contract (**2.70**).

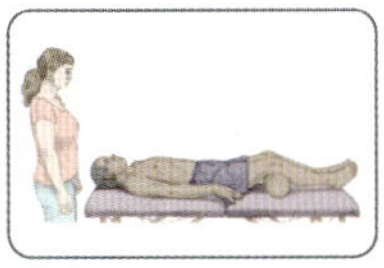

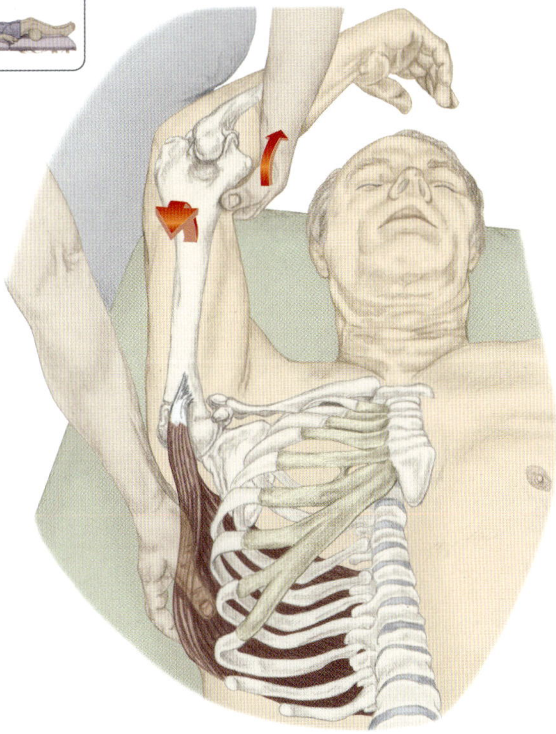

2.70 Partner supine, pressing his elbow toward his hip against your resistance while you palpate the latissimus

Teres major

1. Partner prone with the arm off the side of the table. Locate and grasp the latissimus dorsi fibers between your fingers and thumb.
2. Move your fingers and thumb medially to where you feel the scapula's lateral border. The muscle fibers that lie medial to the latissimus and attach to the lateral border will be the teres major.
3. Follow these fibers toward the axilla where they blend with the latissimus dorsi.

*Lay your thumb on the inferior aspect of the lateral border and have your partner medially rotate the shoulder joint to distinguish the teres major from the latissimus dorsi (**2.71**). The fibers of both muscles will contract. Those that attach directly to the lateral border belong to teres major; the more lateral fibers belong to latissimus dorsi.*

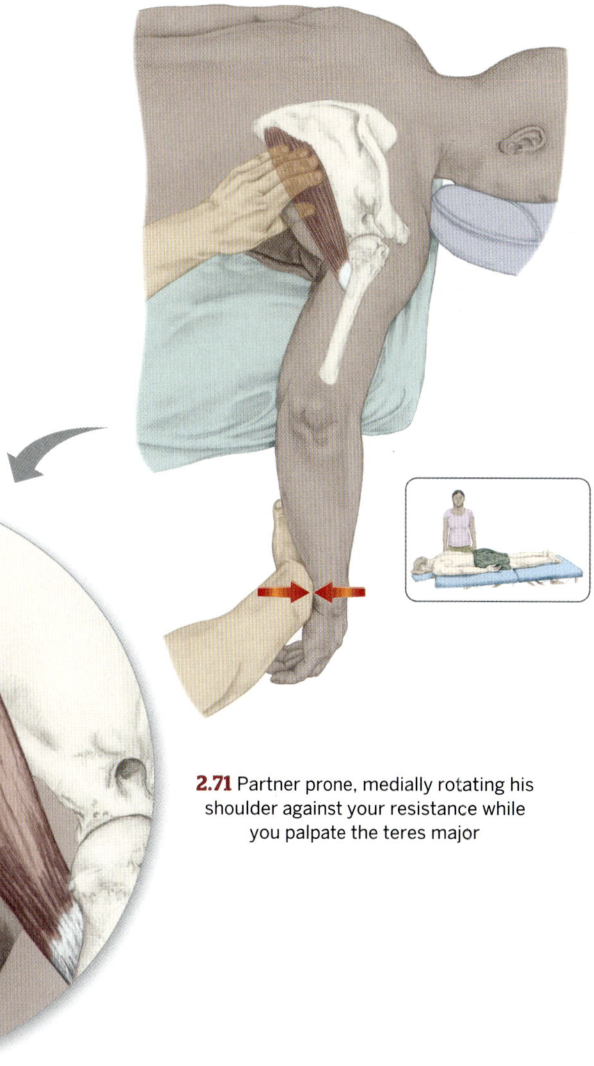

2.71 Partner prone, medially rotating his shoulder against your resistance while you palpate the teres major

Rotator Cuff Muscles ▸

Supraspinatus
Infraspinatus
Teres Minor
Subscapularis

Supraspinatus, infraspinatus, teres minor, and subscapularis are known as the rotator cuff muscles. Together they encompass, and therefore stabilize, the glenohumeral joint. All of the rotator cuff muscles are accessible, including their tendons, which attach to the head of the humerus.

The chunky **supraspinatus** is located in the supraspinous fossa, deep to the trapezius's upper fibers. Its belly runs underneath the acromion and attaches to the humerus's greater tubercle (**2.72**, **2.76**). The supraspinatus assists the deltoid with abduction of the shoulder and is the only muscle of the group not involved in shoulder rotation.

The flat, convergent belly of the **infraspinatus** is located in the infraspinous fossa. Most of its belly is superficial with a medial portion deep to the trapezius and a lateral portion beneath the deltoid (p. 63). The infraspinatus attaches immediately posterior to the supraspinatus on the greater tubercle (**2.73**, **2.76**) and is a synergist with the teres minor in lateral rotation of the shoulder. The unique, dense quality of the infraspinatus muscle is due to its multipennate fibers and thick, superficial fascia.

The **teres minor** is a small muscle squeezed between the infraspinatus and teres major. It is located high in the axilla and can be challenging to grasp (**2.74**, **2.76**). The teres minor and teres major are antagonists in rotation of the humerus.

The deep **subscapularis** (**2.75**, **2.79**), located on the scapula's anterior surface, is sandwiched between the subscapular fossa and serratus anterior muscle (p. 82). With only a small portion of its muscle belly accessible, the subscapularis is the only rotator cuff muscle that attaches to the humerus's lesser tubercle (**2.77**). It rotates the shoulder medially.

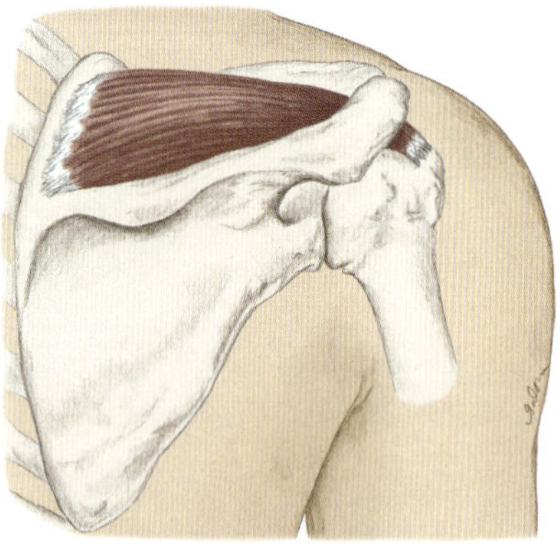

2.72 Posterior view of right shoulder, showing supraspinatus

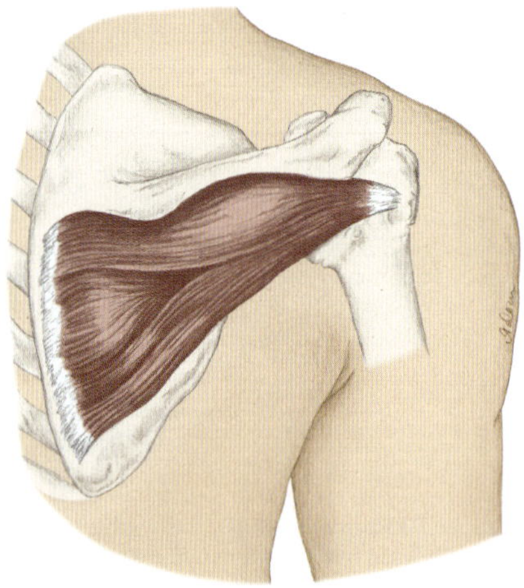

2.73 Posterior view of right shoulder, showing infraspinatus

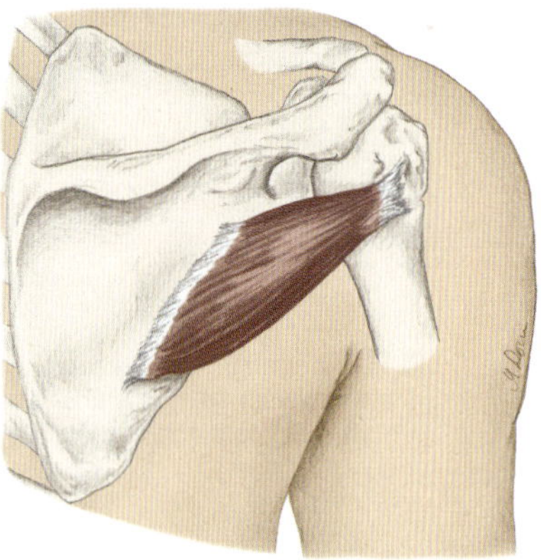

2.74 Posterior view of right shoulder, showing teres minor

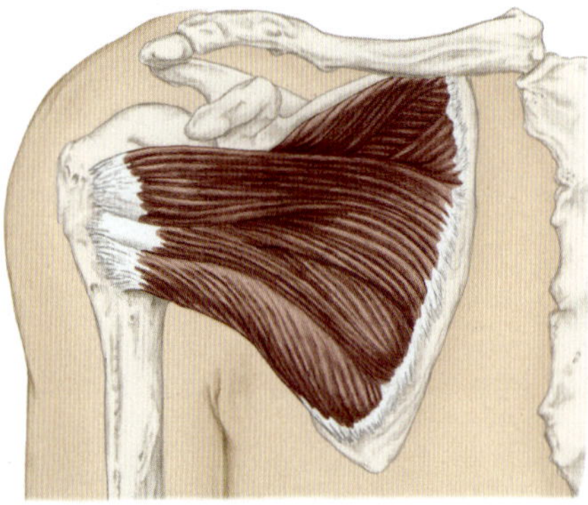

2.75 Anterior view of right shoulder, with rib removed, showing subscapularis

infraspinatus	*in*-fra-spi-***na***-tus
subscapularis	sub-***skap***-u-***lar***-is
supraspinatus	***soo***-pra-spi-***na***-tus

SUPRASPINATUS

A **Abduct** the shoulder (glenohumeral joint)
Stabilize the head of humerus in glenoid cavity

O Supraspinous fossa of the scapula

I Greater tubercle of the humerus

N Suprascapular C4, **5**, **6**

When Do You Use Your Supraspinatus?

- Conducting an orchestra
- Installing ceiling tiles overhead

INFRASPINATUS

A **Laterally rotate** the shoulder (glenohumeral joint)
Adduct the shoulder (G/H joint)
Stabilize the head of humerus in glenoid cavity

O Infraspinous fossa of the scapula

I Greater tubercle of the humerus

N Suprascapular C(4), **5**, **6**

When Do You Use Your Infraspinatus?

- Starting a pull-cord lawnmower
- Fanning a smoke-filled room with your arms

TERES MINOR

A **Laterally rotate** the shoulder (glenohumeral joint)
Adduct the shoulder (G/H joint)
Stabilize the head of humerus in glenoid cavity

O Upper two-thirds of lateral border of the scapula

I Greater tubercle of the humerus

N Axillary C**5**, **6**

When Do You Use Your Teres Minor?

- Starting a pull-cord lawnmower
- Fanning a smoke-filled room with your arms

SUBSCAPULARIS

A **Medially rotate** the shoulder (glenohumeral joint)
Stabilize the head of humerus in glenoid cavity

O Subscapular fossa of the scapula

I Lesser tubercle of the humerus

N Upper and lower subscapular C**5**, **6**, 7

When Do You Use Your Subscapularis?

- Reaching your hand around to scratch your back
- Clutching *Trail Guide to the Body* to your chest

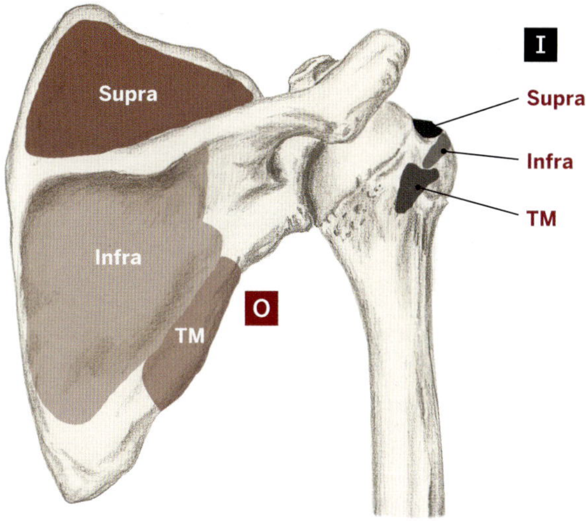

2.76 Posterior view of right shoulder, showing origins and insertions of supraspinatus, infraspinatus, and teres minor

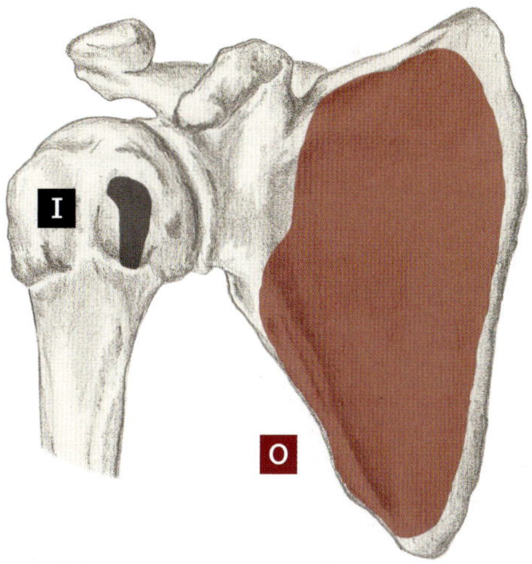

2.77 Anterior view of right shoulder, showing origin and insertion of subscapularis

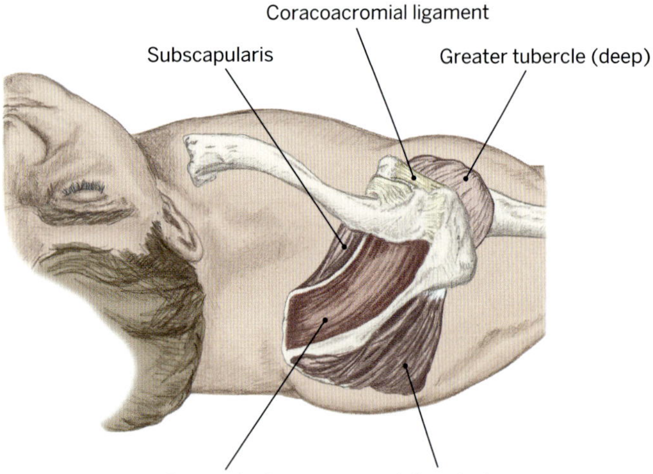

2.78 Superior view of right shoulder, showing rotator cuff muscles

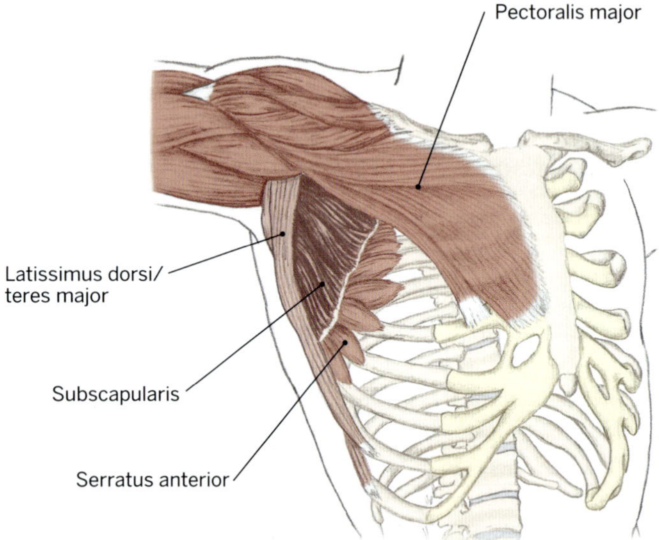

2.79 Lateral/inferior view of right axilla, showing subscapularis

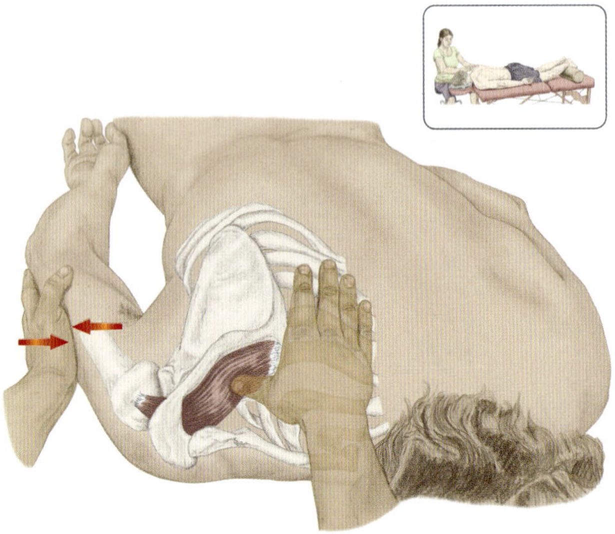

2.80 Partner prone, alternately abducting and relaxing his shoulder while you feel the supraspinatus contract

Supraspinatus

1. Partner prone. Locate the spine of the scapula. Slide your fingers up into the supraspinous fossa.
2. Palpate through the trapezius and onto the supraspinatus fibers. As you palpate, note how the fibers run parallel to the spine.
3. Follow the belly laterally until it tucks under the acromion.

*Can you differentiate the fibers of the trapezius and the deeper supraspinatus? With the arm alongside the body, have your partner alternate between abducting slightly and relaxing the shoulder (**2.80**). Can you feel the supraspinatus tighten and soften underneath the inactive trapezius?*

Infraspinatus

1. Partner prone, with the forearm off the side of the table. Locate the spine, medial border, and lateral border of the scapula.
2. Form a triangle around the infraspinatus by laying a finger along each of these landmarks.
3. Palpate in the triangle and strum across the infraspinatus fibers. Follow them laterally as they converge underneath the deltoid to attach to the humerus.

*With the forearm off the side of the table, ask your partner to alternately raise his elbow one inch toward the ceiling and relax (**2.81**). Do you feel the infraspinatus contract and tighten?*

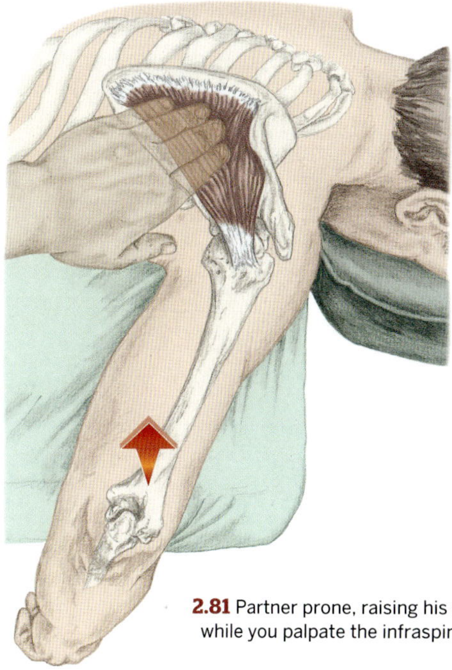

2.81 Partner prone, raising his elbow while you palpate the infraspinatus

Teres minor

1. Partner prone, with the arm off the side of the table. Locate the lateral border of the scapula—specifically, its superior half. Slide laterally off the lateral border onto the surface of the teres minor.
2. Compress into and across its tube-shaped belly. Move inferiorly and compare it in size to the teres major. Also, reach your thumb up into the axilla and grasp the belly of the teres minor as you would a sandwich (**2.82**).
3. Ask your partner to laterally rotate his shoulder. "Swing your hand up toward your head." Bringing the elbow toward the ceiling also forces the teres minor to contract.

Does the muscle you are palpating attach along the superior half of the scapula's lateral border?

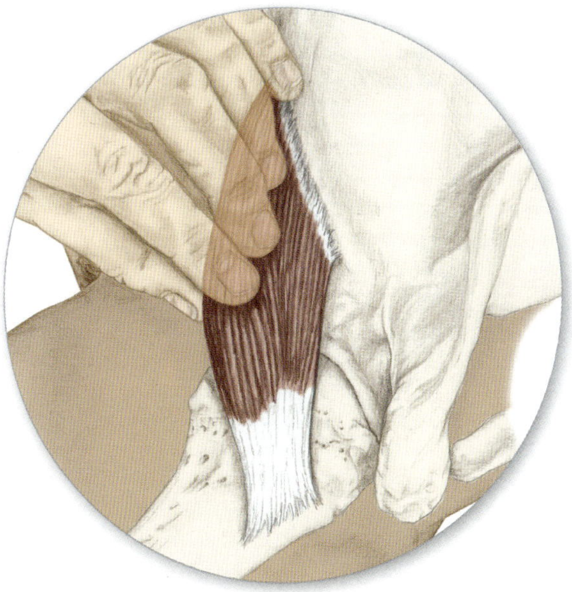

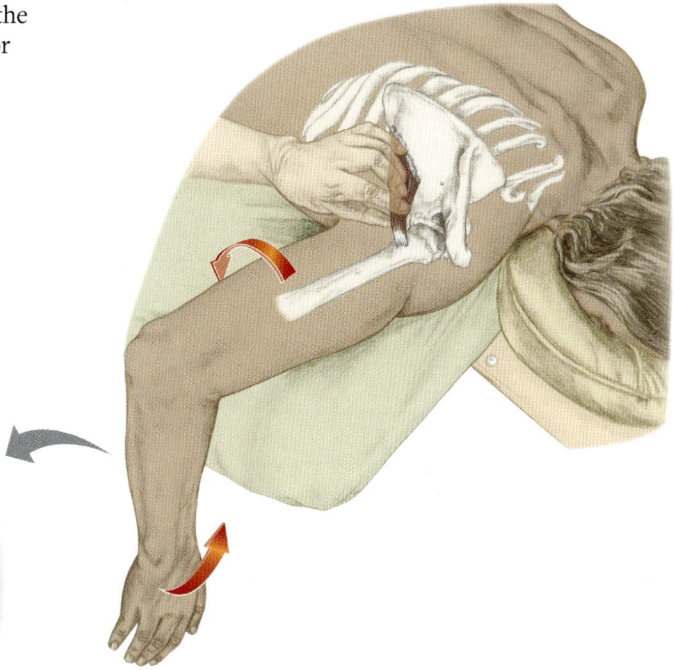

2.82 Partner prone, laterally rotating his shoulder while you grasp the teres minor

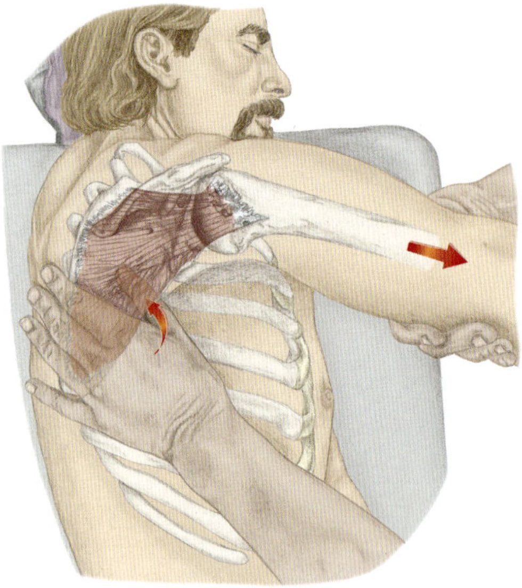

2.83 Partner side lying, as you access the subscapularis

Subscapularis

1. Partner side lying. Flex the shoulder and pull the arm anteriorly as much as possible. This will allow easier access to the scapula's anterior surface.
2. Hold the arm with one hand while the thumb of the other locates the lateral border. Hint: Slide your thumb underneath the latissimus dorsi and teres major fibers instead of going through them (**2.83**).
3. Slowly and gently curl your thumb onto the subscapular fossa. You might not feel the subscapularis fibers immediately, but if your thumb is on the anterior surface of the scapula, you will be accessing a portion of the fibers.

Ask your partner to gently rotate his shoulder medially. Can you feel the subscapularis fibers contract beneath your thumb? Explore the subscapularis by moving your thumb more superiorly or inferiorly.

Partner supine. Cradle the arm in a flexed position and locate the lateral border. Slowly sink your thumbpad onto the subscapular fossa, adjusting the arm and scapula as you progress (**2.84**).

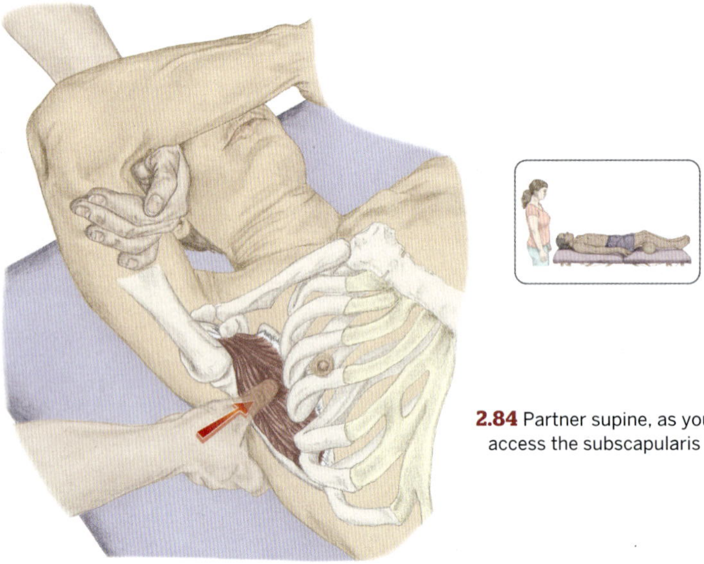

2.84 Partner supine, as you access the subscapularis

Palpation Plus

Here is a fun way to experience the opposite rotational capabilities of the teres major and teres minor. With your partner prone, lay your hand on the surfaces of the teres major and minor. Ask your partner to alternately medially and laterally rotate his arm. (Be sure he does not raise his elbow, because then they both contract.)

Can you feel the teres major contract while the teres minor softens upon medial rotation? Vice versa for lateral rotation?

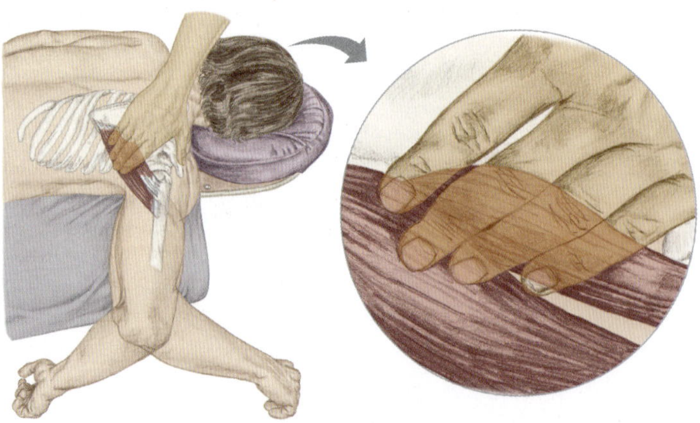

Rotator Cuff Tendons

The tendons of the rotator cuff muscles can be difficult to access in anatomical position (**2.85**). The supraspinatus and infraspinatus tendons are situated deep to the acromion, while the tendons of the subscapularis and teres minor lie deep to the thick belly of the deltoid.

This dilemma can be overcome, however, and the individual tendons isolated by placing the humerus in the positions outlined below. Since the rotator cuff tendons lie against the surface of the greater or lesser tubercles of the humerus, they cannot be separated from the underlying bone.

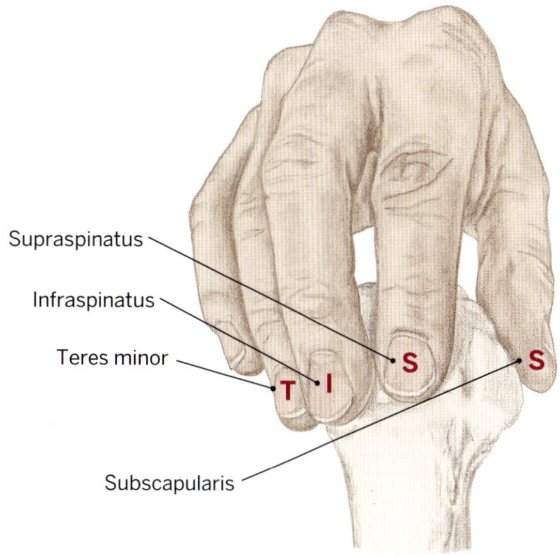

2.85 Anterior/lateral view of right humerus, showing rotator cuff tendon attachment sites

Supraspinatus tendon

1. The attachment of the tendon will be located just distal to the acromion on the greater tubercle.
2. Partner supine or seated, with the arm at the side of the body. Locate the acromion and slide inferiorly onto the surface of the greater tubercle (**2.86**). Between these two landmarks will be a palpable portion of the tendon.
3. Sink your thumb tip through the deltoid fibers. Using firm pressure, roll your thumb across the small mound of the supraspinatus tendon.

Are you palpating on the surface of the greater tubercle or on the superficial deltoid fibers?

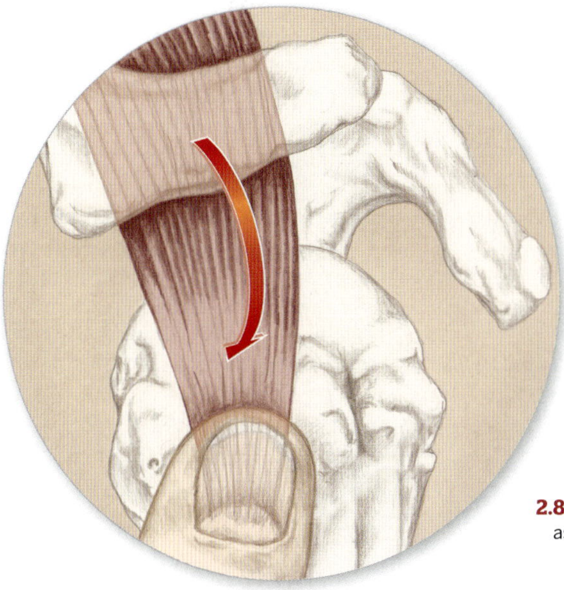

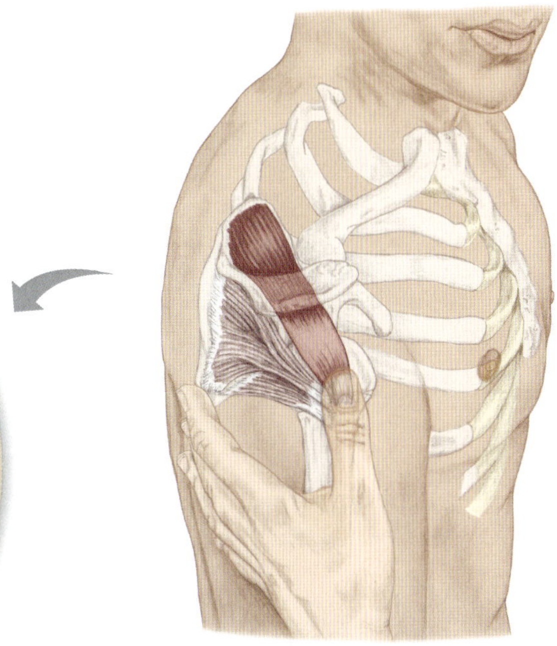

2.86 Anterior/lateral view of right shoulder, as you access the supraspinatus tendon

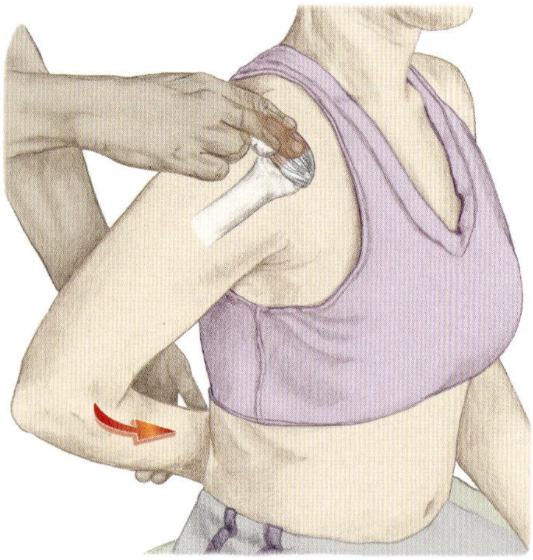

2.87 Partner seated with forearm behind her back, as you palpate the supraspinatus tendon

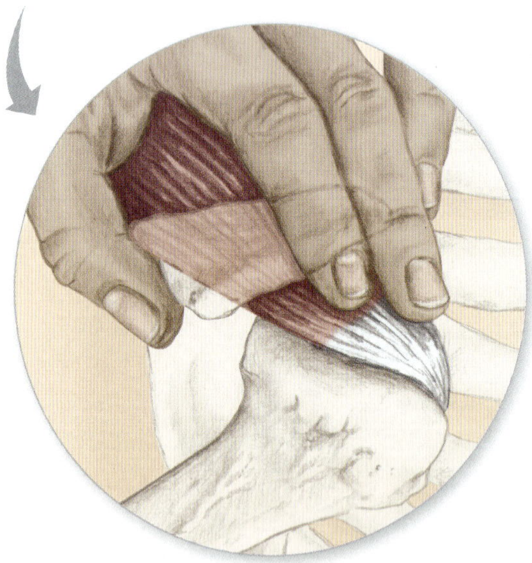

Supraspinatus tendon

1. Partner seated. Place your partner's arm behind her back (**2.87**). This position will medially rotate and extend the humerus.
2. Passively extend the arm as far as is comfortable for your partner. This position brings the supraspinatus tendon out from under the acromion, just anterior and inferior to the acromioclavicular (A/C) joint.

Is the arm medially rotated and extended as far as comfortably possible? Are you palpating inferior to the A/C joint?

Discover More

The supraspinatus was long thought to be a mere "spark plug" for shoulder abduction, initiating the movement before the stronger deltoid took over. Research shows, however, that the supraspinatus contracts through the full movement of abduction and can single-handedly bring the arm to 90˚.

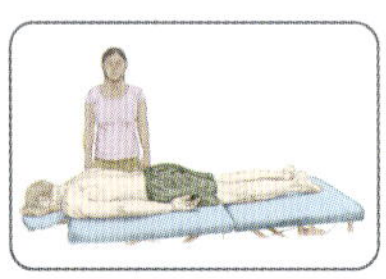

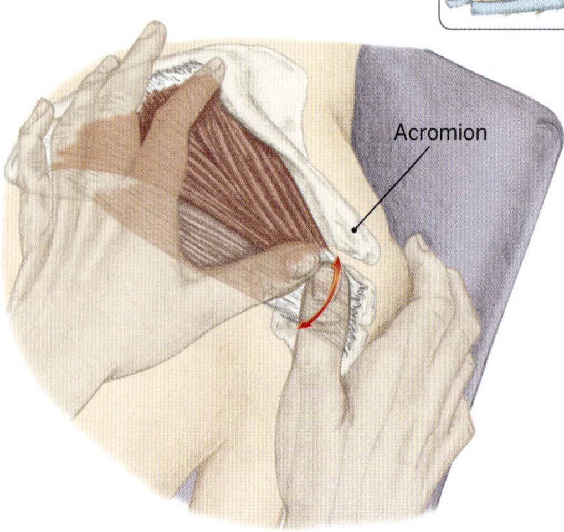

2.88 Partner prone, as you palpate the infraspinatus and teres minor tendons

Infraspinatus and teres minor tendons

1. Partner prone, with arm off the side of the table. Locate the bellies of these muscles.
2. Strumming across their fibers, follow their bellies laterally as they pass inferior to the acromion. Palpating through the deltoid, roll across their slender tendinous attachments at the greater tubercle (**2.88**).
3. Turn your partner supine. Locate the tendinous attachment of supraspinatus. Move posteriorly along the greater tubercle and feel for the small tendinous attachments of the infraspinatus and teres minor.

Are you palpating deep to the deltoid fibers? Do you feel the solid surface of the greater tubercle beneath your fingers?

Infraspinatus and teres minor tendons

1. Partner supine or seated. Flex the shoulder to 90°. Then horizontally adduct and laterally rotate slightly (10°–20°).
2. Although the infraspinatus tendon is deep to the posterior deltoid, this position causes it to move below the acromion and be accessible (**2.89**).
3. Locate the acromial angle. Drop inferiorly off the angle and explore this region.

Is the shoulder flexed, adducted, and laterally rotated? Do you feel the solid surface of the greater tubercle beneath your fingers? Return the arm to a neutral position and notice how the posterior humerus slides back under the acromion.

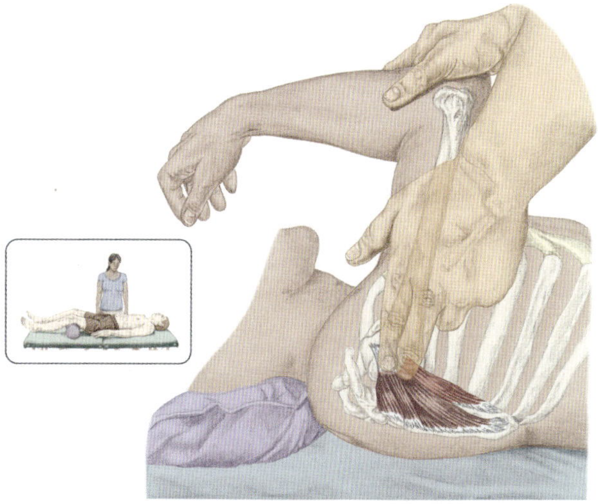

2.89 Lateral view of right shoulder, as you access the infraspinatus and teres minor tendons

Subscapularis tendon

1. Partner seated or supine. Place the arm next to the trunk in anatomical position.
2. Locate the coracoid process of the scapula. Slide one inch inferiorly and laterally from the coracoid. You will be between the two tendons of the biceps brachii.
3. Palpate through the deltoid fibers, exploring the deeper tissue that lies along the lesser tubercle of the humerus (**2.90**). This is the location of the subscapularis tendon. Explore for more of the tendon by moving medially off the lesser tubercle.

Is the arm positioned next to the body? Are you palpating deep to the deltoid fibers? Can you feel the solid surface of the lesser tubercle?

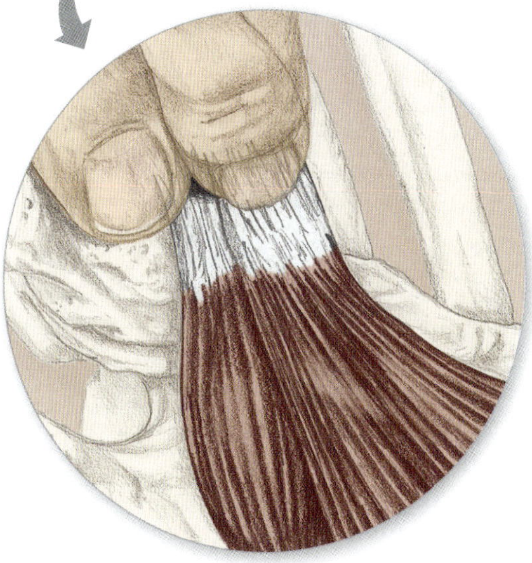

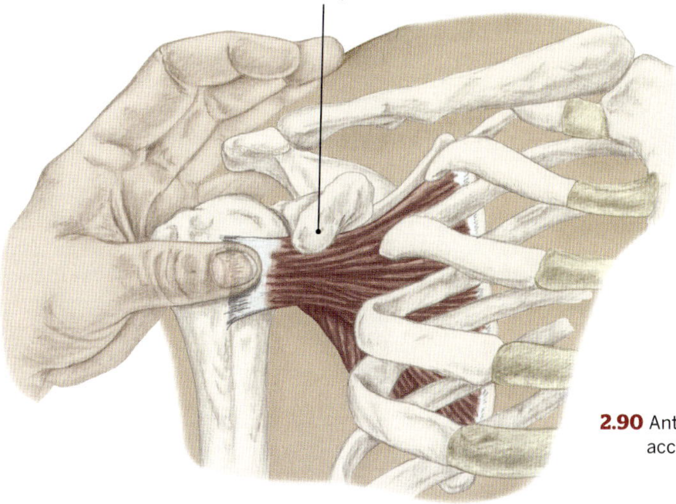

2.90 Anterior view of right shoulder, as you access the subscapularis tendon

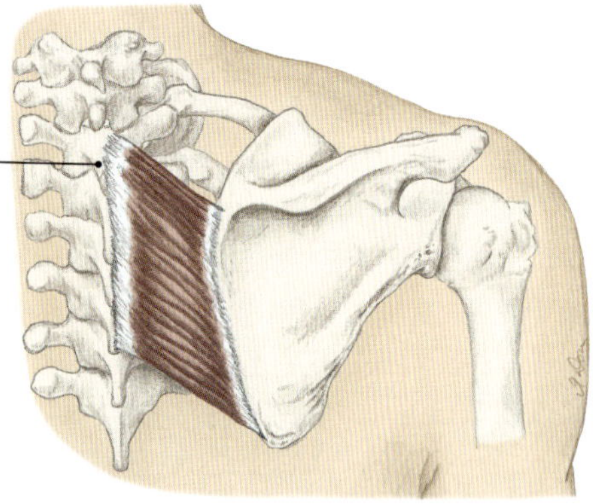

2.91 Posterior view of right shoulder, showing rhomboid major

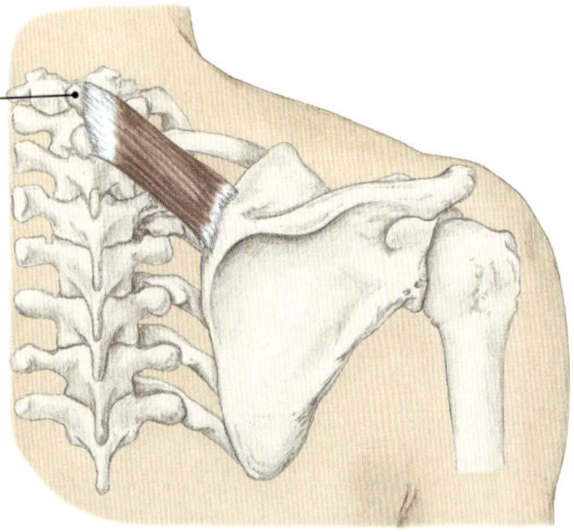

2.92 Posterior view of right shoulder, showing rhomboid minor

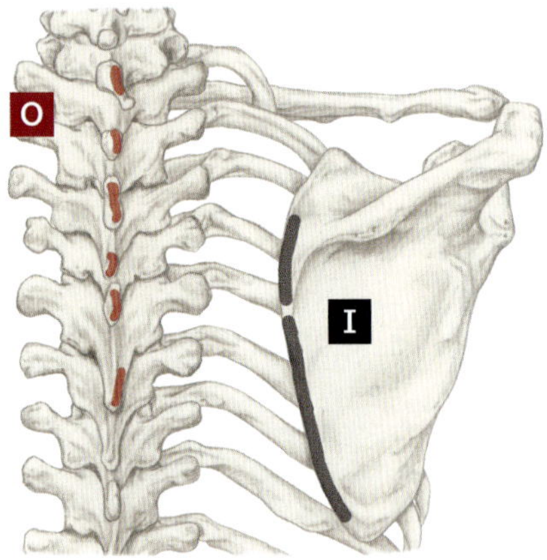

2.93 Posterior view of right shoulder, showing origins and insertions of rhomboids

Rhomboid Major and Minor ▶

The rhomboid muscles are located between the scapula and vertebral column (**2.91-2.93**). Named for their geometric shape, the major is larger than the minor. The muscles are difficult to distinguish individually. They have thin fibers that lie deep to the trapezius and superficial to the erector spinae muscles (p. 196).

RHOMBOID MAJOR AND MINOR	
A	**Adduct** the scapula (scapulothoracic joint) **Elevate** the scapula (S/T joint) **Downwardly rotate** the scapula (S/T joint)
O	*Major:* Spinous processes of T-2 to T-5 *Minor:* Spinous processes of C-7 and T-1
I	*Major:* Medial border of the scapula between the spine of the scapula and inferior angle *Minor:* Upper portion of medial border of the scapula, across from spine of the scapula
N	Dorsal scapular C4, **5**

When Do You Use Your Rhomboid Major and Minor?

- Sticking out your chest (pressing the scapulae together)
- Shrugging your shoulders when uncertain
- Squeezing through the entrance of a small cave

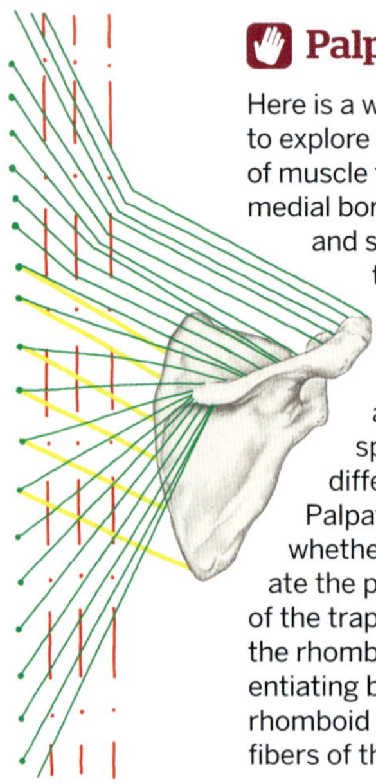

Palpation Plus

Here is a wonderful opportunity to explore the different layers of muscle tissue between the medial border of the scapula and spinous processes of the thoracic vertebrae. The superficial trapezius, intermediate rhomboids, and deep erector spinae muscles all have different fiber directions. Palpate in this area to see whether you can differentiate the perpendicular fibers of the trapezius from those of the rhomboids. Also try differentiating between the diagonal rhomboid fibers and the vertical fibers of the erector spinae.

rhomboid	*rom*-boyd	Grk. in geometry, a parallelogram with oblique angles and only the opposite sides equal

Rhomboids

1. Partner prone. Locate the scapula's medial border and the spinous processes of C-7 through T-5 (p. 178).
2. Palpating through the thin trapezius, explore the area you have identified and strum vertically across the fibers of the rhomboids. Palpate all sides of the rhomboids. On some individuals you can press your fingers into the lower border of the rhomboid major and locate its edge.

*Are you deep to the trapezius fibers? Do the fibers you are palpating run at an oblique angle? Place your partner's hand in the small of his back and ask him to slightly raise his elbow toward the ceiling (**2.94**). Although this action will engage the superficial trapezius, can you feel the deeper rhomboids contract?*

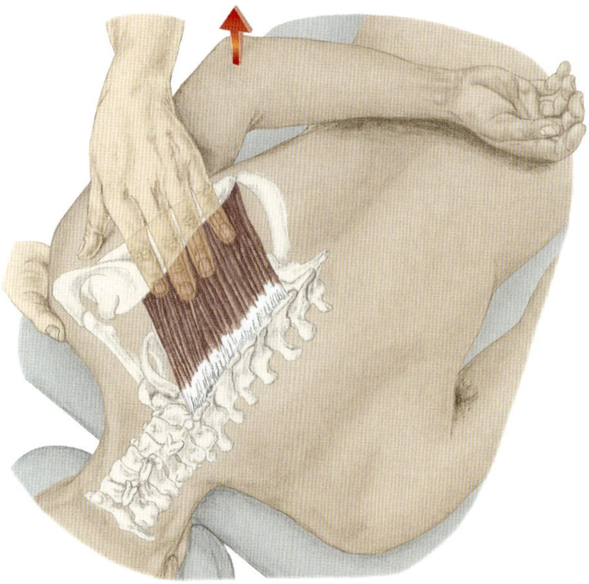

2.94 Partner prone, raising his elbow toward the ceiling while you feel the rhomboids contract

Levator Scapula ▶

The levator scapula is located along the lateral and posterior sides of the neck. Its inferior portion is deep to the upper trapezius; however, as the levator ascends the lateral side of the neck, its fibers come out from under the trapezius and become superficial (**2.96**). Its belly is approximately two fingers wide with fibers that naturally twist around themselves (**2.95**).

The levator scapula attaches to the transverse processes of the cervical vertebrae (**2.97**). Located on the lateral side of the neck, all of these small protuberances extend laterally at approximately the same width, except for the processes of C-1, which are broader (p. 180).

The brachial plexus, a large group of nerves that innervates the arm, exits from the transverse processes of the cervical vertebrae (p. 274). When accessing the processes to locate the origin of the levator scapula, begin by using your soft fingerpads to avoid compressing a nerve.

The levator is completely accessible by palpating either through the upper fibers of the trapezius or directly from the side of the neck.

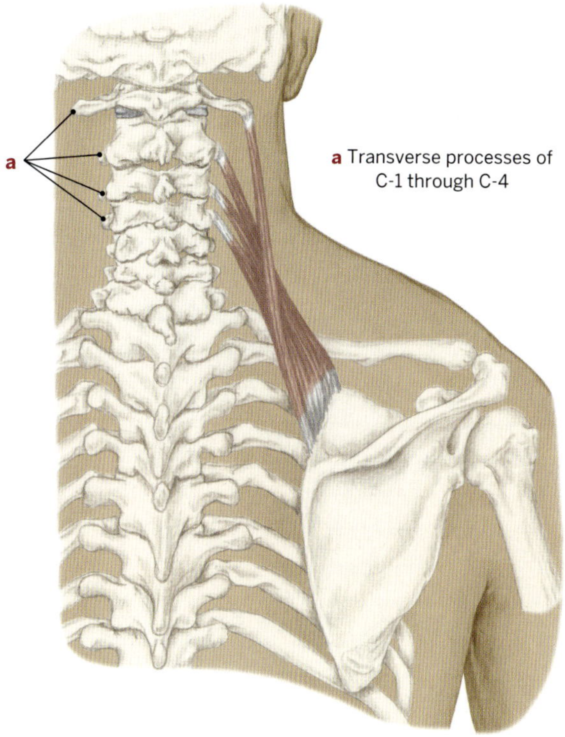

2.95 Posterior view of right shoulder and neck, showing levator scapula

levator leh-*va*-tor L. lifter

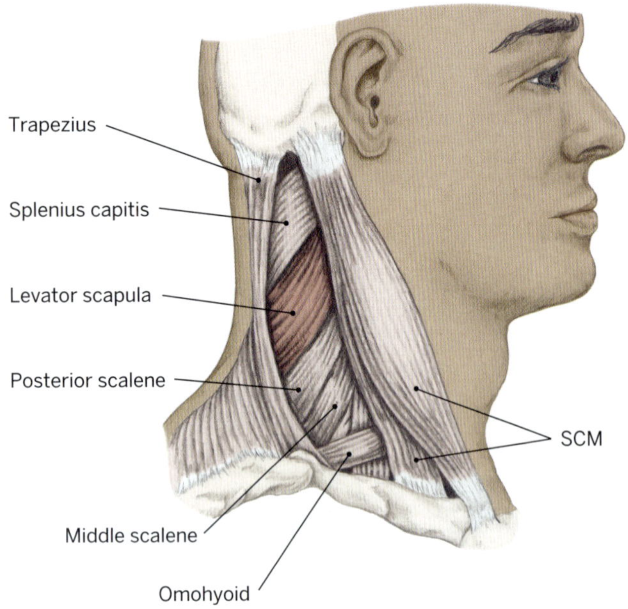

2.96 Lateral view of neck, showing levator scapula and surrounding muscles

LEVATOR SCAPULA

A

Unilaterally:

Elevate the scapula (scapulothoracic joint)
Downwardly rotate the scapula (S/T joint)
Laterally flex the head and neck
Rotate the head and neck to the same side

Bilaterally:

Extend the head and neck

O Transverse processes of first through fourth cervical vertebrae

I Medial border of scapula, between superior angle and superior portion of spine of scapula

N Cervical **3**, **4**, and dorsal scapular C**4**, **5**

When Do You Use Your Levator Scapula?

- Rotating head when changing lanes in traffic
- Scratching your ear with your shoulder
- Lying on your side, snuggling your head into your pillow

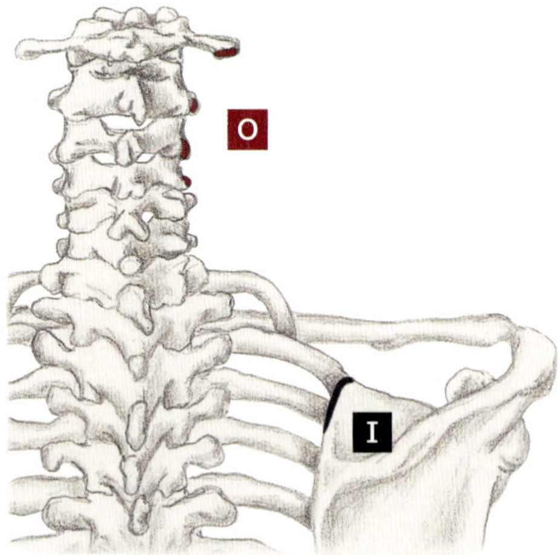

2.97 Posterior view of right shoulder and neck, showing origin and insertion of levator scapula

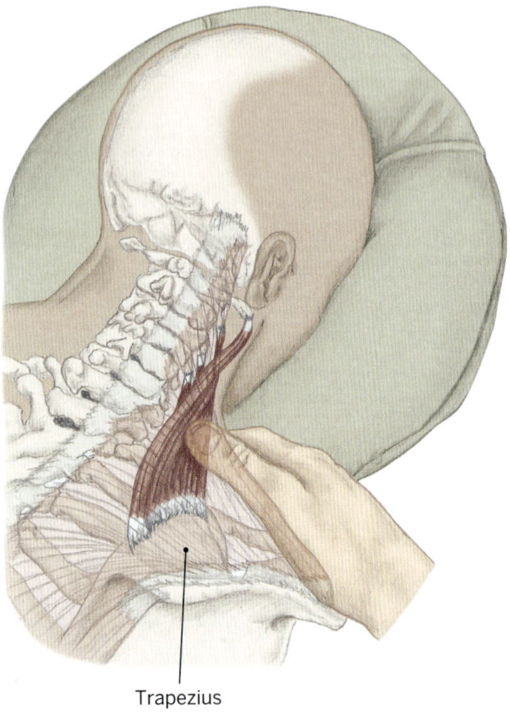

2.98 Partner prone, as you strum across the belly of the levator

Levator scapula

1. Partner prone, supine, or side lying. Palpating through the trapezius, locate the superior angle of the scapula (p. 49) and the upper region of the medial border.
2. Place your fingers just off the superior angle and firmly strum across the belly of the levator. The fibers will likely have a ropy texture (**2.98**).
3. Follow these fibers superiorly as they extend to the lateral side of the neck to the transverse processes of the cervical vertebrae (p. 180).

Can you differentiate the levator fibers from the trapezius fibers? Do the fibers you are palpating lead toward the lateral side of the neck?

Here is an alternate route for palpating the levator's superficial fibers on the lateral side of the neck.

1. Partner prone, supine, or side lying. Locate the upper fibers of the trapezius.
2. Roll two fingers anteriorly off the trapezius and press into the tissue of the neck.
3. Gently strum your fingers anteriorly and posteriorly across the levator fibers (**2.99**). Often you will feel a distinct band of tissue that leads superiorly toward the lateral neck and inferiorly under the trapezius.
4. Place your fingertips on the levator and ask your partner to alternately elevate and relax his scapula. Do you feel the levator scapula contract and relax beneath your fingertips?

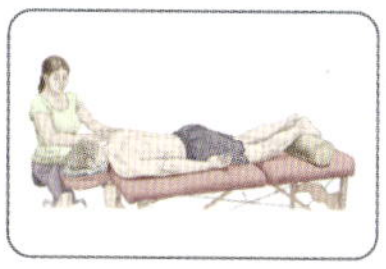

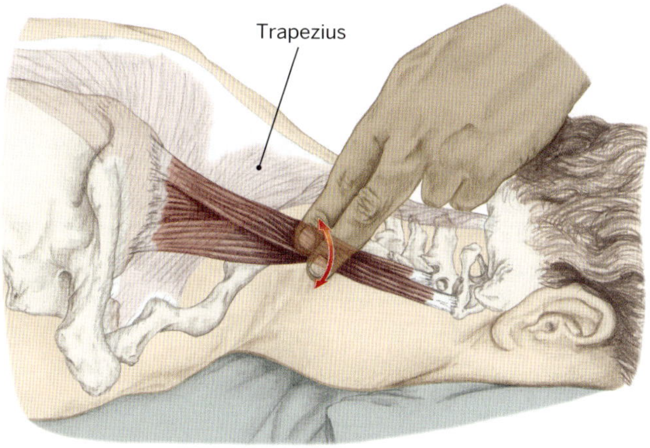

2.99 Partner prone, lateral view of neck, as you strum across the superficial fibers of levator scapula

Palpation Plus

The levator scapula is situated between the splenius capitis and posterior scalene muscles on the lateral side of the neck (**2.96**). The levator can be distinguished from these neighboring muscles during palpation because it moves the scapula. No other muscle deep to the upper trapezius or attaching to the lateral cervical vertebrae is capable of this action.

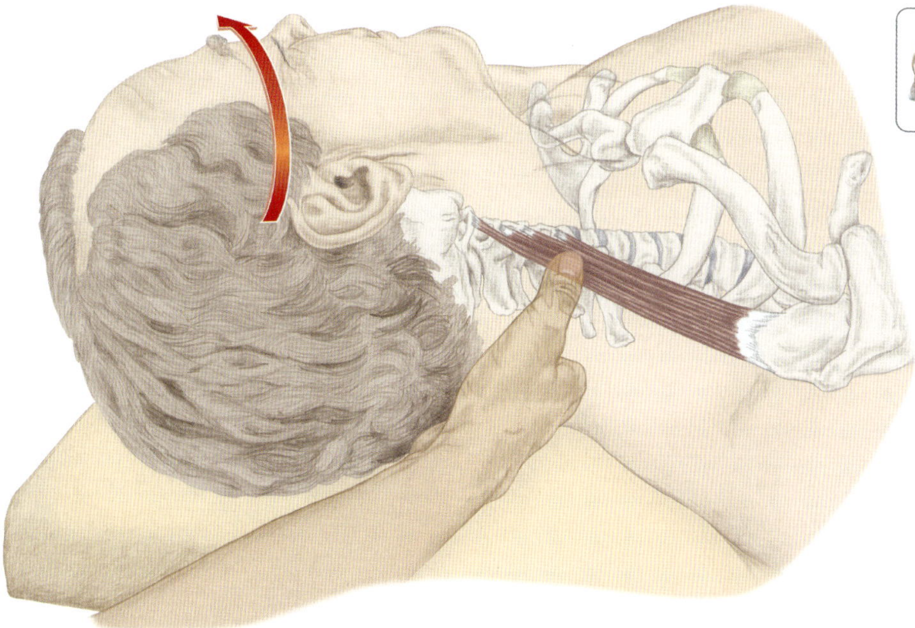

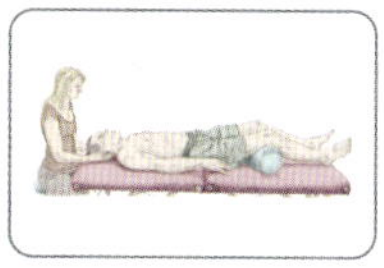

2.100 Partner supine. Passively rotating the head 45° away from the side you are palpating shifts the cervical transverse processes further anteriorly. Also, it gives the levator scapula more palpable tension. Conversely, this position shortens and softens the overlying trapezius fibers.

Serratus Anterior ▶

Always well-developed on superheroes, the serratus anterior lies along the posterior and lateral rib cage. Its oblique fibers extend from the ribs underneath the scapula and attach to its medial border (**2.101**, **2.102**). Most of the serratus anterior is deep to the scapula, latissimus dorsi, or pectoralis major; however, the portion of the serratus below the axilla (armpit) is superficial and easily accessible (**2.103**). This muscle is unique in its ability to abduct the scapula, making it an antagonist to the rhomboids.

Palpating along the sides of the ribs can tickle, so use slow, firm pressure. Also, if you are accessing the right serratus, it may be easier to stand on the left side of the table.

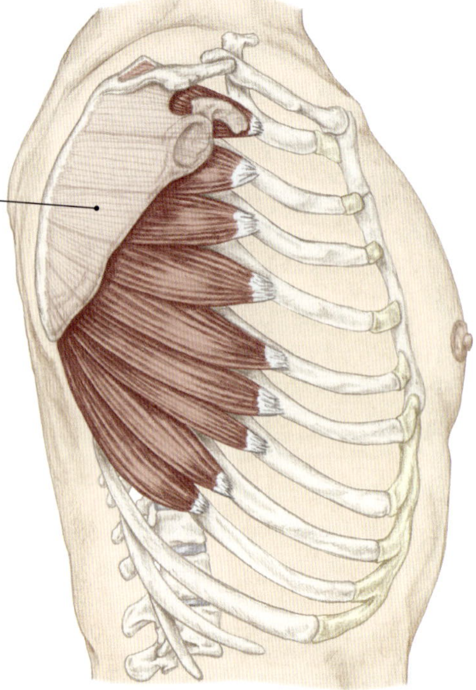

2.101 Lateral view of right shoulder and rib cage, showing serratus anterior

SERRATUS ANTERIOR

A *With the origin fixed:*
Abduct the scapula (scapulothoracic joint)
Upwardly rotate the scapula (S/T joint)
Depress the scapula (S/T joint)
Hold the medial border of the scapula against the rib cage

With the scapula fixed:
May act to **elevate** the thorax during forced inhalation

O External surfaces of upper eight or nine ribs

I Anterior surface of medial border of the scapula

N Long thoracic C**5**, **6**, **7**, 8

When Do You Use Your Serratus Anterior?

- Doing a push-up
- Throwing a punch
- Pushing open a swinging door

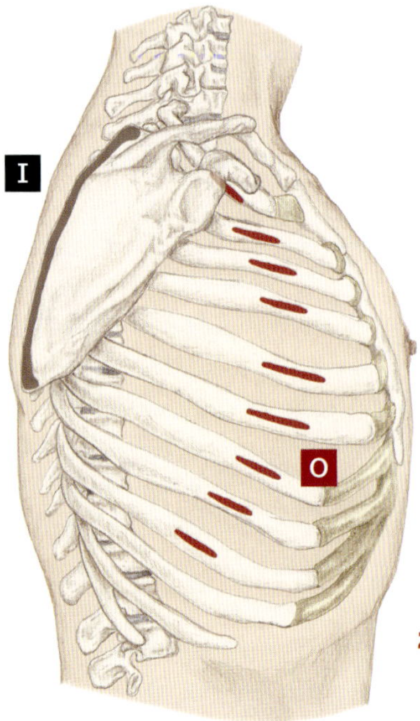

2.102 Lateral view of right shoulder and rib cage, showing origin and insertion of serratus anterior

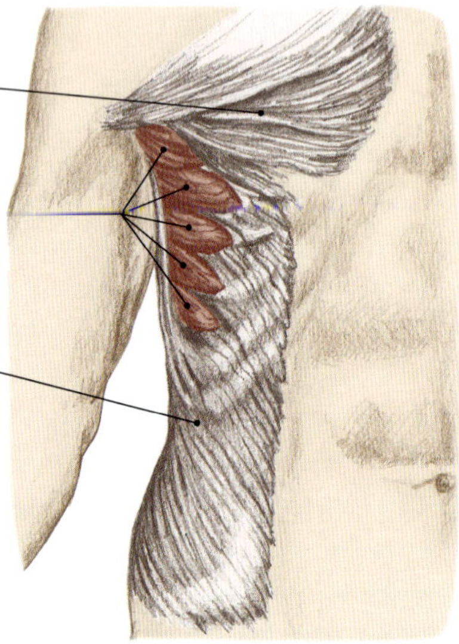

2.103 Anterior view of right arm and torso, showing serratus anterior (highlighted in red)

serratus ser-*a*-tus L. notched

Serratus anterior

1. Partner supine. Isolate the location of the serratus by abducting the arm slightly and locating the lower edge of the pectoralis major (p. 85). Then locate the anterior border of the latissimus dorsi.
2. Place your fingerpads along the side of the ribs between the pectoralis major and latissimus dorsi.
3. Strum your fingers across the ribs and palpate for the serratus anterior fibers. To differentiate between the ribs and the serratus fibers (both have a similar "speed bump" shape), remember that the ribs are deep and have a solid texture while the serratus fibers are superficial and malleable.

*To feel the serratus anterior contract (**2.104**): Ask your partner to flex his shoulder so his fist is raised toward the ceiling. Place one hand on the serratus fibers and your other hand on top of his raised fist. Ask him to alternately abduct his scapula and relax. "Reach toward the ceiling and then relax." Do you feel the serratus fibers contract and soften? Can you follow the fibers along the ribs to where they tuck underneath the latissimus dorsi?*

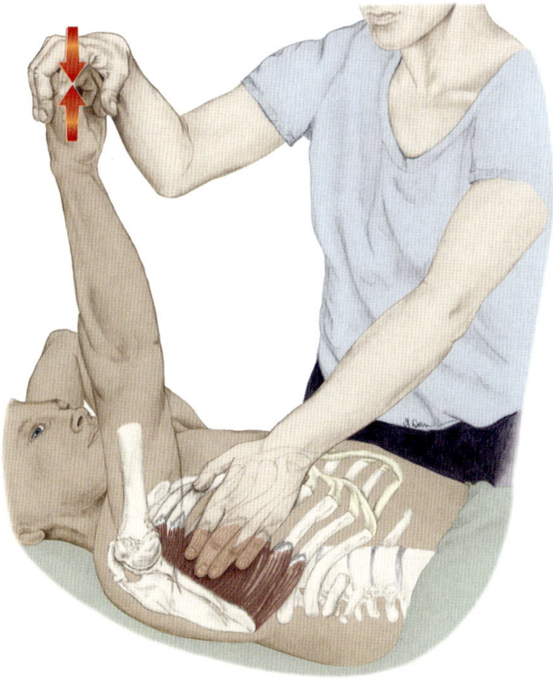

2.104 Partner supine, reaching his hand toward the ceiling while you isolate the serratus

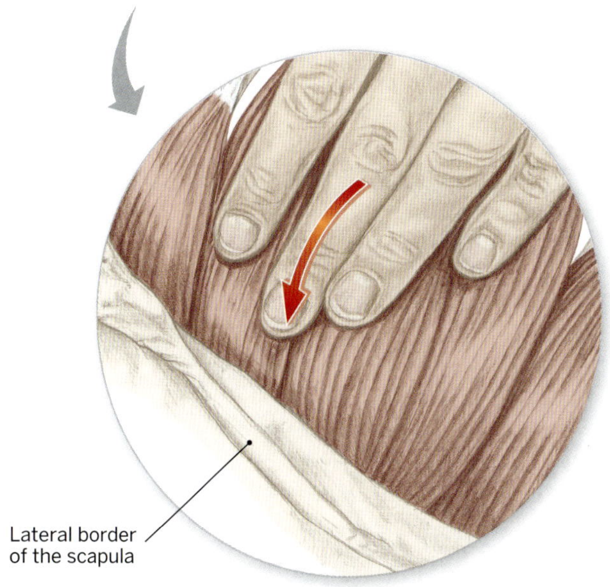

Discover More

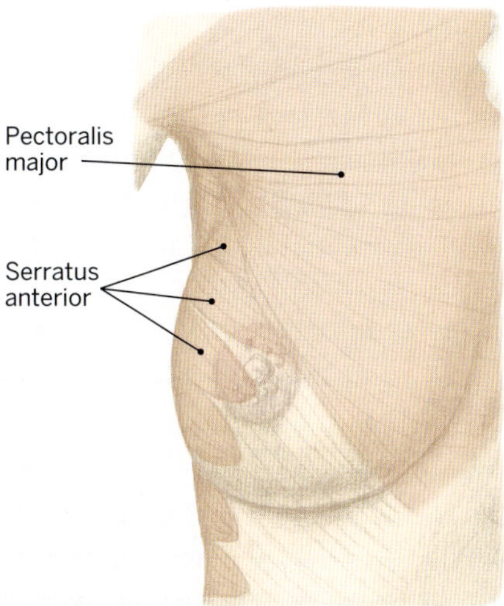

The breast is essentially made up of subcutaneous fat and is primarily supported by suspensory ligaments connecting the skin with the deep fascia over the pectoralis major. Although it varies widely in shape and size, the breast generally extends inferiorly from the second to the sixth ribs, medially to the sternum and laterally to the anterior axilla. Nearly two-thirds of the breast covers the pectoralis major while the inferior/lateral aspect covers the serratus anterior.

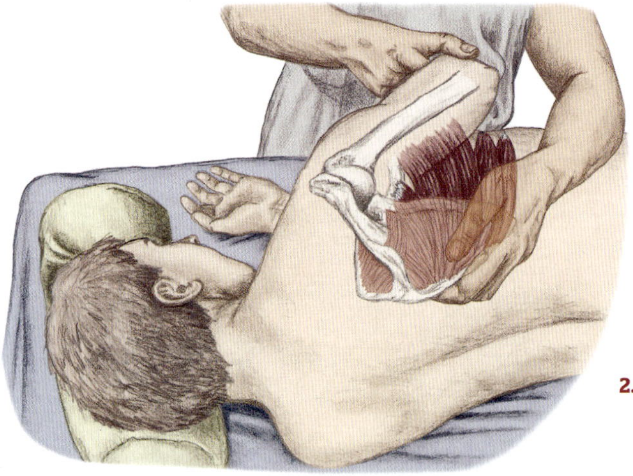

Serratus anterior

Turn your partner side lying with his arm at his side. Locate the medial border of the scapula to access the insertion of the serratus anterior. Curl your fingers beneath the medial border (and through the trapezius and rhomboid fibers) onto the beginnings of the subscapular fossa and explore the area where the serratus attaches (**2.105**).

2.105 Partner side lying, as you curl your fingers under the medial border of the scapula

Comparative Anatomy

The serratus anterior plays a different role on a quadruped than on an upright, bipedal human. For us, the serratus is primarily responsible for abducting the scapula or resisting a push against the shoulder.

But for a four-legged animal such as a dog (right, anterior view), which carries part of its body weight on its front legs, the serratus muscles ("serratus ventralis" in quadrupeds) form a sling from the scapula to the thorax. This cradles and supports the weight of the trunk and stabilizes the limb against the thorax. Get down on your hands to do a push-up and you will see (and feel) how this position forces your serratus anterior muscles to function as a dog's would.

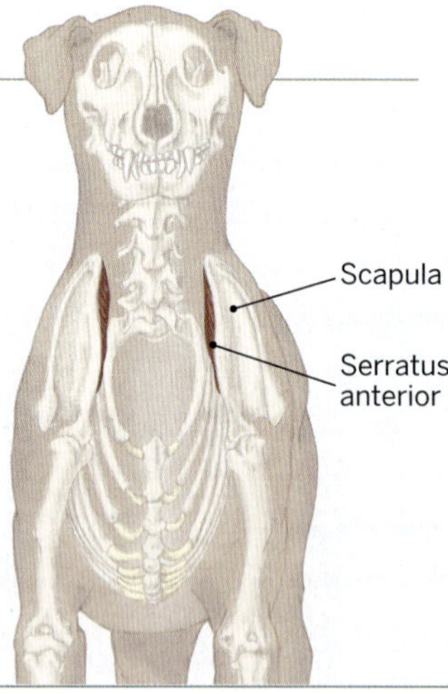

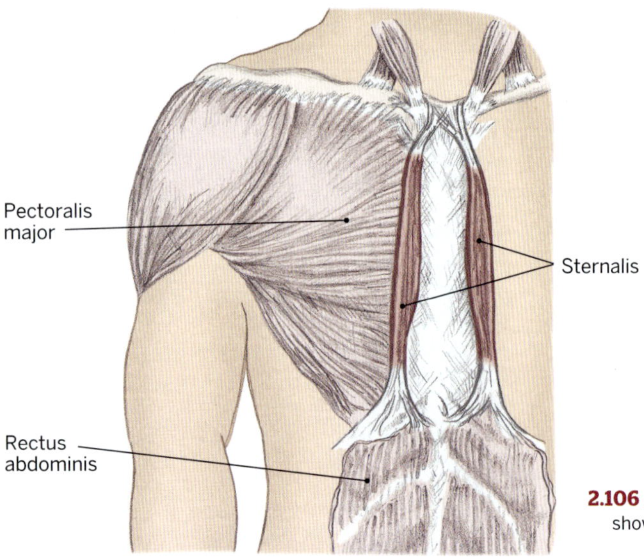

Sternalis

Present in roughly 5% of the population, the sternalis is a thin, superficial muscle lying on the sternum (**2.106**). Its vertical fibers run from the manubrium down to the level of the seventh costal cartilage. The function of the sternalis is unknown. Palpate the surface of your partner's sternum and explore for a sternalis.

2.106 Anterior view of right shoulder and torso, showing sternalis (highlighted in dark red)

Pectoralis Major ▶

The pectoralis major is a broad, powerful muscle located on the chest. Except for the part beneath breast tissue, its convergent, superficial fibers are accessible. Pectoralis major is divided into three segments: the clavicular, sternal, and costal fibers (**2.107**). The upper and lower fibers perform opposing actions at the shoulder joint—flexion and extension, respectively—making this muscle an antagonist to itself.

PECTORALIS MAJOR

A

All fibers:

Adduct the shoulder (glenohumeral joint)

Medially rotate the shoulder (G/H joint)

Assist to **elevate** the thorax during forced inhalation (with the arm fixed)

Upper fibers:

Flex the shoulder (G/H joint)

Horizontally adduct the shoulder (G/H joint)

Lower fibers:

Extend the shoulder (G/H joint)

O

Medial half of clavicle, sternum, and cartilage of first through sixth ribs

I

Crest of greater tubercle of humerus

N

Upper fibers:

Lateral pectoral C**5**, **6**, **7**

Lower fibers:

Lateral and medial pectoral C**6**, **7**, **8**, T**1**

When Do You Use Your Pectoralis Major?

- Doing a chin-up
- Using almost any swim stroke ever invented
- Sawing a piece of wood (both directions)

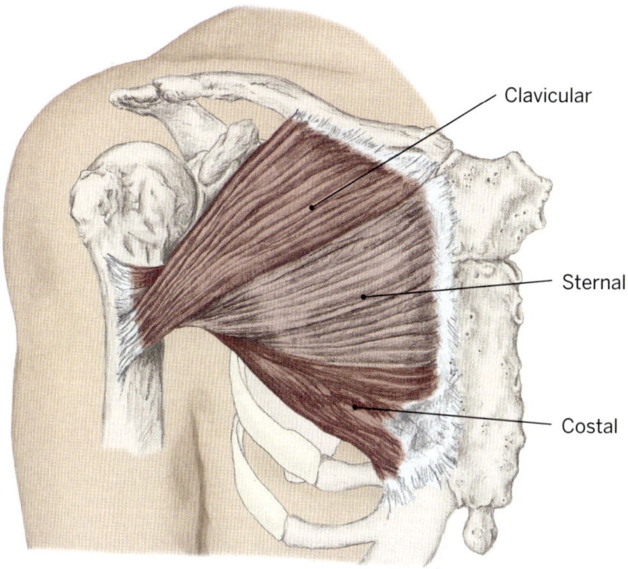

2.107 Anterior view of right shoulder, showing the three segments of pectoralis major

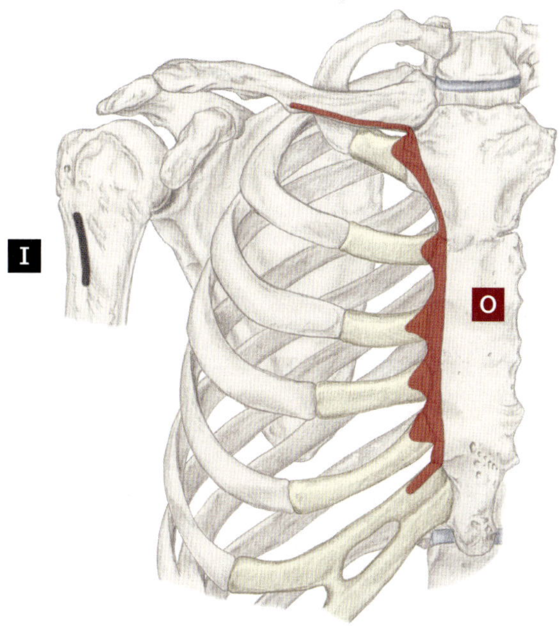

2.108 Anterior view of right shoulder, showing origin and insertion of pectoralis major

pectoralis *pek*-to-*ra*-lis L. chest

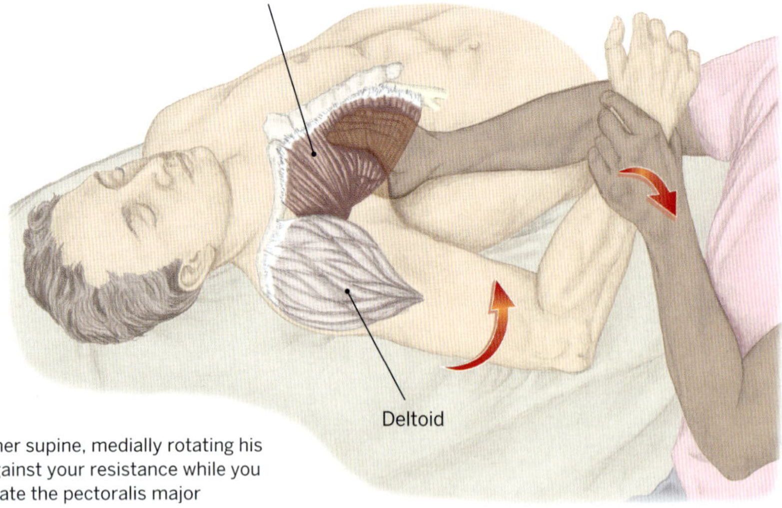

2.109 Partner supine, medially rotating his shoulder against your resistance while you palpate the pectoralis major

Pectoralis major

1. Partner supine. With your partner's shoulder slightly abducted, sit or stand facing him.
2. Locate the medial shaft of the clavicle and move inferiorly onto the clavicular fibers.
3. Explore the surface of the pectoralis major. Follow the fibers laterally as they blend with the deltoid and attach at the greater tubercle.
4. Grasp the belly of the pectoralis by sinking your thumb into the axilla. Ask your partner to medially rotate his shoulder against your resistance. "Press your hand toward your belly" (**2.109**). Note the contraction of the pectoralis.

Do the clavicular fibers run parallel with the anterior deltoid? As you grasp the belly, do you sense its thickness and how it lies across the rib cage?

Palpation Plus ▶

When exploring the pectoralis major and minor, it is advisable to palpate around breast tissue and not directly into it. This raises the question, "When palpating on a female, how do you access these and other chest muscles without contacting breast tissue?"

The most important aspect when palpating near breast tissue is communicating your intentions to your partner. Also, encourage her to let you know if at any time she wishes to stop.

Assuming your partner is draped with a sheet or wearing a sports bra, the key to safe and comfortable palpation around breast tissue is positioning your client so the breast tissue will naturally shift away from where you are accessing. For instance, in a supine position (above), the breast will shift laterally, allowing easier access to the sternal and upper pectoral regions. In this position, however, larger breasts may crowd the axillary region. In such situations you could either ask your partner to shift and hold her breast medially, allowing you to access the axilla, or use the back of your own hand to push the tissue medially.

In a side lying position (left), the breast will fall medially, opening up the axillary region. The axilla can be opened up further by passively shifting the shoulder anteriorly.

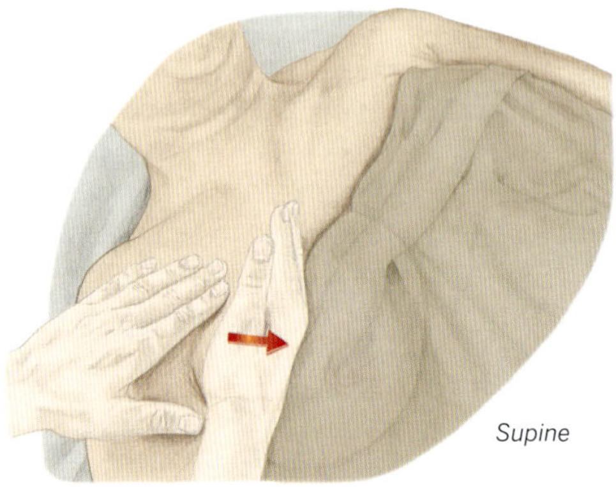

Supine

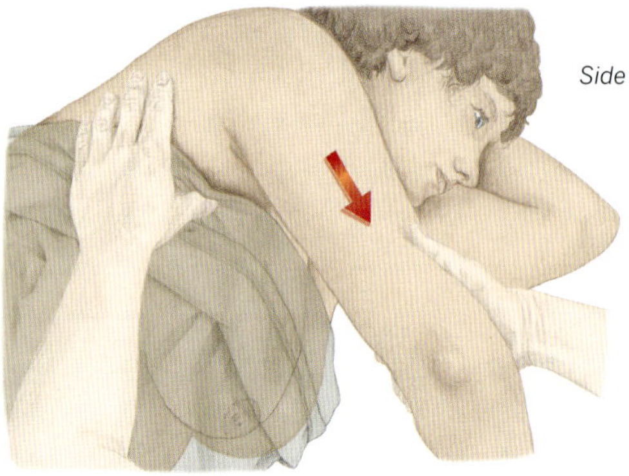

Side lying

1. Partner side lying. Supporting your partner's arm, flex the shoulder and pull it anteriorly toward you. This position not only brings the pectoralis major off the chest wall, but also allows the breast tissue to fall away from the area you are palpating.
2. Grasping the pectoralis major, explore its mass from the ribs to the humerus (**2.110**). Passively flex and extend the shoulder, perceiving the changes in the tension of the tissues.

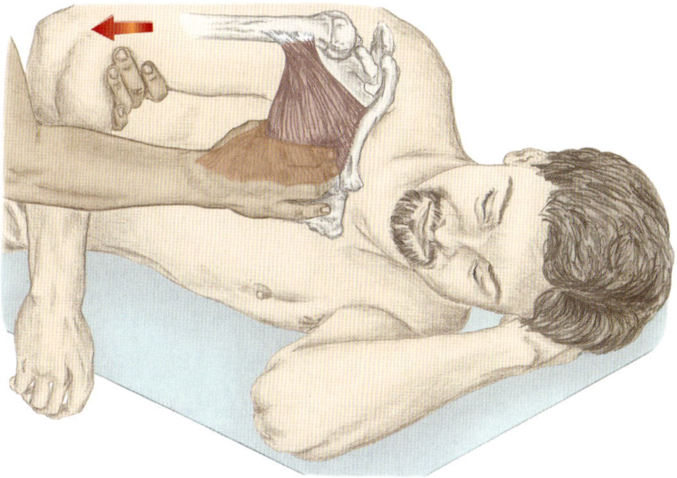

2.110 Partner side lying, as you explore the mass of the pectoralis major

Here is a way to get a sense of the antagonistic movements of the pectoralis major's upper and lower fibers.

1. Partner supine. Begin with your partner's hand raised up toward the ceiling. As you create resistance, ask your partner to flex his shoulder. "Meeting my resistance, try to bring your hand over your head." The upper fibers will contract while the lower fibers remain lax.
2. Ask him to extend against your resistance. "Now try to bring your hand toward your hips." Here the lower fibers will contract while the upper fibers relax (**2.111**).

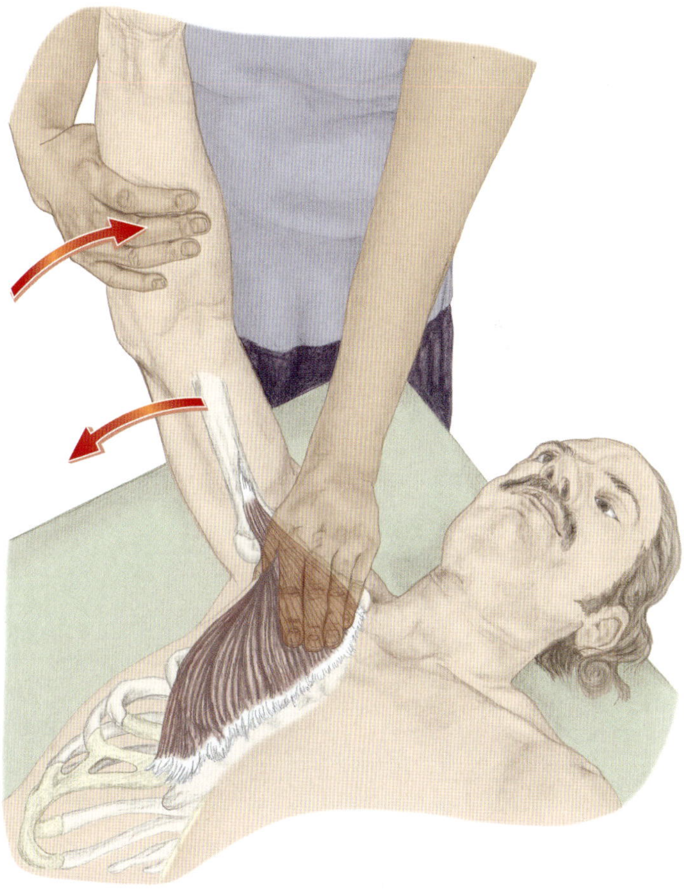

2.111 Partner supine, extending his shoulder against your resistance while you feel the lower fibers of the pectoralis major contract

Pectoralis Minor ▶

The pectoralis minor lies next to the rib cage deep to the pectoralis major (**2.112**, **2.113**). Its fibers run perpendicular to the pectoralis major fibers from the scapula's coracoid process to the upper ribs. During aerobic activity the pectoralis minor helps to elevate the rib cage for inhalation. The major vessels serving the arm—the brachial plexus, axillary artery and vein—cross underneath the pectoralis minor, creating the potential for neurovascular compression by this muscle (**2.114**).

Access to the pectoralis minor can be achieved by either pressing through or sliding underneath the thick pectoralis major. The second method is more specific and will be outlined here. The pectoralis minor can be sensitive, so palpate slowly, allowing your fingers or thumb to sink into the tissue.

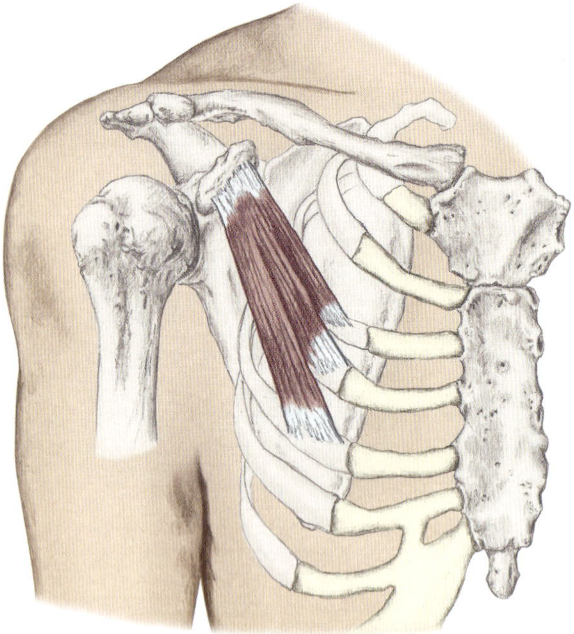

2.112 Anterior view of right shoulder, showing pectoralis minor

	PECTORALIS MINOR
A	**Depress** the scapula (scapulothoracic joint) **Abduct** the scapula (S/T joint) **Downwardly rotate** the scapula (S/T joint) ***With the scapula fixed:*** Assist to **elevate** the thorax during forced inhalation
O	Third, fourth, and fifth ribs
I	Medial surface of coracoid process of the scapula
N	Medial pectoral, with fibers from a communicating branch of the lateral pectoral C(6), **7**, **8**, T1

When Do You Use Your Pectoralis Minor?

- Throwing a punch
- Reaching into a deep front pocket
- Taking a deep inhalation

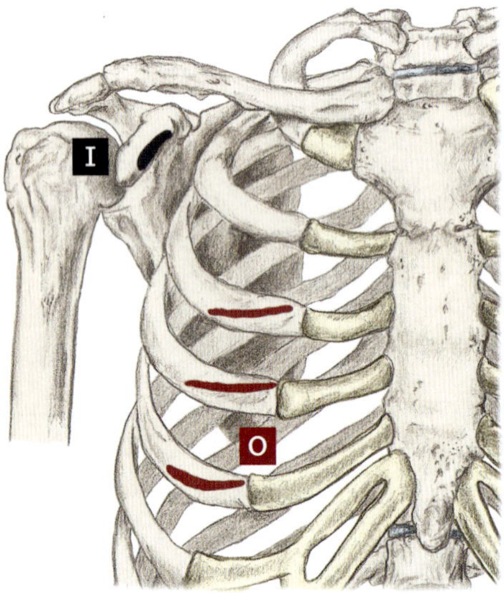

2.113 Anterior view of right shoulder, showing origin and insertion of pectoralis minor

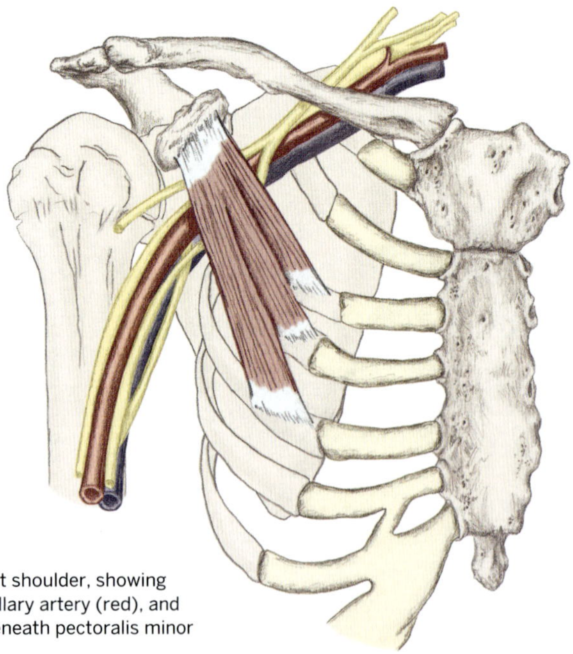

2.114 Anterior view of right shoulder, showing brachial plexus (yellow), axillary artery (red), and axillary vein (blue) passing beneath pectoralis minor

Pectoralis minor

1. Partner supine. Abduct the arm and place your fingerpads at the lateral edge of the pectoralis major.
2. Slowly and gently slide under the pectoralis major, following along the surface of the ribs.
3. Eventually your fingerpads will come in contact with the small wall of muscle lying next to the ribs (**2.115**). This is the side of the pectoralis minor. If you do not feel its tissue, visualize its location next to the ribs.

Ask your partner to depress his scapula. "Ever so slightly press your shoulder down toward your hip." When he depresses, do you feel the pectoralis minor contract? Do the fibers you feel run toward the coracoid process?

1. Partner side lying. Support the arm in a flexed position and pull it anteriorly. This brings the pectoralis major off the chest wall and allows the breast tissue to fall away from the area you are palpating.
2. Slowly slide your thumb under the pectoralis major, following along the surface of the ribs (**2.116**). Your thumb will press into the side and onto the surface of the pectoralis minor. Then ask your partner to gently depress his scapula while you feel for the minor's contraction.

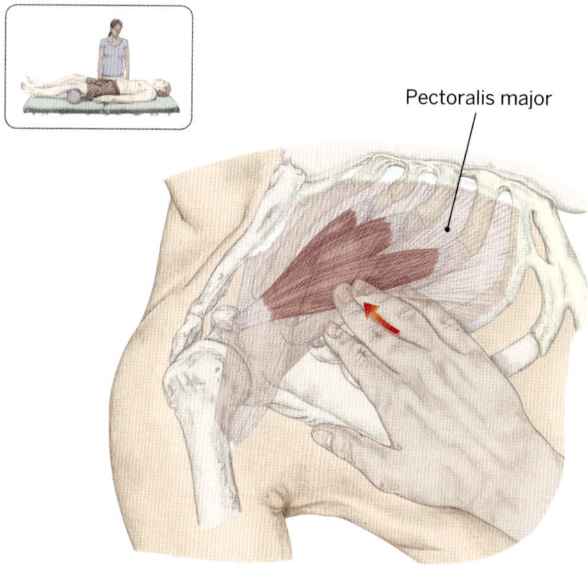

2.115 Partner supine, as you slide your fingerpads under the pectoralis major to access the pectoralis minor

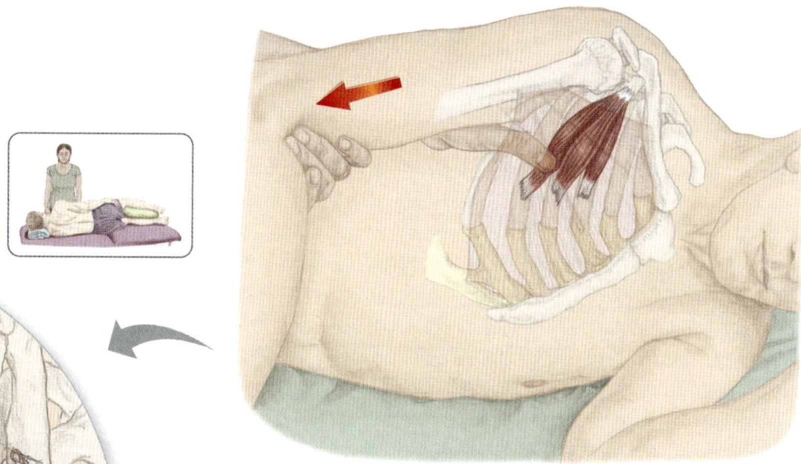
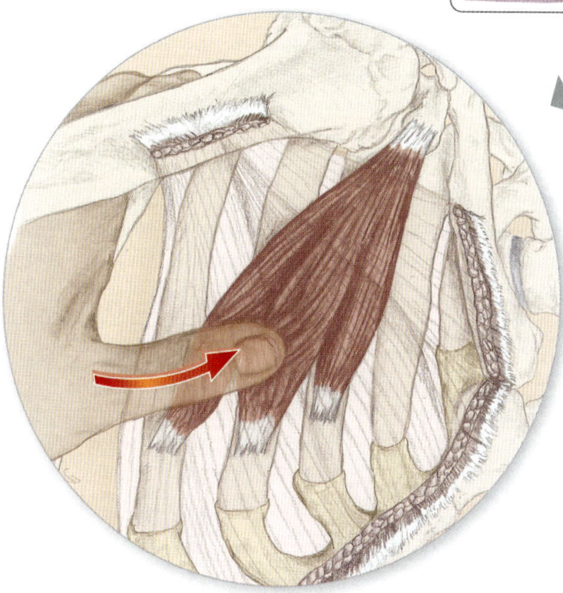

2.116 Partner side lying with arm in flexed position, as you palpate the pectoralis minor

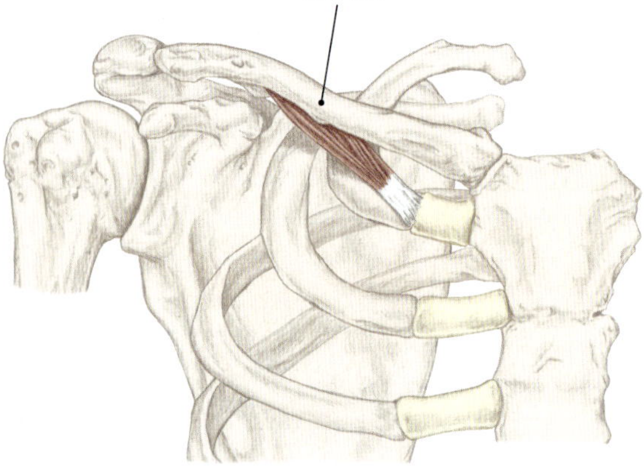

2.117 Anterior view of right shoulder, showing subclavius

Subclavius

As its name suggests, the subclavius is located underneath the clavicle. Its fibers run parallel to the clavicle, deep to the pectoralis major, and can be challenging to truly isolate (**2.117**).

On quadrupeds (four-legged animals), the subclavius is quite large and plays an important role in stabilizing the clavicle and shoulder girdle during locomotion. A human's subclavius, on the other hand, is a small, secondary muscle.

	SUBCLAVIUS
A	**Depress** the clavicle and draw it anteriorly **Elevate** the first rib (to assist during inhalation) **Stabilize** the sternoclavicular joint
O	First rib and cartilage
I	Inferior surface of middle one-third of clavicle
N	Subclavian C**5**, **6**
	When Do You Use Your Subclavius? • Stabilizes clavicle during movements of pectoral girdle • Protects major nerves and blood vessels when clavicle is broken (by shifting shoulder anterior and inferior)

Subclavius

1. Partner side lying. Support the arm in a flexed position and pull it anteriorly. This position brings the clavicle and pectoralis major off the rib cage and allows your thumb to curl even further around the clavicle.
2. Place your thumb and fingers at the center of the clavicle. Slowly curl your thumb around the clavicle's underside, trying to access the subclavius (**2.118**). You might not access a muscle belly, but might feel instead some slightly dense tissue tucked under the clavicle.
3. Try this method with your partner in a supine position.

Can you detect a slender strip of tissue deep to the clavicle? Can you distinguish between the superficial pectoralis major fibers (heading toward the axilla) and the subclavius fibers (parallel to the clavicle)?

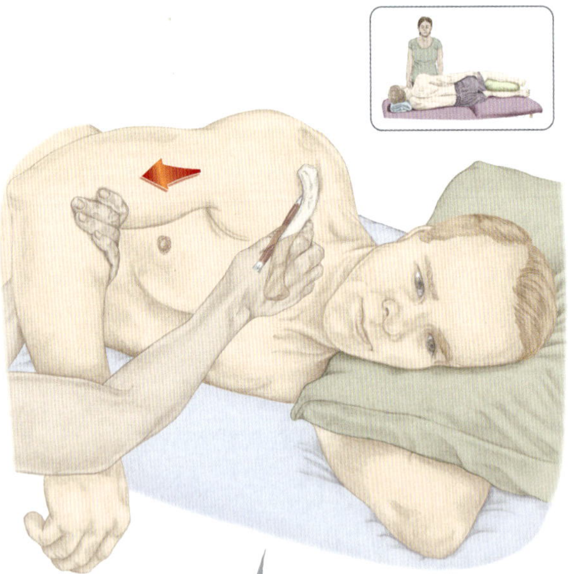

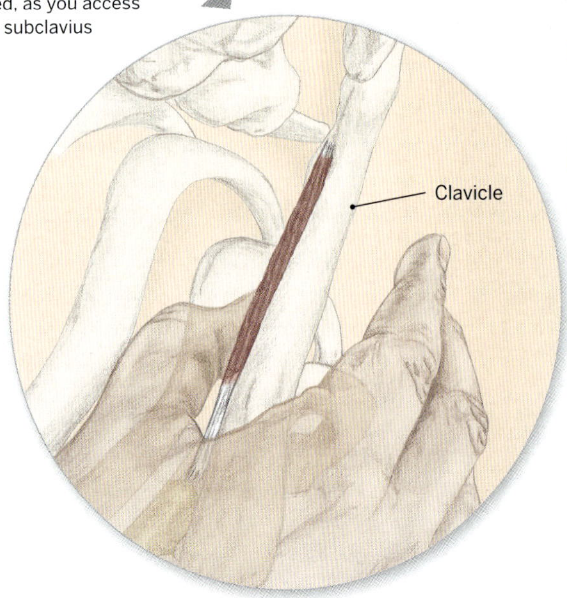

2.118 Partner side lying with arm flexed, as you access the subclavius

subclavius sub-***klay***-vee-us

Biceps Brachii ▶

The biceps brachii lies superficially on the anterior arm. It has a long head and a short head, which merge to form a long, oval belly. The tendon of the long head passes through the intertubercular groove of the humerus (p. 56). This groove helps to stabilize the tendon as it rises over the top of the shoulder (**2.119**).

The distal tendon of the biceps dives into the antecubital space (inner elbow) to attach at the radius, allowing this muscle to be the primary muscle of forearm supination (**2.120**). The majority of the biceps brachii is easily palpable.

	BICEPS BRACHII
A	**Flex** the elbow (humeroulnar joint) **Supinate** the forearm (radioulnar joints) **Flex** the shoulder (glenohumeral joint)
O	*Short head:* Coracoid process of scapula *Long head:* Supraglenoid tubercle of scapula
I	Tuberosity of the radius and aponeurosis of the biceps brachii
N	Musculocutaneous C**5**, **6**

When Do You Use Your Biceps Brachii?

- Holding a heavy hymnal while singing in the church choir
- With your right arm, using a screwdriver to tighten a screw
- Carrying an infant in your arms in a cradled position

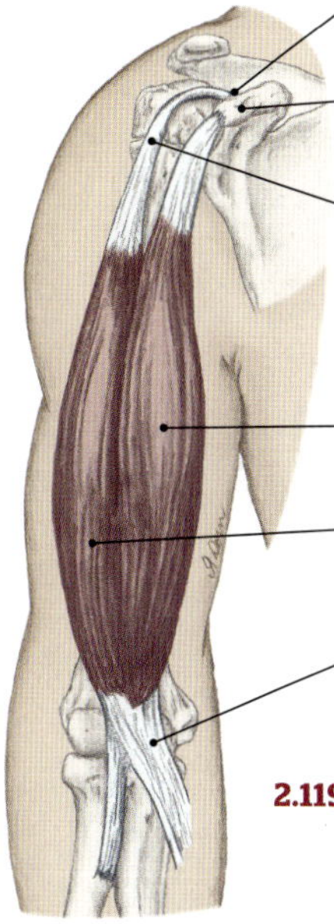

2.119 Anterior view of right arm, showing biceps brachii

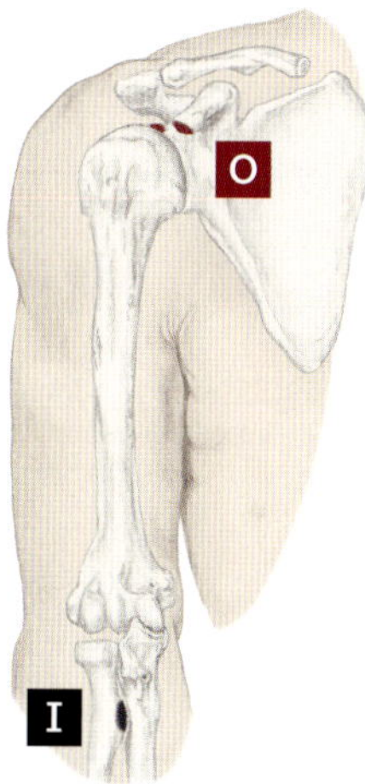

2.120 Anterior view of right arm, showing origin and insertion of biceps brachii

Biceps brachii

1. Partner supine or seated. Bend the elbow and shake hands with your partner.
2. Ask your partner to flex his elbow against your resistance. Palpate the anterior surface of the arm and locate the hard, round belly of the biceps (**2.121**).
3. Follow the belly distally to the inner elbow. Note how the muscle belly thins, becoming a solid, distinct tendon. Then follow the biceps proximally to where it tucks beneath the anterior fibers of the deltoid.

Ask your partner to flex his elbow and see if you can sculpt out the biceps's distal tendon and distinguish it from the deeper brachialis muscle (p. 130). Also, shake hands with your partner and ask him to alternately pronate and supinate his forearm against your resistance. Do you feel the muscle belly and tendon contract upon supination?

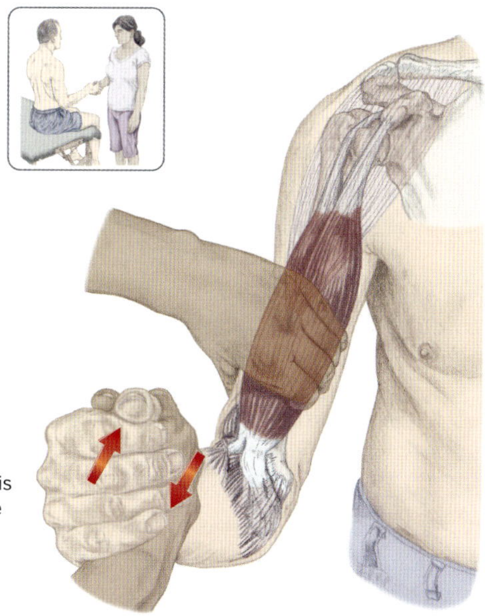

2.121 Partner seated, flexing his elbow against your resistance while you palpate the biceps

biceps brachii *bi*-seps ***bray***-key-i L. two-headed muscle of the arm

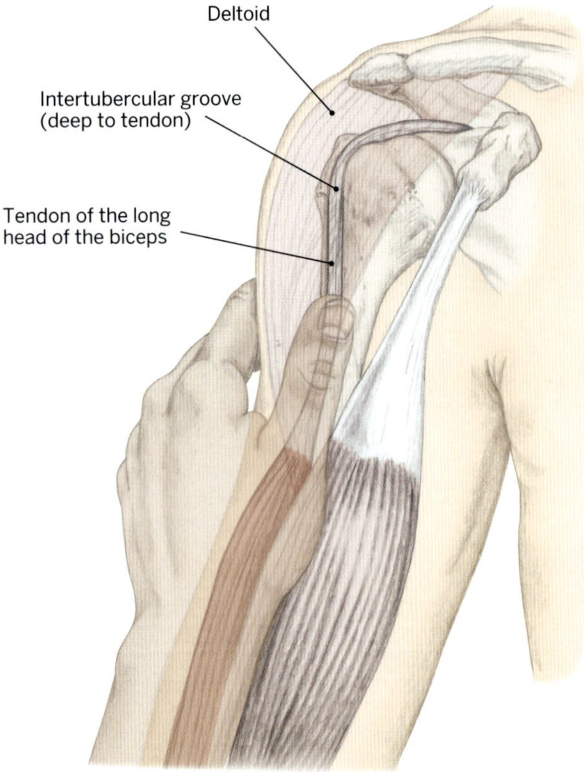

2.122 Anterior view of right shoulder, as you palpate the tendon of the long head of the biceps

Tendon of the Long Head of the Biceps Brachii

Because the biceps tendon is situated in the intertubercular groove of the humerus and runs parallel to the superficial deltoid fibers, it can be difficult to truly isolate.

Tendon of the long head of the biceps brachii

1. Partner supine or seated. Locate the intertubercular groove (p. 56). Laterally rotating the arm may make it easier to pinpoint the tendon (**2.122**).
2. Ask your partner to gently flex his elbow against your resistance in order to feel the biceps tendon become taut in the intertubercular groove. Be aware that the deltoid's anterior fibers will also contract upon flexion of the shoulder.

Discover More

In addition to a long head and a short head, the biceps may have a head that attaches to the humerus. Reported in less than 10% of the population, this extra head originates along the medial humerus next to the coracobrachialis before joining the short head.

Palpation Plus

Distal tendon of the biceps

In exploring the distal tendon of the biceps, you may notice a smaller tendon-like band that expands off it medially. This is the bicipital aponeurosis, a thin sheet of fascia that curves around the forearm flexors and blends into the antebrachial fascia. It stabilizes the ulna during flexion and supination, and—similar to a "tennis elbow" armband—supports the forearm flexors.

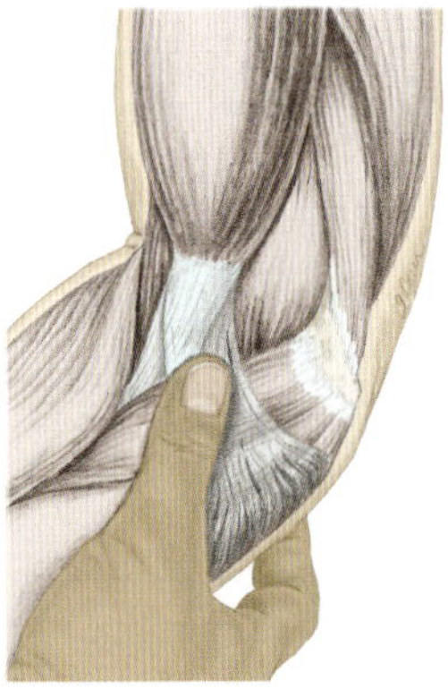

Medial view of right elbow

1. With the elbow flexed, shake hands with your partner. As you locate the biceps's distal tendon, ask your partner to flex her elbow against your resistance, making the tendon more discernible.
2. Slide over to the tendon's medial aspect and explore for the aponeurosis. When the biceps contracts, it is sometimes visible. Follow this fascial strip as far as you can around the medial forearm.

Triceps Brachii ▶

The triceps brachii is the only muscle located on the posterior arm. Creating extension at the elbow and shoulder, it is an antagonist at both these joints to the biceps brachii.

The triceps has three heads: long, lateral, and medial (**2.123**, **2.124**). The long head extends off the infraglenoid tubercle of the scapula (p. 50), weaving between the teres major and minor. The lateral head lies superficially beside the deltoid while the medial head lies mostly underneath the long head. All three heads converge into a thick, distal tendon proximal to the elbow.

Aside from its proximal portion, which is deep to the deltoid, the triceps is superficial and easily accessible.

TRICEPS BRACHII	
A	*All heads:* **Extend** the elbow (humeroulnar joint) *Long head:* **Extend** the shoulder (glenohumeral joint) **Adduct** the shoulder (G/H joint)
O	*Long head:* Infraglenoid tubercle of the scapula *Lateral head:* Posterior surface of proximal half of the humerus *Medial head:* Posterior surface of distal half of the humerus
I	Olecranon process of the ulna
N	Radial C6, **7**, **8**, T1

When Do You Use Your Triceps Brachii?

- Slamming the trunk of a car
- Pounding in large nails with a big ol' hammer
- Raising your body during the up phase of a push-up
- Dribbling a basketball

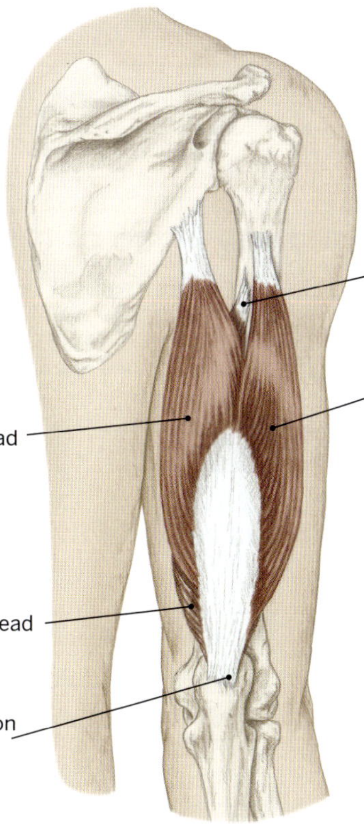

2.123 Posterior view of right shoulder, showing triceps brachii

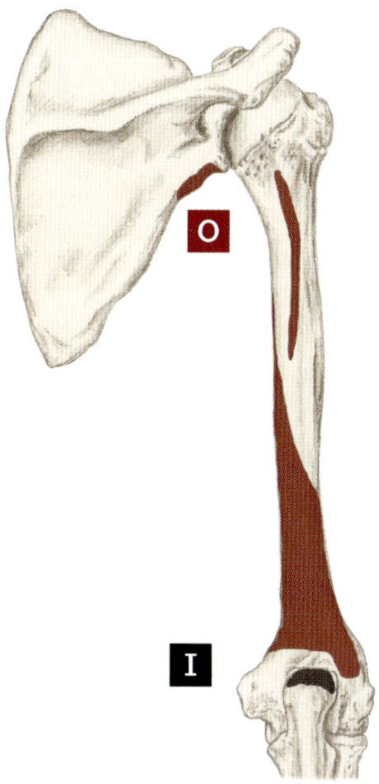

2.125 Posterior view of right shoulder, showing origin and insertion of triceps brachii

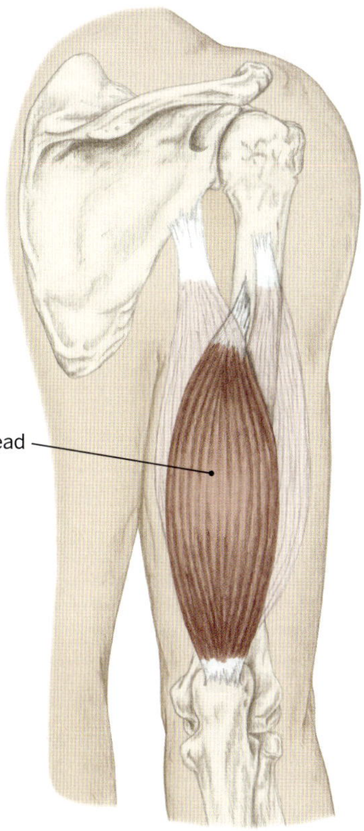

2.124 Posterior view of right shoulder, showing the medial head of triceps brachii, deep to the lateral and long heads

triceps brachii *tri*-seps *bray*-key-i L. three-headed muscle of the arm

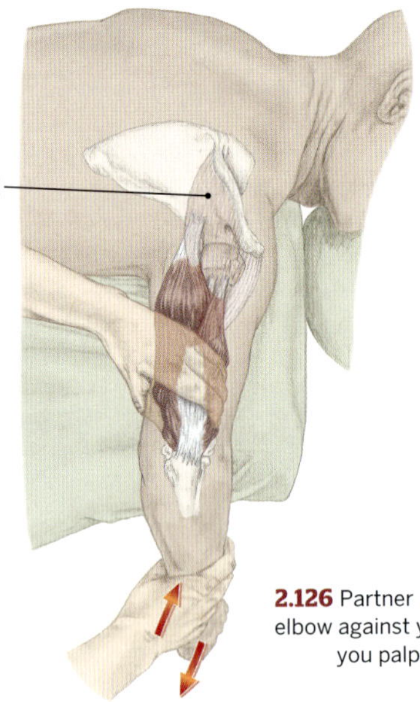

2.126 Partner prone, extending the elbow against your resistance while you palpate the triceps

Triceps brachii

1. Partner prone. Bring the arm off the side of the table and palpate the posterior aspect of the arm. Outline the edge of the posterior deltoid and then explore the size and shape of the triceps.
2. Locate the olecranon process to outline the distal tendon of the triceps. Then ask your partner to extend his elbow as you apply resistance at his forearm (**2.126**). Slide your other hand off the olecranon process proximally and onto the broad triceps tendon.
3. With your partner still contracting, widen your fingers and palpate the medial and lateral heads on either side of the tendon.

Does the muscle tighten when your partner extends his elbow? Can you feel the medial and lateral triceps heads bulge on either side of the distal tendon?

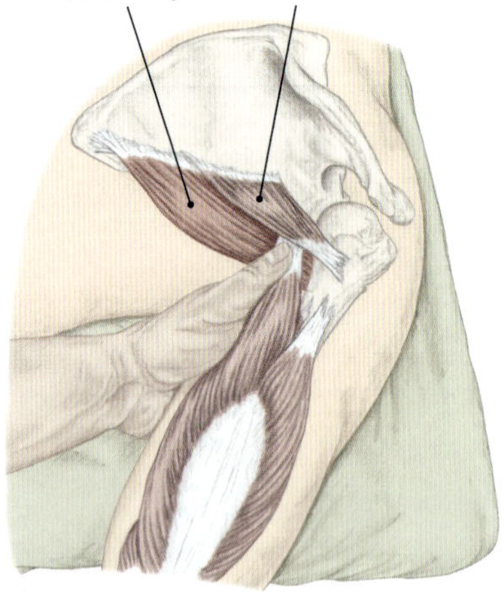

2.127 Partner prone, as you isolate the tendon of the long head of the triceps

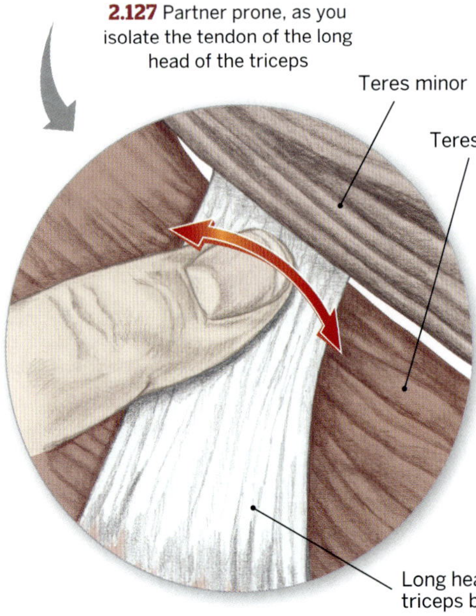

Tendon of the Long Head of the Triceps Brachii

A helpful hint for locating the long head of the triceps is the fact that it is the only band of muscle on the posterior arm that runs superiorly along the proximal and medial aspect of the arm. The deltoid fibers run at a more diagonal direction than the long head of the triceps.

Tendon of the long head of the triceps brachii

1. Partner prone. Place one hand on the proximal elbow and ask your partner to bring his elbow toward the ceiling against your resistance. This action will contract the long head of the triceps.
2. Locate its belly along the proximal and medial aspect of the arm. Follow the muscle proximally by strumming across the belly. Note how it disappears underneath the posterior deltoid toward the infraglenoid tubercle.
3. With the arm relaxed, press through the posterior deltoid and strum across its skinny tendon as it attaches to the infraglenoid tubercle.

*The long head of the triceps crosses over the teres major and under the teres minor (**2.127**). Can you follow the long head up to the division of the teres muscles? Have your partner medially and laterally rotate his shoulder to differentiate the teres muscles (pp. 67, 70).*

Coracobrachialis ▶

The coracobrachialis is a small, tubular muscle located in the axilla (**2.128**, **2.129**). Sometimes known as the "armpit" muscle, it is a secondary flexor and adductor of the shoulder. In anatomical position, the coracobrachialis is deep to the pectoralis major and anterior deltoid and lies anterior to the axillary artery and brachial plexus. Abducting the shoulder (opening up the axilla) brings the belly of the coracobrachialis to a superficial and palpable position.

	CORACOBRACHIALIS
A	**Flex** the shoulder (glenohumeral joint) **Adduct** the shoulder (G/H joint)
O	Coracoid process of the scapula
I	Medial surface of mid-humeral shaft
N	Musculocutaneous C**6**, **7**

When Do You Use Your Coracobrachialis?

- Reaching around your face to scratch your opposite ear
- Weightlifting—doing a bench press
- In martial arts—a forearm block in front of your chest

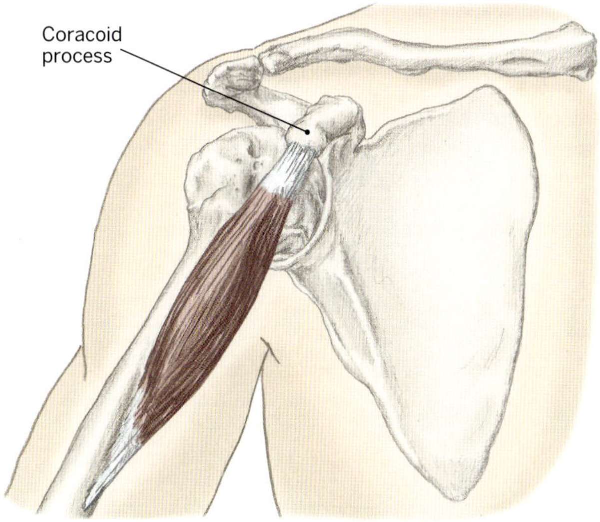

2.128 Anterior view of right shoulder, showing coracobrachialis

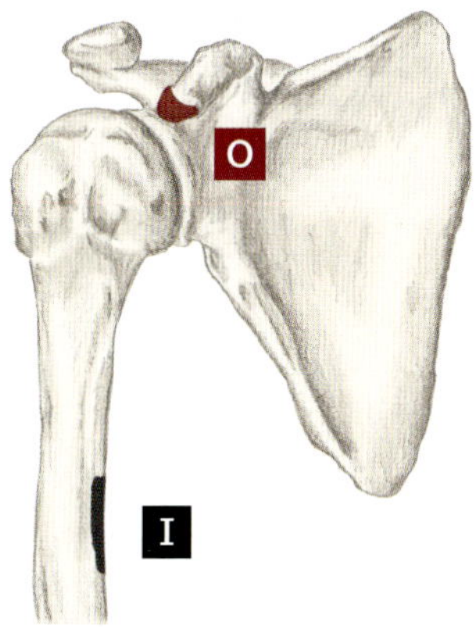

2.129 Anterior view of right shoulder, showing origin and insertion of coracobrachialis

Coracobrachialis

1. Partner supine. Laterally rotate and abduct the shoulder to 45°. Locate the fibers of the pectoralis major. This tissue forms the axilla's anterior wall and will be a reference point for locating coracobrachialis.
2. Lay one hand along the medial side of the arm and move your fingerpads into the armpit.
3. Have your partner horizontally adduct gently against your resistance (**2.130**). Isolate the solid edge of the pectoralis major, then slide off the pectoralis major fibers posteriorly (into the axilla) and explore for the slender, contracting belly of the coracobrachialis. Its belly may be visible upon adduction.

Is the muscle you are palpating on the medial side of the upper arm? Does its belly lie posterior to the overlying flap of the pectoralis major? Can you strum along its cylindrical belly?

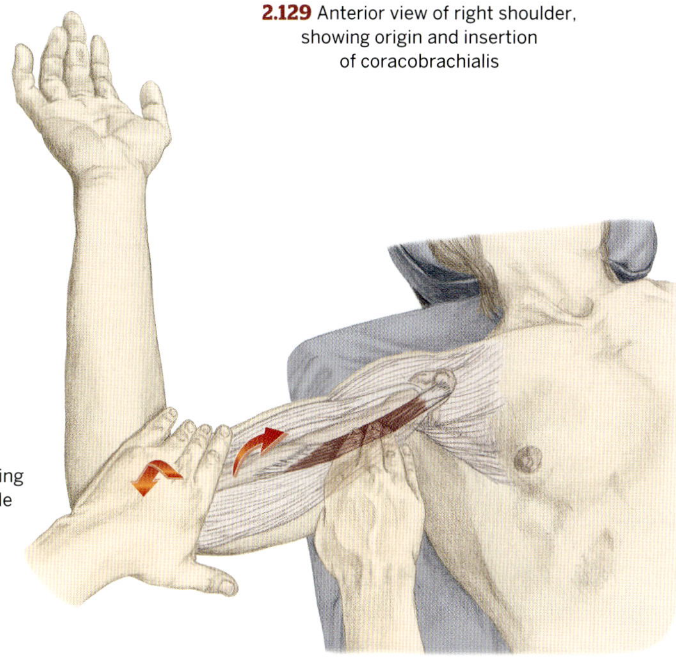

2.130 Partner supine, horizontally adducting the shoulder against your resistance while you palpate coracobrachialis

coracobrachialis *kor*-a-ko-***bra***-kee-***al***-is

Ligaments and Other Structures of the Shoulder and Arm

Axilla

The axilla is the cone-shaped area commonly called the armpit (**2.131**). It is formed by four walls: (**a**) the lateral wall (biceps brachii and coracobrachialis), (**b**) the posterior wall (subscapularis and latissimus dorsi), (**c**) the anterior wall (pectoralis major), and (**d**) the medial wall (rib cage and serratus anterior). Several important vessels pass through the axillary region (**2.132**), including the brachial artery and the brachial plexus (nerves).

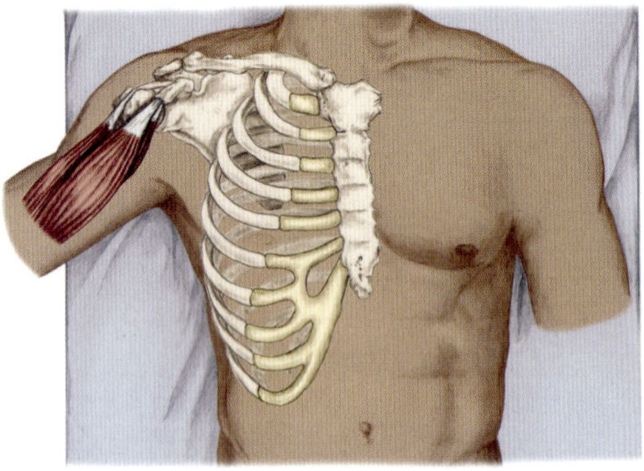

a Anterior view of right shoulder and rib cage, showing biceps brachii and coracobrachialis

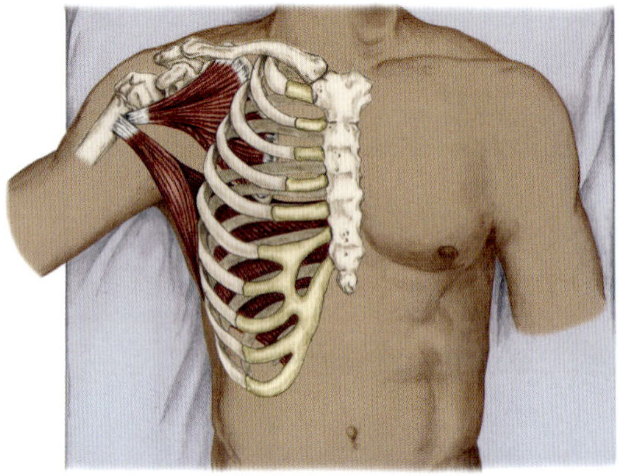

b Anterior view of right shoulder and rib cage, showing subscapularis and latissimus dorsi

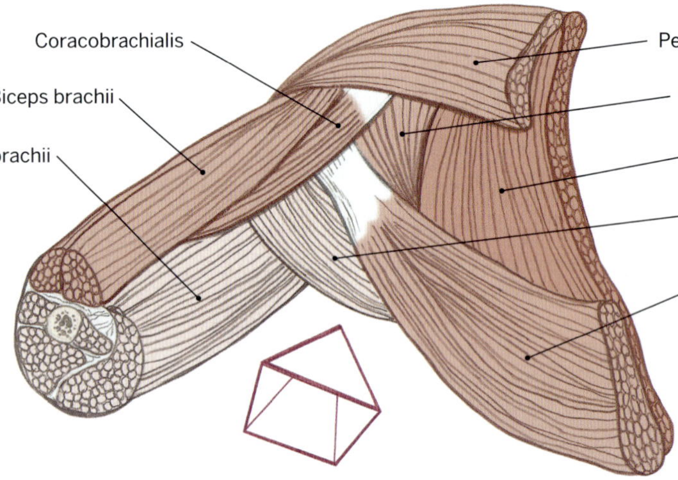

2.131 Inferior view of right axilla, showing the muscles that form the axilla's four walls

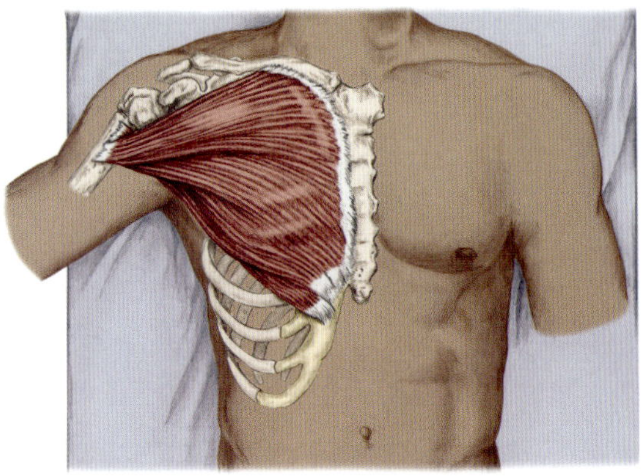

c Anterior view of right shoulder and rib cage, showing pectoralis major

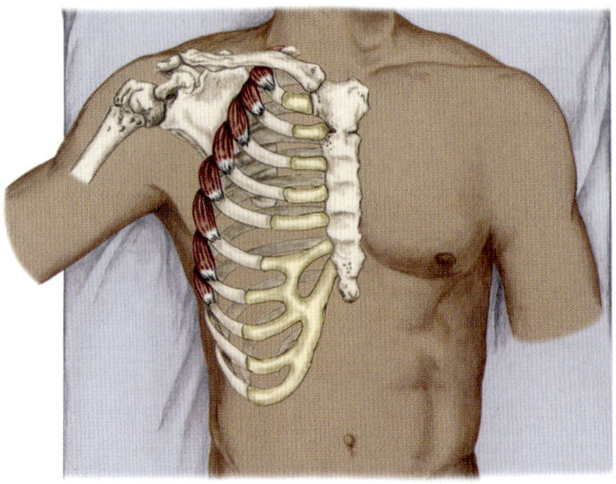

d Anterior view of right shoulder and rib cage, showing serratus anterior

axilla	***ak**-sil-a*	L. armpit
axillary	***ak**-si-**lar**-ee*	

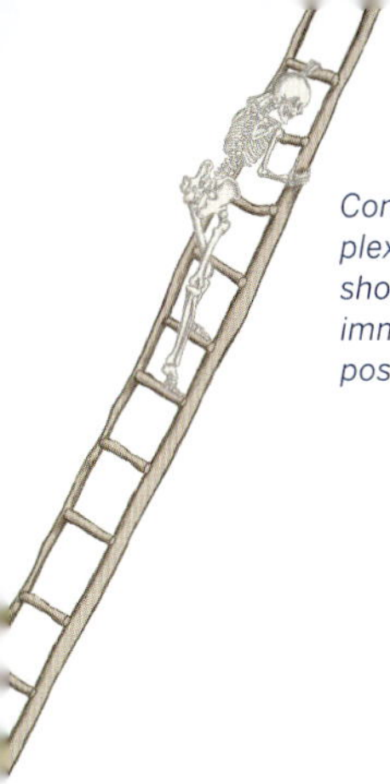

Compression or impingement of the brachial plexus or one of its nerves can create a sharp, shooting sensation down the arm. If this occurs, immediately release and adjust your position posteriorly. Also, ask your partner for feedback.

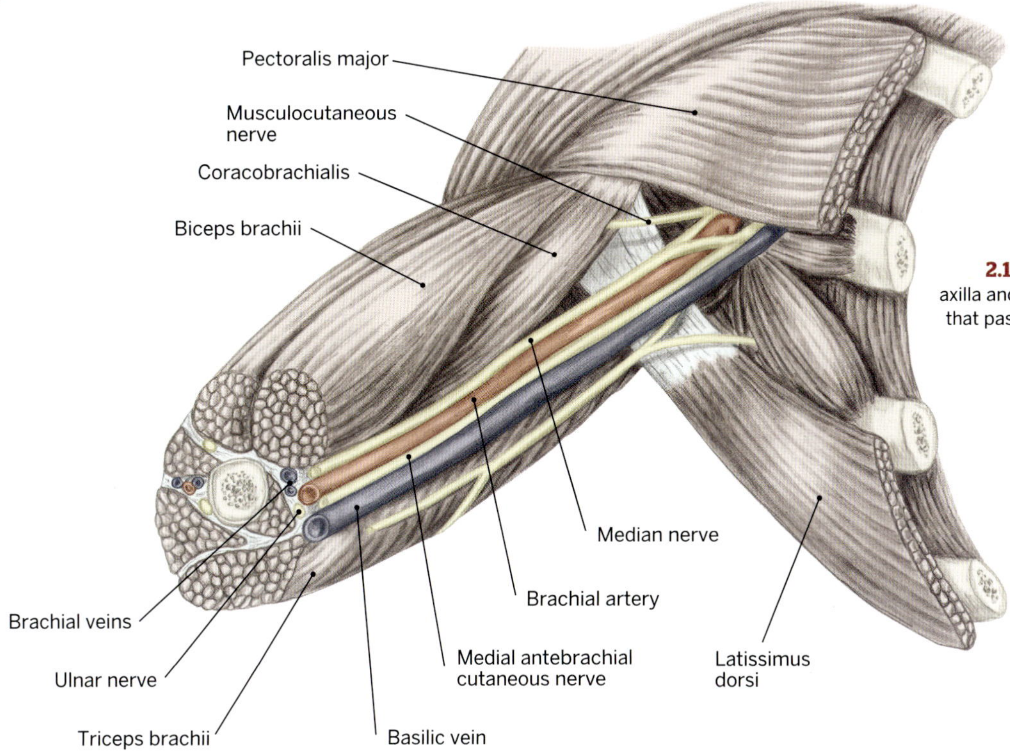

2.132 Inferior view of right axilla and upper arm, showing vessels that pass through the axillary region

Sternoclavicular Joint

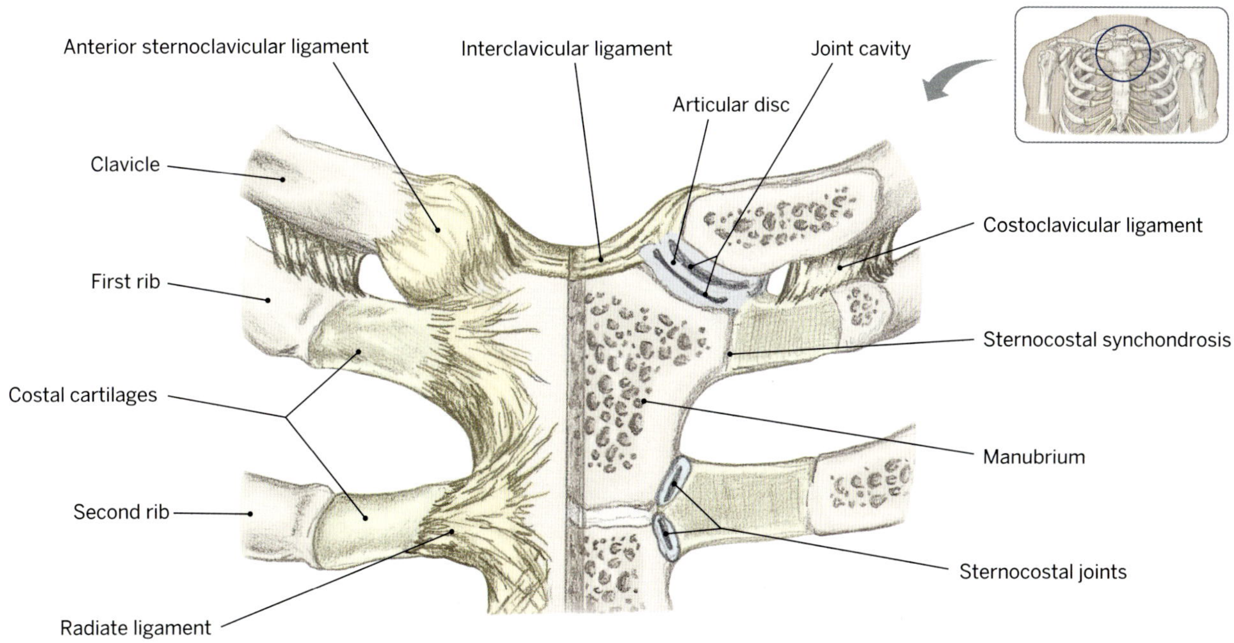

2.133 Anterior view of sternoclavicular joint and superior portion of sternum, right side shown in coronal section

brachial	***bray***-key-al	L. relating to the arm
synchondrosis	*sin*-con-***dro***-sis	

Ligaments of the Shoulder

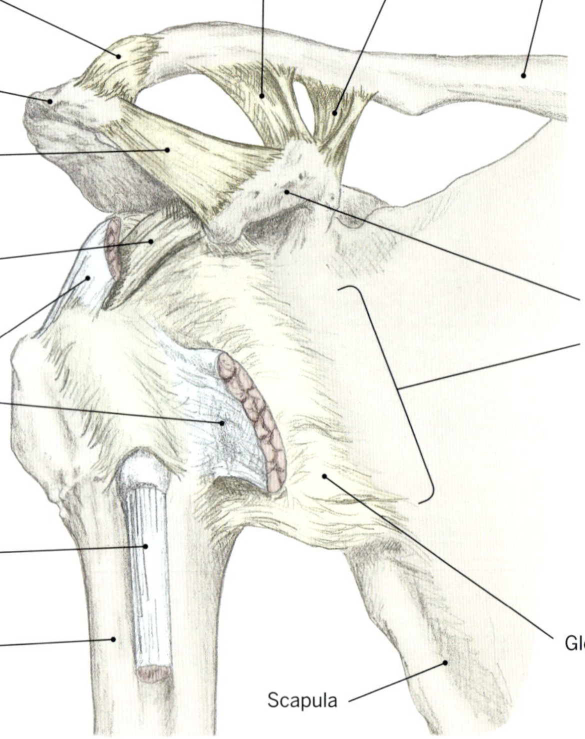

2.134 Anterior view of right shoulder, showing ligaments and tendons

See p. 55 for more information about the ligaments and tendons that attach to the coracoid process.

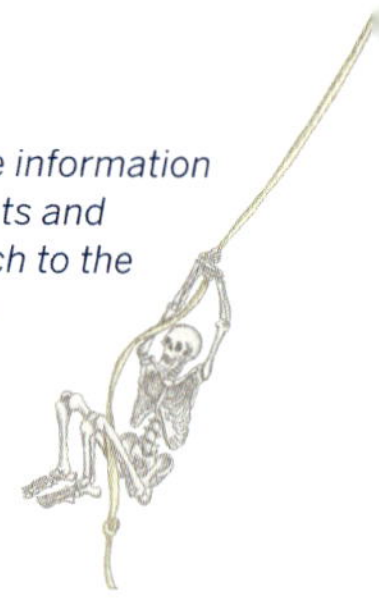

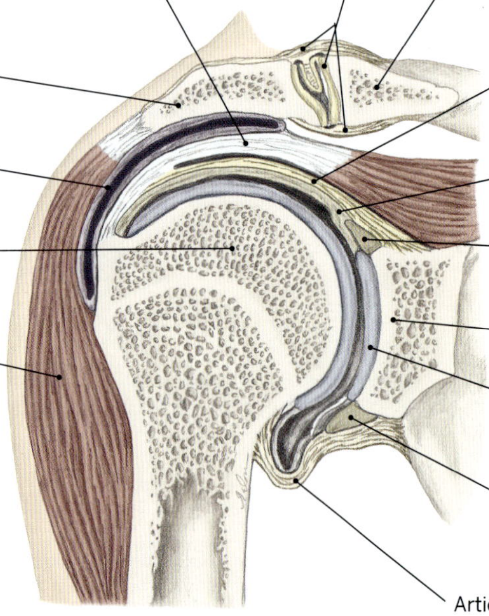

2.135 Cross-section anterior view of right shoulder, showing acromioclavicular and glenohumeral joints

coracoacromial	***kor***-a-***ko***-a-***kro***-mi-ul	
coracoclavicular	***kor***-a-***ko***-cla-***vic***-u-lar	
ligament	***lig***-a-ment	L. a band

Glenohumeral Joint

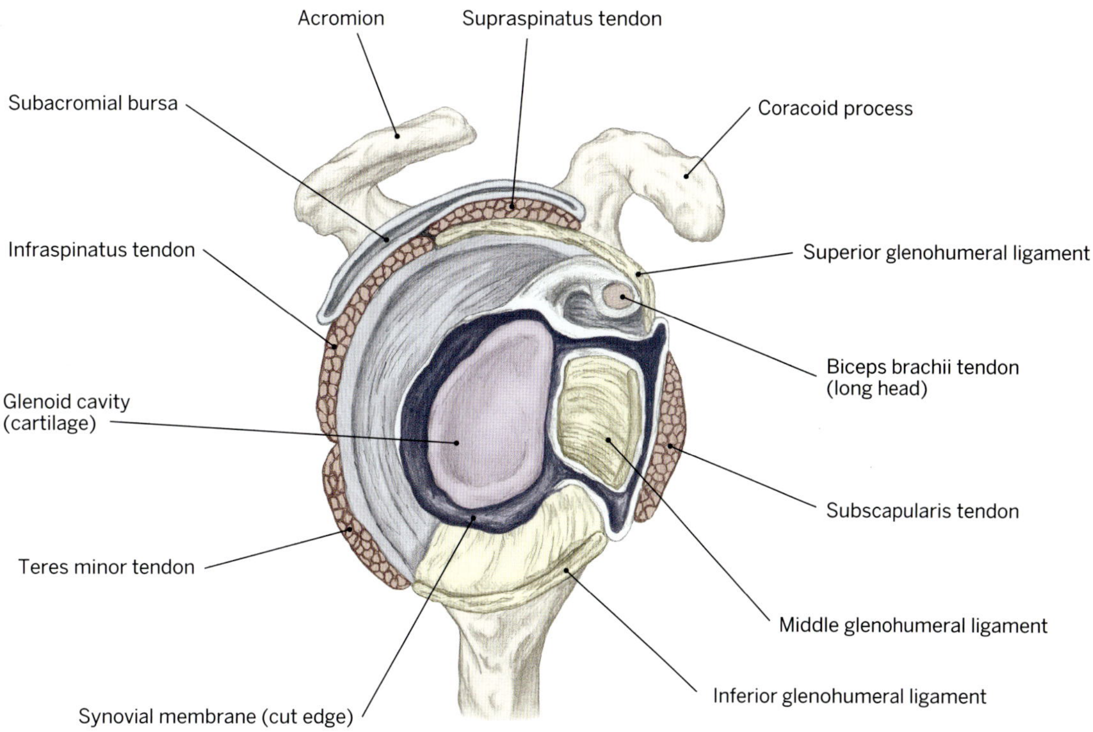

2.136 Lateral view of right shoulder, glenohumeral joint opened and humerus removed

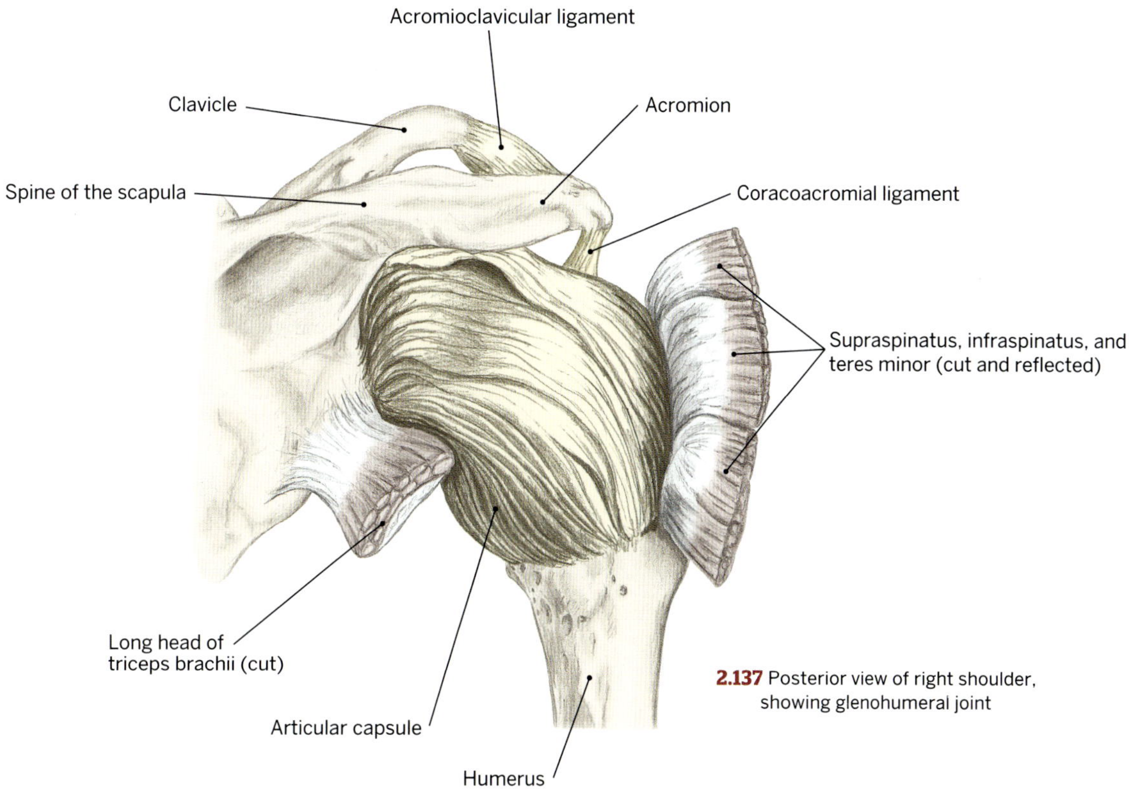

2.137 Posterior view of right shoulder, showing glenohumeral joint

labrum	*lay*-brum	L. lip
conoid	*ko*-noid	Grk. cone-shaped

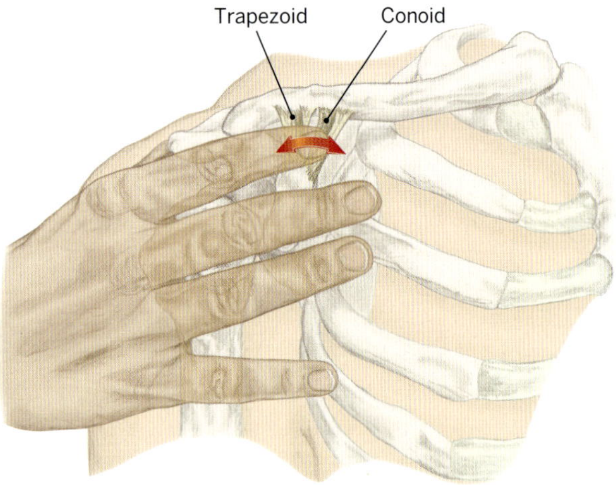

2.138 Anterior view of right shoulder, as you palpate the coracoclavicular ligament

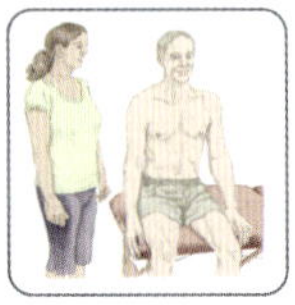

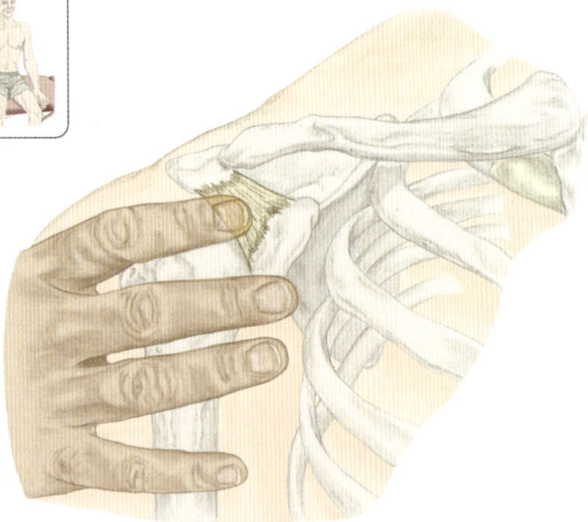

2.139 Anterior view of right shoulder, as you palpate the coracoacromial ligament

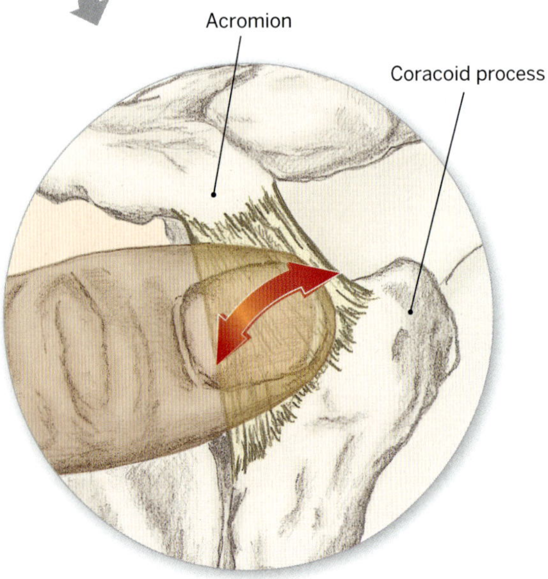

Coracoclavicular Ligament

The coracoclavicular ligament is composed of two smaller ligaments: the trapezoid and conoid. Both ligaments stretch from the coracoid process of the scapula to the inferior surface of the clavicle (see **2.134**, p. 98). Together they provide stability for the acromioclavicular joint and form a strong bridge between the scapula and clavicle.

The coracoclavicular ligament can be accessed by palpating between the clavicle and coracoid process or curling under the anterior aspect of the clavicle.

Coracoclavicular ligament

1. Partner seated or supine. Abduct and medially rotate the shoulder. This position brings the ligaments more to the surface.
2. Locate the coracoid process of the scapula and the shaft of the clavicle.
3. Palpate in the space between these landmarks. Roll your thumbpad across its fibers (**2.138**). Unlike the superficial pectoralis major fibers, the ligaments will feel like solid, taut bands.

Passively move the shoulder girdle in several directions and see if a particular position allows you greater access to the ligaments.

Coracoacromial Ligament

Unlike most ligaments that hold two bones together, the coracoacromial ligament attaches the scapula's coracoid process to its acromion (**2.139**). Along with the acromion, this ligament forms the coracoacromial arch across the top of the shoulder. This arch helps to protect the rotator cuff tendons and subacromial bursa from direct trauma by the acromion. The wide band of the coracoacromial ligament lies deep to the deltoid but is still accessible.

Coracoacromial ligament

1. Partner supine or seated. Locate the coracoid process. Then locate the anterior edge of the acromion.
2. Palpating deep to the deltoid fibers, explore between these landmarks for the wide band of the coracoacromial ligament. Strum your finger across its fibers (**2.139**).
3. To bring the ligament closer to the surface, try extending the arm. This position will roll the humeral head anteriorly and press the ligament forward.

Are you between the acromion and the coracoid process? Place one finger on the ligament and passively move the shoulder girdle in various positions. Can you feel how the ligament's relationship to the surrounding tissues changes as the position of the shoulder changes?

Subacromial Bursa

Also known as the subdeltoid bursa, this sizable fluid sac has two major sections (**2.140**). The lateral portion creates a smooth surface for the acromion and deltoid to glide over the head of the humerus and rotator cuff tendons. The medial part cushions the coracoacromial ligament from the supraspinatus tendon.

With the arm at the side, most of the bursa is underneath the acromion and inaccessible. Extending the shoulder joint, however, will bring the bursa forward. Since abduction of the shoulder compresses the bursa, this action (when accompanied by pain and tenderness) can be used as an indicator of subacromial bursitis.

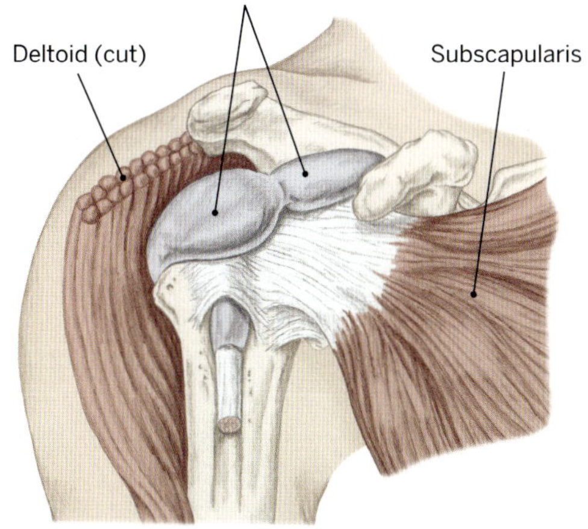

2.140 Anterior view of right shoulder, showing subacromial bursa

Subacromial bursa

1. With your partner seated, stand behind him and locate the acromion.
2. Drop your fingers off the anterior edge of the acromion. Then, with your other hand, slowly extend the shoulder by pulling the elbow posteriorly; this will bring the bursa out from under the acromion. You will be palpating at the depth between the deltoid and rotator cuff tendons (**2.141**).
3. A little hint—palpate gently. Bursae are delicate structures and best accessed with a soft touch. If it is inflamed, it will be acutely tender.

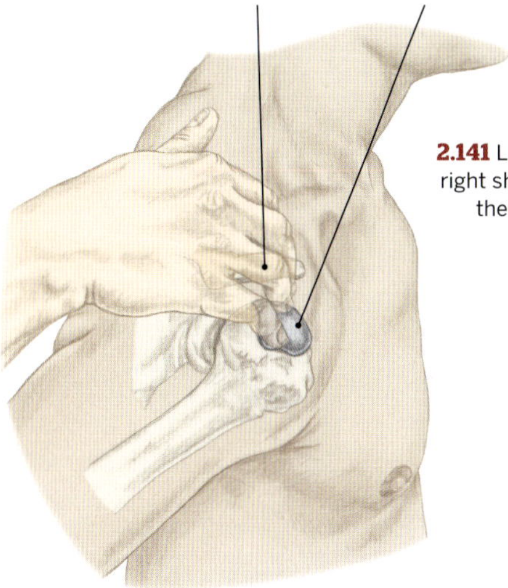

2.141 Lateral view of extended right shoulder, as you palpate the subacromial bursa

Axillary Lymph Nodes

The axillary lymph nodes are located in the axilla. When palpating in the axillary region, use a deliberate yet gentle touch to avoid tickling your partner. Also, move slowly, using gentle pressure to avoid impinging the artery and nerves.

Axillary lymph nodes

1. Partner supine or seated. Abduct the arm and slowly sink two fingers up into the axilla. Then bring the arm back to the side of the body to soften the axillary tissue further.
2. Slide your fingers up to the top of the axilla and then medially toward the rib cage. Often there will be a few lymph nodes located against the ribs (**2.142**).
3. Move to the lateral side of the axilla and use light pressure against the humerus to locate the strong pulse of the brachial artery. The vessel will be positioned between the stringy coracobrachialis and long head of the triceps brachii muscle.

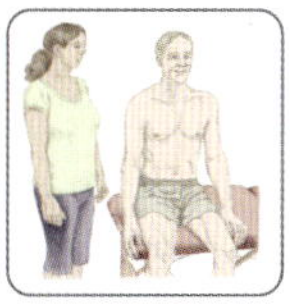

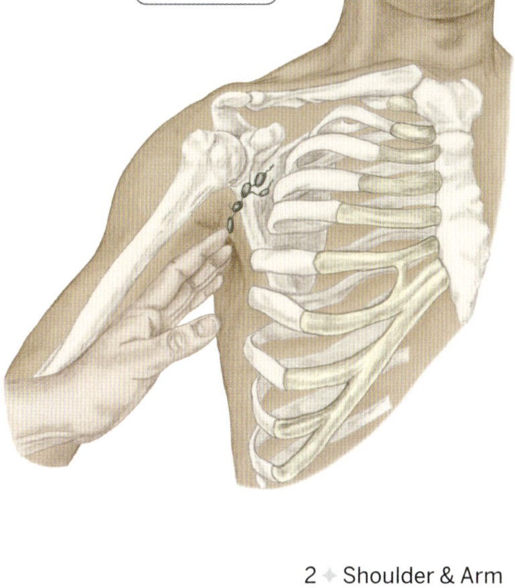

2.142 Anterior view of right shoulder, as you access the axillary lymph nodes

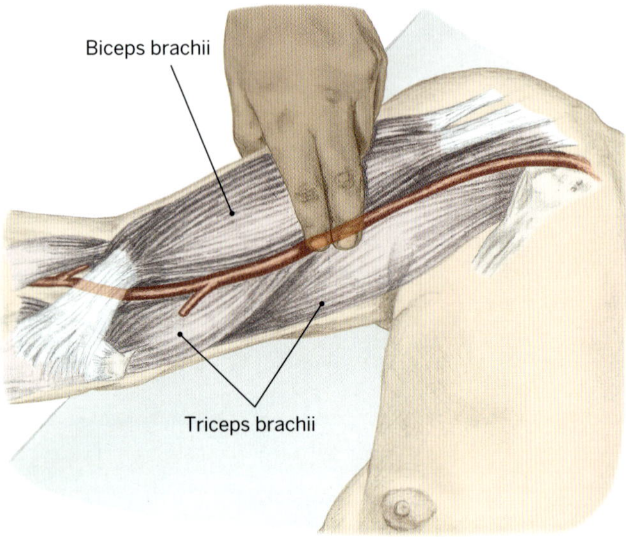

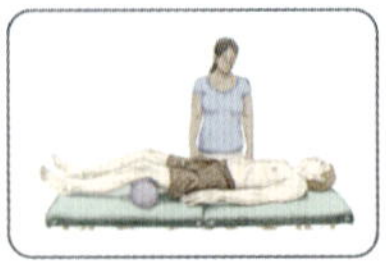

2.143 Anterior/medial view of right arm, as you palpate the brachial pulse between the biceps and triceps brachii

Brachial Artery

The brachial artery is a continuation of the axillary artery and runs between the biceps and triceps brachii. Its pulse can be felt between these muscles on the medial side of the arm (see p. 97). Before the brachial artery branches off to the radial and ulnar arteries, its pulse can be felt at the elbow, just medial to the biceps brachii tendon.

Brachial artery

1. Partner supine or seated. Abduct the arm and place your fingerpads on the medial side of the arm. A helpful guide is the shallow dip that forms between the biceps and triceps (**2.143**).
2. Gently press your fingers toward the shaft of the humerus to feel the brachial pulse.
3. The brachial pulse can also be detected just medial to the distal tendon of the biceps brachii.

On to the forearm and hand, where we'll find flexors, extensors, and an "anatomical snuffbox."

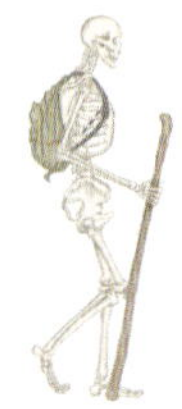

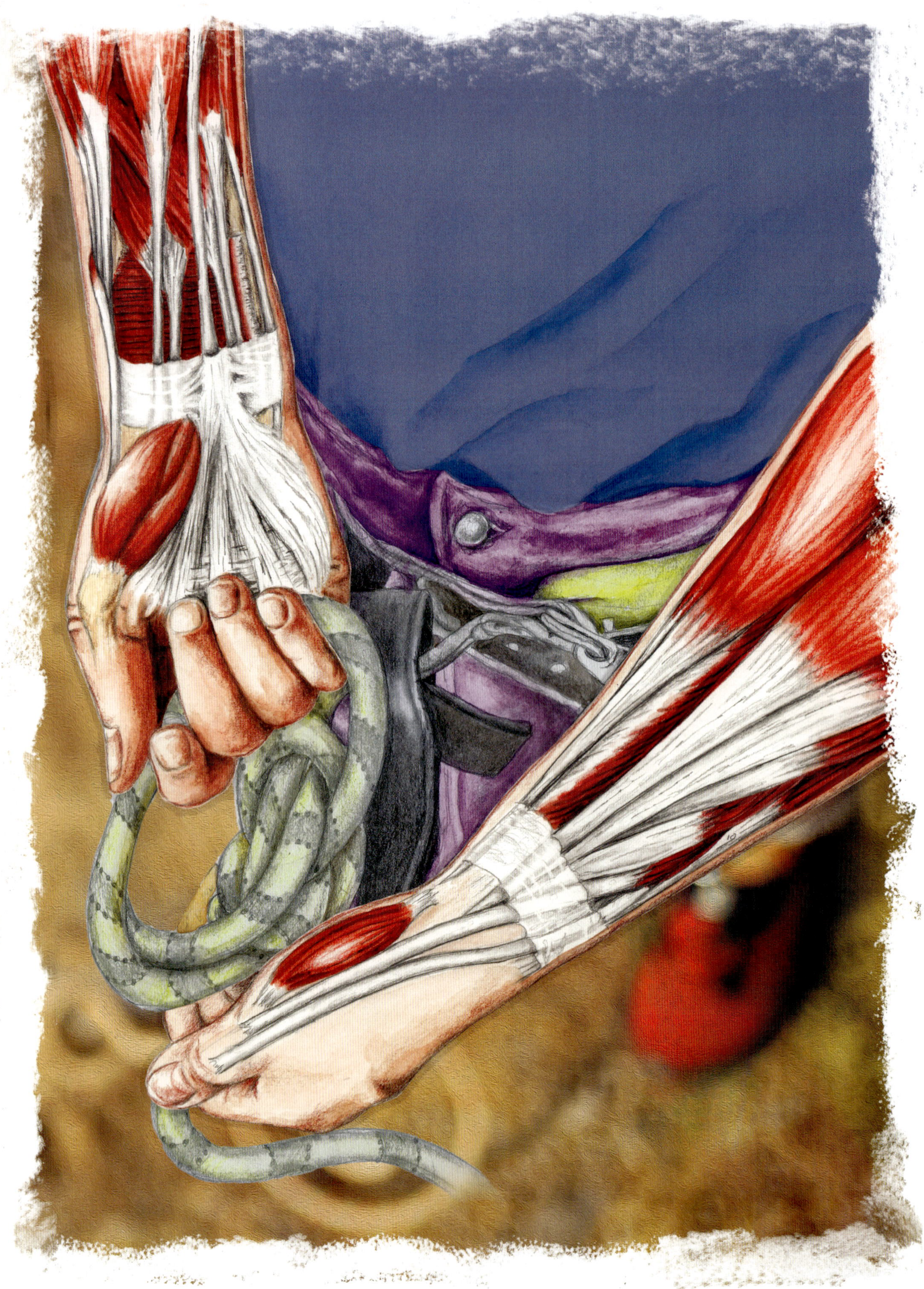

3

Forearm & Hand

Hold your phone, pick up a water bottle, or open this book, and try to imagine doing these actions without the use of your hands. Incredibly, most of the muscle tissue used to perform these simple feats are located nowhere near your fingers, but in the forearm. Your digits mostly contain attaching tendons.

Look at the picture of the climber's hands on the previous page. Using the movement terms you've learned, how would you describe the position of the fingers holding the rope? When the climber holds the rope tightly and the wrist and finger flexor muscles contract, do you think that those muscles are shortening or lengthening?

See for yourself:

- Pick up a pencil, letting it rest across the palm of your hand like the rope is positioned in the picture. Close your fingers around it gently. Now squeeze the pencil tightly, making a fist around it, then release. Repeat this several times. When you tighten your grasp, can you see the tissue in your forearm move? It's true: Making a fist involves muscle bellies located close to the elbow!
- Now place your right hand on a table and slowly, but dramatically, move your fingers as if you're playing a massive piano. Use your left hand to explore the right forearm—and especially the wrist—to feel all the contractions of the various muscles. Follow a muscle or tendon to the elbow or past the wrist.

Topographical Views

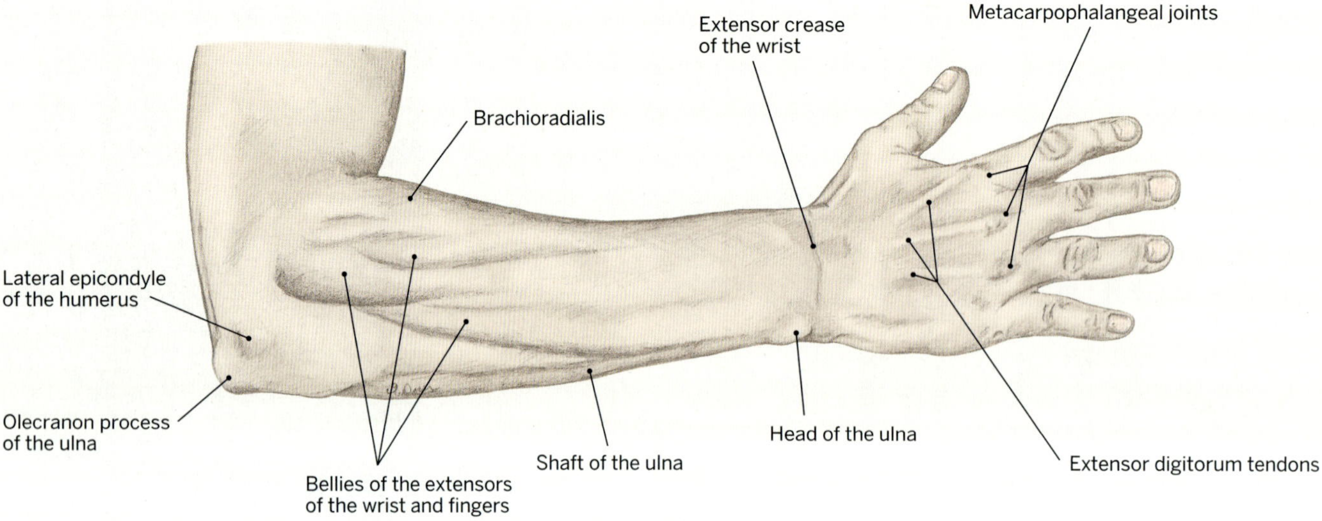

3.1 Lateral view of right forearm and hand

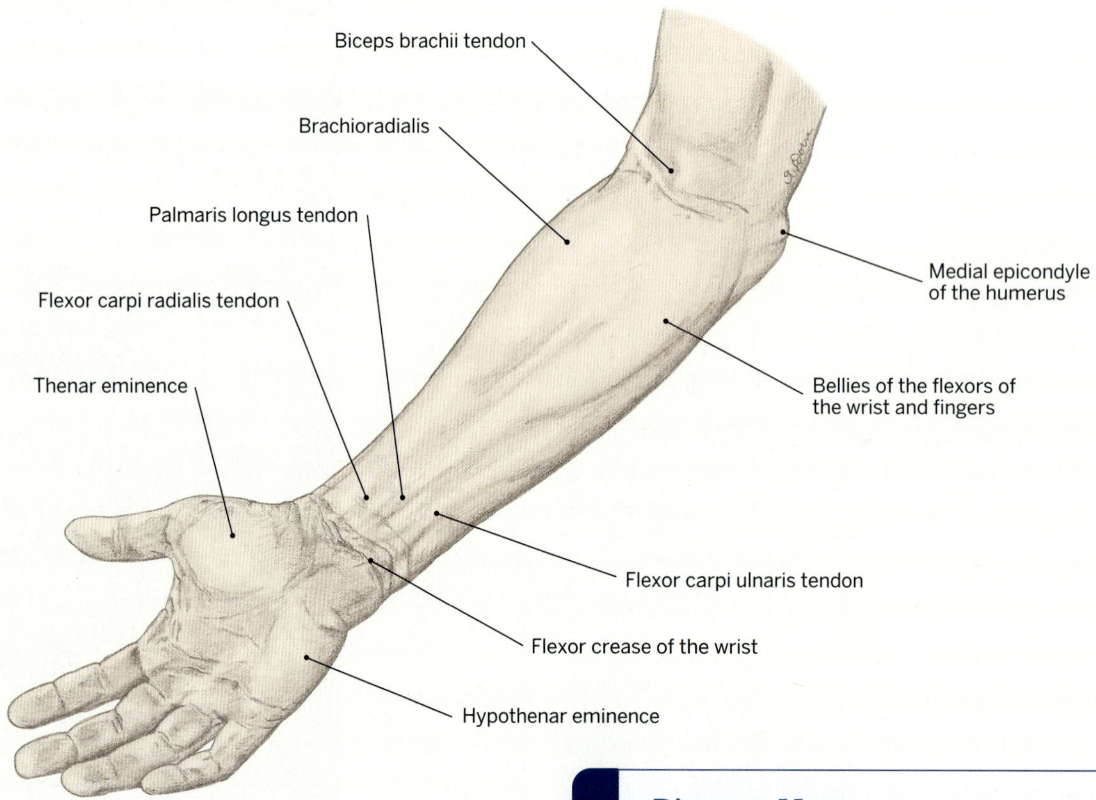

3.2 Anterior view of right forearm and hand

Discover More

In everyday speech, "arm" usually refers to the region between the shoulder and wrist. As an anatomical term, however, "arm" refers to the region between the shoulder and elbow. The portion between the elbow and wrist is called the "forearm."

thenar	***thee***-nar	Grk. palm, flat of the hand
hypothenar	***hi***-po-***thee***-nar	Grk. *hypo*, under or below

Exploring the Skin and Fascia

Forearm

1. Partner seated. Begin by gently lifting the skin and fascia of the forearm. Compare the thickness and elasticity of the posterior (hairy) side to the anterior (hairless) side (**3.3**).
2. Explore the length of the forearm. Note how the tissue along the shaft of the forearm might be more challenging to grasp than the tissue at the wrist and elbow regions.

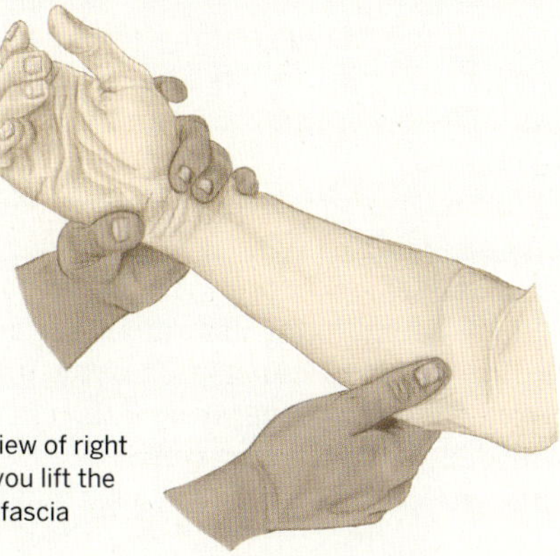

3.3 Anterior view of right forearm, as you lift the skin and fascia

Forearm

1. Using one hand to stabilize the forearm, use your other hand to gently twist the skin and fascia around the forearm's shaft (**3.4**).
2. Now try to tug the skin superiorly and inferiorly. Often the tissue will have more elasticity in a horizontal direction (around the forearm's shaft) than in a vertical one.

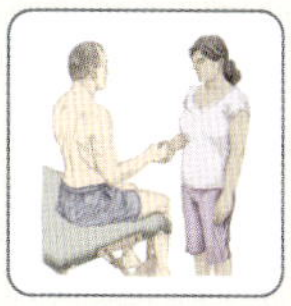

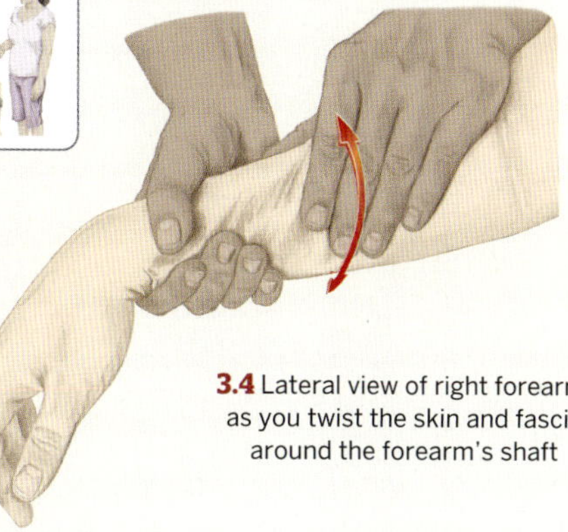

3.4 Lateral view of right forearm, as you twist the skin and fascia around the forearm's shaft

Wrist

1. Here is an opportunity to feel your partner's skin and fascia stretch during passive movement. Grasp the tissue near the wrist and *passively* flex and extend the wrist joint (**3.5**–**3.7**). Feel how supple and plentiful the tissue is when the wrist is flexed. As the wrist is extended, however, the skin may be pulled from between your fingers.
2. Continue to move the wrist while grasping the tissue on all sides of the forearm. Supinate and pronate the forearm, feeling how these actions cause the tissue to move differently.
3. Ask your partner to *actively* move his wrist and fingers while you grasp the skin and fascia. Encourage him to move slowly. Play with isolating specific actions—for instance, extension of the wrist as opposed to extension of the fingers—to feel the tissues shift with different actions.

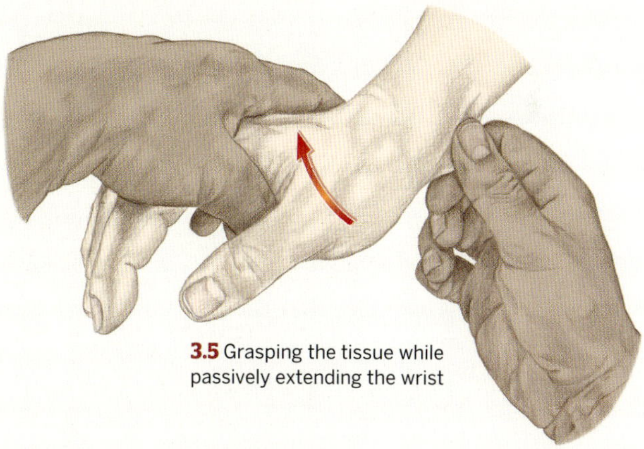

3.5 Grasping the tissue while passively extending the wrist

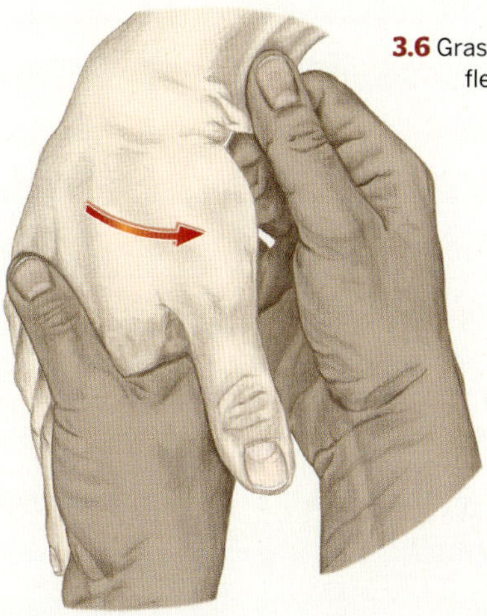

3.6 Grasping the tissue while flexing the wrist

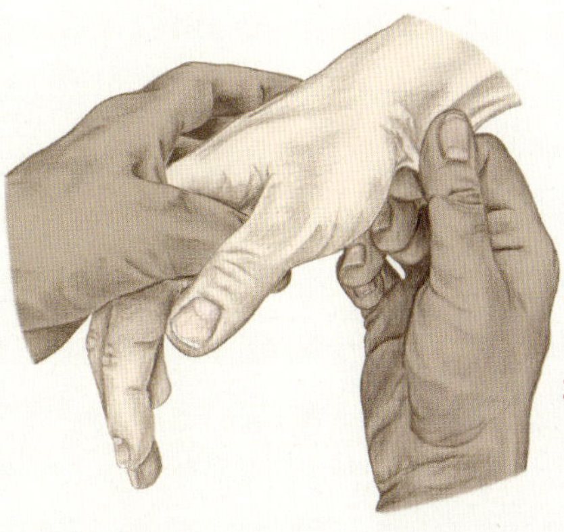

3.7 Grasping the tissue while wrist in neutral

Bones of the Forearm and Hand

The **humerus** is the bone of the arm. Its proximal end articulates with the scapula to form the glenohumeral joint. Its distal end joins with the ulna and radius at the elbow (**3.8**). The elbow has two joints: the humeroulnar and humeroradial.

The **radius** and **ulna** make up the bones of the forearm. The ulna is superficial and has a palpable edge that extends from the elbow to the wrist. The radius (on the thumb side) is lateral to the ulna and is partially buried in muscle. Pronation and supination of the forearm are created by the radius pivoting around the ulna at the proximal and distal radioulnar joints.

The three groups of bones in the wrist and hand are the carpals, metacarpals, and phalanges. The **carpals** are eight pebble-sized bones that form two rows (proximal and distal), each containing four carpal bones (**3.9**). Located distal to the flexor crease of the wrist, the carpals are accessible from all sides—the palmar, dorsal, radial, and ulnar surfaces of the hand.

The **metacarpals** are five long bones spanning the palm of the hand. The metacarpals' proximal end is the base, the long midsection is the shaft, and the distal end is the head (**3.10**). The metacarpals are easily palpable along the hand's dorsal surface. They are deep to the muscles on the palmar side.

The **phalanges** are the bones of the fingers. The thumb has two phalanx bones and the fingers have three. All sides of the phalanges are accessible (**3.11**).

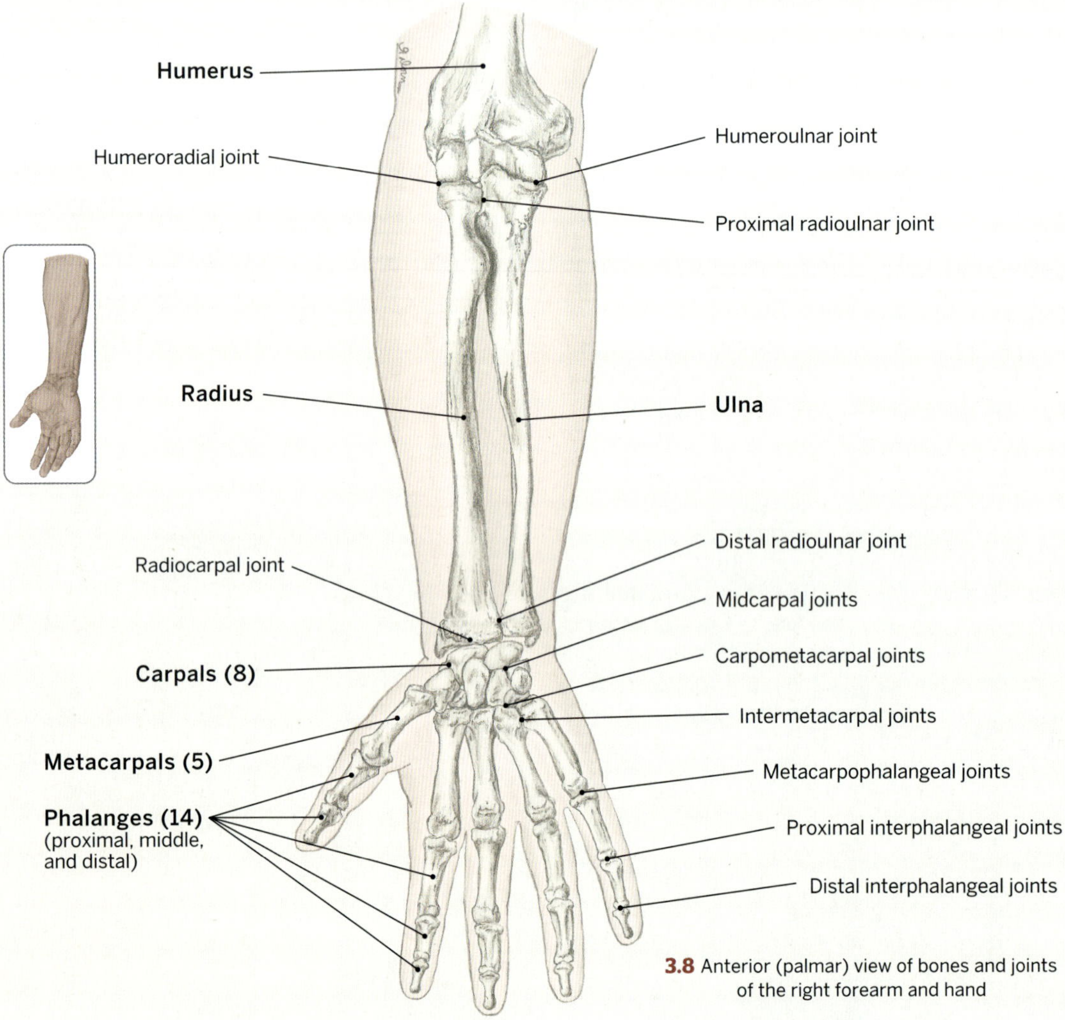

3.8 Anterior (palmar) view of bones and joints of the right forearm and hand

Discover More

Let's talk joints! The **radiocarpal** joint (wrist), formed by the radius and proximal carpals, is an ellipsoid joint. The gliding joints at the **midcarpal** and second to fifth **carpometacarpal** joints allow for only small, shifting movements.

The first **carpometacarpal** joint of the thumb is an ellipsoid-shaped saddle joint. The **metacarpophalangeal** joints, the large "knuckles" of the hand, are also ellipsoid joints. The **interphalangeal** joints of the fingers are hinge joints.

humerus	***hu***-mer-us	L. upper arm
radius	***ray***-dee-us	L. staff, spoke of a wheel
ulna	***ul***-na	L. elbow, arm

Bony Landmarks of the Forearm and Hand

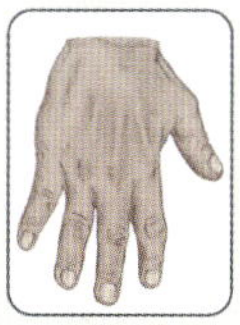

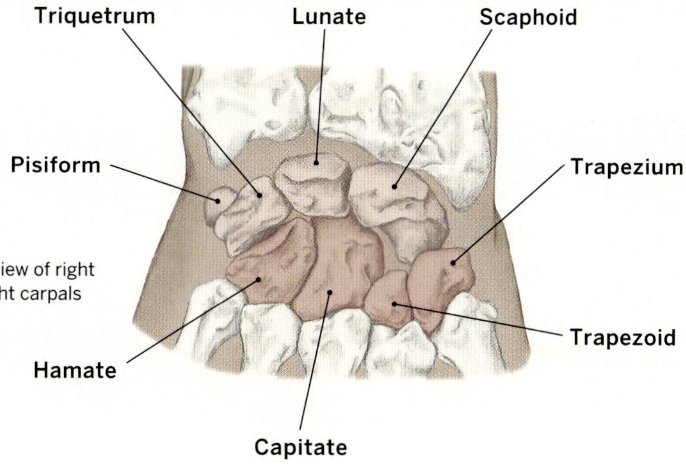

3.9 Posterior (dorsal) view of right wrist, showing the eight carpals

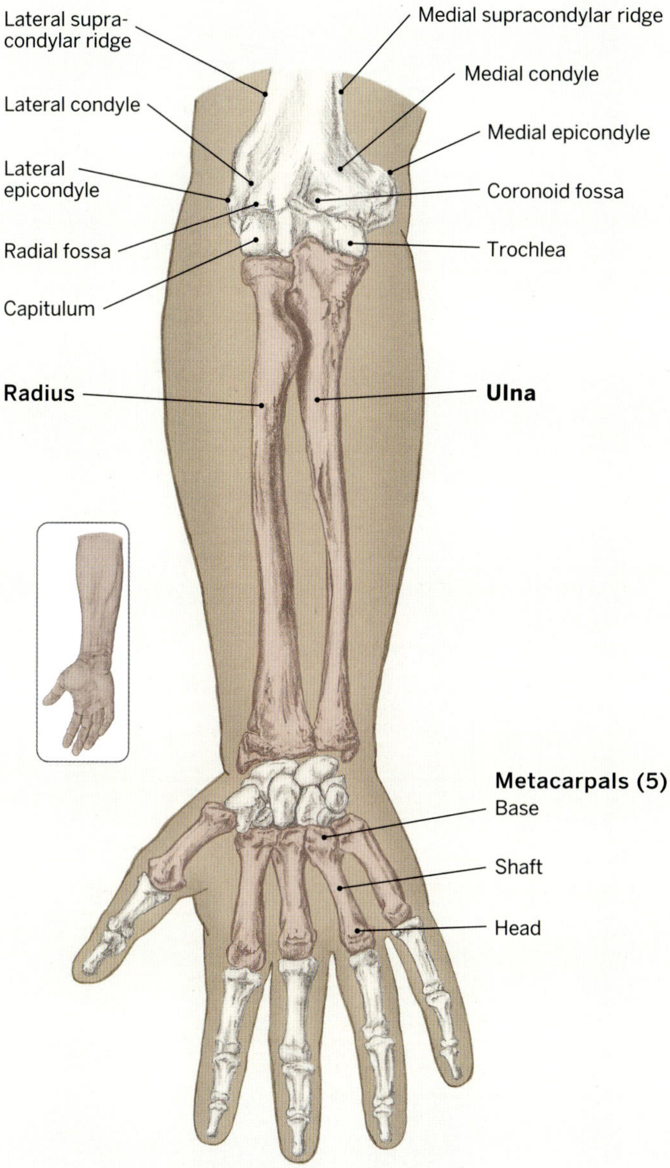

3.10 Anterior (palmar) view of right forearm and hand, showing bony landmarks

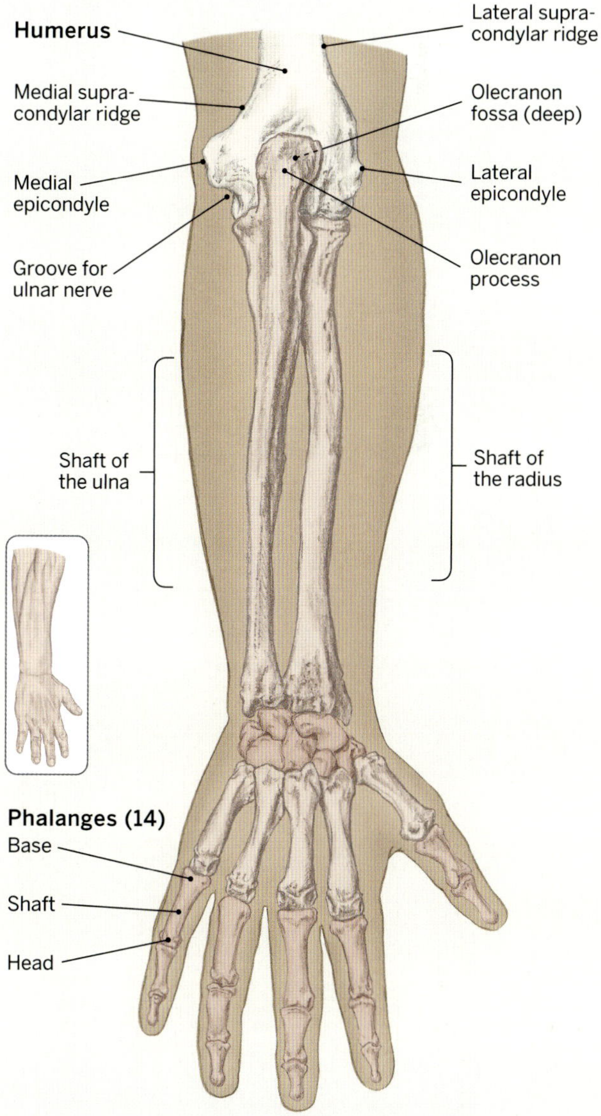

3.11 Posterior (dorsal) view of right forearm and hand, showing bony landmarks

carpal	***kar*-pul**	Grk. pertaining to the wrist
metacarpal	*met*-a-***kar***-pul	Grk. *meta*, after, beyond
phalanges	fa-***lan***-jeez	

The Ulna and Radius

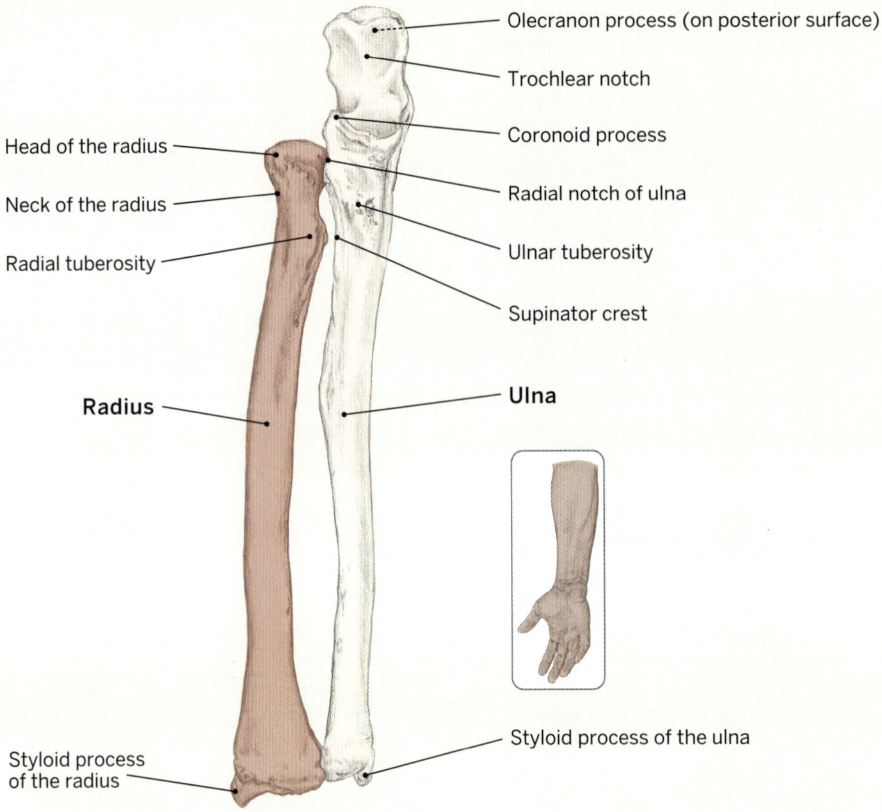

3.12 Anterior view of right radius and ulna

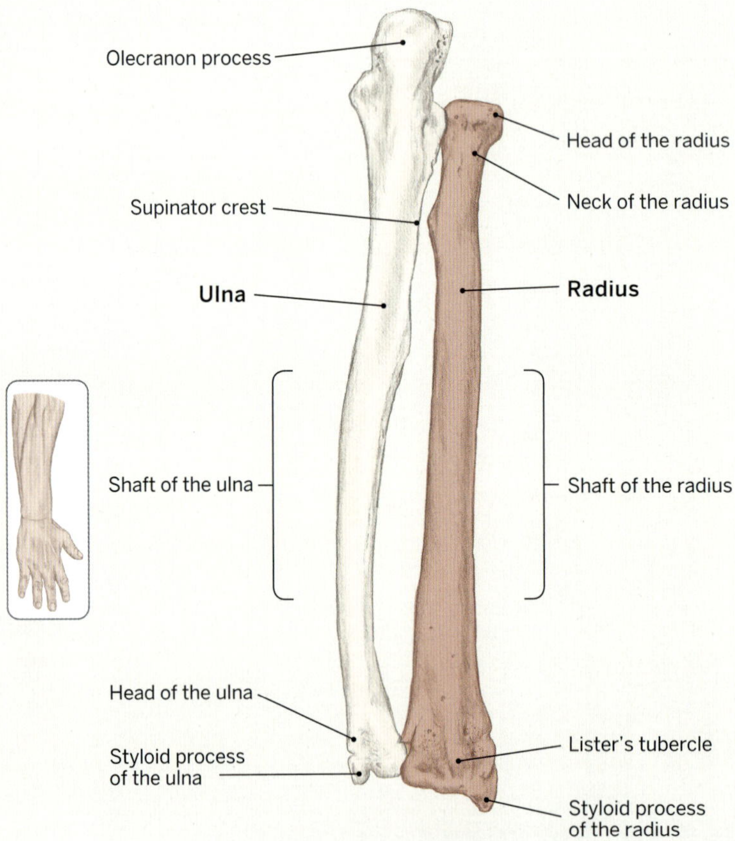

3.13 Posterior view of right radius and ulna

Overview: Bony Landmark Trails

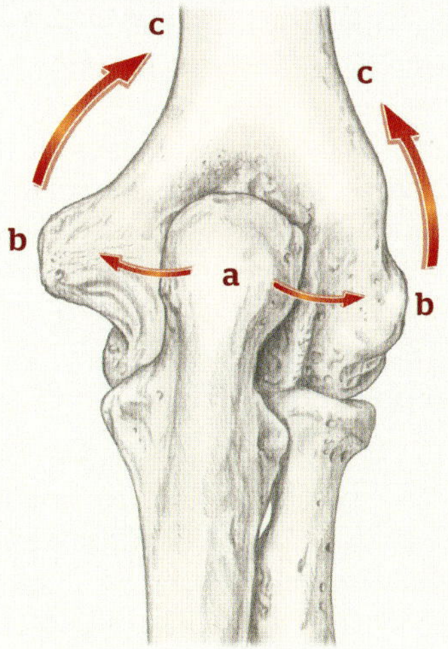

Trail 1 Knob Hill explores the elbow and distal humerus.

a Olecranon process and fossa
b Epicondyles of the humerus
c Supracondylar ridges of the humerus

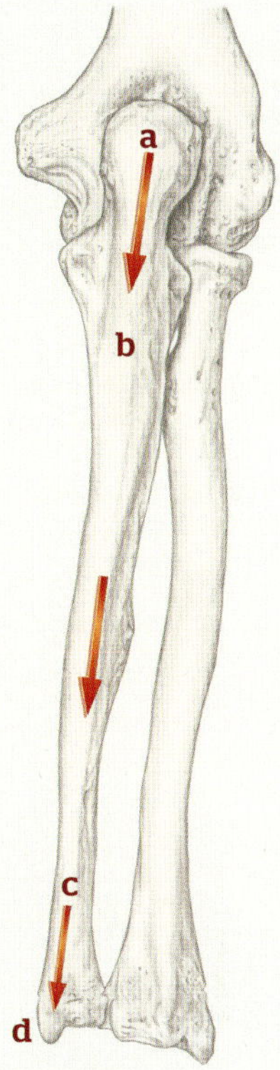

Trail 2 The Razor's Edge follows along the length of the superficial ulna.

a Olecranon process
b Shaft of the ulna
c Head of the ulna
d Styloid process of the ulna

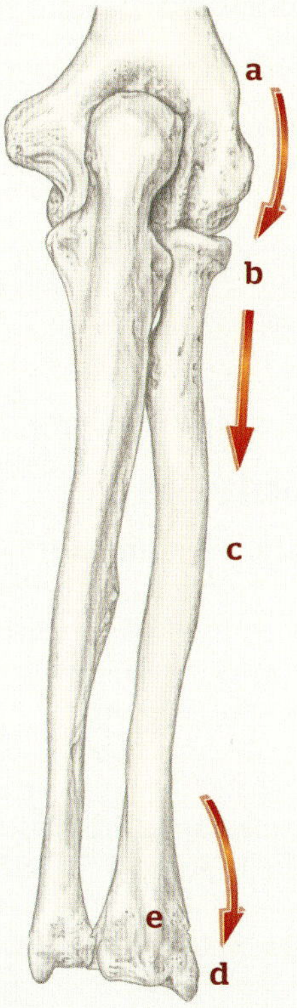

Trail 3 Pivot Pass travels the length of the radius, the bone that creates the pivoting action of the forearm.

a Lateral epicondyle of the humerus
b Head of the radius
c Shaft of the radius
d Styloid process of the radius
e Lister's tubercle

Trail 4 Walking on Your Hands explores the small carpal bones of the wrist as well as the bones and joints of the hand.

Discover More

Some translations for the names of bones may cause you to scratch your head and wonder what early anatomists were thinking. The carpals, luckily, cause no such puzzlement.

capitate	L. head-shaped
hamate	L. hooked
lunate	L. crescent-shaped
pisiform	L. pea-shaped
scaphoid	L. boat-shaped
trapezium	Grk. little table
trapezoid	Grk. table-shaped
triquetrum	L. three-cornered

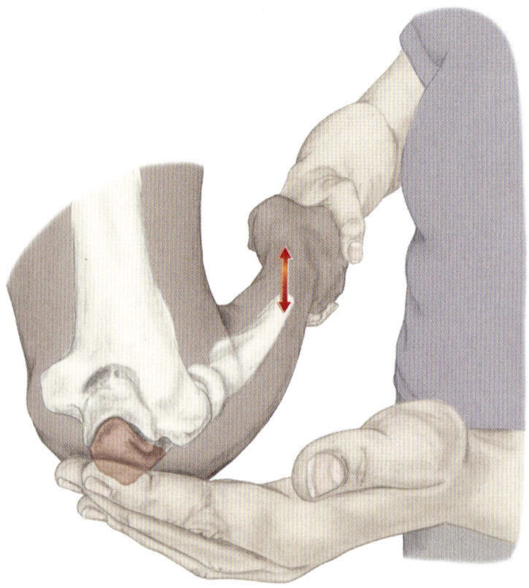

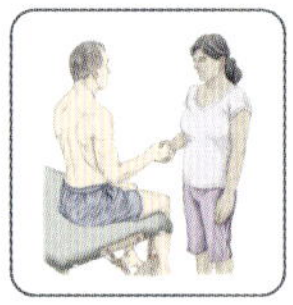

3.14 Posterior view of right elbow, as you palpate the olecranon process

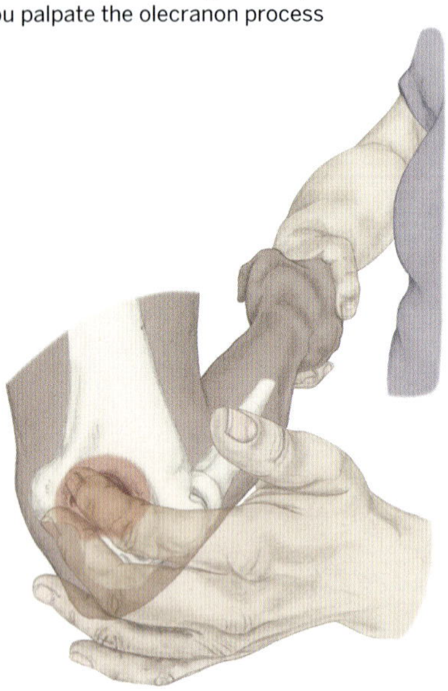

3.15 Posterior view of right elbow, as you locate the olecranon fossa

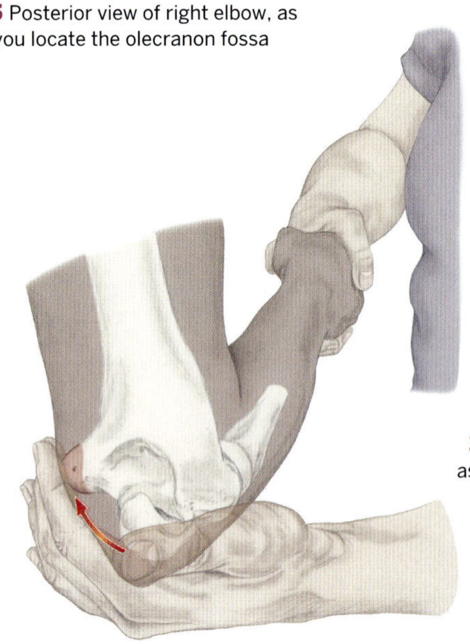

3.16 Posterior view of right elbow, as you palpate the medial epicondyle

Olecranon Process and Fossa

The olecranon process (or elbow) is located on the proximal end of the ulna and articulates with the distal humerus. Its large surface is the attachment site for the triceps brachii muscle. It forms the "point" of the elbow and is easily located.

The olecranon fossa is a large cavity on the posterior, distal end of the humerus designed to accommodate the olecranon process when the elbow is extended. Located deep to the triceps brachii tendon, the fossa is only partially accessible.

Olecranon process

1. Partner seated. Shake hands with your partner and explore the large, superficial knob at the elbow. Palpate and explore its angular surface and sides.
2. Passively flex and extend the elbow, noticing how the olecranon process feels in various positions (**3.14**).

Olecranon fossa

1. Partner seated. Flex the elbow and locate the olecranon process.
2. Roll your finger proximally around the top of the process, pressing through the triceps tendon and into the fossa.
3. Because of the presence of the triceps brachii tendon and the proximity of the olecranon process, only a small, crescent-shaped ditch will be accessible (**3.15**).

✔ *When locating the fossa, are you proximal to the tip of the olecranon process? If you flex and extend the elbow slightly, do you feel a change in the fossa's shape and size?*

Epicondyles of the Humerus

As the humerus extends down the arm, its distal end broadens medially and laterally. Directly medial from the olecranon process is the medial epicondyle (**3.16**). It is superficial and has a protruding, spherical shape designed to accommodate the tendons of the wrist and finger flexors.

The lateral epicondyle is smaller than its medial counterpart and is located lateral to the olecranon process. It is an attachment site for the tendons of the wrist and finger extensors.

fossa	*fos*-a	L. a shallow depression
olecranon	o-*lek*-ran-on	Grk. elbow
process	*pros*-es	L. going forth

Epicondyles of the humerus

1. With your partner seated, shake hands and locate the olecranon process.
2. Slide your finger medially off the olecranon. You will encounter a small ditch before rising up onto the large, superficial medial epicondyle. Explore its bulbous shape (**3.16**).
3. Return to the olecranon. Slide laterally to the lateral epicondyle. Note that it is smaller than the medial epicondyle (**3.17**).

Set a finger on each epicondyle and slowly flex and extend the elbow. The surrounding muscle tissue might move, but the epicondyles should remain stationary. Do they?

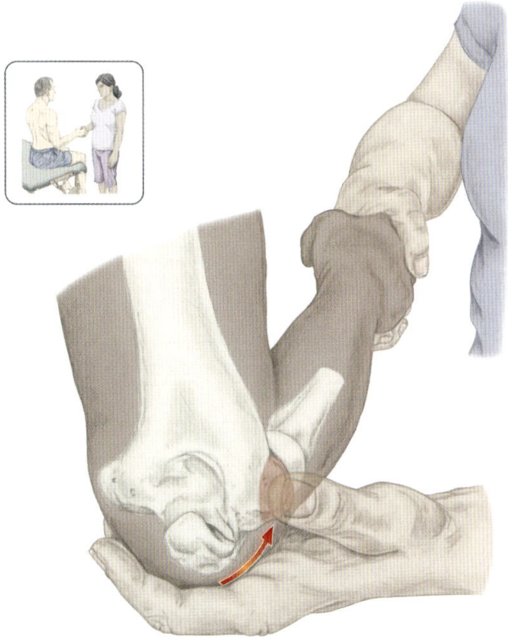

3.17 Posterior view of right elbow, as you palpate the lateral epicondyle

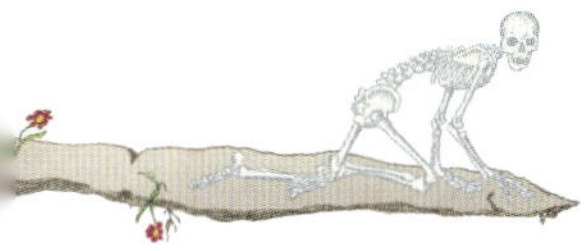

The ulnar nerve (p. 160), which creates the "funny bone" sensation when struck, courses between the medial epicondyle and the olecranon process.

Supracondylar Ridges of the Humerus

These two ridges extend proximally from the respective epicondyles of the humerus. Both serve as attachment sites for the forearm muscles. The lateral supracondylar ridge is located superficially, while the medial ridge sinks into the arm and is situated close to the ulnar nerve.

Supracondylar ridges of the humerus

1. With your partner seated, shake hands and locate the medial epicondyle.
2. Move proximally from the medial epicondyle. The bony ridge that extends from the epicondyle is the medial supracondylar ridge (**3.18**). Roll your fingers back and forth across the ridge to sense its distinct edge.
3. Explore the lateral supracondylar ridge.

Can you follow the ridges proximally a few inches before they disappear under the muscles of the arm?

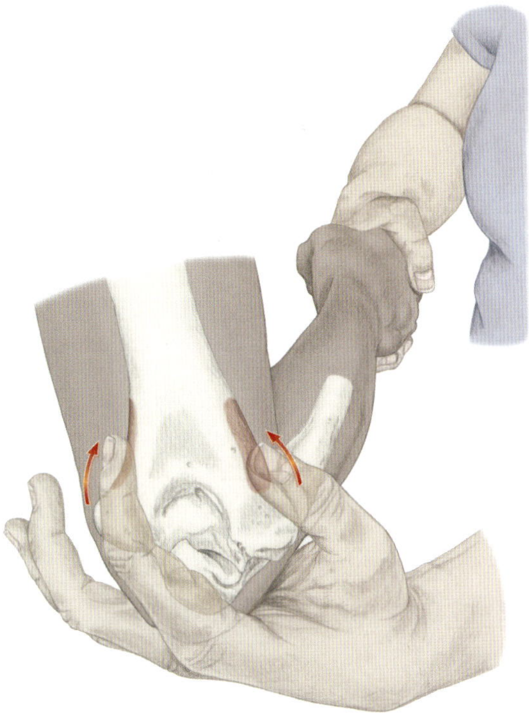

3.18 Posterior view of right elbow, as you explore the supracondylar ridges

condyle	***kon***-dial	Grk. knuckle
epi-	***eh***-pee	Grk. above, upon
lateral	***lat***-er-al	L. to the side

Trail 2 The Razor's Edge ▶

Shaft of the Ulna

The long, straight shaft of the ulna extends from the olecranon process to the head of the ulna. Although numerous muscles lie beside the shaft, it has a superficial, palpable edge that runs along the forearm's posterior/medial aspect.

Shaft of the ulna

1. Shaking hands with your partner, locate the olecranon process. Slide your fingers distally along the shaft.
2. To define its shape and location, roll your fingers across its edge. Follow it down the length of the forearm.

*Is the bone you are palpating superficial? Does it stretch the length of the forearm (**3.19**)?*

Head of the Ulna

The shaft of the ulna swells to form the head of the ulna. The head is the superficial knob visible along the posterior/medial side of the wrist that can disrupt the placement of a watchband.

Head of the ulna

1. Slide your fingers distally along the ulnar shaft.
2. Just proximal to the wrist, the shaft will bulge to become the head of the ulna. Palpate all sides of the bulbous head (**3.20**).

Is the knob you are palpating connected to the shaft of the ulna? In a neutral position, is it on the posterior/medial side of the forearm?

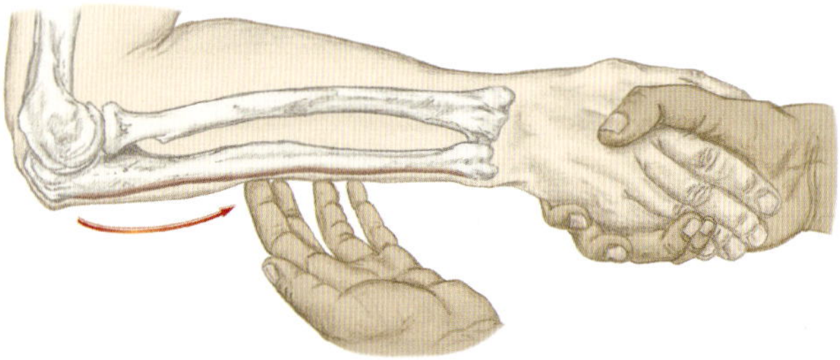

3.19 View of right forearm with elbow flexed, as you palpate the shaft of the ulna

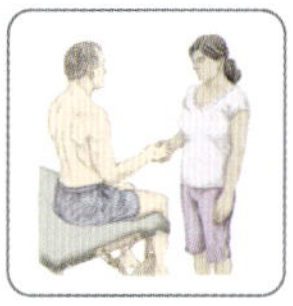

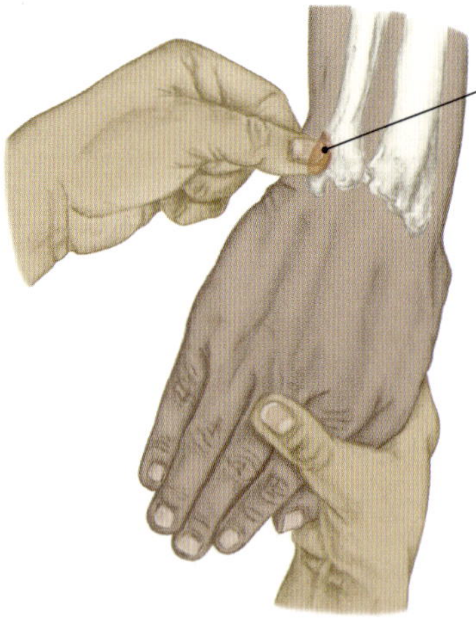

3.20 Posterior (dorsal) view of right wrist, as you palpate the head of the ulna

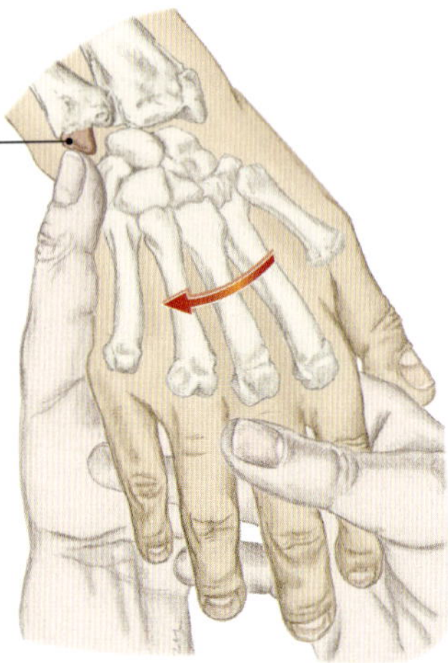

3.21 Posterior (dorsal) view of right wrist and hand, as you palpate the styloid process of the ulna

Styloid Process of the Ulna

Both the ulna and the radius have styloid processes at their distal ends. The radius's styloid process (p. 116) is larger and extends farther distally. The ulna's styloid process is sharper and more pronounced. It is a toothlike projection pointing distally off the head of the ulna. It is located on the posterior/medial side of the wrist. Both styloid processes are superficial, and the tendons of the forearm muscles pass beside them.

Styloid process of the ulna

1. Shake hands with your partner. Passively adduct the wrist to soften the surrounding tendons.
2. Use your thumb to locate the posterior aspect of the ulnar head. Slide distally off the head to palpate the small tip of the styloid process (**3.21**).

Is the bone you are palpating connected to the ulnar head (as opposed to a separate carpal bone)? If you slowly flex and extend the wrist, does it remain stationary?

Head of the Radius

The head of the radius is distal to the humerus's lateral epicondyle. It forms the radius's proximal end and has a circular, bell shape. The head is stabilized by the annular ligament (p. 159) and is a pivoting point for supination and pronation of the forearm. Although it is deep to the supinator and extensor muscles, the head's posterior, lateral aspect can be accessed.

Head of the radius

1. Shake hands with your partner and locate the lateral epicondyle.
2. Slide distally off the lateral epicondyle, across the small ditch between the humerus and radius and onto the head of the radius (**3.22**).
3. The head of the radius is the only bony structure in this vicinity. Explore its ring-shaped, superficial surface.

*Are you distal to the lateral epicondyle? Place your thumb on the head and, with your other hand, slowly supinate and pronate the forearm (**3.23**). Do you feel the head's rotating movement under your thumb?*

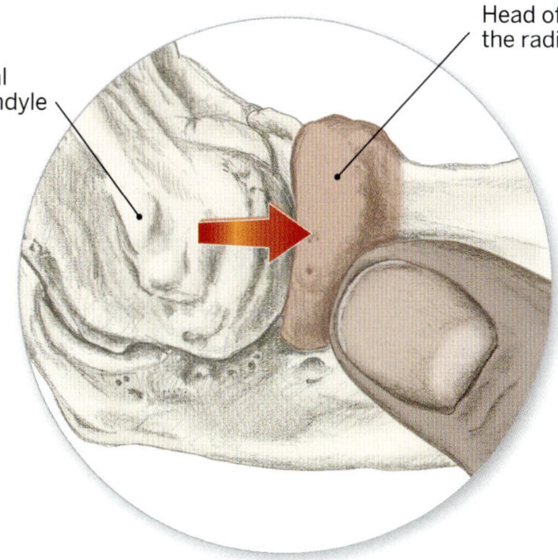

3.22 Lateral view of right elbow, as you explore the head of the radius

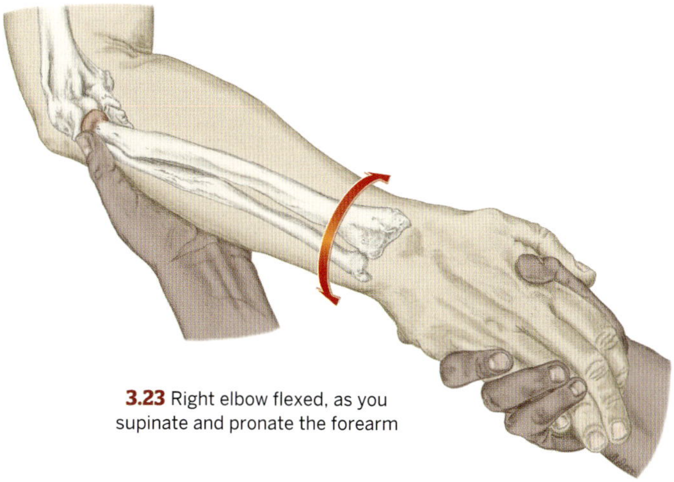

3.23 Right elbow flexed, as you supinate and pronate the forearm

Shaft of the Radius

The shaft of the radius is located on the lateral side (thumb side) of the forearm. Unlike the superficial edge of the ulnar shaft, most of the shaft of the radius is buried under muscle tissue. Its distal portion, however, is superficial and can be directly accessed.

Shaft of the radius

1. Flex the elbow to 90° and put the forearm in a neutral "handshake" position.
2. Locate the head of the radius. Slide distally off the head, noting how the radius sinks beneath the forearm muscles. Continue down the forearm and feel the radius become superficial near the wrist (**3.24**).
3. Along the distal forearm, explore all sides of the superficial shaft of the radius.

Is the bone you are palpating along the lateral side of the forearm? Place one hand on the radial shaft, while the other hand slowly supinates and pronates the forearm. Do you feel the shaft of the radius pivot around the shaft of the ulna?

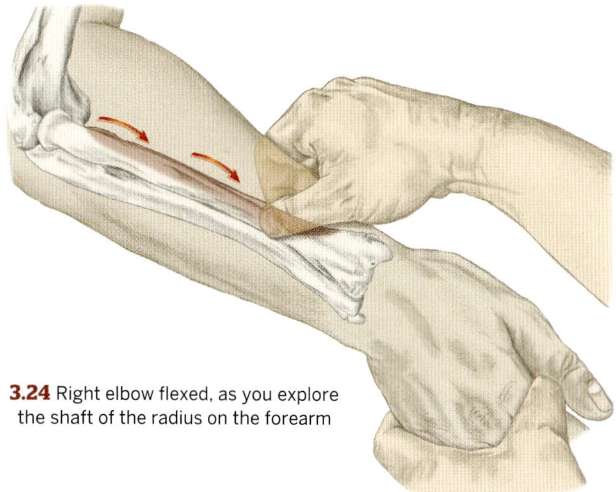

3.24 Right elbow flexed, as you explore the shaft of the radius on the forearm

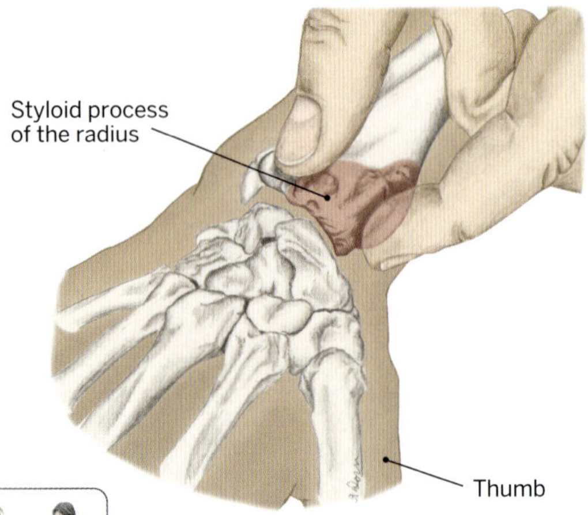

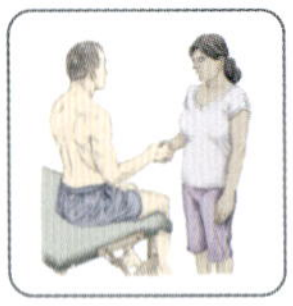

3.25 Dorsal/medial view of right wrist, as you palpate the styloid process of the radius

Styloid Process of the Radius

The styloid process of the radius, in comparison to the toothlike styloid process of the ulna, is a wider, more substantial mound of bone. Located on the lateral side of the radius, the styloid process is surrounded by the extensor tendons and is the attachment site for the brachioradialis (p. 131).

Styloid process of the radius

1. Begin by grasping the distal radial shaft between your thumb and finger. Slide distally, noting how the radius broadens in all directions.
2. Palpate along the lateral side (thumb side) of the radius to the tip of the styloid process (**3.25**).

Are you proximal to the flexor crease of the wrist? Is the portion of bone you are palpating surrounded by several thin tendons? If you passively flex and extend the wrist, the styloid process should remain stationary. Does it?

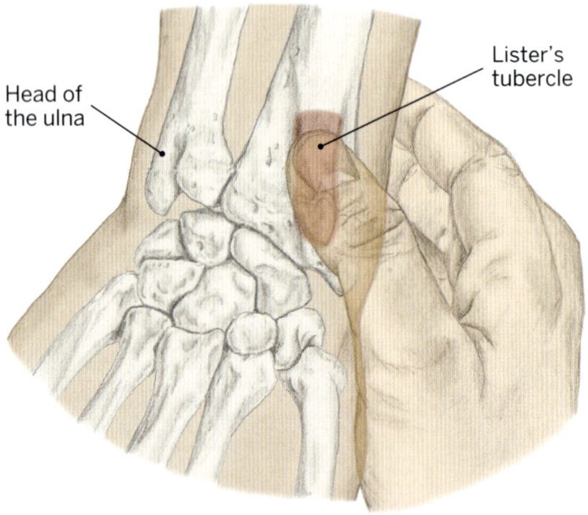

3.26 Dorsal view of right wrist, as you palpate Lister's tubercle

Lister's Tubercle

Named in honor of Joseph Lister, father of modern antiseptic surgery, this superficial knob is located on the dorsal surface of the radial styloid process. With its oblong shape, Lister's tubercle (also known as the dorsal tubercle) acts as a hook for the extensor pollicis longus tendon (p. 149). For our purposes, however, it will serve as a trail marker for finding two of the carpals—the lunate and capitate.

Lister's tubercle

1. Using your thumb, locate the dorsal surface of the styloid process of the radius.
2. Slide your thumb in the direction of the head of the ulna and explore for the oblong knob of Lister's tubercle.
3. The tubercle will be felt directly across from the head of the ulna—perhaps an inch away (**3.26**).

Are you on the dorsal surface of the radius? Is the bump you feel superficial, oval, and across from the head of the ulna? If you passively flex and extend the wrist, the tissue over the tubercle should move, yet the tubercle itself should stay stationary. Does it?

Palpation Plus

The styloid processes of the radius and ulna serve as important jumping-off points for locating the carpals. Locate both processes and determine if the radial styloid process extends farther distally than the ulnar. (It should.) Then explore just distal to the processes, noting how your fingers naturally sink into the tissue of the wrist. This is the general location of the proximal row of carpals.

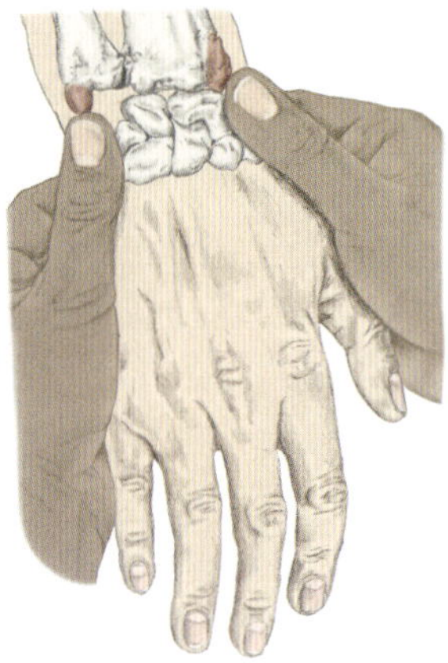

styloid *sti*-loyd Grk. a pillar

Carpals

There are eight carpal bones located at the wrist (**3.27**, **3.28**). Small and uniquely shaped, the carpals are closely wedged together between the distal radius and ulna and the metacarpals. The carpals form two rows, each composed of four bones (**3.29**).

Located distal to the flexor crease at the wrist, under the heel of the hand, the carpals lie deep to numerous flexor and extensor tendons. These overlying tendons, combined with the carpals' compact arrangement, make isolating individual bones a challenge.

The next few pages present the carpals in pairs. We will begin by exploring the carpals as one large group. We will then access the pisiform, triquetrum, and the hamate, as these are possibly the easiest to isolate.

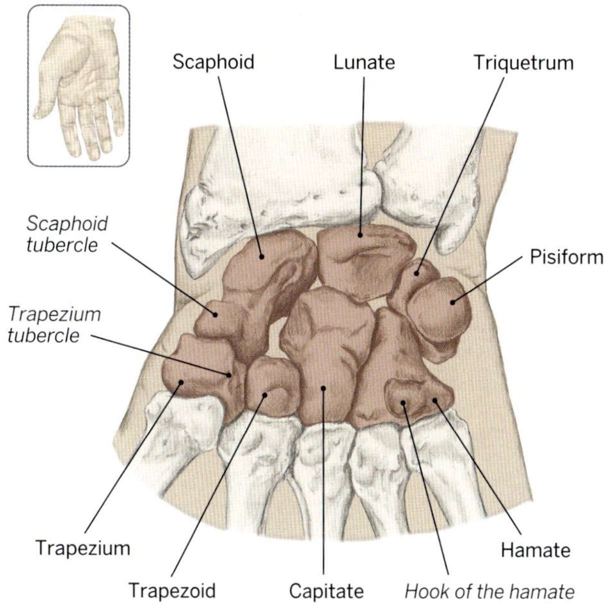

3.27 Palmar view of right wrist

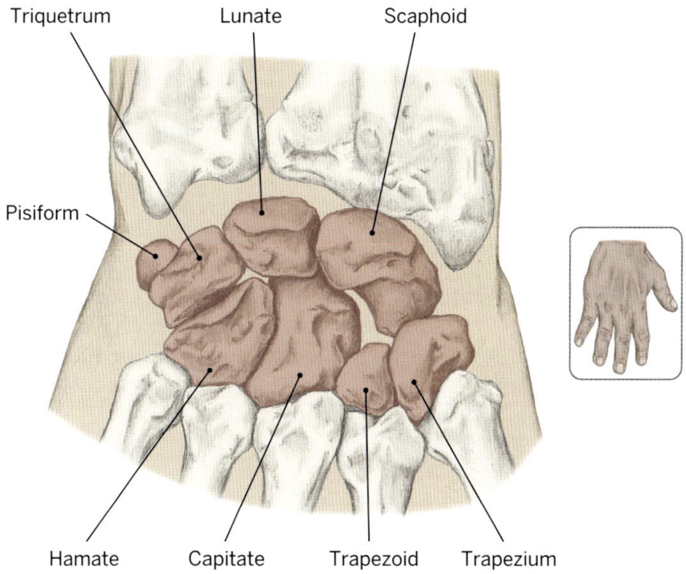

3.28 Dorsal view of right wrist

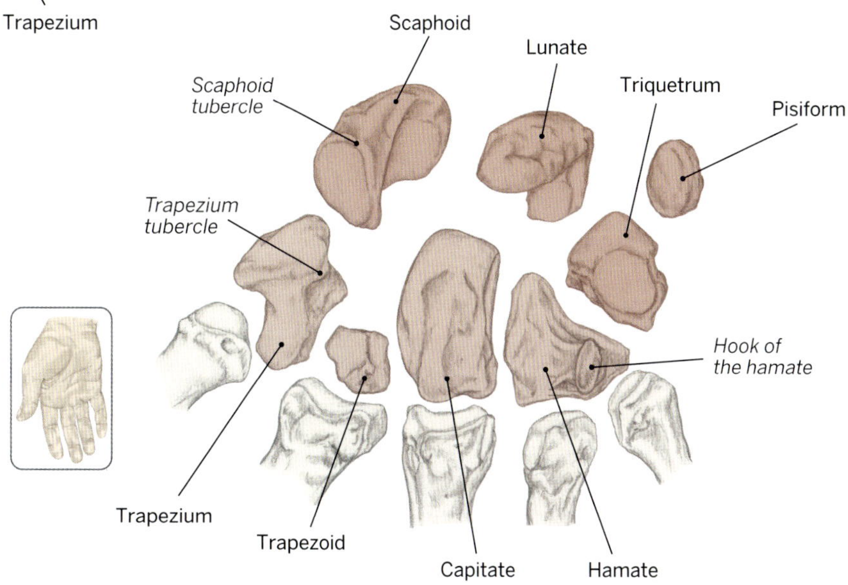

3.29 Palmar view of right hand, showing the expanded carpals. The scaphoid, lunate, triquetrum, and pisiform form the proximal row, while the trapezium, trapezoid, capitate, and hamate make up the distal row.

carpal *kar*-pul
metacarpal *met*-a-*kar*-pul

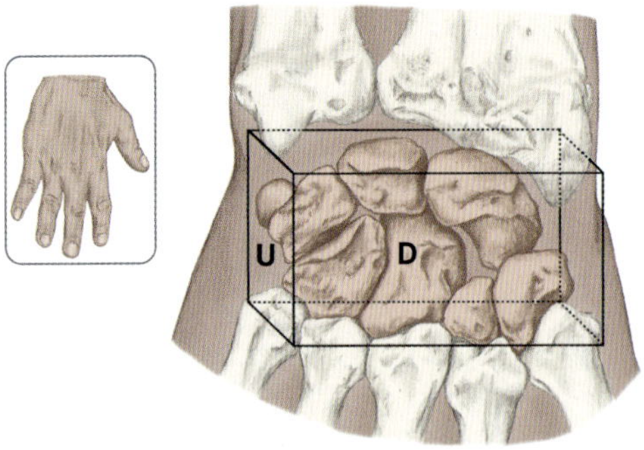

Ulnar/dorsal view of right wrist

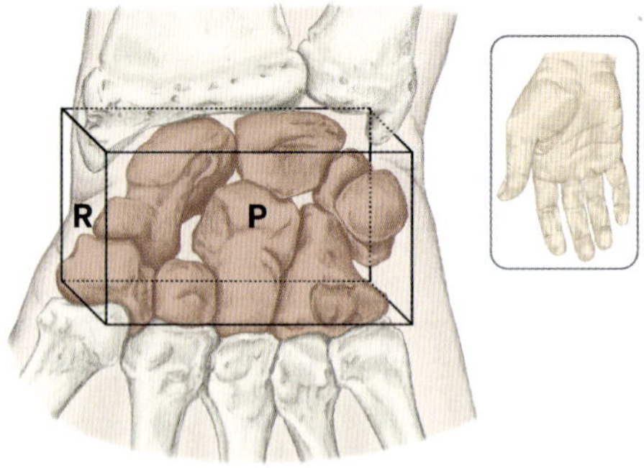

Radial/palmar view of right wrist

3.30 Luckily, the wrist has four surfaces from which to explore—the **P**almar, **D**orsal, **R**adial, and **U**lnar sides. Some carpals are accessible from one side of the wrist, while others can be explored from a few sides. In any case, exploring all of the wrist's surfaces will allow you to feel at least a portion of each carpal.

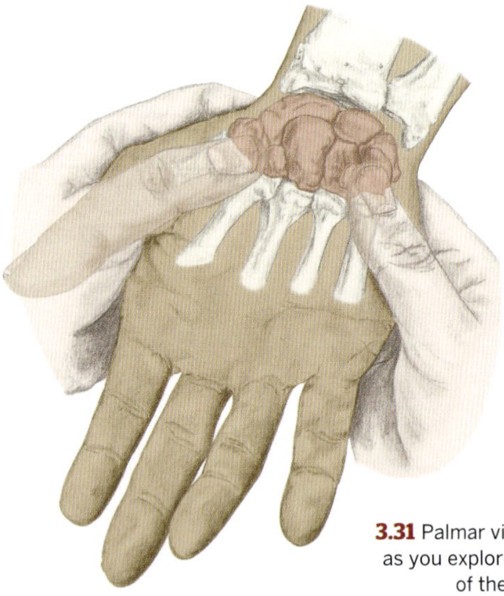

3.31 Palmar view of right hand, as you explore the movement of the carpals

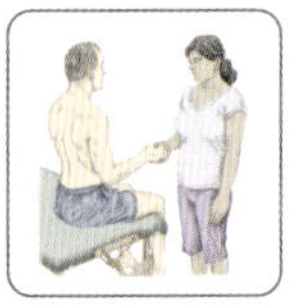

Carpals as a group

1. Position the hand with the palm up and locate the styloid processes of the ulna and radius.
2. Sliding just distal from the styloid processes, explore the palmar surface for the carpals.
3. Rest your thumbpads on the heel of the hand and then passively move the wrist in all directions (**3.31**). Note how the carpals shift and undulate slightly, like small stones in a pouch. Turn the hand over and explore the dorsal surface (**3.32**).

Are you distal to the wrist's flexor crease? When the wrist is flexed, can you sense how the carpals press into the palm of the hand? When the wrist is extended, can you feel the carpals shift and become more prominent on the hand's dorsal surface?

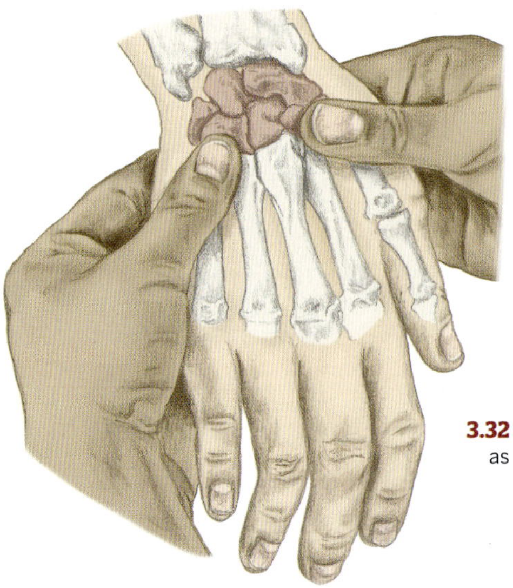

3.32 Dorsal view of right hand, as you explore the carpals

Pisiform

The knobby pisiform is an attachment site for the flexor carpi ulnaris (p. 138). Protruding along the ulnar/palmar surface of the wrist, the pisiform is just distal to the flexor crease.

Pisiform

1. Locate the flexor crease of your partner's wrist. Then slide over to the pinkie side of the crease.
2. Move slightly distal to the crease, rolling your thumbpad in small circles. Explore under the thick tissue of the palm for the nugget-like pisiform (**3.33**).

*Passively flex the wrist and notice how the pisiform can be wiggled from side to side (**3.34**). Extend the wrist and observe how it becomes immobile. (This immobility is due to the tension created by the flexor carpi ulnaris tendon.) Then ask your partner to actively adduct her wrist. Can you feel the tendon of flexor carpi ulnaris as it comes down the medial wrist and attaches to the pisiform?*

Triquetrum

This pyramid-shaped bone is located on the dorsal surface of the pisiform, just distal to the styloid process of the ulna. In a neutral position, only the dorsal surface of the triquetrum is palpable; however, abduction shifts the triquetrum so it is accessible on the wrist's ulnar surface.

Triquetrum

1. With the palm of your partner's hand facing away from you, locate the styloid process of the ulna. Slide distally, noting a slender ditch, before rising to the surface of the triquetrum (**3.35**).
2. Keeping your finger stationary, abduct the wrist and note how the triqetrum protrudes to the side (**3.36**). Adduct and feel the bone disappear back into the wrist.

During abduction and adduction, do you feel the triquetrum protrude and then disappear? Locate the pisiform on the wrist's palmar surface. Can you locate the triquetrum by beginning at the pisiform and slowly sliding around to the ulnar side of the wrist?

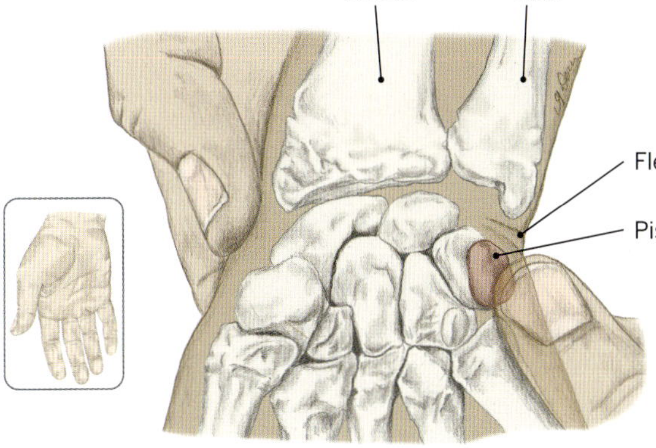

3.33 Palmar surface of right hand, as you locate the pisiform

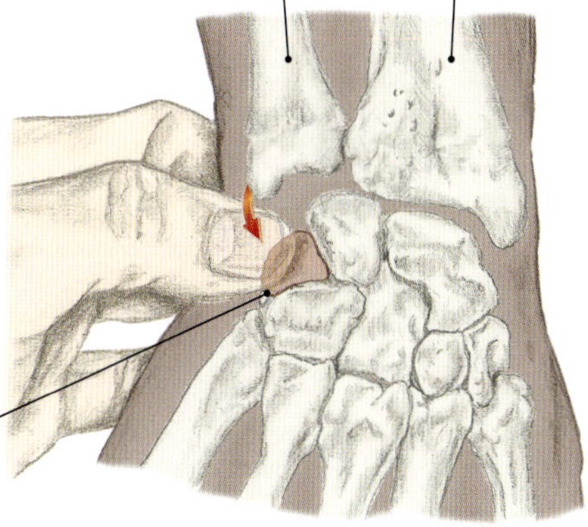

3.35 Dorsal view of right hand with wrist in neutral, as you access the triquetrum

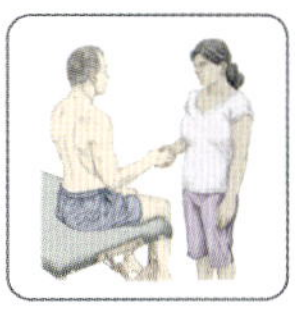

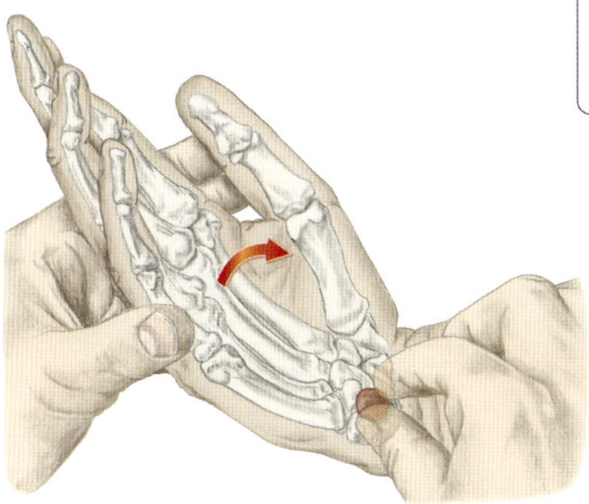

3.34 Ulnar view of right hand, as you isolate the pisiform

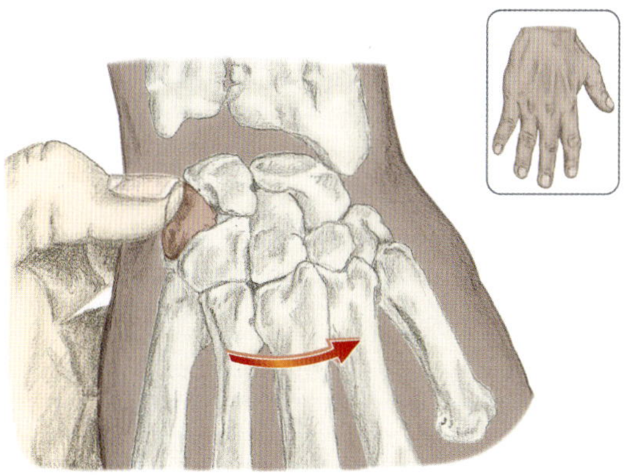

3.36 Dorsal view of right hand with wrist abducted, as you palpate the triquetrum

pisiform ***pi***-si-form
triquetrum tri-***kwe***-trum

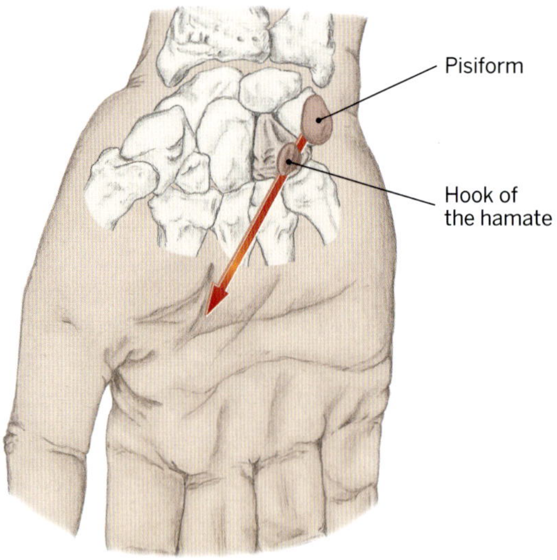

3.37 Palmar view of right hand, indicating an imaginary line from the pisiform toward the index finger

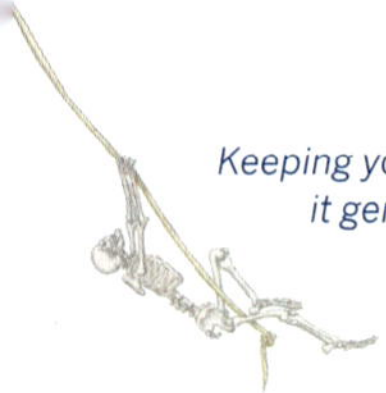

Keeping your thumbpad in place and rolling it gently around the hook will give you the best sense of its shape and locale!

Hamate

Located distal to the pisiform, the hamate has a small protuberance or "hook" that is palpable on the hand's palmar surface. The pisiform and the hook of the hamate serve as medial attachment sites for the flexor retinaculum, the connective tissue band that forms the "roof" of the carpal tunnel. The flat surface of the hamate's body is accessible on the hand's dorsal surface where the bases of the fourth and fifth metacarpals merge. When palpated, the hook is often tender.

Hamate

1. Locate your partner's pisiform. Draw an imaginary line from the pisiform to the base of the index finger (**3.37**).
2. Using your thumbpad, slide off the pisiform along this line. Approximately half of an inch from the pisiform, explore for this subtle mound beneath the padding of the hand (**3.38**).

Are you between the pisiform and the base of the index finger? Using gentle pressure, can you sense a small ditch between the pisiform and the hook of the hamate?

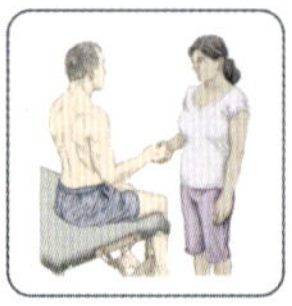

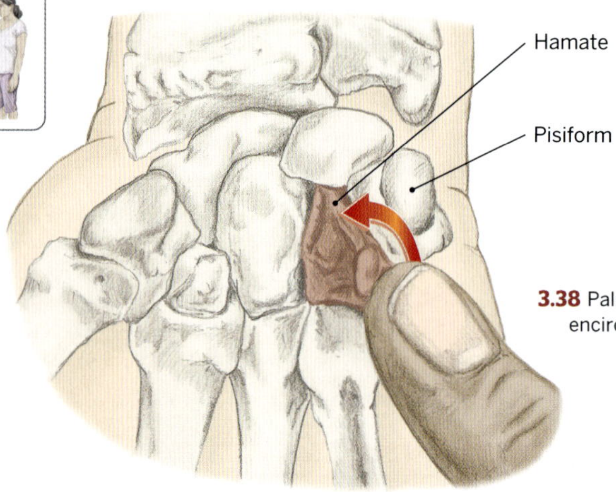

3.38 Palmar view of right wrist, as you encircle the hook of the hamate

Discover More

The pisiform and hook of the hamate form a small channel called the Tunnel of Guyon. The ulnar nerve and artery pass through this canal, under shelter of its roof—the pisohamate ligament (p. 163). The ulnar nerve is particularly vulnerable in the vicinity of the Tunnel of Guyon to compression injuries. Activities such as repeated use of a pneumatic jackhammer or leaning on the handlebars during long-distance bicycling can put chronic pressure on the nerve.

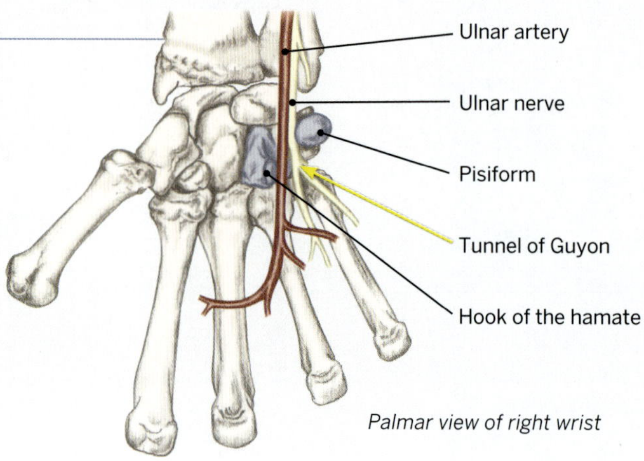

Palmar view of right wrist

hamate *ham*-ate

Scaphoid

The peanut-shaped scaphoid (or navicular) is the most commonly fractured carpal. It is located on the radial side of the hand, distal to the styloid process of the radius. Although the scaphoid forms the floor of the tendinous "anatomical snuffbox" (p. 151), it is still accessible from the dorsal, palmar, and radial sides of the wrist.

Scaphoid

1. Beginning on the wrist's radial surface, locate the radius's styloid process. Slide your thumb distally off the process, falling between the superficial tendons and into the natural ditch where the scaphoid will be found (**3.39**).
2. Maintain your position and passively adduct the wrist. As you do so, feel for the scaphoid to bulge into your thumb (**3.40**). Now abduct the wrist and feel how the scaphoid disappears back into the wrist.
3. From here, explore the scaphoid's dorsal and palmar surfaces. On the palmar surface, along the flexor crease, is the scaphoid tubercle (p. 122).

Are you distal to the end of the styloid process of the radius? During adduction and abduction, do you feel the scaphoid protrude and then disappear?

Trapezium

Located distal to the scaphoid, the small trapezium articulates with the base of the first metacarpal. This articulation, the first carpometacarpal joint, is the source of the thumb's unique movements.

The trapezium is most accessible on its radial or dorsal side and can be isolated either distally from the scaphoid or proximally from the first metacarpal.

Trapezium

1. Palpating along the hand's radial/dorsal side, locate the scaphoid. Then slide distally (**3.41**).
2. You might, by accident, pass the trapezium and ride up onto the base of the first metacarpal. If so, simply slide back proximally to the trapezium.

To check if you are indeed feeling the base of the first metacarpal instead of the trapezium, ask your partner to slowly flex and extend his thumb. With this action, the base of the first metacarpal should clearly move. To check for the trapezium: Are you distal to the scaphoid and proximal to the base of the first metacarpal?

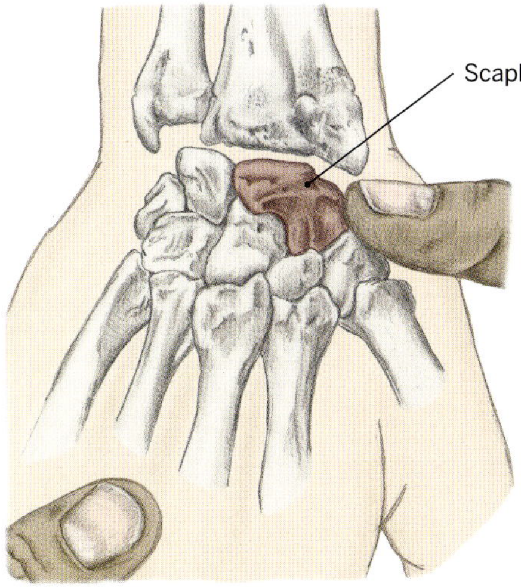

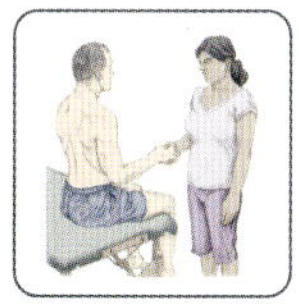

3.39 Dorsal view of right hand with wrist in neutral, as you locate the scaphoid

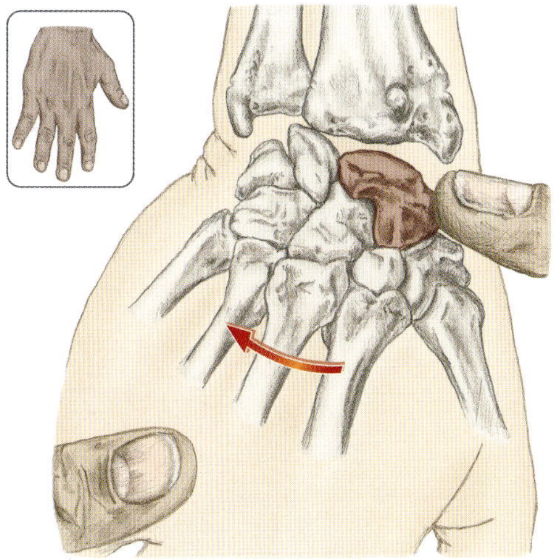

3.40 Dorsal view of right hand with wrist adducted, as you palpate the scaphoid

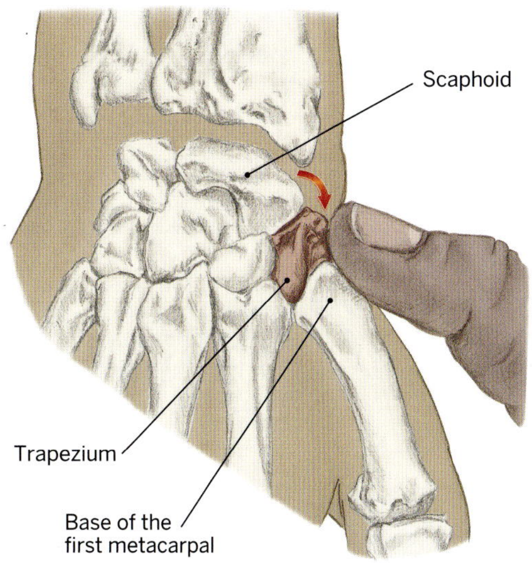

3.41 Dorsal view of right hand, as you locate the trapezium

trapezium tra-***pee***-ze-um
scaphoid ***skaf***-oyd

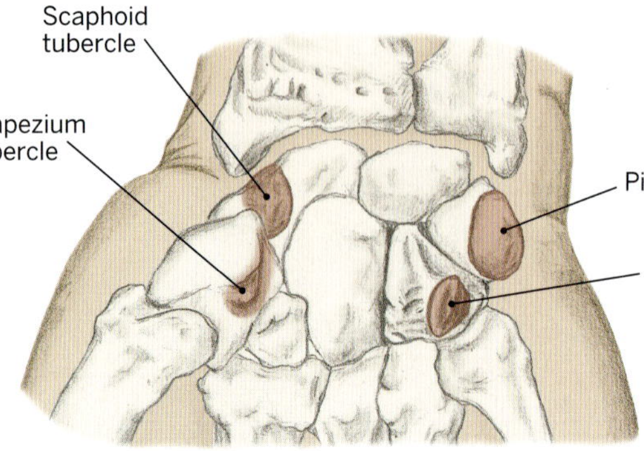

3.42 Palmar view of right wrist, showing the four attachment sites of the flexor retinaculum

Scaphoid and Trapezium Tubercles

The scaphoid and trapezium tubercles serve as lateral attachment sites for the flexor retinaculum (p. 161), the connective tissue band that forms the "roof" of the carpal tunnel (**3.42**). Both tubercles are located on the palmar surface of the wrist, near the flexor crease. Oftentimes, the tubercles are situated so closely to each other that they are difficult to distinguish individually. The two, however, are palpable, either separately or together.

Scaphoid and trapezium tubercles

1. Locate the radial surface of the scaphoid, along the flexor crease. Then walk your thumb around to the palmar side of the scaphoid.
2. Using your thumbpad, explore just distal to the flexor crease for a prominent, bony knob (**3.43**).
3. Flex the wrist slightly to soften the surrounding tissue (**3.44**).

Are you distal to the end of the styloid process of the radius?

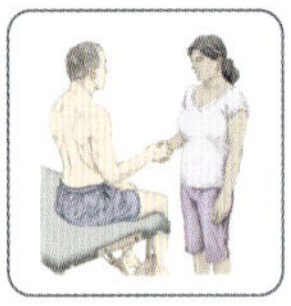

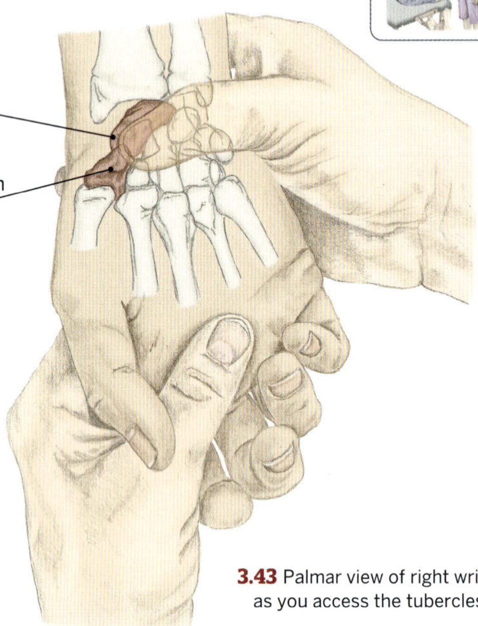

3.43 Palmar view of right wrist, as you access the tubercles

Comparative Anatomy

The pisiform is much larger on quadrupeds such as dogs (right), on whom it protrudes posteriorly above the heel of the front paw. This arrangement allows the flexor carpi ulnaris muscle that attaches to the pisiform greater leverage and power to flex the wrist when running on all fours. A human's pisiform is only a pea-sized knob. It is, nevertheless, still useful for kneading bread dough.

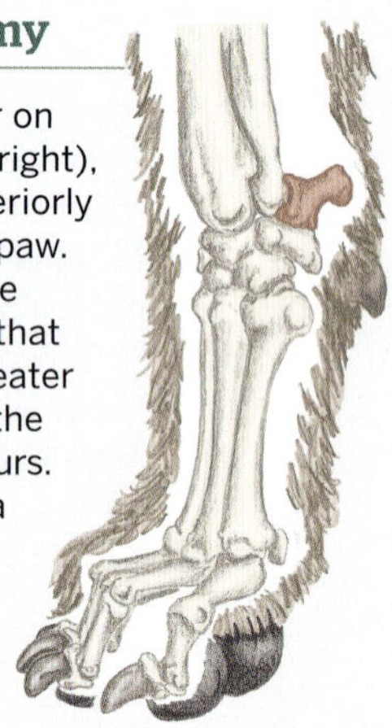

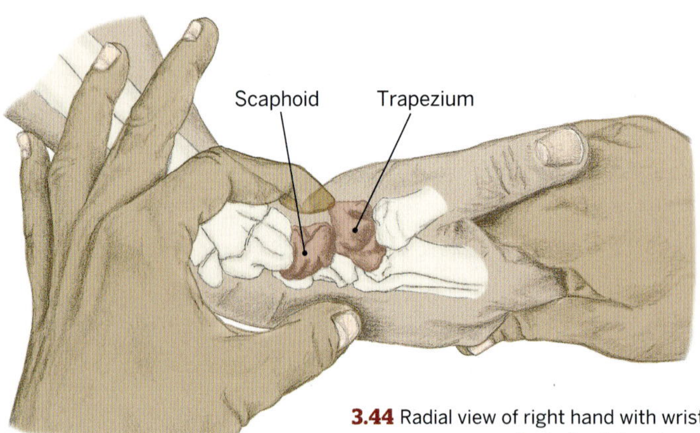

3.44 Radial view of right hand with wrist flexed, as you palpate the tubercles

Lunate and Capitate

The **lunate** is the most frequently dislocated carpal. Located distal and medial to Lister's tubercle (p. 116), it is relatively inaccessible when the wrist is in a neutral position; flexing the wrist, however, will slide the lunate to the dorsal surface.

The **capitate** is the largest of the carpals and is located distal to the lunate. It has a shallow ditch on its dorsal surface that can be easily palpated.

Although the lunate and capitate lie deep to the extensor tendons, both carpals are accessible on their dorsal surfaces and can be isolated between Lister's tubercle and the shaft of the third metacarpal (**3.45**).

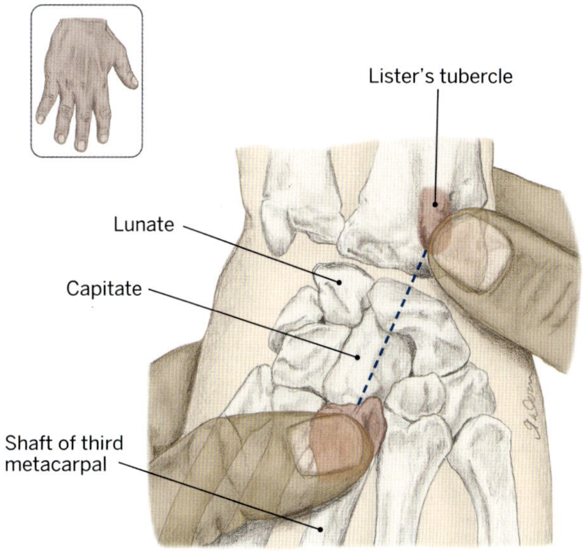

3.45 Dorsal view of right wrist. With the wrist in neutral, draw an imaginary line between Lister's tubercle and the base of the third metacarpal, marking out the location of the capitate.

Lunate and capitate

1. Locate Lister's tubercle and the base of the third metacarpal. With the wrist slightly extended, lay your thumb between these points and notice how it falls into a small cavity. This is the location of the lunate and capitate (**3.46**).
2. Set your thumb at the proximal end of this cavity. Then flex the wrist and feel the lunate press into your finger (**3.47**). Next, extend the wrist and feel this carpal disappear back into the wrist.
3. Shift your thumb to the distal end of the cavity and notice how it bumps into the base of the third metacarpal. Passively flex the wrist, noting how the capitate rolls into your finger, "filling" its own cavity.

Are you between Lister's tubercle and the shaft of the third metacarpal? When isolating the lunate, are you distal and lateral to the edge of Lister's tubercle? Do you feel a small knob press into your thumb upon flexion?

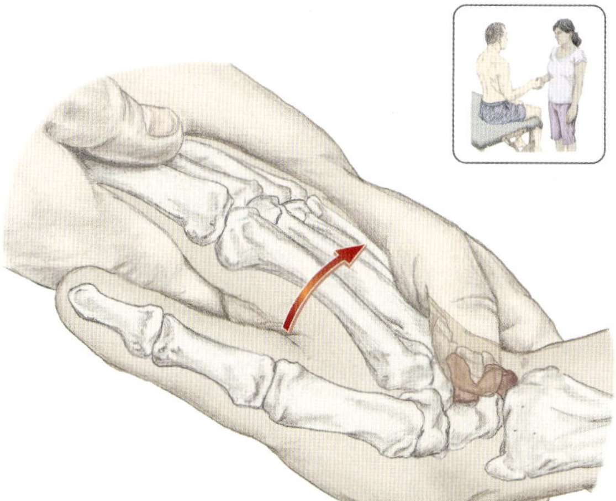

3.46 Radial view of right hand with wrist extended, as you locate the lunate and capitate

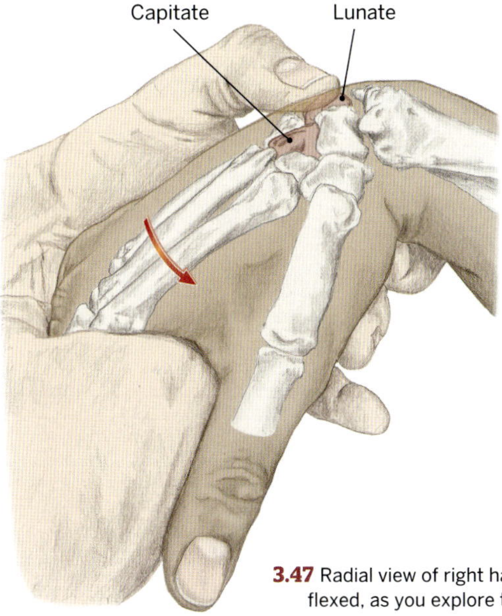

3.47 Radial view of right hand with wrist flexed, as you explore the lunate

capitate *kap*-i-tate L. head-shaped
lunate *lu*-nate L. crescent-shaped

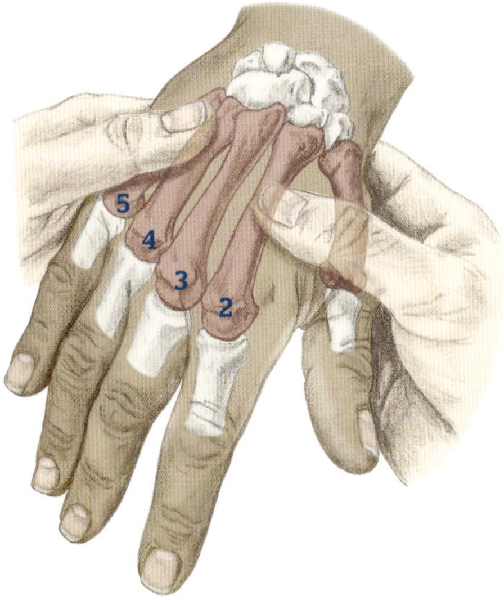

3.48 Notice how the fourth and fifth metacarpals allow for more movement between them than the second and third metacarpals

Metacarpals and phalanges

The fingers contain no muscles, only the tendons of the digitorum muscles and strong ligaments that hold together the phalanges of each finger.

1. Palpate the dorsal surface of your partner's hand and feel the superficial metacarpal shafts. Explore the space between the metacarpals for the interossei muscles (p. 155). Then gently undulate the metacarpals up and down (**3.48**).
2. Turn the hand over, and explore the metacarpals and phalanges from the palmar surface, noting how they lie deep to the tissues of the palm (**3.49**).
3. Move distally and explore where the heads of the metacarpals join with the phalanges to form the large metacarpophalangeal (knuckle) joints (**3.50**). Passively flex a metacarpophalangeal joint and distinguish between the head of the metacarpal and the base of the proximal phalange.
4. Move distally to the phalanges and isolate the slender tendons, ligaments, and connective tissue of the fingers. Also note the absence of any muscle tissue.

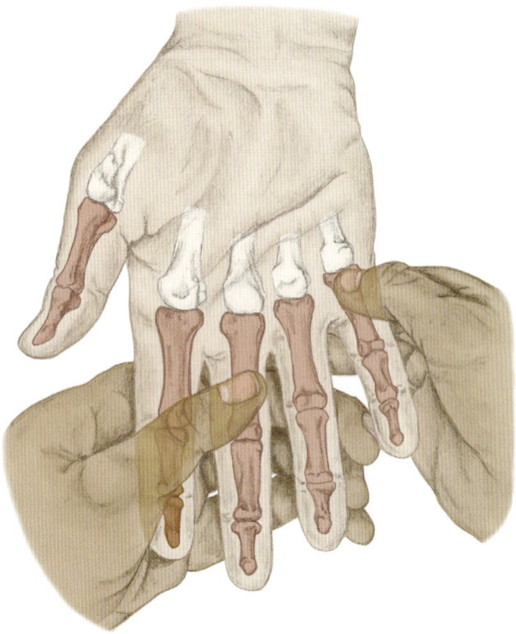

3.49 Palmar view of right hand, as you explore the metacarpals and phalanges

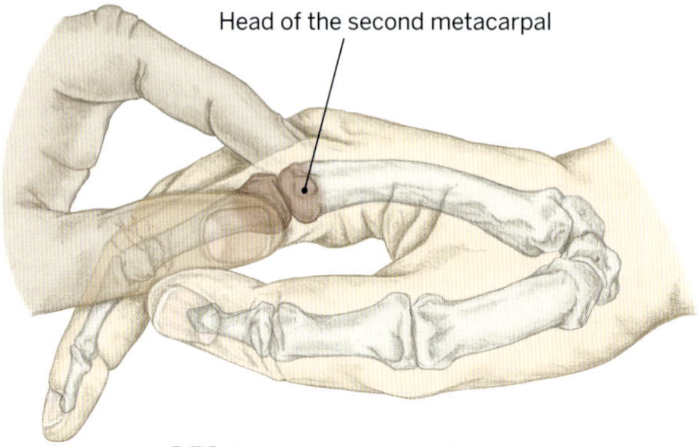

3.50 Radial view of second finger, as you explore the knuckle joints

Palpation Plus

To locate the carpometacarpal joints (right), ask your partner to flex her fingers and wrist. Roughly an inch or two distal to the extensor crease at the wrist will be a series of bumps across the dorsal surface of the hand. These bumps are the bases of the metacarpals, which articulate with the carpals to form the carpometacarpal joints.

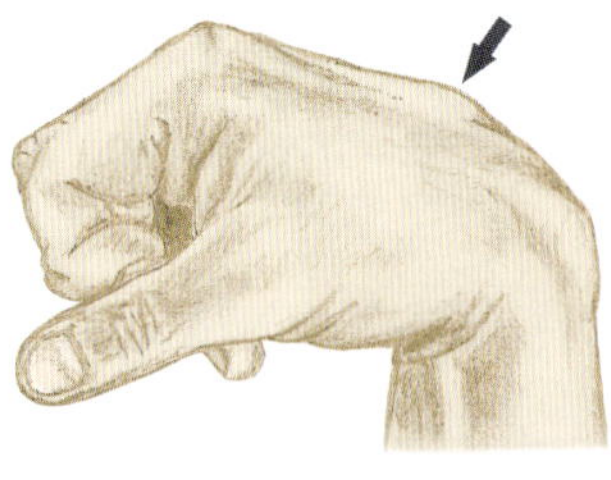

metacarpophalangeal ***met***-a-***kar***-po-***fa***-lan-***jee***-al

Overview: **Muscles of the Forearm and Hand**

The muscles of the forearm primarily create movement at the wrist and fingers (**3.51–3.56**). Many have small, fusiform bellies that connect to space-efficient tendons in the lower forearm. These tendons extend distally into the wrist, hand, and fingers. The crowded muscle bellies and tendons of the forearm can be challenging to isolate. To simplify matters, the muscles of this chapter have been arranged into four primary groups:

a. Muscles that act primarily at the **elbow**:
   Brachialis
   Brachioradialis

b. Muscles that move the **wrist and/or fingers** (*carpi*, *digitorum*, or *palmaris* muscles). This group can be further subdivided into four smaller groups:
   Extensors of the wrist and fingers
   Flexors of the wrist and fingers
   Adductors of the wrist
   Abductors of the wrist

   (Some muscles that act upon the wrist can actually move it in two directions. Flexor carpi ulnaris, for example, both flexes and adducts the wrist.)

c. Muscles that create the pivoting action between the **radius and ulna**:
   Pronator teres
   Pronator quadratus
   Supinator

d. Short and long muscles that maneuver the **thumb** (*pollicis* muscles).

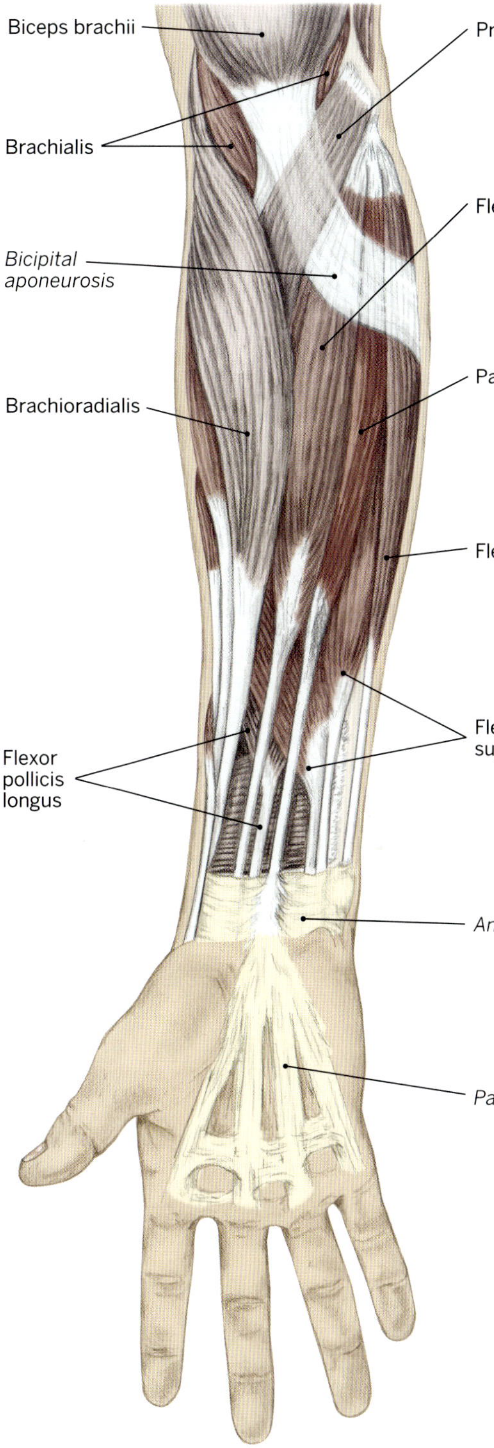

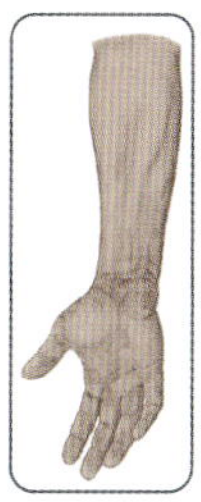

3.51 Anterior view of muscles of right forearm and hand, skin removed from palm of hand

Discover More

Distinguishing between **abduction** (left) and **adduction** (right) of the wrist can be confusing if the forearm is pronated or supinated. For instance, if you pronate your forearm (palm toward the floor) and then adduct at the wrist, your hand will move away from the centerline of your body and it will appear as though you have abducted your wrist. Not so: Both adduction and abduction remain the same regardless of the forearm's position.

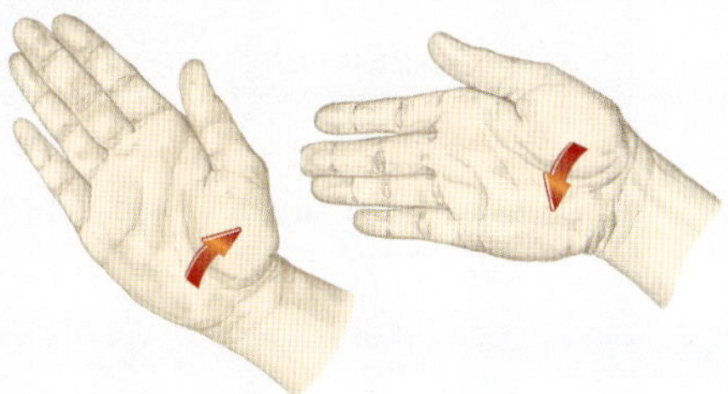

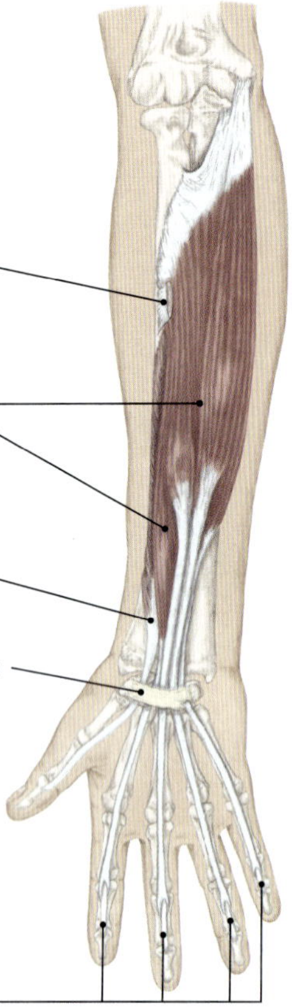

3.52 Anterior view of right forearm and hand, showing intermediate layer of muscles

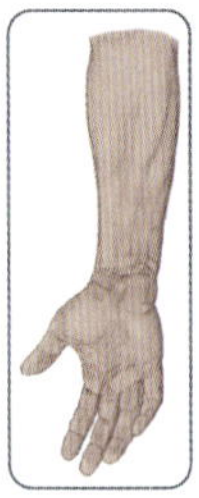

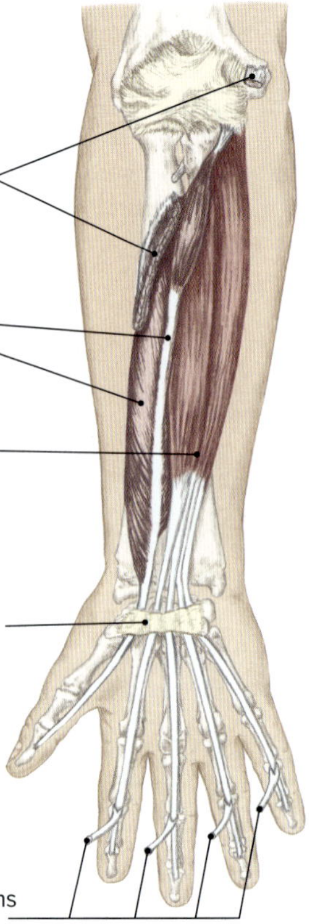

3.53 Anterior view of right forearm and hand, showing deep layer of muscles

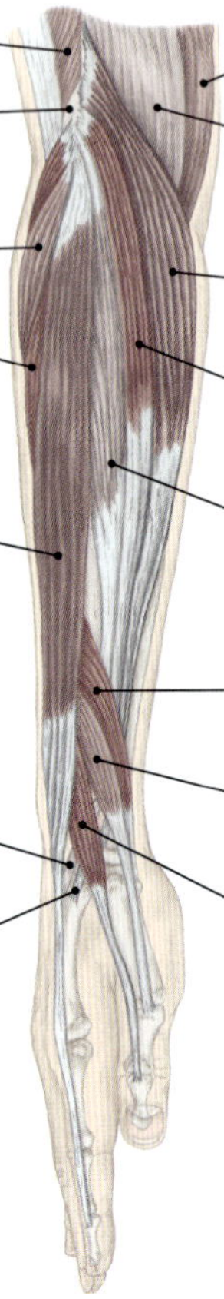

3.54 Lateral view of muscles of right forearm

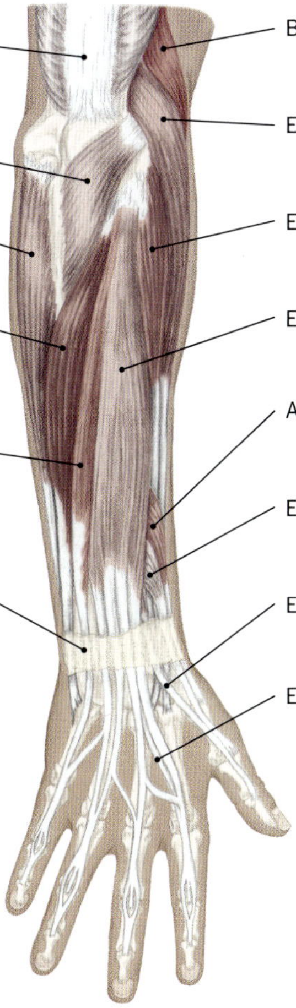

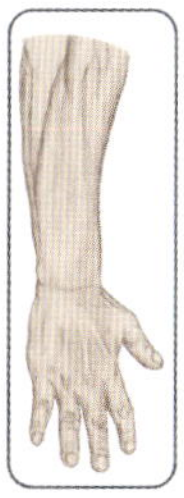

3.55 Posterior view of right forearm and hand, showing superficial layer of muscles

Discover More

The names of the forearm muscles can be a mouthful. Nevertheless, these same names can be very helpful when it comes to understanding a muscle's function, location, and more. Take, for example, the muscle **extensor carpi radialis longus**. What does its name reveal?

1. It is specified as an *extensor*, so it extends. This also indicates that there is a *flexor* carpi radialis.
2. *Carpi* means it extends the carpals (wrist joint). This indicates there is also a different muscle that moves the *digits*—extensor digitorum.
3. It runs along the *radial* side of the forearm. This indicates that there is also an extensor carpi ulnaris on the *ulnar* side.
4. If there is a *longus*, there must also be a *brevis*—extensor carpi radialis brevis.

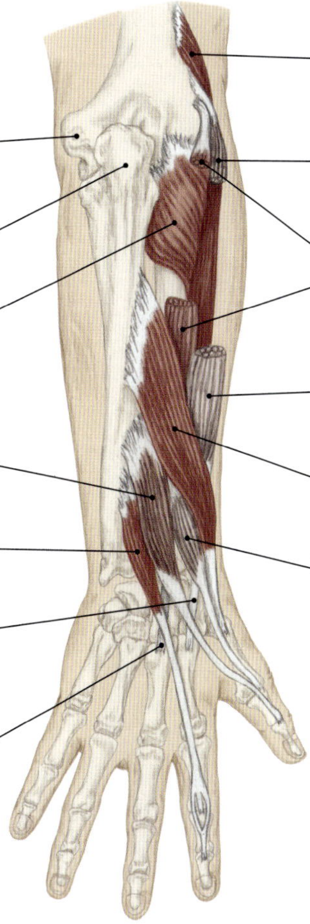

3.56 Posterior view of right forearm and hand, showing deep layer of muscles

Discover More

The next time a hooligan threatens to punch you in the schnoz, catch him off guard by inquiring, "Will you deliver that blow with your *extrinsic* or *intrinsic* muscles?" The long muscles with bellies in the forearm are the extrinsics, while the short muscles with bellies in the body of the hand are the intrinsics (p. 155). While the ruffian ponders your query (the correct answer would be "both"), you will have hopefully used the extrinsic and intrinsic muscles of your legs and feet—the same relationship applies—to tiptoe away.

extrinsic L. without
intrinsic L. within

Synergists—Muscles Working Together

Muscles are listed in the order of their ability to create the movement. Asterisk indicates muscles not shown.

Elbow

(humeroulnar and humeroradial joints)

Flexion

(antagonists on extension)

Biceps brachii
Brachialis
Brachioradialis
Flexor carpi radialis (assists)
Flexor carpi ulnaris (assists)
Palmaris longus (assists)
Pronator teres (assists)
Extensor carpi radialis longus (assists)*
Extensor carpi radialis brevis (assists)*

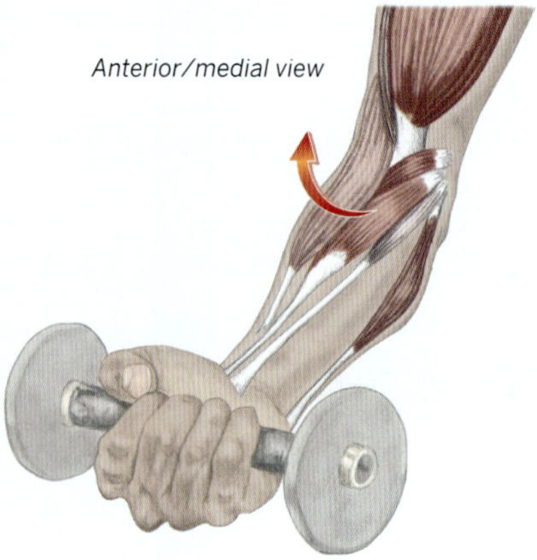

3.57 Flexion of the elbow

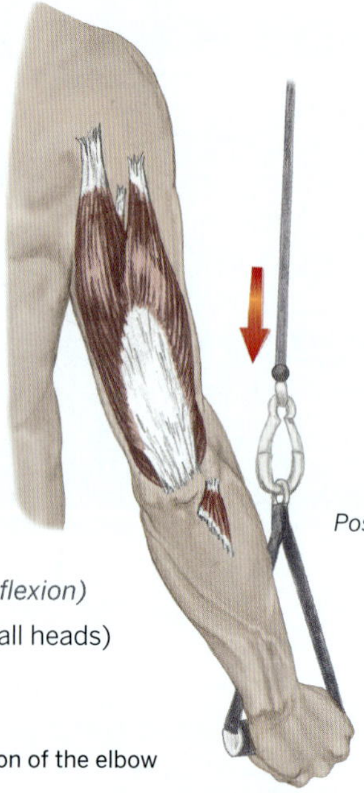

Extension

(antagonists on flexion)

Triceps brachii (all heads)
Anconeus

3.58 Extension of the elbow

Forearm

(proximal and distal radioulnar joints)

Supination

(antagonists on pronation)

Biceps brachii
Supinator
Brachioradialis (assists)

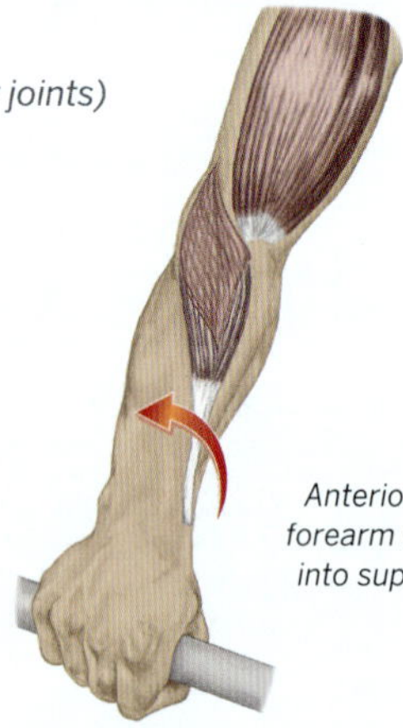

3.59 Supination of the forearm

Pronation

(antagonists on supination)

Pronator teres
Pronator quadratus
Brachioradialis (assists)

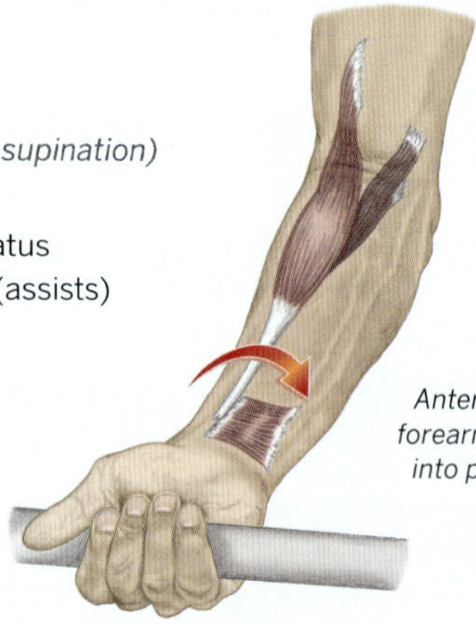

3.60 Pronation of the forearm

Wrist

(radiocarpal joint)

Extension

(antagonists on flexion)

Extensor carpi radialis longus
Extensor carpi radialis brevis
Extensor carpi ulnaris
Extensor digitorum (assists)
Extensor indicis (assists)

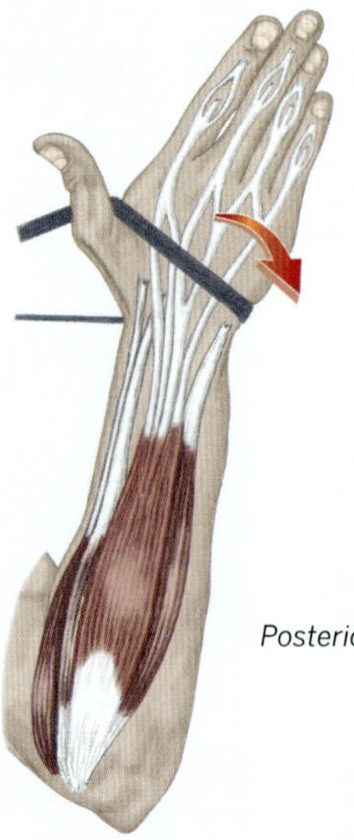

3.61 Extension of the wrist

Flexion

(antagonists on extension)

Flexor carpi radialis
Flexor carpi ulnaris
Palmaris longus
Flexor digitorum superficialis
Flexor digitorum profundus (assists)*
Flexor pollicis longus (assists)*

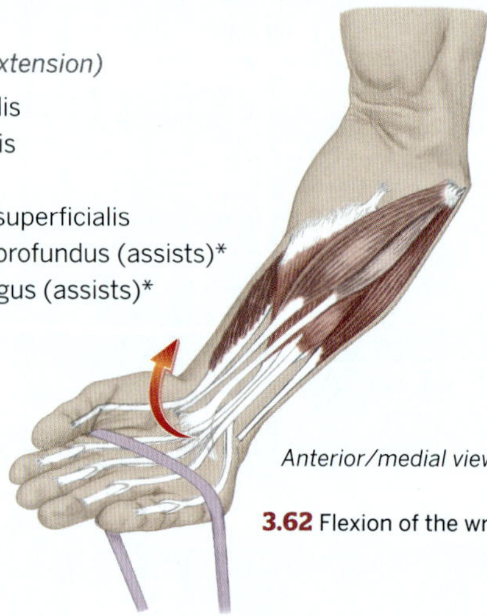

3.62 Flexion of the wrist

Wrist

(radiocarpal joint)

Abduction (radial deviation)

(antagonists on adduction)

Extensor carpi radialis longus
Extensor carpi radialis brevis
Extensor pollicis longus
Extensor pollicis brevis
Flexor carpi radialis
Abductor pollicis longus

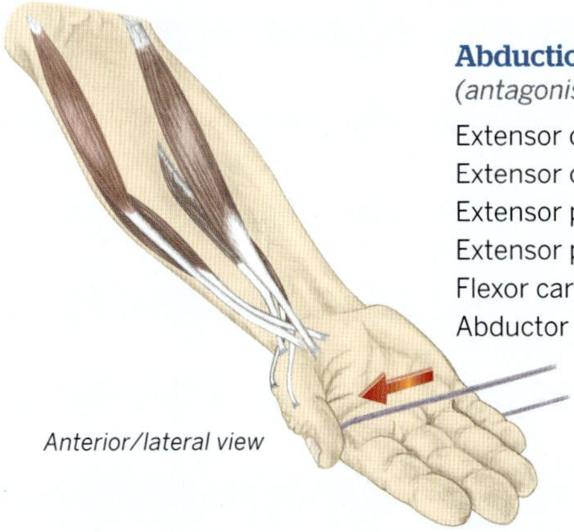

3.63 Abduction (radial deviation) of the wrist

Adduction (ulnar deviation)

(antagonists on abduction)

Extensor carpi ulnaris
Flexor carpi ulnaris

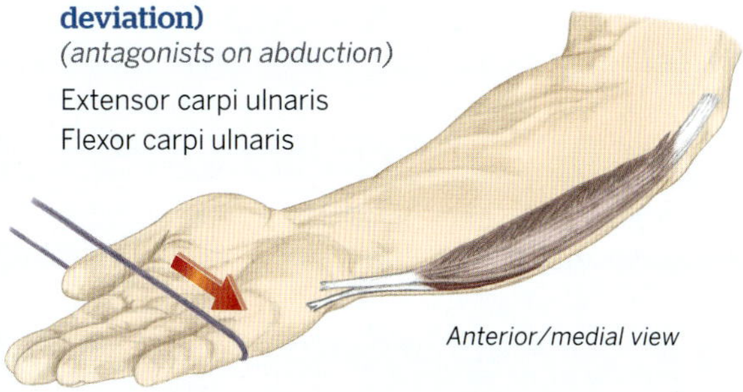

3.64 Adduction (ulnar deviation) of the wrist

Hand and Fingers

(metacarpophalangeal, proximal and distal interphalangeal joints)

Extension of the Second through Fifth Fingers

(antagonists on flexion)

Extensor digitorum
Lumbricals
Dorsal interossei
(2nd–4th, assists)
Palmar interossei
(2nd, 4th, 5th, assists)
Extensor indicis (2nd)*

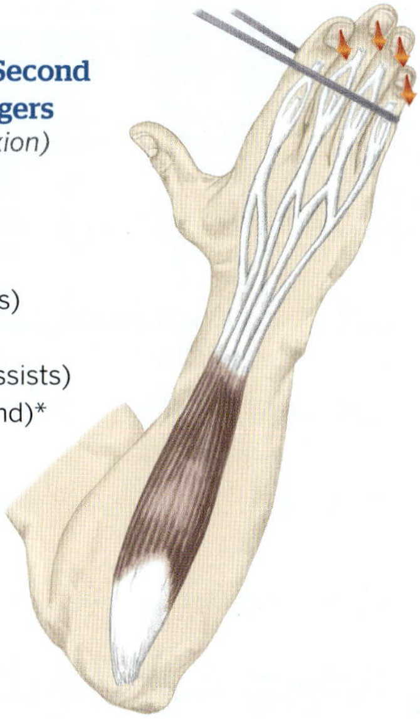

3.65 Extension of the second through fifth fingers

Flexion of the Second through Fifth Fingers

(antagonists on extension)

Flexor digitorum superficialis
Flexor digitorum profundus
Flexor digiti minimi brevis (5th)*
Lumbricals
Dorsal interossei (2nd–4th, assists)
Palmar interossei (2nd, 4th, 5th, assists)

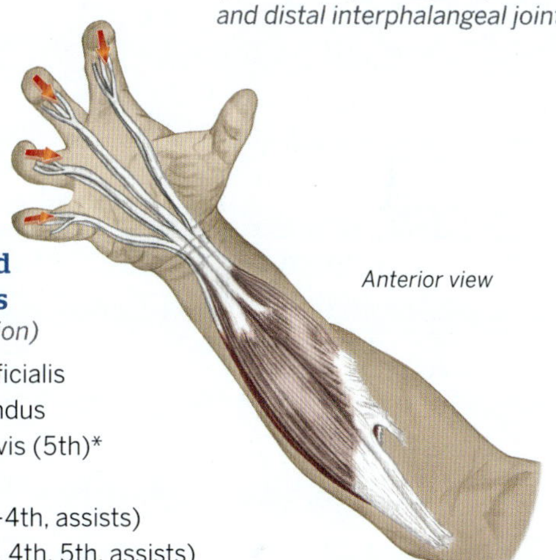

3.66 Flexion of the second through fifth fingers

Thumb

(first carpometacarpal and metacarpophalangeal joints)

Flexion

(antagonists on extension)

Flexor pollicis longus
Flexor pollicis brevis*
Adductor pollicis (assists)
Palmar interossei (1st, assists)*

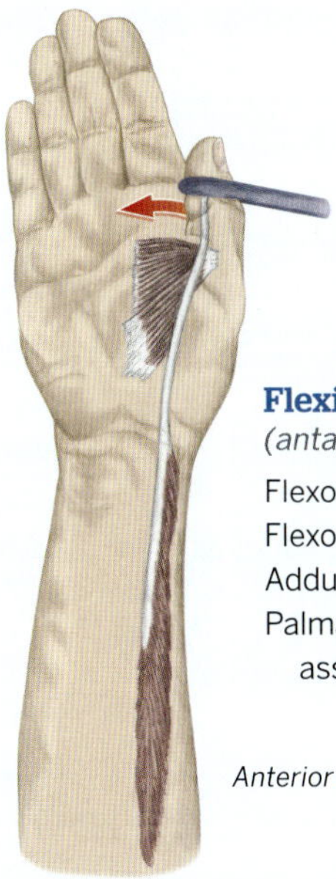

3.67 Flexion of the thumb

Opposition

Opponens pollicis
Flexor pollicis brevis (assists)*
Abductor pollicis brevis (assists)*

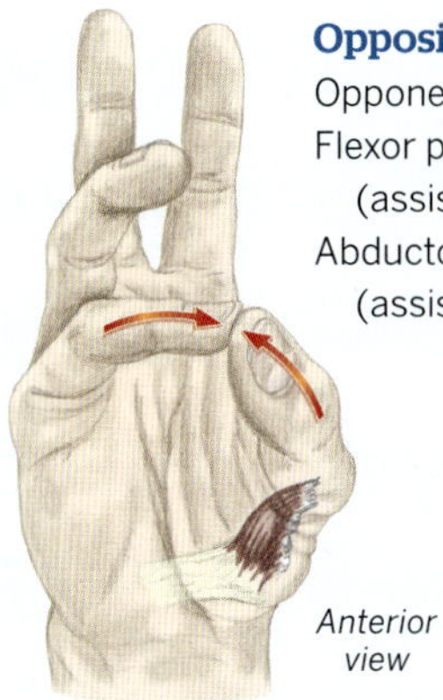

3.68 Opposition of the thumb

Extension

(antagonists on flexion)

Extensor pollicis longus
Extensor pollicis brevis
Abductor pollicis longus
Palmar interossei (1st, assists)

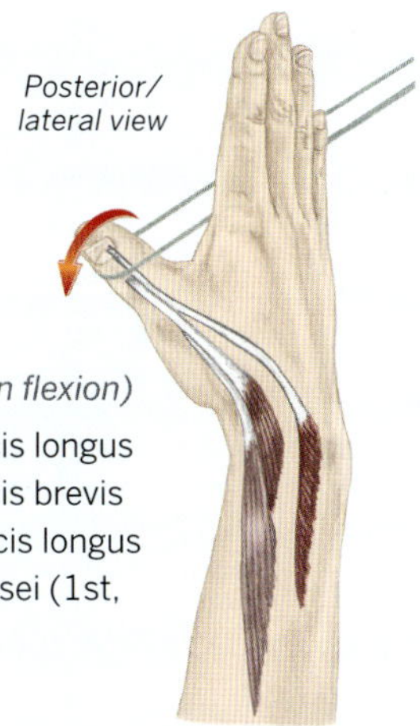

3.69 Extension of the thumb

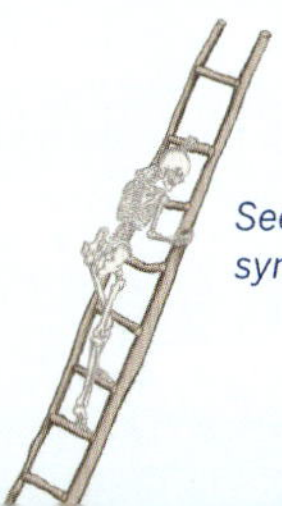

See pp. 431 for a complete list of synergists for the fingers and thumb.

Muscles of the Forearm and Hand

Brachialis ▶

The brachialis is a strong elbow flexor that lies deep to the biceps brachii (p. 91) on the anterior arm (**3.70**, **3.71**). It has a flat yet thick belly. Ironically, however, the brachialis's girth only helps the biceps to bulge further from the arm, making brachialis the biceps's best friend.

Although it lies underneath the biceps, portions of the brachialis are accessible. Its lateral edge, sandwiched between the biceps and triceps brachii, is superficial and palpable. The distal aspect of the brachialis is also accessible as it passes along either side of the biceps tendon.

	BRACHIALIS
A	**Flex** the elbow (humeroulnar joint)
O	Distal half of anterior surface of humerus
I	Tuberosity and coronoid process of ulna
N	Musculocutaneous, small branch from radial C**5**, **6**

When Do You Use Your Brachialis?

- Bringing food from the plate to your mouth
- Picking up a load of anatomy books
- Carrying a baby's car seat

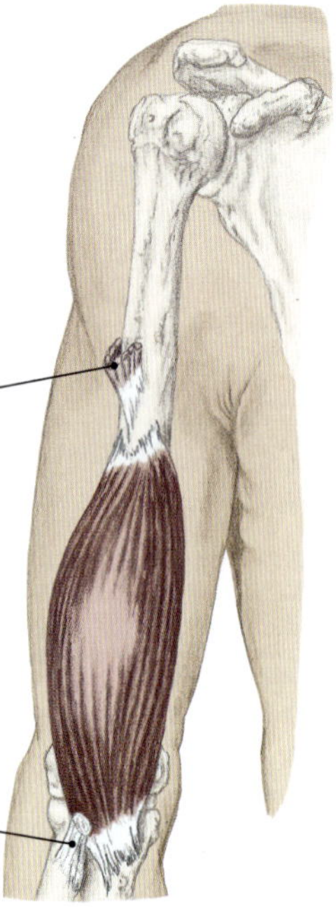

3.70 Anterior view of right arm, showing brachialis

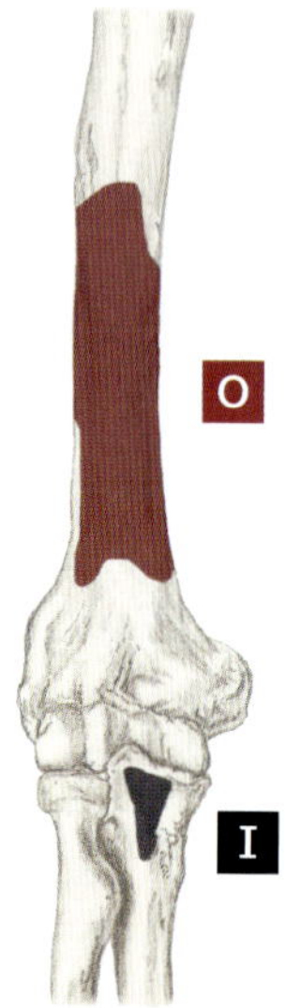

3.71 Anterior view of right arm, showing origin and insertion of brachialis

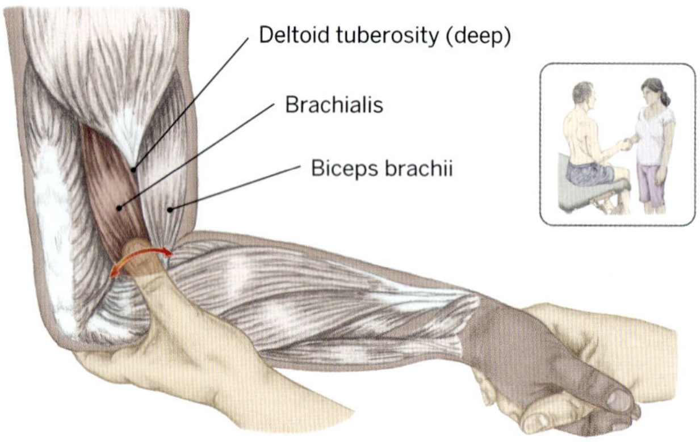

3.72 Lateral view of right forearm, as you strum across the edge of brachialis

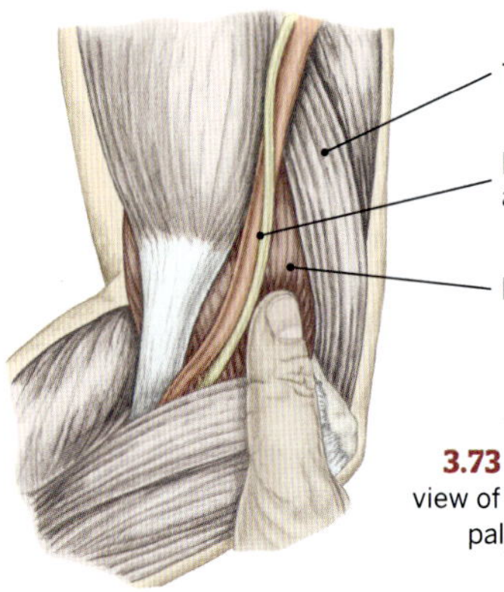

3.73 Anterior/medial view of right elbow, as you palpate brachialis

Brachialis

1. Shake hands with your partner and flex the elbow to 90°. Distinguishing the muscle tissue of the biceps brachii from that of the brachialis is important. Ask your partner to flex her elbow against your resistance and isolate the edges of the round biceps brachii belly.
2. With the arm relaxed, slide laterally half an inch off the distal biceps. The edge of the brachialis can be detected by rolling your fingers across its surface. As you strum across its solid edge, you will feel a pronounced "thump" (**3.72**).
3. Continuing to strum across its edge, follow it distally to where it disappears into the elbow.
4. Locate the distal biceps tendon. Palpate along either side of the tendon for portions of the deeper brachialis (**3.73**).

Can you roll across a distinct wad of muscle on the lateral side of the arm? Can you follow it distally toward the inner elbow? Locate the triceps and biceps brachii. Are the brachialis fibers between them on the lateral arm?

Locate the deltoid tuberosity. Slide distally straight down the lateral side of the arm and explore for the edge of the brachialis.

brachial	***bray**-key-al*	L. relating to the arm
brachialis	***bray**-key-**al**-is*	

Brachioradialis ▶

The brachioradialis is superficial on the lateral side of the forearm (**3.74–3.76**). It has a long, oval belly, which forms a helpful dividing line between the flexors and extensors of the wrist and fingers. Its muscle belly becomes tendinous halfway down the forearm. It is the only muscle that runs the length of the forearm but does not cross the wrist joint. Resisted flexion of the elbow causes brachioradialis to visibly protrude on the forearm and become readily palpable.

BRACHIORADIALIS	
A	**Flex** the elbow (humeroulnar joint) Assist to **pronate** and **supinate** the forearm when these movements are resisted (humeroradial joints)
O	Proximal two-thirds of the lateral supracondylar ridge of humerus
I	Styloid process of radius
N	Radial C**5**, **6**

When Do You Use Your Brachioradialis?

- Turning a door handle or screwdriver
- Bringing a beer stein up to your mouth
- Whisking cream in a bowl

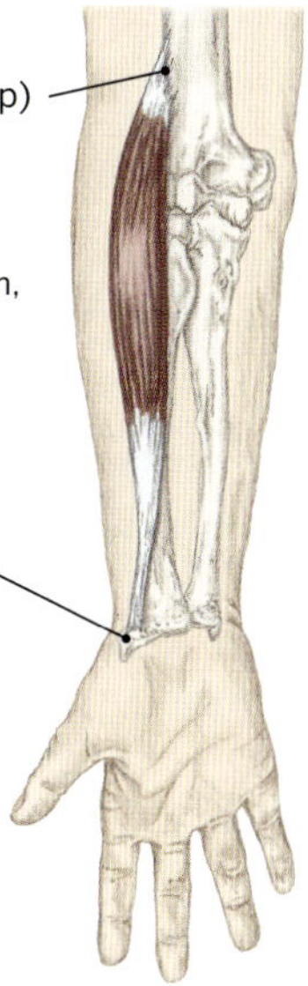

3.74 Anterior view of right forearm, showing brachioradialis

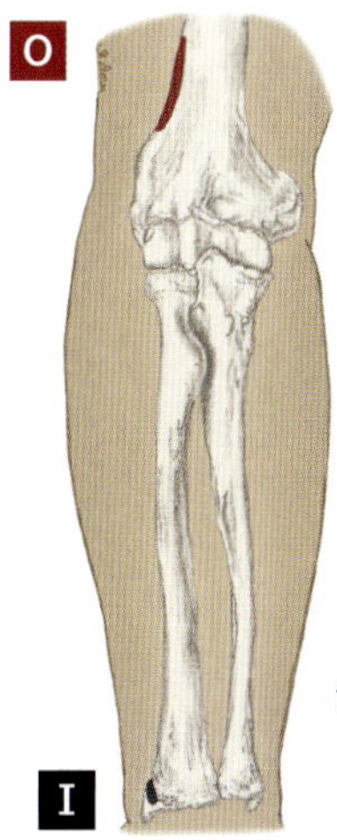

3.75 Anterior view of right forearm, showing origin and insertion of brachioradialis

Brachioradialis

1. Shake hands with your partner and flex the elbow to 90°. With the forearm in a neutral position (thumb toward the ceiling), ask your partner to flex her elbow against your resistance.
2. Look for the brachioradialis bulging out on the lateral side of the elbow. If it is not visible, locate the lateral supracondylar ridge of the humerus and slide distally.
3. With your partner still contracting, use your other hand to palpate its superficial, tubular belly (**3.77**). Try to pinch its belly between your fingers and follow it as far distally as possible. As it becomes more tendinous, strum across its distal tendon toward the styloid process of the radius.

✓ *Upon resisted flexion of the elbow, does the belly you are palpating contract and bulge out? Is it superficial? Does it extend off the lateral supracondylar ridge of the humerus?*

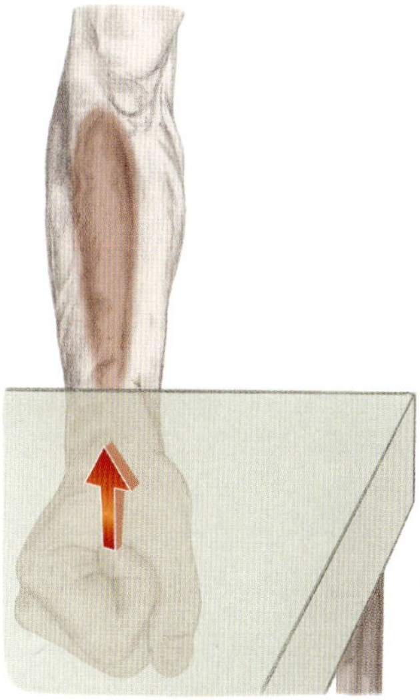

3.76 Pressing your fist up into a table is a great way to get the brachioradialis to pop out.

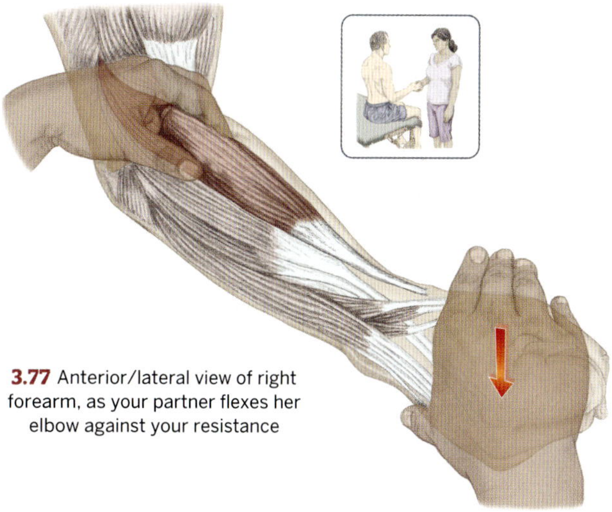

3.77 Anterior/lateral view of right forearm, as your partner flexes her elbow against your resistance

brachioradialis *bray*-key-o-*ra*-de-*a*-lis

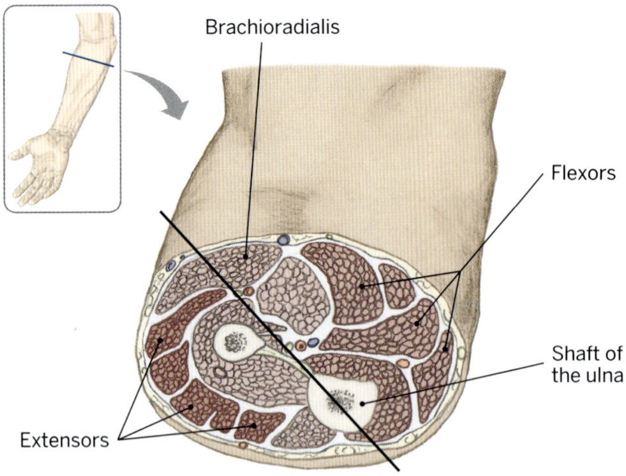

3.78 Cross section of the right forearm, diagonal line dividing the flexors and extensors

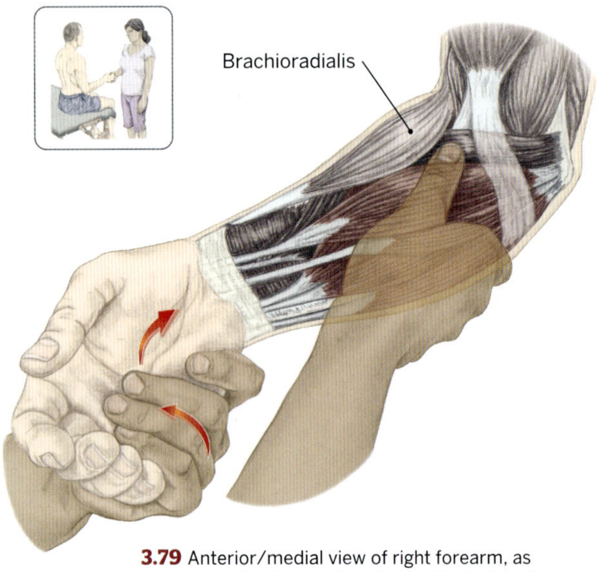

3.79 Anterior/medial view of right forearm, as you palpate the flexors (highlighted in dark red)

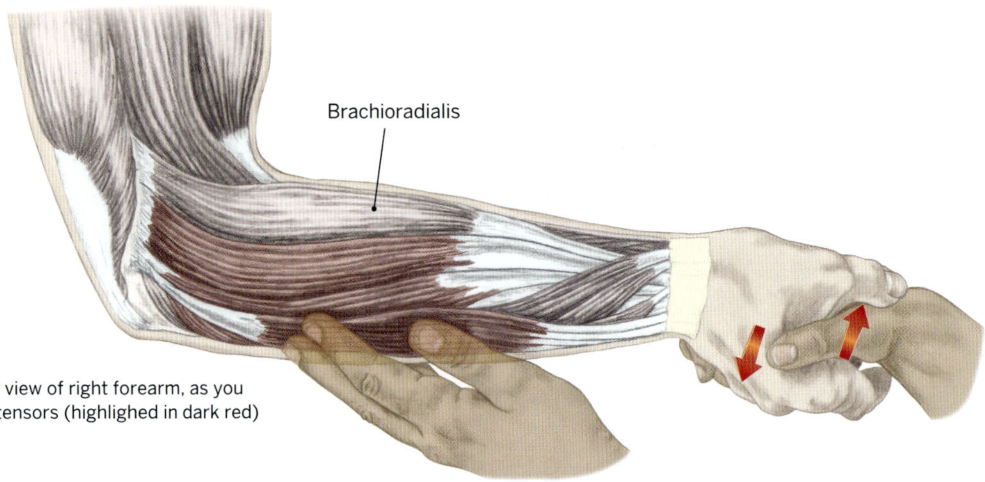

3.80 Lateral view of right forearm, as you explore the extensors (highlighed in dark red)

Distinguishing between the Flexor and Extensor Groups of the Forearm ▶

Before we isolate specific flexors and extensors, let us first determine the location of these two muscle groups. The flexors and extensors of the hand and wrist are located in the forearm. In anatomical position, the flexors are located on the anterior/medial (hairless) side of the forearm, while the extensors are positioned on the posterior/lateral (hairy) side.

The brachioradialis and shaft of the ulna can be used as clear dividing lines between these muscle groups (**3.78**). Both of these structures run superficially down the opposite sides of the forearm, separating the flexors and extensors.

Flexors and extensors

1. Shake hands with your partner and flex the elbow to 90°. Locate the brachioradialis and shaft of the ulna (p. 114). Palpate the length of these structures, observing how they divide the forearm into two halves.
2. Move medially from the shaft of the ulna onto the flexors of the forearm. Explore this half of the forearm, noting the girth of these muscles.
3. Ask your partner to slightly flex her wrist against your resistance (**3.79**). Note the contraction of the flexors.
4. Move to the lateral side of the shaft of the ulna and explore the extensor bellies (**3.80**). Notice how they are smaller and more sinewy than the flexor bellies. Ask your partner to extend her wrist against your resistance, feeling the extensors contract.

When your partner curls (flexes) her wrist, do the muscles on the hairless side of the forearm contract? Do the extensors contract when the hand moves in the opposite direction (extension)?

Extensors of the Wrist and Fingers ▶

Extensor Carpi Radialis Longus
Extensor Carpi Radialis Brevis
Extensor Carpi Ulnaris
Extensor Digitorum

The four extensors create extension primarily at the wrist and fingers. They are situated between the brachioradialis and the shaft of the ulna along the forearm's lateral, posterior surface. All of these muscles are superficial and accessible, though challenging to truly isolate. Originating on the lateral side of the humerus, the bellies of the extensors become tendinous approximately two inches proximal to the wrist joint (**3.81**). As a group, they are smaller and more sinewy than the forearm flexors.

Extensor carpi radialis longus and **brevis** are lateral/posterior to the brachioradialis (**3.82**, **3.83**). **Extensor carpi ulnaris**, as its name suggests, lies beside the ulnar shaft (**3.84**). **Extensor digitorum** is located between these muscles and has four long, superficial tendons stretching along the dorsal surface of the hand and fingers (**3.85**). The *extensor digiti minimi* is sometimes classified as a separate muscle, but in reality it is just the most medial portion of the extensor digitorum with a tendon attaching to the fifth finger.

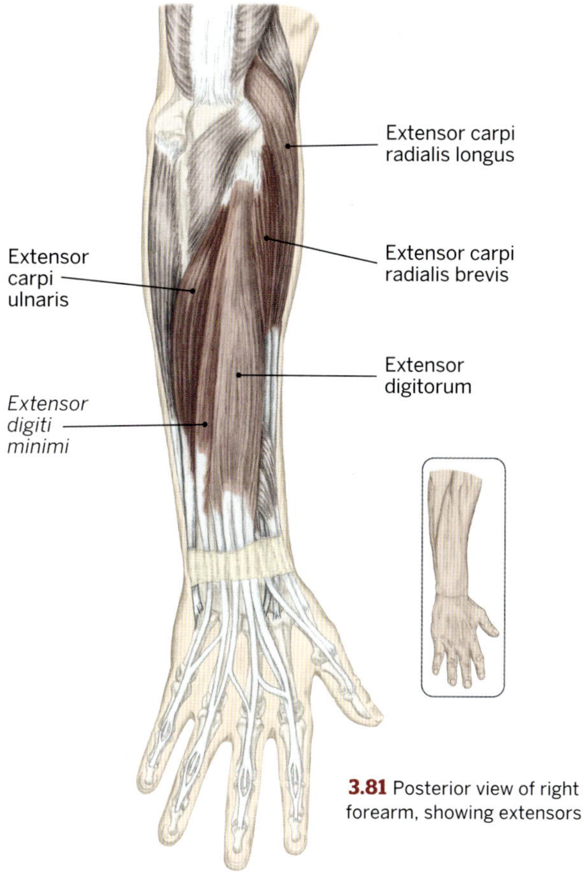

3.81 Posterior view of right forearm, showing extensors

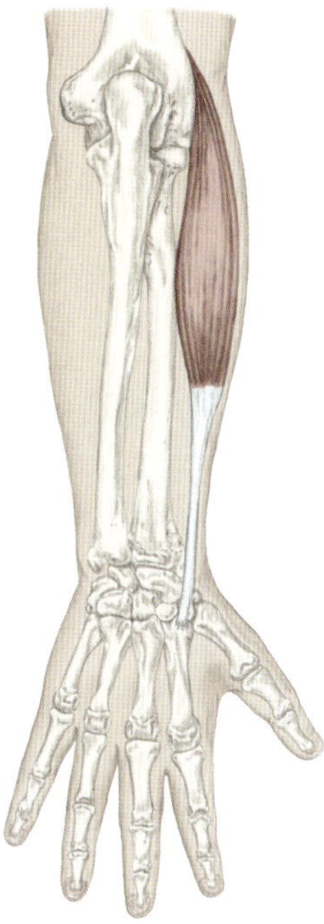

3.82 Posterior view of right forearm, showing extensor carpi radialis longus

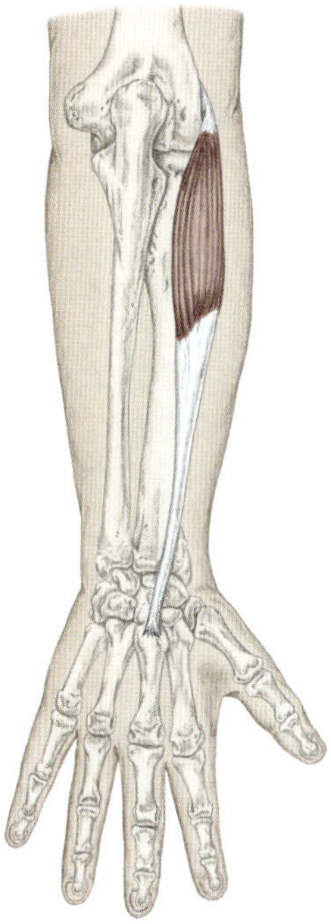

3.83 Posterior view of right forearm, showing extensor carpi radialis brevis

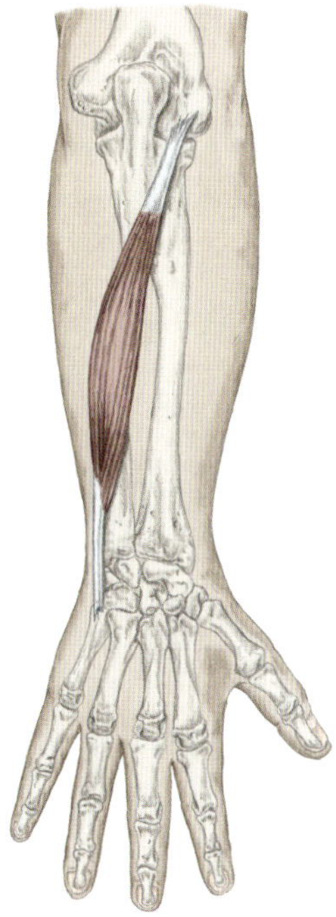

3.84 Posterior view of right forearm, showing extensor carpi ulnaris

brevis	***breh**-vis*	L. short
carpi	***kar**-pi*	L. of the wrist
digit	***di**-jit*	L. finger

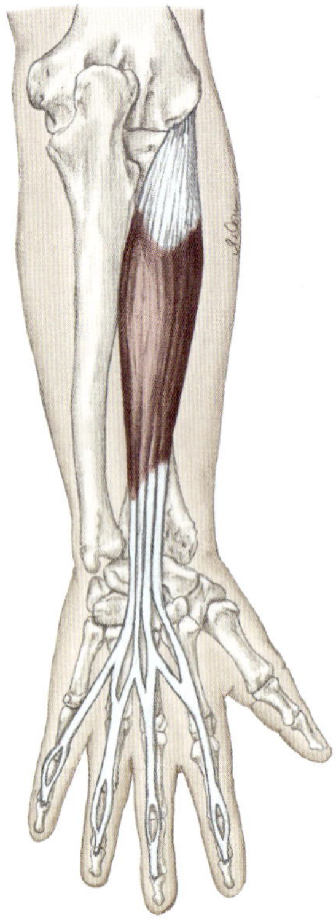

3.85 Posterior view of right forearm, showing extensor digitorum

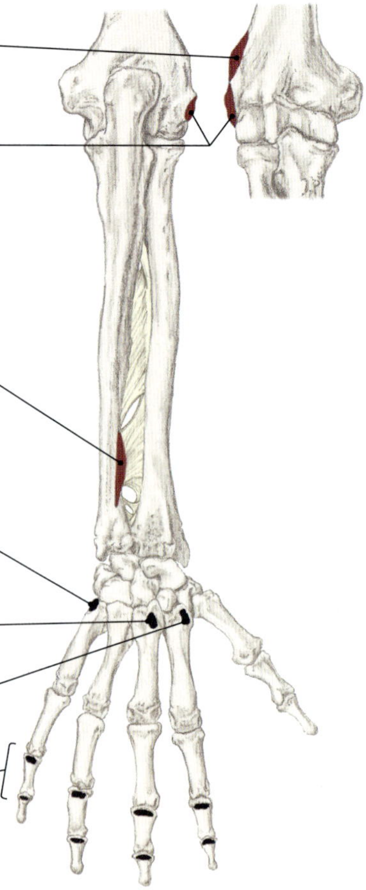

3.86 Posterior view of right forearm (left) and anterior view of right elbow (right), showing origins and insertions of extensors

EXTENSOR CARPI RADIALIS LONGUS AND BREVIS

A **Extend** the wrist (radiocarpal joint)
Abduct the wrist (radiocarpal joint)
Assist to **flex** the elbow (humeroulnar joint)

O *Longus:* Distal one-third of the lateral supracondylar ridge of humerus
Brevis: Common extensor tendon from the lateral epicondyle of humerus

I *Longus:* Base of second metacarpal
Brevis: Base of third metacarpal

N *Longus:* Radial C5, **6**, **7**, 8
Brevis: Radial C**6**, **7**, 8

When Do You Use Your Extensor Carpi Radialis Longus and Brevis?

- Stabilizing the wrist while gripping (opening a jar)
- Washing the dishes
- Turning off a faucet

EXTENSOR CARPI ULNARIS

A **Extend** the wrist (radiocarpal joint)
Adduct the wrist (radiocarpal joint)

O Common extensor tendon from the lateral epicondyle of humerus

I Base of fifth metacarpal

N Radial C6, **7**, **8**

When Do You Use Your Extensor Carpi Ulnaris?

- Shaping soft clay for an art project
- Pulling a book off a tall library shelf
- Reaching into the back seat of your car

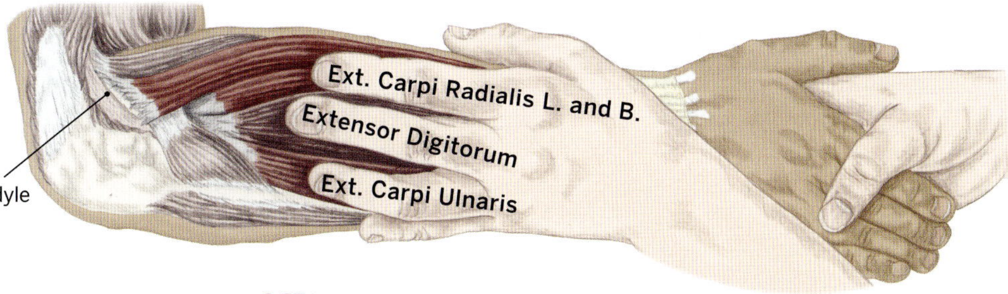

3.87 Lateral view of right forearm, with fingers showing order of extensors

EXTENSOR DIGITORUM

A	**Extend** the second through fifth fingers (metacarpophalangeal and interphalangeal joints) Assist to **extend** the wrist (radiocarpal joint)
O	Common extensor tendon from the lateral epicondyle of humerus
I	Bases of middle and distal phalanges of second through fifth fingers
N	Radial C**6**, **7**, **8**

When Do You Use Your Extensor Digitorum?

- Playing the piano or trumpet
- Holding your hand up to give the Vulcan hand greeting (extension of wrist and fingers)
- Releasing a handshake

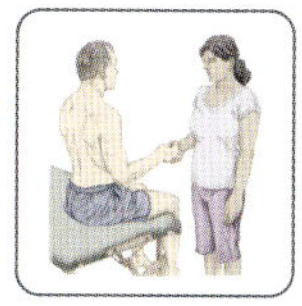

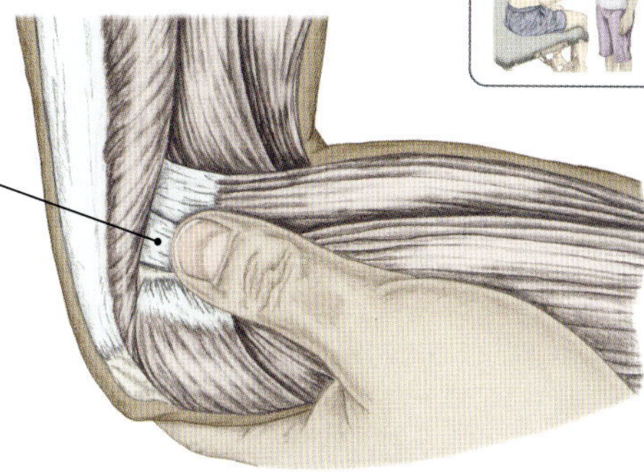

3.88 Lateral view of right elbow, as you palpate the common extensor tendon located at the lateral epicondyle

Extensor group

1. Shake hands with your partner and flex the elbow to 90°. Locate the brachioradialis and shaft of the ulna (see p. 132).
2. Lay the flat of your hand between these landmarks and ask your partner to alternately extend and relax her wrist against your resistance.
3. Explore the slender, sinewy fibers of these muscles and note how they contract upon extension. Access their origin at the lateral epicondyle (**3.88**).

Are you between the brachioradialis and ulnar shaft? Do the muscles contract on extension of the wrist?

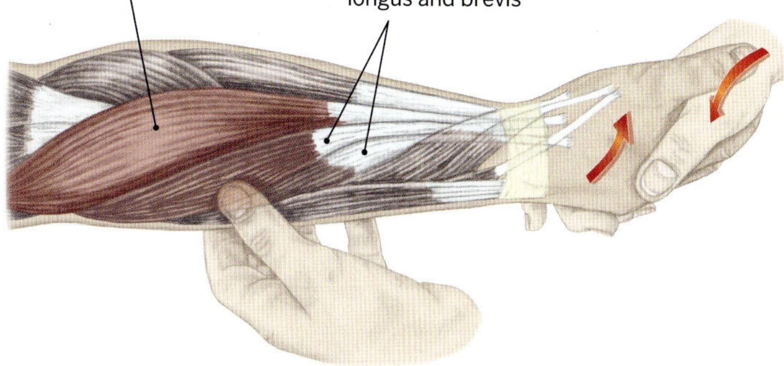

3.89 Lateral view of right forearm, as you explore the extensor carpi radialis longus and brevis

Extensor carpi radialis longus and brevis

1. Shake hands with your partner and flex the elbow to 90°. Locate the brachioradialis. Slide laterally off its belly onto the extensor carpi radialis fibers.
2. Ask your partner to alternately abduct and relax her wrist against your resistance. Sense how the fibers tighten with this movement (**3.89**).
3. Follow their muscle fibers distally as far as possible to where they become tendinous.

Differentiate between the extensor carpi radialis muscles and brachioradialis by asking your partner to alternately abduct and relax her wrist against your resistance. The brachioradialis, which does not cross the wrist joint, will remain slack throughout this action while the extensor carpi radialis muscles will contract.

Extensor digitorum

1. Shake hands with your partner and flex her elbow to 90°. Slide laterally off the extensor carpi radialis fibers.
2. As you move around the forearm, palpate the digitorum's flat surface and roll across its fibers.
3. Isolate its belly by asking your partner to extend her wrist and fingers. Follow the belly distally as it transforms into tendons. The tendons will be palpable as they pass beneath the extensor retinaculum and continue along the dorsal surface of the hand.

*Ask your partner to wiggle her fingers as if she were typing (**3.90**). Do you feel an undulating contraction of the extensor digitorum?*

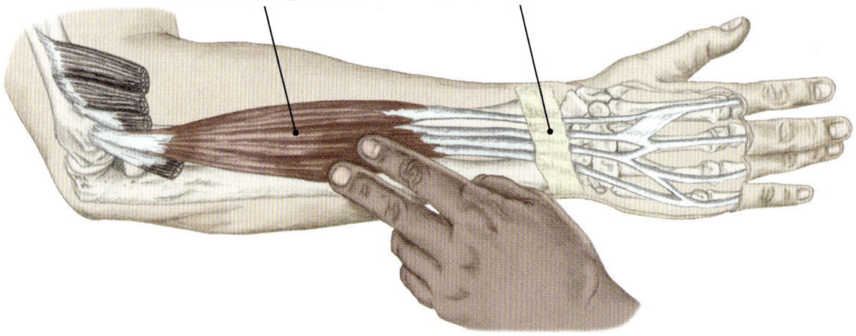

3.90 Lateral view of posterior surface of right forearm, partner wiggling her fingers while you palpate extensor digitorum

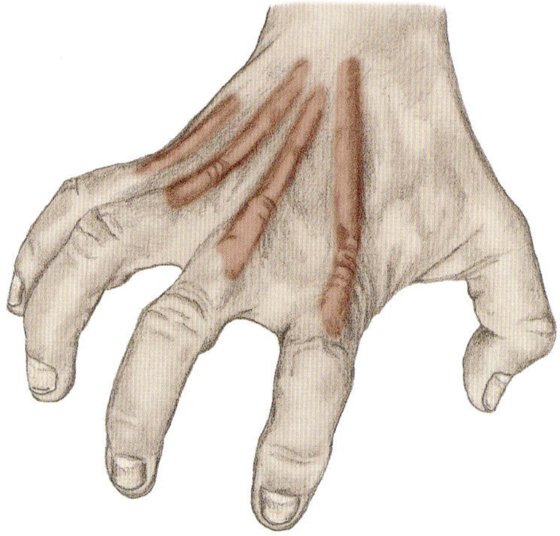

3.91 Making the infamous "death claw" gesture will bring your extensor digitorum tendons to the surface.

Extensor carpi ulnaris

1. Shake hands with your partner and flex the elbow to 90°. Locate the shaft of the ulna.
2. Slide laterally off the shaft onto the slender belly of the extensor carpi ulnaris.
3. Ask your partner to adduct her wrist against your resistance (**3.92**). Note how the tissue directly lateral to the ulna tightens with this movement.
4. Follow the tendon distally past the head of the ulna.

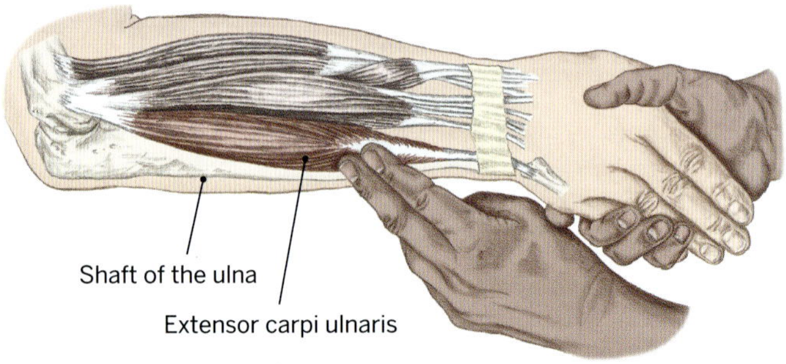

3.92 Lateral view of posterior surface of right forearm, as you explore the extensor carpi ulnaris

Palpation Plus

Brachioradialis and extensor carpi radialis longus and brevis are sometimes known collectively as the "wad of three." Together they form a long mass of muscle that extends distally from the lateral supracondylar ridge of the humerus.

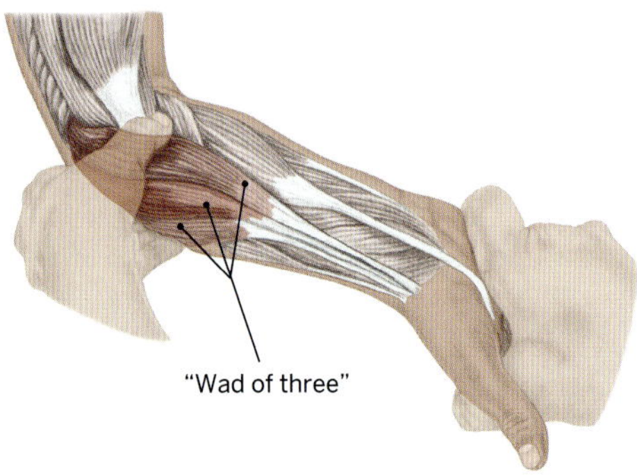

To locate the wad, shake hands with your partner and palpate just lateral to the inner elbow. The wad will be the thick, mobile tissue that can be easily grasped between your fingers and thumb. Follow it distally as far as possible.

Anconeus ▶

The anconeus is a weak elbow extensor located lateral to the olecranon process. Triangular-shaped, it originates at the lateral epicondyle of the humerus and fans out to attach on the shaft of the ulna (**3.93**, **3.94**). The anconeus is superficial, yet it can be difficult to differentiate from the surrounding extensors.

ANCONEUS	
A	**Extend** the elbow (humeroulnar joint)
O	Lateral epicondyle of the humerus
I	Olecranon process and posterior, proximal surface of ulna
N	Radial C**7**, **8**

When Do You Use Your Anconeus?

- Steering a kayak with a paddle
- Unzipping the back of your dress

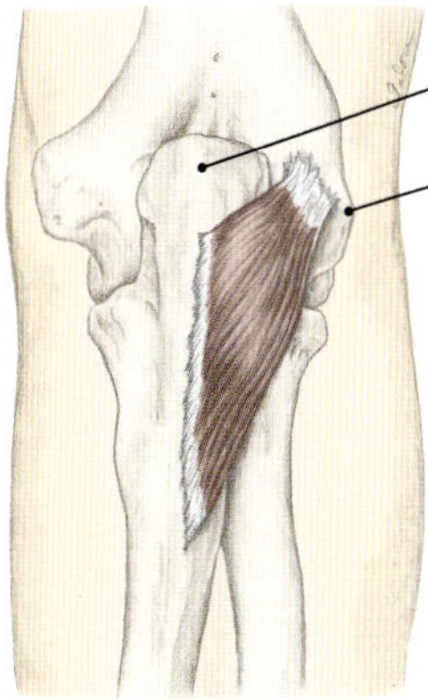

3.93 Posterior view of right elbow, showing anconeus

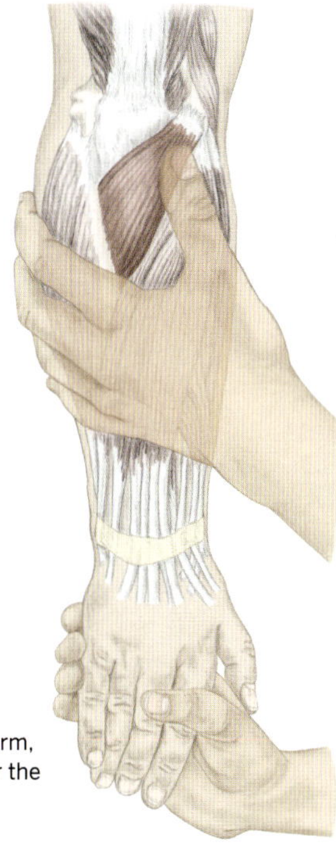

3.94 Posterior view of right arm, as you strum your thumb over the belly of the anconeus

Anconeus

1. Locate the olecranon process, the proximal shaft of the ulna, and the lateral epicondyle of the humerus.
2. Then lay your index finger along the proximal ulna and the tip of your middle finger on the lateral epicondyle. The V formed by your fingers is the outline of the anconeus.

Extensor Indicis

Located deep to the extensor digitorum and extensor carpi ulnaris, this small but crucial muscle assists the digitorum in specifically extending the index finger. Its tendon runs diagonally across the wrist and hand, sheathed with the extensor digitorum tendon (**3.95**). If you extend your index finger at the metacarpophalangeal joint, you might see two side-by-side tendons passing across the top of the knuckle (**3.96**). The medial tendon (closer to the middle finger) is the extensor indicis tendon.

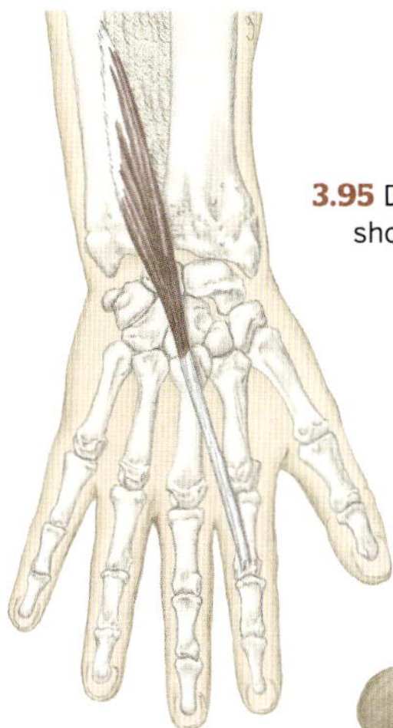

3.95 Dorsal view of right hand, showing extensor indicis

EXTENSOR INDICIS	
A	**Extend** the second finger (metacarpophalangeal joint) **Adduct** the second finger May assist to **extend** the wrist (radiocarpal joint)
O	Posterior surface of distal shaft of ulna and interosseous membrane
I	Tendon of the extensor digitorum at the level of the second metacarpal
N	Radial C6, **7**, **8**

When Do You Use Your Extensor Indicis?

- Holding up a small rock between the index finger and thumb to examine all sides of it more closely

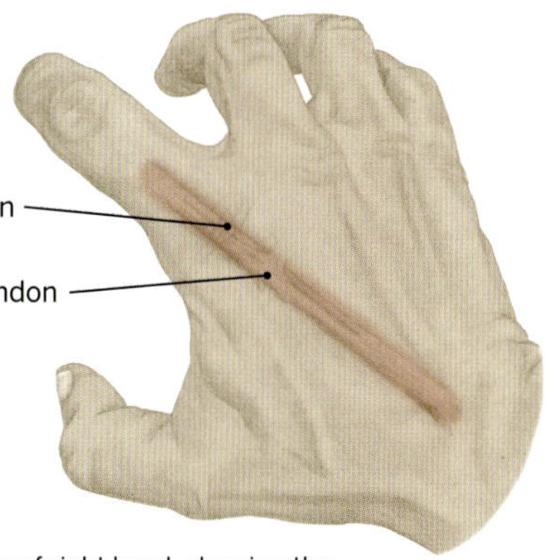

3.96 Dorsal view of right hand, showing the positions of the extensor indicis tendon and the extensor digitorum tendon

anconeus an-*ko*-nee-us Grk. elbow
indicis *in*-di-kis

Flexors of the Wrist and Fingers ▶

Flexor Carpi Radialis
Palmaris Longus
Flexor Carpi Ulnaris
Flexor Digitorum Superficialis
Flexor Digitorum Profundus

The five flexors included in this section create flexion primarily at the wrist or fingers (**3.97**, **3.98**). They are located on the forearm's anterior/medial surface between the brachioradialis and the ulnar shaft. Most of the flexors originate as one mass from the common flexor tendon at the medial epicondyle of the humerus (**3.99**). The bellies of the flexors extend down the forearm, becoming thin tendons roughly two inches proximal to the wrist.

As a group, the flexors are thicker and more pliable than the extensors. Although the flexors are easily accessed as a group, isolating specific muscle bellies can be challenging.

The flexors are arranged in three layers. The superficial layer is formed by the long bellies of flexor carpi radialis, palmaris longus, and flexor carpi ulnaris (**3.98**). **Flexor carpi radialis** is medial to the pronator teres and brachioradialis (**3.100**). **Flexor carpi ulnaris** lies close to the ulnar shaft and has a distinct tendon attaching to the pisiform (**3.101**). The **palmaris longus** (**3.102**), which is sometimes absent, runs between flexor carpi radialis and flexor carpi ulnaris and attaches to the palmar aponeurosis (p. 161). Portions of all three muscles can be isolated for palpation purposes.

The middle and deep layers contain the wide bellies of **flexor digitorum superficialis** and **flexor digitorum profundus**, respectively (**3.104**, **3.105**). Each digitorum muscle has four thin tendons that pass through the carpal tunnel (p. 161) and attach at the phalanges. The bellies of the digitorums are difficult to access directly, but their density can be felt beneath the superficial flexors.

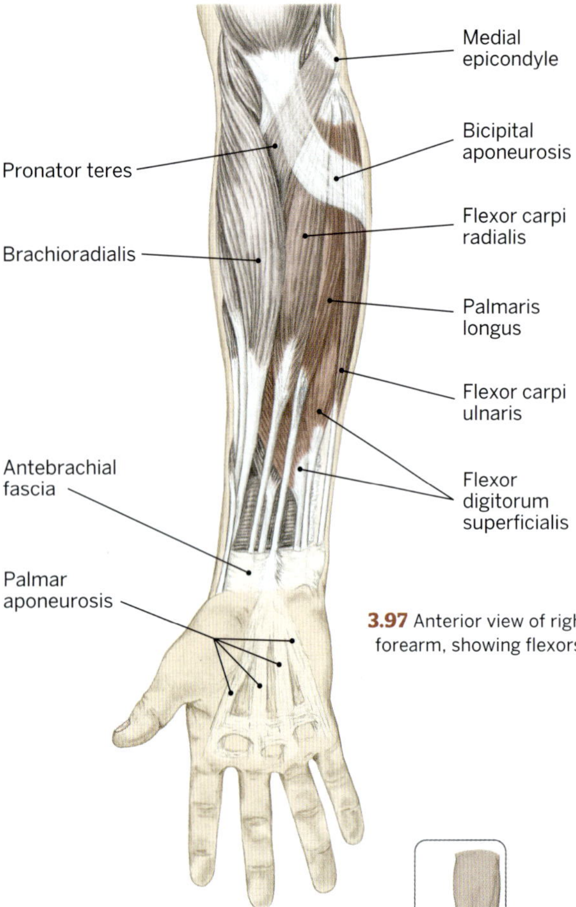

3.97 Anterior view of right forearm, showing flexors

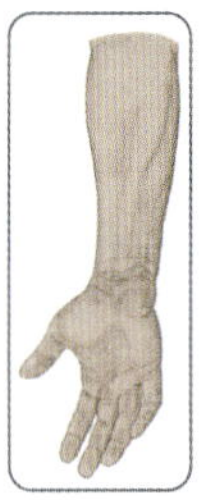

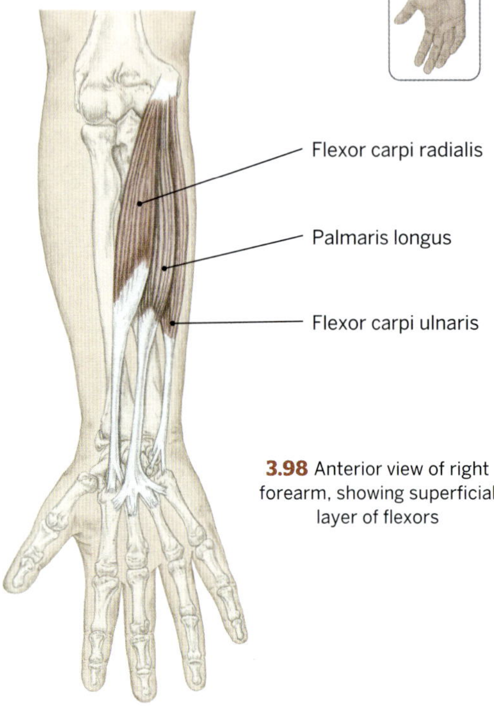

3.98 Anterior view of right forearm, showing superficial layer of flexors

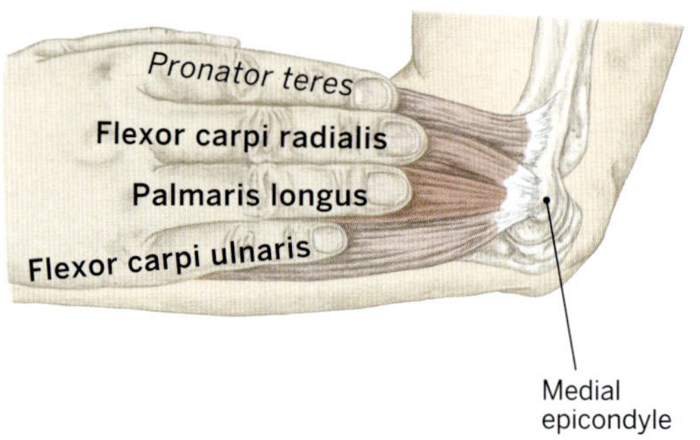

3.99 Medial view of right forearm with fingers showing order of muscles

superficialis	soo-per-***fish***-ee-***a***-lis	L. on the surface
profundus	pro-***fun***-dus	L. deep

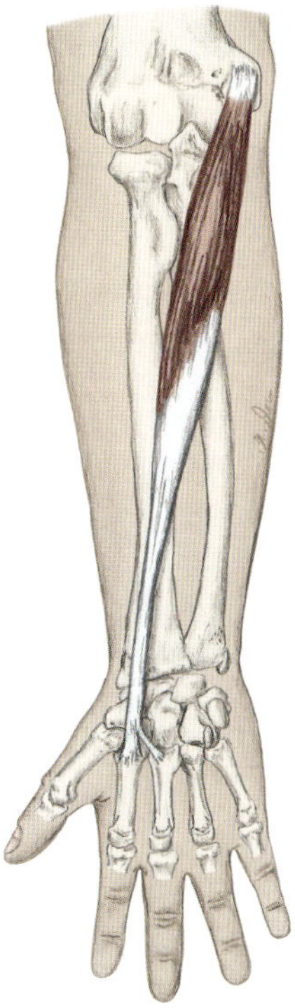

3.100 Anterior view of right forearm, showing flexor carpi radialis

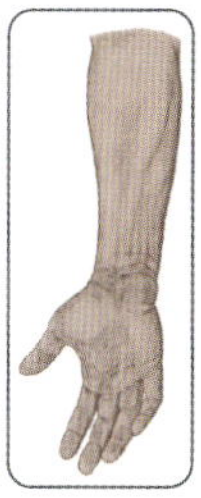

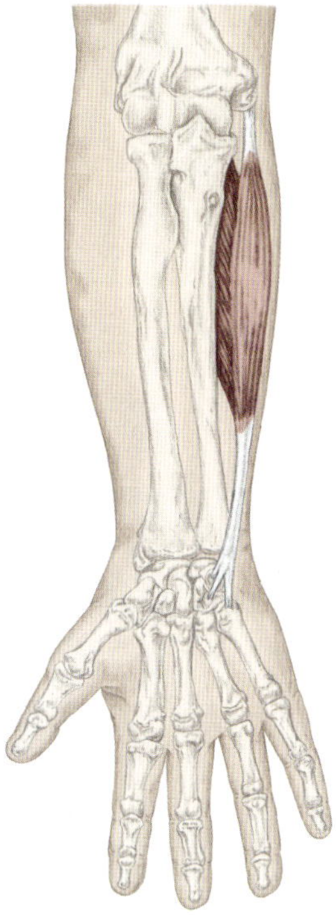

3.101 Anterior view of right forearm, showing flexor carpi ulnaris

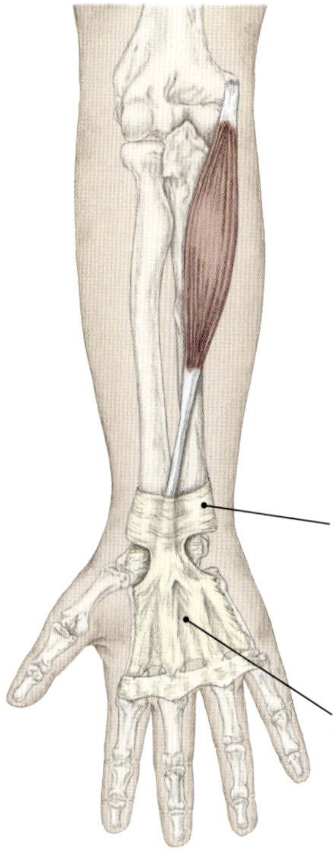

3.102 Anterior view of right forearm, showing palmaris longus

FLEXOR CARPI RADIALIS

A **Flex** the wrist (radiocarpal joint)
Abduct the wrist (radiocarpal joint)
May assist to **flex** the elbow (humeroulnar joint)

O Common flexor tendon from medial epicondyle of humerus

I Bases of second and third metacarpals

N Median C**6**, **7**, 8

When Do You Use Your Flexor Carpi Radialis?

- Squeezing the hand strap of a fast-moving train
- Turning a water valve
- Holding a cell phone

PALMARIS LONGUS

A **Tense** the palmar fascia
Flex the wrist (radiocarpal joint)
May assist to **flex** the elbow (humeroulnar joint)

O Common flexor tendon from medial epicondyle of humerus

I Flexor retinaculum and palmar aponeurosis

N Median C(6), **7**, **8**, T1

When Do You Use Your Palmaris Longus?

- Palming a large grapefruit
- Doing fingertip push-ups
- Making a snowball

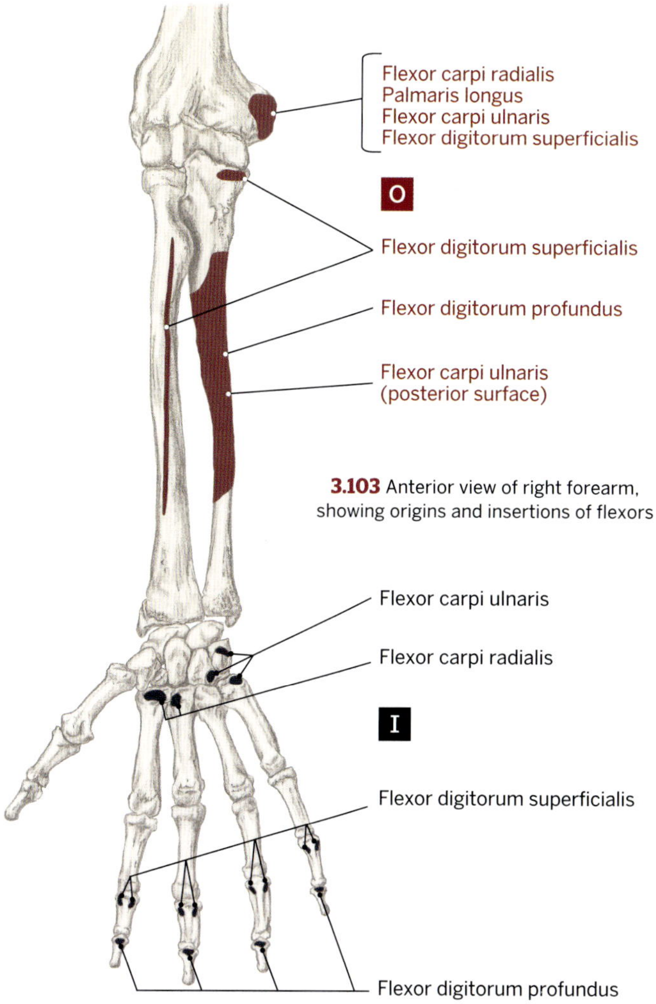

3.103 Anterior view of right forearm, showing origins and insertions of flexors

FLEXOR CARPI ULNARIS

A
- **Flex** the wrist (radiocarpal joint)
- **Adduct** the wrist (radiocarpal joint)
- Assist to **flex** the elbow (humeroulnar joint)

O

Humeral head:

Common flexor tendon from medial epicondyle of humerus

Ulnar head:

Posterior surface of proximal two-thirds of ulna

I Pisiform, hook of the hamate, and base of fifth metacarpal

N Ulnar C7, **8**, T1

When Do You Use Your Flexor Carpi Ulnaris?

- Using your hand to brush food off a kitchen table
- Unscrewing a tight lid on a jar
- Delivering an incredible judo chop

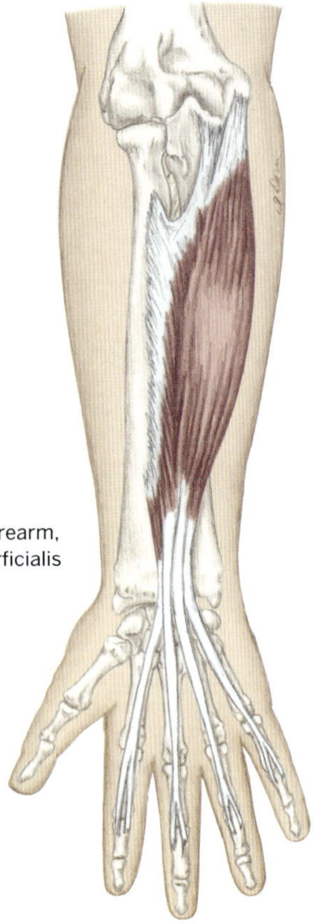

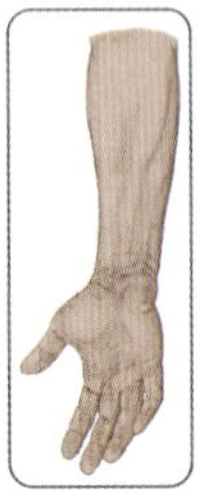

3.104 Anterior view of right forearm, showing flexor digitorum superficialis

FLEXOR DIGITORUM SUPERFICIALIS

A
- **Flex** the second through fifth fingers (metacarpophalangeal and proximal interphalangeal joints)
- **Flex** the wrist (radiocarpal joint)

O Common flexor tendon from medial epicondyle of humerus, ulnar collateral ligament, coronoid process of ulna, interosseous membrane, and proximal shaft of radius

I Sides of middle phalanges of second through fifth fingers

N Median C**7**, **8**, T**1**

When Do You Use Your Flexor Digitorum Superficialis?

- Picking up small objects such as crumbs, needles, or coins
- Playing a guitar
- Typing a letter

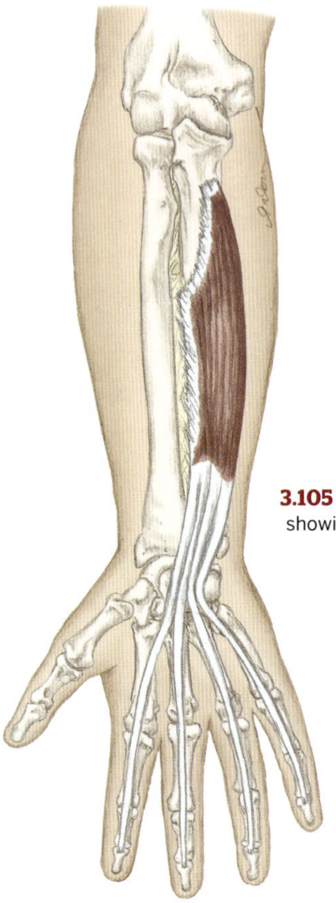

3.105 Anterior view of right forearm, showing flexor digitorum profundus

FLEXOR DIGITORUM PROFUNDUS

A
- **Flex** the second through fifth fingers (metacarpophalangeal and distal interphalangeal joints)
- Assist to **flex** the wrist (radiocarpal joint)

O Anterior and medial surfaces of proximal three-quarters of ulna

I Bases of distal phalanges, palmar surface of second through fifth fingers

N

Second and third fingers: Median C7, **8**, T**1**

Fourth and fifth fingers: Ulnar C7, **8**, T**1**

When Do You Use Your Flexor Digitorum Profundus?

- Typing a letter
- Tying your shoelaces
- Buttoning your shirt

Flexor group

1. Shake hands with your partner and flex the elbow to 90°. Locate the brachioradialis and shaft of the ulna (see p. 114).
2. Lay the flat of your hand between these landmarks on the forearm's anterior surface and ask your partner to alternately flex and relax her wrist against your resistance (see p. 132).
3. Explore the chubby bellies from their origin at the medial epicondyle to their distal tendons at the wrist (**3.106**).

Are you between the brachioradialis and ulnar shaft? Do the muscles contract on flexion of the wrist?

Flexor carpi radialis and palmaris longus

1. Flex your partner's elbow to 90° and supinate the forearm. Begin at the distal tendons. Ask your partner to flex her wrist against your resistance.
2. At the center of the wrist will be two superficial tendons, flexor carpi radialis and palmaris longus (**3.107**). The palmaris longus may be absent, but if both tendons are present, the palmaris will be the most medial.
3. As your partner contracts, roll across the tendons and follow them proximally as they expand into muscle bellies (**3.108**). Ask your partner to alternately abduct and relax her wrist to create a distinct contraction of flexor carpi radialis (**3.109**).

Are the tendons/muscle bellies superficial? If you palpate the belly of flexor carpi radialis, is it superficial and medial to the pronator teres (p. 144)? Is the palmaris longus medial to the flexor carpi radialis? Follow the bellies toward the elbow. Do they merge at the medial epicondyle of the humerus?

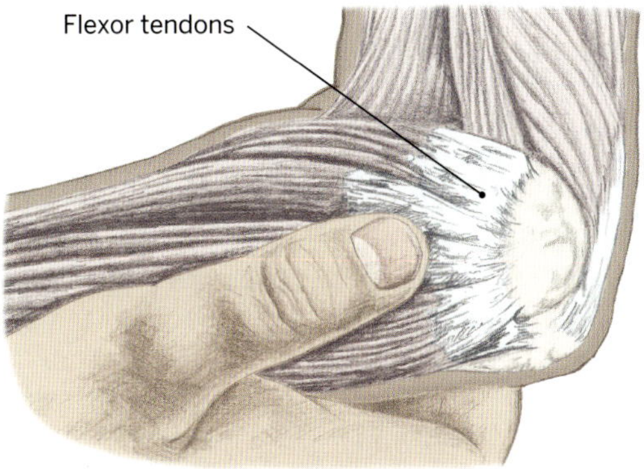

3.106 Medial view of right elbow, as you palpate the common flexor tendon located at the medial epicondyle

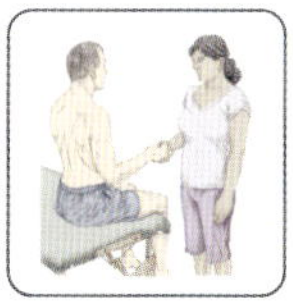

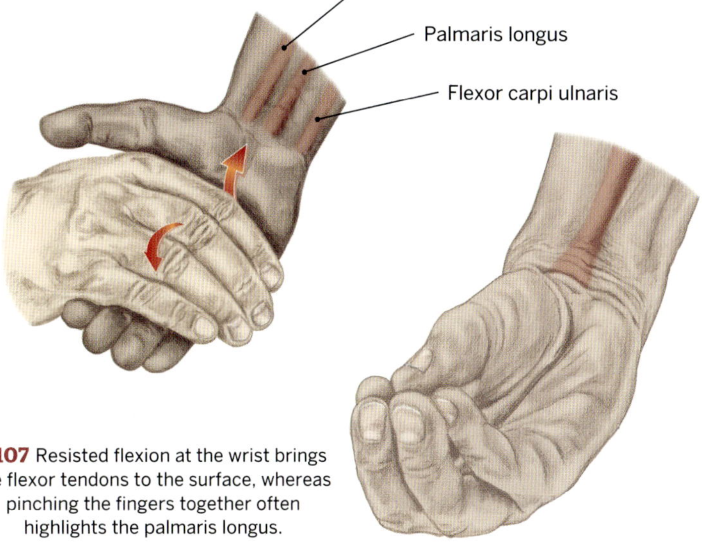

3.107 Resisted flexion at the wrist brings the flexor tendons to the surface, whereas pinching the fingers together often highlights the palmaris longus.

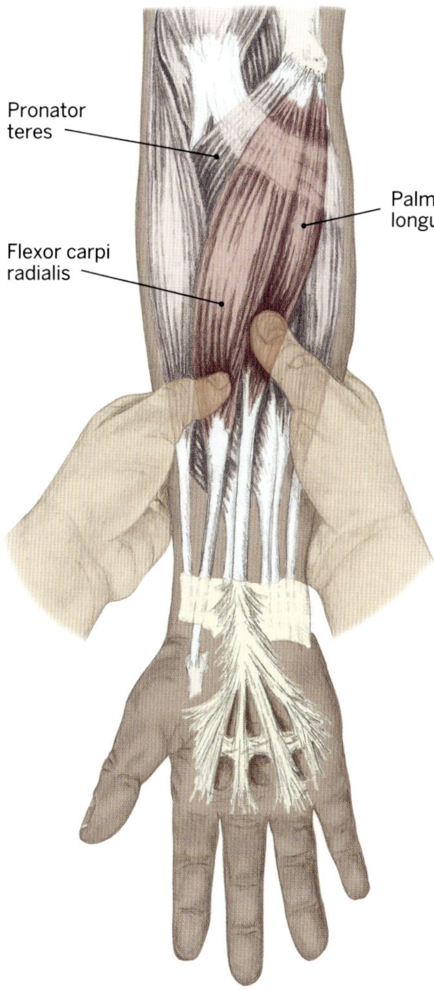

3.108 Anterior view of right forearm, as you palpate flexor carpi radialis and palmaris longus

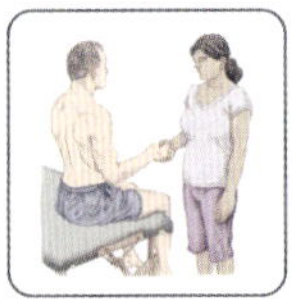

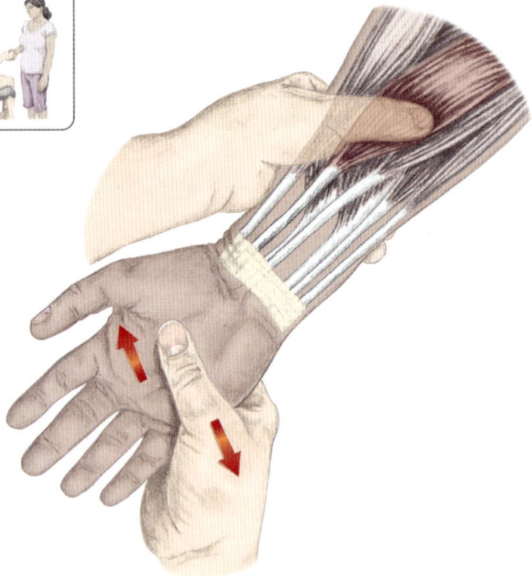

3.109 Anterior view of right forearm, as your partner abducts the wrist against your resistance while you palpate flexor carpi radialis

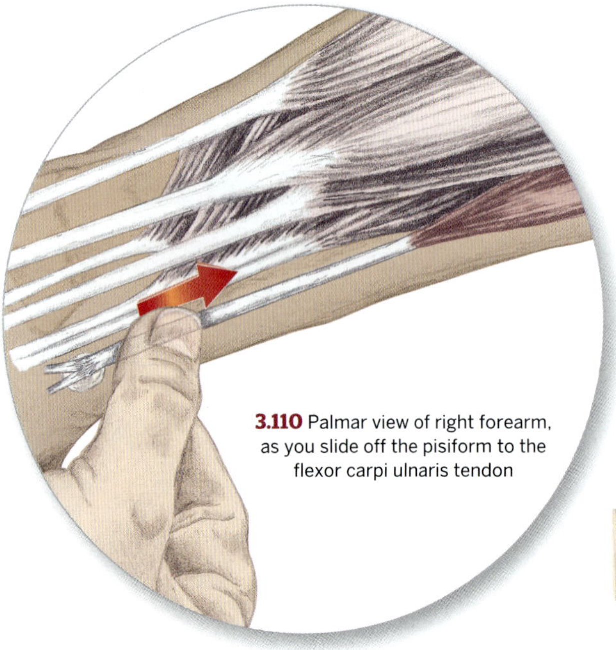

3.110 Palmar view of right forearm, as you slide off the pisiform to the flexor carpi ulnaris tendon

Discover More

The palmaris longus is absent in about 11% of the population. The palmar aponeurosis, however, is always present. The palmaris longus may vary from a mere tendinous band to a distal muscle belly with a long, proximal tendon. On occasion, there may be two palmaris longus muscles. The insertion site is also variable. It may attach to the fascia of the forearm, the tendon of the flexor carpi ulnaris, the flexor retinaculum, the pisiform, or the scaphoid.

Flexor carpi ulnaris

1. Shaking hands with your partner, flex the elbow to 90° and supinate the forearm. Begin at the distal tendon by locating the pisiform (p. 119).
2. Slide proximally off the pisiform to the slender, superficial tendon of flexor carpi ulnaris (**3.110**).
3. As your partner alternately adducts and relaxes her wrist against your resistance, follow the tendon proximally, strumming across its surface (**3.111**). Feel how it widens into a muscle belly and heads toward the medial epicondyle. (Note: Unlike the extensor carpi ulnaris, the flexor carpi ulnaris lies roughly a finger's width away from the ulnar shaft.)

Do you feel the muscle contract upon adduction? Is the tendon/muscle belly superficial and along the forearm's anterior/medial surface? Is it medial to the palmaris longus?

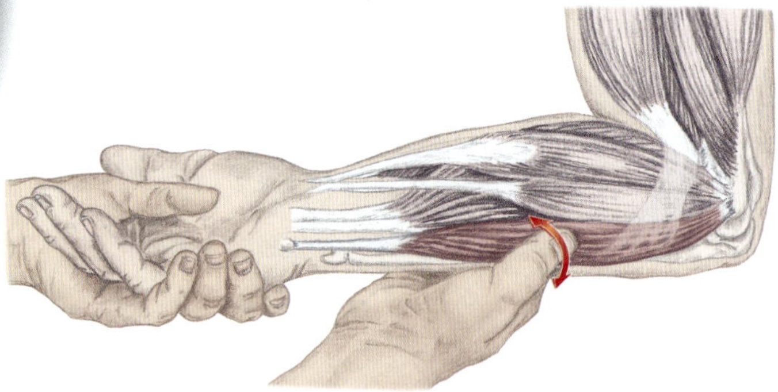

3.111 Medial view of right forearm, as you strum across the flexor carpi ulnaris

Flexor digitorum superficialis and profundus

1. Beginning at the wrist, locate the tendons of the superficial flexors (carpi ulnaris, carpi radialis, and palmaris longus). Passive flexion of the wrist will soften the tendons and allow for easier access.
2. Slowly work your thumb between the superficial tendons for the deeper digitorum tendons and bellies (**3.112**).

Is the tissue you are accessing deep to the first layer of flexors? If your partner wiggles the tips of her fingers, can you detect any small, undulating contractions in the forearm?

Flexor digitorum superficialis

1. Although the digitorum muscles are deep, their contractions are palpable along the medial side of the ulnar shaft. Ask your partner to simultaneously flex her elbow and wrist to 90°.
2. Locate the ulnar shaft, sliding just off its edge into the flexors. Ask your partner to squeeze the tips of her fifth finger and thumb together and then relax. You should feel the small but distinct contraction of the digitorum muscles as they bulge into your fingers (**3.113**).
3. Try squeezing the ring, middle, and index fingers together with the thumb and note how this changes the contraction.

Discover More

There are two primary supinators (biceps brachii and supinator) and two primary pronators (pronator teres and pronator quadratus). You might assume that this structural symmetry would mean a balance of strength between the pronators and supinators, but in reality, the size and power of the biceps brachii cause the scales to tip in favor of the supinators. The expression "righty-tighty, lefty-loosey" is not only a reminder of the direction in which to turn a screw, but also applies to the hand that holds the screwdriver. We have more power to supinate than to pronate and the world is dominated by right-handed individuals, so screws have been designed to be tightened by right forearm supination. This, of course, leaves "southpaws" to tighten with either weak pronators or the undeveloped supinators of the right forearm.

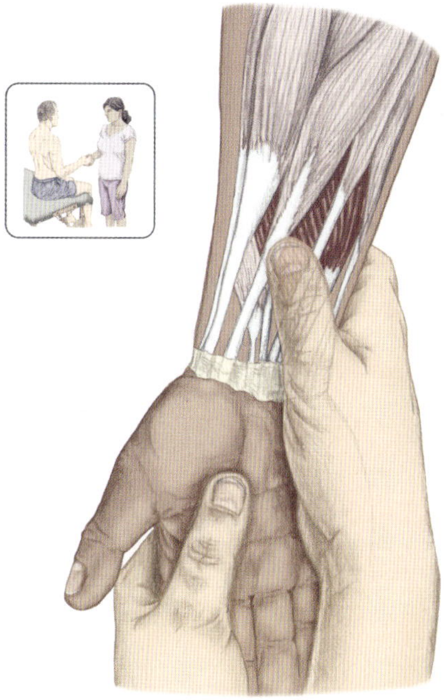

3.112 Anterior view of right forearm, as you palpate between the superficial flexors for the flexor digitorum muscles

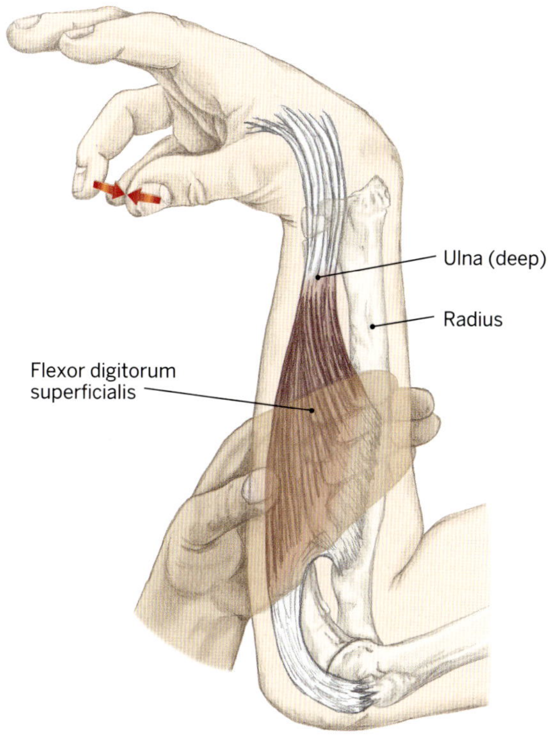

3.113 Medial view of right forearm, as your partner presses the fifth finger and thumb together while you palpate flexor digitorum superficialis

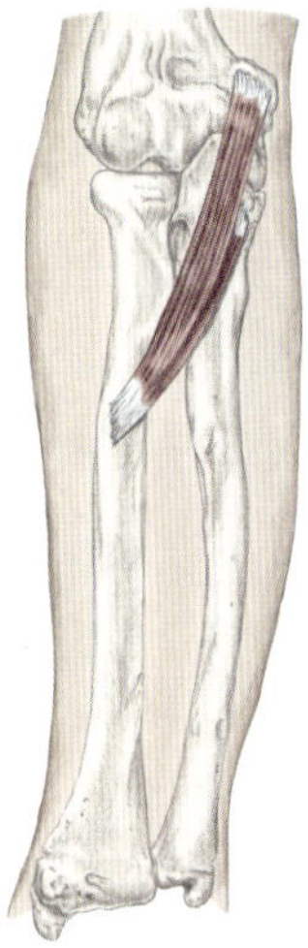

3.114 Anterior view of right forearm, showing pronator teres

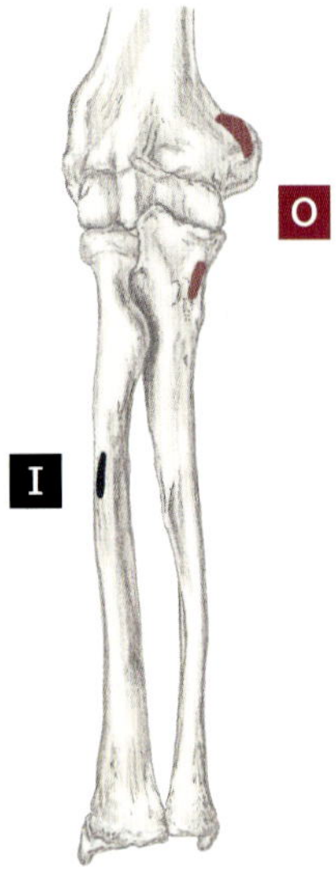

3.115 Anterior view of right forearm, showing origin and insertion of pronator teres

Pronator Teres ▶

Located on the anterior surface of the forearm, the round pronator teres is tucked between the brachioradialis and forearm flexors (p. 138). It is partially superficial and the only muscle in this vicinity with oblique fibers (**3.114**). The pronator teres is an antagonist to the biceps brachii and supinator ("carrying a bowl of soup") muscles and creates pronation of the forearm ("prone to spill it"). The distal tendon of biceps brachii, situated just lateral to the pronator teres, is a good landmark for locating its fibers.

	PRONATOR TERES
A	**Pronate** the forearm (radioulnar joints) Assist to **flex** the elbow (humeroulnar joint)
O	Common flexor tendon from medial epicondyle of humerus and coronoid process of the ulna
I	Middle of lateral surface of the radius
N	Median C**6**, **7**

When Do You Use Your Pronator Teres?

- Turning a doorknob
- Arranging cups in the dishwasher
- Swimming the breaststroke (forearms pronated)

Pronator teres

1. Shake hands with your partner and flex the elbow to 90°. Locate the distal tendon of the biceps brachii. For assistance, ask your partner to flex her elbow against your resistance.
2. Slide distally off the tendon into the valley between the brachioradialis and forearm flexors. Sink your thumb into this space.
3. Explore for the finger-wide pronator belly running obliquely from the medial elbow across to the radius. Strum across its oblique fibers (**3.116**, **3.117**).
4. Follow it toward the medial epicondyle (noting how it blends into the other flexors) and the middle radius (feeling how it tucks under the brachioradialis).

✓ *Shake hands and ask your partner to pronate against your resistance. Does the belly of the muscle you are palpating form a solid contraction? Do the fibers you are palpating run diagonally toward the middle of the radius?*

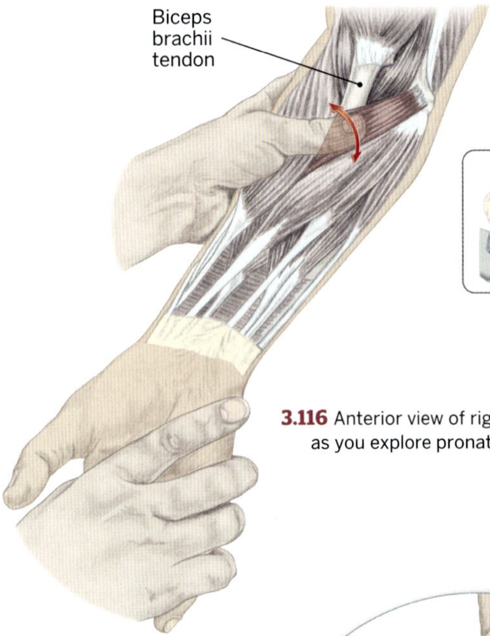

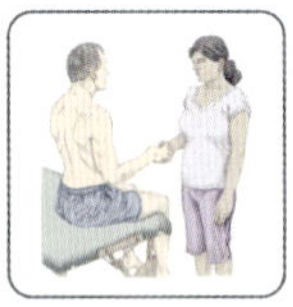

3.116 Anterior view of right forearm, as you explore pronator teres

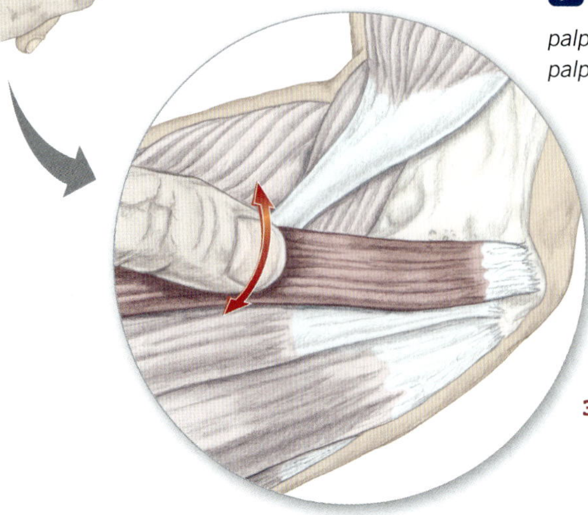

3.117 Anterior/medial view of right elbow, as you strum across the pronator belly

pronate *pro*-nate L. bent forward

Pronator Quadratus

Although it lacks the pronator teres's power and speed, the small quadratus is still a capable pronator. It has transverse fibers that lie deep to the flexor tendons and the major nerve and blood vessels of the anterior forearm (**3.118**). The majority of the muscle is inaccessible, except for its most lateral portion. This small palpatory window, however, is also the location of the radial artery—so explore gently.

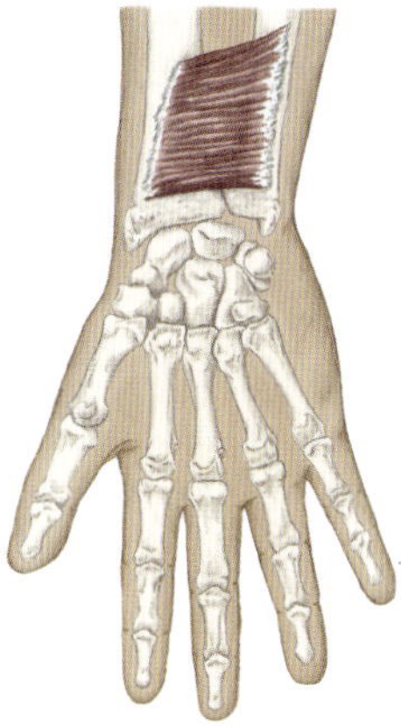

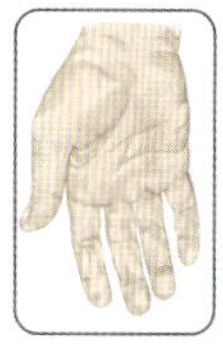

3.118 Palmar view of right hand, showing pronator quadratus

	PRONATOR QUADRATUS
A	**Pronate** the forearm (radioulnar joints)
O	Medial, anterior surface of distal ulna
I	Lateral, anterior surface of distal radius
N	Median C7, **8**, T**1**

When Do You Use Your Pronator Quadratus?

- Receiving the pitch as the catcher in baseball
- Unzipping the back of your dress
- Walking with crutches

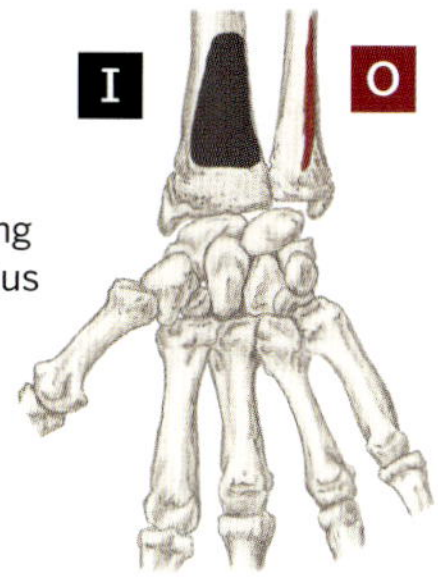

3.119 Palmar view of right hand, showing origin and insertion of pronator quadratus

Pronator quadratus

1. Shake hands with your partner. First, isolate the pulse of the radial artery (p. 162). Then locate the radius's styloid process, sliding around to its anterior surface.
2. Before accessing the quadratus, flex and pronate the wrist slightly, softening the overlying flexor tendons. Then use your thumb to explore the thin band of tissue between the radius and the tendons (**3.120**).
3. You might not feel the fibers specifically, but asking your partner to pronate ever so gently can elicit a small contraction.

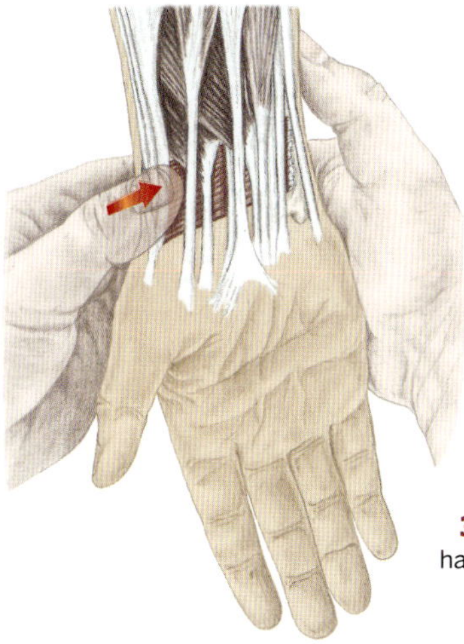

3.120 Palmar view of right hand and wrist, as you explore pronator quadratus

Supinator ▶

Located on the lateral side of the elbow, the short supinator is deep to the forearm extensors and superficial to the head of the radius (**3.121**, **3.122**). As its name suggests, it supinates the forearm and is an antagonist to the pronator teres. It has a slender muscle belly that can be difficult to truly isolate.

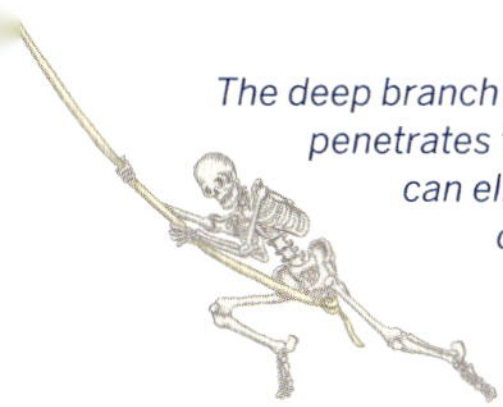

The deep branch of the radial nerve penetrates the supinator's belly and can elicit a sharp, shooting sensation down the forearm when compressed.

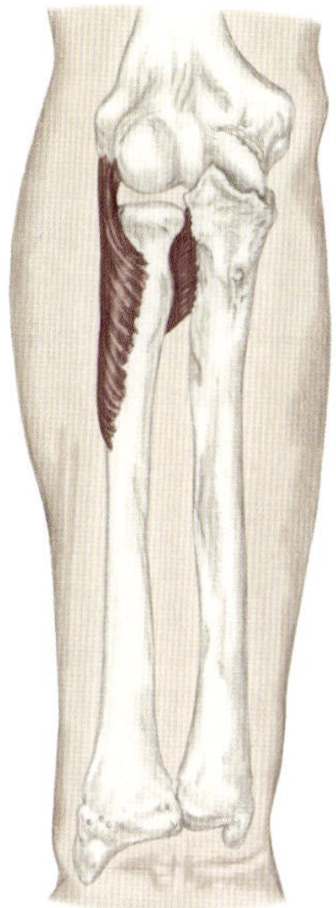

3.121 Anterior view of right forearm, showing supinator

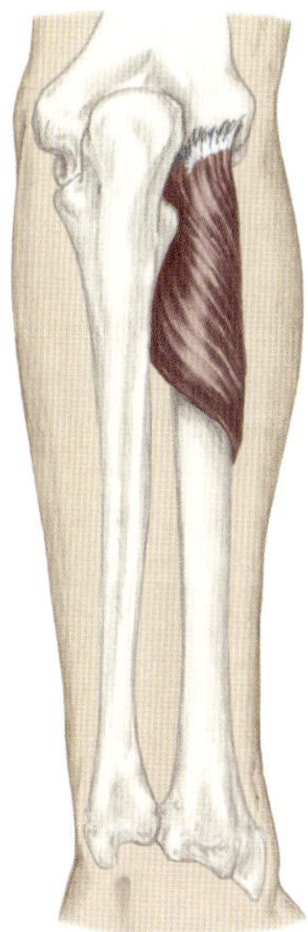

3.122 Posterior view of right forearm, showing supinator

supinate *su*-pi-nate L. bent backward

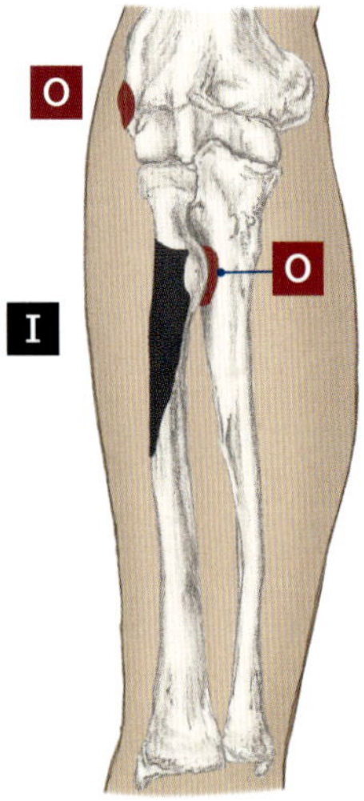

3.123 Anterior view of right forearm, showing origin and insertion of supinator

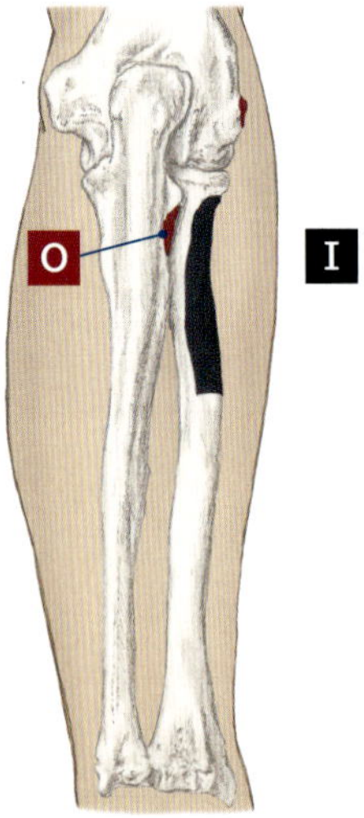

3.124 Posterior view of right forearm, showing origin and insertion of supinator

	SUPINATOR
A	**Supinate** the forearm (radioulnar joints)
O	Lateral epicondyle of humerus, radial collateral ligament, annular ligament, and supinator crest of the ulna
I	Anterior, lateral surface of proximal one-third of radial shaft
N	Radial C5, **6**, (7)

When Do You Use Your Supinator?

- Digging out a big scoop of ice cream
- Swirling the water in a bathtub
- Folding your clothes

Supinator

1. Shake hands with your partner and flex the elbow to 90°. Locate the lateral epicondyle of the humerus and the proximal shaft of the radius.
2. Place your fingerpads between these landmarks and palpate through the extensor fibers for the deep supinator belly (**3.125**).
3. Ask your partner to alternately supinate and relax her forearm against your resistance. The brachioradialis may contract with this movement, but it will be felt superficially, while the supinator is deep to the extensors.

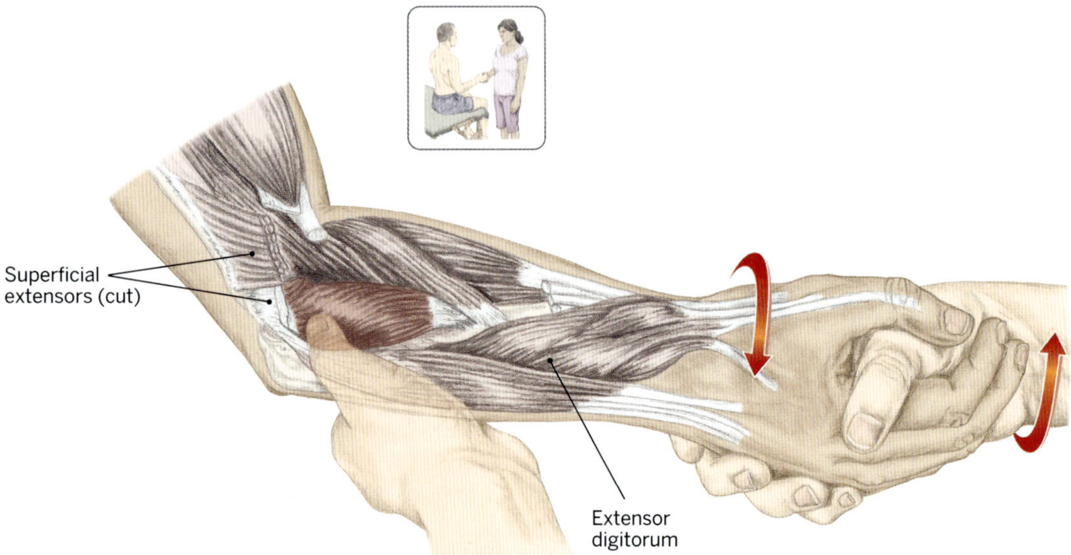

3.125 Lateral view of right forearm, as your partner supinates against your resistance while you access the supinator

Overview: **Muscles of the Thumb and Hand**

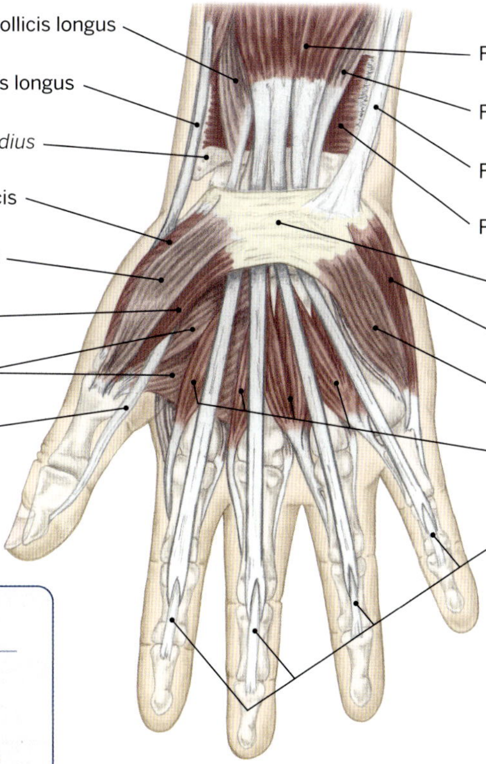

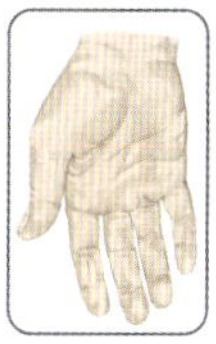

3.126 Palmar view of right hand and wrist, showing superficial layer of muscles

Discover More

The eight muscles that move the thumb can be divided into two groups: short and long muscles. The four *short* muscles (p. 152) are located at the thenar eminence (the fleshy mass at the thumb's base).

Abductor pollicis brevis
Flexor pollicis brevis
Opponens pollicis
Adductor pollicis

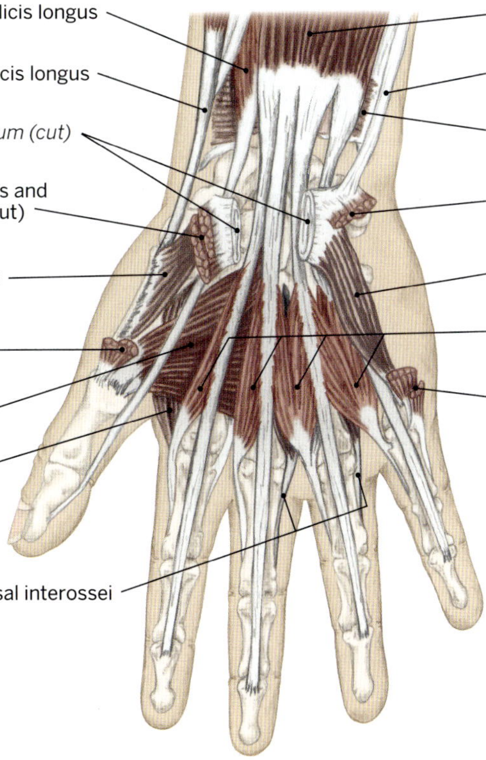

3.127 Palmar view of right hand and wrist, showing intermediate layer of muscles

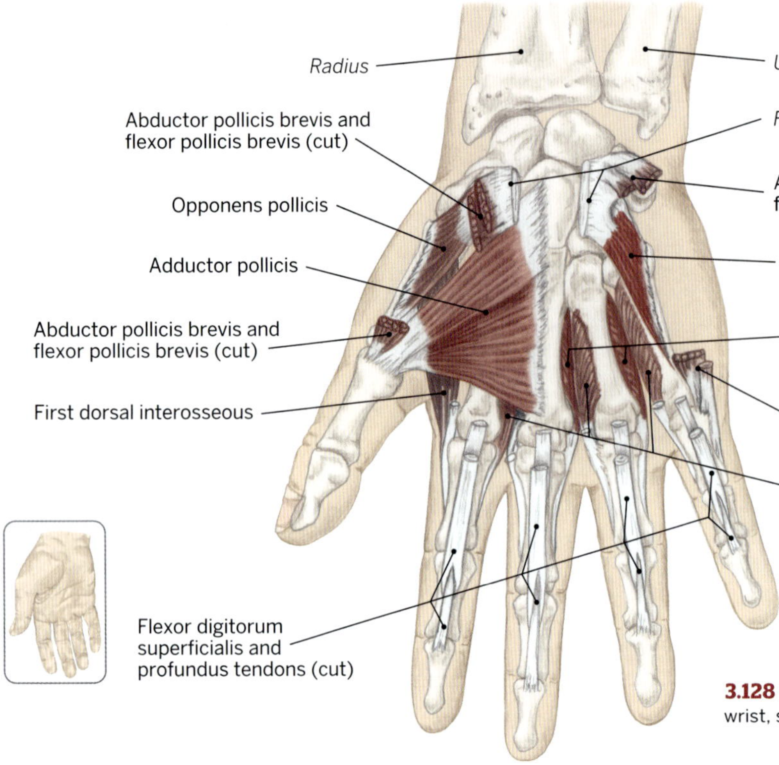

3.128 Palmar view of right hand and wrist, showing deep layer of muscles

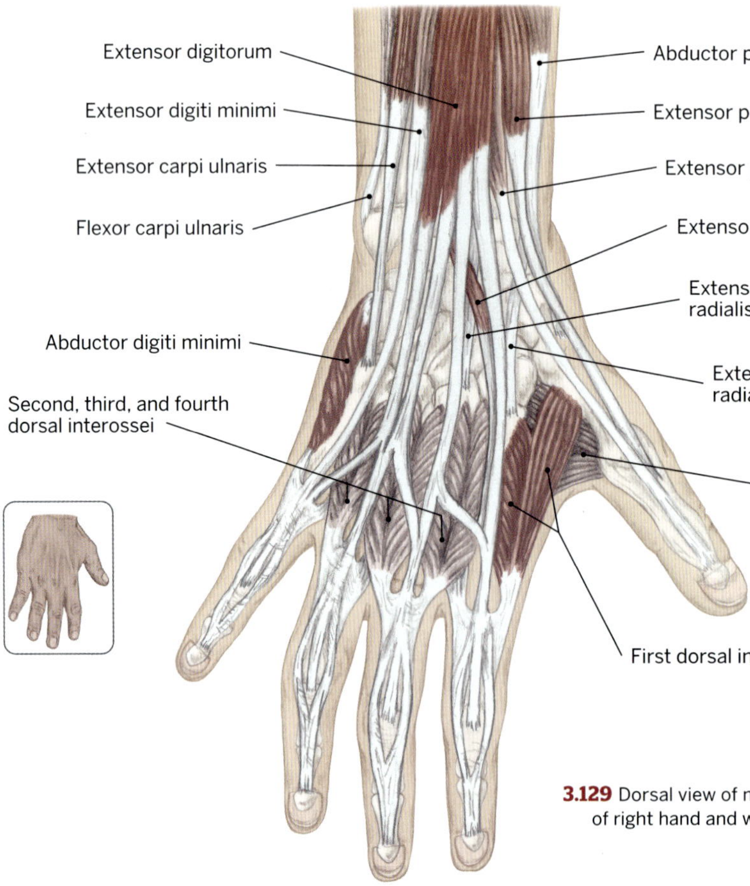

3.129 Dorsal view of muscles of right hand and wrist

Long Muscles of the Thumb

The bellies of **abductor pollicis longus** and **extensor pollicis longus** and **brevis** lie along the posterior aspect of the forearm, deep to the wrist extensors (**3.130–3.134**). Their distal tendons, however, are superficial and form the "anatomical snuffbox." Used historically as a platform for inhaling a variety of substances, this small cavity is located along the dorsal surface of the hand, just distal to the styloid process of the radius.

The belly of the **flexor pollicis longus** lies on the forearm's anterior surface, deep to the wrist flexors, and is inaccessible. Its long, distal tendon travels through the carpal tunnel between the thenar eminence muscles to the distal phalanx of the thumb (**3.135, 3.136**).

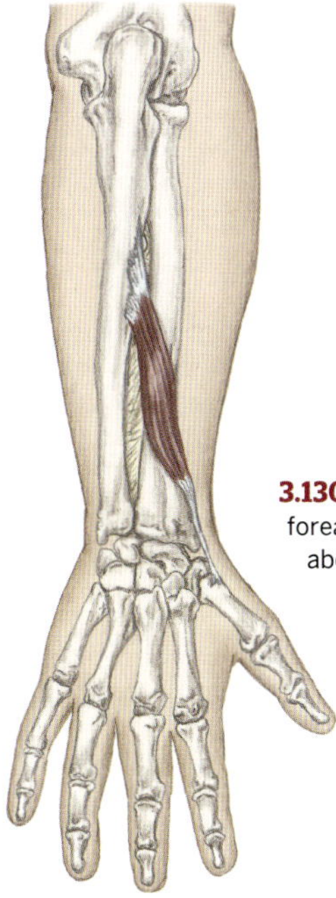

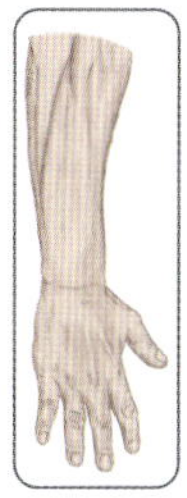

3.130 Posterior view of right forearm and hand, showing abductor pollicis longus

ABDUCTOR POLLICIS LONGUS

A **Abduct** the thumb (carpometacarpal joint)
Extend the thumb (carpometacarpal joint)
Abduct the wrist (radiocarpal joint)

O Posterior surface of radius and ulna, and interosseous membrane

I Base of first metacarpal

N Radial C6, **7**, **8**

When Do You Use Your Abductor Pollicis Longus?

- Giving a thumbs-up gesture
- Pulling one's pinned thumb out from the bottom position during thumb wrestling

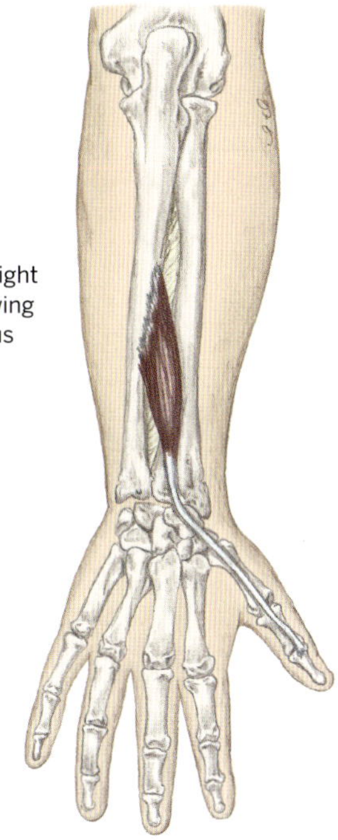

3.131 Posterior view of right forearm and hand, showing extensor pollicis longus

EXTENSOR POLLICIS LONGUS AND BREVIS

A **Extend** the thumb (interphalangeal joint), EPL only
Extend the thumb (metacarpophalangeal and carpometacarpal joints)
Abduct the wrist (radiocarpal joint)

O *Longus:* Posterior surface of ulna and interosseous membrane
Brevis: Posterior surface of radius and interosseous membrane

I *Longus:* Base of distal phalanx of thumb
Brevis: Base of proximal phalanx of thumb

N Radial C6, **7**, **8**

When Do You Use Your Extensor Pollicis Longus and Brevis?

- Giving a thumbs-up gesture
- Pulling one's pinned thumb out from the bottom position during thumb wrestling

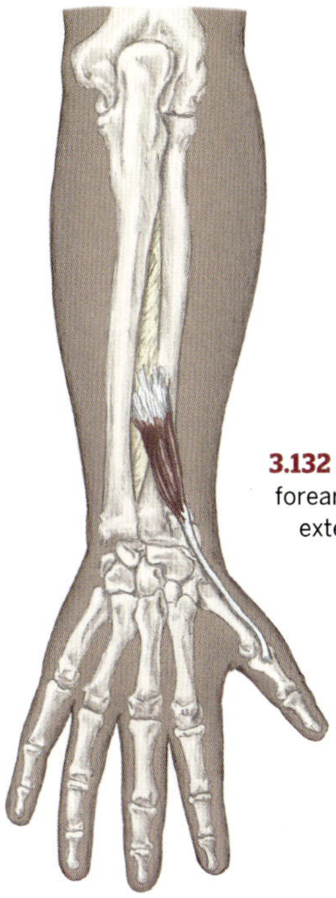

3.132 Posterior view of right forearm and hand, showing extensor pollicis brevis

Discover More

The four *long* muscles of the thumb are tendinous and originate along the shafts of the radius or ulna.

Abductor pollicis longus	*Flexor pollicis longus*
Extensor pollicis longus	*Extensor pollicis brevis*

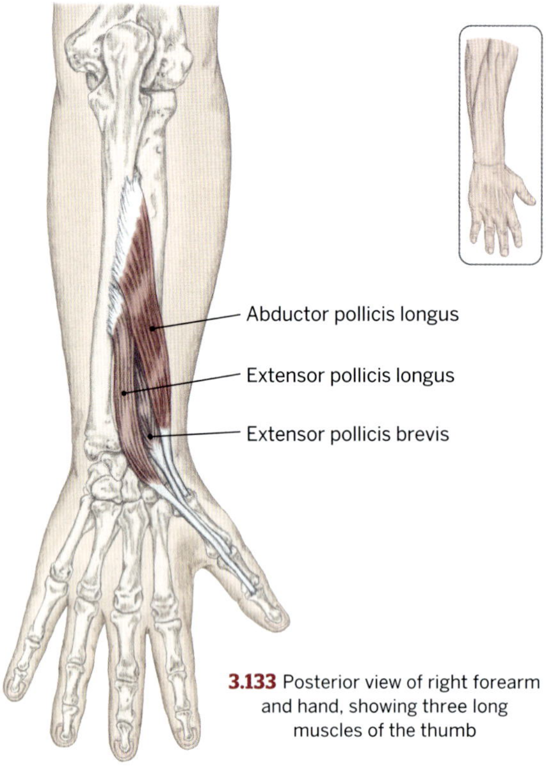

3.133 Posterior view of right forearm and hand, showing three long muscles of the thumb

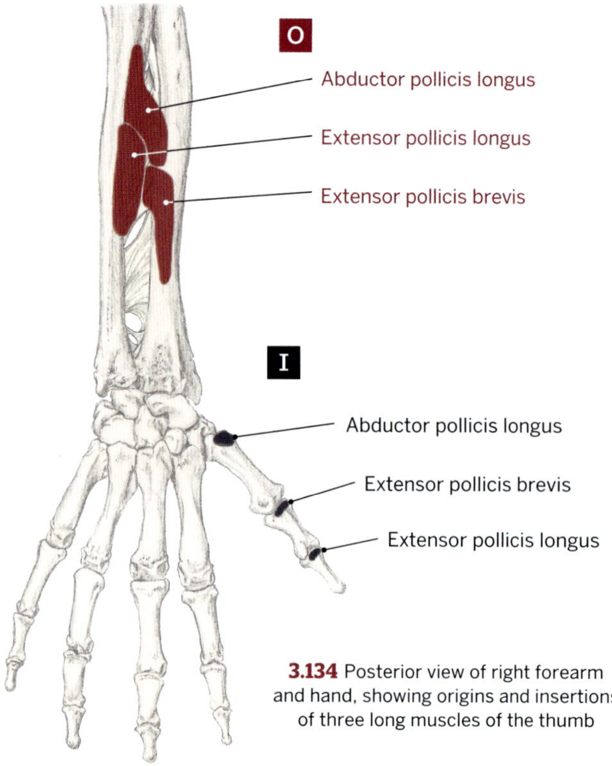

3.134 Posterior view of right forearm and hand, showing origins and insertions of three long muscles of the thumb

FLEXOR POLLICIS LONGUS

A
- **Flex** the thumb (interphalangeal joint)
- **Flex** the thumb (metacarpophalangeal and carpometacarpal joints)
- Assist to **flex** the wrist (radiocarpal joint)

O Anterior surface of radius and interosseous membrane

I Base of distal phalanx of thumb

N Median C(6), 7, **8**, T**1**

When Do You Use Your Flexor Pollicis Longus?

- Grasping the handle of a teacup
- Making a fist
- Holding the key while unlocking the door

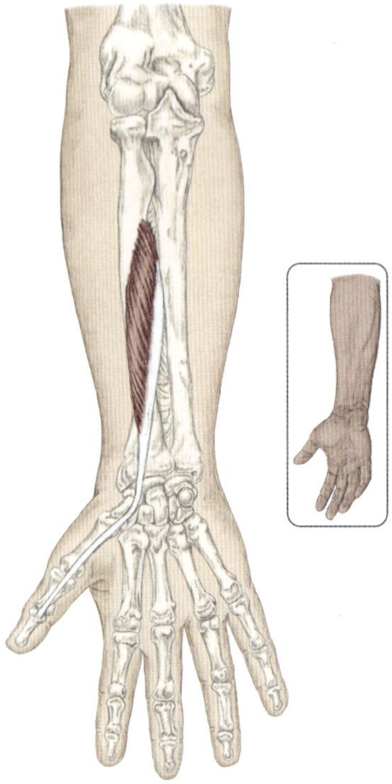

3.135 Anterior view of right forearm and hand, showing flexor pollicis longus

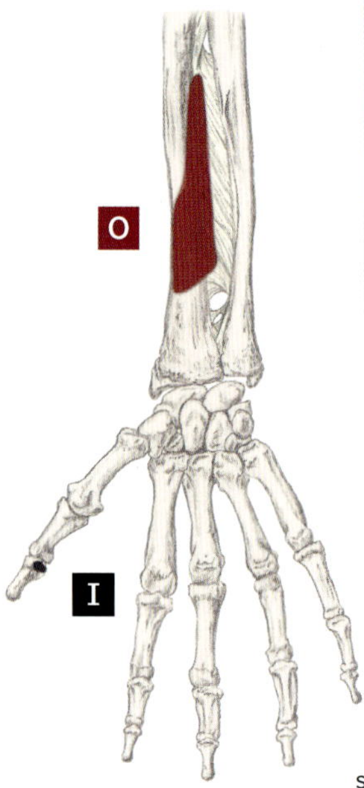

3.136 Anterior view of right forearm and hand, showing origin and insertion of flexor pollicis longus

Anatomical snuffbox and long muscles of the thumb

1. With your partner's wrist in a neutral position, ask her to extend her thumb. "Bring your thumbnail toward your inner elbow" (**3.137**).
2. Just distal to the styloid process of the radius will be a small trough formed by the surrounding tendons. This is the anatomical snuffbox. If not seen immediately, change the angle of the thumb.
3. Follow the tendons that form the snuffbox (extensor pollicis longus and brevis, and abductor pollicis) proximally as they slide over the posterior surface of the radius. Lay your fingers along the posterior surface of the radius as your partner circumducts her thumb in order to feel a portion of these muscles contract (**3.138**).

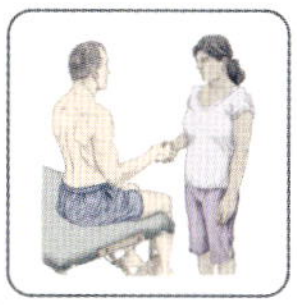

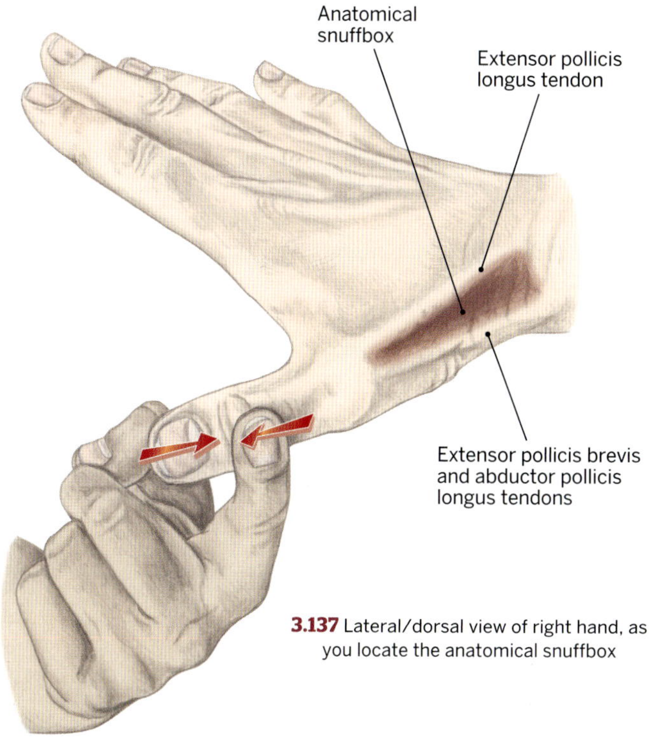

3.137 Lateral/dorsal view of right hand, as you locate the anatomical snuffbox

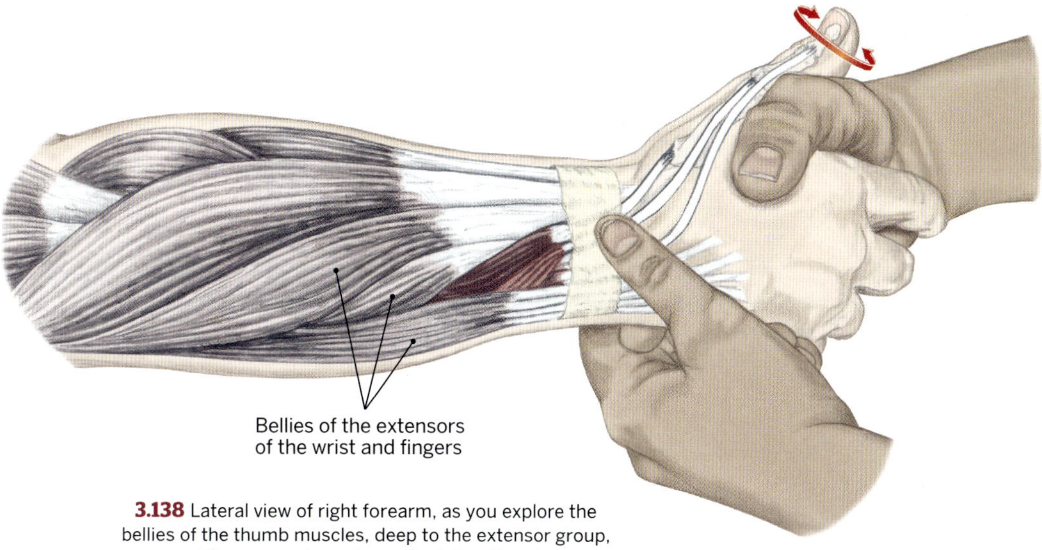

3.138 Lateral view of right forearm, as you explore the bellies of the thumb muscles, deep to the extensor group, while your partner circumducts her thumb

Discover More

The term *anatomical snuffbox* originates from the 16th- to 19th-century European habit of sniffing powdered tobacco, or snuff, from the natural cavity formed between the tendons of the thumb.

Short Muscles of the Thumb

The **abductor pollicis brevis** and **flexor pollicis brevis** (**3.139**, **3.140**) are the superficial and intermediate muscles of the thenar eminence (from a palmar view). As their names suggest, they are short, intrinsic muscles that help to abduct and flex the thumb.

Deep to these two muscles is the **opponens pollicis** (**3.141**). It performs the important task of pulling the thumb across the palm in opposition.

The mass of these three muscles can be easily felt in the thenar eminence, but their specific bellies are difficult to isolate.

The largest of the thumb's short muscles is the strong **adductor pollicis** (**3.142**). It lies deep along the palmar surface and draws the thumb toward the index and middle fingers (adduction). It can sometimes be felt in the web of the hand between the thumb and first finger.

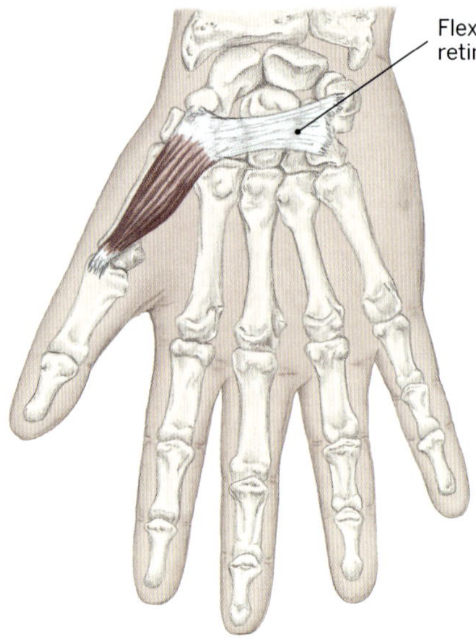

3.139 Palmar view of right hand, showing abductor pollicis brevis

ABDUCTOR POLLICIS BREVIS

A	**Abduct** the thumb (carpometacarpal and metacarpophalangeal joints) Assist in **opposition** of the thumb
O	Flexor retinaculum, trapezium and scaphoid tubercles
I	Base of proximal phalanx of thumb
N	Median C6, 7, 8, T1

When Do You Use Your Abductor Pollicis Brevis?

- Spreading one's fingers apart from each other

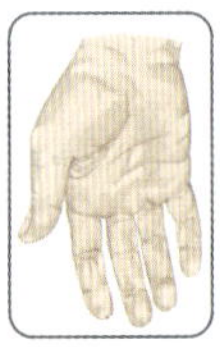

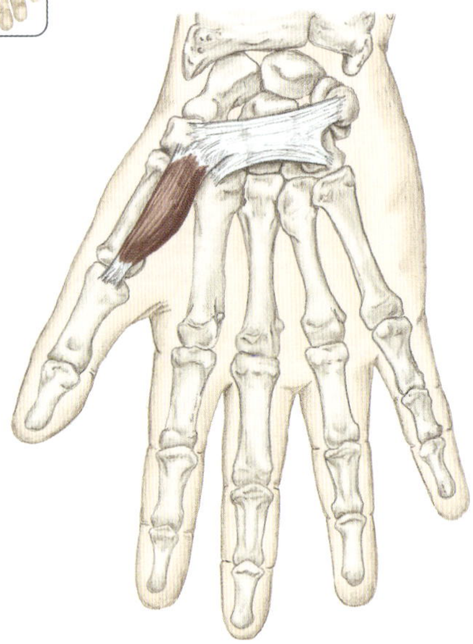

3.140 Palmar view of right hand, showing flexor pollicis brevis

FLEXOR POLLICIS BREVIS

A	**Flex** the thumb (carpometacarpal and metacarpophalangeal joints) Assist in **opposition** of the thumb
O	*Superficial head:* Flexor retinaculum *Deep head:* Trapezium, trapezoid, and capitate
I	Base of proximal phalanx of thumb
N	*Superficial head:* Median C6, 7, 8, T1 *Deep head:* Ulnar C**8**, **T1**

When Do You Use Your Flexor Pollicis Brevis?

- Touching one's thumb to one's pinkie finger

opponens	o-*po*-nens	L. opposing
pollicis	*pol*-li-sis	L. thumb

OPPONENS POLLICIS

A **Opposition** of the thumb at the carpometacarpal joint (bringing the pads of the thumb and fifth finger together)

O Flexor retinaculum and tubercle of the trapezium

I Entire length of first metacarpal bone, radial surface

N Median C6, 7, 8, T1

When Do You Use Your Opponens Pollicis?

- Bringing all one's fingertips together

ADDUCTOR POLLICIS

A **Adduct** the thumb (carpometacarpal and metacarpophalangeal joints)
Assist to **flex** the thumb (metacarpophalangeal joint)

O Capitate, second and third metacarpals

I Base of proximal phalanx of thumb

N Ulnar C**8**, T**1**

When Do You Use Your Adductor Pollicis?

- Snapping one's thumb and finger

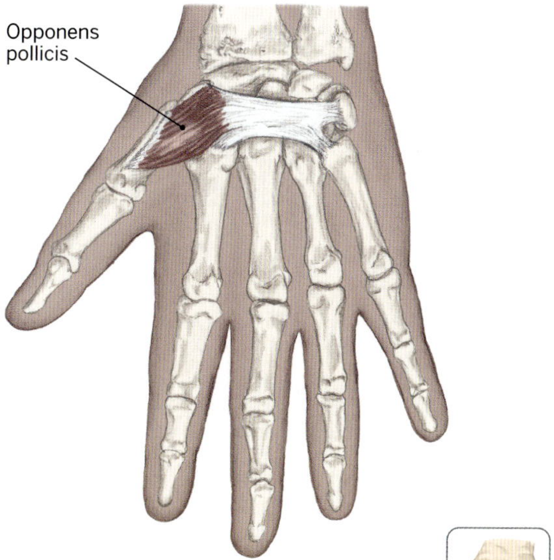

3.141 Palmar view of right hand, showing opponens pollicis

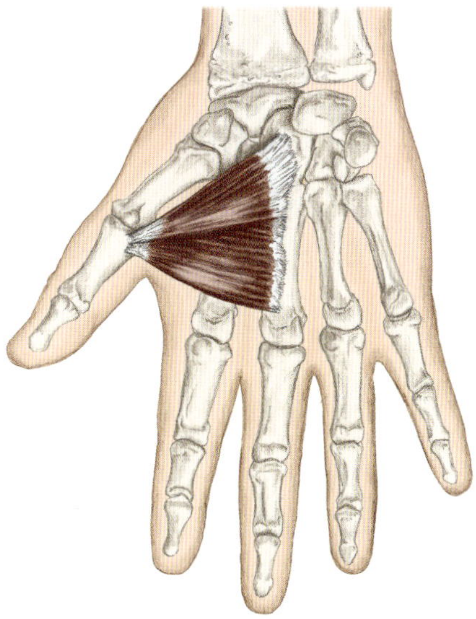

3.142 Palmar view of right hand, showing adductor pollicis

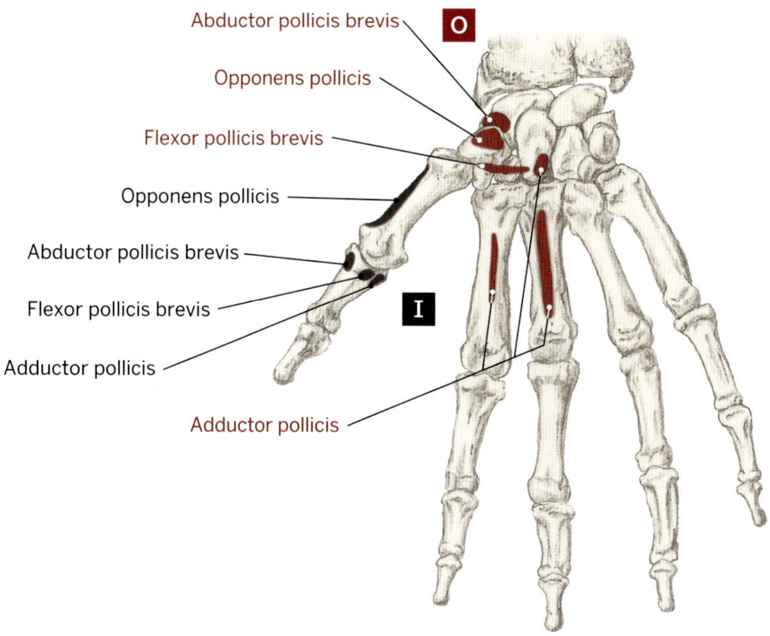

3.143 Palmar view of right hand, showing origins and insertions of short muscles of the thumb

thenar *thee*-nar Grk. palm, flat of the hand

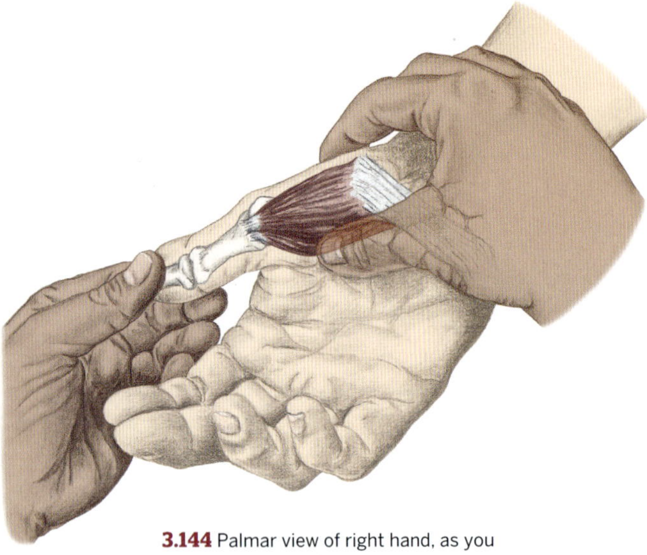

3.144 Palmar view of right hand, as you explore the thenar eminence

Short muscles of the thumb

1. Locate the base of your partner's thumb and explore all sides of the thenar eminence's thick, movable tissue. Palpate from the shaft of the first metacarpal to the webbing between the thumb and finger (**3.144**).
2. Ask your partner to gently squeeze her thumb and fifth fingerpads together. Note how the thenar eminence becomes dense and compact (**3.145**).

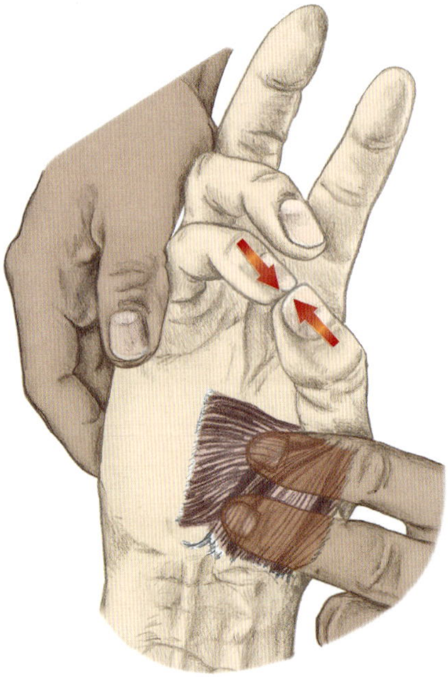

3.145 Palmar view of right hand, as you feel the thenar muscles contract during opposition

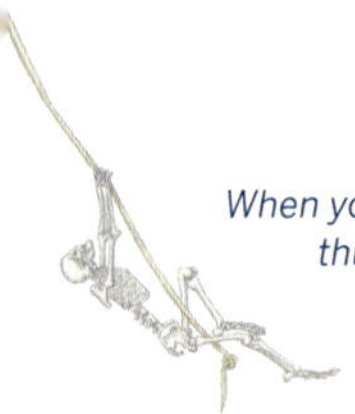

When your partner performs an action with her thumb, be sure the contractions are small and repetitive. More forceful contractions will tighten all the surrounding muscles.

Comparative Anatomy

The human thumb has several unique qualities that distinguish it from the thumbs of other primates. One characteristic that is not distinctly human is the saddle joint of the first carpometacarpal joint. The joint's shape allows for opposition of the thumb and fingers, a skill shared by many higher primates including chimpanzees, orangutans, and gorillas.

One reason for the dexterity of the human thumb is the separation between the flexor pollicis longus and flexor digitorum profundus muscles. In other primates these muscles are united, restricting the ability of the fingers and thumb to move independently. A human is also capable of applying a strong, precise grip with the thumb and fingertips, as when one tightens the lid on a jar. A human's thumb is quite long in proportion to the fingers, whereas the thumbs of many other primates are much shorter than the fingers. Additionally, the muscles on a human's thenar eminence are larger than those on a primate's thenar pad, which is typically flat and lacking in thick musculature.

Chimpanzees, gorillas, and other primates can grasp with terrific force by curling their digits around an object, but opposing the thumb and finger for a specific, detailed task is something only humans can do.

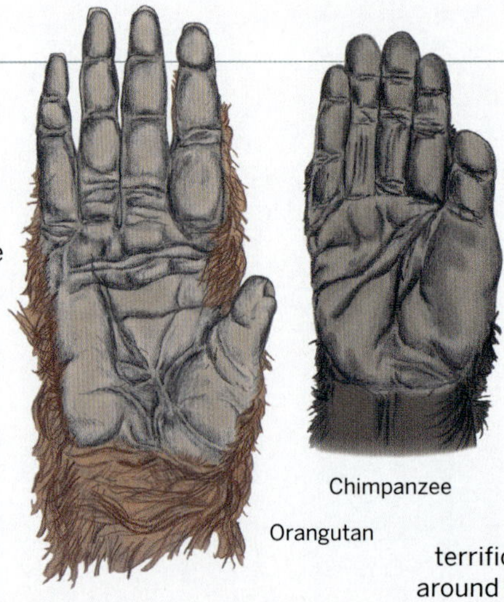

Lumbricals and Interossei

The **lumbricals** sprout from the sides of the flexor digitorum profundus tendons on the palmar side of the hand (**3.146**). Deep to the lumbricals, the **palmar interossei** (**3.147**) are located between the metacarpals and hence are difficult to access. The **dorsal interossei** (**3.148**), however, are accessible between the metacarpals from the hand's dorsal surface (**3.149**).

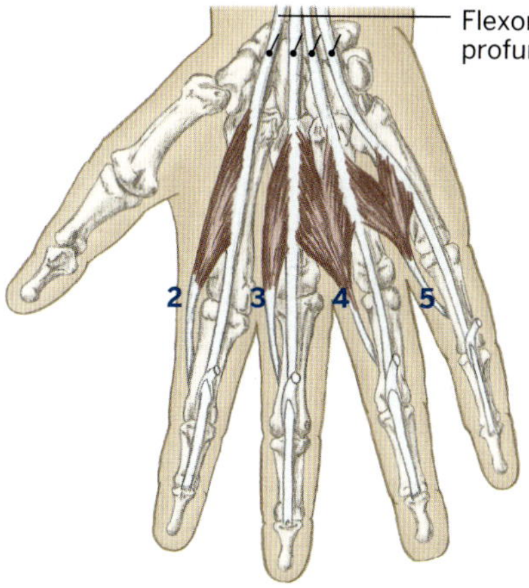

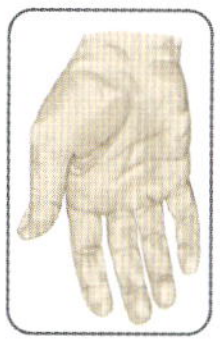

3.146 Palmar view of right hand, showing lumbricals

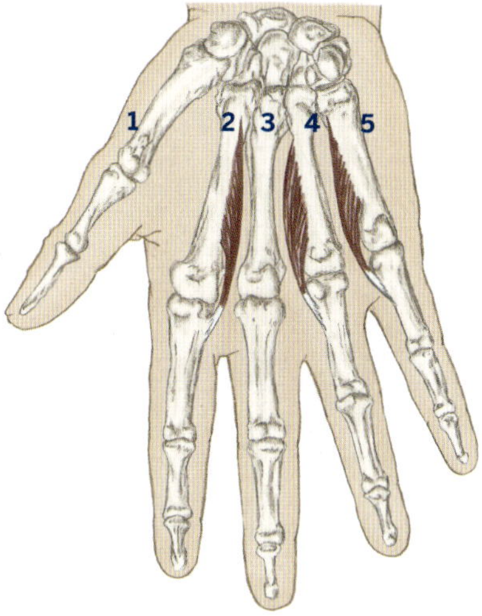

3.147 Palmar view of right hand, showing palmar interossei

LUMBRICALS OF THE HAND

A — **Extend** the second through fifth fingers at the interphalangeal joints

Flex the second through fifth fingers at the metacarpophalangeal joints

O — Surfaces of the flexor digitorum profundus tendons

I — Extensor aponeurosis on dorsal surface of phalanges

N — *Second and third fingers:* Median C(6), 7, **8**, **T1**

Fourth and fifth fingers: Ulnar C(7), **8**, **T1**

When Do You Use Your Lumbricals?

- Fingering chords on a guitar
- Knuckle rolling a coin

PALMAR INTEROSSEI

A — **Adduct** the thumb and second, fourth, and fifth fingers toward the third finger

Assist to **flex** the thumb and second, fourth, and fifth fingers at the metacarpophalangeal joints

Assist to **extend** the thumb and second, fourth, and fifth fingers at the interphalangeal joints

O — Base of first, second, fourth, and fifth metacarpals

I — Base of the proximal phalanx of the related finger and the extensor aponeurosis

N — Ulnar C**8**, **T1**

When Do You Use Your Palmar Interossei?

- Fingering chords on a guitar
- Knuckle rolling a coin

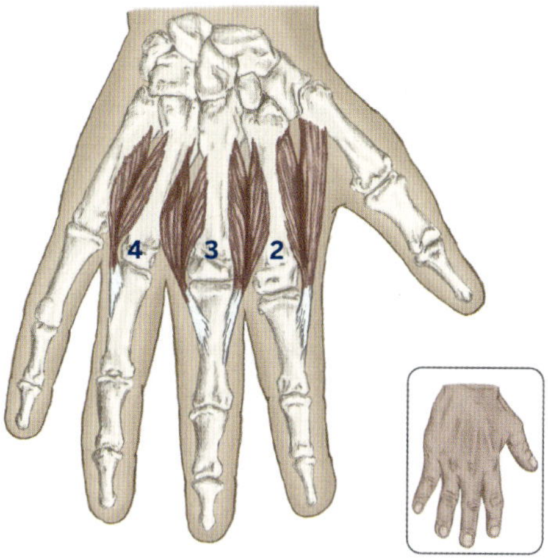

3.148 Dorsal view of right hand, showing dorsal interossei

DORSAL INTEROSSEI

A — **Abduct** the second, third, and fourth fingers at the metacarpophalangeal joints

Assist to **flex** the second, third, and fourth fingers at the metacarpophalangeal joints

Assist to **extend** the second, third, and fourth fingers at the interphalangeal joints

O — Adjacent sides of all metacarpals

I — Base of the proximal phalanx of the second, third, and fourth fingers and the extensor aponeurosis

N — Ulnar C**8**, **T1**

When Do You Use Your Dorsal Interossei?

- Fingering chords on a guitar
- Knuckle rolling a coin

lumbrical	*lum*-bri-kal	L. earthworm
interosseous	*in*-ter-*ah*-see-us	L. between bones

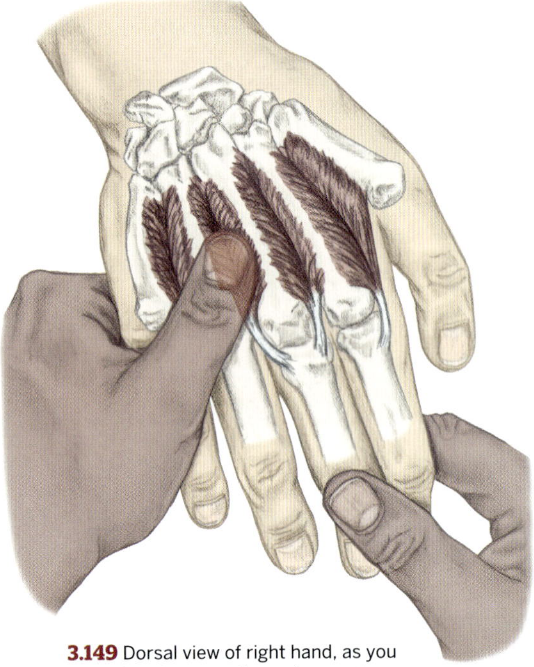

3.149 Dorsal view of right hand, as you explore between the metacarpals for the dorsal interossei

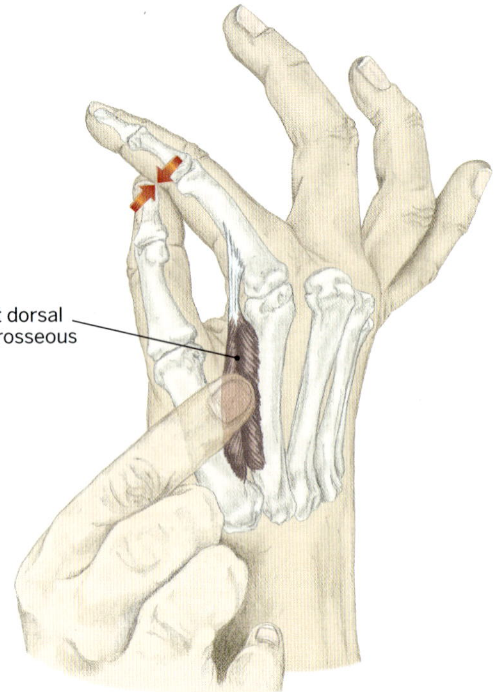

3.150 Dorsal/radial view of right hand. Ask your partner to adduct her thumb. "Press the side of your thumb into the side of your index finger." Note how the muscles of the thenar eminence may soften, but the muscles in the hand's webbing (adductor pollicis and first dorsal interosseous) become taut.

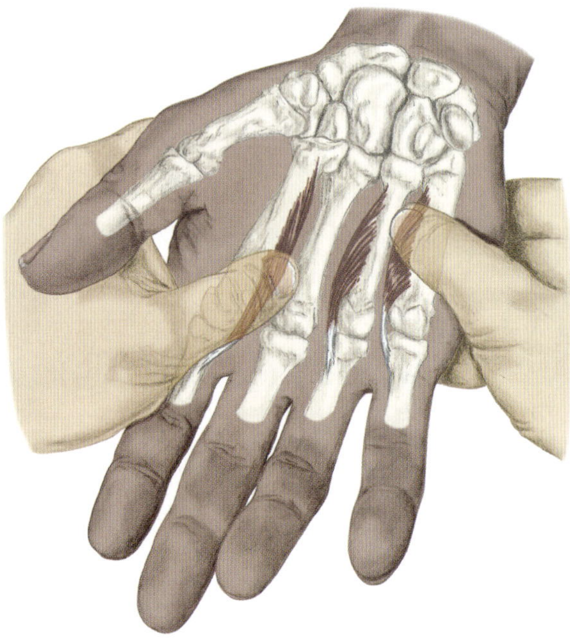

3.151 Palmar view of right hand, as you access the palmar interossei muscles

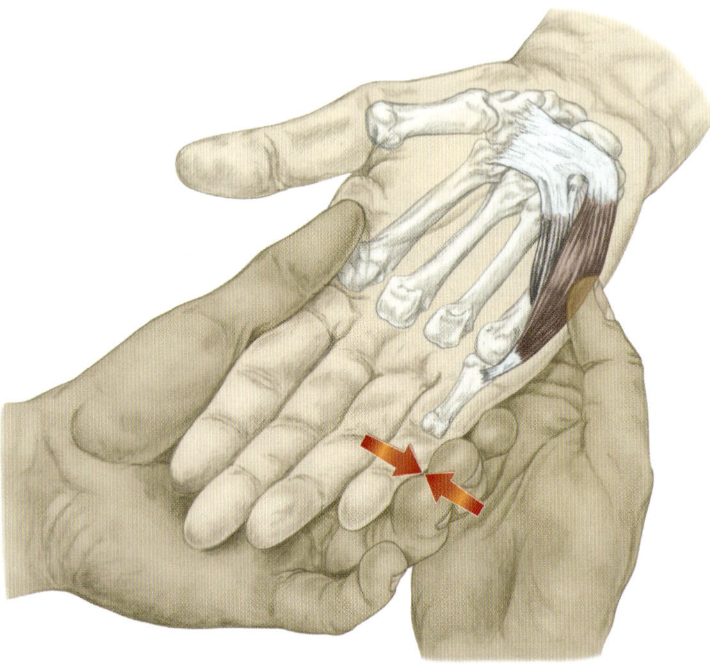

3.152 Palmar view of right hand, as you feel the hypothenar muscles contract when your partner abducts her fifth finger against your resistance

Hypothenar Eminence

Opposite the thenar eminence, along the ulnar side of the palm, is the hypothenar eminence. This oblong mound of flesh is composed of three short muscles: **abductor digiti minimi**, **flexor digiti minimi brevis**, and **opponens digiti minimi** (**3.153–3.156**).

The abductor digiti minimi is superficial and extends from the pisiform to the base of the fifth finger. To isolate it, ask your partner to abduct her fifth finger as you apply a little resistance. The solid belly of the digiti minimi will become immediately apparent next to the shaft of the fifth metacarpal (see **3.152**).

ABDUCTOR DIGITI MINIMI	
A	**Abduct** the fifth finger (metacarpophalangeal joint) Assist in **opposition** of the fifth finger toward the thumb (metacarpophalangeal joint)
O	Pisiform and tendon of flexor carpi ulnaris
I	Base of proximal phalanx of fifth finger, ulnar surface
N	Ulnar C(7), **8**, T**1**

When Do You Use Your Abductor Digiti Minimi?

- Spreading one's fingers apart
- Knuckle rolling a coin

FLEXOR DIGITI MINIMI BREVIS	
A	**Flex** the fifth finger (metacarpophalangeal joint) Assist in **opposition** of the fifth finger toward the thumb
O	Hook of hamate and flexor retinaculum
I	Base of proximal phalanx of fifth finger, palmar surface
N	Ulnar C(7), **8**, T**1**

When Do You Use Your Flexor Digiti Minimi Brevis?

- Playing a saxophone
- Knuckle rolling a coin

OPPONENS DIGITI MINIMI	
A	**Opposition** of the fifth finger at the carpometacarpal joint
O	Hook of hamate and flexor retinaculum
I	Shaft of fifth metacarpal, ulnar surface
N	Ulnar C(7), **8**, T**1**

When Do You Use Your Opponens Digiti Minimi?

- Playing a saxophone
- Knuckle rolling a coin

hypothenar *hi*-po-*thee*-nar Grk. *hypo*, under or below
Grk. *thenar*, palm, flat of the hand

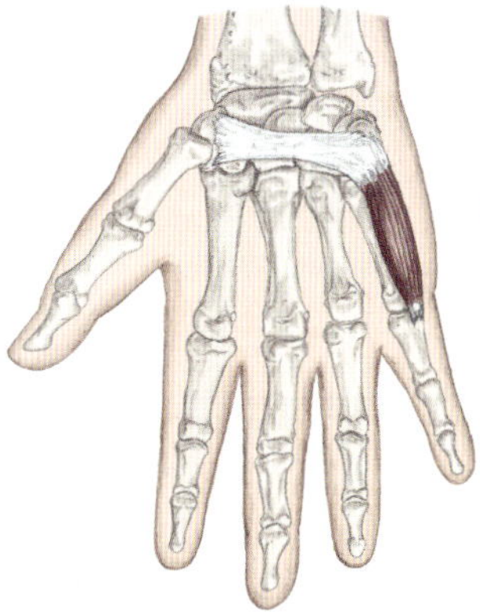

3.153 Palmar view of right hand, showing abductor digiti minimi

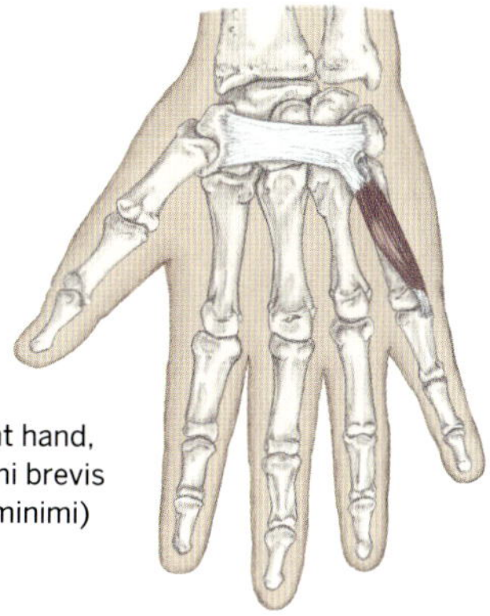

3.154 Palmar view of right hand, showing flexor digiti minimi brevis (deep to abductor digiti minimi)

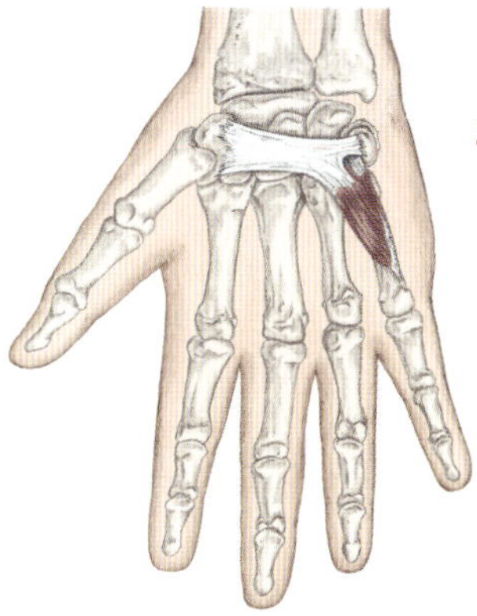

3.155 Palmar view of right hand, showing opponens digiti minimi (deep to flexor digiti minimi brevis)

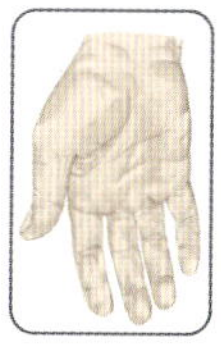

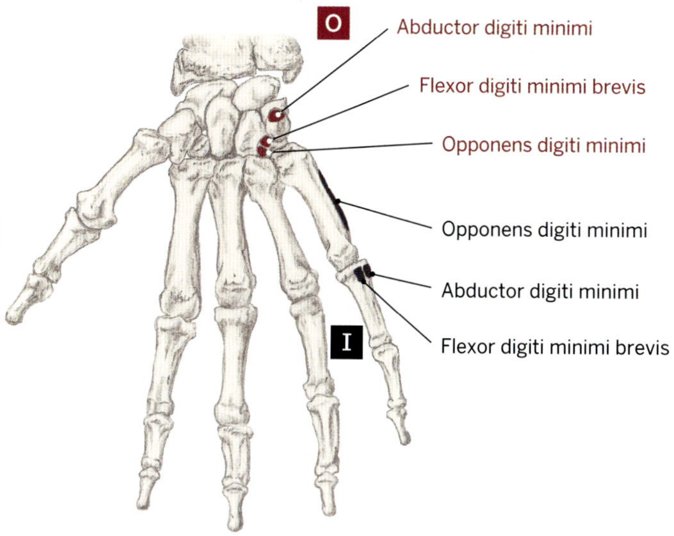

3.156 Palmar view of right hand, showing origins and insertions of muscles of the hypothenar eminence

Ligaments and Other Structures of the Forearm and Hand

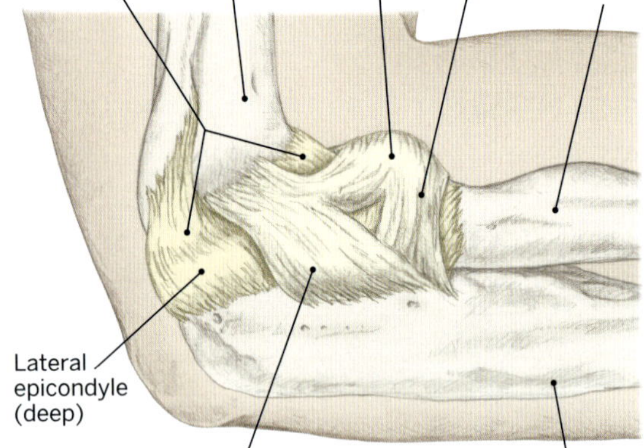

3.157 Lateral view of right elbow, showing humeroulnar and proximal radioulnar joints

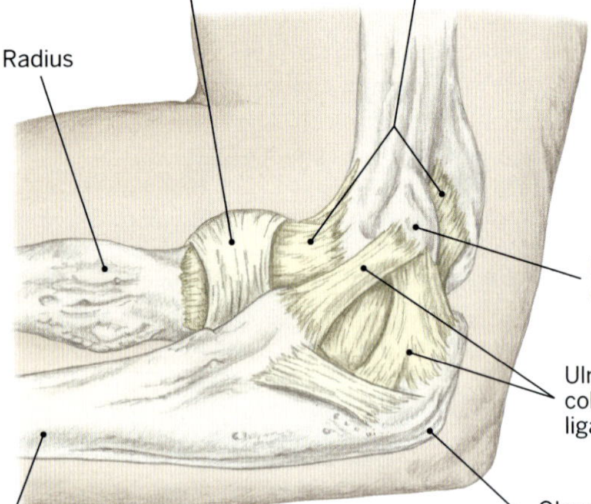

3.158 Medial view of right elbow, showing humeroulnar and proximal radioulnar joints

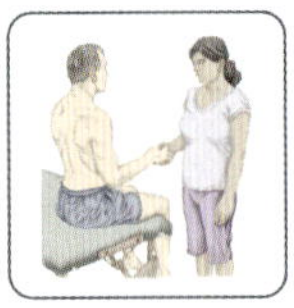

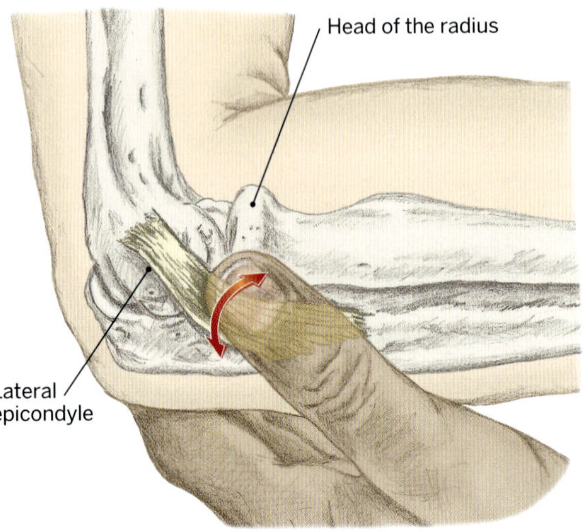

3.159 Lateral view of right elbow, as you palpate the radial collateral ligament

Radial Collateral Ligament

The radial collateral ligament is a cord-like band that stretches from the lateral epicondyle of the humerus to the annular ligament and lateral side of the ulna (**3.157**). The ligament is deep to the supinator and extensors of the forearm.

Radial collateral ligament

1. Shaking hands with your partner, locate the lateral epicondyle of the humerus and head of the radius.
2. Between these landmarks will be a slight ditch. Place your fingertip in this space. Visualize the ligament spanning across the ditch and gently roll your finger across the ligament's slender surface. It may feel like a thin strip of duct tape (**3.159**).

Are you between the head of the radius and the lateral epicondyle? With the elbow flexed, do the fibers of the ligament run parallel to the forearm?

annular	***an***-u-ler	L. ringlike
collateral	ko-***lat***-er-al	L. of both sides

Annular Ligament

The annular ligament wraps around the head and neck of the radius, stabilizing the proximal radius against the ulna during pronation and supination (see **3.158**). It lies deep to the supinator and the extensor muscles of the forearm. Although the annular ligament cannot be palpated separately, its location can be isolated.

Annular ligament

1. With your partner's elbow flexed, place your thumbpad on the head of the radius.
2. While passively pronating and supinating the forearm, allow the head and neck of the radius to pivot under your thumb (**3.160, 3.161**). You may not feel the annular ligament separately, but visualize it stabilizing the head of the radius to the ulna.

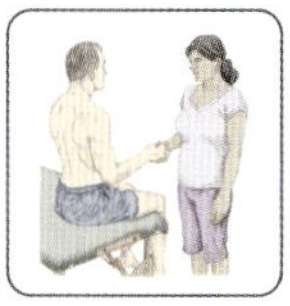

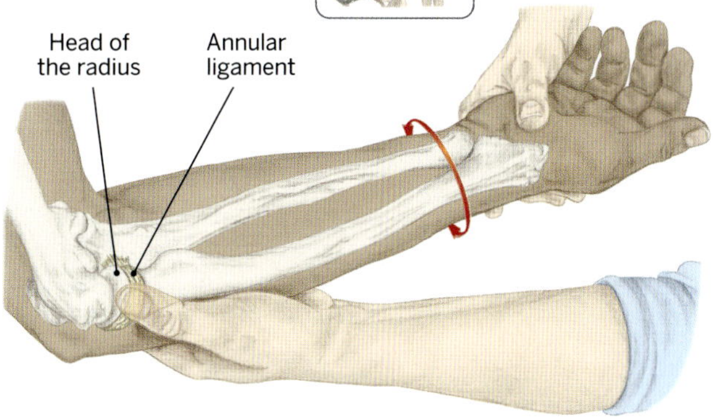

3.160 Posterior/lateral view of right forearm, as you palpate the annular ligament

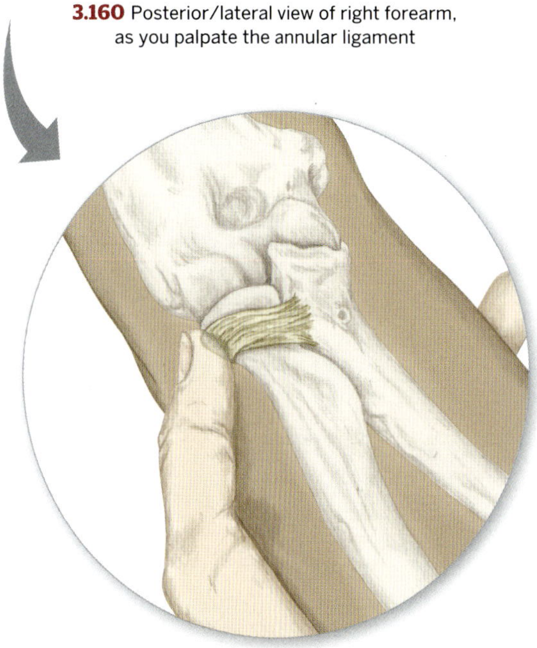

3.161 Anterior/lateral view of right elbow, as you palpate the annular ligament

Ulnar Collateral Ligament

The ulnar collateral ligament is a strong, triangular-shaped ligament that originates on the humerus's medial epicondyle (see **3.158**). Its fibers spread out and attach to the coronoid process of the ulna and to the olecranon process. The collateral ligament is deep to the common flexor tendon and the ulnar nerve.

Ulnar collateral ligament

1. With the elbow flexed, locate the medial epicondyle of the humerus and the medial aspect of the olecranon process.
2. Place your thumb between these landmarks.
3. Palpating through the overlying muscle tissue, explore the ligament's thin fibers, which run transversely to the fibers of the muscles (**3.162**). You may not feel something distinct, but if you are between the stated landmarks, you are in the right location.

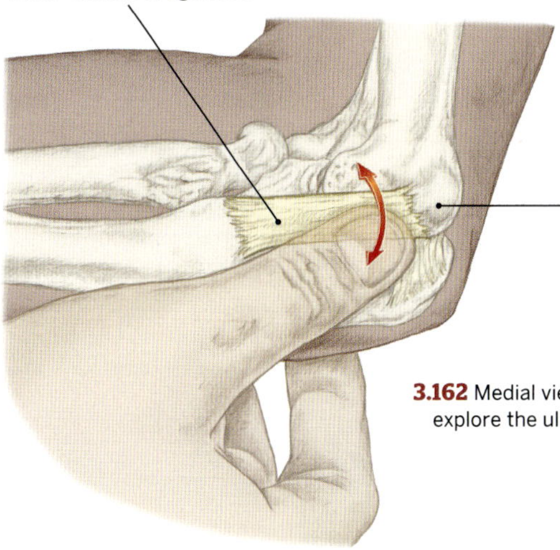

3.162 Medial view of right elbow, as you explore the ulnar collateral ligament

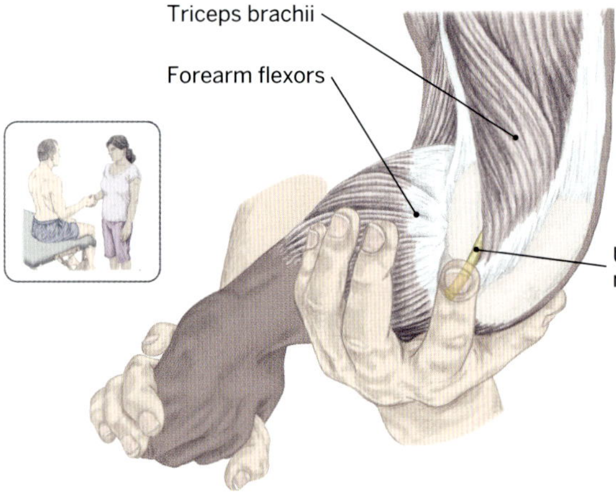

3.163 Medial/posterior view of right elbow, as you gently palpate the ulnar nerve

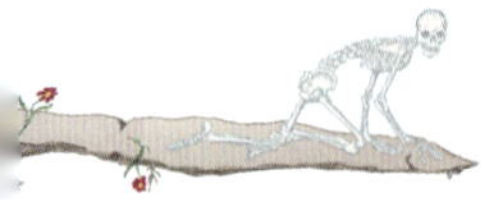

When palpating, be sure not to press too hard and impinge on the ulnar nerve, which can create tingling or numbness in the forearm or hand.

Ulnar Nerve

The ulnar nerve passes between the medial epicondyle and olecranon process as it extends down the forearm. Between these two landmarks the nerve is superficial and easily accessible. Hence, bumping your elbow can irritate the ulnar nerve and create the annoying "funny bone" sensation down the forearm.

Ulnar nerve

1. With the elbow flexed, locate the medial epicondyle and olecranon process. Using gentle pressure, slide your finger into the space between these landmarks and palpate for the tube-shaped nerve (**3.163**).
2. Explore its location in relation to the triceps brachii tendon and common flexor tendon.

Is the structure you feel soft and movable? Are you palpating the ulnar nerve or the triceps brachii's fibrous tendon? Ask your partner to extend her elbow. Does the tendon tighten and the nerve "disappear" into the tissue?

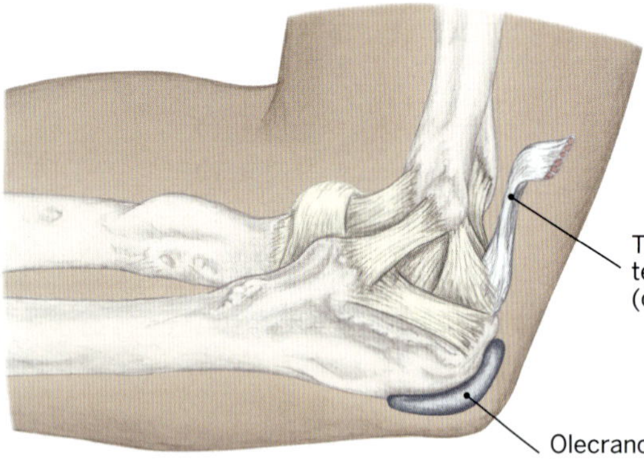

3.164 Medial view of right elbow, showing olecranon bursa

Olecranon Bursa

Just distal to the triceps brachii tendon, this small bursa pads the space between the olecranon process and skin of the elbow (**3.164**). Due to its location, the bursa can become inflamed when the elbow is irritated or struck by an external object. This condition, olecranon bursitis (or "student's elbow"), is readily observable by the distinct, localized ballooning of the elbow.

Olecranon bursa

1. Flex the elbow to 90° and locate the olecranon process.
2. Palpating just distally to the process, gently explore the elbow's thin, malleable tissue. Then let the elbow extend and note how the skin and fascia become even more lax.
3. If the bursa is inflamed, the elbow will present a "goose egg" swelling with localized tenderness. In a healthy state, the bursa is not palpable.

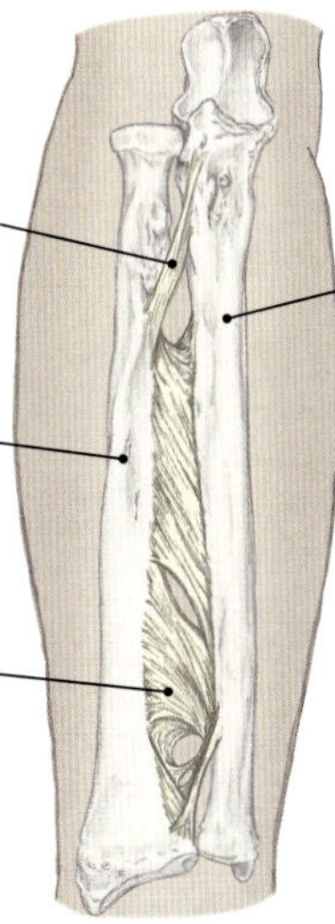

3.165 Anterior view of right forearm, showing interosseous membrane

Interosseous Membrane

This thin but strong fibrous sheet binds together the forearm bones and serves as an attachment site for several muscles (**3.165**). Its oblique cord strengthens the membrane's proximal end. During stress, it is not uncommon for the bones to fracture before the interosseous membrane tears.

Because of its deep location, the membrane is not directly accessible. Exploration between the bones at the distal half of the forearm, however, can give you a sense of its presence and tensile firmness.

Retinacula of the Wrist and Palmar Aponeurosis

The **flexor retinaculum** is located on the palmar surface of the wrist just distal to the flexor crease. Its transverse fibers lie deep to the palmaris longus tendon and superficial to the other flexor tendons and median nerve. The flexor retinaculum and carpal bones form the carpal tunnel, in which the flexor tendons and median nerve pass (**3.166**).

Isolating the thin flexor retinaculum can be difficult, but its transverse fibers (which are perpendicular to the deeper tendons) help to distinguish it. Also, if the retinaculum is "tight," the tissue of the anterior wrist might have an inflexible feel.

The thick **palmar aponeurosis** is a continuation of the antebrachial fascia that stretches superficially across the palm of the hand and is an attachment site for the palmaris longus tendon. It is shaped in a similar way to the plantar aponeurosis (p. 408) on the sole of the foot. Although it might not be easy to palpate, nevertheless, like the flexor retinaculum, its tensile quality can be felt.

The **extensor retinaculum** is superficial and located on the posterior wrist. Like the flexor retinaculum, it is a thickening of fascia that has transverse fibers stretching across the wrist to attach to underlying bones. It stabilizes the wrist and thumb extensors. It is roughly three-quarters of an inch wide and located distal to the head of the ulna and the styloid process of the radius.

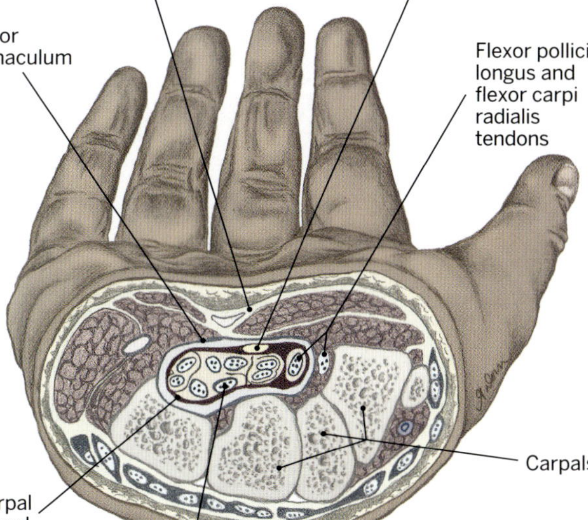

3.166 Cross section of the right wrist

Flexor retinaculum and palmar aponeurosis

1. Cradle your partner's hand so your thumbpad is on the flexor crease of the wrist. Slide half an inch distally to the crease and sink into the thick tissues of the "heel" of the hand (**3.167**).
2. As you explore the carpal space, visualize the retinaculum spanning across the carpals. Passively flex and extend the wrist and feel the tension in the retinaculum change.
3. Slide distally onto the palm of the hand and palpate for the thick, superficial palmar aponeurosis.

*When palpating the flexor retinaculum, are you distal to the level of the pisiform (p. 119)? To highlight the palmar aponeurosis, ask your partner to tighten his hand as if he were "palming a basketball" (**3.168**). Note how this action also brings the palmaris longus tendon into view.*

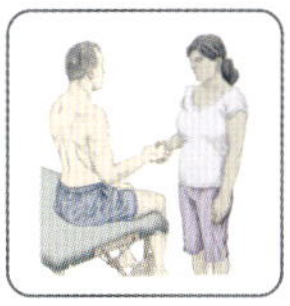

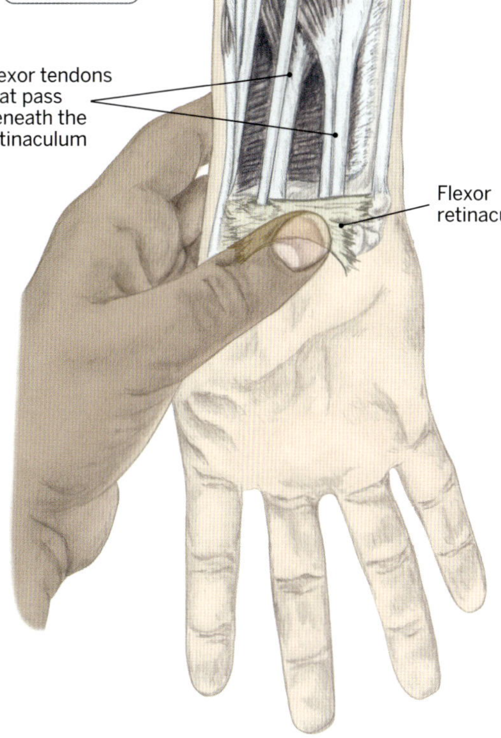

3.167 Palmar view of right hand and wrist, as you palpate the flexor retinaculum

retinaculum	*ret*-i-*nak*-u-lum	L. halter, band, rope
aponeurosis	*ap*-o-nu-*ro*-sis	Grk. *apo*, from + *neuron*, nerve or tendon

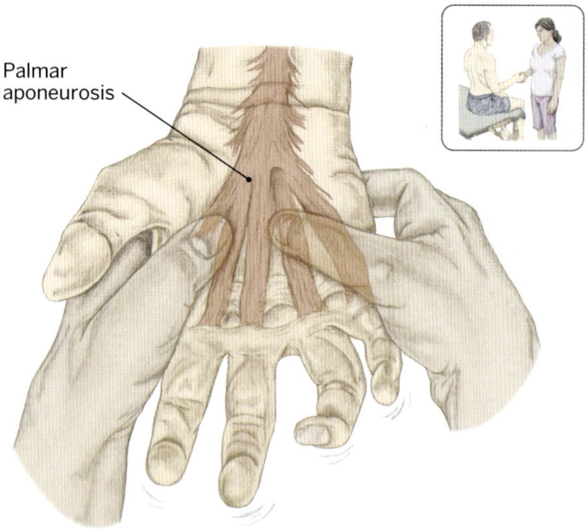

3.168 Palmar view of right hand and wrist, as you palpate the palmar aponeurosis

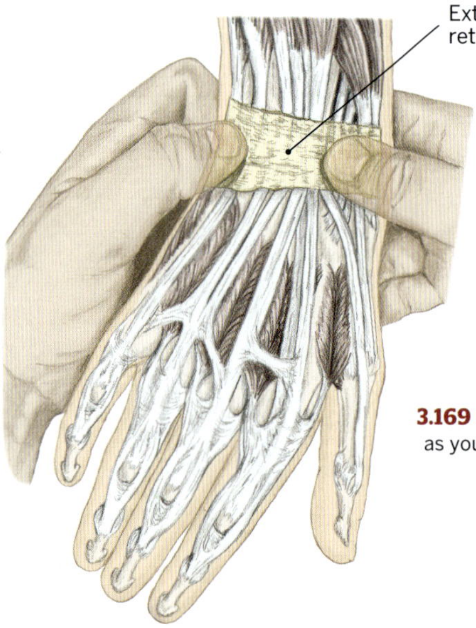

3.169 Dorsal view of right hand and wrist, as you palpate the extensor retinaculum

Extensor retinaculum

1. Ask your partner to extend her fingers and wrist. The pressure from the bulging extensor tendons will make the retinaculum more distinct.
2. Locate the head of the ulna and the styloid process of the radius.
3. Palpate just distal to these landmarks by sliding across the transverse fibers of the thin retinaculum (**3.169**).

Are you distal to the head of the ulna and the styloid process of the radius? Can you distinguish superficial, transverse fibers?

Radial and Ulnar Arteries

The radial and ulnar arteries branch off the brachial artery and travel down the forearm to the hand. The **radial artery** is often used for taking a pulse. It is detectable on the anterior wrist between the tendon of the flexor carpi radialis and the shaft of the radius.

The **ulnar artery** is found proximal to the pisiform and medial to the palmaris longus tendon. Its pulse may not be as easily accessible as the radial pulse.

Radial and ulnar arteries

1. Locate the radial pulse by placing two fingerpads on the flexor side of the wrist. Move laterally and gently press to feel the pulse (**3.170**).
2. Locate the ulnar pulse by moving your fingerpads to the medial side of the flexor surface (**3.171**).

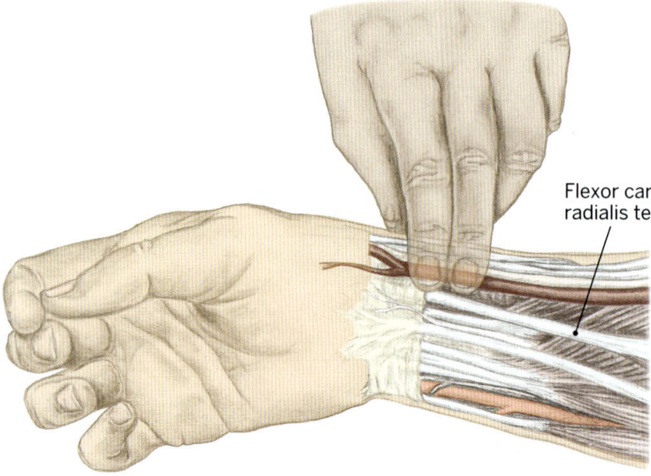

3.170 Palmar view of right wrist, as you feel the pulse of the radial artery

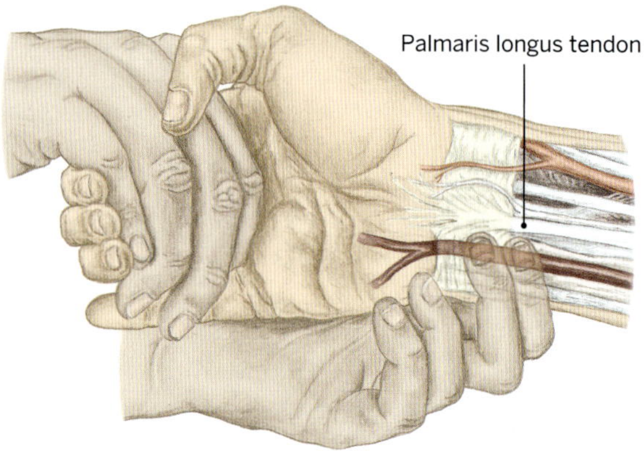

3.171 Palmar view of right wrist, as you feel the pulse of the ulnar artery

Ligaments of the Wrist, Hand, and Fingers

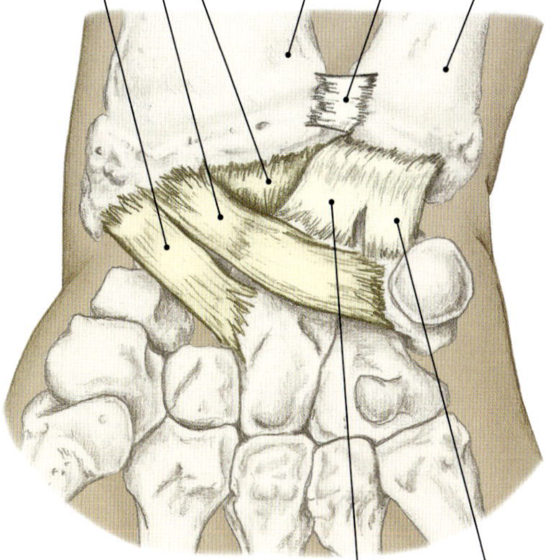

3.172 Palmar view of right wrist, showing ligaments of radiocarpal joints

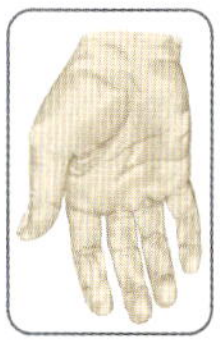

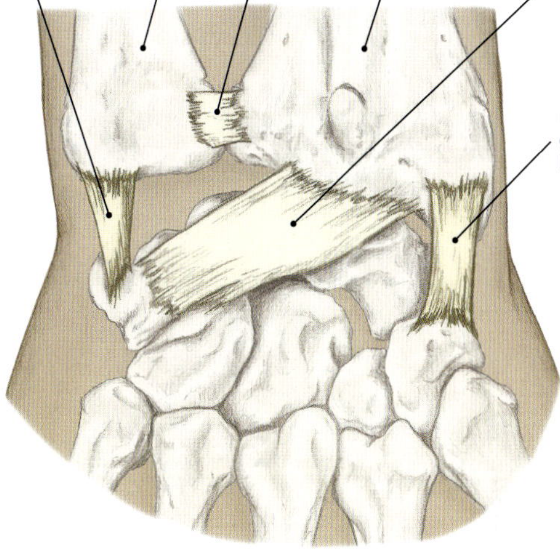

3.173 Dorsal view of right wrist, showing ligaments of radiocarpal joints

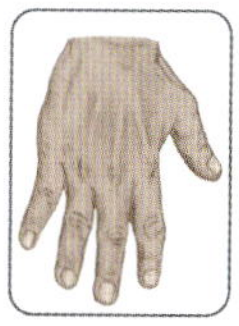

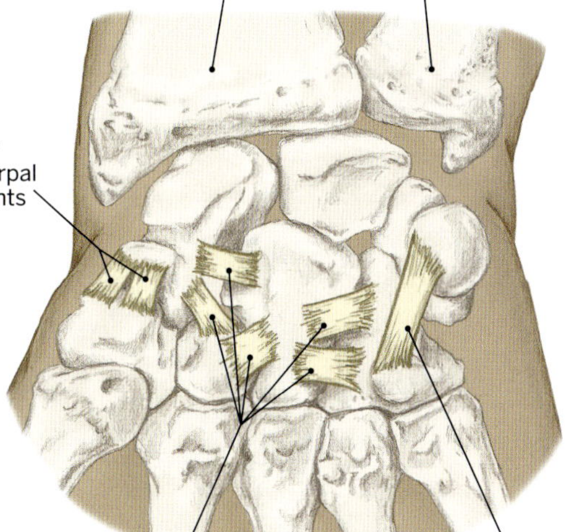

3.174 Palmar view of right wrist, showing ligaments of intercarpal joints

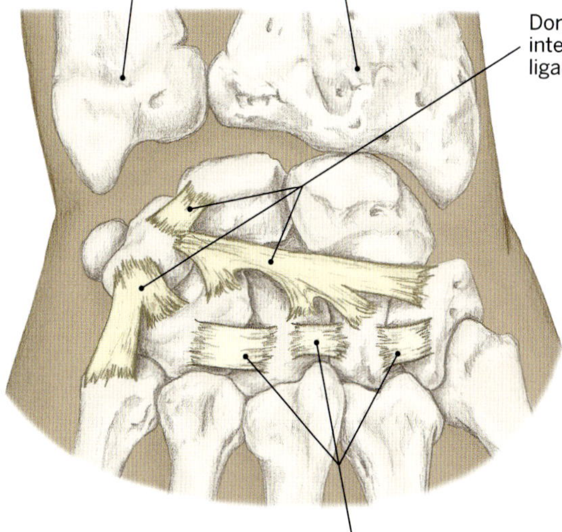

3.175 Dorsal view of right wrist, showing ligaments of intercarpal joints

radioscapholunate	*ray*-dee-o-***skaf***-o-***loo***-nate
radiotriquetrum	*ray*-dee-o-tri-***kwe***-trum
radiocapitate	*ray*-dee-o-***kap***-i-tate
ulnolunate	*ul*-no-***lu***-nate
ulnotriquetrum	*ul*-no-tri-***kwe***-trum

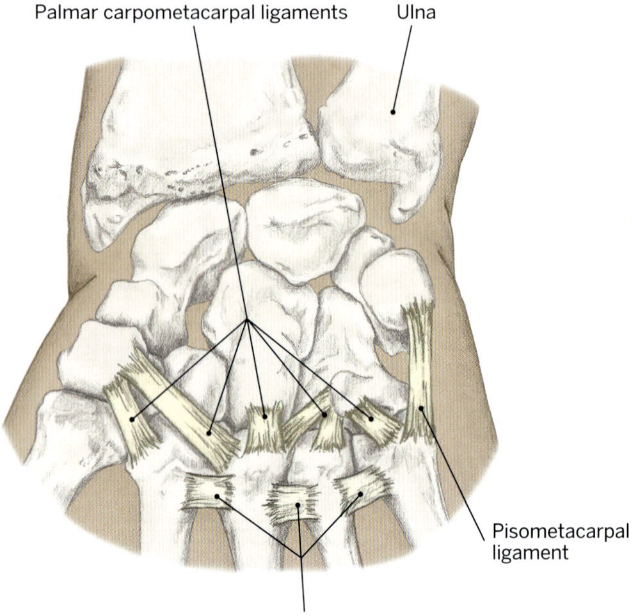

3.176 Palmar view of right wrist, showing ligaments of carpometacarpal and metacarpal joints

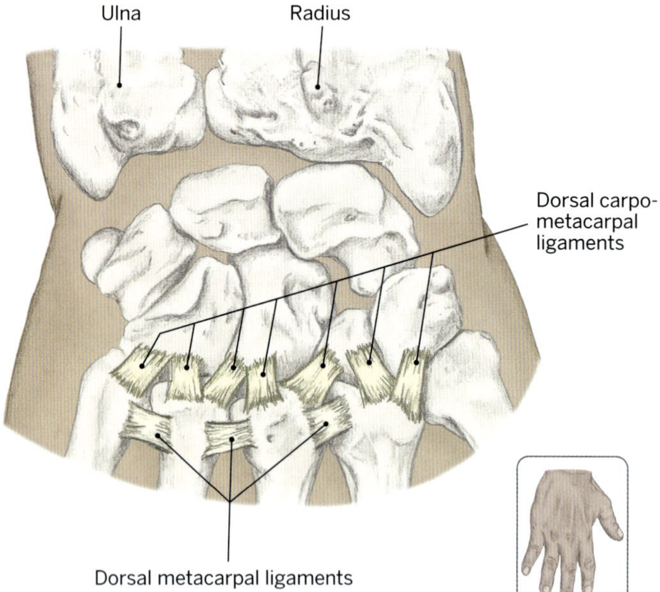

3.177 Dorsal view of right wrist, showing ligaments of carpometacarpal and metacarpal joints

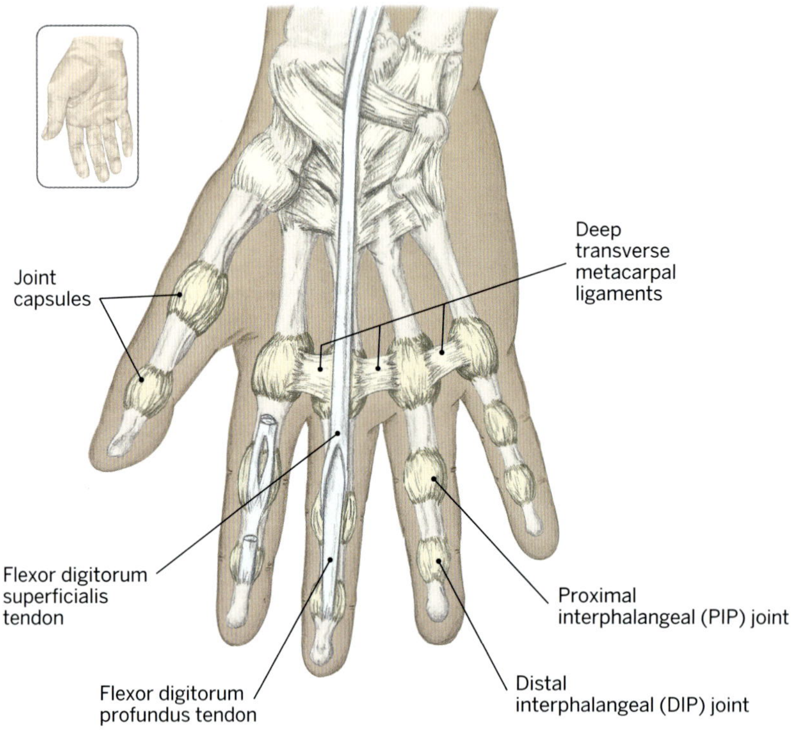

3.178 Palmar view of right wrist and hand, showing interphalangeal joints

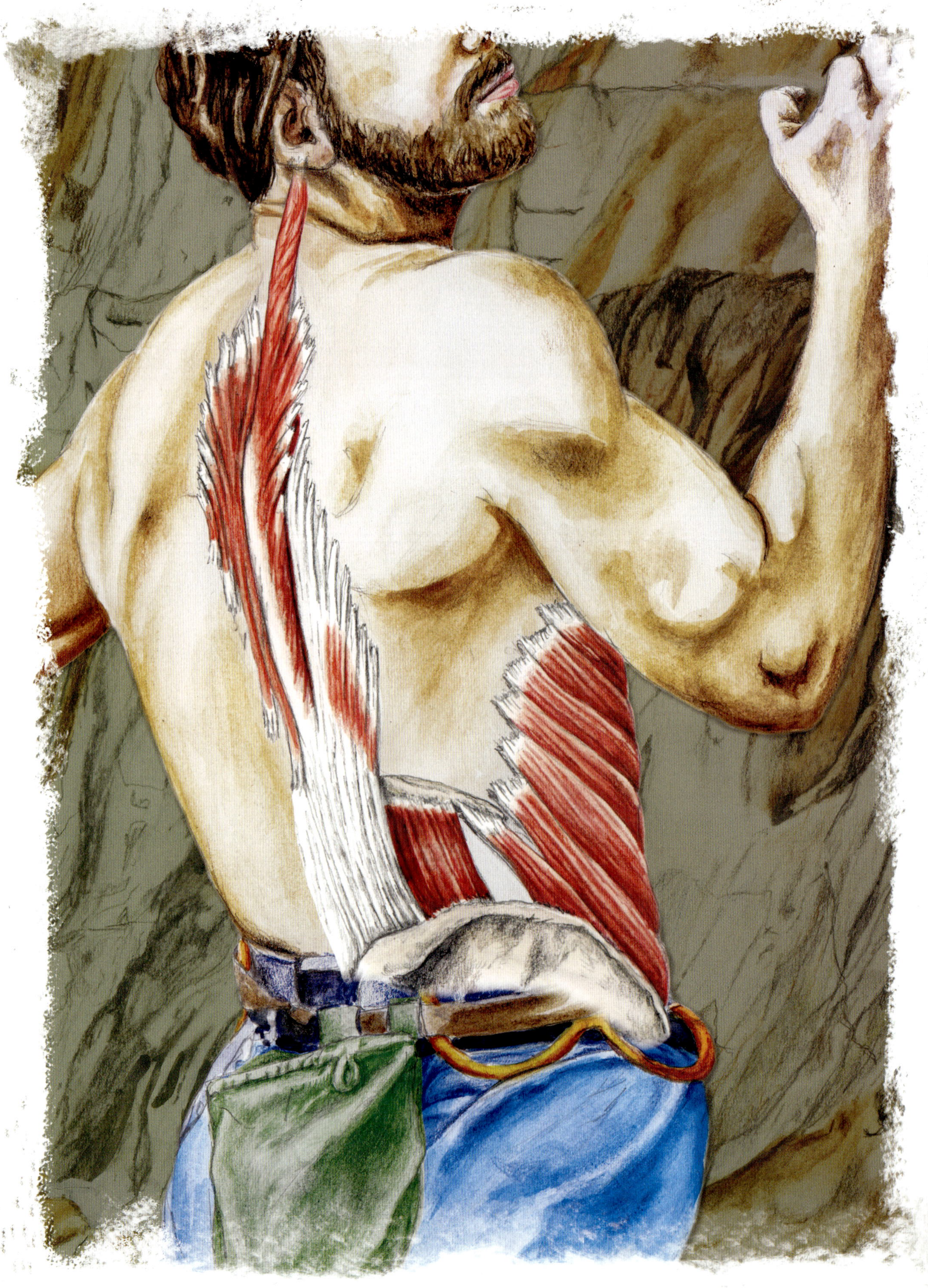

4

Spine & Thorax

If you're breathing, laughing, standing in line, or doing sit-ups, give a shout-out to your spine and thorax. Composing the core of your body, they provide support and stability and play a role in virtually every movement. They also offer important safeguards; the vertebral column protects the spinal cord, while the rib cage and pelvic girdle shield your vital organs.

This region includes some of your largest and smallest muscles. In the picture on the previous page, you might notice that some muscles orient vertically, diagonally, or horizontally. Some reach from the low back all the way to the head and neck. Others wrap from the anterior side of the body to the posterior side.

Since we rely on the spine and thorax muscles for a variety of actions—and often at the same time—they can be prone to injury. For instance, how are the climber's muscles working together to hold his torso facing one direction while his hips are being twisted in another direction?

See for yourself:

- Place both of your hands around your rib cage and take some slow, deep breaths. In which directions do your ribs move?
- Now slide your hands down off the ribs and onto the sides of your abdomen. Exhale fully, pushing all the air out. Hold this position and palpate around the front, sides, and back of your lower torso. Can you feel how your abdominals form a "muscular shield" around the front, sides, and back of your lower torso—as well as down to the groin area?

Topographical Views

Comparative Anatomy

A vertebrate is an animal that has a spinal column. Vertebrates include fishes, amphibians, reptiles, birds, mammals, and humans. An insect or a mollusk has no spinal column and is therefore called an invertebrate. Animals that walk on four legs are called quadrupeds, whereas humans are bipeds.

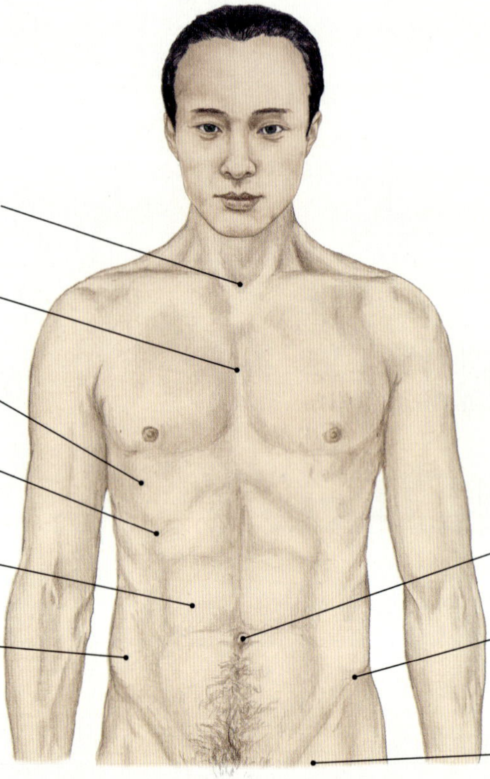

4.1 Anterior view of upper body

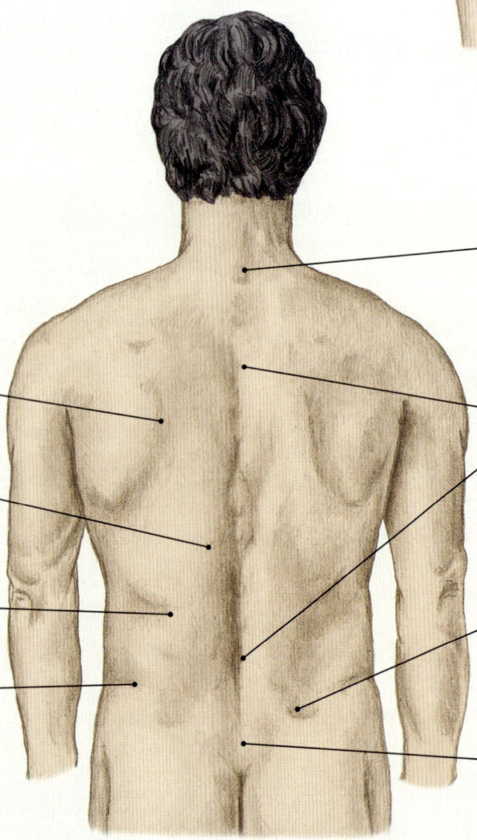

4.2 Posterior view of upper body

Comparative Anatomy

The vertebrae, sternum, and pelvis of a bird are usually air-filled, or pneumatized. A bone becomes pneumatized, it is believed, when its surface comes in contact with an air sac. The bone tissue that rests against the air sac becomes thin before it disappears entirely, leaving behind a cavity that is then penetrated by the air sac. In such a way, the tiny air-filled outgrowths or sacs that extend off the lungs of a bird fill its bones and body cavities, thereby reducing its total body weight.

Exploring the Skin and Fascia

Spine

1. Partner prone. Begin by laying your hands on your partner's middle and lower back and sensing the temperature of the tissue. Explore the sides of the torso as well.
2. Begin to gently lift the skin and fascia superficial to the spinal column in the low back region (**4.3**). Often this tissue can be quite dense and impliable. Move a few inches laterally and compare it to the tissue superficial to the large erector muscles.
3. Continue further laterally to the sides of the trunk (between the axilla and pelvis). As you move more laterally, can you detect any differences in the tissue's elasticity or thickness?

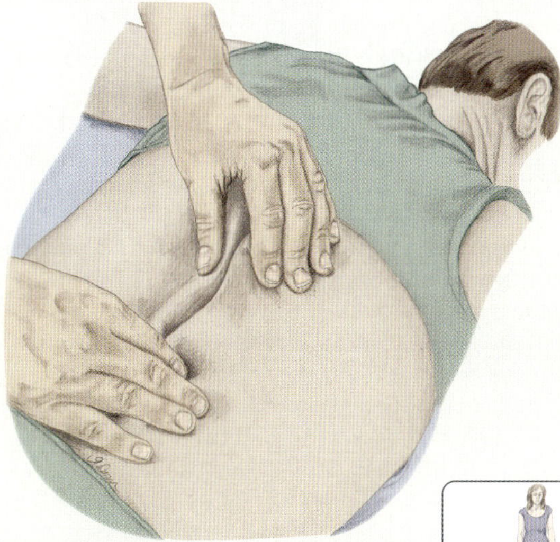
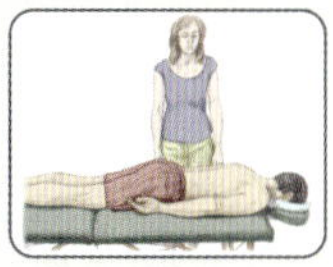

4.3 Partner prone, as you lift the skin and fascia in the low back region

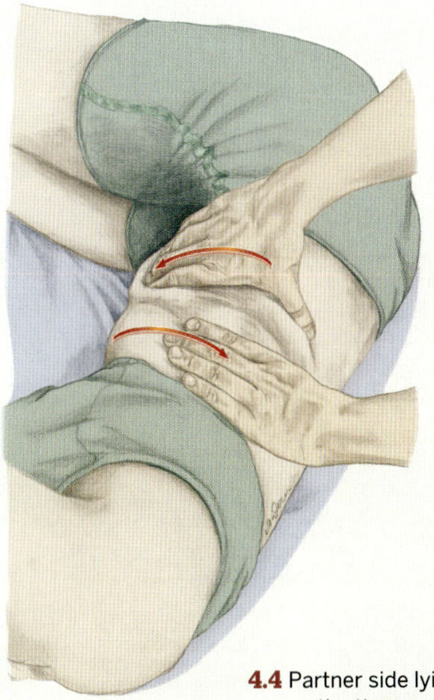
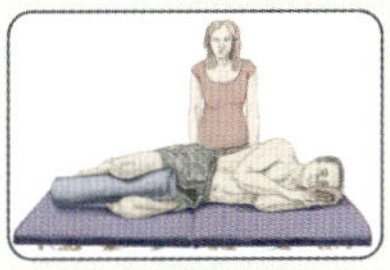

4.4 Partner side lying, as you explore the tissue of the thorax

Trunk

When thinking about the thorax (the trunk of the body), most of us consider the "belly and back" surfaces and neglect the sides. Side lying position will allow you to see that the sides of the thorax connect the "belly and back" together and that the thorax is actually one three-dimensional unit.

1. Partner side lying. Lay both hands on the side of the thorax. See and feel how the anterior, lateral, and posterior sides of the thorax form one continuous surface.
2. Gently wring your hands in opposite directions (**4.4**), sensing the tissue's pliability or resistance. Try to move it in all directions.

Abdomen

The abdomen can be ticklish or sensitive when palpated. Be sure to move slowly and gently, checking in with your partner.

1. Partner supine. Begin with your hands on the sides of the abdomen to sense the temperature of the tissue. Then explore toward the center of the abdomen, up to the edge of the ribs and just below the umbilicus.
2. Begin by gently lifting the skin and fascia of the lateral abdomen and proceed further toward the body's midline (**4.5**). If some areas may be particularly challenging to grasp, it may be an indication that such action is unwelcome by the body at this time.
3. While grasping a portion of tissue, ask your partner to perform a small "crunch." As the deeper abdominal muscles contract, notice how the tissue may come right out from between your fingers.

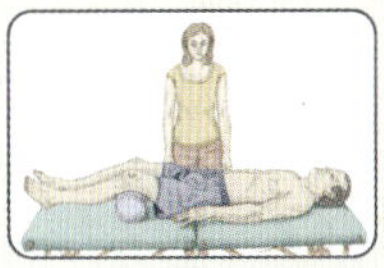
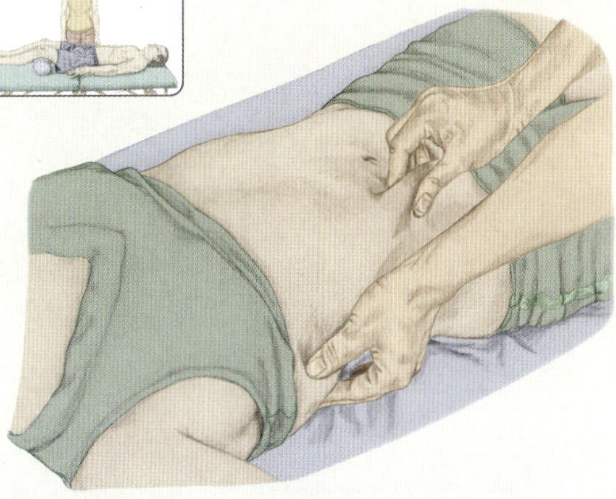

4.5 Partner supine, as you explore the tissue of the abdomen

Bones of the Spine and Thorax

The **vertebral column** (or spine) consists of twenty-four vertebrae: seven **cervical** in the neck, twelve **thoracic** of the thorax and five **lumbar** in the lower back (**4.6**). The sacrum and coccyx are composed of fused vertebrae and are also considered part of the vertebral column. For the purposes of palpation and clarity, the sacrum and coccyx are included in Chapter 6, *Pelvis and Thigh*.

The **cervical vertebrae** are the most mobile and accessible of the twenty-four spinal bones. The twelve **thoracic vertebrae** articulate with the twelve pairs of ribs. Designed for minimal movement, they help to stabilize the thoracic area and protect the internal organs. In contrast, the larger, stockier **lumbar vertebrae**, located between the twelfth rib and posterior iliac crest, are designed to support the weight of the upper body.

As you palpate along the back, all twenty-four vertebrae will be deep to the layers of muscle tissue. However, the spinous and transverse processes protrude from each vertebra and can be helpful location points.

The **thorax** includes the sternum and rib cage (**4.7**). The superficial **sternum** (breastbone) is located along the midline of the chest. The **rib cage** consists of costal cartilage and twelve pairs of ribs. The costal cartilage is identical in shape and size to the ribs and serves as a bridge between them and the sternum.

Ribs 1–7 are known as "true ribs" because they attach directly to the sternum. Ribs 8–12 are referred to as "false ribs" because they attach indirectly to the sternum by means of the costal cartilage. Aside from being false ribs, the eleventh and twelfth ribs are also considered "floating ribs," as they do not attach to the sternum or costal cartilage at all.

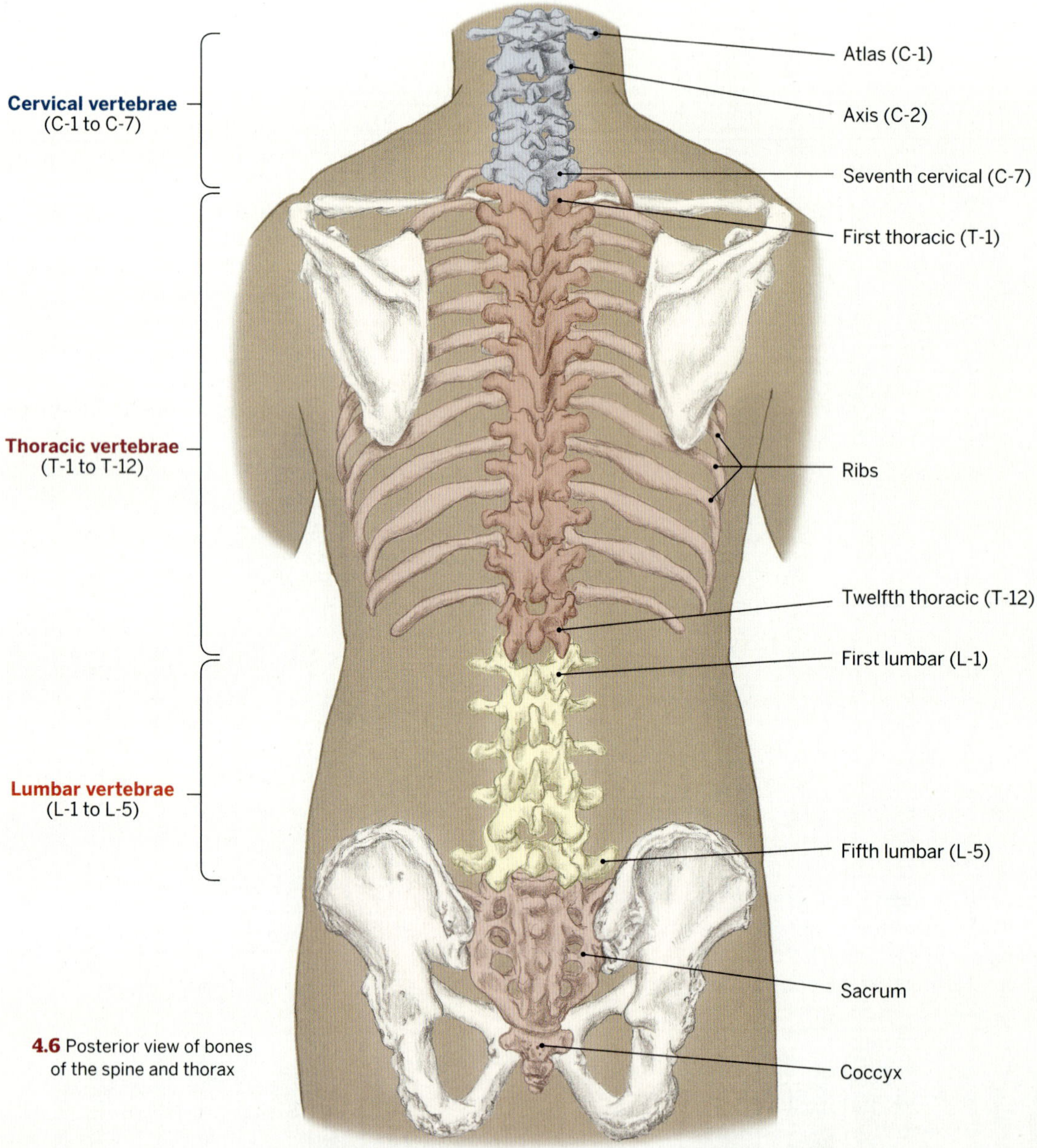

4.6 Posterior view of bones of the spine and thorax

Bony Landmarks of the Spine and Thorax

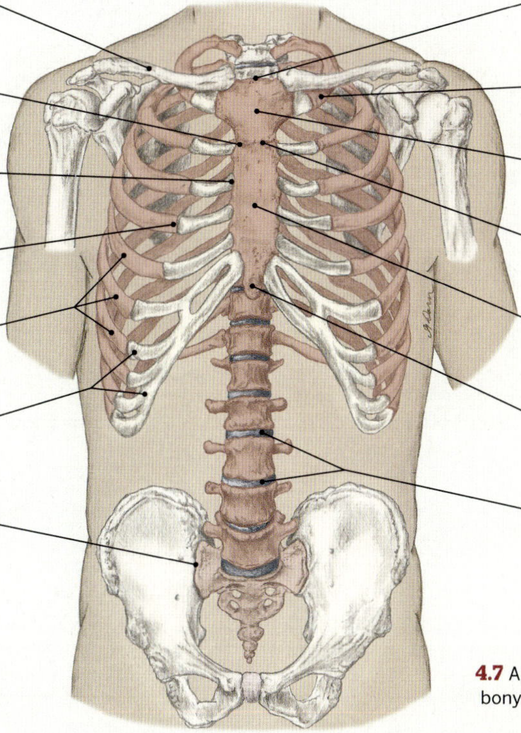

4.7 Anterior view of bones and bony landmarks of the thorax

Atlas (C-1)

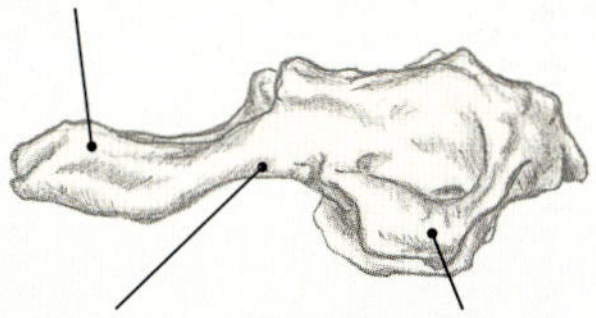

4.8 Lateral view of atlas

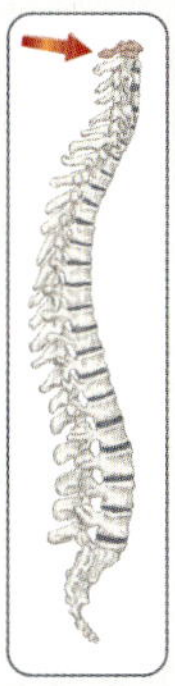

Lateral view of vertebral column

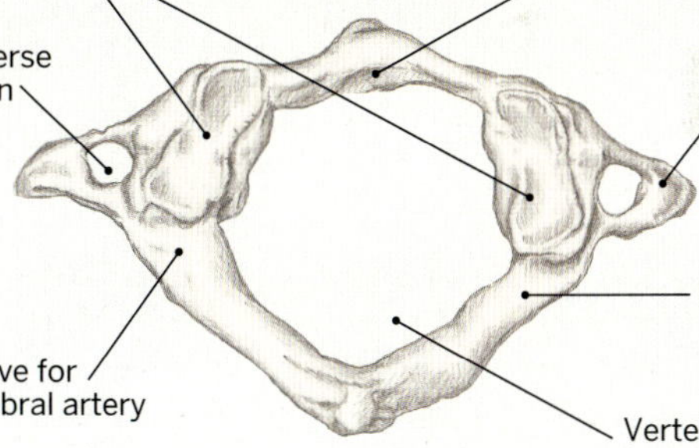

4.9 Superior view of atlas

Axis (C-2)

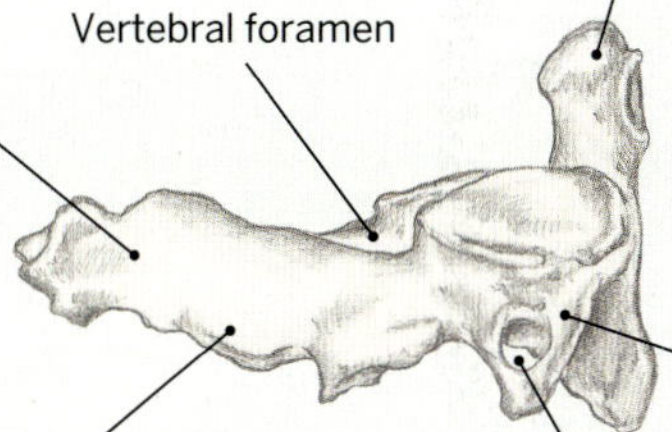

4.10 Lateral view of axis

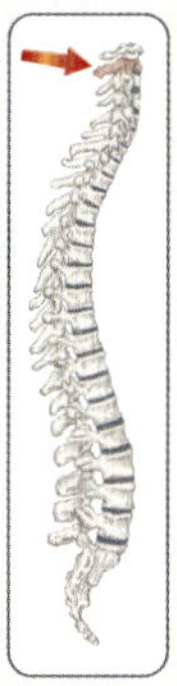

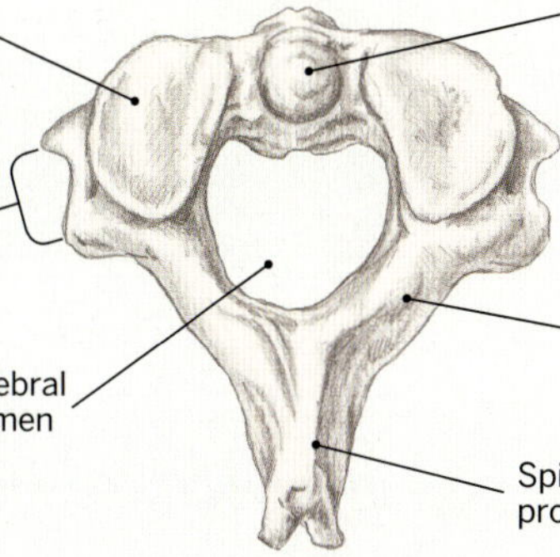

4.11 Superior view of axis

odontoid o-***don***-toyd Grk. toothlike

Cervical

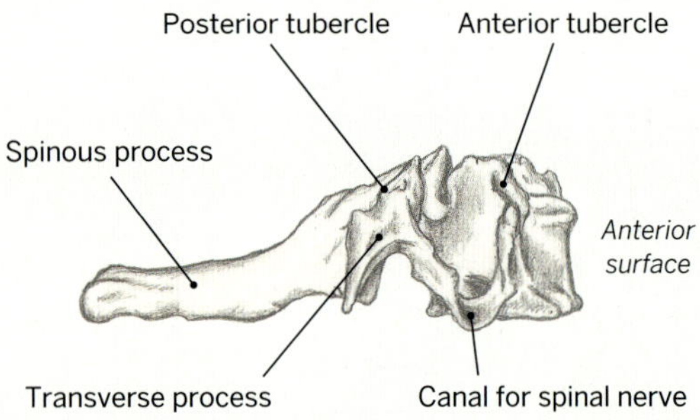

4.12 Lateral view of cervical vertebra

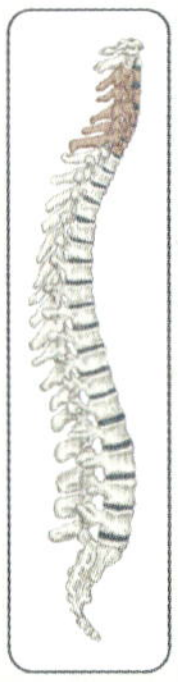

Lateral view of vertebral column

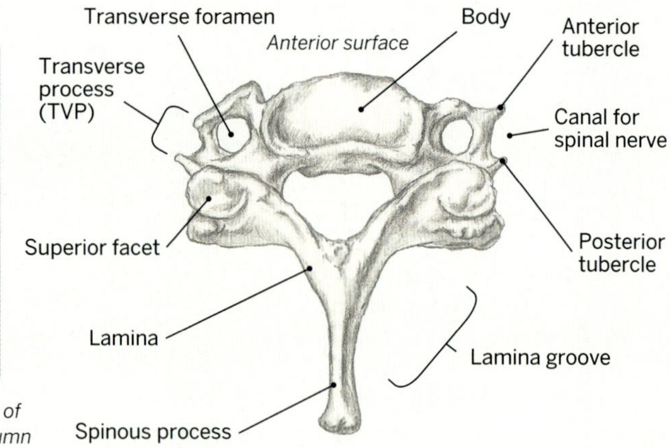

4.13 Superior view of cervical vertebra

Thoracic

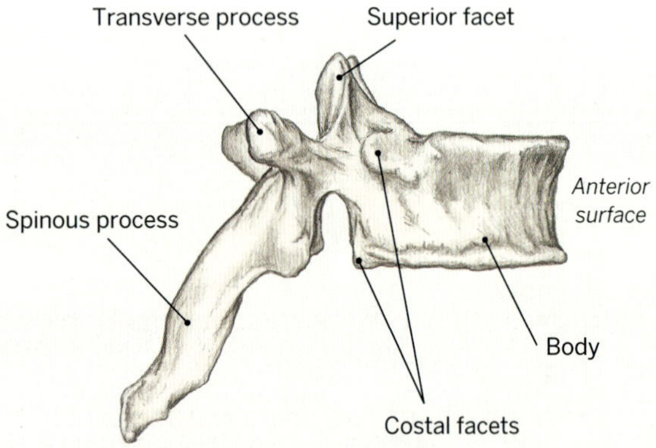

4.14 Lateral view of thoracic vertebra

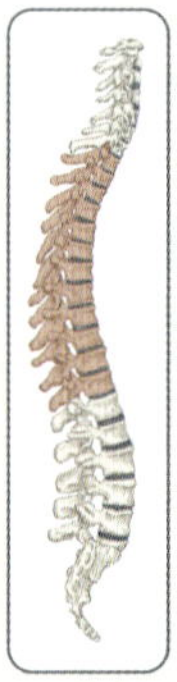

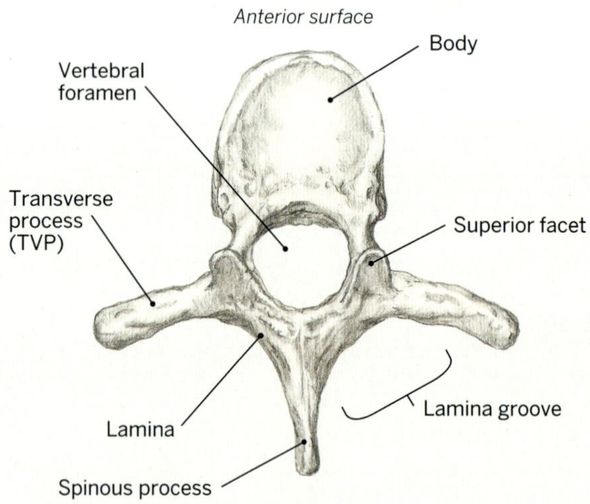

4.15 Superior view of thoracic vertebra

Lumbar

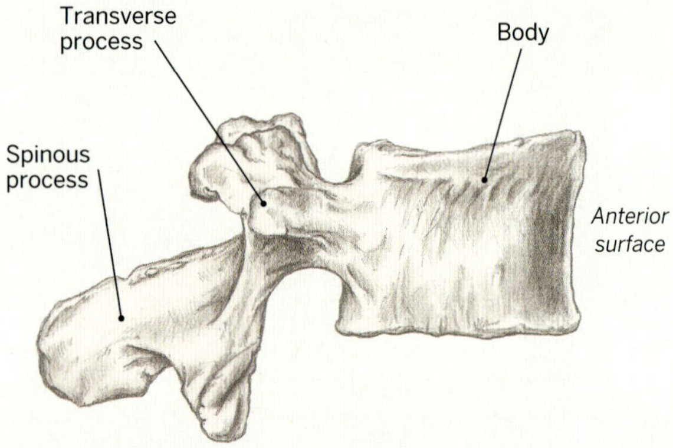

4.16 Lateral view of lumbar vertebra

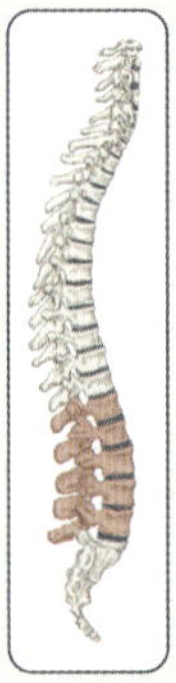

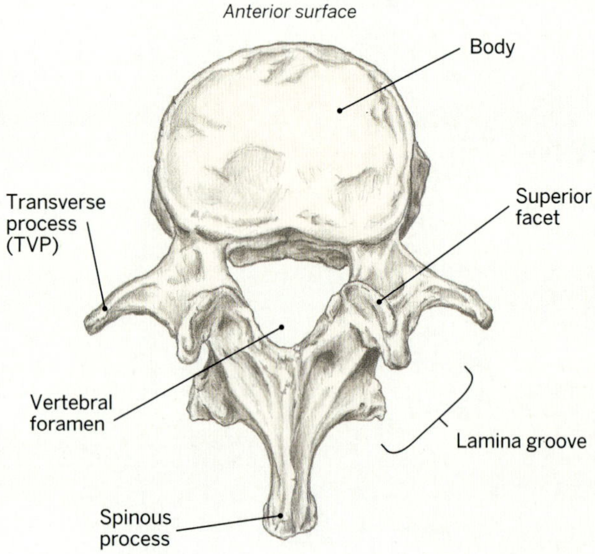

4.17 Superior view of lumbar vertebra

facet	***fas**-et*	Fr. small face
foramen	for-***aye**-men*	L. a passage or opening

Additional Bony Landmarks

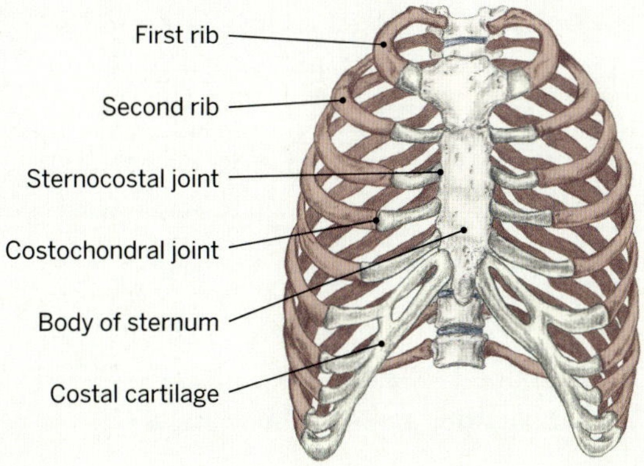

4.18 Anterior view of thorax

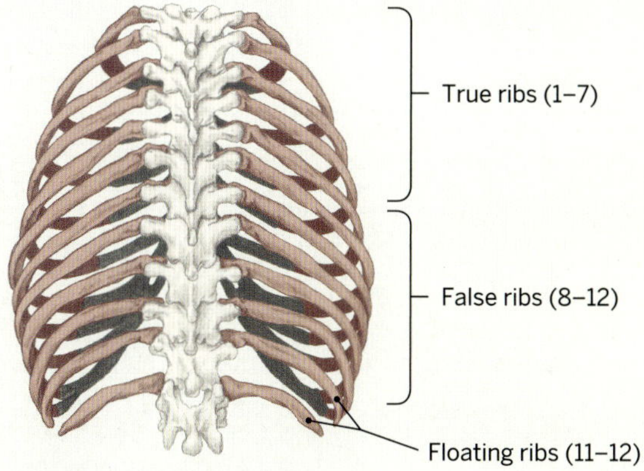

4.19 Posterior view of thorax

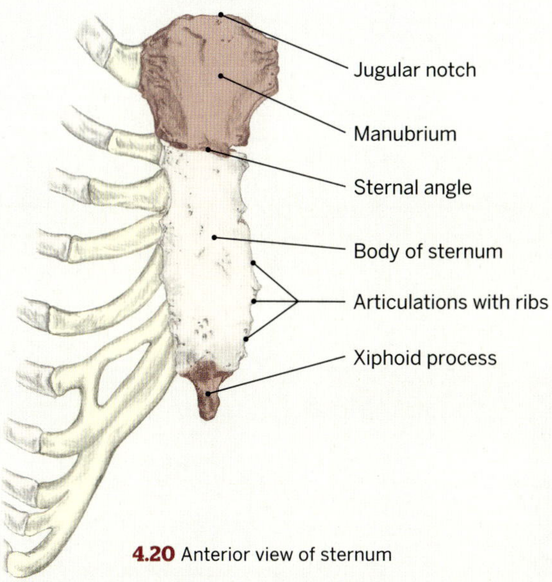

4.20 Anterior view of sternum

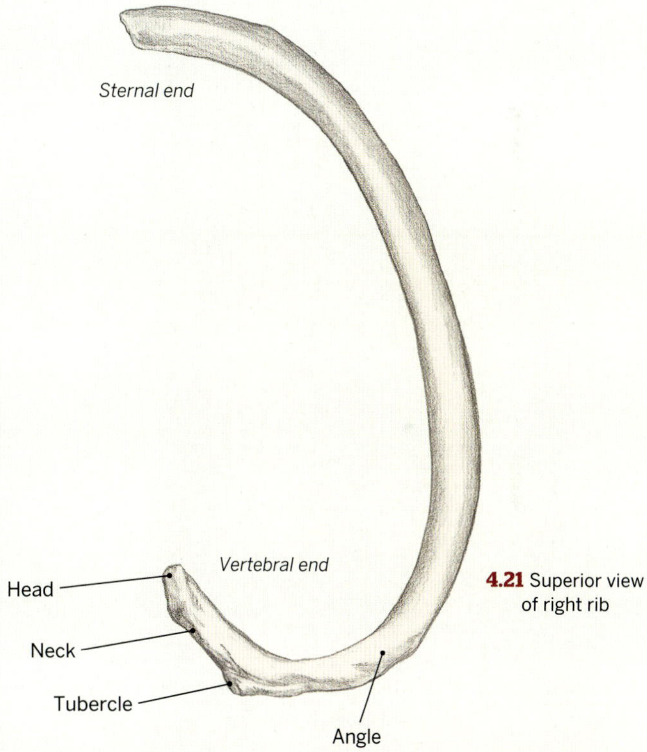

4.21 Superior view of right rib

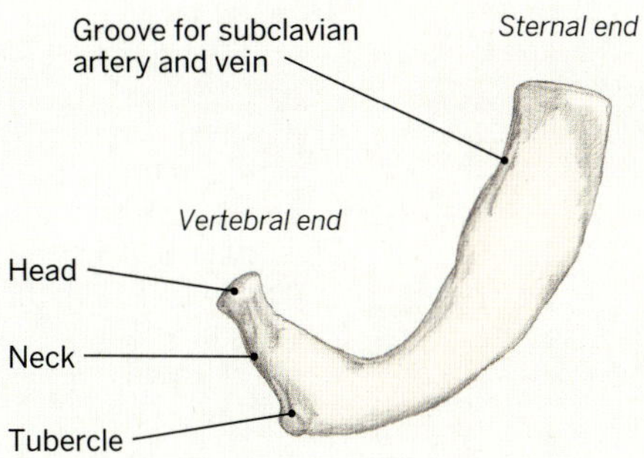

4.22 Superior view of right first rib

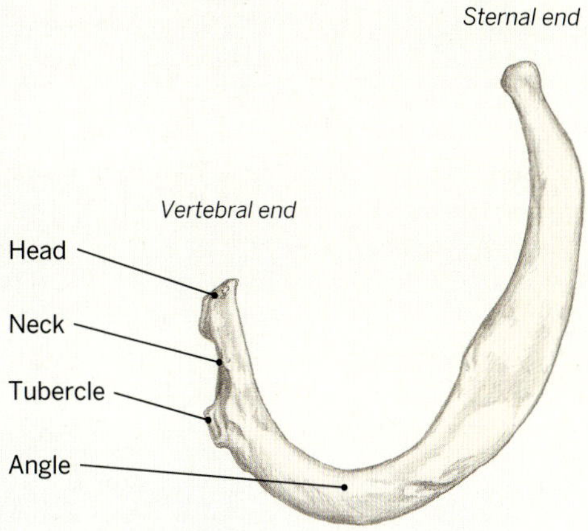

4.23 Superior view of right second rib

Overview: **Bony Landmark Trails**

Trail 1 Midline Ridge explores the spinous processes of the vertebrae and the spaces between them as they run down the middle of the back.

Trail 2 Crossing Paths describes surrounding bony landmarks that intersect with specific spinous processes.

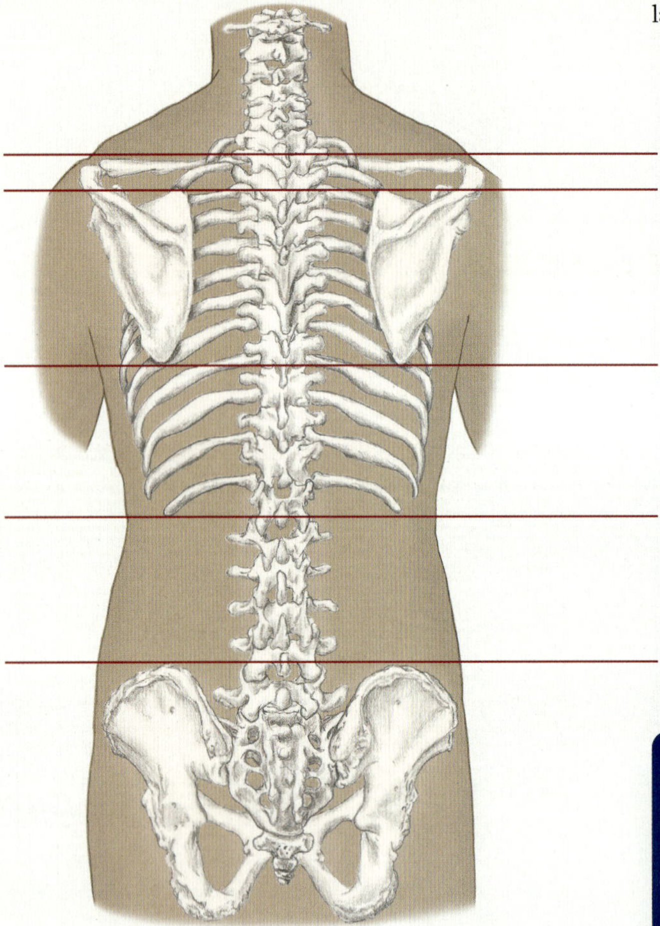

Posterior view, Trail #2

Discover More

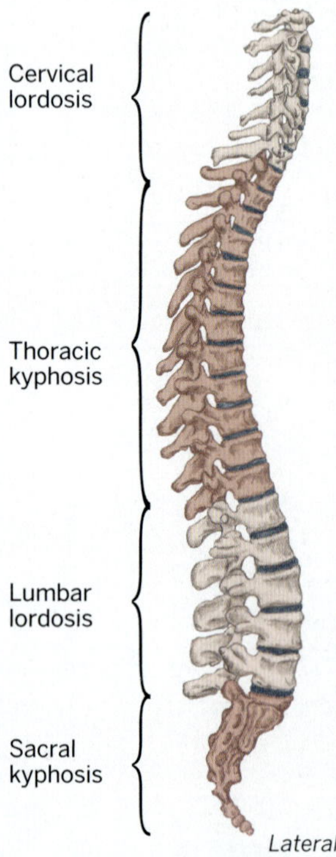

Lateral view

When viewed from the side, the vertebral column has four natural curvatures. The cervical and lumbar regions bend anteriorly to form lordotic curves, while the thoracic and sacral sections bow posteriorly, creating kyphotic curves. An abnormal lateral curvature of the spine is called scoliosis.

At birth, the spine has a single kyphotic curvature. The cervical lordosis develops when an infant begins to hold his head erect. As he begins to stand and walk, the lumbar lordosis evolves.

kyphosis	ki-***fo***-sis	Grk. bent, curved, or stooped
lordosis	lor-***doh***-sis	Grk. bent backward

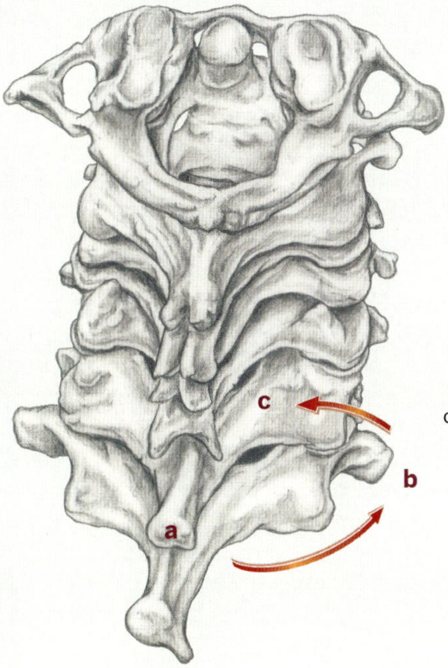

Posterior view of cervical vertebrae

Trail 3 **Nape Lane** locates the landmarks of the cervical vertebrae.

a Spinous processes of the cervicals
b Transverse processes of the cervicals
c Lamina groove of the cervicals

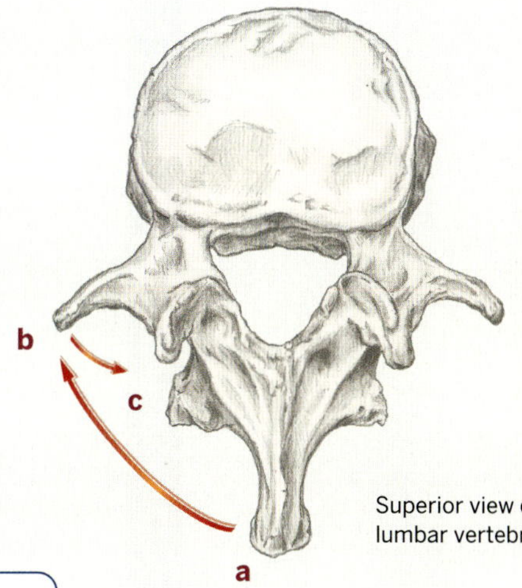

Superior view of lumbar vertebra

Trail 4 **Buried Boulevard** delves into the middle and low back regions to locate landmarks of the thoracic and lumbar vertebrae.

a Spinous processes
b Transverse processes
c Lamina grooves

Discover More

When you are standing, the entire weight of your trunk, head, and arms is transferred through the bodies of the vertebrae. The lumbar vertebrae at the base of the spine bear the brunt of this weight.

Fortunately, between the bodies of the vertebrae are intervertebral discs that cushion some of this shock. The discs are composed of a tough outer layer, the annulus fibrosus, and a liquid center called the nucleus pulposus. When weight is placed on a disc, the annulus fibrosus supports the nucleus pulposus in compressing and distributing the pressure. The nucleus is mostly water, some of which is squeezed out in the course of the day.

When you are asleep, the pressure is off the spine and the discs are able to fully restore themselves—so you wake up in the morning half an inch taller than you were the night before.

Trail 5 **Breastbone Ridge** explores the sternum and its landmarks.

a Jugular notch
b Manubrium
c Body of the sternum
d Xiphoid process

Trail 6 **One Bumpy Road** explores the ribs, the rib cage, and the costal cartilage.

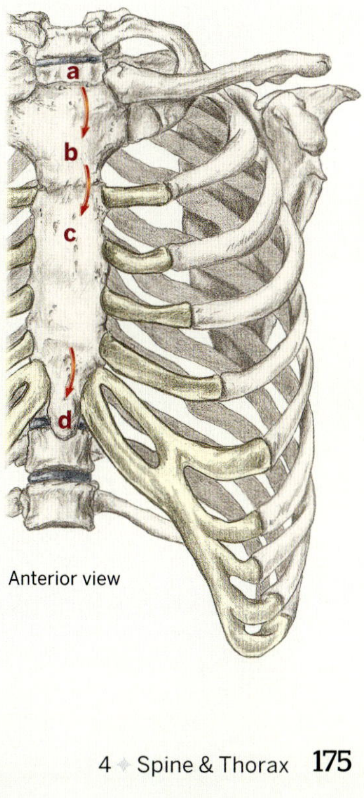

Anterior view

Trail 1 Midline Ridge ▸

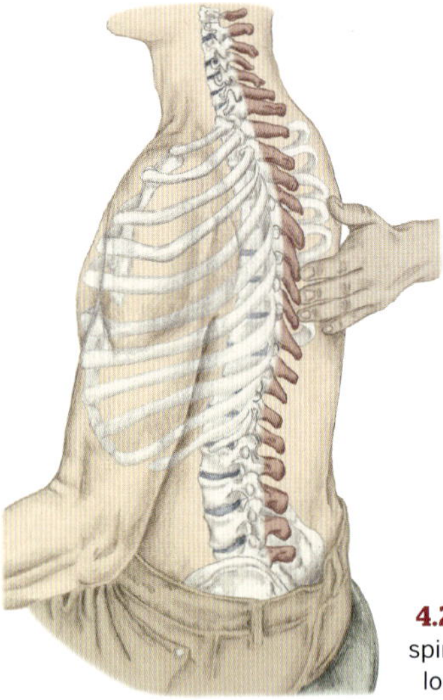

4.24 Lateral/posterior view of spine in neutral position, as you locate the spinous processes

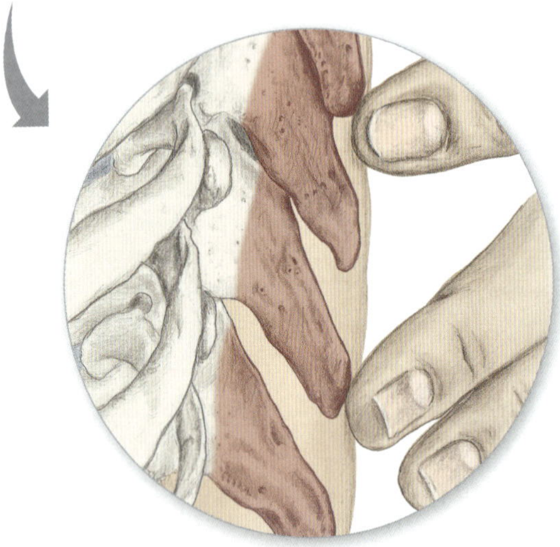

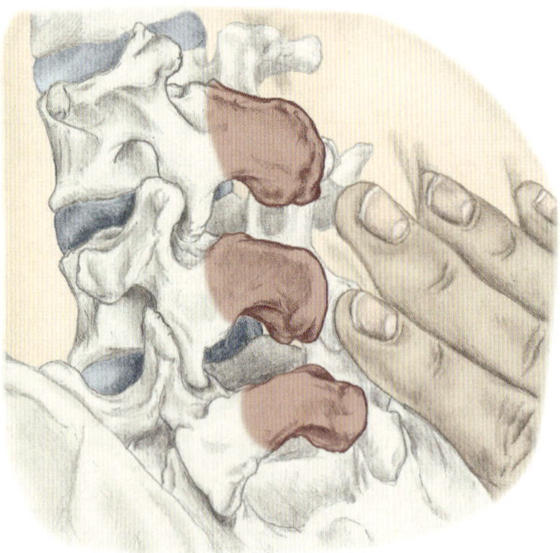

4.25 Posterior/lateral view of vertebrae, as you palpate the lumbar spinous processes

Spinous Processes of the Vertebrae

A spinous process is a vertebra's posterior projection. As a group, the spinous processes form the visible row of bumps that run down the center of the back. They are designed as attachment sites for layers of muscles, ligaments, and fasciae.

The lumbar, thoracic, and cervical spinous processes differ from one another in several respects. The **spinous processes of the lumbar vertebrae** are much larger than the thoracic or cervical processes. Tall and stocky, the tips of the lumbar processes may feel more like short strips than points. The bodies of these vertebrae are quite massive and tall; they may have a finger's width of space between their processes. The **thoracic spinous processes** are smaller and closer together than their lumbar counterparts and angle downward.

The **cervical spinous processes** are shorter and smaller than the thoracic processes. Because of the lordotic curve in the cervical spine and the overlying ligamentum nuchae, the cervical spinous processes are actually deeper than the thoracic and lumbar vertebrae. The first cervical vertebra (C-1), or atlas, is the only vertebra that does not have a spinous process.

Spinous processes of the vertebrae

1. Partner seated, with trunk and neck slightly flexed (this will stretch the overlying tissues and allow the processes to move posteriorly for easier access). Place your fingers along the midline of the back and locate the long line of processes (**4.24**, **4.25**).
2. Slide your fingers slowly up and down the spine, palpating the different sizes, prominences, and spaces between processes. Some processes might present themselves immediately, while others might be more difficult to find. Ask your partner to slowly flex and extend his spine, noting the movement of the processes.
3. Try this same method with your partner prone.

Can you sculpt out the sides of the processes as you palpate them? Is there a dip superior and inferior to the point you feel? Can you line up three fingers on a series of processes or in the spaces between the processes?

Partner prone or seated. Palpate the entire spinal column and count the spinous processes. How many can you feel? All the vertebrae (except C-1) have spinous processes, making a total of twenty-three. Use the intersecting spinous processes, such as C-7, T-12, and L-4, to check your accuracy.

L-4 and Top of the Iliac Crest

Several spinous processes can be located with the help of intersecting bony landmarks. For example, a line drawn between the tops of the two iliac crests will cross the spinous process of L-4, which, in turn, leads you to its neighboring processes. Because everyone's body is unique, these intersecting landmarks are not definitive; they are best used as guides.

L-4 and top of the iliac crest

1. With your partner either prone or standing, locate the lateral aspects of both iliac crests (p. 287).
2. With your index fingers along the top of the crests, slide your thumbs medially, meeting at the spine (**4.26**).
3. Isolate the large knob of L-4. Explore superiorly and inferiorly for the adjacent lumbar processes.

Are you at the level of the iliac crests? Can you feel a firm protuberance at the midline of the body?

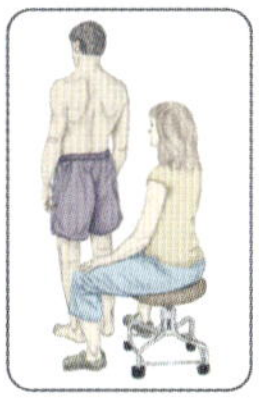

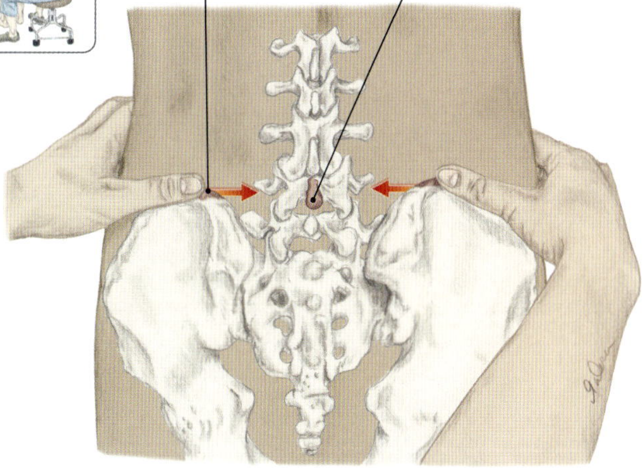

4.26 Partner standing, posterior view, as you palpate the iliac crests

T-12 and the Twelfth Rib

The eleventh and twelfth ribs do not attach to the costal cartilage and are therefore considered "floating ribs." The twelfth rib has a slender, spear-like shape and angles inferiorly. It may vary in length between three to six inches and can be used as a locator for the spinous process of T-12. (See p. 187 for more information about the twelfth rib.)

T-12 and the twelfth rib

1. Partner prone or standing. The strategy is to locate the tip of the twelfth rib and follow its shaft to the spinous process. Reaching across to the opposite side of the body, place your hand along the lateral edge of the ribs.
2. Slide inferiorly to the bottom of the rib cage and explore for the tip of the twelfth rib (**4.27**).
3. With the tip isolated, gently follow the shaft of the rib medially, noting how it lies at an angle. As the rib lies deep to the erector spinae muscles, you might lose contact with its most medial portion. Continue to slide your fingers in the direction of the shaft, palpating for the spinous process.

If you have located L-4, can you now count the processes up to T-12?

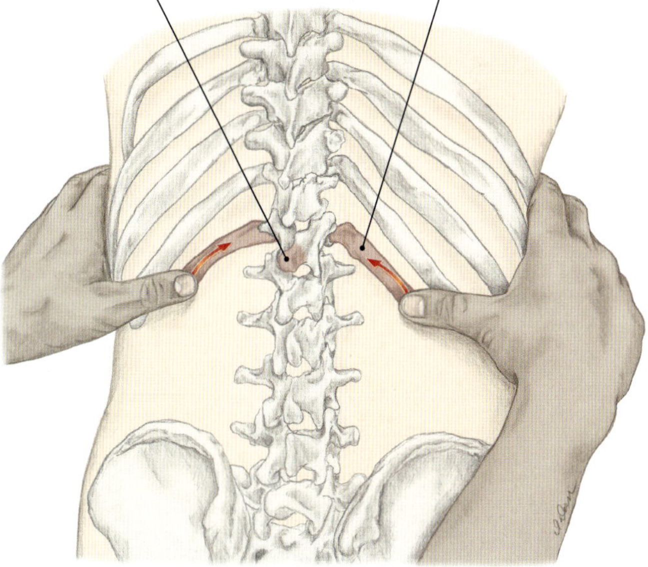

4.27 Partner standing, posterior view, as you explore the twelfth rib

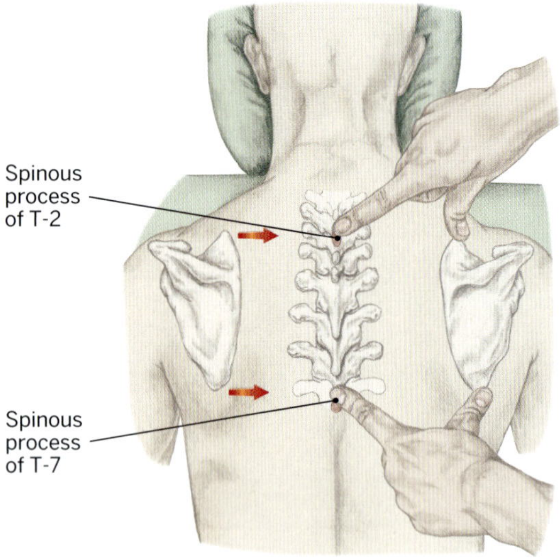

4.28 Partner prone, as you locate the inferior and superior angles

T-7 and Inferior Angle T-2 and Superior Angle

Body type, muscular contraction, and other factors affect the positioning of the scapulae. The inferior angle of the scapula will generally lie at the level of the spinous process of T-7, while the superior angle is at the level of T-2.

T-7 and inferior angle, T-2 and superior angle

1. Partner prone or standing. Locate the inferior angle (p. 49). Keep one hand at the angle while sliding the other medially to the vertebral column.
2. Locate the superior angle. Keep one hand at the angle while sliding the other medially toward the vertebrae (**4.28**).

From T-7, can you count the processes down to T-12? Can you count them up to T-2? From T-2, can you count down to T-7?

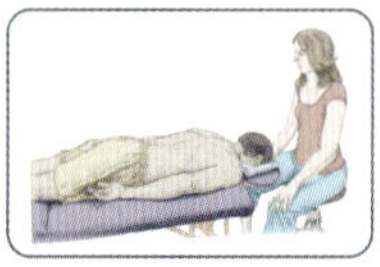

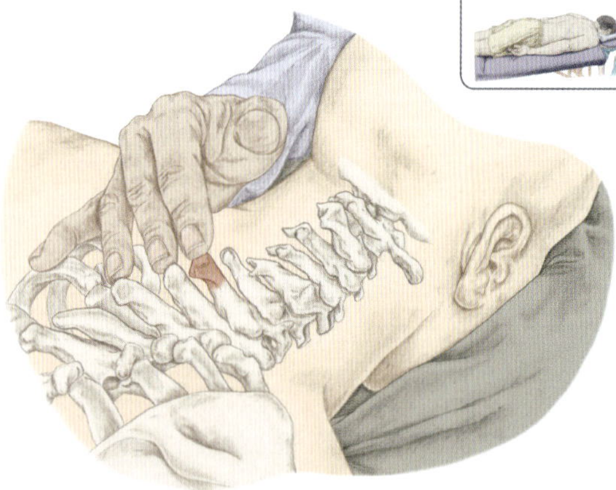

4.29 Partner prone, as you locate the spinous process of C-7

C-7 and Base of the Neck

The spinous process of C-7 is located at the base of the neck. It protrudes further than C-6, C-5, and C-4—a helpful distinction when locating structures in the upper back and neck.

C-7 and base of the neck

1. Partner prone. Place your fingerpad superior to the base of the neck along the midline of the body.
2. Slide inferiorly. At the base of the neck, your finger will bump into the process of C-7 (**4.29**).
3. Explore its edges and neighboring processes and then try to locate it from a supine position (**4.30**).

Are you at the base of the neck? Is the process superior to your finger smaller than the process you are palpating? Is there an equally protruding process (T-1) immediately inferior?

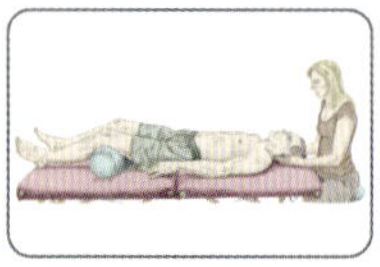

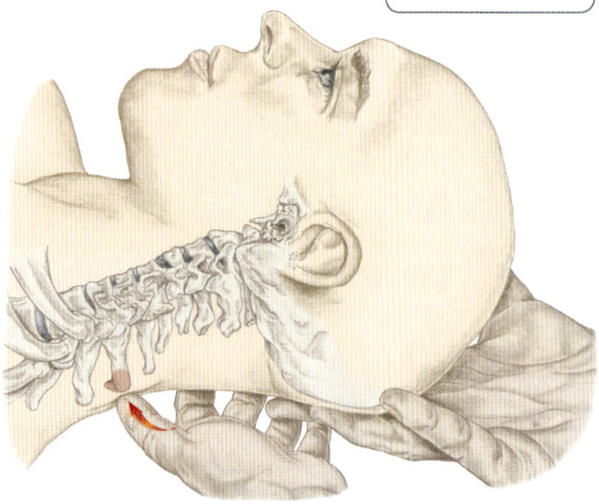

4.30 Partner supine, as you palpate spinous process of C-7

Palpation Plus

When the neck is flexed, the spinous process of C-7 shifts superiorly. T-1, however, is buckled in by the first ribs and does not move. With your partner seated, place a finger on the spinous processes of C-7 and T-1. Have your partner slowly flex his neck and observe both processes. Does C-7 tilt superiorly while T-1 is stationary?

Spinous Processes of the Cervicals

The spinous processes of C-3 to C-6 protrude posteriorly to approximately the same extent. The process of C-2, however, is larger and more distinct. The tips of the cervical spinous processes are all deep to the ligamentum nuchae (p. 218), a flat ligament attaching to the processes and running superiorly to the occiput (p. 231).

Spinous processes of the cervicals

1. Partner supine. Locate the spinous process of C-7.
2. Using gentle pressure, explore the tips and sides of the other cervical processes (**4.31**). Strum transversely across the dense ligamentum nuchae that spans the tips of the spinous processes.
3. Continue superiorly until you reach the prominence of C-2. As you explore the spinous processes, passively flex, extend, and rotate the neck.

Can you feel the subtle ridge formed by the processes along the back of the neck? When exploring the spinous process of C-2, are you inferior to the level of the earlobes? Is the process of C-2 larger and more pronounced than that of the other cervicals?

1. Being able to differentiate between the spinous process of C-2 and the external occipital protuberance (p. 232) can be helpful when navigating the posterior neck. Begin by laying your fingers horizontally along the base of your partner's head.
2. Place your ring finger at the external occipital protuberance while locating the spinous process of C-2 with your index finger (**4.32**). Your middle finger will lie between these two structures at the level of C-1. Explore the distance between these prominent landmarks.

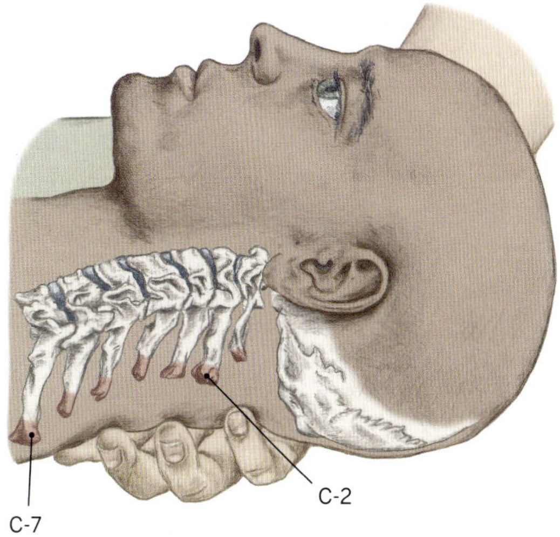

4.31 Partner supine, as you explore the cervical processes

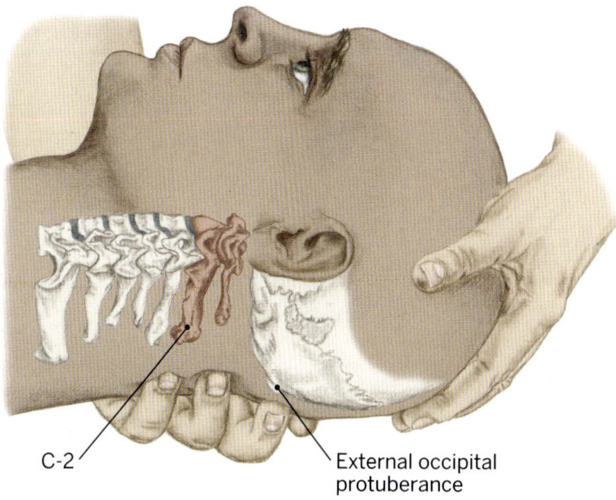

4.32 Partner supine, as you locate the spinous process of C-2

Discover More

Some bony landmarks serve as attachment sites for multiple tendons and connective tissues. Whether palpating with your fingers or dissecting with a scalpel, these tissues are often difficult to distinguish from one another. The transverse processes of the cervical vertebrae are a case in point. Tendons come from several different directions to attach to their surfaces while nerves pass between the tendons, complicating matters further. To coordinate the tendons and the spinal nerves of the cervical and brachial plexuses, the TVPs of C-2 through C-7 have anterior and posterior tubercles (left). The tubercles are small tips situated on either side of the canal (or sulcus) that channels the cervical nerves. The anterior tubercle is an attachment site for the anterior scalene and other muscles. The middle and posterior scalenes, levator scapula, and other posterior muscles attach to the posterior tubercles. It can be difficult initially to palpate individual tubercles, but with experience you will be able to detect them more easily.

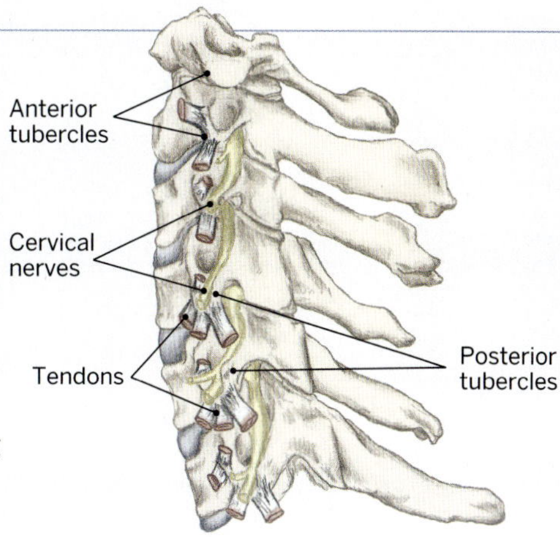

nape ME. the back of the neck

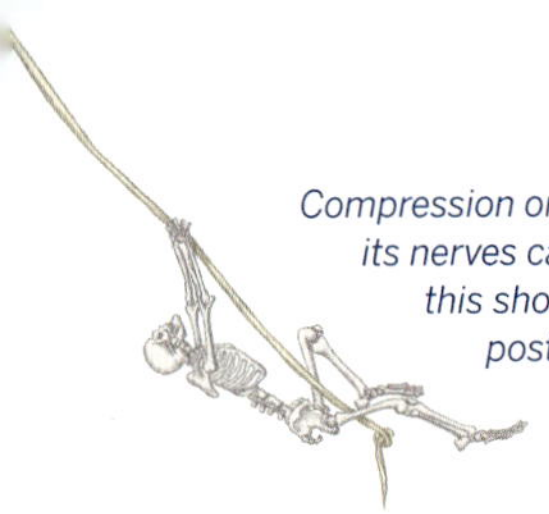

Compression or impingement of the brachial plexus (p. 274) or one of its nerves can create a sharp, shooting sensation down the arm. If this should occur, immediately release and adjust your position posteriorly. As always, ask your partner for feedback.

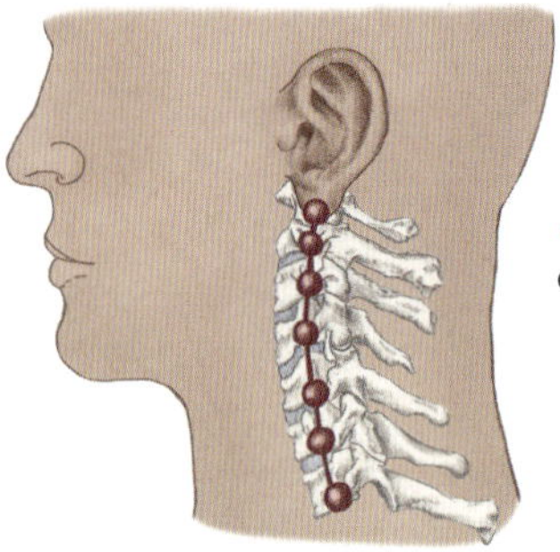

4.33 The arrangement of the cervical TVPs simulate that of a long, dangling earring.

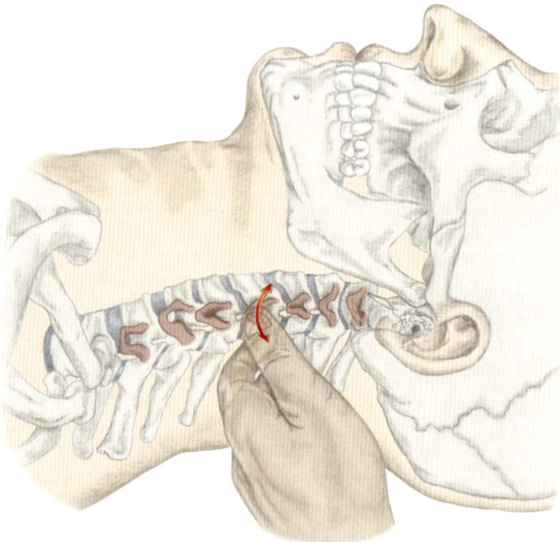

4.34 Partner supine, lateral view of neck with head *in neutral*, as you explore the length of the neck

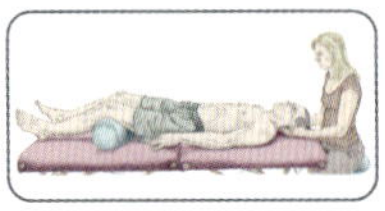

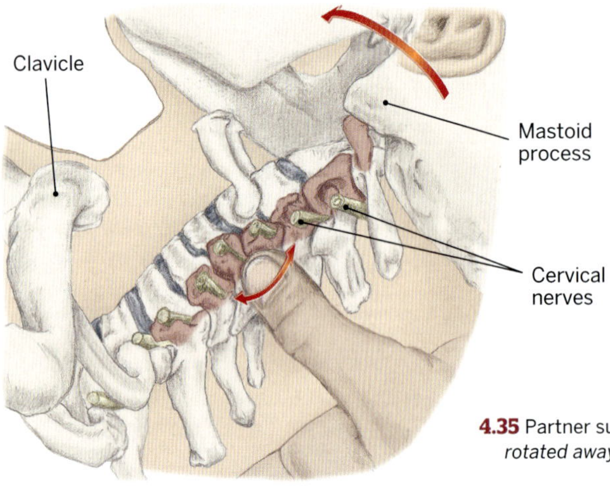

4.35 Partner supine, lateral view of neck with head *rotated away* from the side you are palpating

Transverse Processes of the Cervicals

The transverse processes (TVPs) of the cervical vertebrae are located on the side of the neck (**4.33**). Old Hollywood films put the Frankenstein monster's neck bolts into his TVPs!

The TVPs extend inferiorly from the mastoid process and many are deep to the sternocleidomastoid muscle (p. 244). All of the TVPs are the same width except for the TVPs of C-1, which are much wider.

The TVPs of C-1 are located just distal and anterior to the tip of the mastoid process (p. 233) and are relatively accessible.

All of the TVPs serve as attachment sites for various muscles, including the scalenes and levator scapulae. The brachial plexus, a large group of nerves that innervates the arm, exits between the TVPs. When first accessing the TVPs, use the flat of your thumb or fingerpads. As your palpation skills improve, explore the TVPs' surfaces more specifically.

TVPs of cervicals

1. Partner supine. Place your fingers on the side of the neck below the earlobes.
2. Using your flat thumbpads, slide anteriorly and posteriorly to feel the ridge of TVPs. Explore the length of the neck (**4.34**).
3. You might not feel the tips of individual processes, but the ridge formed by the TVPs beneath the overlying tissue instead.

Are you palpating inferior to the earlobe? Do you feel a subtle ridge running down the side of the neck? If you passively flex, laterally flex, or rotate the neck, can you feel the TVPs move individually?

1. Partner supine. Rotate the head 45° to the right. With the head in this position, the TVPs form a line from the left mastoid process to the center of the shaft of the clavicle (**4.35**).
2. Draw an imaginary line from these two landmarks and visualize and palpate the TVPs along the path.

Transverse process of C-1

1. Partner supine or seated. Locate the left mastoid process of the temporal bone (p. 233) and rotate the head 45° to the right.
2. Using your broad fingerpad, slide slightly inferior and anterior from the mastoid process. Explore deep to the sternocleidomastoid muscle for the solid bump of the transverse process of C-1 (**4.36**). Even pressing gently on these points can be uncomfortable for your partner, so use a soft touch.
3. For reference, locate the other transverse process of C-1.

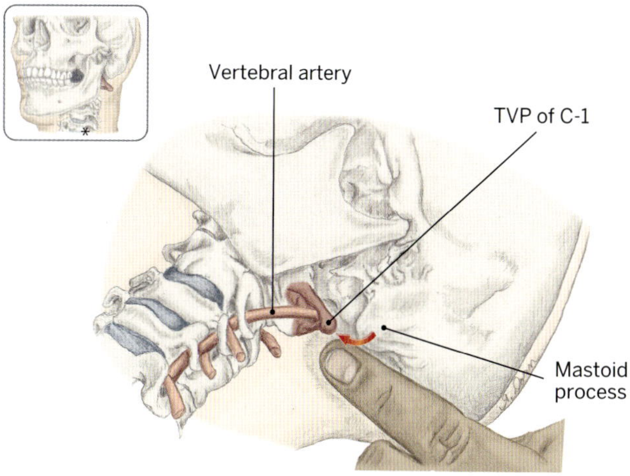

4.36 Partner supine, anterior/lateral view of neck with head rotated away from the side you are palpating

Cervical Lamina Groove

The lamina groove is the trough-like space between the spinous and transverse processes of the vertebrae (**4.37**). Although sizable on a skeleton, the lamina groove of your partner is filled with layers of muscles, which renders it almost inaccessible. The lamina groove is best thought of as a helpful region for locating muscle bellies.

Cervical lamina groove

1. Partner supine. Scoop the head with one hand, and with your other hand, locate the cervical transverse processes.
2. Slide posteriorly off the TVPs. Explore the space between the transverse and spinous processes, which constitutes the lamina groove of the cervical vertebrae (**4.38**). Again, since the groove is filled with muscles, the bone that forms the groove is impalpable.

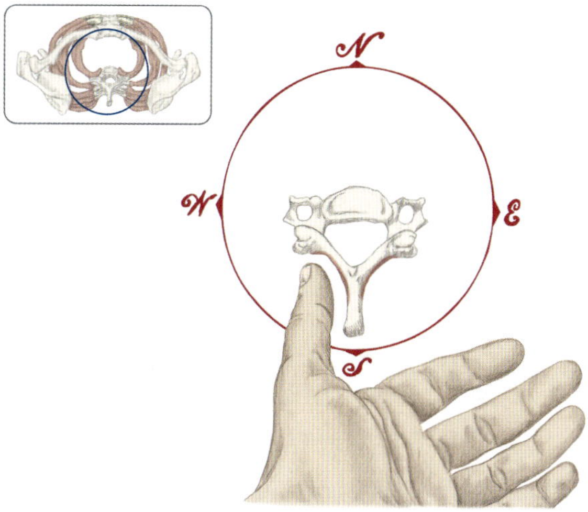

4.37 A schematic cross section of the neck as if your partner were supine. The lamina grooves can be thought of as being in the neck's southeast and southwest quadrants.

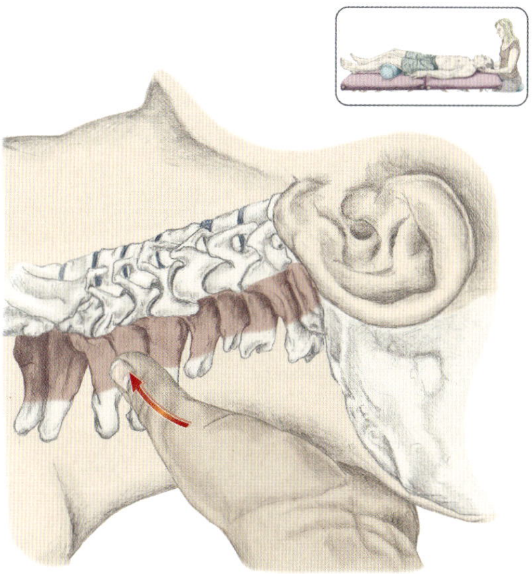

4.38 Partner supine, lateral view of neck, as you palpate in the lamina groove

Discover More

C-6 has a large anterior tubercle called the carotid tubercle. Its name corresponds to the carotid artery (p. 271) that passes immediately lateral to it. Although you would not want to, you can occlude the carotid artery by placing your finger lateral to the cricoid cartilage and pressing in a posterior direction against the carotid tubercle. Long ago this dramatic maneuver was used in emergency rooms as a last-ditch effort to stem hemorrhaging inside the skull.

cricoid *kri*-koyd Grk. ring-shaped
lamina *lam*-i-na L. thin plate, leaf

Transverse Processes of the Thoracic and Lumbar Vertebrae

The TVPs of the thoracic vertebrae are shorter and do not extend as far laterally as the TVPs of the lumbar vertebrae. They are palpable deep to the erector spinae muscles (p. 196) and superficial to the connecting aspect of the ribs. The TVPs of the lumbar vertebrae are also deep to the erector spinae. Extending an inch or two laterally, their solid presence can be felt beneath the overlying muscle tissue.

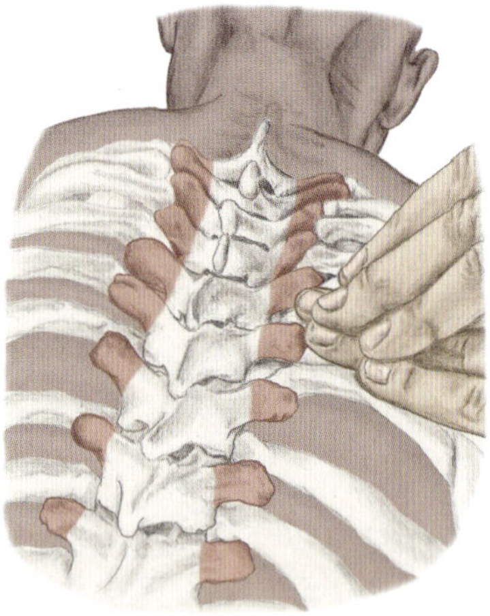

4.39 Partner prone, as you isolate the TVPs of the thoracic vertebrae

Thoracic transverse processes

1. Partner prone. Locate a portion of the thoracic spinous processes. Move roughly one inch laterally and sink your fingers through the thick erector spinae muscles.
2. Roll your fingers superiorly and inferiorly, palpating for the TVPs' subtle, knobby shapes (**4.39**).

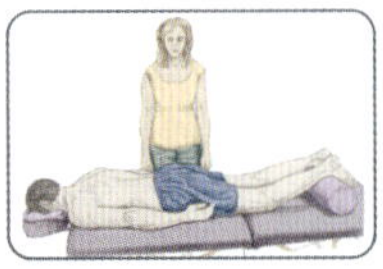

Slide further laterally from the thoracic transverse processes and onto the posterior ribs. Can you determine where the ribs and transverse processes meet? Can you feel the short processes beneath the erector spinae fibers?

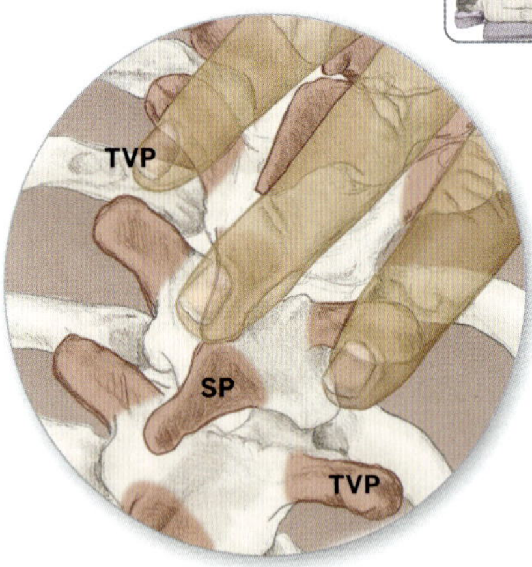

4.40 Try using three fingerpads to span between the TVPs, with your middle finger falling on the spinous process.

Lumbar transverse processes

1. Partner prone. Locate the lumbar spinous processes. Slide roughly two inches laterally to avoid the thick mound of the erector spinae muscles (p. 196).
2. Slowly sink your fingers through the muscle tissue. Directing your pressure at a medial/anterior angle (as if toward the navel), explore for the tips of the TVPs (**4.41**). Because of the thick overlying tissue, the individual processes might not be directly palpable, but try to sense the solid ridge they form.

Ask your partner to raise her feet slightly to determine whether you are lateral to the erector spinae muscles. Can you feel the hard surface of the processes running horizontally?

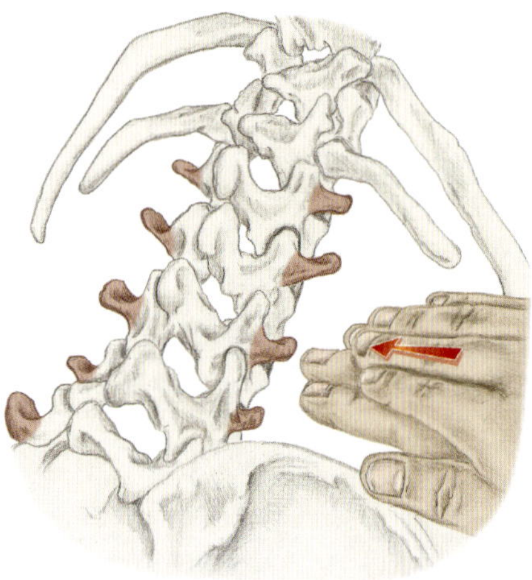

4.41 Partner prone, as you palpate the TVPs of the lumbar vertebrae

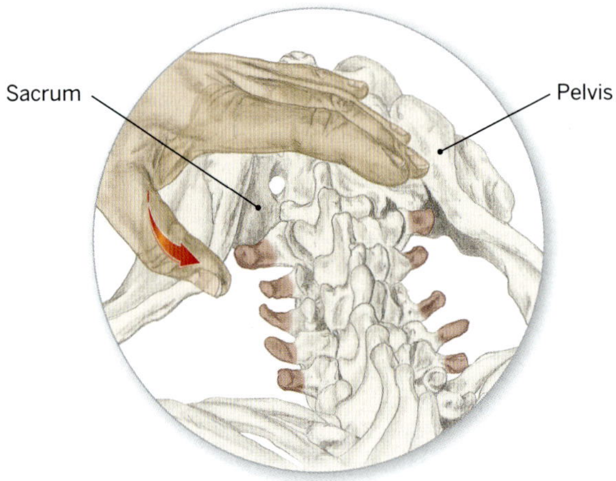

4.42 Superior view looking down the spine, as you access lumbar TVPs with your thumb

Lamina Groove of the Thoracic and Lumbar Vertebrae

The lamina groove of the thoracic and lumbar vertebrae is located between their spinous and transverse processes. Shaped like a long, vertical trough, the lamina groove expands in depth and width as it progresses down the spine. In the thoracic and lumbar vertebrae, the lamina groove is filled with the layers of the erector spinae and transversospinalis muscles. Because of this overlying tissue, the lamina groove is difficult to access directly, but its borders (the spinous and transverse processes) are palpable.

Lamina groove of the thoracic and lumbar vertebrae

1. Partner prone. Locate the spinous processes of the thoracic vertebrae. With the other hand, locate the TVPs of the thoracic vertebrae.
2. Using firm pressure, explore between these landmarks in the lamina groove (**4.43**). Note the thick muscle tissue that lies in this groove.
3. Try this same method in the lumbar region (**4.44**). Observe how the lamina groove widens and deepens and how the muscle tissue is thicker in this region compared with the muscle tissue in the thoracic region.

Are you between the transverse and spinous processes of the vertebrae? Can you slide your fingers between the muscle fibers and sink into the lamina groove?

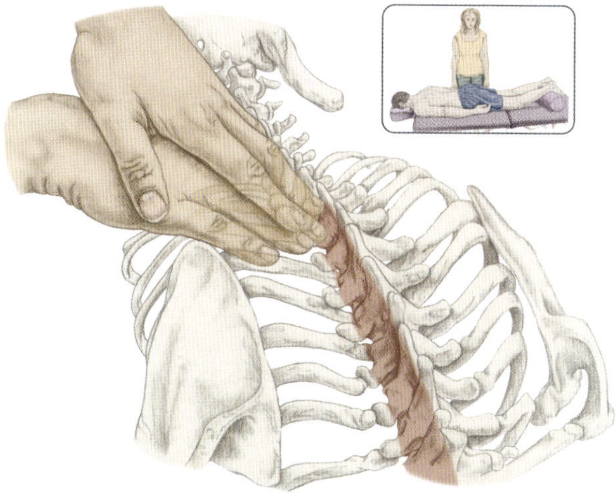

4.43 Lateral/superior view of spine, as you access the lamina groove of the thoracic vertebrae. Muscles overlying the groove are shown below.

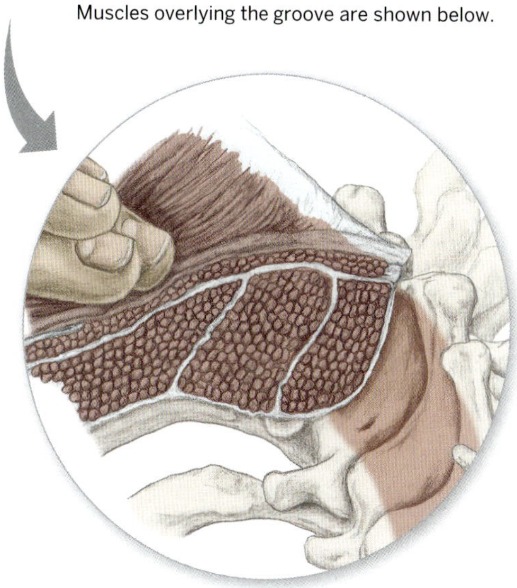

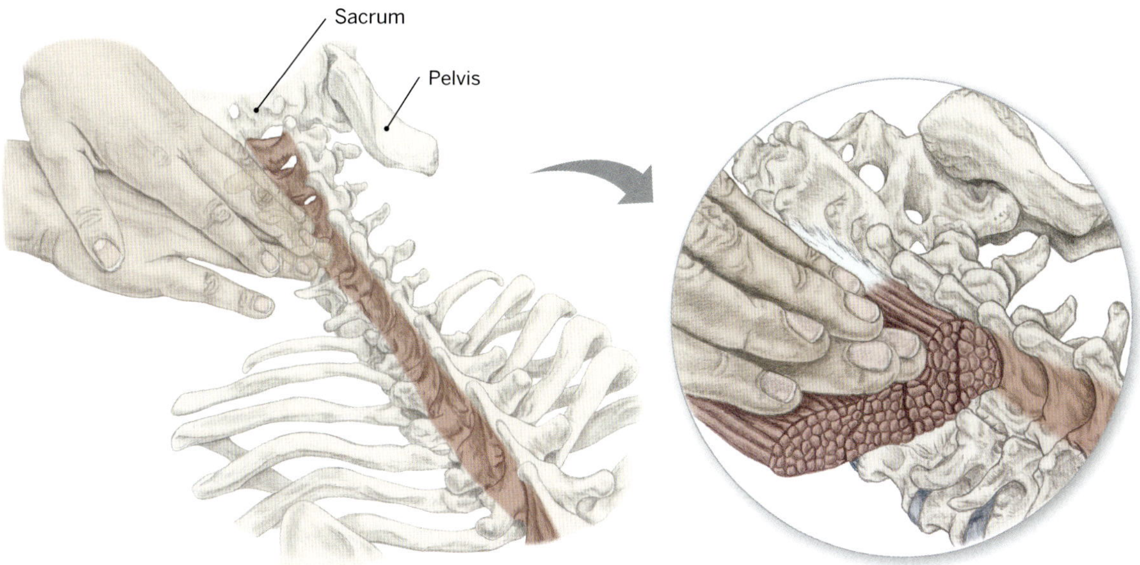

4.44 Lateral/superior view of spine (left), as you access the lamina groove of the lumbar vertebrae. Muscles overlying the groove are shown at right.

Trail 5 Breastbone Ridge ▶

Sternum

The sternum features several landmarks (p. 173). At the top of the sternum, the **jugular notch** is between the sternal heads of the clavicles. It may be flat or bowl-shaped, and although no muscles attach directly to it, the sternocleidomastoids pass superficially to it while the infrahyoids attach deep to it.

The **manubrium**, the superior portion of the sternum, articulates with the clavicles, the first rib, and the second rib. The **body of the sternum** is located inferior to the manubrium and forms the major portion of the sternum. The junction between the manubrium and body of the sternum is called the **sternal angle**.

Extending off the bottom of the sternum, the **xiphoid process** can be an inch in length or completely absent. It is an attachment site for the rectus sheath. The manubrium and the body and xiphoid process of the sternum are superficial, covered only by fasciae and the pectoralis major tendon.

Jugular notch, manubrium, and sternum

1. Partner supine. Place your finger on the sternum at the center of your partner's chest.
2. Slide superiorly until you reach the jugular notch at the top of the sternum. Explore the notch and its location next to the sternoclavicular joints.
3. Move your fingers inferiorly off the jugular notch onto the manubrium and body of the sternum. Explore any crevices or hills on this "flat" bone. Also, palpate laterally toward its attachments with the costal cartilage.

Xiphoid process

Partner supine. Slide your fingers inferiorly until they drop off the sternum and fall into the muscles of the abdomen. Now backtrack to the most inferior tip of the sternum, which will be the xiphoid process (**4.45**). Gently sculpt this tip.

✔ *Are you at the most inferior point of the sternum?*

Spine & Thorax

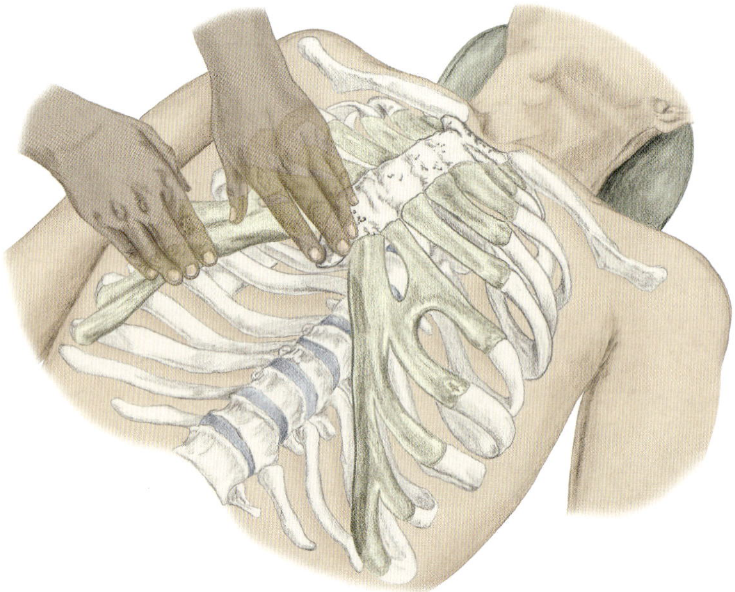

4.45 Partner supine, as you palpate the sternum, xiphoid process, and edge of the rib cage

Palpation Plus

Partner supine. The **sternal angle** is the junction point between the manubrium and sternum. Stretching horizontally, it might feel like a small speed bump or a dip. Locate the jugular notch and glide inferiorly along the surface of the manubrium. Palpate within an inch or two for a ridge or ditch that stretches horizontally across the sternum.

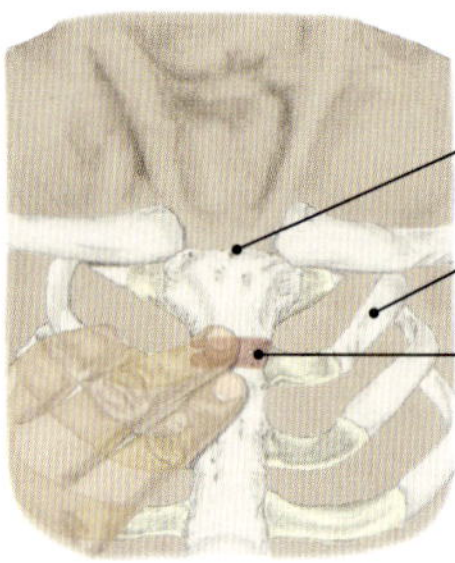

✔ *The second rib attaches to the sternum at the level of the sternal angle. Slide your fingers laterally off the angle. Can you feel the round surface of this rib?*

abdomen	***ab***-do-men	L. belly	**sternum**	***ster***-num	Grk. chest
costal	***kos***-tal	L. rib	**xiphoid**	***zif***-oyd	Grk. sword-shaped

Ribs and Costal Cartilage

The **ribs** articulate posteriorly with the thoracic vertebrae and then curve around the thorax to the anterior chest (p. 173). Extending off the ribs is the **costal cartilage** that attaches them to the sternum. There are six or seven costal branches, all of which are identical in shape and similar in feel to the ribs. The ribs, with their costal cartilage, run at varying angles around the trunk of the body.

The entire rib cage is deep to muscle tissue; however, the ribs along the sides of the trunk are easily accessed. The spaces between the ribs are filled with thin intercostal muscles that can be easily palpated.

When exploring the thorax, consider its three-dimensional quality. Often the thorax is viewed as having only a front and back, leaving its lateral portions neglected. As you explore the body's trunk, try to connect all of its sides together in your mind and with your hands. Note how several muscles, such as the deeper abdominals and intercostals, literally enwrap the thorax.

As you explore the thorax, avoid accessing mammary (breast) tissue. Ask your partner, male or female, whether you may palpate the surrounding areas.

Trail 6 One Bumpy Road ▸

Ribs and costal cartilage

1. Partner supine. Slide laterally from the sternum onto the costal cartilage. Use your fingertips to locate one costal branch and palpate its rounded surface.
2. Roll off the cartilage into the space between the branches. Explore this groove as it extends laterally. Continue along the length of the sternum, locating and exploring each branch of rib/cartilage and the spaces between them (**4.46**).

Can you determine how the angle of the ribs changes as you move around the body? Can you differentiate the round shafts of the ribs from the ditch-like spaces between them? Ask your partner to breathe deeply and note any change in the amount of space you can feel between the ribs.

Spine & Thorax

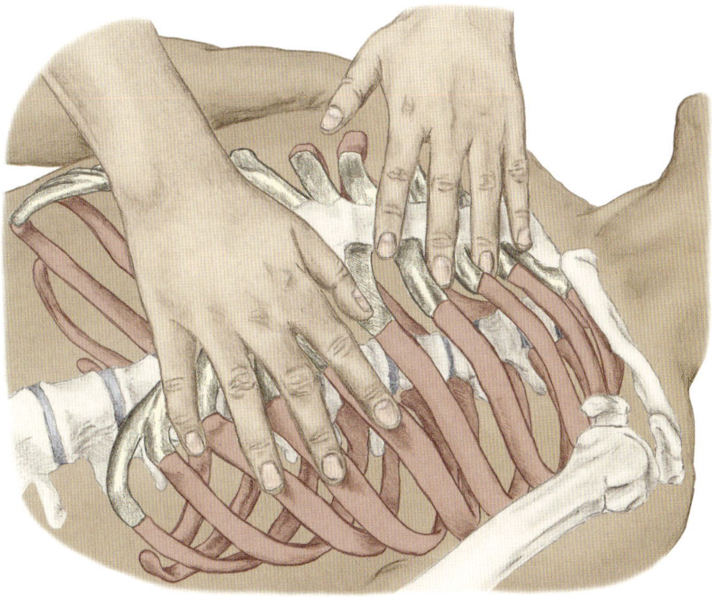

4.46 Partner supine, as you explore the ribs

Palpation Plus

The jugular notch, sternal angle, and xiphoid process can be guidemarks along the vertebral column. The jugular notch lies on the same transverse plane as the spinous process of T-2 (**a**). The sternal angle lines up with the spinous process of T-4 (**b**), while the xiphoid process is directly across from the body of T-10 (**c**). Of course, many factors, such as posture and body type, will affect the placement of the ribs, so use these correlations only as guides.

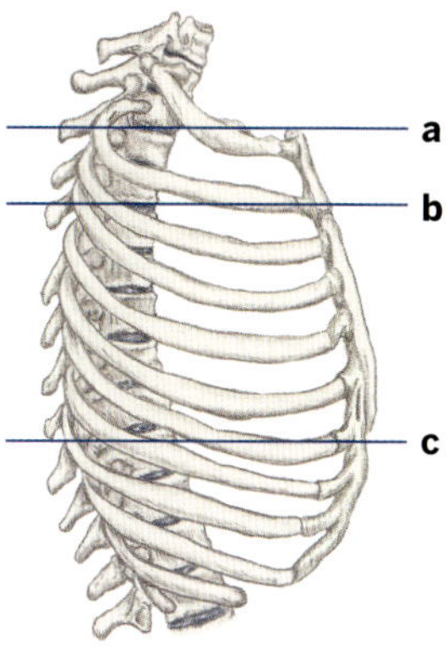

With your partner standing, palpate the jugular notch with one hand while your other hand locates the spinous process of T-2. Note whether you can see or feel a difference in the levels of these landmarks. Follow the same procedure for T-4 and T-10.

jugular	*jug*-u-lar	L. throat
manubrium	ma-*nu*-bree-um	L. handle

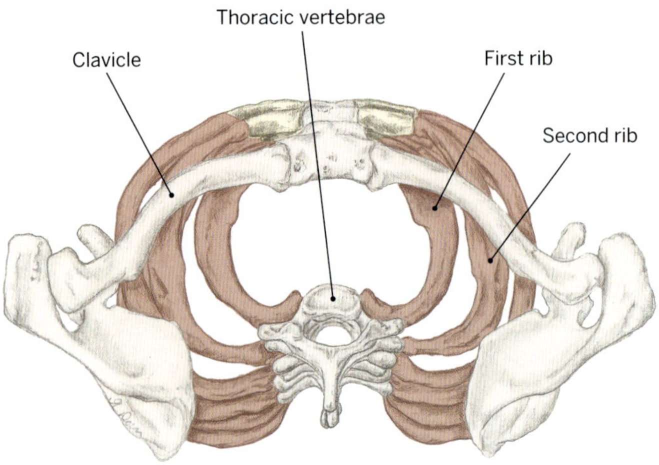

4.47 Superior view of thorax

First Rib

Unlike its cohorts, the first rib is difficult to isolate along the anterior thorax. It lies directly beneath the clavicle and then quickly curves toward the back (**4.47**). It can, however, be accessed in the posterior triangle (p. 226) of the neck, which is formed by the clavicle and the sternocleidomastoid and trapezius muscles.

The scalene muscles (p. 246) fan across the posterior triangle and attach to the first and second ribs. To access the first rib, you must palpate through the scalenes. The brachial plexus (p. 274) and subclavian artery pass between the first rib and the clavicle.

First rib

1. Partner supine. Soften the overlying tissue by passively elevating your partner's shoulder.
2. Locate the clavicle and upper flap of the trapezius to identify the posterior triangle. Place your thumbpad between these structures.
3. Slowly sink into the tissue of the scalene muscles, directing your fingers straight in an inferior direction toward your partner's feet (**4.48**). As your fingers sink into the tissue, you will meet the solid resistance of the shaft of the first rib.

Ask your partner to take a slow, deep breath into the upper chest. Can you feel the rib rise?

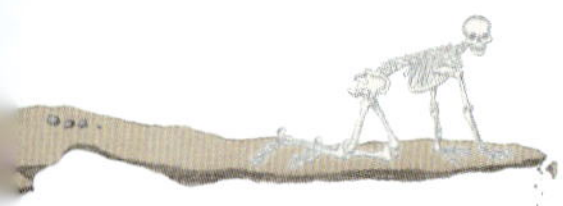

Compression or impingement of the brachial plexus or one of its nerves can create a sharp, shooting sensation down the arm. If this should occur, adjust your position to one side. Also, ask your partner for feedback.

Partner supine. When palpating in the posterior triangle of the neck, the posterior aspect of the first rib can sometimes be confused with the superior angle of the scapula. Distinguish between these structures by palpating in the posterior triangle and locating what you believe to be the first rib. Check it by passively elevating and depressing the scapula. The first rib should remain stationary during this movement.

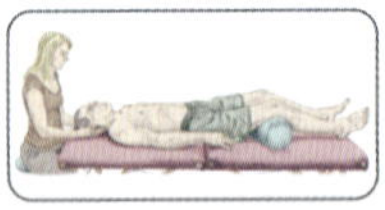

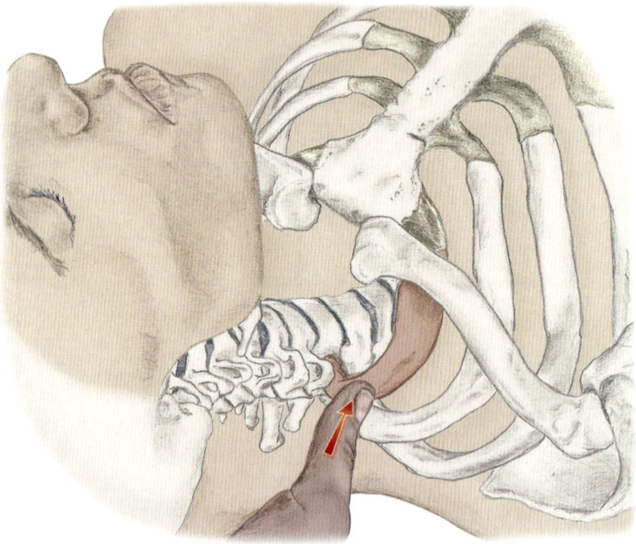

4.48 Partner supine, as you palpate the first rib

Discover More

It is not uncommon for the number of ribs to vary from person to person. There are ordinarily twelve pairs of ribs, but on some people, eleven or thirteen pairs can be found. If there is an extra rib, it may be bilateral or merely unilateral and will be found in either the cervical or lumbar area. A cervical rib often articulates with C-7 and can be felt in the posterior triangle region of the neck at the level of the clavicle. An extra rib in the lumbar will extend off L-1.

thorax ***tho***-raks Grk. chest

Palpation Plus

Ideally, the ribs are designed to expand in three directions during inhalation: anterior/posterior, lateral, and superior. Yet, for reasons ranging from posture to emotional trauma, few people truly breathe in this manner. Often the breath becomes restricted to a portion of the thorax, and the ribs will move in only one or two directions.

1. With this in mind, ask your partner to stand and breathe normally. Observe any changes in the shape or movement of the thorax, shoulders, and abdomen.

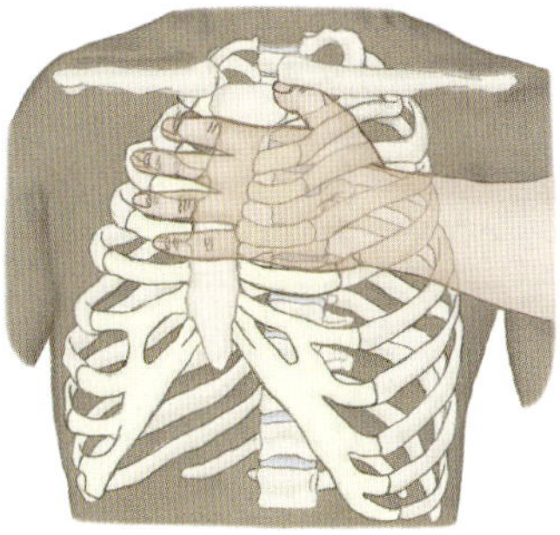

Position of the ribs during exhalation

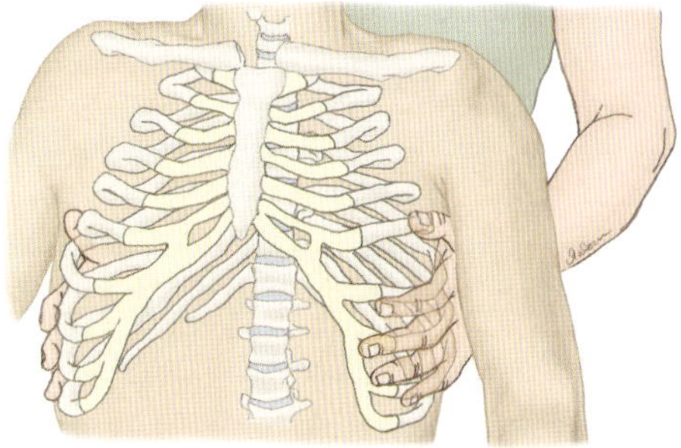

Position of the ribs during inhalation

2. Then lay your hands on all sides of the rib cage and feel for activity in the thorax. Do the ribs move in all three directions? Do some move individually?
3. Ask your partner to inhale deeply and exhale fully. Explore the ribs and anterior neck muscles (scalenes and sternocleidomastoid) during inhalation. These muscles will tighten to elevate the upper ribs. Try these exercises with your partner seated, prone, and supine.

Spine & Thorax

Eleventh and Twelfth Ribs

The eleventh and twelfth ribs are called floating ribs because they do not attach to the costal cartilage. Both ribs have a slender, spear-like shape and lie at roughly a 45° angle. Their medial portions lie deep to the thick erector spinae muscles; however, their lateral aspects and tips are palpable.

The eleventh rib is six to eight inches in length and extends halfway around the body. The twelfth rib can vary in length from three to six inches. Since anomalies are common in either the length or number of ribs, your partner's ribs might not match this description. (See p. 177 for more information about finding the twelfth rib.)

Eleventh and twelfth ribs

1. Partner prone. Reaching across to the body's opposite side, place your hand along the lateral portion of the ribs.
2. Slide inferiorly to the bottom of the rib cage, allowing your hand to sink into the soft abdominal tissue. Compressing your fingerpads into the side of the thorax, explore this region for the tips of the eleventh and twelfth ribs (**4.49**).
3. With the tips isolated, gently follow the shafts of the ribs medially, noting how they run at an angle.

Can you feel two tips, one of which is more lateral than the other? Ask your partner to take a slow, deep breath and note whether the tips or the bodies of the ribs press into your hand.

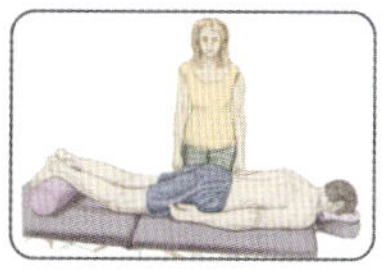

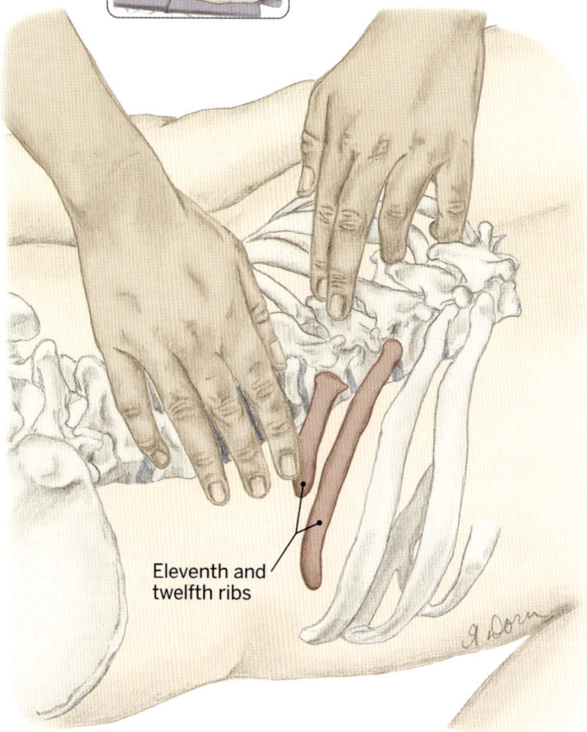

4.49 Partner prone, as you explore the eleventh and twelfth ribs

Overview: Muscles of the Spine and Thorax

The muscles of the spine and thorax are situated along the posterior and abdominal regions and create movement of the vertebral column and rib cage (**4.50**).

The muscles of the spine are uniquely arranged. Unlike the limb muscles that can often be distinguished individually, the spinal muscles are composed of numerous bands of densely interwoven fibers that make it difficult to isolate a particular portion of muscle.

The muscles of the spine may be divided into small, individual sections or separated into a few major groups. For our purposes, the muscles of the spine will be divided into four groups:

1. The large **erector spinae group** is the most superficial of the spinal muscles and has three major branches.
2. The smaller **transversospinalis group** also has three branches but lies deep to the erectors. Its name refers to its muscle fibers, which extend at varying lengths from the transverse and spinous processes of the vertebrae.
3. The two **splenii** muscles are located along the posterior neck, deep to the trapezius.
4. The eight short **suboccipitals** are the deepest muscles. They are located at the base of the head.

Other muscles affecting the thorax, most notably the sternocleidomastoid and scalenes, are presented in Chapter 5, *Head, Neck, and Face.*

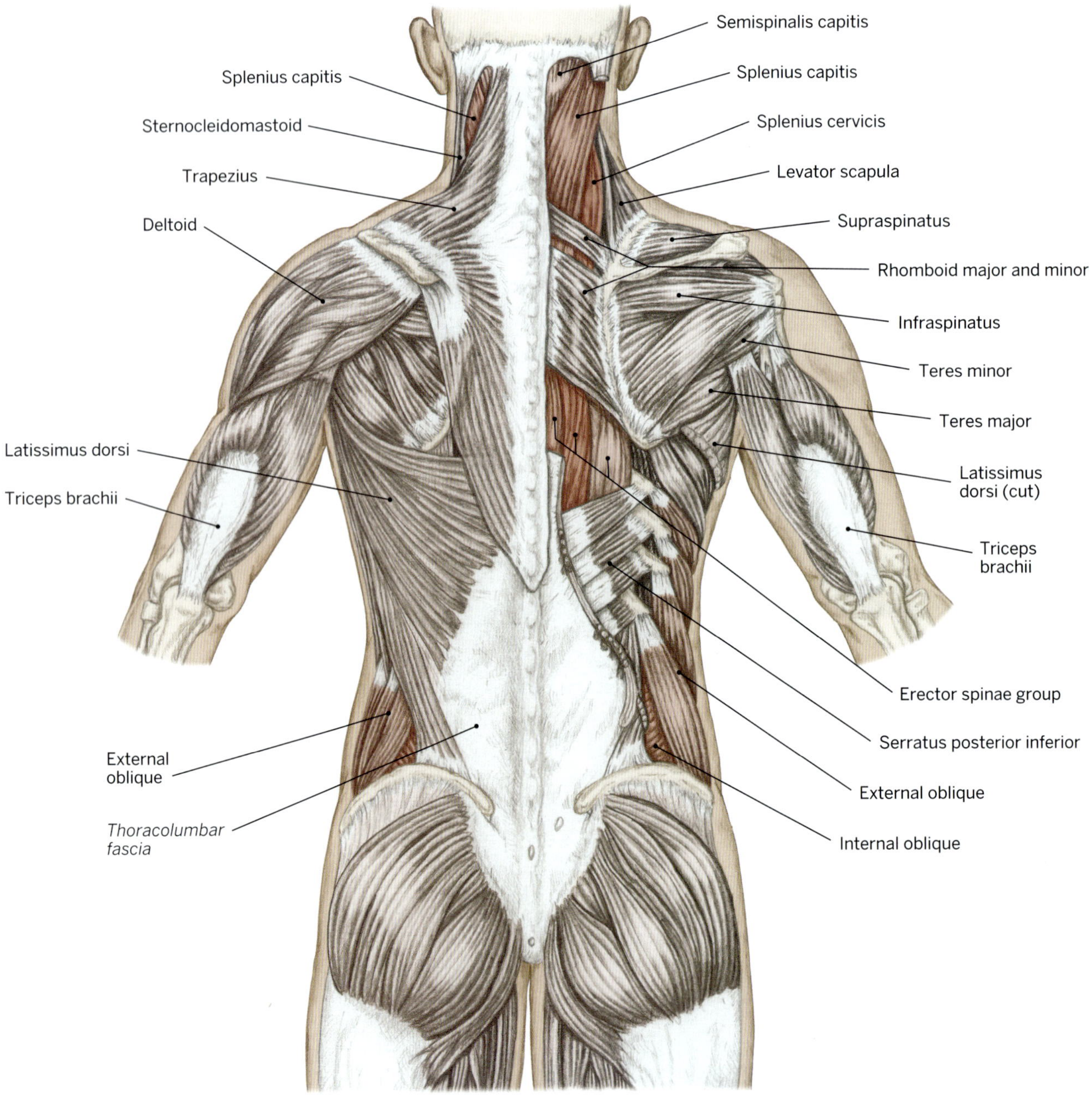

4.50 Posterior view of superficial muscles of the back. The deltoid, trapezius, and latissimus dorsi are removed on the right side.

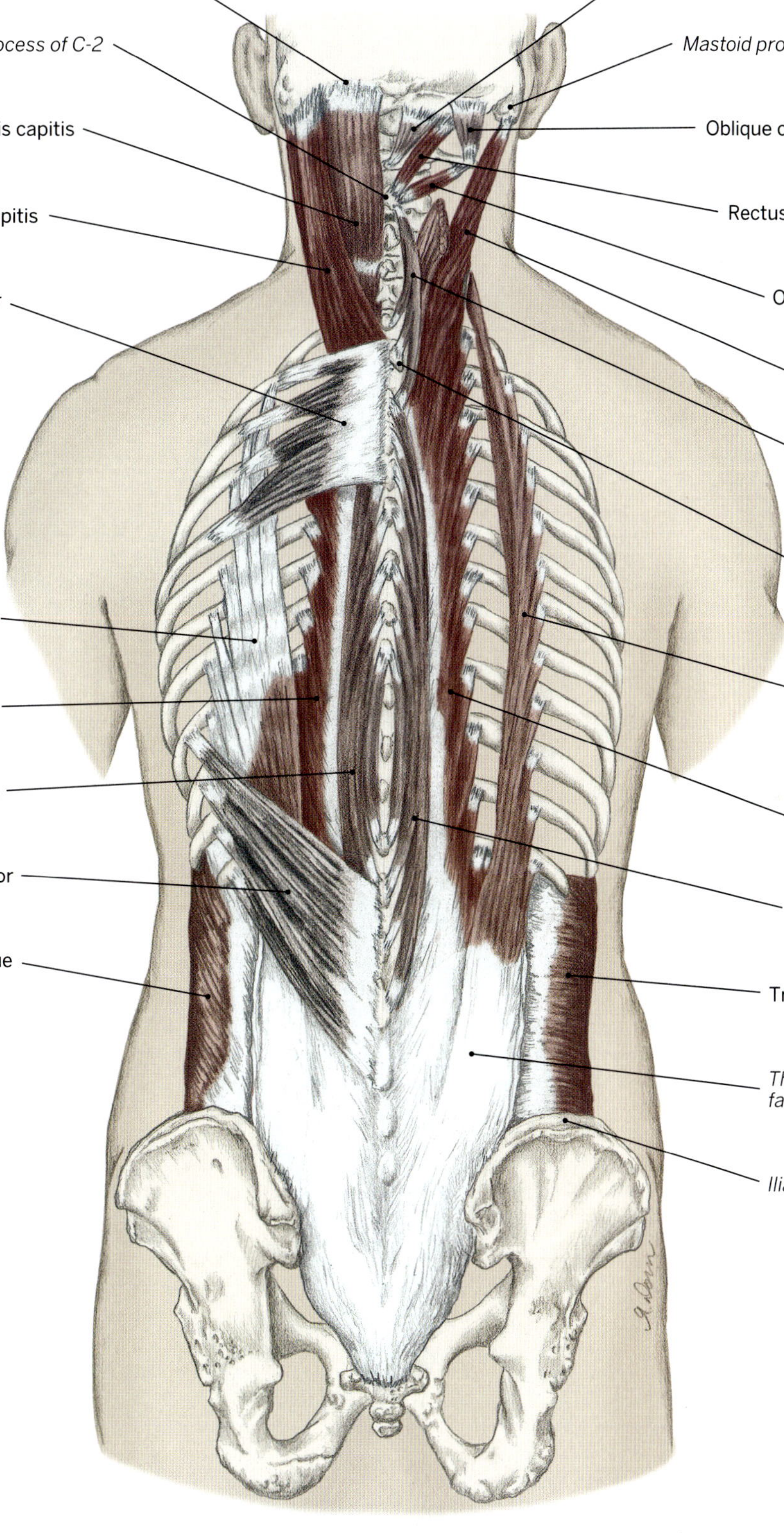

4.51 Posterior view of intermediate muscles of the back

abdominis ab-***dah***-min-is

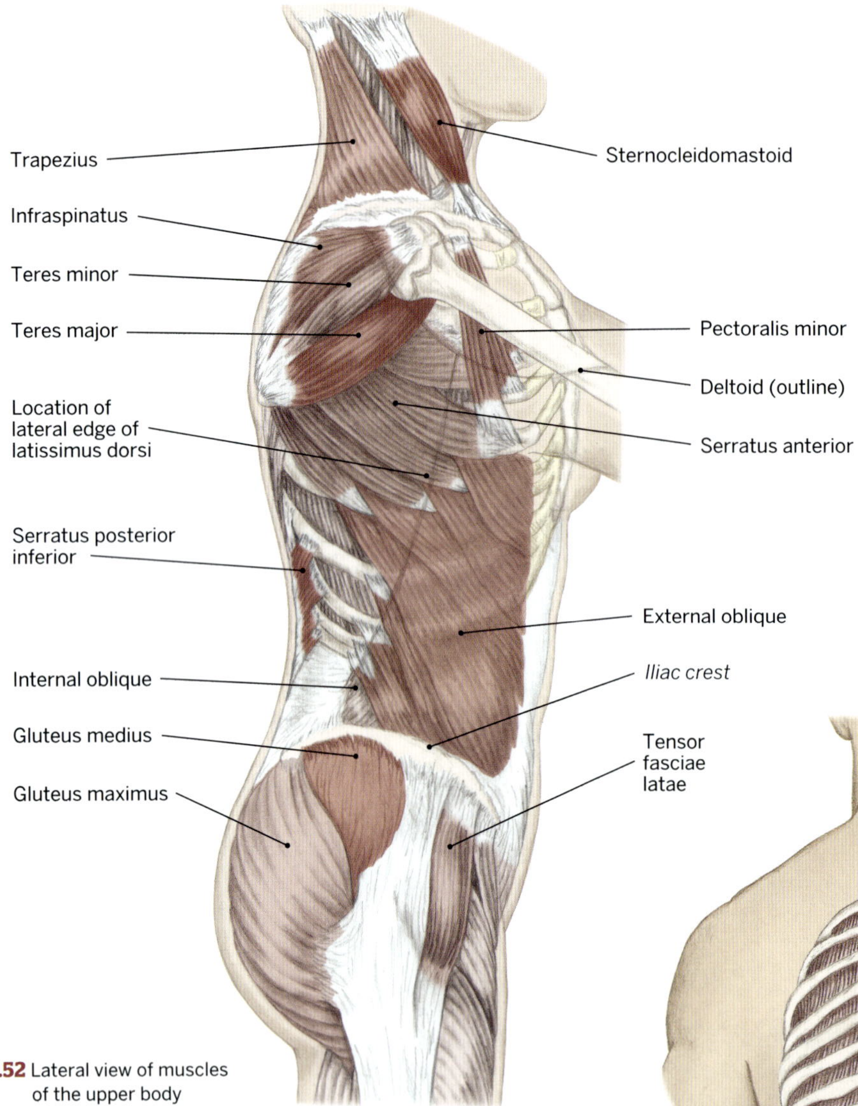

4.52 Lateral view of muscles of the upper body

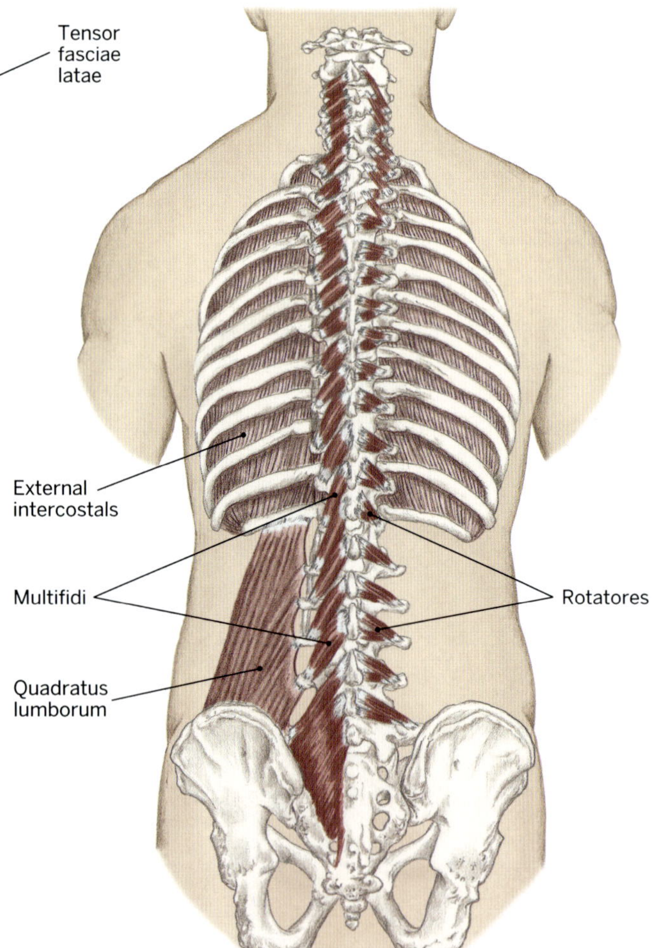

4.53 Posterior view of deep muscles of the back

Discover More

Here is a schematic cross-section view of the muscles of the spine. The transversospinalis muscles (rotatores, multifidi, and semispinalis) are located within the lamina groove, while the erector spinae muscles (spinalis, longissimus, and iliocostalis) extend from the tip of the spinous process to the body of the rib.

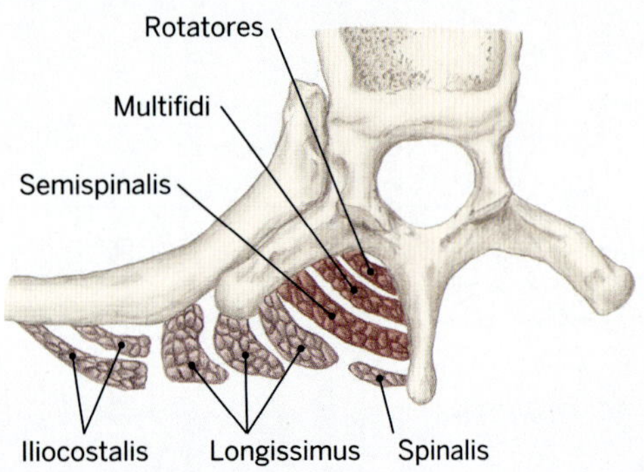

Muscle Layers of the Posterior Neck

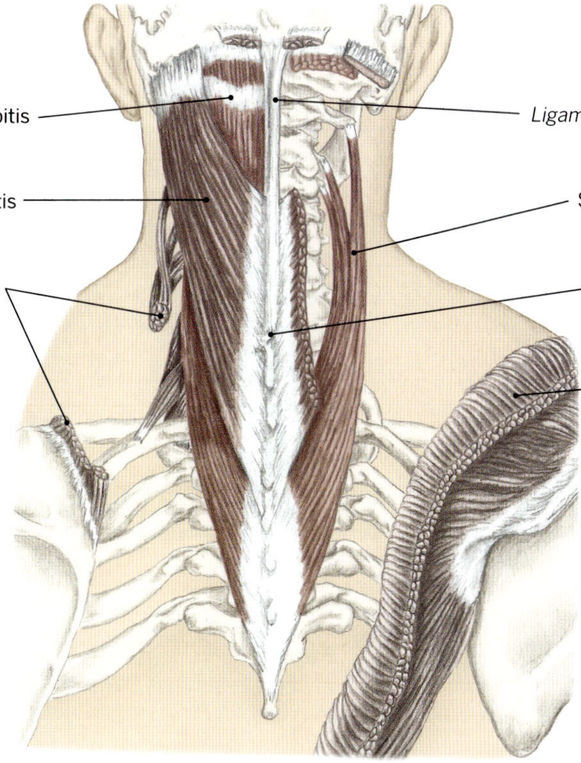

4.54 Posterior view of upper back and neck, showing superficial layer of spinal muscles

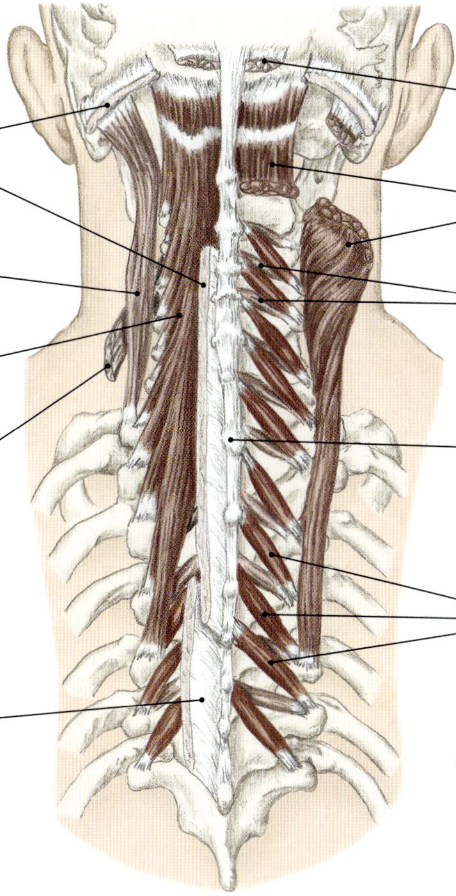

4.55 Posterior view of upper back and neck, showing intermediate layer of spinal muscles

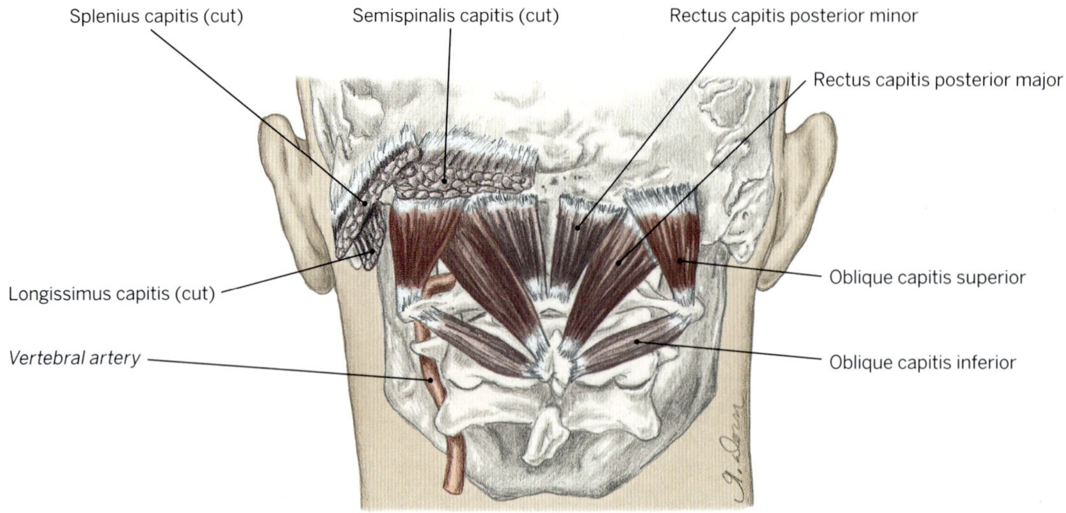

4.56 Posterior view of upper neck, showing deepest layer of spinal muscles

Cross Section of the Neck

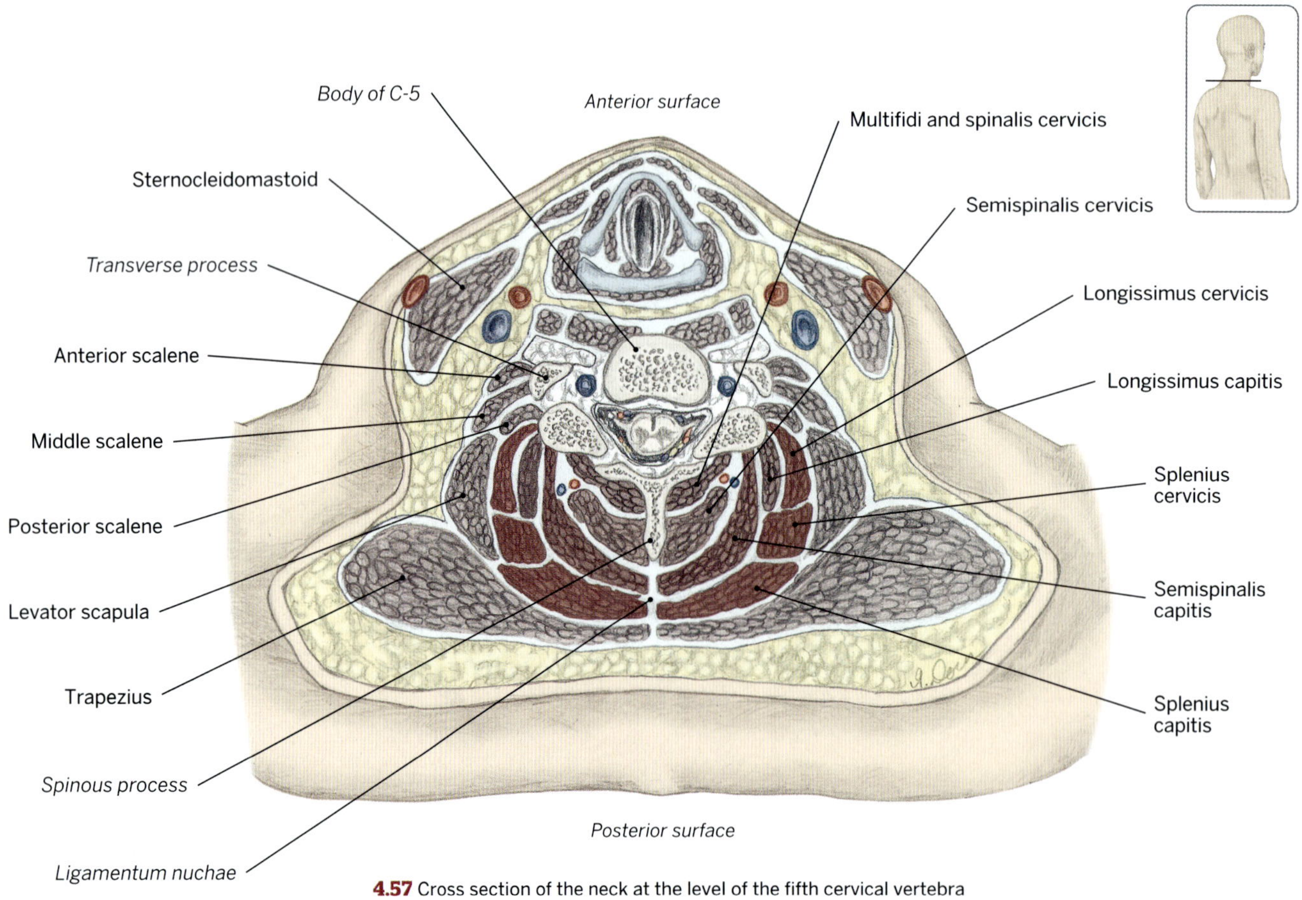

4.57 Cross section of the neck at the level of the fifth cervical vertebra

Cross Sections of the Thorax

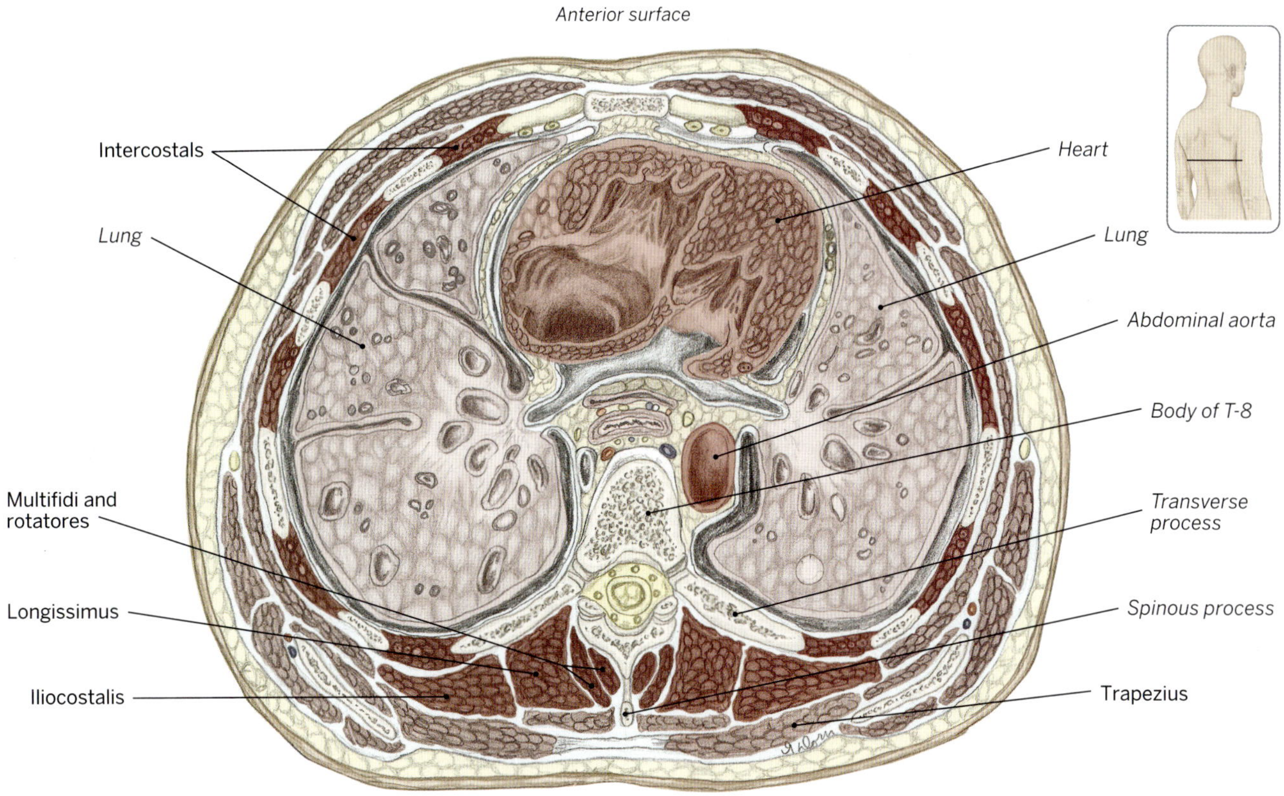

4.58 Cross section of the thorax at the level of the eighth thoracic vertebra

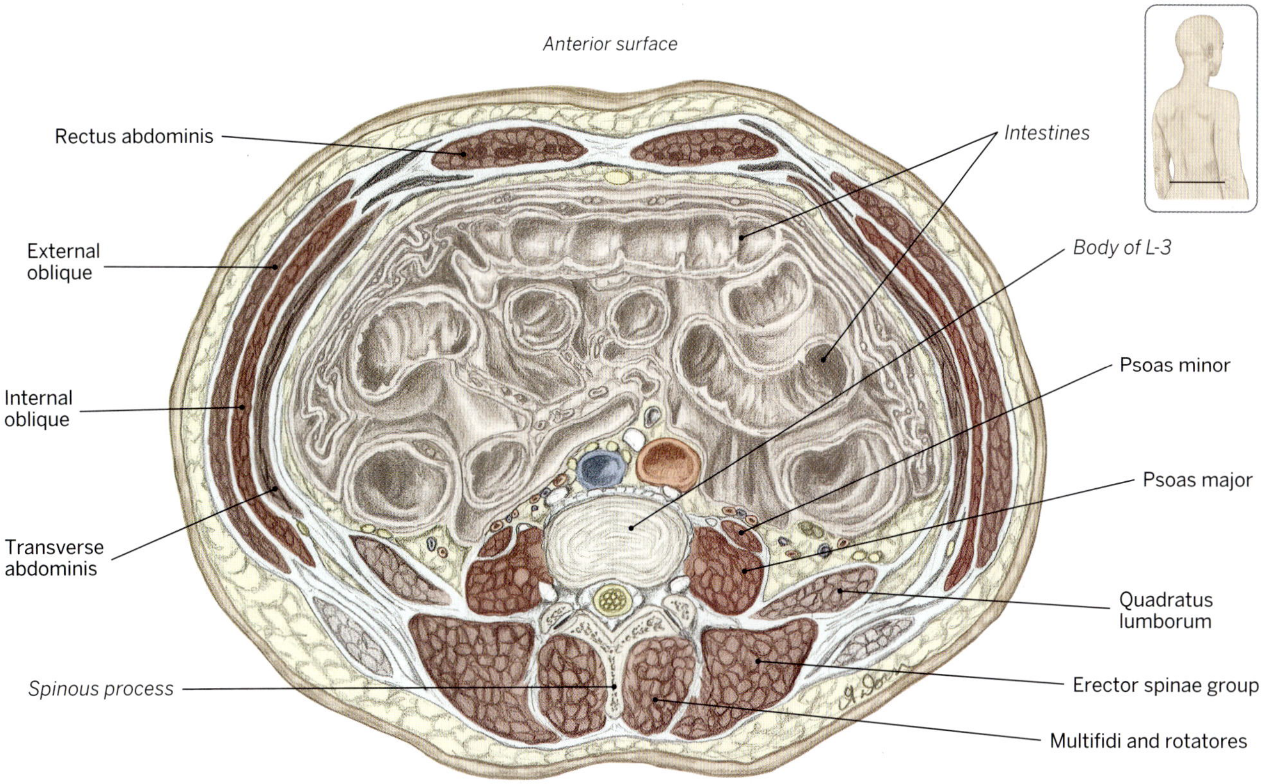

4.59 Cross section of the abdomen at the level of the third lumbar vertebra

Synergists—Muscles Working Together

Muscles are listed in the order of their ability to create the movement. Asterisk indicates muscles not shown.

Vertebral Column

Flexion

(antagonists on extension)

Rectus abdominis
External oblique (bilaterally)
Internal oblique (bilaterally)
Psoas major (with the insertion fixed)
Iliacus (with the insertion fixed)

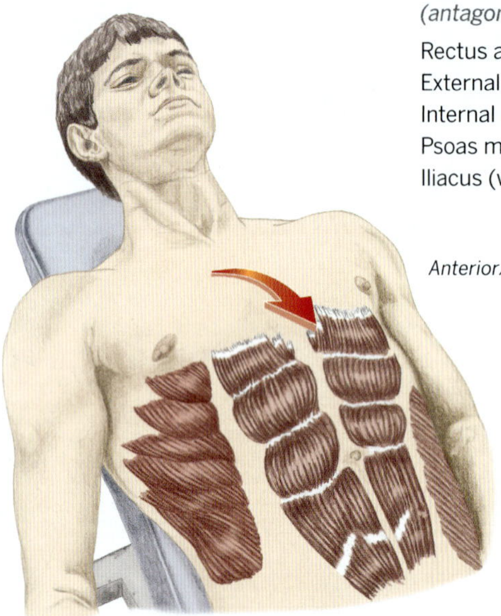

4.60 Flexion of the vertebral column

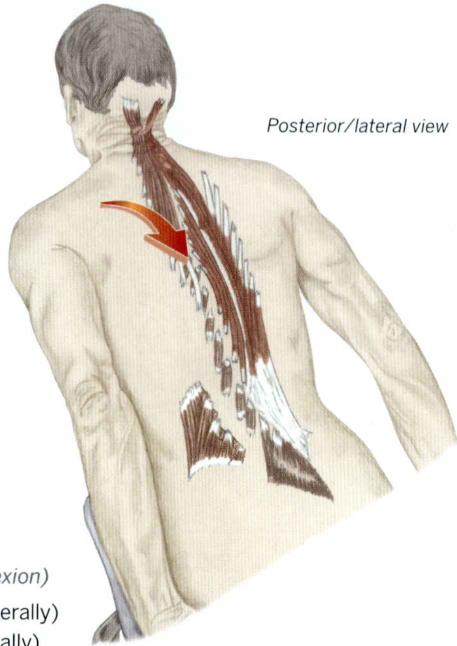

4.61 Extension of the vertebral column

Extension

(antagonists on flexion)

Longissimus (bilaterally)
Iliocostalis (bilaterally)
Multifidi (bilaterally)
Rotatores (bilaterally)*
Semispinalis capitis
Spinalis (bilaterally)
Quadratus lumborum (assists)
Interspinalis*
Intertransversarii (bilaterally)*
Latissimus dorsi (assists, when arm is fixed)*

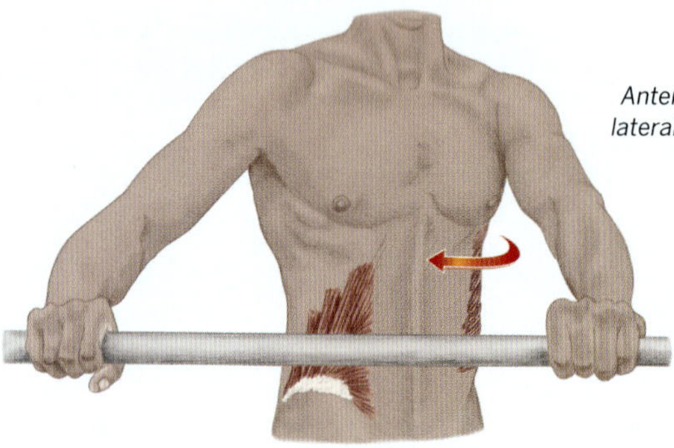

4.62 Rotation of the vertebral column

Rotation

(all unilaterally)

External oblique (to the opposite side)
Internal oblique (to the same side)
Multifidi (to the opposite side)
Rotatores (to the opposite side)

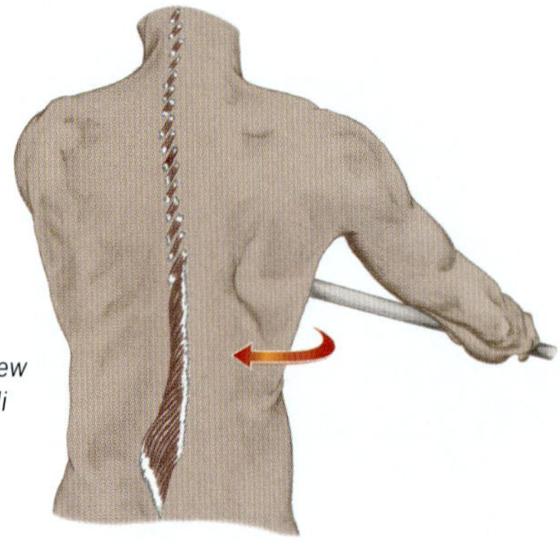

4.63 Rotation of the vertebral column

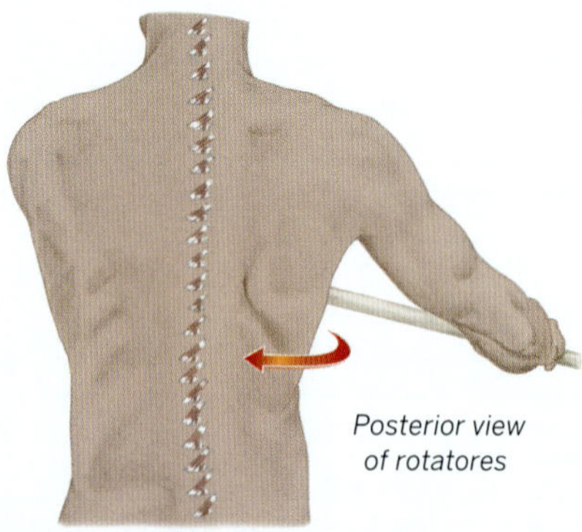

4.64 Rotation of the vertebral column

Vertebral Column

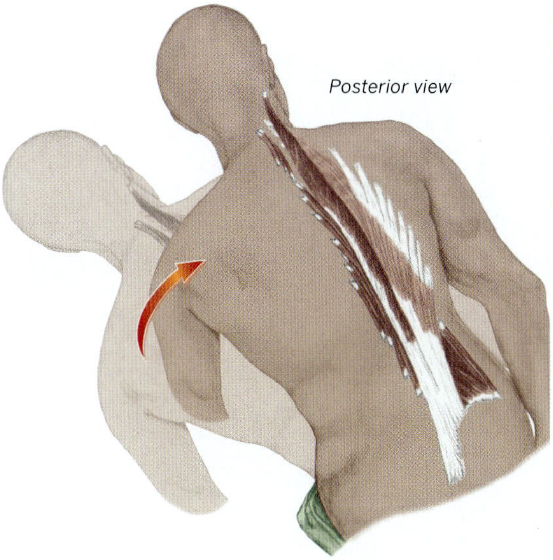

4.65 Lateral flexion of the vertebral column

Lateral Flexion
(unilaterally to the same side)

Iliocostalis
External oblique
Internal oblique
Longissimus
Quadratus lumborum
Psoas major (assists)*
Intertransversarii*
Spinalis
Latissimus dorsi (assists)

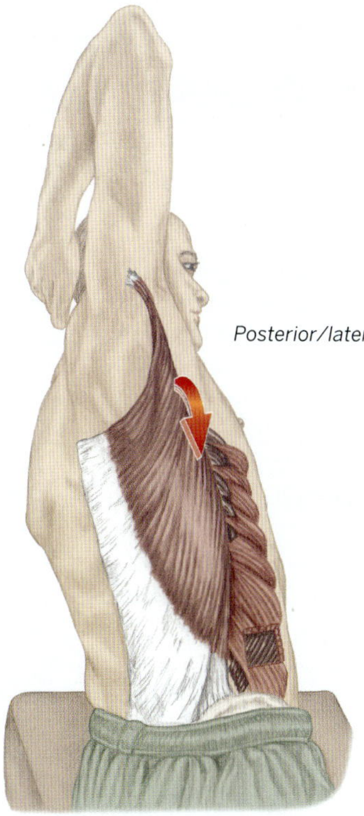

4.66 Lateral flexion of the vertebral column

Ribs/Thorax

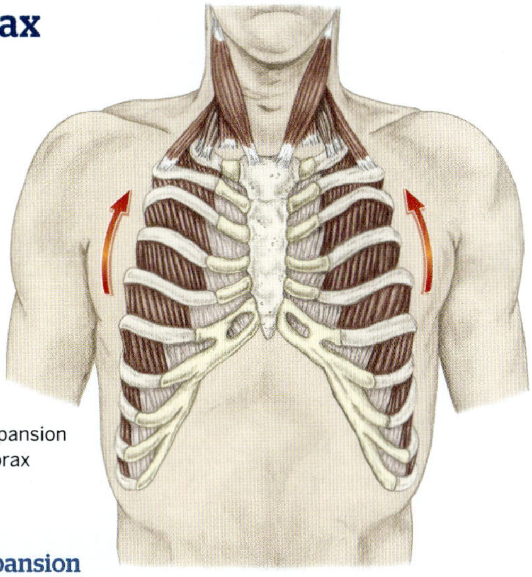

4.67 Elevation/expansion of the ribs/thorax

Elevation/Expansion (involved with inhalation)
(antagonists on depression)

Anterior scalene (bilaterally)
Middle scalene (bilaterally)
Posterior scalene (bilaterally)
Sternocleidomastoid (assists)
External intercostals (assists)
Serratus posterior superior*
Pectoralis major (all fibers may assist if arm is fixed)*
Pectoralis minor (if scapula is fixed)*
Serratus anterior (if scapula is fixed)*
Subclavius (first rib)*

Depression/Collapse (involved with exhalation)
(antagonists on elevation)

Internal intercostals (assists)
Serratus posterior inferior*

Anterior views

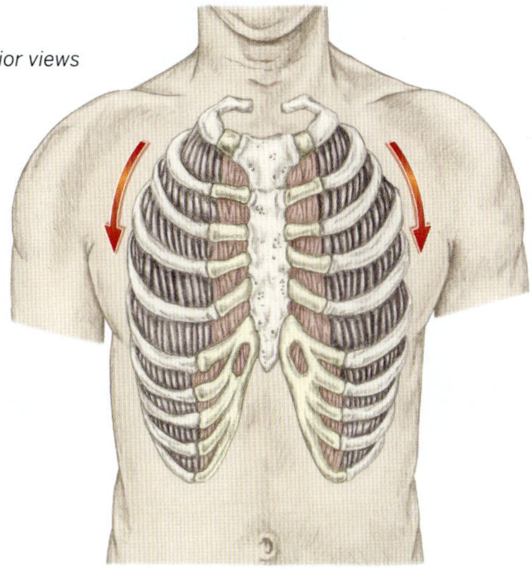

4.68 Depression/collapse of the ribs/thorax

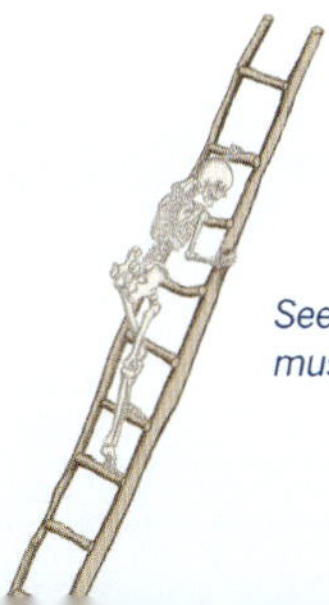

See p. 431 for a list of the muscles of respiration.

Muscles of the Spine and Thorax

Erector Spinae Group ▶

Spinalis
Longissimus
Iliocostalis

The erector spinae group runs from the sacrum to the occiput along the posterior aspect of the vertebral column. Its musculature has a dense, layered arrangement that can be difficult to visualize. It might simplify matters if you imagine the erector spinae muscles as a tall poplar tree (**4.69**) with three main branches—the spinalis, longissimus, and iliocostalis (**4.70**). These branches can then be subdivided into numerous smaller branches such as spinalis thoracis, longissimus capitis, iliocostalis lumborum, and more.

The **spinalis** is the smallest of the three muscles and lies closest to the spine in the lamina groove (**4.71**, **4.72**). The thick **longissimus** (**4.73**, **4.75**) and lateral **iliocostalis** (**4.74**, **4.76**) form a visible mound alongside the lumbar and thoracic spine. The long tendons of iliocostalis extend laterally beneath the scapula.

In the lumbar region, the erectors lie deep to the thin but dense thoracolumbar fascia (p. 220). In the thoracic and cervical areas, they are deep to the trapezius, the rhomboids, and the serratus posterior superior and inferior. As a group, the erectors are easily palpated along the entire length of the back and neck; locating a specific branch of the erectors, however, can be challenging.

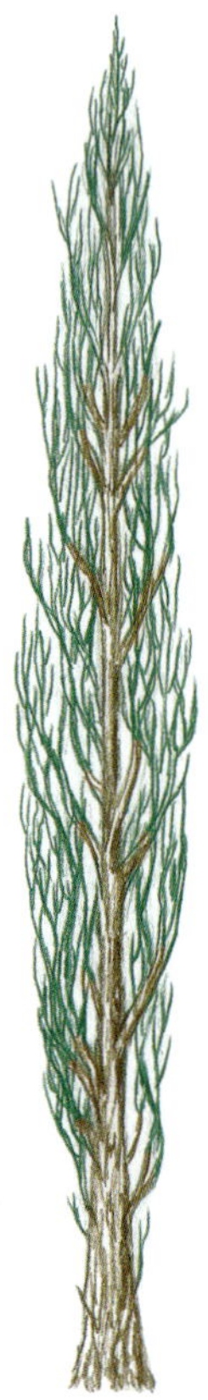

4.69 Poplar tree

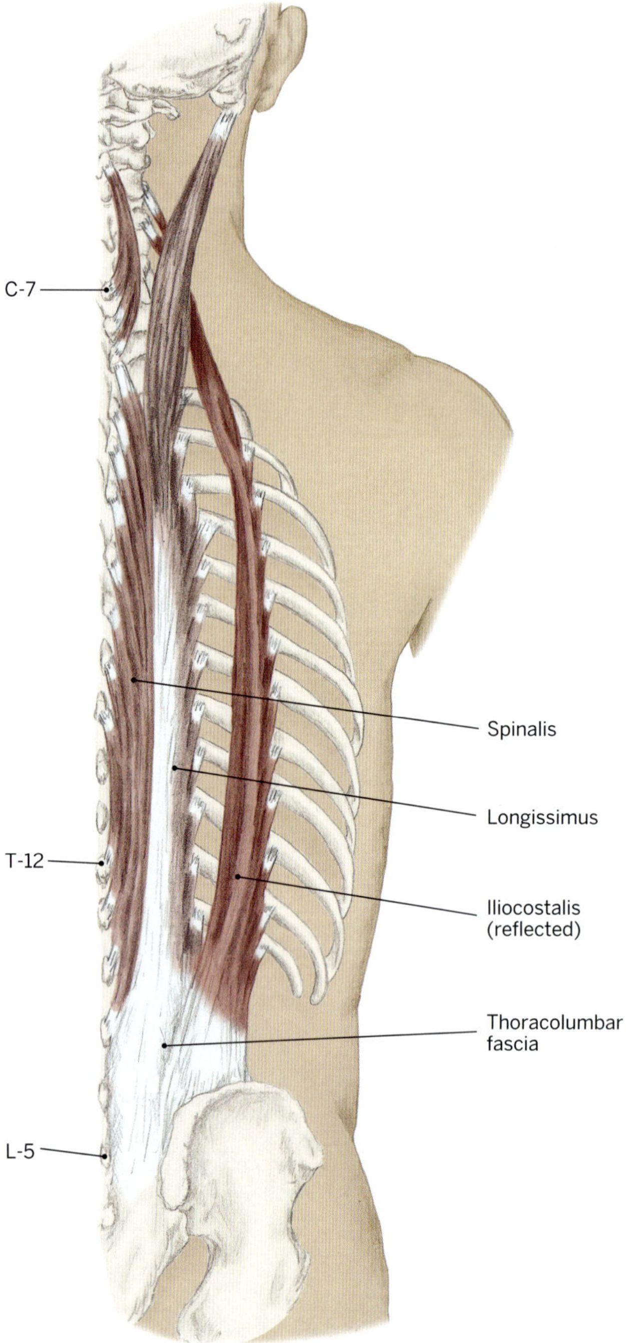

4.70 Posterior view of right side, showing erector spinae group

iliocostalis	*il*-ee-o-kos-***ta***-lis	L. from hip to rib
longissimus	lon-***jis***-i-mus	L. longest

ERECTOR SPINAE GROUP

A *Unilaterally:* **Laterally flex** vertebral column to the same side

Bilaterally: **Extend** the vertebral column

O Common tendon (thoracolumbar fascia) that attaches to the posterior surface of sacrum, iliac crest, spinous processes of the lumbar and last two thoracic vertebrae

I Various attachments at the posterior ribs, spinous and transverse processes of thoracic and cervical vertebrae, and mastoid process of temporal bone

N Spinal

When Do You Use Your Erectors?

- Maintaining an upright posture
- Returning to anatomical position after tying your shoes
- Picking up a heavy suitcase (lateral flexion)

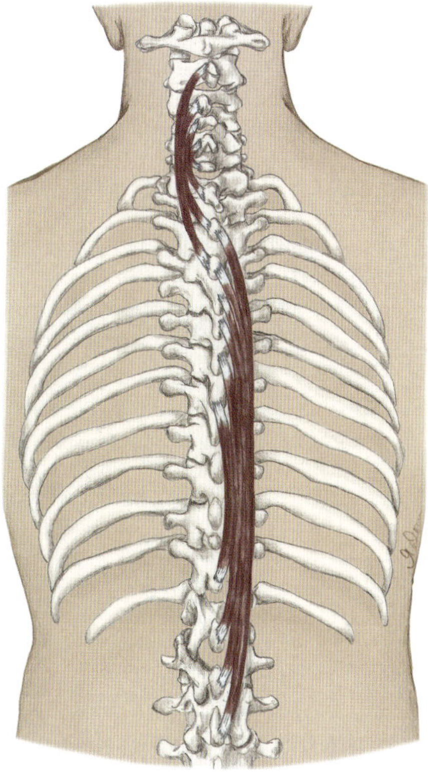

4.71 Posterior view of thorax, showing spinalis

Discover More

The upper fibers of longissimus and iliocostalis muscles (longissimus cervicis and capitis, iliocostalis cervicis) assist in extension, lateral flexion, and rotation of the head and neck to the same side.

Branches of the Erector Spinae Group

SPINALIS

O Spinous processes of the upper lumbar and lower thoracic vertebrae **(thoracis)**

Ligamentum nuchae, spinous process of C-7 **(cervicis)**

I Spinous processes of upper thoracic **(thoracis)**

Spinous processes of cervicals, except C-1 **(cervicis)**

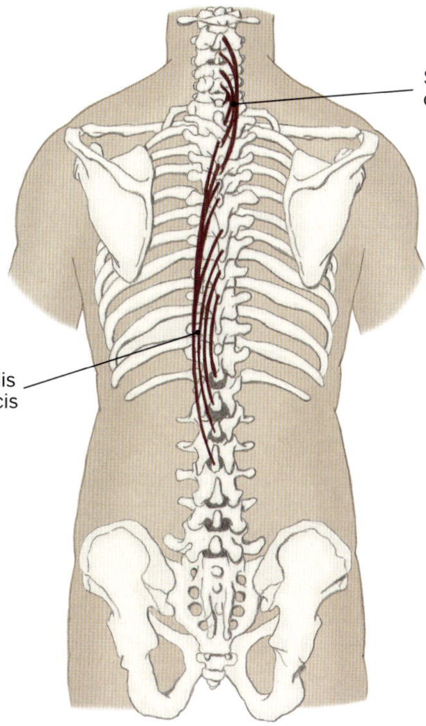

4.72 Posterior view of thorax, showing branches of the spinalis

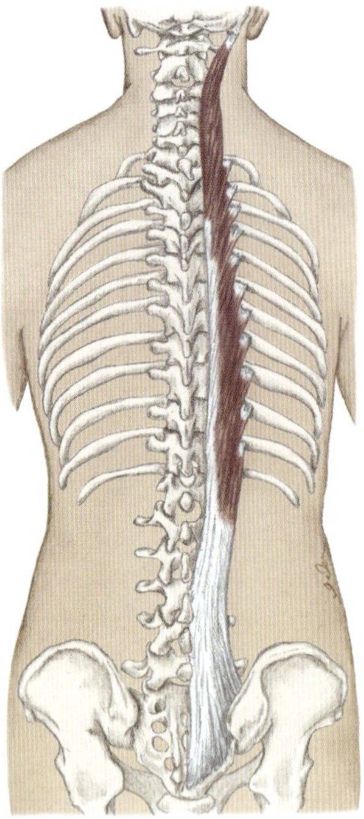

4.73 Posterior view of thorax, showing longissimus

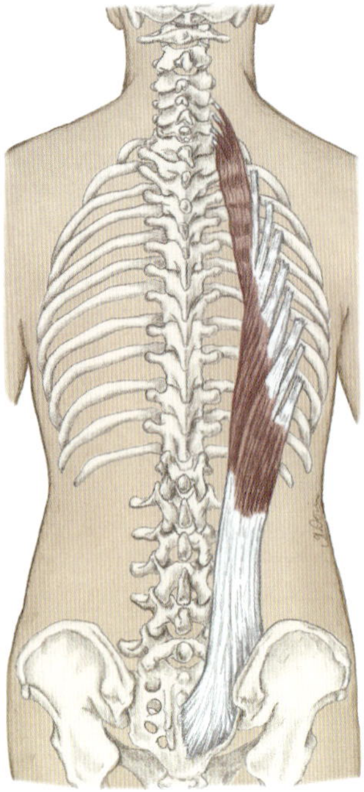

4.74 Posterior view of thorax, showing iliocostalis

LONGISSIMUS

O	Common tendon **(thoracis)** Transverse processes of upper five thoracic vertebrae **(cervicis and capitis)**
I	Lower nine ribs and transverse processes of thoracic vertebrae **(thoracis)** Transverse processes of cervical vertebrae **(cervicis)** Mastoid process of temporal bone **(capitis)**

ILIOCOSTALIS

O	Common tendon **(lumborum)** Posterior surface of ribs 1–12 **(thoracis and cervicis)**
I	Transverse processes of lumbar vertebrae 1–3 and posterior surface of ribs 6–12 **(lumborum)** Posterior surface of ribs 1–6 **(thoracis)** Transverse processes of lower cervicals **(cervicis)**

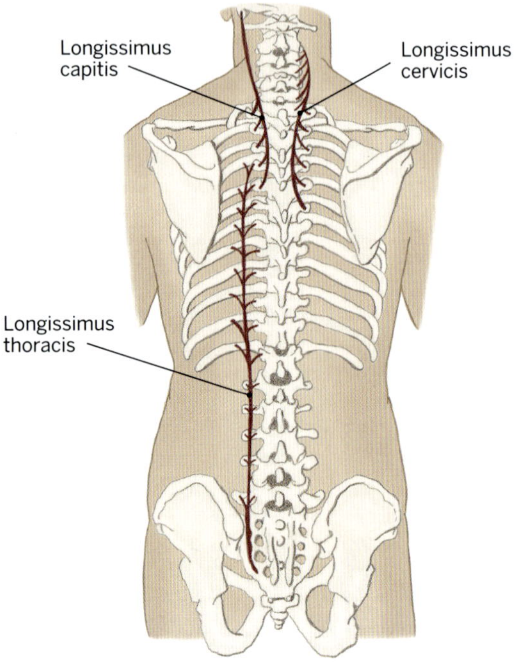

4.75 Branches of the longissimus

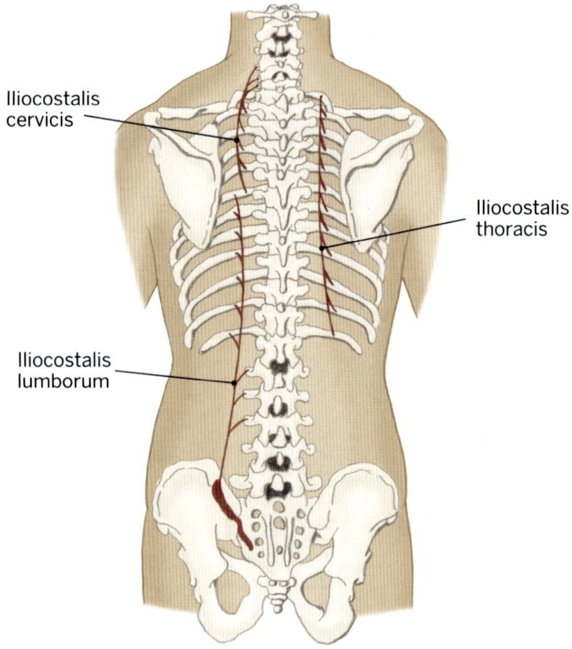

4.76 Branches of the iliocostalis

Erector spinae group

1. Partner prone. Lay both hands along either side of the lumbar vertebrae. Locate the region of the lower erectors by asking your partner to alternately raise and lower his feet slightly. The erectors do not, of course, raise the feet, but they will contract in order to stabilize the pelvis. Notice how the strong, rounded erector fibers tighten and relax with this action (**4.77**).
2. As your partner maintains this contraction, palpate inferiorly onto the sacrum and then superiorly along the thoracic vertebrae. Ask your partner to extend his spine and neck slightly in order to contract the erectors in the thoracic region (**4.78**).
3. Follow the ropy fibers of the erectors between the scapulae and along the back of the neck. These fibers are smallest in the cervical region and are primarily situated lateral to the lamina groove.
4. With your partner relaxed, sink your fingers into the erector fibers, feeling their ropy texture and vertical direction (**4.79**).

Is the tissue you are palpating directly beside the spinous processes of the vertebrae? Do the fibers run parallel to the spine? When the muscles are contracted, can you locate the lateral edge of the erector group? Can you distinguish the fiber direction of the middle trapezius, rhomboids, and erectors between the scapulae?

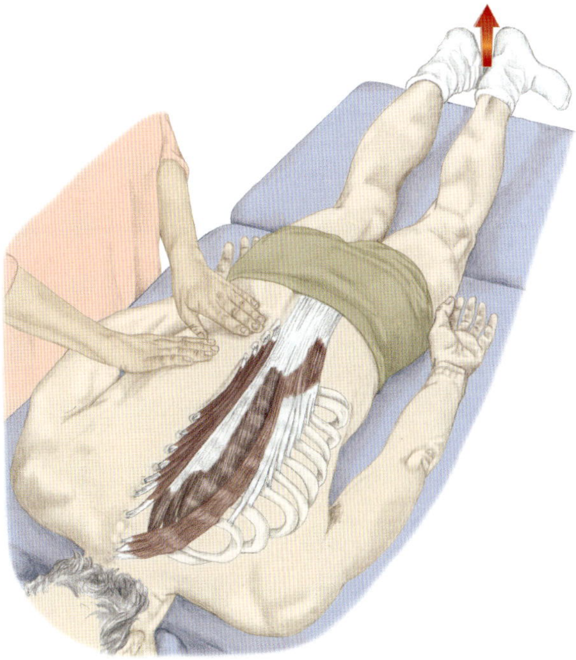

4.77 Partner prone, raising his feet while you palpate the lower erectors

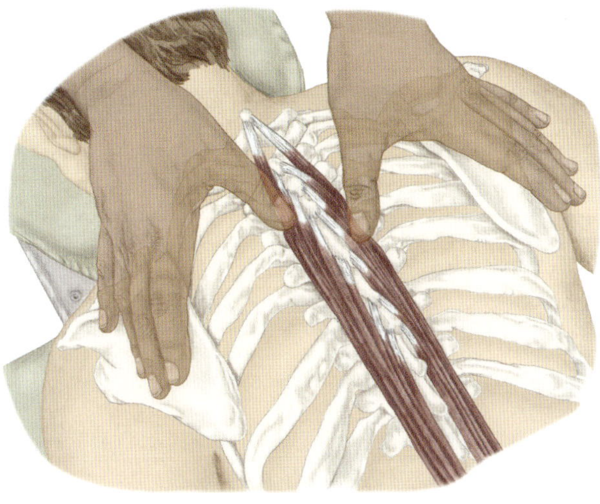

4.78 Partner prone, as you strum your thumbs across the fibers of the spinalis

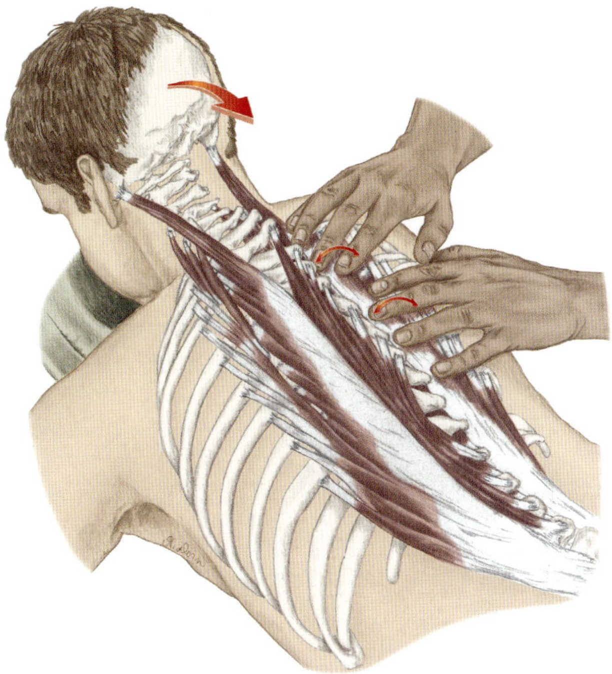

4.79 Partner prone, extending his spine while you palpate the upper erectors

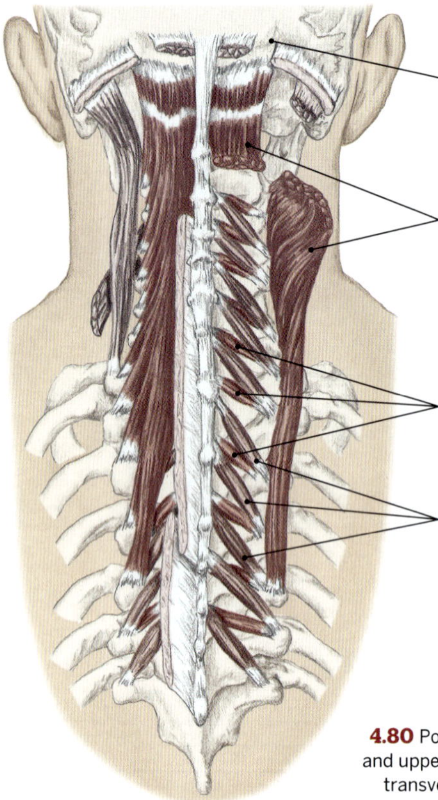

4.80 Posterior view of neck and upper vertebrae, showing transversospinalis group

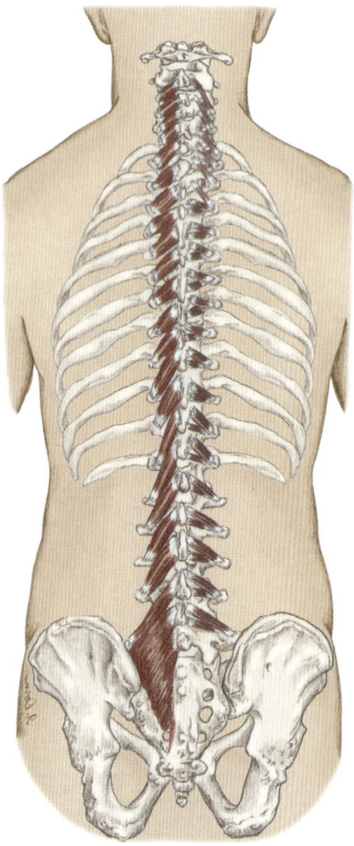

4.81 Posterior view of vertebral column, with the multifidi on the left and the rotatores on the right

Transversospinalis Group ▶

Multifidi
Rotatores
Semispinalis Capitis

Deep to the erector spinae muscle group is the transversospinalis muscle group (**4.80**). The transversospinalis is composed of three branches—multifidi, rotatores, and semispinalis—and extends the length of the vertebral column. Unlike the long, vertical erector fibers, the branches of the transversospinalis consist of many short, diagonal fibers. These fibers form an intricate stitchlike design that links the vertebrae together. The name "transversospinalis" refers to the fact that the fibers of this muscle group extend at varying lengths from the transverse and spinous processes of the vertebrae.

The surprisingly thick **multifidi** are directly accessible in the lumbar spine. They are the only muscles with fibers that lie across the posterior surface of the sacrum. The shorter, smaller **rotatores** lie deep to the multifidi (**4.81–4.83**). The **semispinalis capitis** is located along the thoracic and cervical vertebrae and ultimately reaches the cranium (**4.84**). Both semispinalis muscles form the twin "speed bumps" easily seen on the posterior neck when the neck is extended against resistance.

It can be difficult to isolate the individual bellies of the transversospinalis muscles, as they are closely interwoven; however, as a group, their mass or density can be easily felt along the lamina groove of the thoracic and lumbar vertebrae.

MULTIFIDI AND ROTATORES

A *Unilaterally:* **Rotate** the vertebral column to the opposite side

Bilaterally: **Extend** the vertebral column

O *Multifidi:* Sacrum and transverse processes of lumbar through cervical vertebrae

Rotatores: Transverse processes of lumbar through cervical vertebrae

I Spinous processes of lumbar vertebrae through second cervical vertebra

(Multifidi span two to four vertebrae; rotatores span one to two vertebrae.)

N Spinal

When Do You Use Your Multifidi and Rotatores?

- Rotating your torso to strap on a seat belt
- Arching and rotating your spine during a big "power yawn"
- Heaving dirt off a shovel (extension and rotation of spine)

multifidi	mul-***tif***-i-di	L. *fidi*, to split
rotatores	***ro***-ta-***tor***-ays	L. plural for rotator

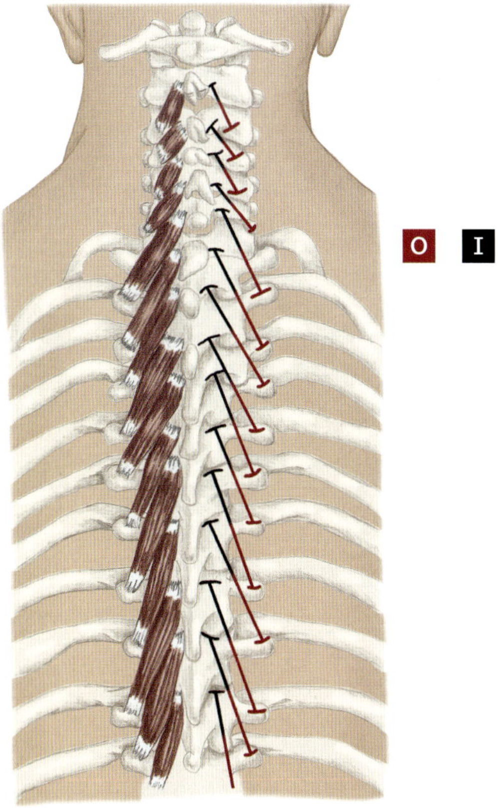

4.82 Posterior view of upper vertebrae, showing origins and insertions of the upper multifidi

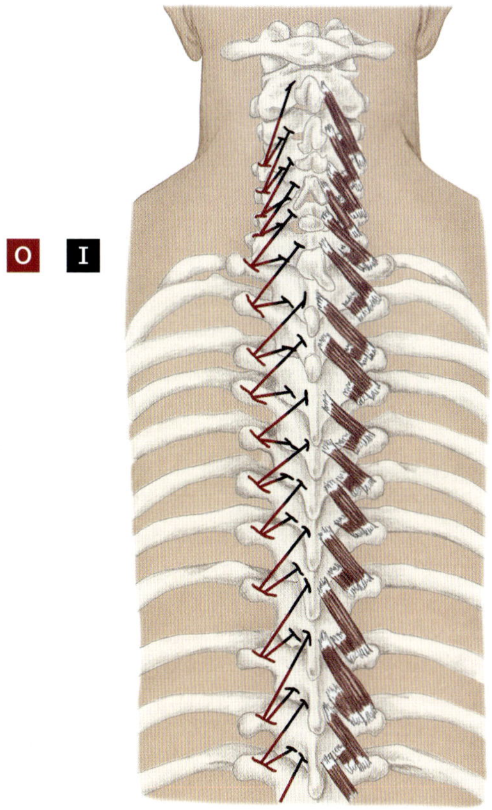

4.83 Posterior view of upper vertebrae, showing origins and insertions of the upper rotatores

SEMISPINALIS CAPITIS

A	**Extend** the vertebral column and head
O	Transverse processes of C-4 to T-5
I	Between the superior and inferior nuchal lines of the occiput
N	Cervical

When Do You Use Your Semispinalis Capitis?

- Rotating your torso to strap on a seat belt
- Arching and rotating your spine during a big "power yawn"
- Heaving dirt off a shovel (extension and rotation of spine)

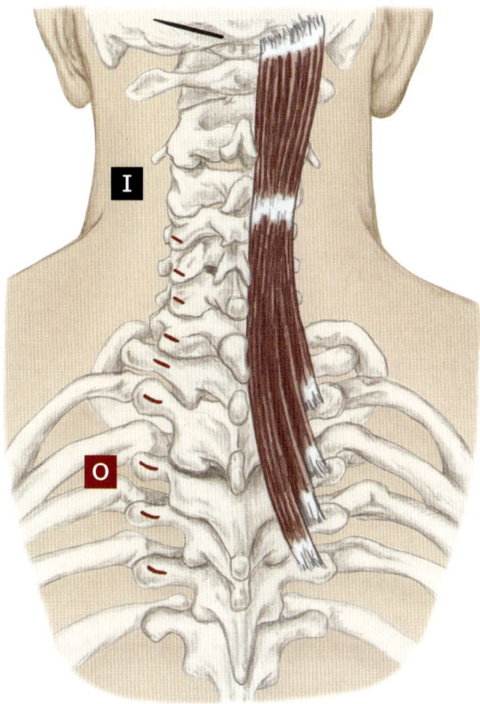

4.84 Posterior view of neck and upper vertebrae, showing origin and insertion of the semispinalis capitis

semispinalis	*sem*-eye-spi-***na***-lis	L. half spinal
transversospinalis	trans-***ver***-so-spi-***nal***-is	

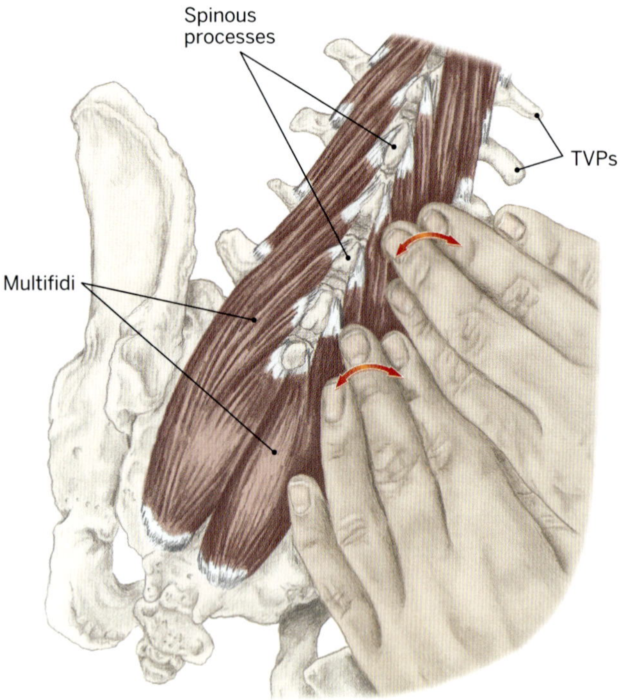

4.85 Partner prone, posterior view of lumbar vertebrae, as you locate the multifidi

Transversospinalis group

1. Partner prone. Locate the spinous processes of the lumbar vertebrae. Slide your fingers laterally off the spinous processes, sinking between them and the erector spinae fibers.
2. Having shifted the erectors laterally out of the way, explore deeply for the dense, diagonal fibers of the multifidi. Progress inferiorly to the sacrum, rolling your fingers in a perpendicular direction to the multifidi fibers (**4.85**).
3. Move superiorly, exploring the lamina groove of the thoracic and cervical areas (**4.86**). Then turn your partner supine and palpate the cervical region.

*Are you between the spinous and transverse processes (**4.87**)? Can you get a sense of these smaller, deeper fibers that stretch at an oblique angle?*

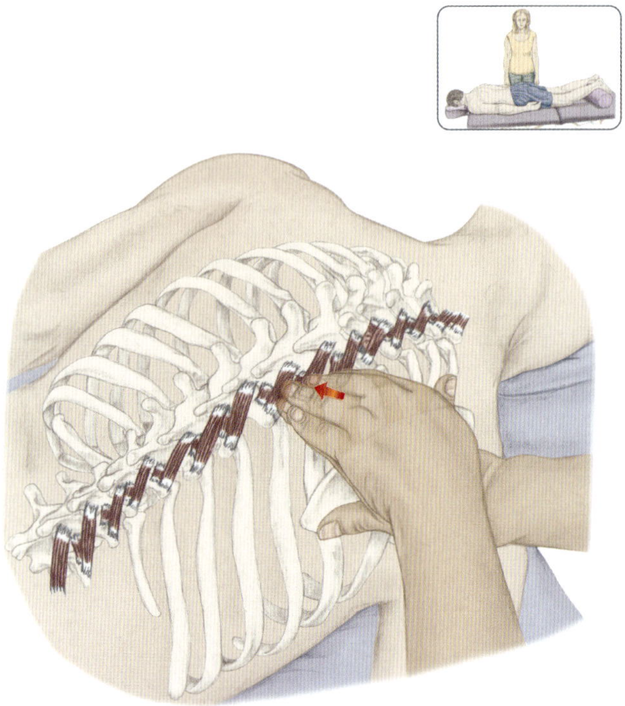

4.86 Partner prone, posterior view of vertebral column with superficial muscles removed, as you access the rotatores by directing your fingers *toward* the vertebrae

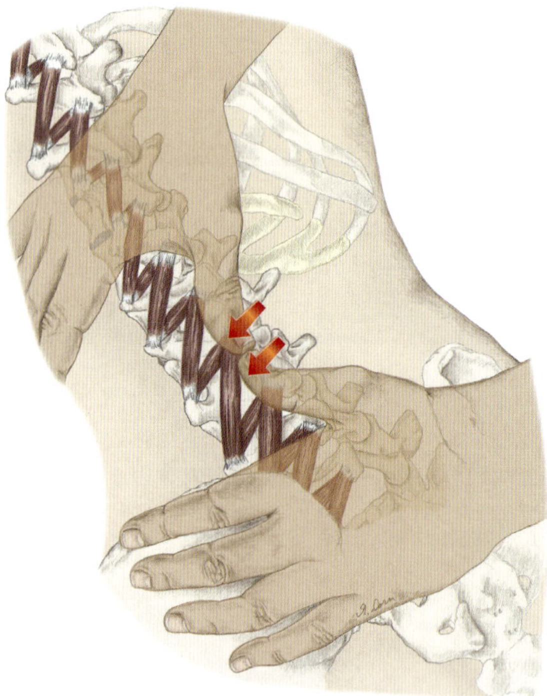

4.87 Partner prone, posterior/lateral view of vertebral column with superficial muscles removed, as you palpate into the lamina groove on opposite side of the body with the thumbs sliding *away* from the vertebrae

Splenius Capitis and Cervicis ▶

The long splenius capitis and splenius cervicis muscles are located along the upper back and posterior neck (**4.88**, **4.89**). In contrast to the other back muscles that run parallel to the spine, the splenii fibers run obliquely. The **splenius capitis** is deep to the trapezius and rhomboids. Its fibers angle toward the mastoid process and are superficial between the trapezius and sternocleidomastoid (**4.90**, **4.91**).

The **splenius cervicis** is deep to the splenius capitis and not as easily isolated; however, its general location can be outlined in the lamina groove of the upper thoracic and cervical spine.

SPLENIUS CAPITIS AND CERVICIS

A *Unilaterally:*
Rotate the head and neck to the same side
Laterally flex the head and neck to the same side

Bilaterally:
Extend the head and neck

O *Capitis:* Inferior one-half of ligamentum nuchae and spinous processes of C-7 to T-4

Cervicis: Spinous processes of T-3 to T-6

I *Capitis:* Mastoid process and lateral portion of superior nuchal line

Cervicis: Transverse processes of C-1 to C-3

N Cervical

When Do You Use Your Splenii?

- Rotating your head and neck before changing lanes in traffic
- Applying ear drops (holding your head in lateral flexion)
- Crouched over in a huddle during a football game (extension of neck)

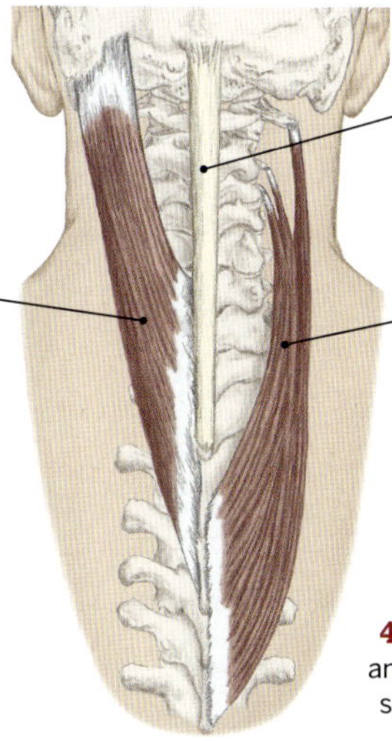

4.88 Posterior view of neck and upper vertebrae, showing splenius capitis and cervicis

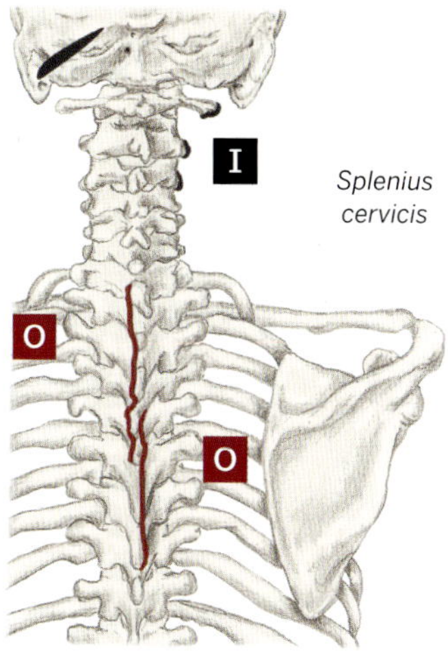

4.89 Posterior view of neck and upper vertebrae, showing origins and insertions of splenius capitis and cervicis

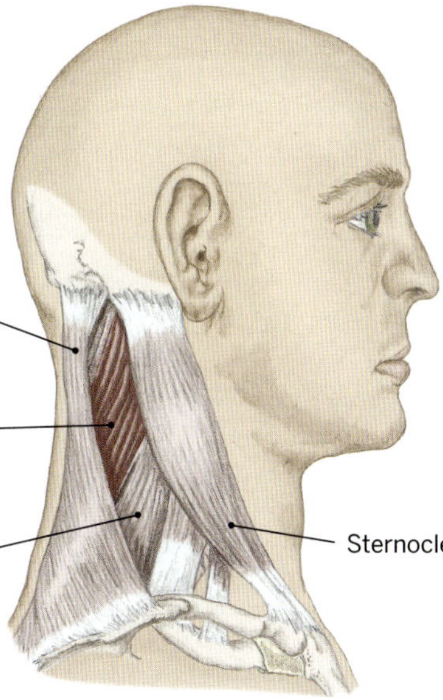

4.90 Lateral view of neck, showing splenius capitis (highlighted in dark red)

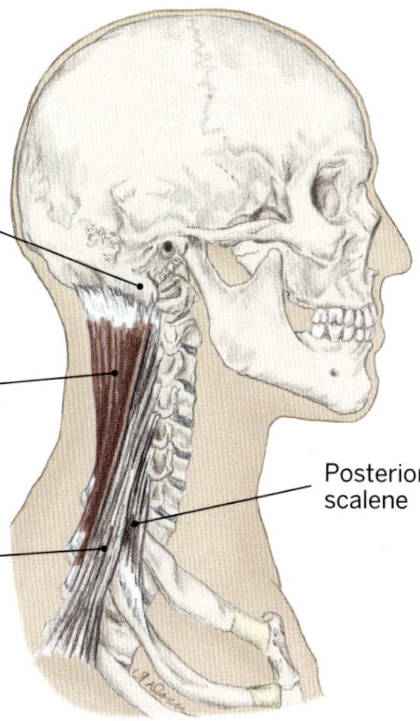

4.91 Lateral view of neck, showing splenius capitis (highlighted in dark red)

splenius capitis *sple*-nee-us ***kap***-i-tis L. bandage-like (muscle) of the head
splenius cervicis *sple*-nee-us ***ser***-vi-sis

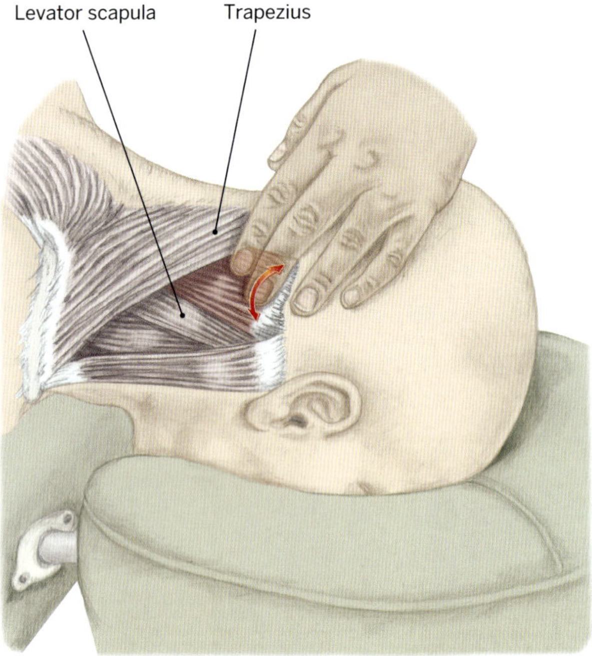

4.92 Partner prone, as you locate splenius capitis

Splenius capitis

1. Partner prone. Locate the upper fibers of the trapezius.
2. Isolate the lateral edge of the trapezius by having your partner extend his head slightly.
3. Ask your partner to relax. Palpate just lateral to the trapezius for the splenius capitis's oblique fibers, following them up to the mastoid process and inferiorly through the trapezius (**4.92**).

Do the fibers you feel lead toward the mastoid process? Distinguish the trapezius fibers from the splenius capitis fibers by asking your partner to rotate his head slightly toward the side you are palpating. Do you feel these oblique fibers contract while the trapezius remains passive?

Locate the mastoid process and slide medially and inferiorly onto the superficial capitis fibers.

Both splenii muscles

1. Partner supine with the head rotated 45° away from the side you are palpating. Cradle the head with one hand while the other hand locates the lamina groove of the upper cervical and thoracic vertebrae (**4.93**).
2. Passively extend the neck slightly to shorten the tissue and palpate through the overlying trapezius fibers. These bellies will not be particularly distinct; however, the density of both splenii can be felt in the lamina groove.

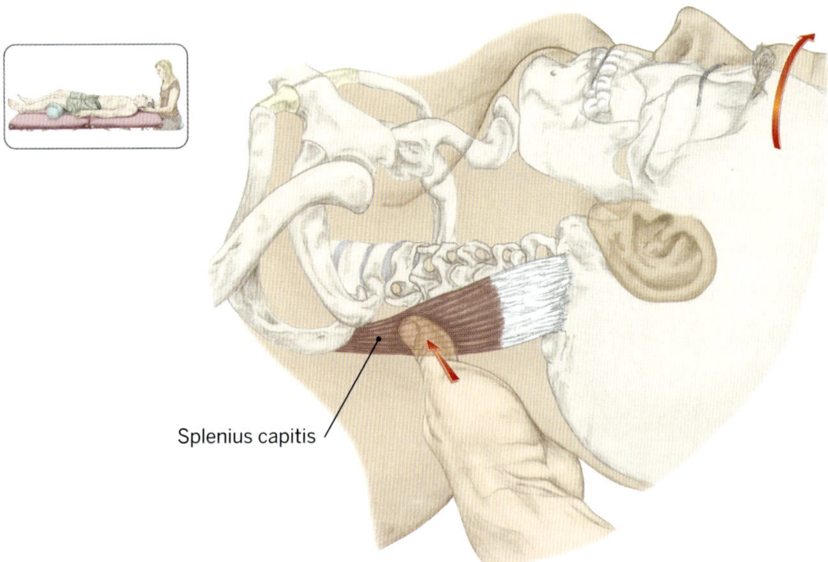

4.93 Partner supine, with head rotated 45° to the right, away from the side you are palpating

capitis	***kap***-i-tis	L. of the head
cervicis	***ser***-vi-sis	L. neck
splenius	***sple***-nee-us	Grk. bandage

Suboccipitals ▶

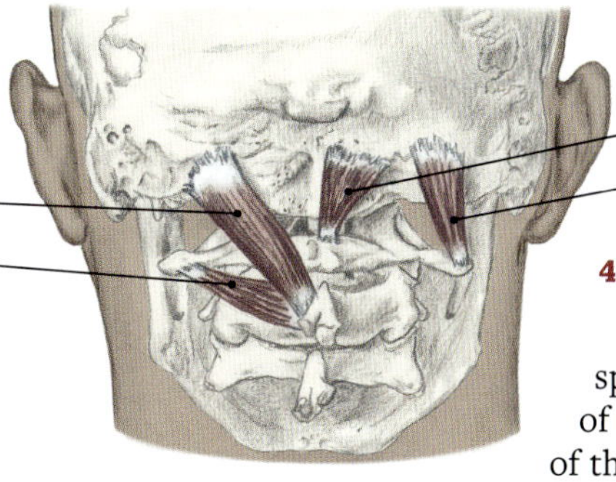

4.94 Posterior view of neck, showing suboccipitals

The eight small suboccipitals are the deepest muscles of the upper posterior neck (**4.94–4.98**). They are involved in stabilizing the axis and atlas and in creating intrinsic movements such as rocking and tilting of the head. To outline the suboccipitals' location, find the spinous process of C-2, the transverse processes of C-1, and the space between the superior nuchal line of the occiput and C-2. The upper fibers of the trapezius can also be used as a marker. The lateral edge of the muscle is the same width as the suboccipitals. The density of the suboccipital bellies can be felt, but accessing specific muscle bellies may be challenging.

A

Rectus capitis posterior major
Rectus capitis posterior minor
Oblique capitis superior

Rock and **tilt** the head back into extension

A

Rectus capitis posterior major
Oblique capitis inferior

Rotate the head to the same side

A

Oblique capitis superior

Laterally flex the head to the same side

RECTUS CAPITIS POSTERIOR MAJOR	
O	Spinous process of the axis (C-2)
I	Inferior nuchal line of the occiput
N	Suboccipital

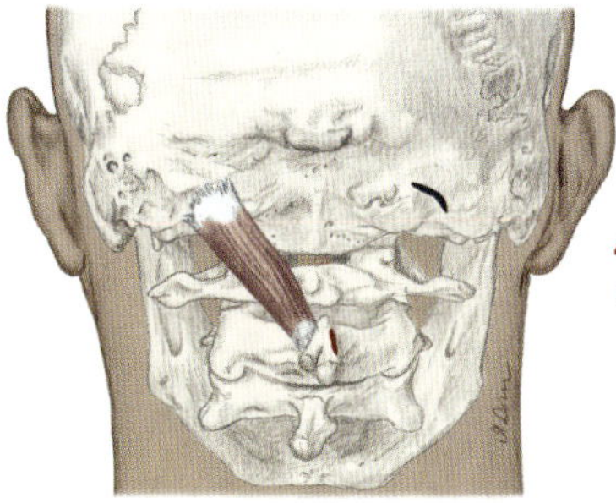

4.95 Posterior view of neck, showing rectus capitis posterior major and its origin **(red)** and insertion **(black)**

RECTUS CAPITIS POSTERIOR MINOR	
O	Tubercle of the posterior arch of the atlas (C-1)
I	Inferior nuchal line of the occiput
N	Suboccipital

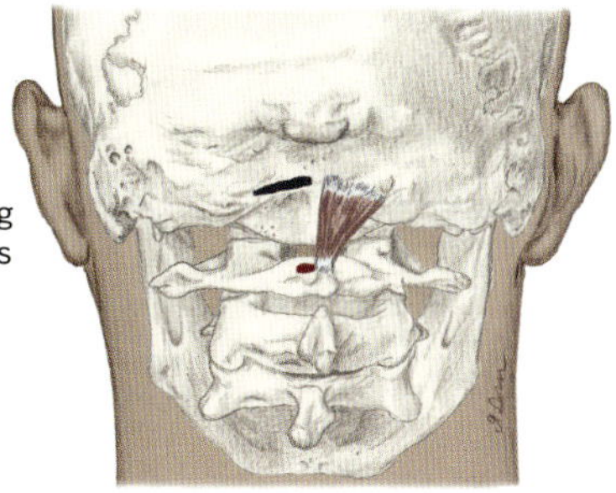

4.96 Posterior view of neck, showing rectus capitis posterior minor and its origin **(red)** and insertion **(black)**

OBLIQUE CAPITIS SUPERIOR	
O	Transverse process of the atlas (C-1)
I	Between the nuchal lines of the occiput
N	Suboccipital

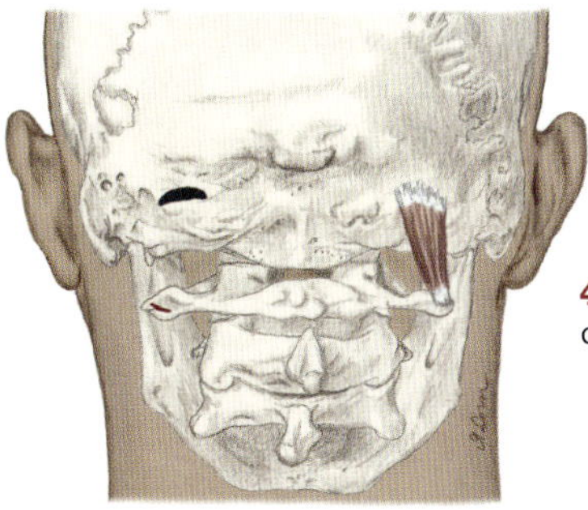

4.97 Posterior view of neck, showing oblique capitis superior and its origin **(red)** and insertion **(black)**

OBLIQUE CAPITIS INFERIOR	
O	Spinous process of the axis (C-2)
I	Transverse process of the atlas (C-1)
N	Suboccipital

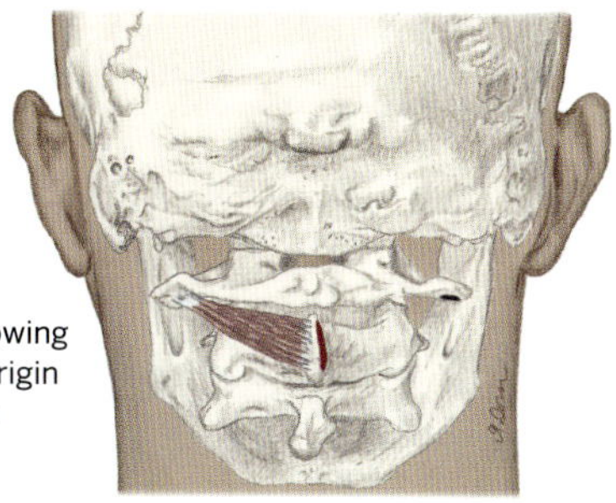

4.98 Posterior view of neck, showing oblique capitis inferior and its origin **(red)** and insertion **(black)**

When Do You Use Your Suboccipitals?

- Shampooing your hair
- Appreciating a large painting from a close proximity (small, fine movements of the head and neck)
- Nodding your head incessantly to a person you wish would just stop talking

occiput *ok*-si-put L. the back of the skull

Suboccipitals

1. Partner supine. Cradle the head in both hands. Passively extending the neck a bit will soften the overlying tissue. Locate the superior nuchal line of the occiput and the spinous process of C-2. The suboccipitals span the area between these two landmarks.
2. Cradle the head with one hand while two fingertips of the other hand palpate slowly through the trapezius, splenius capitis, and semispinalis capitis fibers (**4.99**).
3. Roll your fingers across the suboccipitals' small, short bellies. Again, you may initially feel only the density of these muscles rather than the individual bellies.

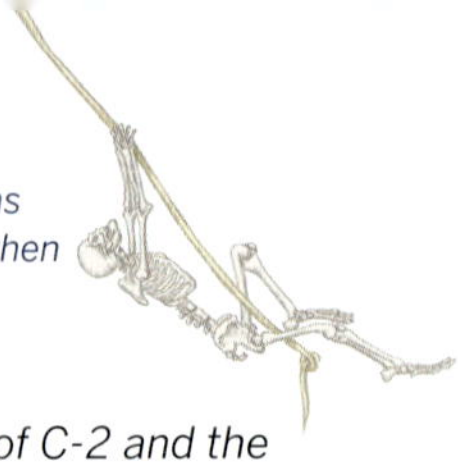

Located deep to the suboccipital bellies are portions of the vertebral artery and suboccipital nerve. So when exploring the muscles, use caution.

Are you between the spinous process of C-2 and the superior nuchal line of the occiput? If you ask your partner to tilt his head back ever so slightly, do you feel some contraction in the deepest layer of tissue?

Partner prone. Locate the lateral edge of the trapezius' upper fibers (**4.100**). Palpating beside the level of C-1, place one finger at the lateral edge of the trapezius. Slowly sink medially into the suboccipitals.

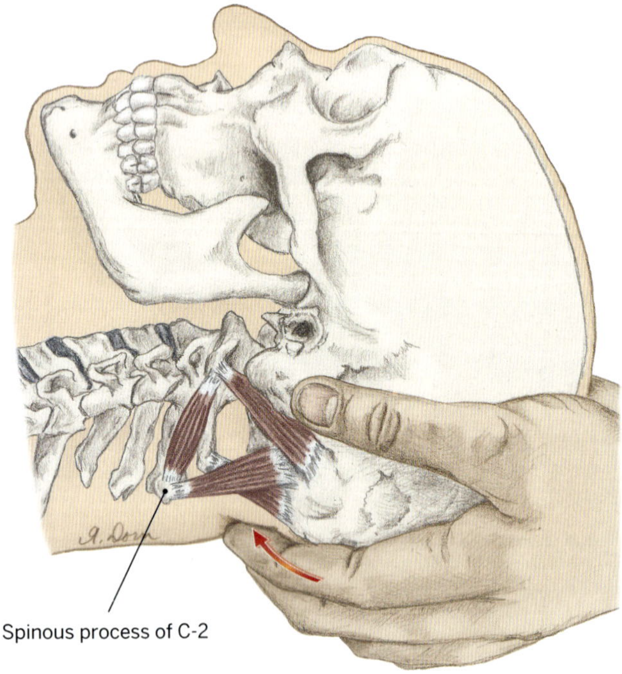

4.99 Partner supine, as you curl your fingers under the occiput

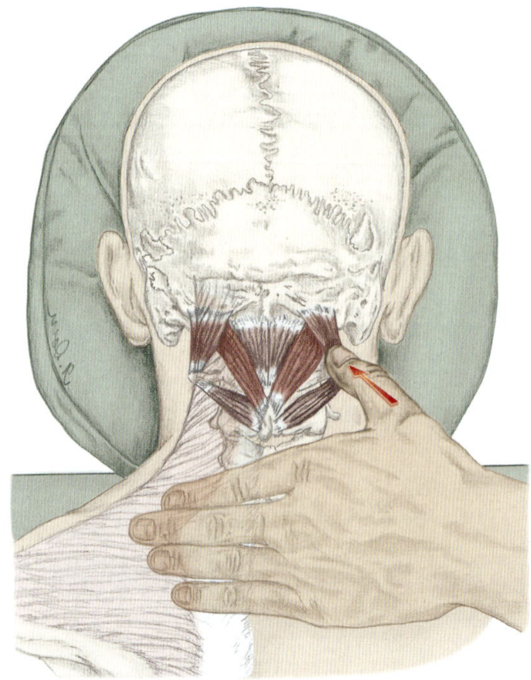

4.100 Partner prone, as you sink your thumb medially, just lateral to the edge of the trapezius

Discover More

Researchers have discovered that the rectus capitis posterior minor attaches not only to the occiput, but also to the dura mater, the connective tissue that surrounds the spinal cord and brain. Because of this connection between the rectus capitis posterior minor and the dura mater, this muscle may cause headaches by disrupting normal cerebrospinal fluid fluctuations and hence the functioning of the vertebral artery and suboccipital nerve.

dura mater *dyoo*-ra *ma*-ter L. tough mother

Quadratus Lumborum ▶

Although it would seem to be the deepest muscle of the low back, the quadratus lumborum is, strangely enough, the deepest muscle of the abdomen (**4.101**, **4.102**). Stretching from the posterior ilium to the transverse processes of the lumbar vertebrae and twelfth rib (**4.103**), this squat muscle is simply an abdominal muscle located on the posterior surface of the thorax.

While the medial portion of the quadratus lumborum is buried beneath the thoracolumbar fascia and the thick erector spinae, its lateral edge is accessible from the side of the torso.

QUADRATUS LUMBORUM

A

Unilaterally:

Laterally tilt (elevate) the pelvis

Laterally flex the vertebral column to the same side

Bilaterally:

Fix the last rib during forced inhalation and exhalation

Assist to **extend** the vertebral column

O Posterior iliac crest

I Last rib and transverse processes of first through fourth lumbar vertebrae

N Lumbar plexus T12, L**1**, **2**, **3**

When Do You Use Your Quadratus Lumborum?

- Hiking up your hip when stepping over a big log
- Raising yourself up from a side lying position (lateral flexion)
- Salsa, tango, and ballroom dancing

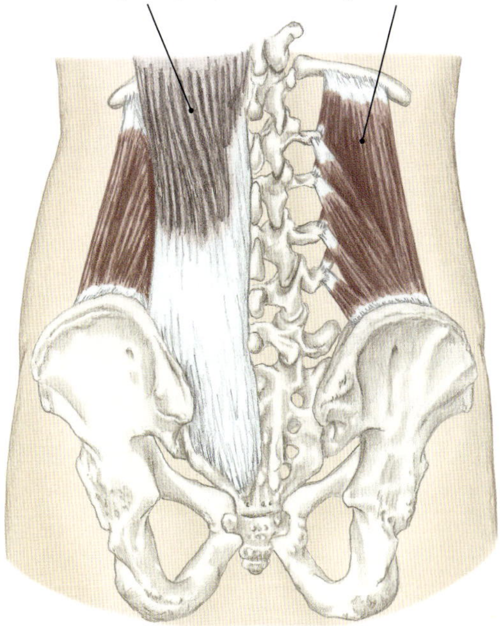

4.101 Posterior view of thorax with erector spinae group removed on right side, showing quadratus lumborum

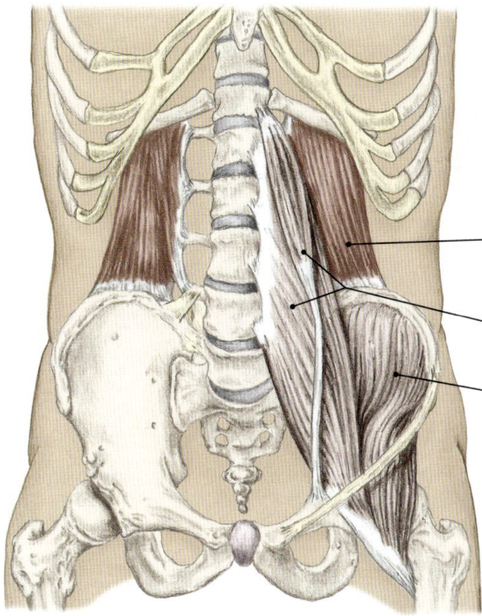

4.102 Anterior view of thorax, showing quadratus lumborum (highlighted in dark red)

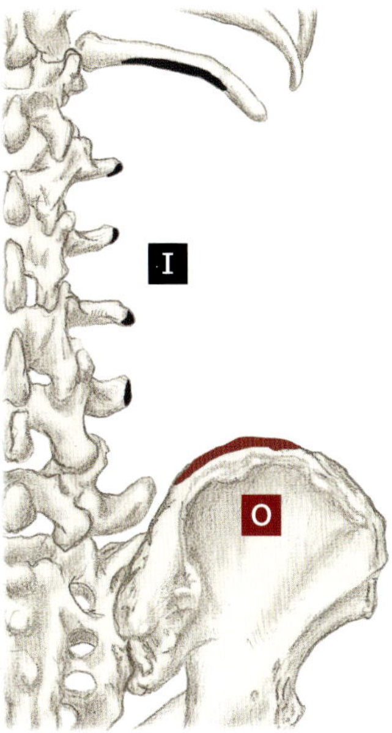

4.103 Posterior view of thorax, showing origin and insertion of quadratus lumborum

The quadratus lumborum is sometimes known as the "hip hiker" because of its capacity to laterally tilt (elevate) the hip.

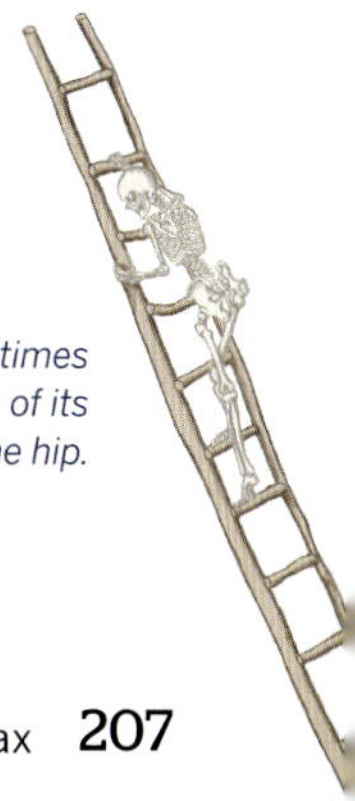

quadratus lumborum *kwod*-rait-us lum-***bor***-um L. four-sided muscle of the lumbar region

Quadratus lumborum

1. Patrner prone. Isolate the borders of the quadratus by locating the twelfth rib, posterior iliac crest, and transverse processes of the lumbar vertebrae.
2. Lay your fingers along these landmarks to outline the edges of the quadratus (**4.104**).
3. Lay your thumbpad along the lateral edge of this square. Using slow, firm pressure, sink your thumb medially toward the lumbar vertebrae and into the edge of the quadratus (**4.105**).
4. Ask your partner to laterally tilt (elevate) his hip toward his shoulder in order to feel its solid contraction. The hip should remain on the table.

As you palpate, be sure you are accessing the deeper tissue in the low back and not just the superficial external oblique fibers. When your partner hikes his hip, can you feel the lateral edge of the quadratus contract? Can you distinguish between the edge of the erector spinae and the quadratus?

Follow the above instructions, only this time with your partner side lying (**4.106**). Placing a bolster between his knees will balance the pelvis and soften the tissue around the quadratus. This position will also allow the abdominal contents to shift away from where you are accessing.

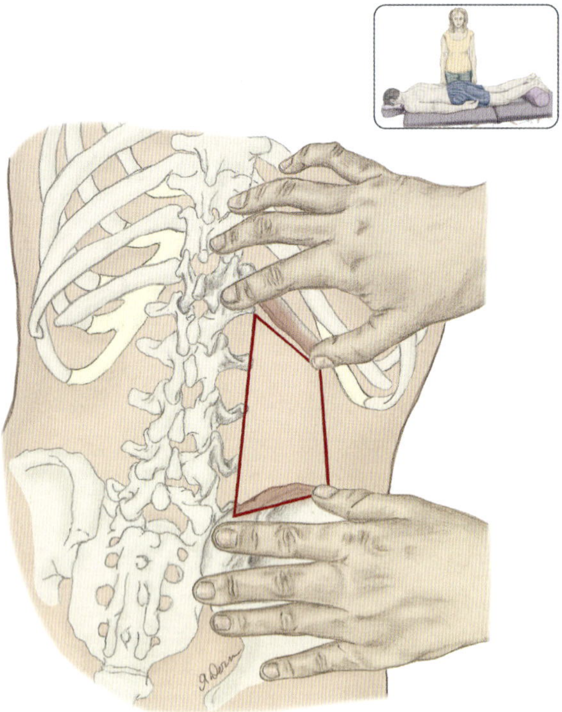

4.104 Partner prone, as you lay your fingers along the corners of the quadratus lumborum

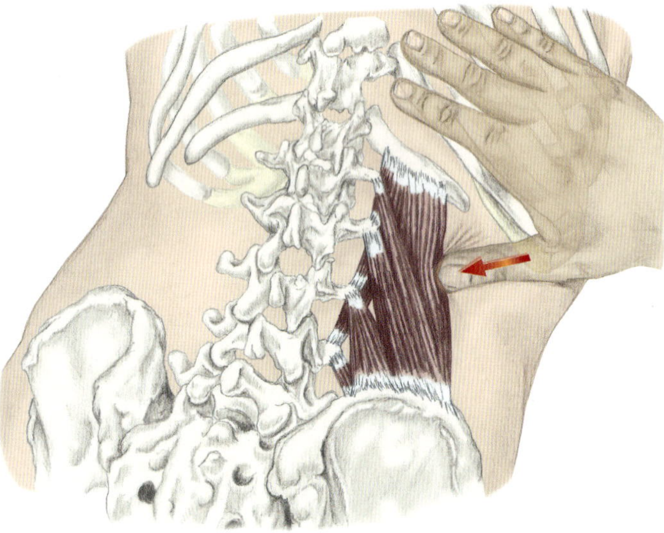

4.105 Partner prone, as you access the quadratus lumborum

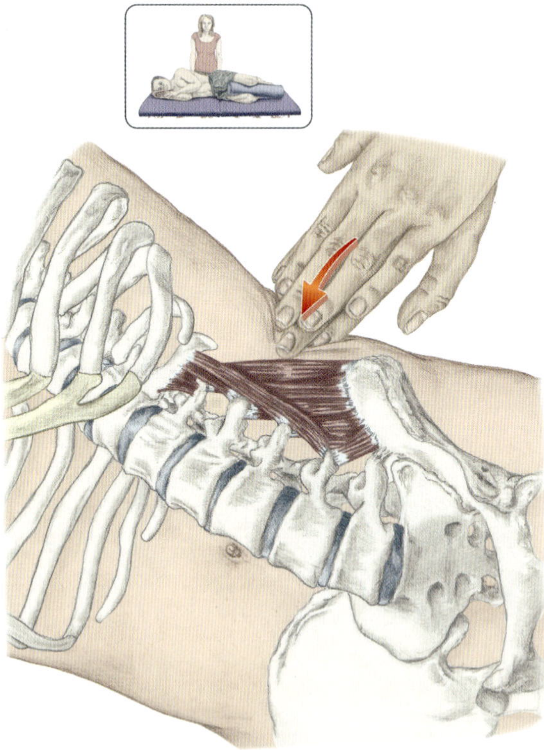

4.106 Partner side lying, anterior/lateral view of thorax, as you palpate the quadratus lumborum

Abdominals ▸

Rectus Abdominis
External Oblique
Internal Oblique
Transverse Abdominis

The four abdominal muscles expand far beyond the stomach region. In fact, they form a muscular girdle that reaches around the sides of the thorax to the thoracolumbar fascia, superiorly to the middle ribs and inferiorly to the inguinal ligament (**4.107**). The immense span of these muscles, with its unique overlapping arrangement and varying fiber direction, helps to stabilize the entire abdominal region.

The revered "washboard belly" is formed by the multiple, superficial bellies of the **rectus abdominis** (**4.108**, **4.109**). Lateral to the rectus abdominis is the **external oblique** (**4.110**, **4.111**). Unlike the round bellies of the rectus abdominis, the external oblique is a broad, superficial muscle, best palpated at its attachments to the lower ribs.

The thin **internal oblique** fibers are deep and perpendicular to the external oblique fibers and can be difficult to distinguish (**4.112**, **4.113**). The **transverse abdominis**, the deepest muscle of the group, plays a major role in forced exhalation. It cannot be specifically palpated (**4.114**, **4.115**).

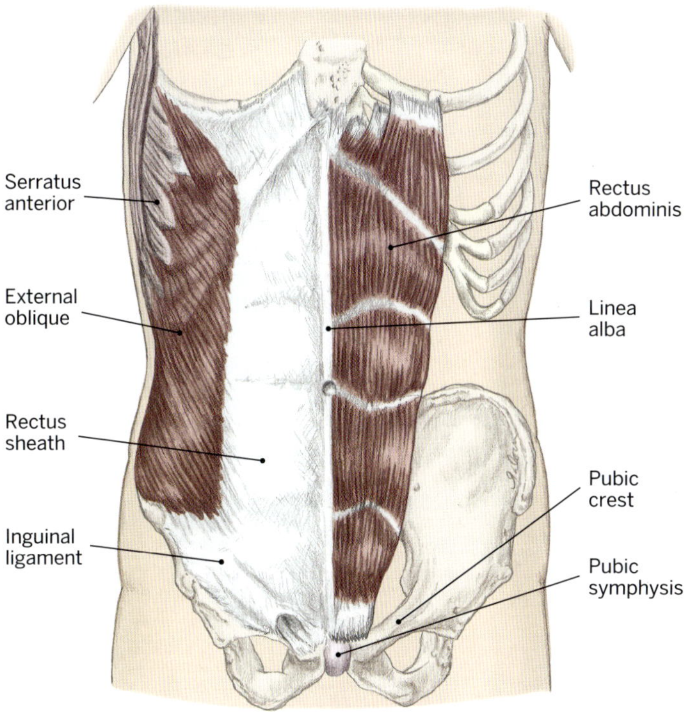

4.107 Anterior view of thorax

Spine & Thorax

Discover More

The organs of the upper thorax are protected by the rib cage, while the viscera of the lower thorax rely on the four abdominal muscles for support and protection. The four abdominal muscles wrap the entire abdomen in vertical, horizontal, and diagonal directions, in the same way packing tape is wrapped around a box going for a long journey.

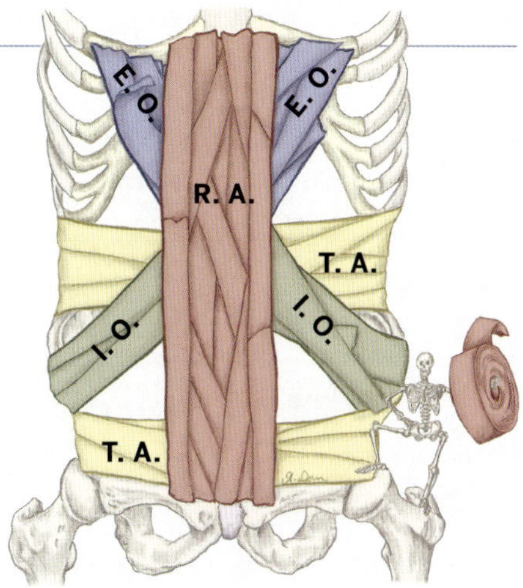

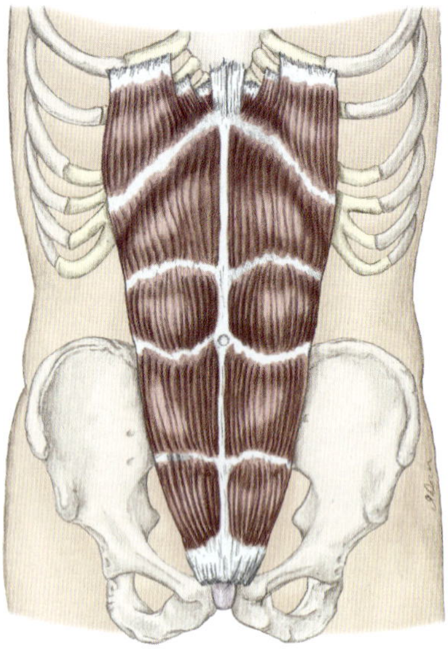

4.108 Anterior view of thorax, showing rectus abdominis

RECTUS ABDOMINIS

A **Flex** the vertebral column
Tilt pelvis posteriorly

O Pubic crest, pubic symphysis

I Cartilage of fifth, sixth, and seventh ribs and xiphoid process

N T5, 6, T**7–11**, T12, ventral rami

When Do You Use Your Rectus Abdominis?

- A sit-up (flexion)
- Belly dancing
- A Navy SEAL sit-up (flexion with rotation)

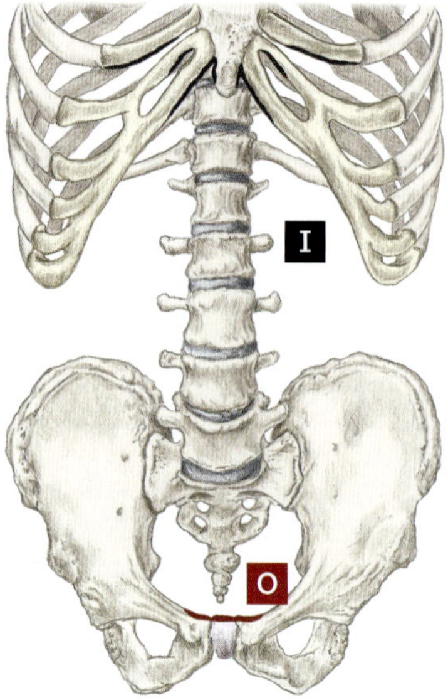

4.109 Anterior view of thorax, showing origin and insertion of rectus abdominis

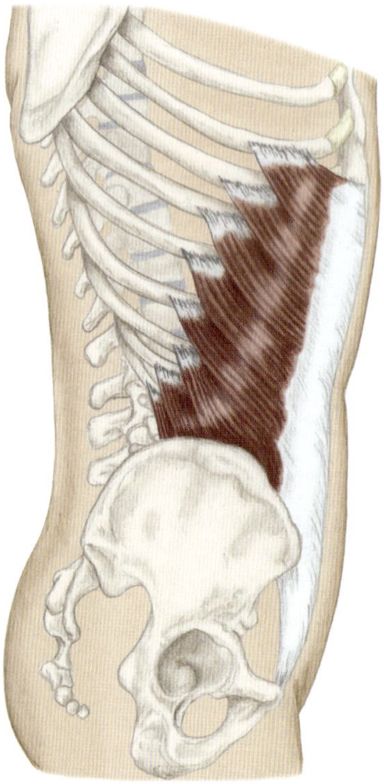

4.110 Lateral view of thorax, showing external oblique

EXTERNAL OBLIQUE

A *Unilaterally:*
Laterally flex vertebral column to the same side
Rotate vertebral column to the opposite side
Bilaterally:
Flex the vertebral column
Compress abdominal contents

O External surfaces of fifth to twelfth ribs

I Anterior part of the iliac crest, rectus sheath to linea alba

N (T5, 6), T**7–11**, T12

When Do You Use Your External Oblique?

- Sitting up in bed and reaching over for the alarm clock (flexion, rotation)
- Coughing, vomiting, defecating (hopefully not at the same time)

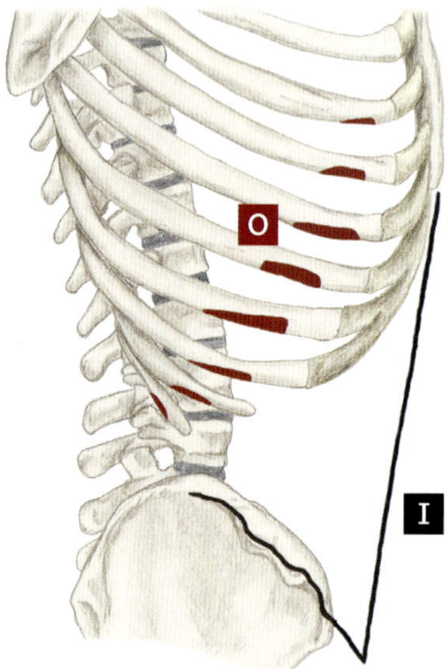

4.111 Lateral view of thorax, showing origin and insertion of external oblique

oblique	o-***bleek***	L. diagonal, slanting
rectus	***rek***-tus	L. straight

Spine & Thorax

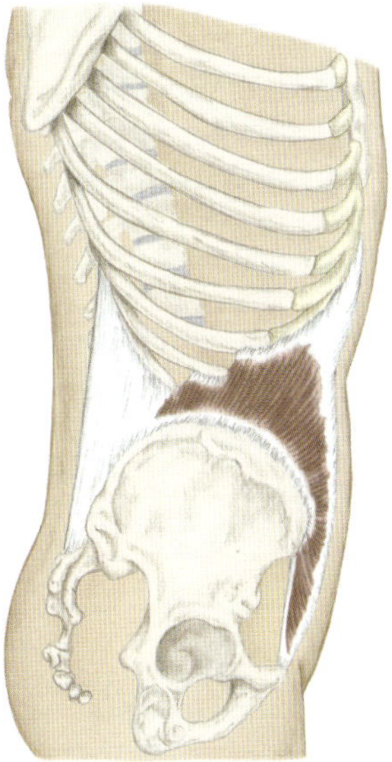

4.112 Lateral view of thorax, showing internal oblique

INTERNAL OBLIQUE

A *Unilaterally:*
Laterally flex vertebral column to the same side
Rotate vertebral column to the same side
Bilaterally:
Flex the vertebral column
Compress abdominal contents

O Lateral inguinal ligament, iliac crest, and thoracolumbar fascia

I Internal surface of lower three ribs, rectus sheath to linea alba

N T7, 8, **T9–12**, **L1**, iliohypogastric and ilioinguinal, ventral rami

When Do You Use Your Internal Oblique?

- A Navy SEAL sit-up (flexion with rotation)
- Sitting up in bed and reaching over for the alarm clock (flexion, rotation)

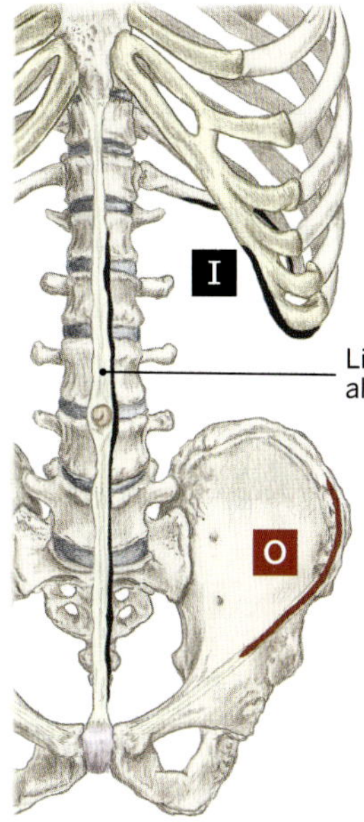

4.113 Anterior view of thorax, showing origin and insertion of internal oblique

TRANSVERSE ABDOMINIS

A **Compress** abdominal contents

O Lateral inguinal ligament, iliac crest, thoracolumbar fascia, and internal surface of lower six ribs

I Rectus sheath to linea alba

N T**7-12**, L**1**, iliohypogastric and ilioinguinal, ventral divisions

When Do You Use Your Transverse Abdominis?

- A sit-up (flexion)
- Coughing, vomiting, defecating (hopefully not at the same time)

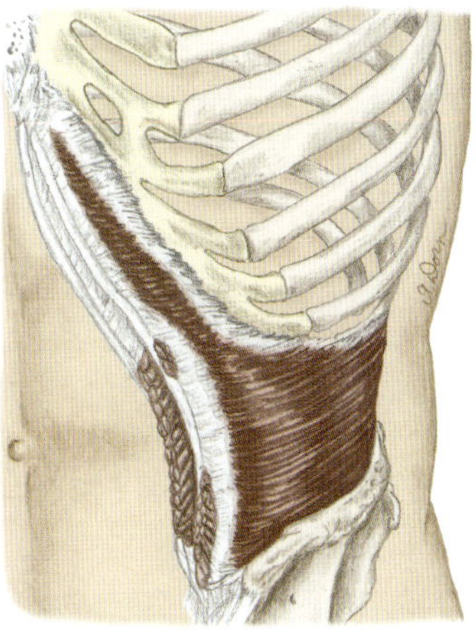

4.114 Anterior view of thorax, showing transverse abdominis (both obliques cut and reflected)

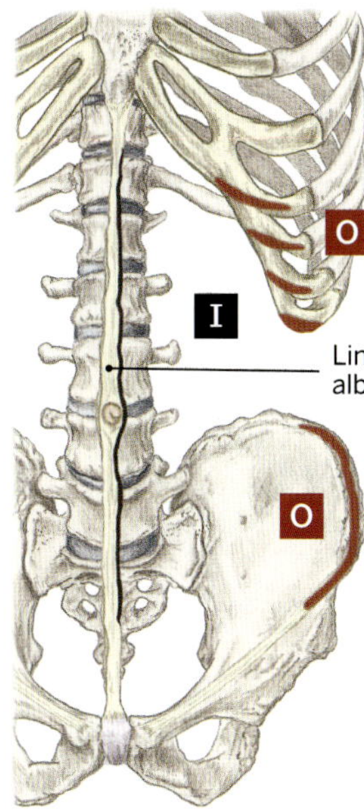

4.115 Anterior view of thorax, showing origin and insertion of transverse abdominis

Discover More

Pyramidalis

Located superficial to the rectus abdominis, this small muscle is absent in roughly 20% of the population.

A **Tenses** the linea alba

O Pubic symphysis

I Linea alba

N Twelfth thoracic nerve

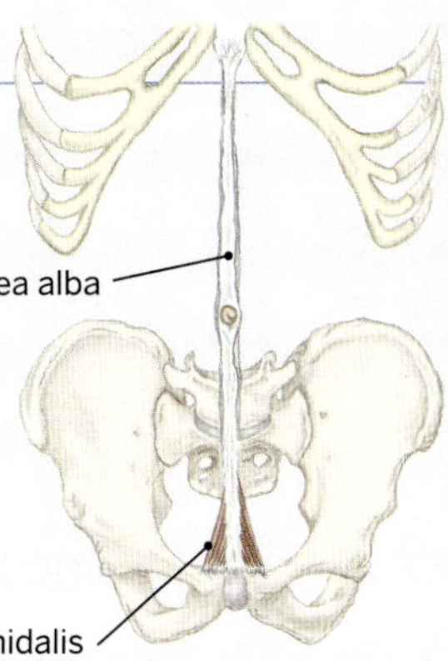

Spine & Thorax

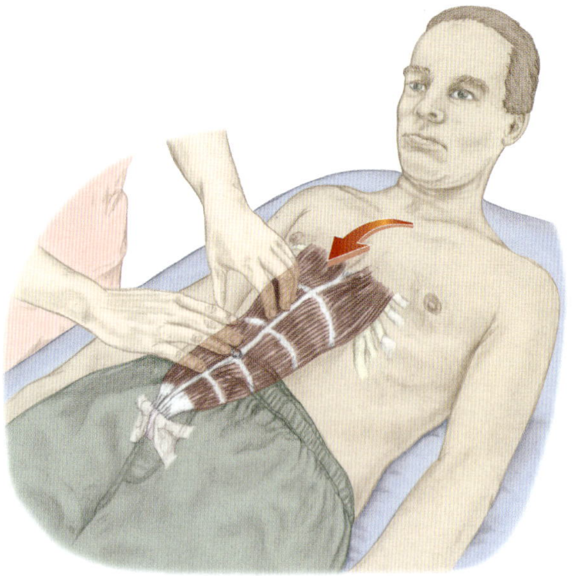

4.116 Partner supine with knees flexed, flexing his trunk while you palpate rectus abdominis

Rectus abdominis

1. Partner supine with knees flexed. Locate the xiphoid process and the ribs just lateral to the xiphoid. Also locate the pubic crest (p. 295).
2. Place your hand between these landmarks and ask your partner to alternately flex and relax his trunk slightly. "Do a small sit-up."
3. Explore the entire length of the rectus and sculpt between its rectangular muscle bellies (**4.116**).

As your partner flexes his trunk, can you palpate the lateral edges of the rectus abdominis?

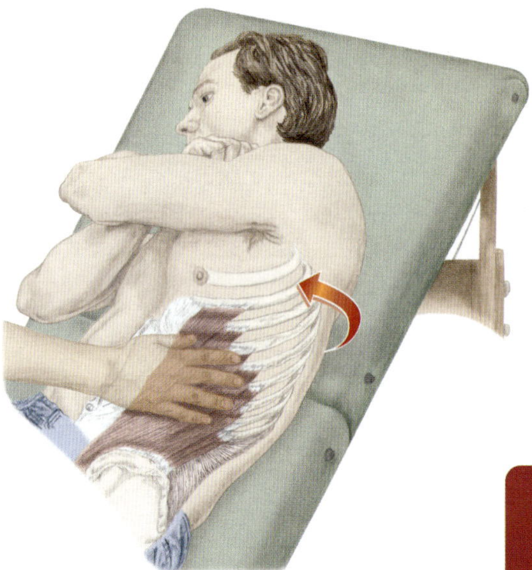

4.117 Partner supine with knees flexed, rotating his trunk toward the opposite side while you access the external oblique

External oblique (left side)

1. Partner supine with his knees flexed. Lay your hand on the left side of the abdomen and lower ribs. Ask your partner to raise his left shoulder toward his right hip (rotating his trunk).
2. Palpate across the superficial fibers of the external oblique, noting their diagonal direction (**4.117**).
3. With the trunk still rotated, follow the fibers superiorly to where they interdigitate with the serratus anterior, then inferiorly to the rectus sheath and, finally, laterally to the iliac crest.

Are you palpating lateral to the edge of rectus abdominis? Are the fibers superficial and running at an angle? Palpate lateral to the rectus abdominis with the abdomen relaxed. Can you distinguish between the fibers of the external oblique and the deeper internal oblique? Their fibers should be virtually perpendicular to each other.

Palpation Plus

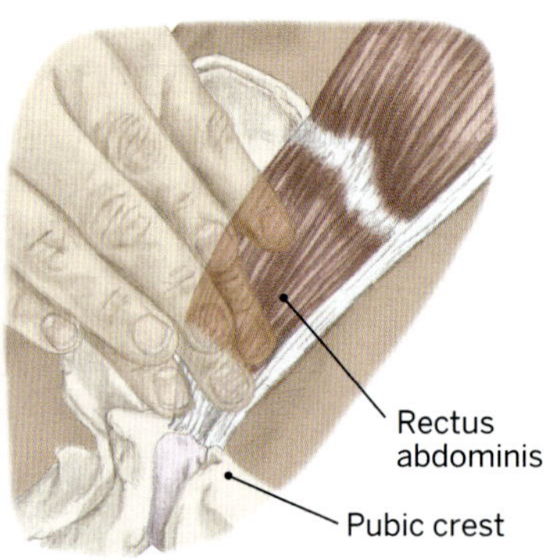

Palpating the inferior attachment of the rectus abdominis requires locating the pubic crest. (See p. 295 for instructions.) Explore the inferior rectus by first locating your partner's umbilicus. As he does a small sit-up, follow the narrowing muscle bellies to the pubic crest. At their insertion site, they are surprisingly slender, perhaps only three inches wide.

interdigitate *in*-ter-*dij*-i-tate L. to interlock, as the fingers of clasped hands

Diaphragm ▶

The diaphragm is the primary muscle of respiration and is unique in both its design and function. Its broad, umbrellalike shape separates the upper and lower thoracic cavities (**4.118**). The diaphragm's muscle fibers attach to the inner surface of the ribs and the lumbar vertebrae and converge at the central tendon (**4.119**).

The diaphragm creates inspiration (inhalation) when its muscle fibers contract and pull the central tendon inferiorly. Because the central tendon is attached to the connective tissue that surrounds the lungs, a vacuum is created in the upper thoracic cavity, pulling air into the lungs. On exhalation, the muscle fibers of the diaphragm relax, releasing the central tendon and allowing the lungs to deflate.

Although only a small portion of the diaphragm is accessible, the muscle's effect on the thorax and breathing is easily felt.

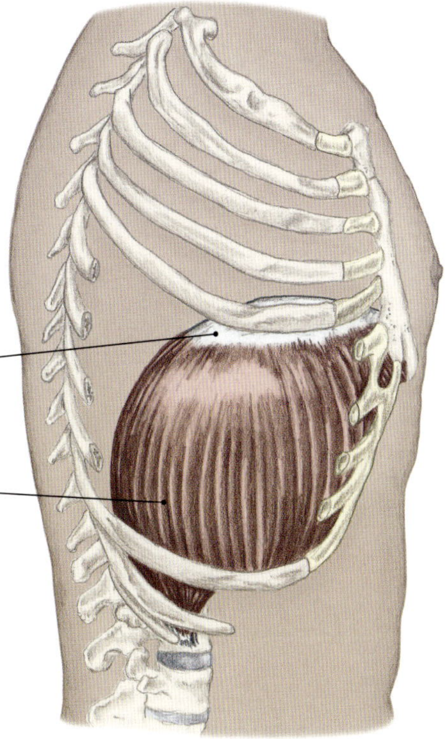

4.118 Lateral view of thorax, showing diaphragm in position of exhalation

DIAPHRAGM	
A	**Draw down** the central tendon of the diaphragm **Increase the volume** of the thoracic cavity during inhalation
O	***Costal attachment:*** Inner surface of lower six ribs ***Lumbar attachment:*** Upper two or three lumbar vertebrae ***Sternal attachment:*** Inner part of xiphoid process
I	Central tendon
N	Phrenic C3, **4**, 5

When Do You Use Your Diaphragm?

- While singing at the Metropolitan Opera
- Blowing up a balloon

Discover More

An involuntary contraction of the diaphragm will cause air to rush into the lungs and the vocal cords to snap shut. The audible result is a hiccup.

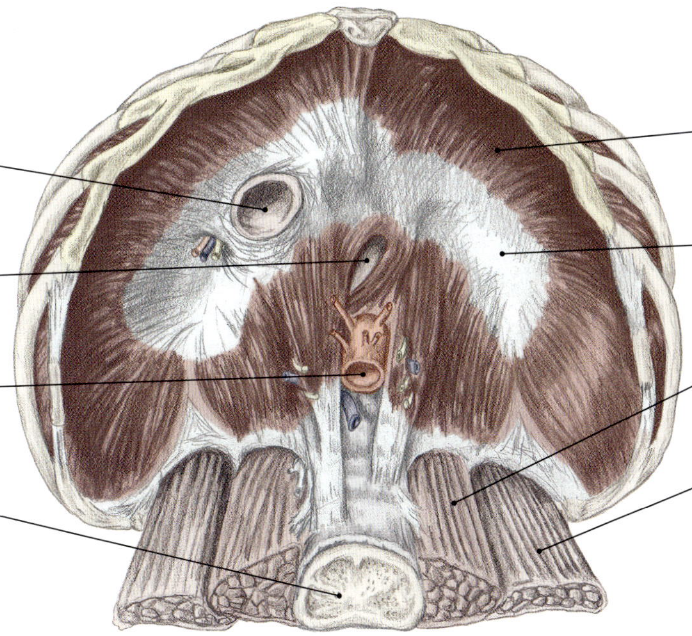

4.119 Inferior view of the diaphragm

diaphragm *di-a-fram* Grk. a partition, wall

Move slowly, communicating with your partner as you palpate. If, at any time, he does not feel safe or comfortable, gently remove your hands.

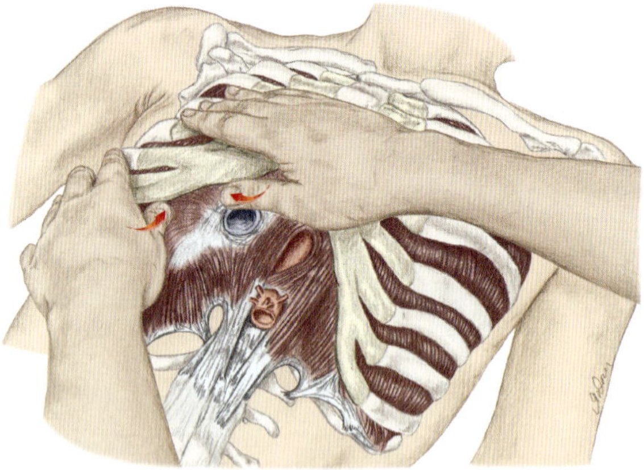

4.120 Partner supine, as you palpate the diaphragm

Diaphragm

1. Partner supine, with knees bolstered. Locate the inferior edge of the rib cage, lateral to the xiphoid process.
2. Lay your thumbpads just inferior to the ribs on the abdomen and ask your partner to take slow, deep breaths.
3. Moving only as your partner exhales, slowly press and curl your thumbpads underneath the edge of the ribs (**4.120**). During inhalation, you may not feel the tissue of the diaphragm, but you will most likely feel its contraction as it pushes other tissues into your thumbpads.

Are your thumbs curling under the ribs rather than sinking into the abdominal organs? Ask your partner to breathe into his belly and notice how the abdominal region expands as the diaphragm contracts.

Try the above procedure with your partner side lying and his trunk flexed slightly. This position will allow the abdominal contents to shift away from where you are accessing (**4.121**).

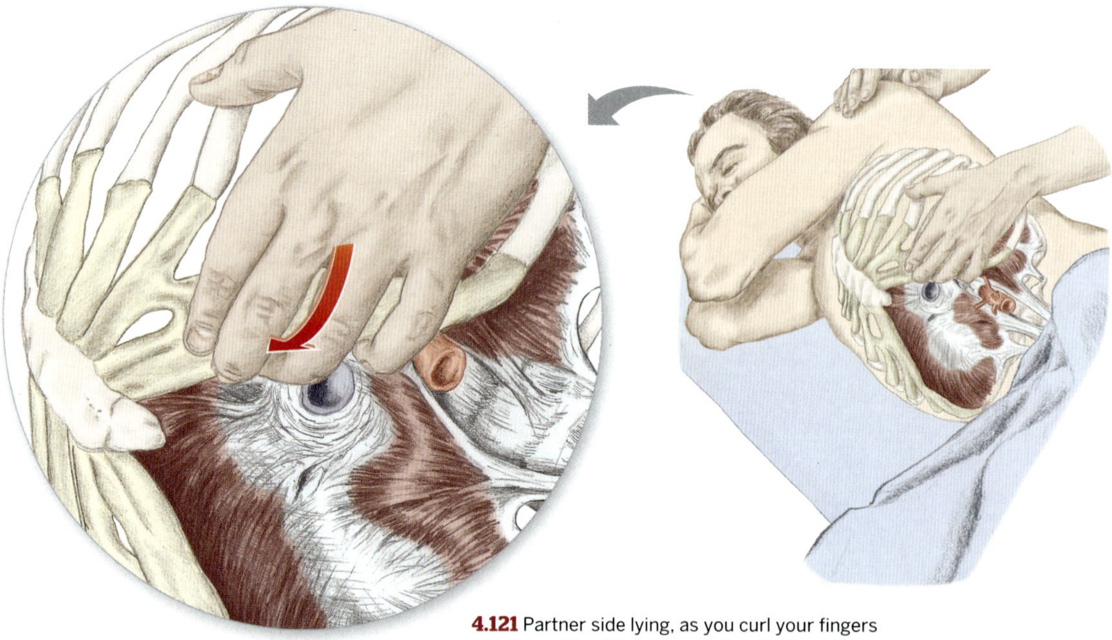

4.121 Partner side lying, as you curl your fingers around the ribs to access the diaphragm

Discover More

The heart is directly affected by the motion of the diaphragm. As the heart's fibrous pericardium is attached to the diaphragm's central tendon by ligaments, the heart literally rides up and down on the diaphragm as you breathe. The yogis were right—breathing can massage the heart!

Intercostals ▶

Better known to carnivores as the meat on spare ribs, the intercostals are the small, slender muscles between the ribs. They are divided into two groups: the external and the internal intercostals (**4.122**). The fibers of these two groups run perpendicular to each other and can be visualized as extensions of the external and internal oblique muscles (pp. 210, 211).

The intercostals help to stabilize the rib cage and assist in respiration, but their specific role is debatable. Although the entire rib cage lies deep to one or more layers of muscle, portions of the intercostals remain easily accessible. It is not possible, however, to distinguish the external intercostals from the internal intercostals.

Since the ribs and the spaces between them can be sensitive areas to access, use slow, firm hand movements.

	INTERCOSTALS
A	***External intercostals:*** Draw the ribs superiorly (increasing the space of the thoracic cavity) to assist with **inhalation** ***Internal intercostals:*** Draw the ribs inferiorly (decreasing the space of the thoracic cavity) to assist with **exhalation**
O	Inferior border of the rib above
I	Superior border of the rib below
N	Thoracic

When Do You Use Your Intercostals?

- Deep breathing during meditation
- During a triathlon—swimming, biking, running

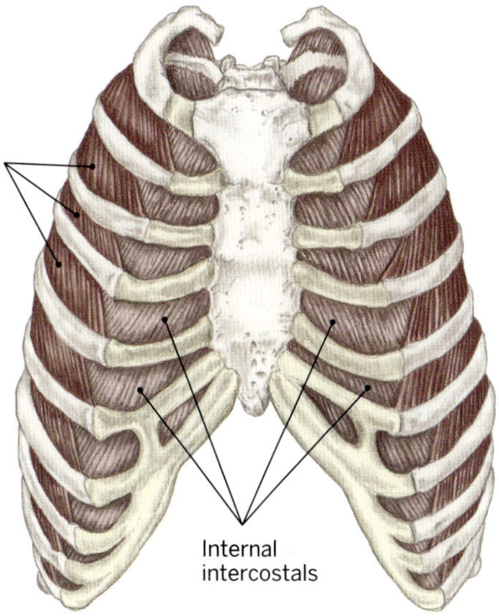

4.122 Anterior view of rib cage, showing intercostals

Spine & Thorax

Intercostals

1. Partner supine. Begin just inferior to the pectoralis major on the side of the rib cage. Working across the body, position your fingers in the spaces between the ribs.
2. With one fingerpad, isolate and palpate the tissue between two ribs. Roll your finger along the rib space and palpate the short, dense intercostals that bridge the ribs (**4.123**).
3. Ask your partner to take several slow, deep breaths. Note any expansion or collapse in the spaces between the ribs. Then turn your partner prone or side lying and continue to explore the intercostals.

Are you between the ribs or just on the surface? Can you roll your fingers across the small intercostal fibers? Can you sink your fingers through the pectoralis major, latissimus dorsi, or external oblique to isolate the intercostals?

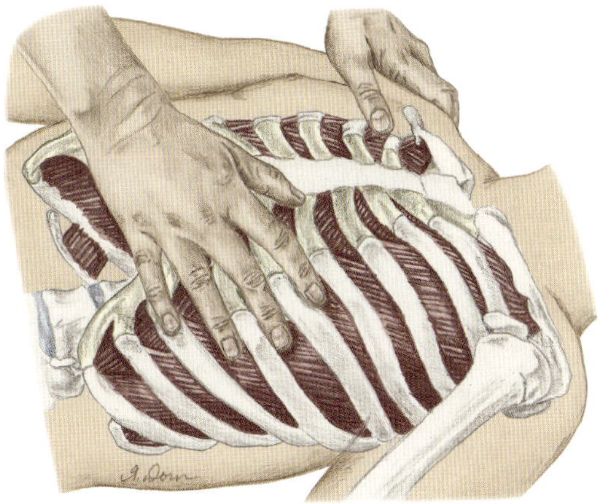

4.123 Partner supine, as you palpate the intercostals

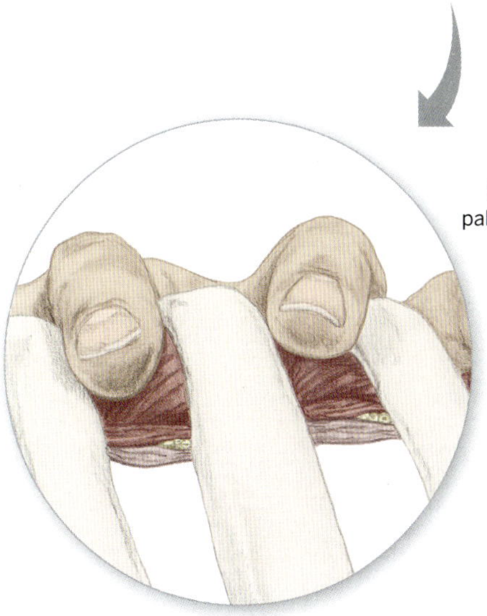

Cross section of palpating intercostals

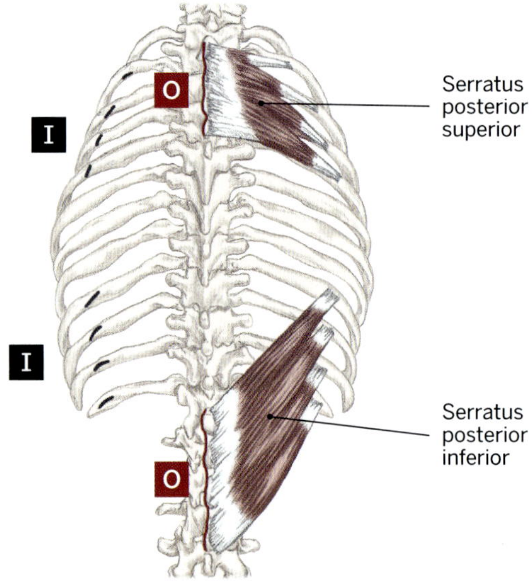

4.124 Posterior view of thorax, showing serratus posterior superior and inferior, with origins and insertions shown on left side

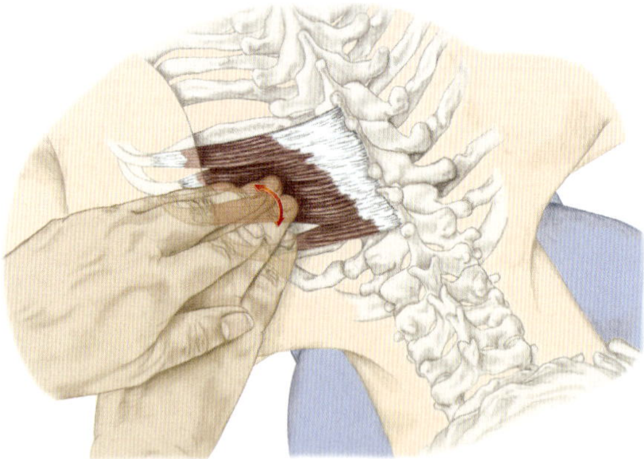

4.125 Partner prone, as you palpate serratus posterior superior

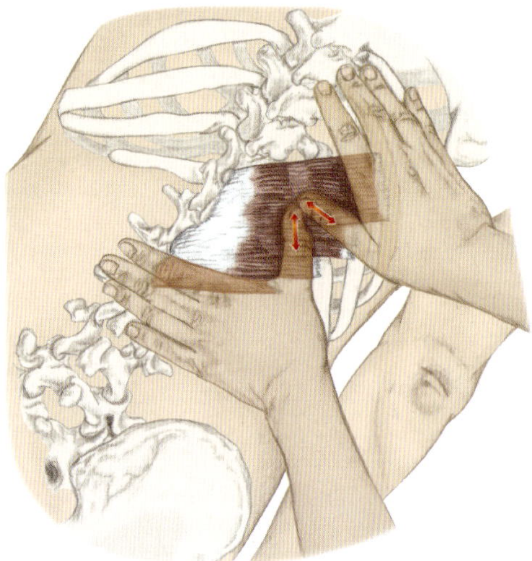

4.126 Partner prone, as you palpate serratus posterior inferior

Serratus Posterior Superior
Serratus Posterior Inferior

Although they are sandwiched between the shoulder muscles and the erector spinae group, these two broad muscles only affect movement of the ribs (**4.124**). The belly of the **superior** is partially deep to the scapula and has fibers that parallel the superficial rhomboids. The **inferior** is deep to the thoracolumbar fascia (p. 220) and, during exhalation, can stabilize the ribs against the pull of the diaphragm.

Both muscles are superficial enough to be accessed, but due to their thin, tendonous bellies, discerning them is a different story.

SERRATUS POSTERIOR SUPERIOR

A	**Elevate** the ribs during inhalation
O	Spinous processes of C-7 to T-3
I	Posterior surface of second through fifth ribs
N	T1, 2, 3, 4

When Do You Use Your Serratus Posterior Superior?

- Respiration
- Stabilizing your rib cage in preparation for a deep breath

SERRATUS POSTERIOR INFERIOR

A	**Depress** the ribs during exhalation
O	Spinous processes of T-12 to L-3
I	Posterior surface of ninth through twelfth ribs
N	T9, 10, 11, (12)

When Do You Use Your Serratus Posterior Inferior?

- Respiration
- Stabilizing your rib cage in preparation for a deep breath

Serratus posterior superior/inferior

1. *Superior*: Partner prone. With the arm off the side of the table (pulling the scapula laterally), locate the upper portion of the medial border of the scapula.
2. Ask your partner to inhale as you sink your fingers deep to the rhomboid fibers (**4.125**). Although you may not feel the belly directly, explore this region for its fibers.
3. *Inferior*: Partner prone. Locate the bottom of the rib cage (eleventh or twelfth rib). Ask your partner to slowly exhale as you begin to roll your fingers across the muscle fibers (**4.126**).

For sandwiched muscles such as these, it can be worthwhile to first identify the muscles that are not the serrati. Then, with a patient and delicate touch, explore the "space between."

serratti plural of serratus

Intertransversarii

As their name suggests, these small, short muscles span between the transverse processes. They are the deepest muscles in the cervical and lumbar regions and, for this reason, are nearly impossible to detect, let alone access (**4.127**).

	INTERTRANSVERSARII
A	*Unilaterally:* **Laterally flex** the vertebral column to the same side *Bilaterally:* **Extend** the vertebral column
O	*Cervical:* Spanning the transverse processes of vertebrae C-2 to C-7
I	*Lumbar:* Spanning the transverse processes of vertebrae L-1 to L-5
N	Spinal

When Do You Use Your Intertransversarii?

- Stabilizing your upper and lower vertebrae through all movements of the spine

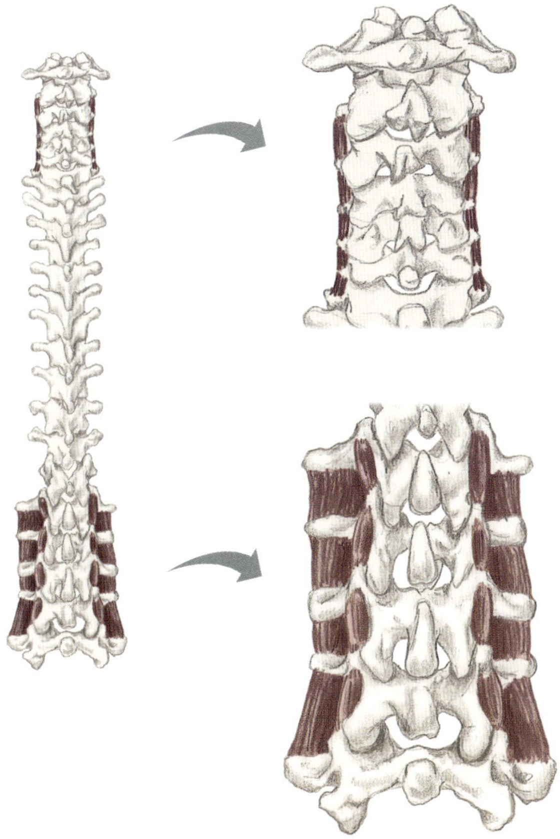

4.127 Posterior views of vertebral column, showing cervical and lumbar intertransversarii

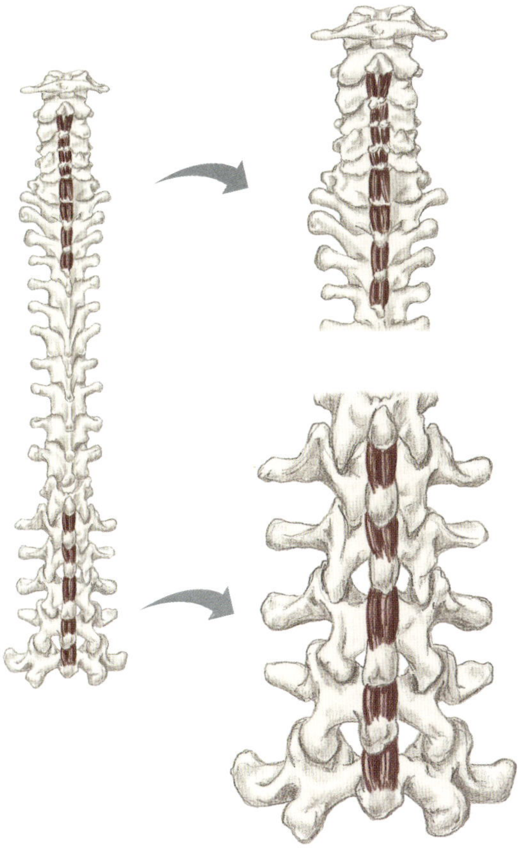

4.128 Posterior views of vertebral column, showing cervical and lumbar interspinalis

Interspinalis

Extending from the spinous processes in the cervical and lumbar regions, these short muscles help extend the spine. The cervical muscles are deep to the ligamentum nuchae, while the lumbar muscles are deep to the interspinous ligament (**4.128**). Like the intertransversarii, these muscles are too deep to isolate.

	INTERSPINALIS
A	**Extend** the vertebral column
O I	*Cervical:* Spanning the spinous processes of C-2 to T-3 *Lumbar:* Spanning the spinous processes of T-12 to L-5
N	Spinal

When Do You Use Your Interspinalis?

- Stabilizing your upper and lower vertebrae through all movements of the spine

intertransversarii *in*-ter-trans-***verse***-er-i
interspinalis *in*-ter-spi-***na***-lis

Ligaments and Other Structures of the Spine and Thorax

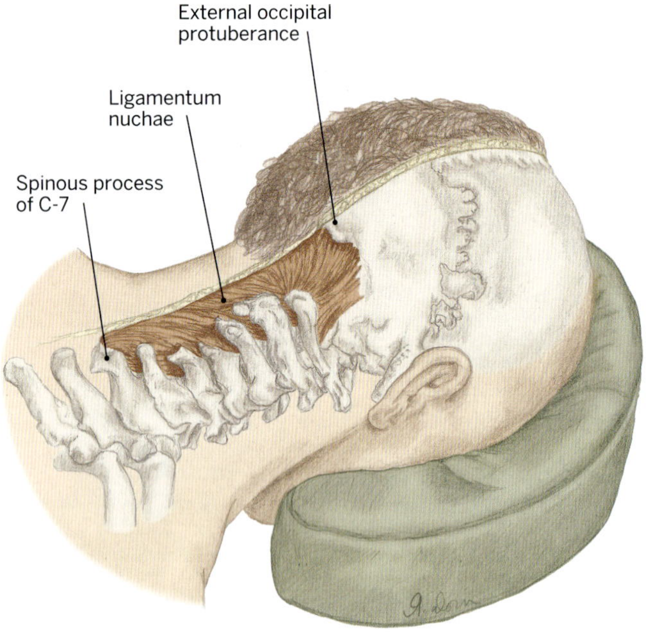

4.129 Posterior/lateral view of neck, with muscles and tissue removed from right side

Ligamentum Nuchae

The ligamentum nuchae is the finlike sheet of connective tissue that runs along the sagittal plane from the external occipital protuberance to the spinous process of C-7 in the neck (**4.129**).

The chief function of the ligamentum nuchae is to help stabilize the head and neck. It is also an attachment site for the superficial muscles of the posterior neck, such as the trapezius and splenius capitis. Since the cervical spinous processes do not extend far enough posteriorly for these superficial muscles to attach, they use the ligamentum nuchae instead.

For palpation purposes, the posterior edge of the ligamentum nuchae is superficial but can be difficult to discern from the surrounding muscle tissue.

Ligamentum nuchae

1. Partner supine. Locate the external occipital protuberance (p. 232) and the spinous process of C-7.
2. Palpate between these landmarks along the midline of the neck. Be sure you are superficial to the spinous processes. It might help to access the ligamentum nuchae if you roll your fingertips across its fiber direction and explore for what may feel like a flap of soft rubber (**4.130**).
3. Slowly and passively flex and extend the head, rolling your fingers across the fibers of the ligamentum nuchae. Note the changing degree of tension in the ligament as the head is moved.

Are you superficial to the spinous processes of the vertebrae as you palpate?

With your partner seated, ask him to flex his head and neck as far as he can comfortably. In this position, the ligamentum nuchae will stretch and rise to the surface. It should feel like a long, thin "speed bump" on the back of the neck.

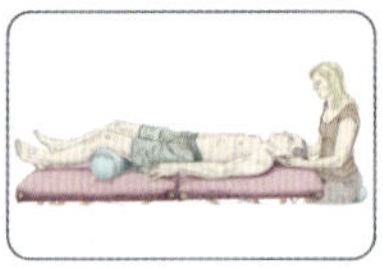

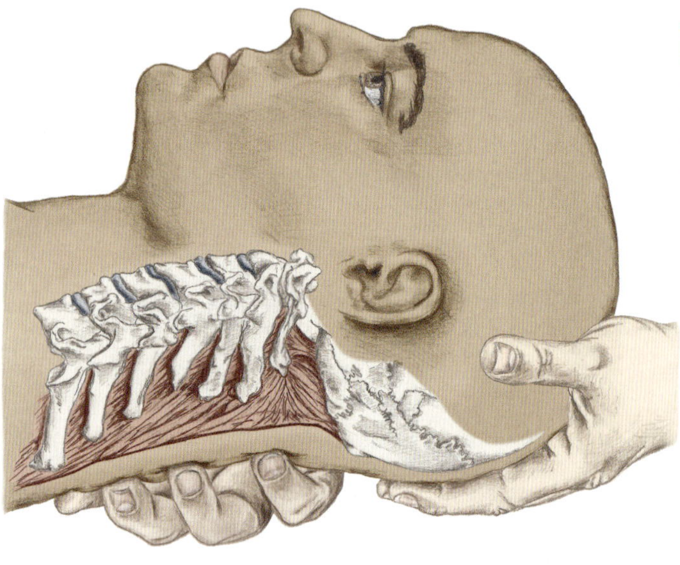

4.130 Partner supine, as you palpate the ligamentum nuchae

nuchae *nu*-kay L. nape of neck

Supraspinous Ligament

The long, thin supraspinous ligament extends inferiorly from the ligamentum nuchae. As it continues down the spine, it attaches to the spinous processes of the thoracic and lumbar vertebrae. It is superficial and easily accessed in the spaces between the spinous processes.

Supraspinous ligament

1. Partner prone. Locate several thoracic or lumbar spinous processes (**4.131**).
2. Palpate between the spinous processes. Feel the slender shape and vertical fiber direction of the ligament by rolling your fingertips across its surface.

With your partner seated, ask her to slowly flex and extend her spine. Can you feel any changes in the tension or prominence of the ligament as she moves it?

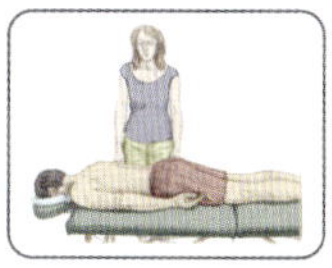

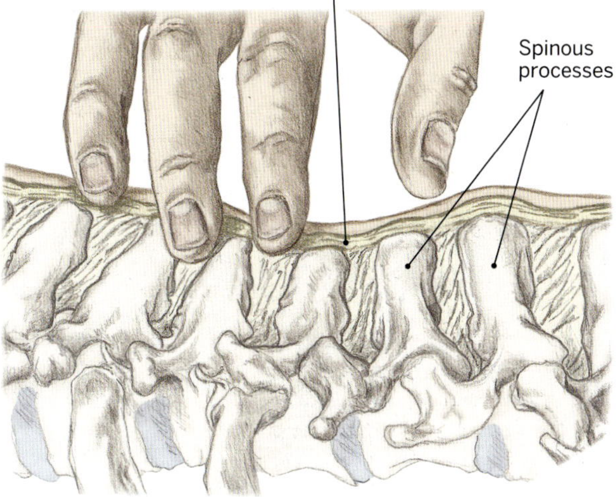

4.131 Partner prone, lateral view of the vertebrae, as you palpate the supraspinous ligament

Abdominal Aorta

Measuring nearly an inch in diameter, the abdominal aorta is the chief artery for carrying blood to the abdominal organs and lower appendages. It lies on the anterior surface of the vertebrae, deep to the small intestines. Lateral to the aorta is the psoas major (p. 334).

Abdominal aorta

1. Partner supine. Locate the umbilicus. Place your fingerpads two inches superior to the umbilicus.
2. Access the pulse of the abdominal aorta by slowly but firmly pressing straight down into the abdomen. Its strong pulse should be easily detectable (**4.132**).

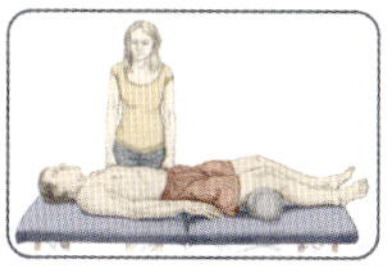

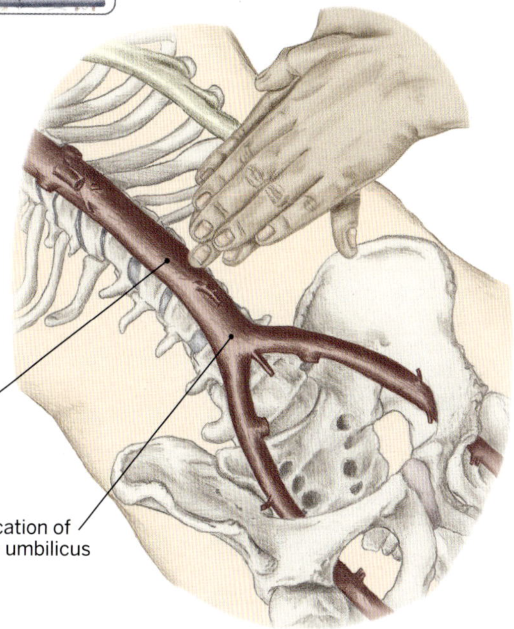

4.132 Partner supine, as you feel the pulse of the abdominal aorta

Comparative Anatomy

A horse's head and neck can weigh up to 300 pounds and require an enormous ligamentum nuchae. Because the head and neck are normally held in a resting posture without any muscular effort, the ligamentum nuchae is primarily an antigravity device. A small muscle contraction brings the head down to the ground, which in turn stretches the ligament. When the muscles relax, the ligament recoils, raising the head.

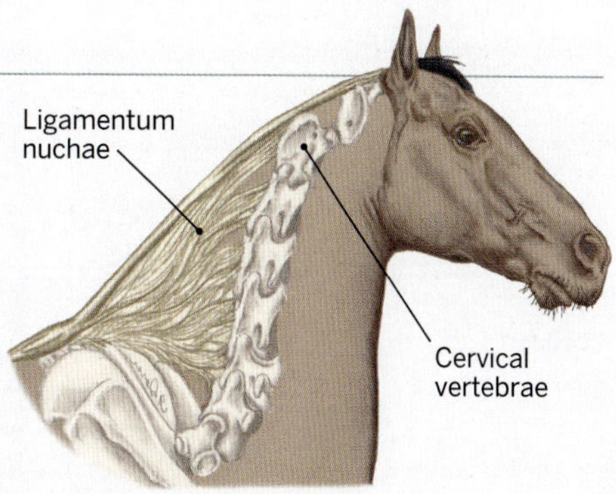

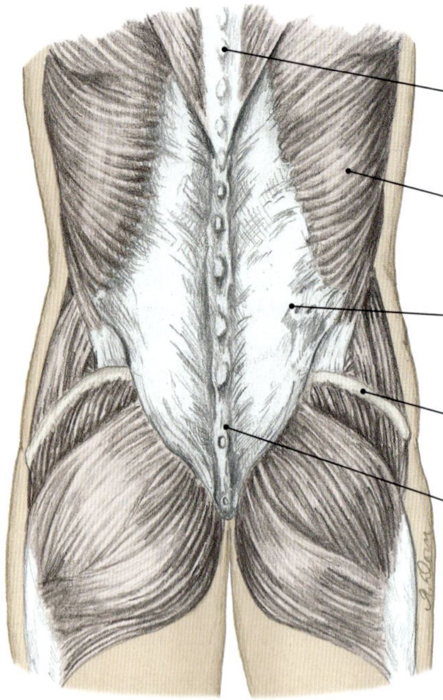

4.133 Posterior view of lower thorax and pelvis, showing thoracolumbar fascia

Thoracolumbar Fascia

Despite its formidable name, the thoracolumbar fascia is just what it says it is: a broad, flat, tendinous sheath stretching across the thorax and lumbar regions. More accurately, the thoracolumbar fascia is a thick, diamond-shaped tendon that lies superficially across the posterior thorax, stretches across the sacrum to the posterior iliac crest, and runs upward to the lower thoracic vertebrae (**4.133**).

The fascia is an anchor for several muscles in the thorax and hips, including the latissimus dorsi and the erector spinae group. It has a flat, dense texture that is difficult to distinguish from the deeper muscles.

Thoracolumbar fascia

1. Partner prone. Draw out the diamond shape of the fascia by locating the posterior iliac crest, the surface of the sacrum, and the lower thoracic vertebrae.
2. Using both hands, firmly grasp and lift the tissue of the low back. Note the thick layer of connective tissue underneath the skin but superficial to the erector spinae muscles. Do not be surprised if the fascia is so dense that you find it difficult to grasp, let alone lift.

*Ask your partner to alternately raise her elbows slightly and relax (this will contract the latissimus dorsi and tighten the fascia). Do you feel any change in the superficial tissue? Then move your hands laterally off the "diamond" and onto the latissimus dorsi muscle belly (**4.134**). Do you notice any textural differences between these two tissues?*

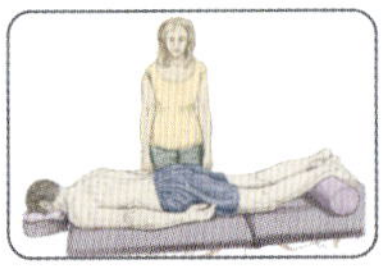

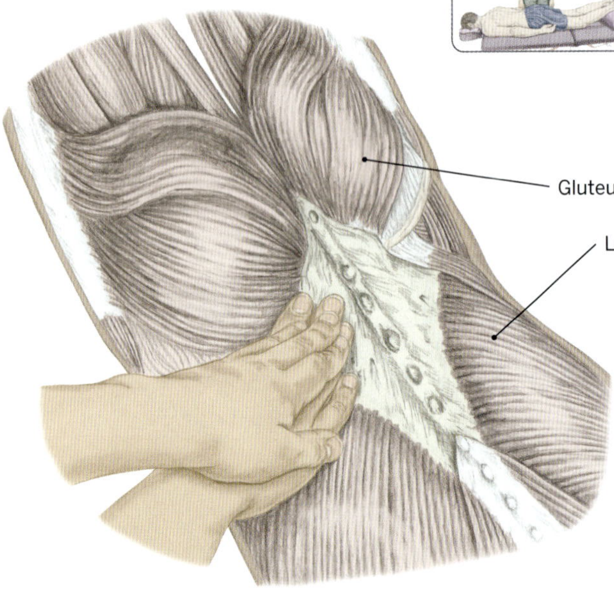

4.134 Partner prone, as you explore the fascia

Comparative Anatomy

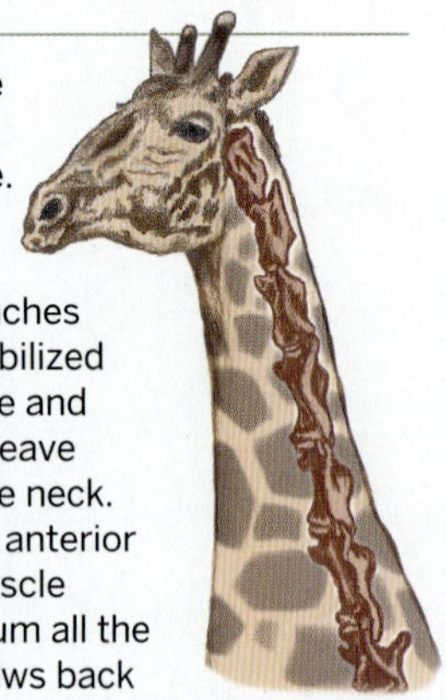

A giraffe's neck is more than five feet in length but nevertheless has just seven cervical vertebrae. The atlas and axis are relatively short, whereas the five cervical vertebrae can measure eleven inches each. The neck and head are stabilized by a massive ligamentum nuchae and an array of short muscles that weave along the posterior surface of the neck. The retractor muscle covers the anterior surface of the cervicals. This muscle extends from the giraffe's sternum all the way up to its hyoid bone and draws back the tongue.

thoracolumbar tho-***rak***-o-***lum***-bar

Craniovertebral Joints–Atlantooccipital and Atlantoaxial Joints

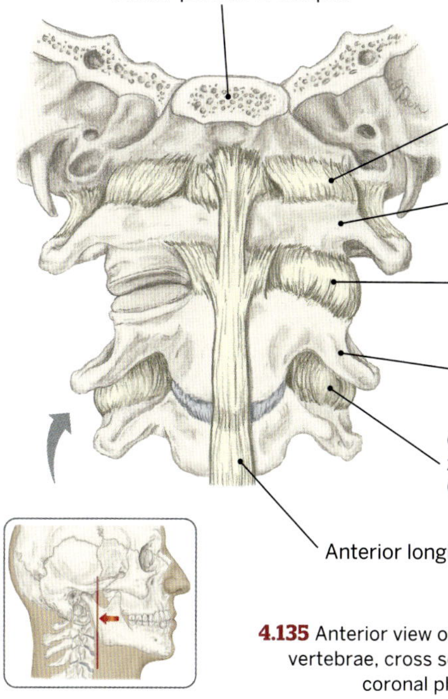

4.135 Anterior view of upper cervical vertebrae, cross section along coronal plane

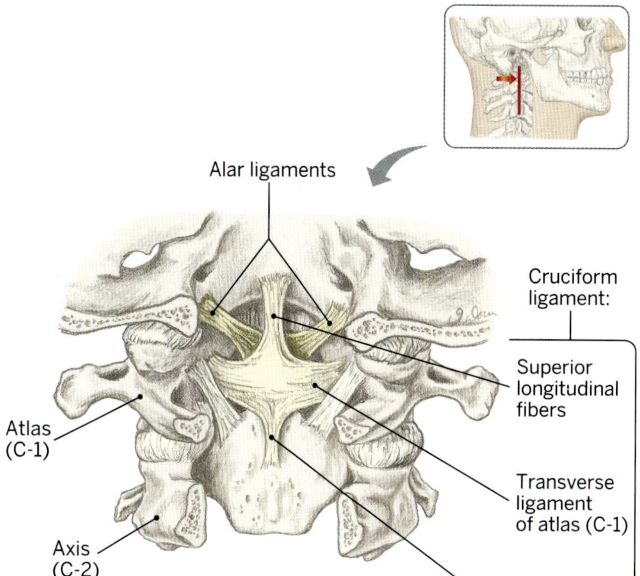

4.136 Posterior view of neck, showing axis, atlas, and occiput, with posterior portion of bones removed

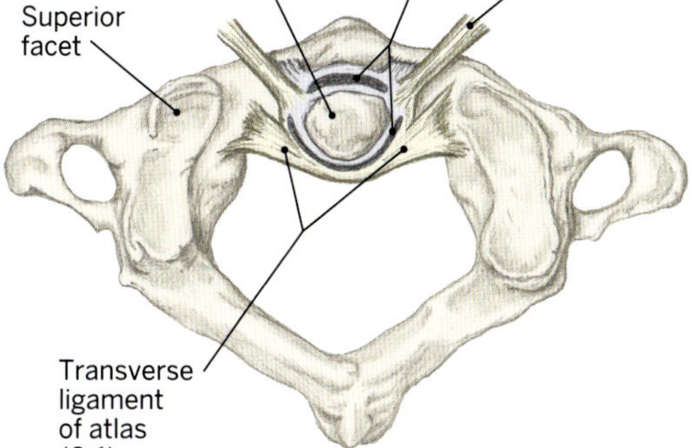

4.137 Superior view of atlas (C-1)

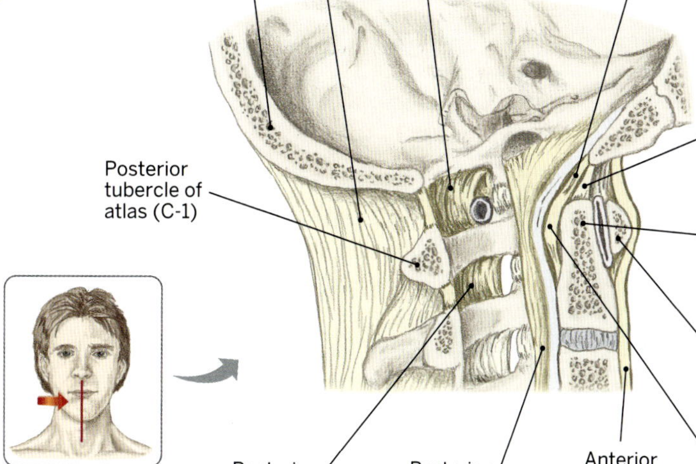

4.138 Lateral view of neck, cross section along the sagittal plane

alar	***ay**-lar*	**atlantoaxial**	at-***lan**-to-**ak**-se-al*
atlantooccipital	at-***lan**-to-ok-**si**-pi-tal*	**zygapophyseal**	***zy**-gah-**pof**-i-se-al*

Intervertebral Joints

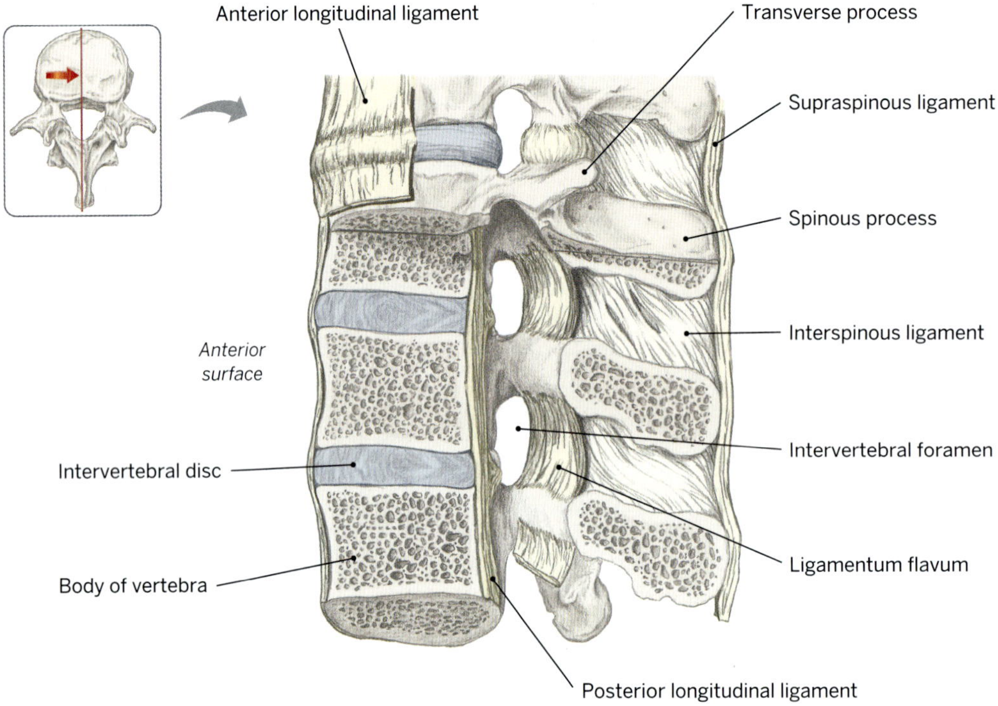

4.139 Lateral view of lumbar vertebrae, partially sectioned

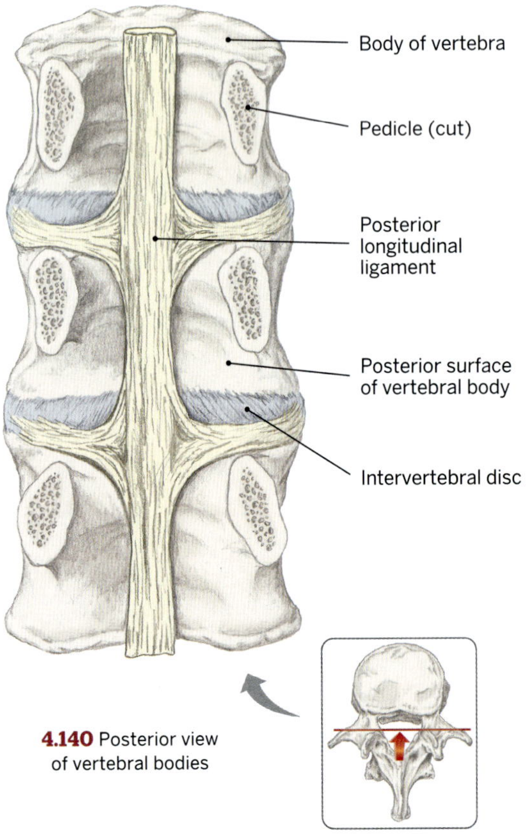

4.140 Posterior view of vertebral bodies

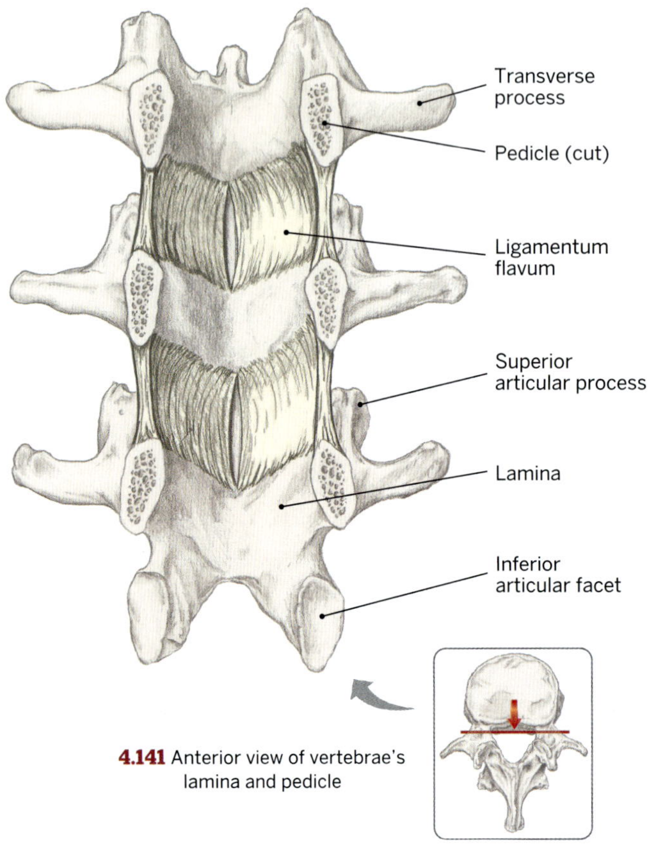

4.141 Anterior view of vertebrae's lamina and pedicle

flavum	***flay***-vum	L. yellow
pedicle	***ped***-i-k'l	L. a little foot

Costovertebral Joints

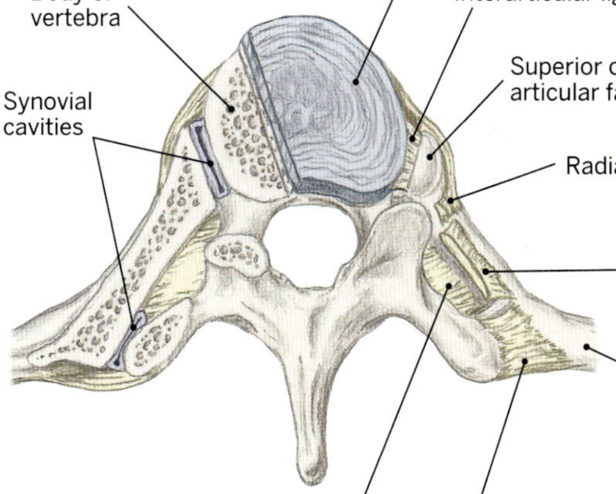

4.142 Superior view of thoracic vertebra, left side of illustration cut in cross section

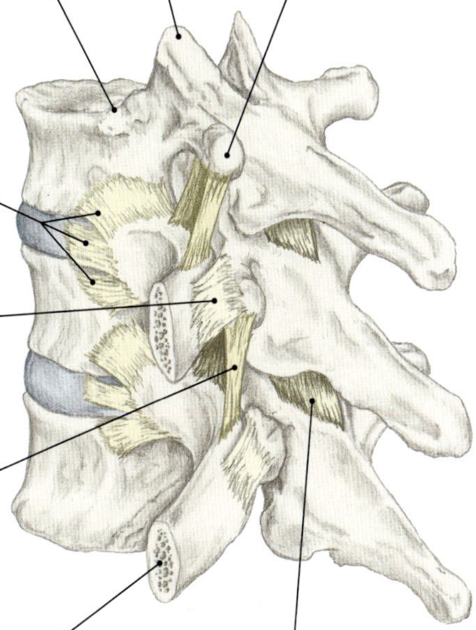

4.143 Lateral/posterior view of vertebrae

Sternocostal Joints

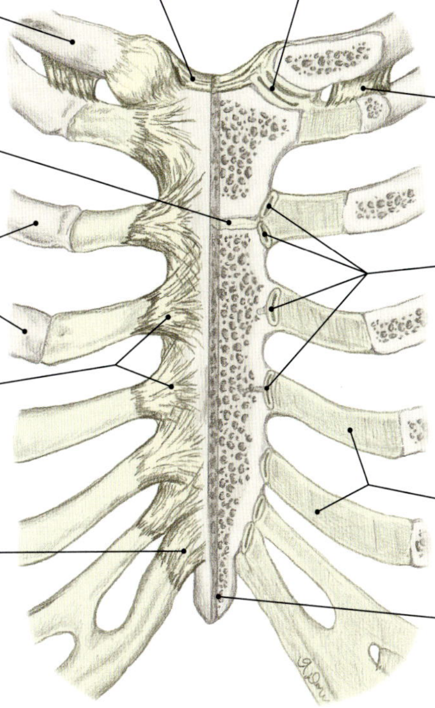

4.144 Anterior view of sternum and ribs, right side of illustration shown in coronal cross section

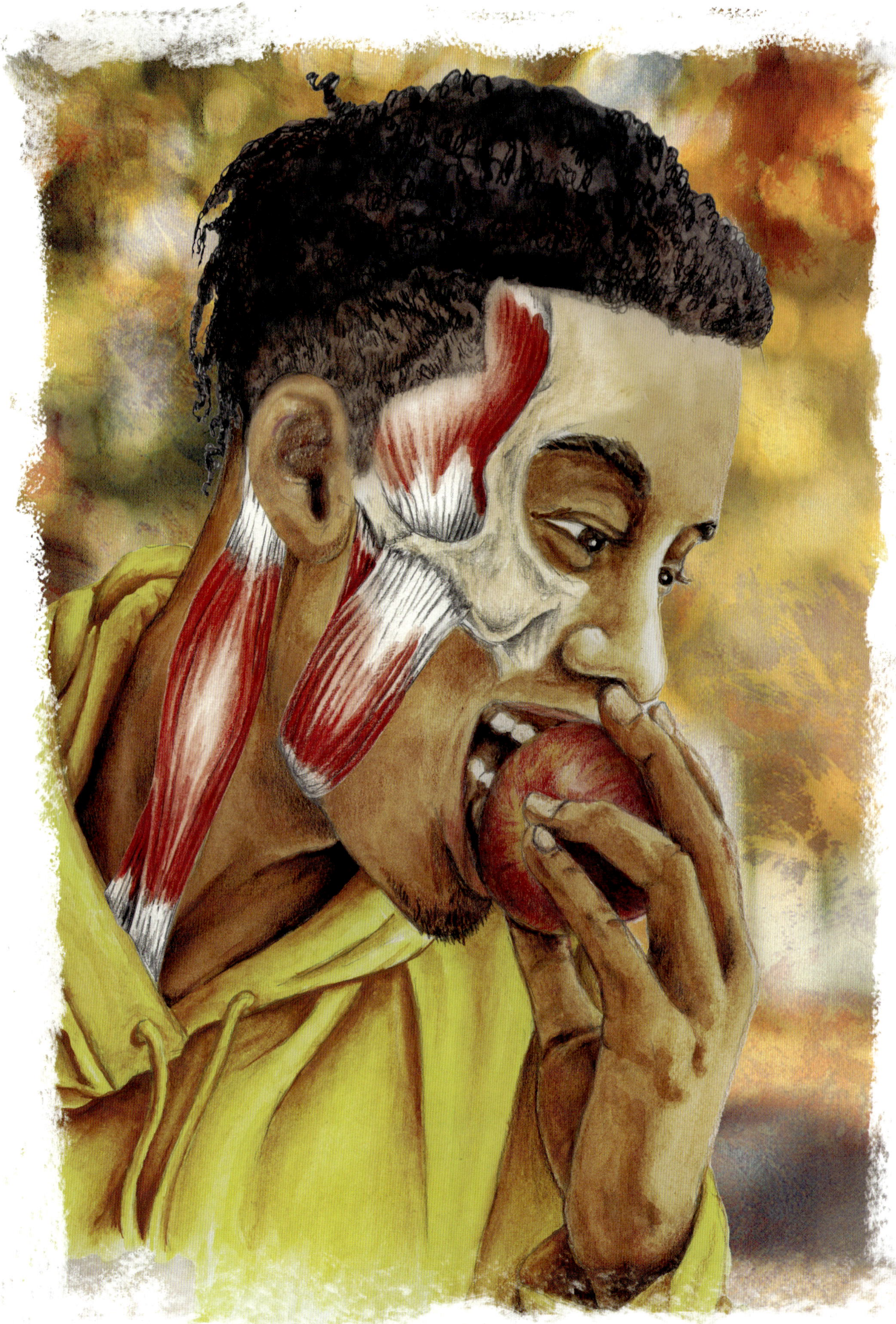

5

Head, Neck & Face

In today's world, we take a lot of selfies with our cell phones. Here's one more reason for a snapshot—and for educational purposes! When set in front of a camera or mirror, your head and face are terrific instructional guides to the muscles of this region and their corresponding expressions. So get ready for your close-up!

See for yourself:

- Pull out your phone and open the camera. Take one selfie with a neutral expression and another where you show a big smile. Toggling between the photos, compare the changes you see. What parts of your face shifted with a smile, especially around the eyes, forehead, or chin? Where do you think the muscles that produced those changes might be on your face?
- With your torso facing the camera, turn your head to the left and take a selfie. Take another shot, but this time open your jaw—as if you are taking a bite of an apple. Reviewing both photos, where can you see muscles at work? Compare your "apple shot" with the picture on the previous page. Feeling your face and head, which of the muscles highlighted in the picture do you think you can locate?
- Experiment with other selfies and movements. Try to raise your eyebrows. Can you raise just one? Can you wink? Flare your nostrils? How about wiggle your ears? Why do you think some people can make these movements while others find it challenging?

Topographical View

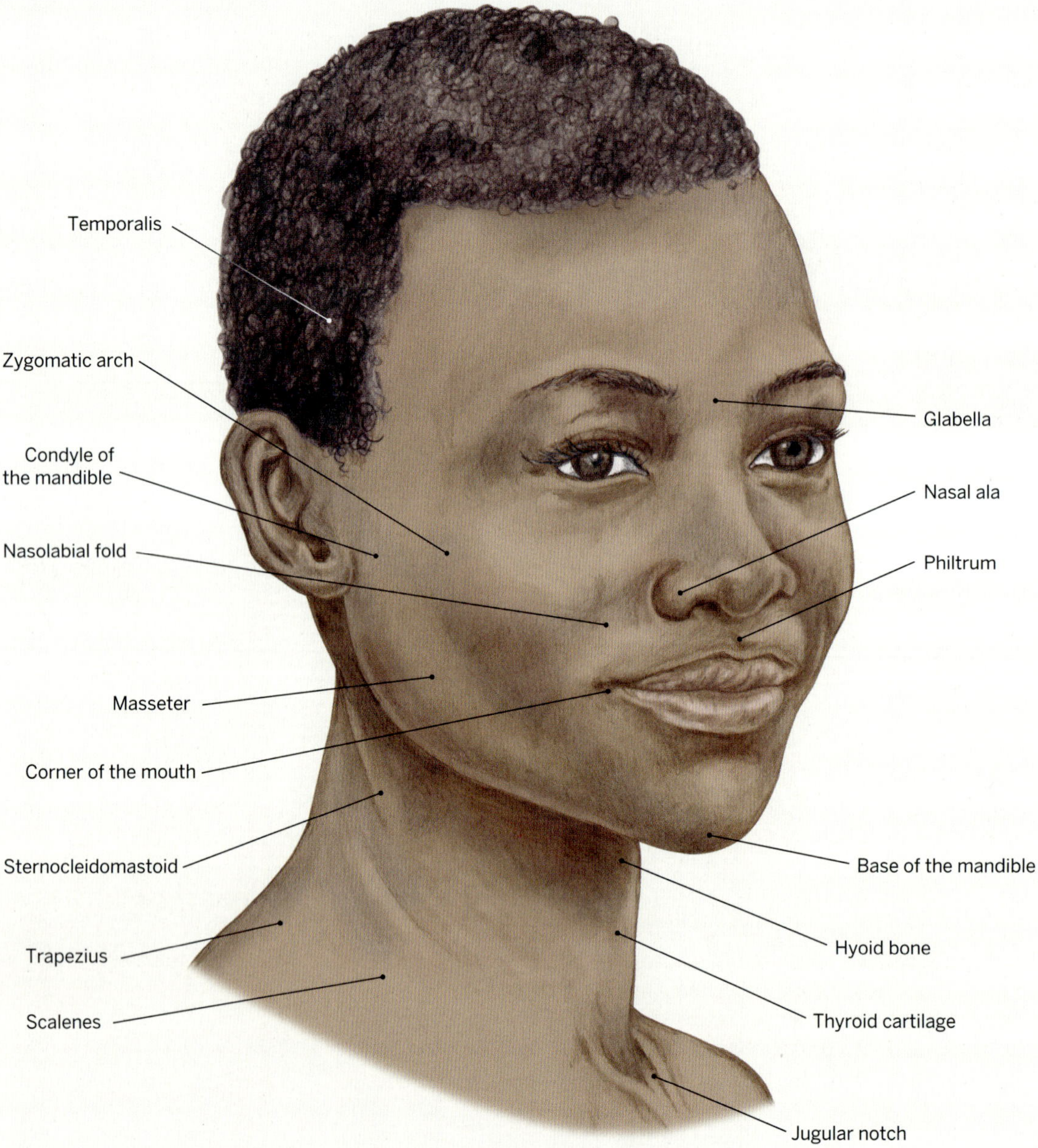

5.1 Anterior/lateral view of head and neck

Discover More

The anterior and lateral sides of the neck can be divided into two triangular regions. The **anterior triangle** (**a**) is bordered by the sternocleidomastoid (SCM), the base of the mandible, and the trachea. The hyoid bone, thyroid gland, carotid artery, submandibular gland, and styloid process of the temporal bone are some of the structures within the anterior triangle.

The **posterior triangle** (**b**) is formed by the sternocleidomastoid (SCM), clavicle, and trapezius and contains, among other structures, the brachial plexus and the external jugular vein.

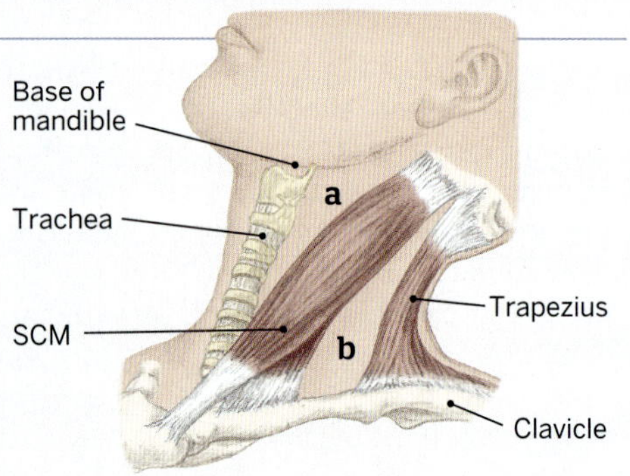

philtrum	***fil***-trum	Grk. to love, to kiss
glabella	gla-***bel***-a	L. *glaber*, smooth

Exploring the Skin and Fascia

Scalp

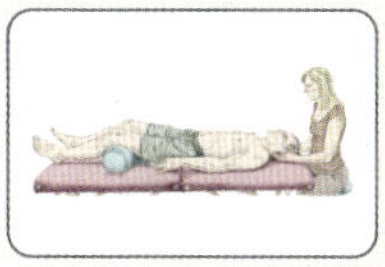

1. Partner supine. Sink your fingers into your partner's hair and onto her scalp. Note the temperature and moisture or oiliness.
2. Using your fingerpads for contact, gently tug the scalp in all directions (**5.2**). Rotate the head to the side to reach behind the ears and at the base of the skull. As you sense the tissue's thickness and mobility, do you notice any regions of the scalp that are more pliable than others?

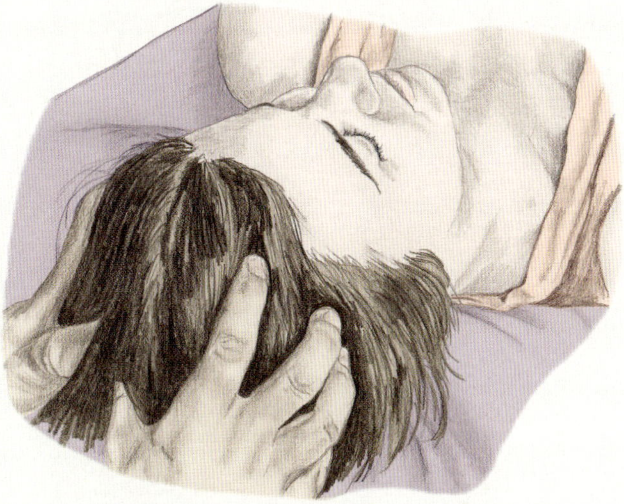

5.2 Partner supine, as you palpate the scalp

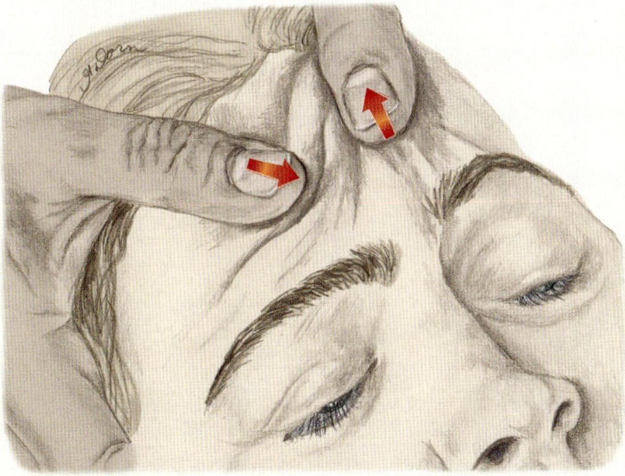

5.3 Partner supine, as you explore the forehead and face

Forehead and face

Partner supine. Using your thumbpads, gently torque the skin and fascia of the forehead and face. Sense the tissue's elasticity and thickness (**5.3**).

Neck

1. Partner supine. Moving to the neck, gently grasp and lift the skin and fascia of the lateral neck (**5.4**). Often the tissue here will be quite thin, almost delicate. Turn your hand 90° and try lifting the tissue in a horizontal direction. Is it more challenging to lift? Next explore the anterior neck, including the tissue under the mandible. Do you notice any restrictions in the skin?
2. Resting the head on the heel of your hand, explore the skin and fascia of the posterior neck. Often this tissue is thicker and denser than the anterior tissue. Is this true of your partner?

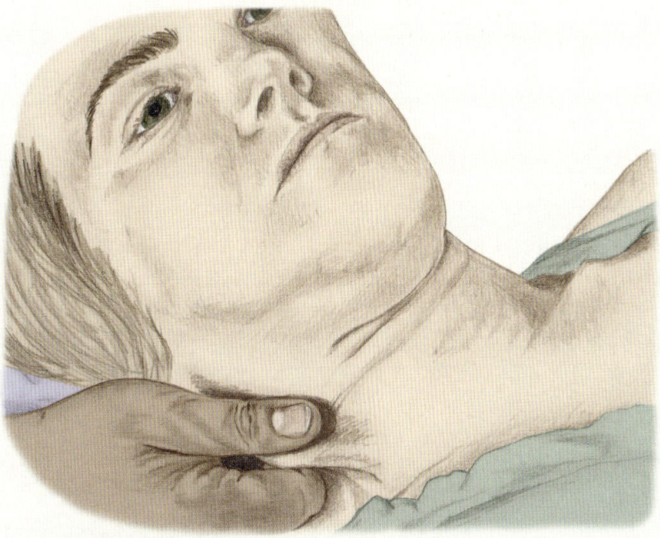

5.4 Partner supine, as you lift the skin and fascia of the neck

Bones and Bony Landmarks of the Head, Neck, and Face

The **skull** is composed of twenty-two bones: eight in the cranium and fourteen in the facial region. Seven of the eight **cranial** bones are directly accessible. The eighth, the ethmoid, is accessible only by way of the nasal cavity. Most of the cranial bones are superficial. Seven of the fourteen **facial** bones are palpable, as are the numerous bony landmarks of the **mandible** (jaw) (**5.5–5.8**).

The articulations of the cranial bones are different from the articulations of the appendages. The joints of the arms and legs have a synovial (mobile) joint structure. The cranial bones, in contrast, have fibrous joints that are woven together to form tight-fitting sutures.

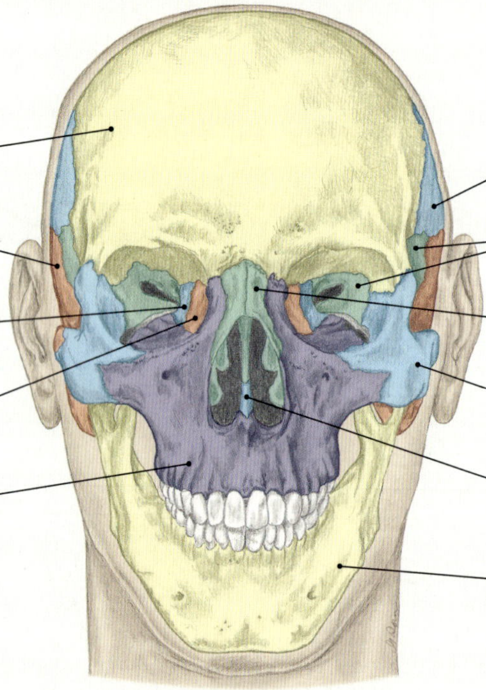

5.5 Anterior view of cranial and facial bones

Discover More

Facial bones (14)
- Inferior nasal concha (2)
- Lacrimal (2)
- Mandible
- Maxilla (2)
- Nasal (2)
- Palatine (2)
- Vomer
- Zygomatic (2)

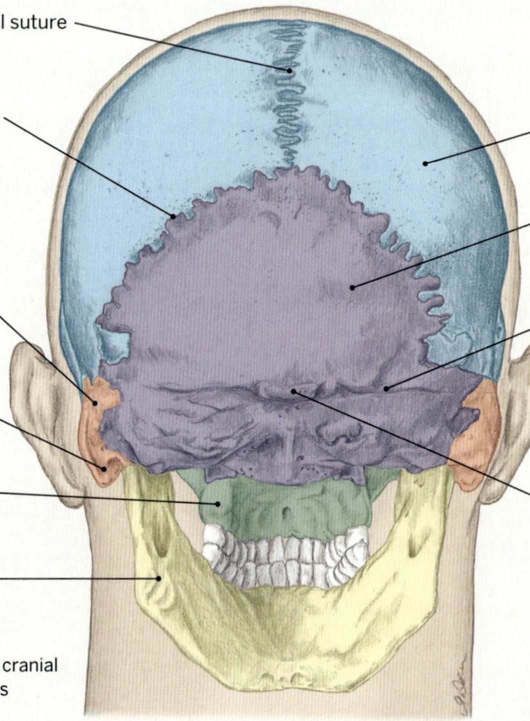

5.6 Posterior view of cranial and facial bones

Discover More

Cranial bones (8)
- Ethmoid
- Frontal
- Occiput
- Parietal (2)
- Sphenoid
- Temporal (2)

cranio-	*cra*-nee-o	Grk. skull
skull		ME. bow
suture	*su*-chur	L. a seam

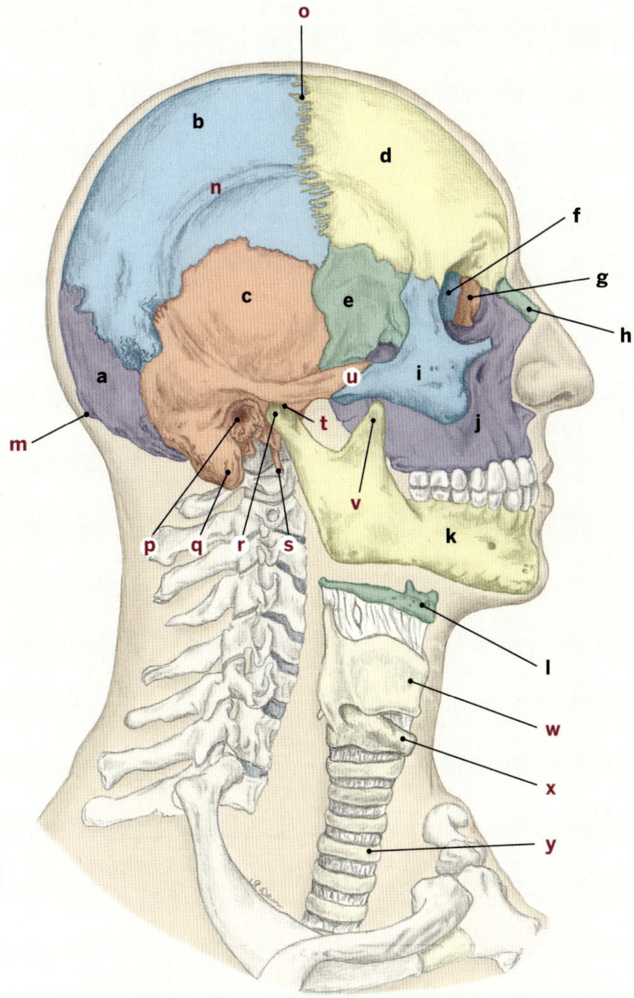

a. Occiput
b. Parietal
c. Temporal
d. Frontal
e. Sphenoid
f. Ethmoid
g. Lacrimal
h. Nasal
i. Zygomatic
j. Maxilla
k. Mandible
l. Hyoid
m. External occipital protuberance
n. Temporal lines of parietal bones
o. Coronal suture
p. External auditory meatus
q. Mastoid process
r. Condyle of the mandible
s. Styloid process of the temporal bone
t. Temporomandibular joint
u. Zygomatic arch
v. Coronoid process
w. Thyroid cartilage
x. Cricoid cartilage
y. Trachea

Black letters indicate bones; **red** letters indicate bony landmarks or other structures.

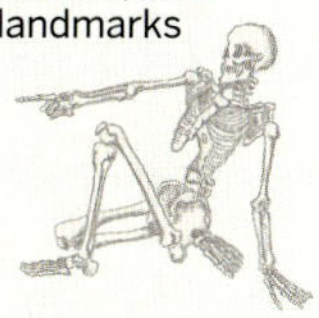

5.7 Lateral view of head and neck, showing bones and bony landmarks

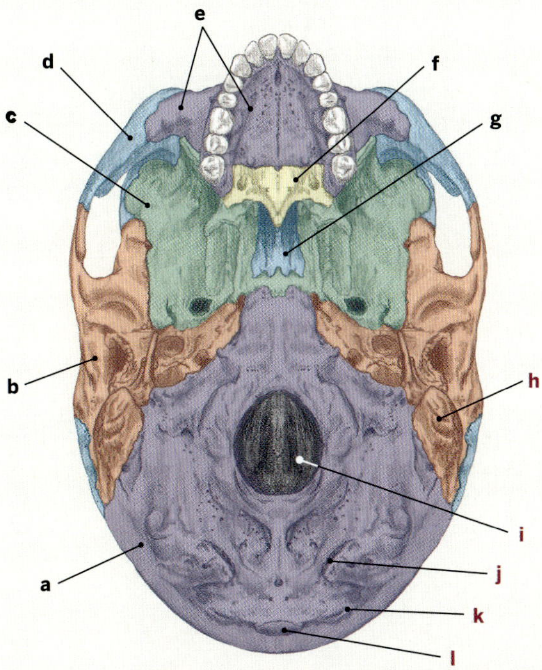

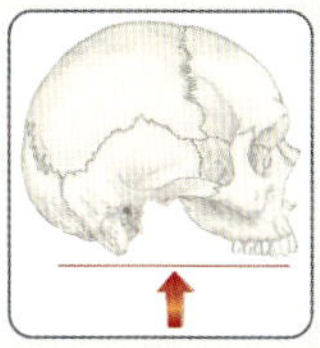

a. Occiput
b. Temporal
c. Sphenoid
d. Zygomatic
e. Maxilla
f. Palatine
g. Vomer
h. Mastoid process
i. Foramen magnum
j. Inferior nuchal line
k. Superior nuchal line
l. External occipital protuberance

5.8 Inferior view of cranium, showing bones and bony landmarks

Overview: **Bony Landmark Trails**

Trail 1 Around the Globe palpates the bones and bony landmarks of the cranium and face.

a Occiput
  External occipital protuberance
  Superior nuchal lines
b Parietal
c Temporal
  Mastoid process
  Zygomatic arch
  Styloid process
d Frontal
e Sphenoid
f Nasal, zygomatic, and maxilla

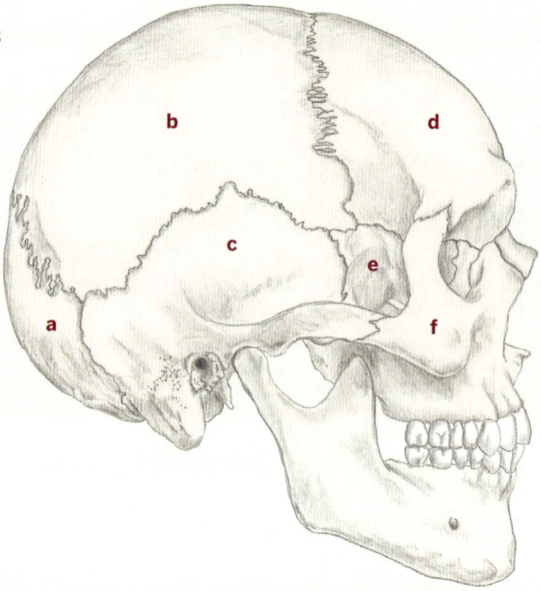

Trail 2 Jaw Jaunt explores the mandible.

a Body
b Base
c Submandibular fossa
d Angle
e Ramus
f Coronoid process
g Condyle

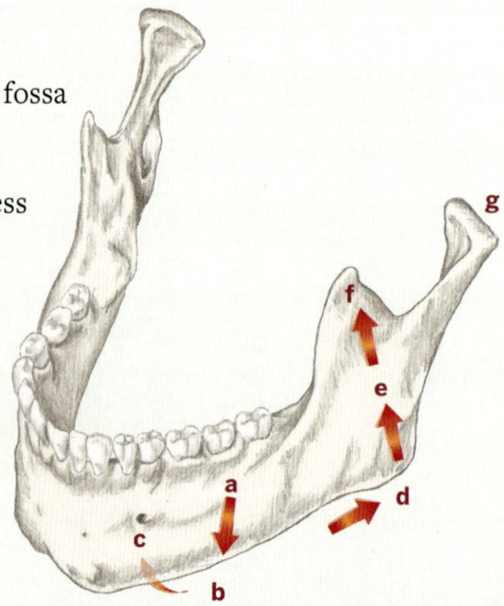

Trail 3 Horseshoe Trek locates the cartilaginous structures of the anterior neck and the horseshoe-shaped hyoid bone.

a Trachea
b Cricoid cartilage
c Thyroid cartilage
d Hyoid bone

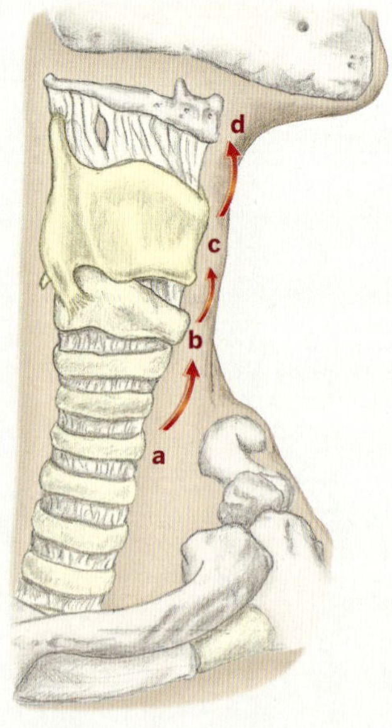

Lateral view of neck

Comparative Anatomy

With the progress of evolution, the skulls of more advanced creatures began to have fewer and fewer bones. For example, some fish have more than one hundred bones in the skull, reptiles may have seventy, and primitive mammals forty. A human skull contains twenty-two bones, eight of which form the cranium. From a design perspective, this makes good sense: Fewer bones mean fewer sutures, and fewer seams mean greater protection.

Occiput

External Occipital Protuberance
Superior Nuchal Lines

The occiput is located at the posterior and inferior aspects of the cranium. It extends superiorly from the external occipital protuberance and laterally to the mastoid processes of the temporal bones. The portion of the occiput superior to the occipital protuberance is superficial and easily palpable. The portion inferior to the protuberance curves in and under the head and is covered by layers of tendon and muscle (**5.9**, **5.10**).

Sometimes called the "bump of knowledge," the **external occipital protuberance** is a small, superficial point located along the back of the head at the center of the occiput. It lies between the attachment sites of both trapezius muscles and is the superior attachment for the ligamentum nuchae. Regardless of people's intelligence, it varies in size.

Located along either side of the occipital protuberance, the **superior nuchal lines** are faint, sometimes bumpy ridges which extend laterally to the mastoid processes. The nuchal lines are attachment sites for the trapezius and splenius capitis muscles.

Occiput (general location)

1. Partner prone. Place your hand on the back of the head between the ears.
2. Explore its surface by sliding your fingers:
   - *superiorly* from the occipital protuberance two or three inches;
   - *inferiorly* where the occiput curves and sinks into the muscles of the neck;
   - *laterally* to the mastoid processes behind the ears.

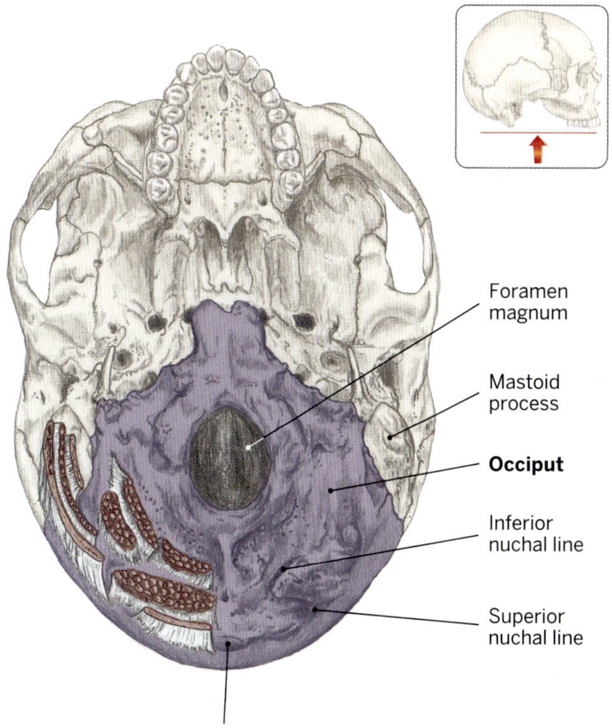

5.9 Inferior view of cranium, showing occiput

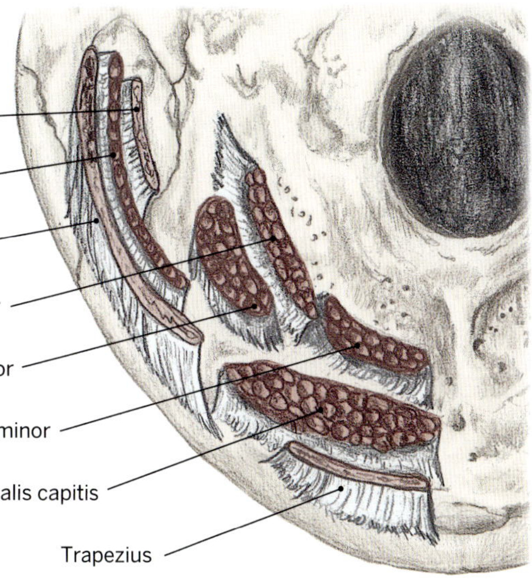

5.10 Inferior view of cranium, showing muscle attachment sites

Discover More

The superior nuchal line is an attachment site for several muscles. Metaphorically, it is the shoreline between the dry land of the cranium and the sea of neck muscles.

nuchal	***nu***-kal	L. the back of the neck
occiput	***ok***-si-put	L. the back of the skull

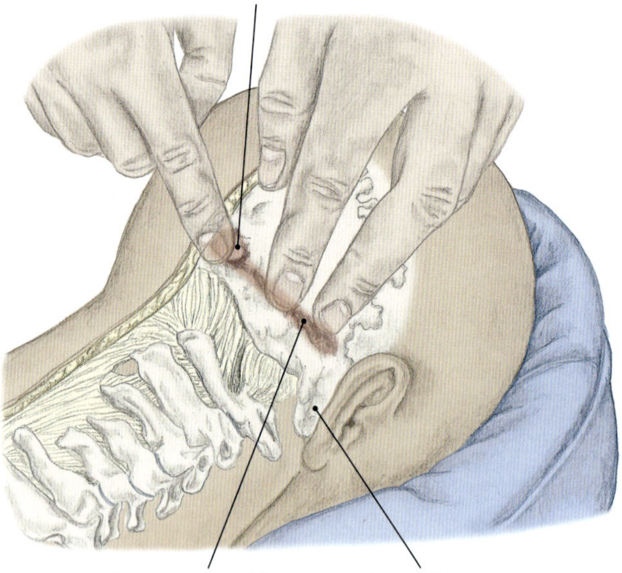

5.11 Partner prone, posterior/lateral view of cranium with superficial tissue removed on right side, as you palpate the external occipital protuberance and superior nuchal line

External occipital protuberance

1. Partner prone or supine. Place your fingers along the back of the neck at the body's midline (**5.11**).
2. Slide superiorly onto the bony surface of the cranium. The protuberance will be at the "shoreline" between the neck muscles and the cranium.

Are you level with the top of the ears? If your partner is prone, ask her to extend her head slightly. Is the bump you feel just superior to where the muscles tighten?

Superior nuchal lines

1. Partner prone or supine. Stand at the head of the table and place both index fingers at the external occipital protuberance.
2. Allow the other fingers to fall in place beside them. Glide your fingerpads up and down and palpate the edge of the superior nuchal lines.
3. Follow these ridges laterally as they extend toward the ear and mastoid processes (**5.11**).

Are you just lateral to the occipital protuberance? Do the ridges lead toward the back of the ears? Can you find them from a prone position? Are you on the cranium as opposed to the muscles of the neck?

Head, Neck & Face

Discover More

At birth, the cranial bones are neither fully developed nor joined. Usually there are six unossified gaps in the skull called fontanels. The name (old French, *little fountain*) perhaps came from the pulse of the blood vessels felt under the skin that reminded physicians of the spurting of a fountain. The fontanels close over a period of between two and twenty-four months.

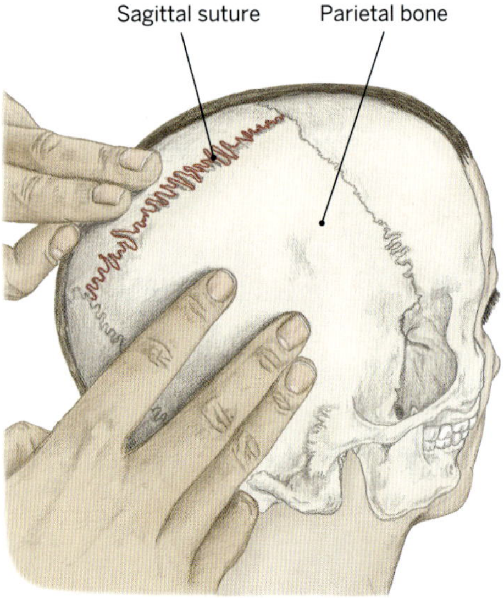

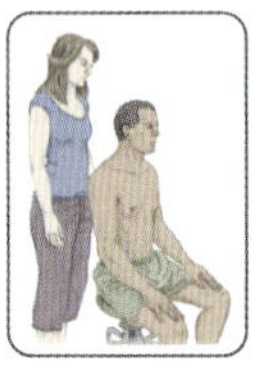

5.12 Partner seated, posterior/lateral view of cranium with superficial tissue removed on right side, as you access the parietals

Parietal Bones

The large, rectangular parietal bones form the top and sides of the cranium. Positioned between the frontal, occipital, and temporal bones, the parietals are saucer-shaped and extend anteriorly to the level of the ear canal. They merge at the body's midline to form the sagittal suture, a slight crest that often can be felt.

Parietals

1. Partner seated, prone or supine. To access the general area of the parietals, place both hands on top of the cranium.
2. Palpate the sagittal suture between the parietals. If you cannot feel its crest, visualize it along the top of the skull.
3. Follow it anteriorly to the level of the ear canal and posteriorly to the occiput (**5.12**).

parietal puh-*ri*-e-tul L. wall

Temporal Bone

Mastoid Process
Styloid Process
Zygomatic Arch

The temporal bone is located on the side of the head, encompassing the area around the ear. It has three important bony landmarks: the mastoid process, the zygomatic arch, and the styloid process (**5.13**). The temporal bone is superficial, except for its superior aspect, which lies deep to the temporalis muscle.

The **mastoid process** (**a**) forms a large, superficial bump directly behind the earlobe. It is an attachment site for the sternocleidomastoid and other muscles. Also, it is larger on males than females and is undeveloped on infants.

The superficial **zygomatic arch** (**c**) (or cheekbone) is formed by the temporal and zygomatic bones. It is an attachment site for the masseter muscle. The space between the zygomatic arch and the cranium is filled by the thick temporalis muscle.

The **styloid process** (**b**) is located behind the earlobe between the mastoid process and the posterior edge of the mandible. Its fang-like shape serves as an attachment site for several ligaments and muscles. The styloid process is deep to overlying muscles and tissue and is not directly palpable; however, its location can be accessed.

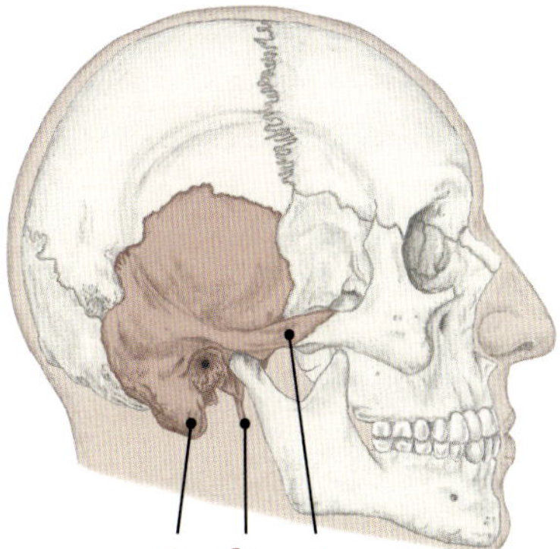

5.13 Lateral view of cranium, showing temporal bone: (**a**) mastoid process, (**b**) styloid process, and (**c**) zygomatic arch

Temporal bone

1. Partner supine. Locate the mastoid process by placing your finger behind the earlobe. Sculpt around its edges, exploring its entire surface (**5.14**).
2. Explore the zygomatic arch by placing your finger anterior to the ear canal. Move anteriorly along the arch, outlining its sides with your thumb and finger (**5.15**). Follow it anteriorly as it merges with the orbit of the eye.

When locating the mastoid, are you behind the earlobe? Is the bone you feel round and superficial? Can you palpate posteriorly onto the superior nuchal line of the occiput? Does the ridge of the zygomatic arch run horizontally? Is it level with the ear canal?

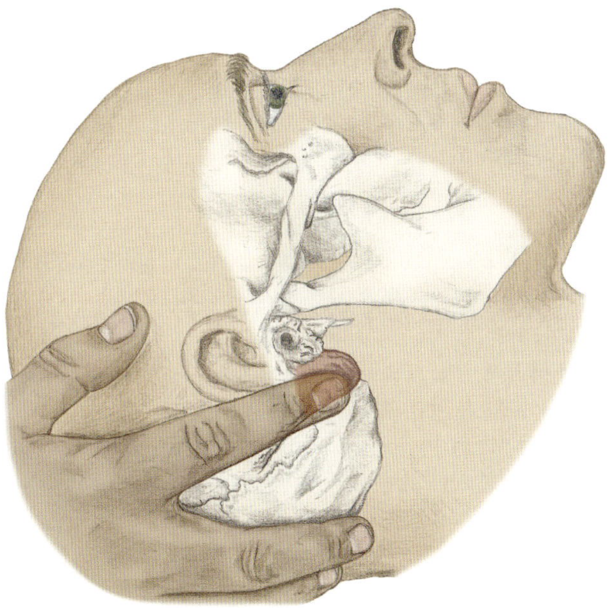

5.14 Partner supine, lateral view of cranium with inferior portion of the ear removed, as you access the mastoid process

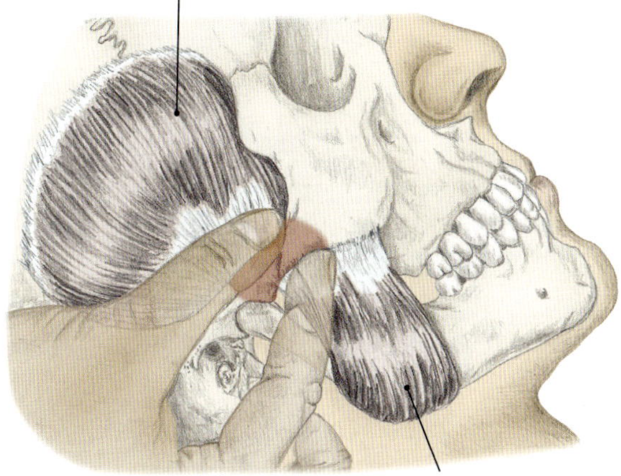

5.15 Partner supine, as you palpate the zygomatic arch

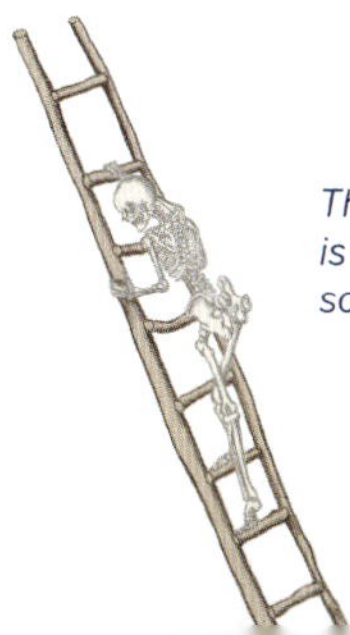

The styloid process of the temporal bone is fragile and is deep to the facial nerve (p. 272), so exploration in this area should be very gentle.

mastoid	*mas*-toyd	Grk. breast-shaped
styloid	*sti*-loyd	Grk. a pillar
zygomatic	*zy*-go-*mat*-ik	Grk. cheekbone

Head, Neck & Face

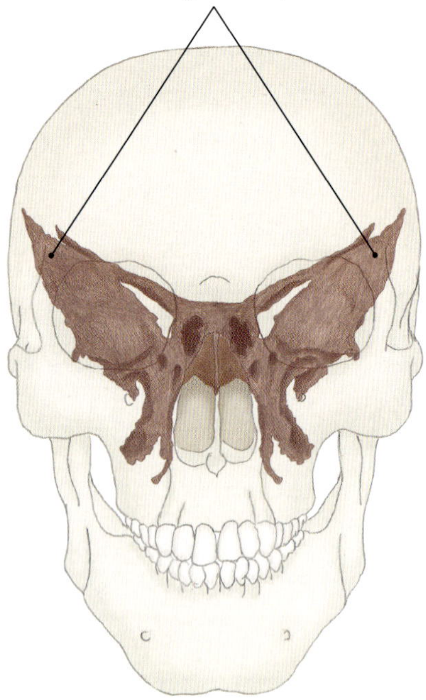

5.16 Anterior view of cranium, showing location of the sphenoid bone

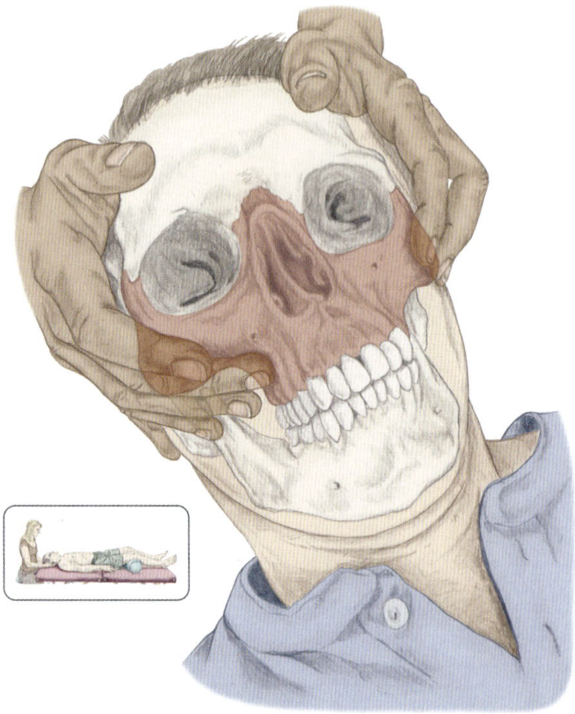

5.17 *Dawn of the Dead*? No, just exploring the facial bones with your partner supine.

Frontal Bone

Located on the anterior aspect of the cranium, the broad frontal bone forms the forehead and upper rim of the eye sockets. It articulates with the parietal bones to form the coronal sutures, which are deep to the occipitofrontalis and lateral edge of the temporalis muscles (p. 251).

Frontal bone

Partner supine. Explore the region of the forehead, moving superiorly to the coronal sutures, inferiorly to the brow, and laterally to the anterior edge of the temporalis muscle.

Sphenoid Bone

The sphenoid bone is located inside the cranium and has major articulations with the fourteen bones of the skull. Located behind the eyeballs and superior to the zygomatic arches, the sphenoid is shaped like a butterfly, and its lateral portions are called the greater wings (**5.16**). The temporalis lies on top of these flat wings, making them inaccessible.

Sphenoid bone

1. Partner supine. Place your fingers at the middle of the zygomatic arch (cheekbone) to locate the greater wings of the sphenoid.
2. Slide your fingers superiorly one inch onto the temporalis muscle belly. The greater wing of the sphenoid is located deep to the thick temporalis belly.

Facial Bones

Nasal

Located at the bridge of the nose, the small nasal bones are positioned between the frontal and maxillary bones (**5.17**; see also p. 228) and are virtually indistinguishable from them.

Zygomatic

Better known as the cheekbone, the zygomatic bone forms the anterior aspect of the zygomatic arch and the lateral portion of the orbit of the eye (**5.17**; see also p. 228). It serves as an attachment site for the masseter muscle.

Maxilla

The maxillary bones form the center of the face, the inferior portion of the orbit of the eye, the surface around the nose, and the upper jaw in which the upper row of teeth articulate (**5.17**; see also p. 228).

maxilla	***max***-il-a	L. jawbone
nasal	***na***-zl	L. nose
sphenoid	***sfe***-noyd	Grk. wedge-shaped

Mandible

Body, Base, Submandibular Fossa, Angle, Ramus, Condyle, and Coronoid Process

The mandible, or jaw, has numerous landmarks that are superficial and accessible (**5.18**). The **body** is the flat surface of the mandible inferior to the lower teeth. The **base**, or jawline, is the edge of the body and an attachment site for the thin platysma muscle. The **submandibular fossa** is located on the underside of the mandible and is an attachment site for the suprahyoid muscles (p. 253).

The superficial **angle** is located at the posterior end of the base. It forms part of the attachment for the masseter. The flat **ramus** is the posterior, vertical portion of the mandible and is deep to the masseter.

The mandible articulates with the cranium at two temporomandibular joints. The superficial **condyle** is located just anterior to the ear canal and inferior to the zygomatic arch. The deeper, inaccessible head of the condyle forms the articulating surface of the mandible at the temporomandibular (TM) joint (**5.19**, **5.20**).

The **coronoid process** is located an inch anterior to the condyle of the mandible and is the attachment site of the temporalis muscle. When the jaw is closed, the coronoid process lies underneath the zygomatic arch and is inaccessible. Opening the mouth fully, however, will bring the coronoid process out from under the arch and allow the process to be accessed.

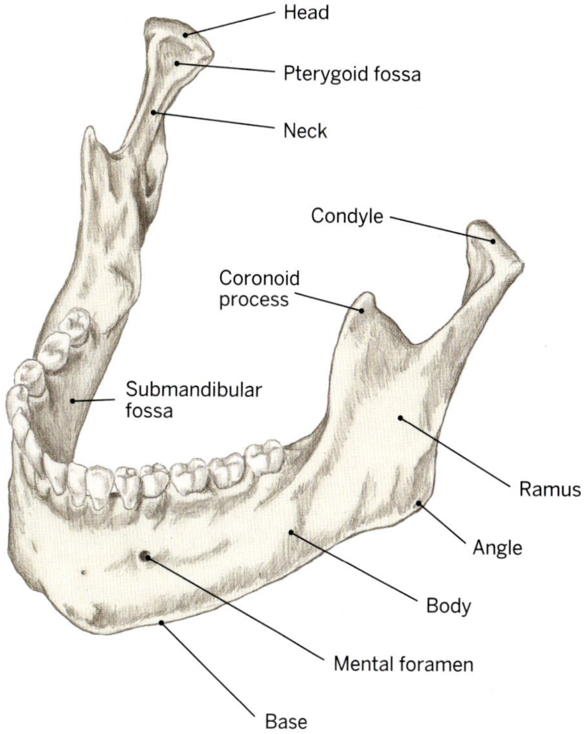

5.18 Anterior/lateral view of mandible

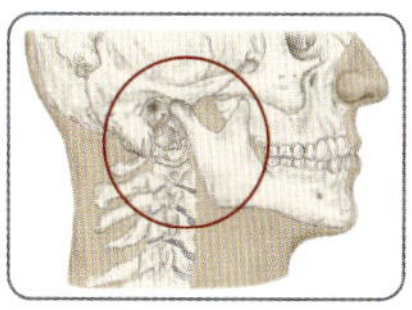

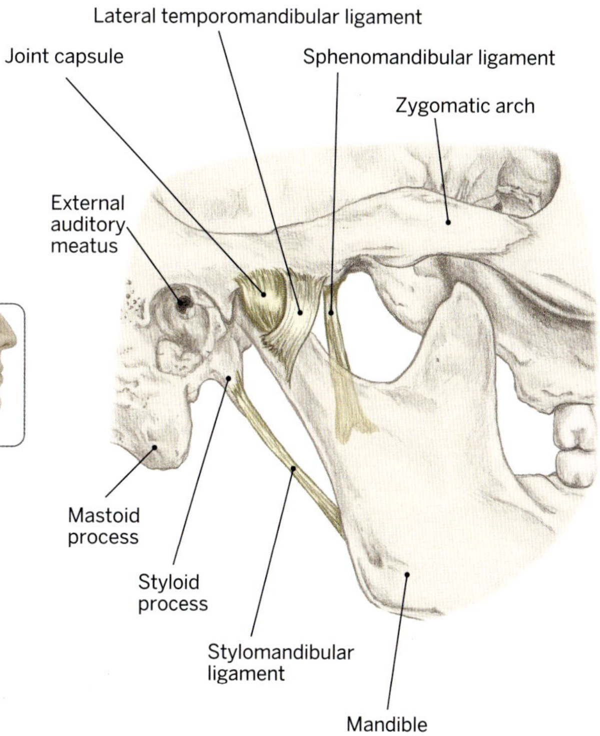

5.19 Lateral view of right temporomandibular (TM) joint

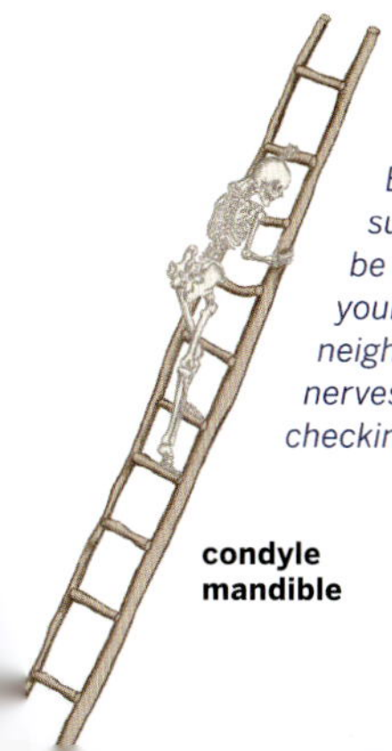

Exploring in the submandibular fossa can be uncomfortable for your partner because of neighboring glands and nerves. Move slowly, checking in as you proceed.

condyle	***kon**-dial*	Grk. knuckle
mandible	***man**-di-ble*	L. lower jawbone

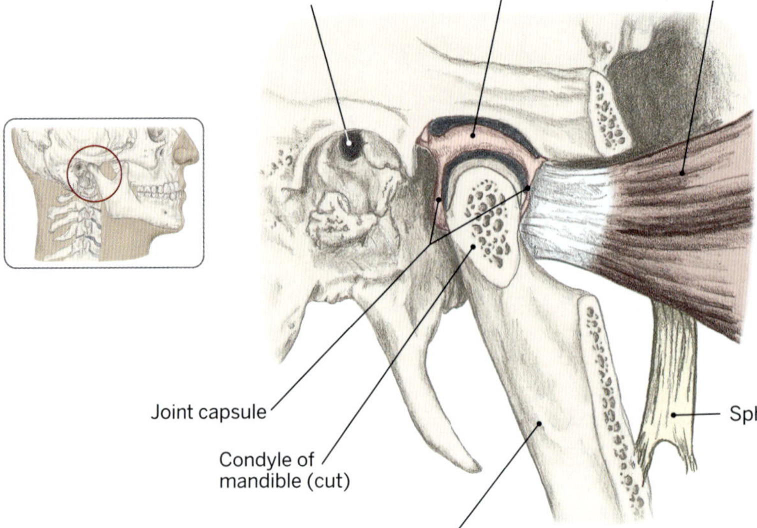

5.20 Lateral view of right temporomandibular (TM) joint

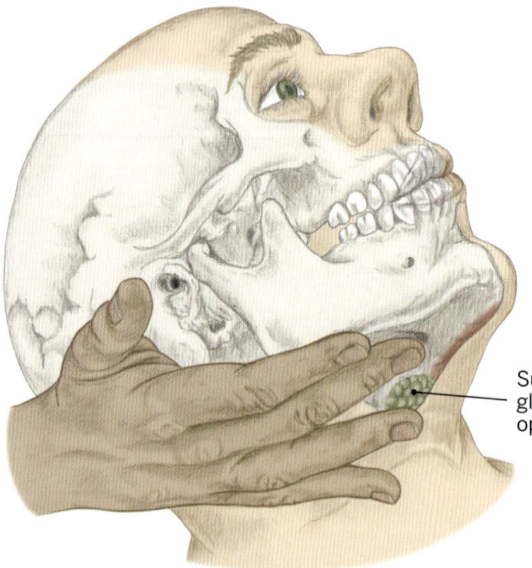

5.21 Partner supine, as you palpate the submandibular fossa

Body, base, and submandibular fossa

1. Partner supine. Place your fingers inferior to the bottom teeth and explore the superficial surface of the body.
2. Move inferiorly and palpate the base or edge of the mandible. Explore its entire length from the chin to the angle of the mandible.
3. With one hand stabilizing the mandible, slowly curl a fingertip underneath its edge and into the submandibular fossa (**5.21**).

Discover More

The temporomandibular joint is the most frequently used joint in the body, moving 2,000–3,000 times a day. This wear and tear is compounded by the incongruity of its joint surfaces, namely the mandibular condyle and its fossa. Luckily, the TM joint is equipped with an articular disc (**1**). Shaped like a Life Saver, this disc lies on top of the condyle and helps to create more congruity between the joint surfaces, reducing the potential for bone deterioration.

When the mandible depresses, the condyle and disc move in tandem, pivoting anteriorly and inferiorly (**2**, **3**). The reverse occurs when the mandible elevates.

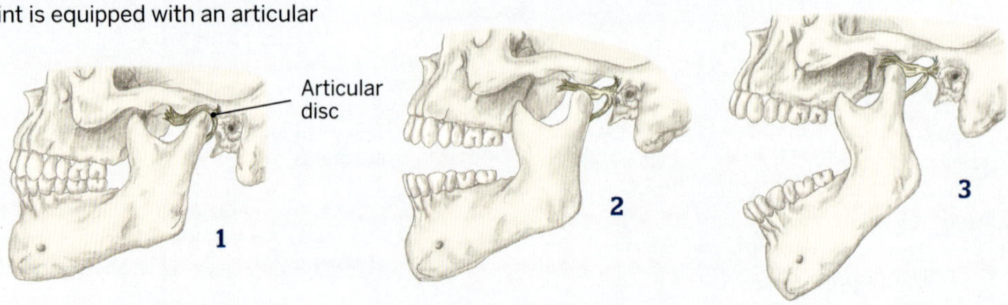

coronoid	***kor***-o-noyd	Grk. crown-shaped
ramus	***ray***-mus	L. branch

Angle and ramus of mandible

1. Partner supine. Slide posteriorly along the base of the mandible to the angle. Clarify your location by asking your partner to open her mouth and note the movement of the angle (**5.22**).
2. Slide superiorly from the angle onto the ramus, which is deep to the masseter muscle.

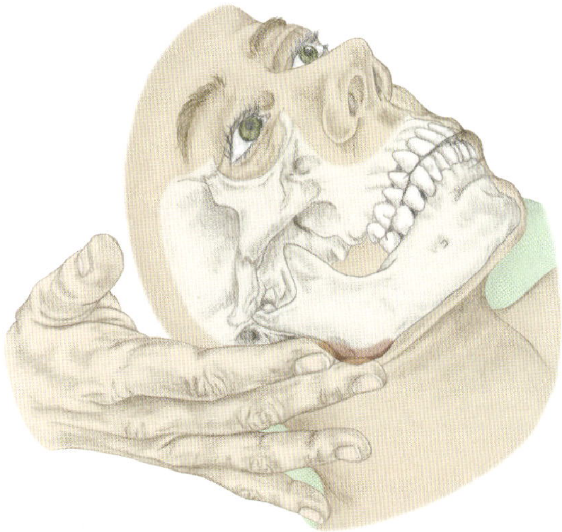

5.22 Partner supine, as you palpate the angle of the mandible

Condyle of mandible

1. Partner supine. Place your fingerpad anterior to the ear canal and below the zygomatic arch.
2. Ask your partner to open her mouth fully. With this action, the condyle will become more palpable as it slides anteriorly and inferiorly (**5.23**).
3. As the jaw closes, follow the condyle to its original position.

Are you anterior to the ear canal, below the zygomatic arch? As your partner opens her mouth, can you palpate both condyles simultaneously?

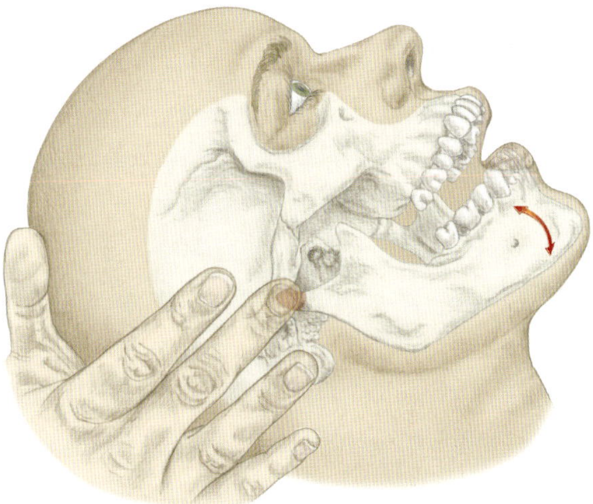

5.23 Partner supine, opening and closing her mouth while you feel the condyle shift

Coronoid process of mandible

1. Partner supine. Place your fingerpad on the middle aspect of the zygomatic arch.
2. Drop half an inch inferiorly and ask your partner to open her mouth fully. As the jaw drops, the large process will press into your finger (**5.24**).
3. With the mouth still open, explore the surfaces of the process.

Are you inferior to the zygomatic arch? When the mouth is open, can you feel the anterior edge of the process?

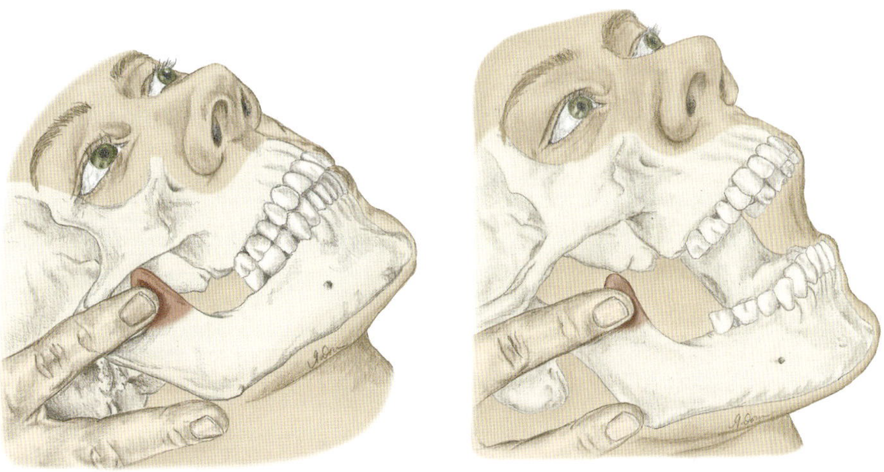

5.24 Partner supine, opening her mouth while you feel the coronoid process come out from under the zygomatic arch

Trail 3 Horseshoe Trek

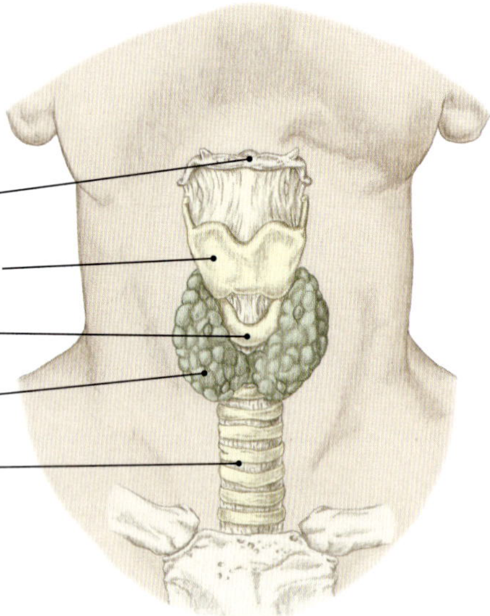

5.25 Anterior view of the neck

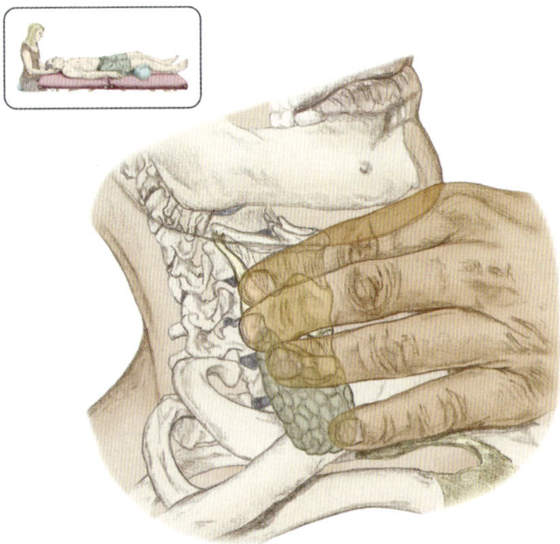

5.26 Partner supine, as you gently access the structures on the front of the neck

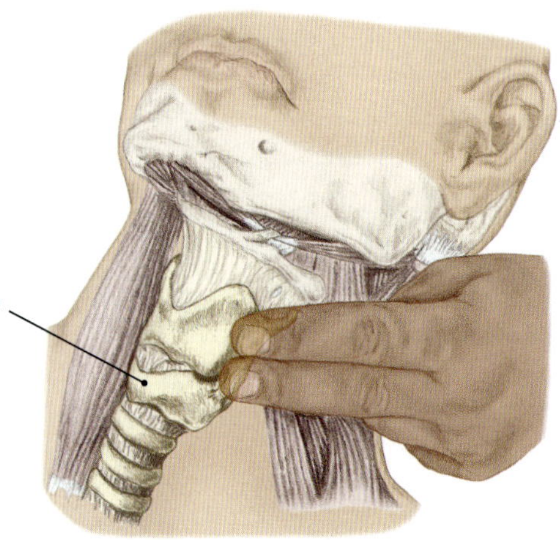

5.27 Partner supine, as you palpate the trachea and cartilages

Trachea

Cricoid Cartilage, Thyroid Cartilage, and Hyoid Bone

The **trachea** (windpipe) is located at the center of the anterior neck (**5.25**). It is a ribbed, cartilaginous tube that is roughly an inch in diameter and deep to the thyroid gland. The **cricoid cartilage** is a slightly larger ring of the trachea superior to the thyroid gland. The **thyroid cartilage** (Adam's apple) is superior to the cricoid cartilage below the level of the chin. Present in both sexes, the thyroid cartilage is larger and more visibly protruding on adult males. The three structures are partially deep to the slender infrahyoid muscles (p. 255), yet are easily palpable.

The horseshoe-shaped **hyoid bone** is located superior to the thyroid cartilage (**5.28**, **5.29**). It is roughly an inch in diameter and lies parallel to the base of the mandible (jawline) and the third or fourth cervical vertebrae. The hyoid bone serves as an attachment site for the suprahyoid and infrahyoid muscles. It is accessible and elevates upon swallowing.

Trachea and cartilages

1. Partner supine or seated. Using a fingerpad and thumbpad to palpate, gently explore the anterior surface of the neck for the tubular trachea.
2. Slide your finger up and down to feel the trachea's ribbed surface, and slowly and gently shift it from side to side, noting its pliability (**5.26**).
3. The cricoid cartilage can be isolated by sliding your finger and thumb superiorly along the trachea to just below the thyroid cartilage. Explore for its large, ringed surface (**5.27**).
4. Slide superiorly from the cricoid cartilage onto the thyroid cartilage. Palpate its sides and central tip.

Are you at the midline of the neck? Can you distinguish any rings along the trachea's surface? Is the trachea roughly an inch in diameter? With your fingerpad on the thyroid cartilage, ask your partner to swallow. Do you feel it move up and down?

Discover More

The thyroid cartilage is sometimes referred to as the "Adam's apple." The name derives from a folk legend that described how the biblical Adam's first bite of apple became stuck halfway down his throat. According to the legend, his male descendants, with their more visibly protruding thyroid cartilage, appear to have carried on his condition.

cricoid	***kri***-koyd	Grk. ring-shaped
hyoid	***hi***-oyd	Grk. U-shaped

Hyoid bone

1. Partner supine or seated. Place your index finger on the thyroid cartilage. Roll your fingerpad superiorly over the thyroid cartilage, onto the hyoid.
2. Then gently palpate the sides of the hyoid with your first finger and thumb (**5.30**). The hyoid will be wider than the trachea.
3. Using gentle pressure, explore the surface of the hyoid as well as its small side-to-side movements. If you have difficulty accessing the hyoid, encourage your partner to relax her tongue and jaw.

*Are you superior to the thyroid cartilage (Adam's apple)? Can you gently move the hyoid from side to side? With your first finger and thumb on either side of the hyoid, ask your partner to swallow. Do you feel the hyoid rise up and then return (**5.31**)?-*

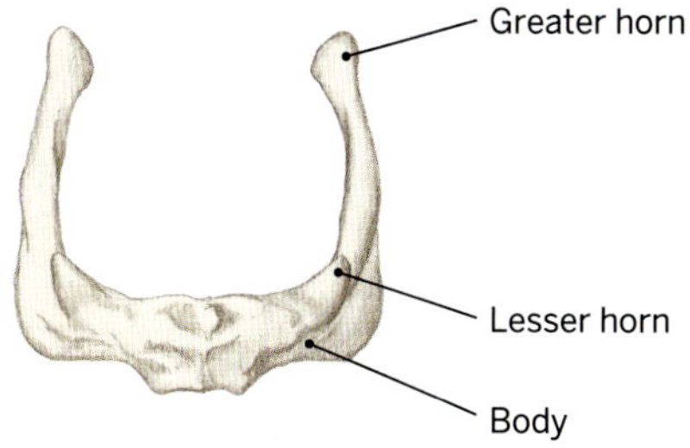

5.28 Superior view of hyoid

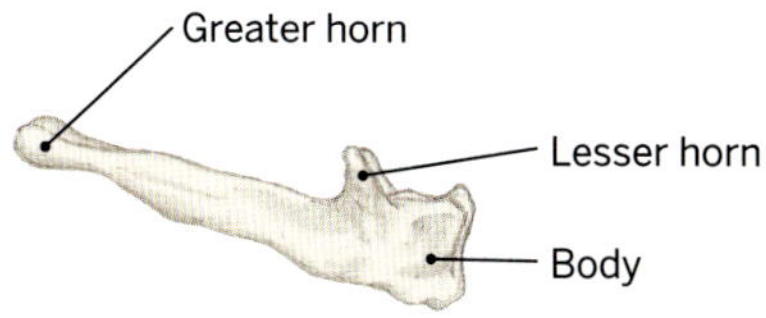

5.29 Lateral view of hyoid

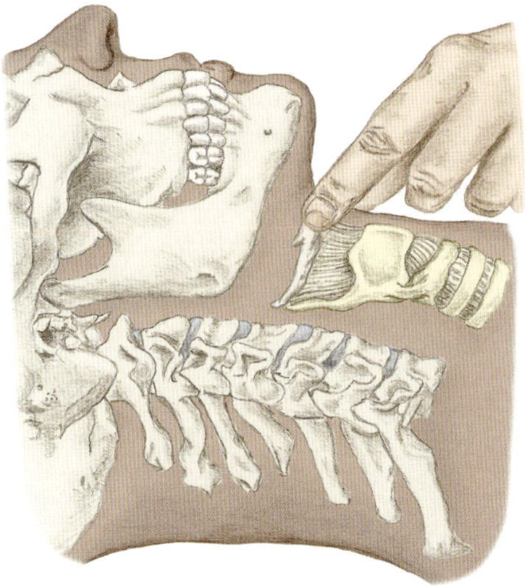

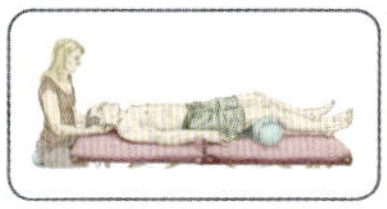

5.30 Partner supine, as you isolate the hyoid bone

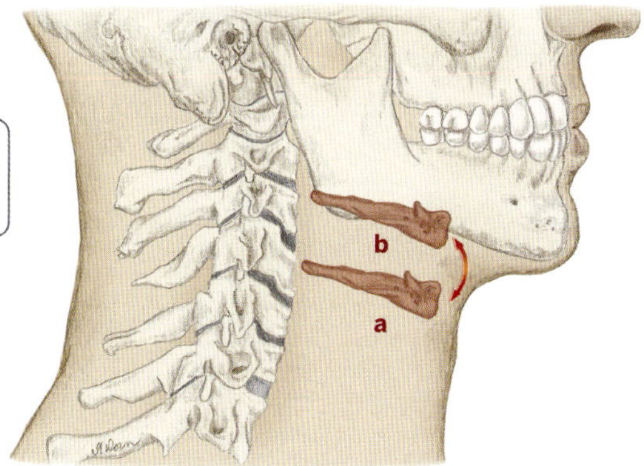

5.31 The hyoid bone at rest (**a**) and its placement during swallowing (**b**)

Comparative Anatomy

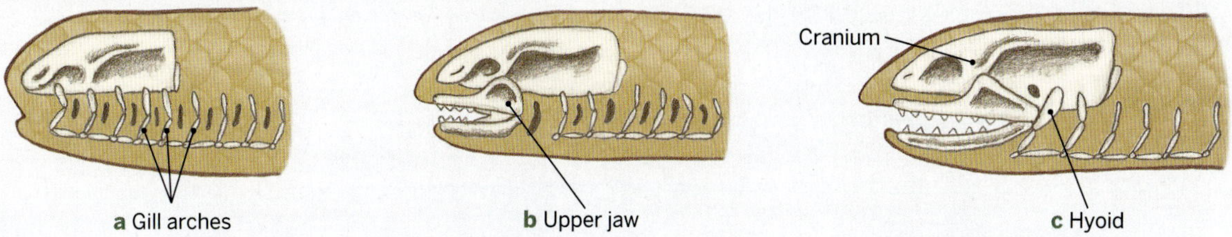

The hyoid bone is an ancestral remnant of the tissue that once formed gills. In the evolution of the jaw, the gill arches (the bones around the gills) (**a**) gravitated toward the head to hold the upper jaw next to the cranium (**b**). For fish, which do not have the long necks we do, the position of the hyoid provides an important link between the jaw and cranium (**c**). For humans, the hyoid lost this function and shifted down the neck to become the only non-articulating bone in the body. It is supported instead by the muscles that attach to its surface, such as the suprahyoids and infrahyoids.

thyroid	***thi***-royd	Grk. shield
trachea	***tray***-ke-a	Grk. rough

Overview: **Muscles of the Head, Neck, and Face**

The head and face contain more than thirty pairs of muscles, many of which are small, thin, and difficult to isolate. Nevertheless, the several muscles that act upon the mandible are easily accessible on the side of the jaw (**5.32**).

The anterior and lateral neck muscles perform a wide variety of tasks, including moving the head and neck, providing assistance in swallowing, and raising the rib cage during inhalation (**5.32**, **5.33**). The posterior neck muscles, which act primarily upon the cervical spine and head, are detailed in Chapter 4, *Spine and Thorax*.

Before you palpate the following muscles on your partner, you are advised to skip to the back of this chapter to familiarize yourself with the arteries, glands, and nerves of the head, neck, and face (p. 270).

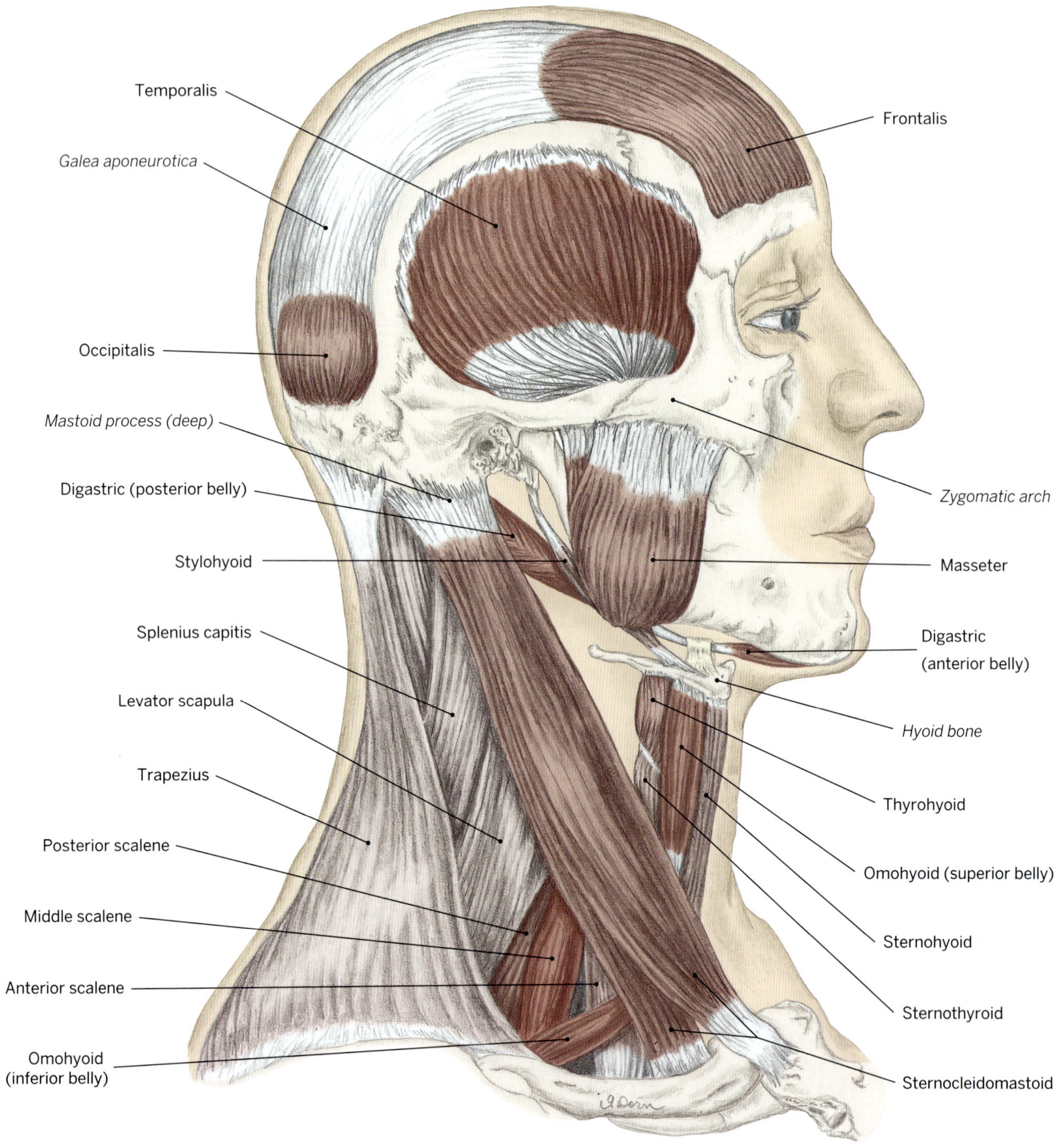

5.32 Lateral view of muscles of the head, neck, and face

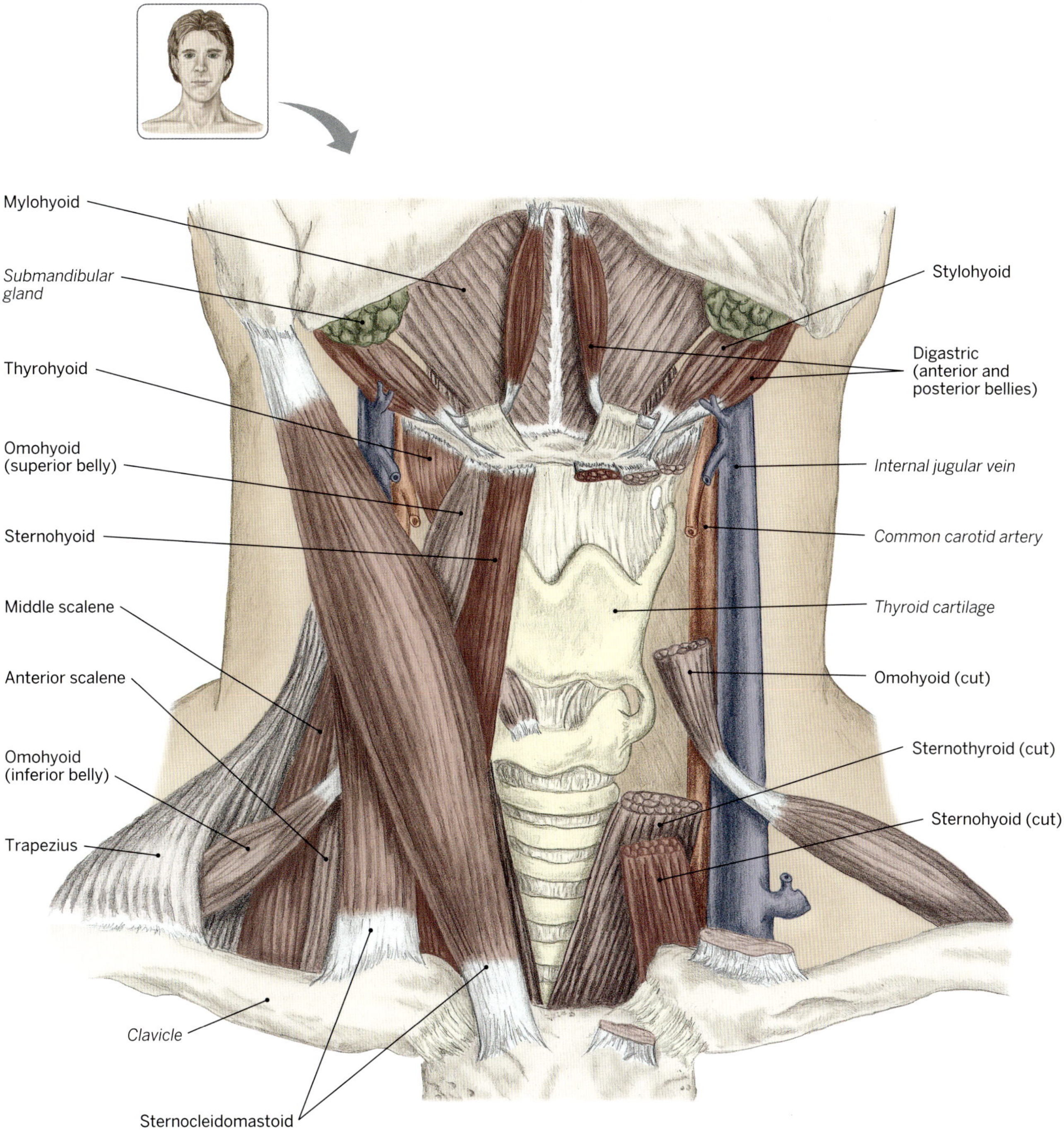

5.33 Anterior view of muscles of the neck, superficial muscles removed on his left side

Discover More

The single smallest muscle in the human body is located in the middle ear. The stapedius muscle measures less than 1/20 of an inch, thinner than a U.S. dime. It activates the stirrup, one of the tiny bones of the ear, which sends vibrations from the eardrum into the inner ear.

The stapedius, however, may not be the absolute shortest muscle in the body. A minuscule involuntary muscle called the arrector pili (p. 8) attaches to every hair follicle on the human body. These microscopic muscles nevertheless have a big responsibility: When you are cold or respond to a strong emotion such as fear, the arrector pili muscles raise the hair, producing goose bumps which help to retain body heat. They are also believed to have given our evolutionary ancestors the hair-raising ability of appearing larger to potential enemies.

arrector pili	a-***rek***-tor ***pee***-li	L. *arrector*, lifter; *pilus*, hair
stapedius	sta-***pe***-de-us	L. stirrup

Synergists—Muscles Working Together

Muscles are listed in the order of their ability to create the movement. Asterisk indicates muscles not shown.

Cervical Spine

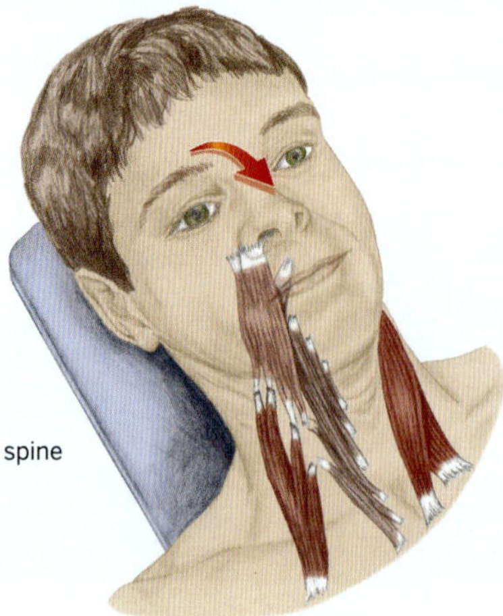

5.34 Flexion of the cervical spine

Flexion
(antagonists on extension)

Sternocleidomastoid (bilaterally)
Anterior scalene (bilaterally)
Longus capitis (bilaterally)
Longus colli (bilaterally)

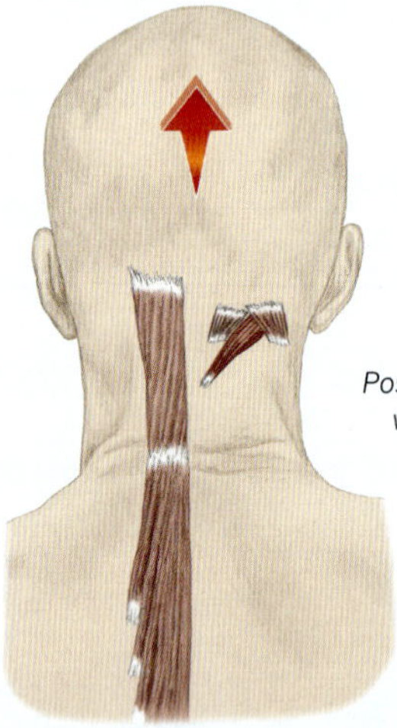

5.35 Extension of the cervical spine

Extension
(antagonists on flexion)

Trapezius (upper fibers, bilaterally)
Levator scapula (bilaterally)
Splenius capitis (bilaterally)
Splenius cervicis (bilaterally)
Rectus capitis posterior major
Rectus capitis posterior minor
Oblique capitis superior
Semispinalis capitis
Longissimus capitis (assists)*
Longissimus cervicis (assists)*
Iliocostalis cervicis (assists)*
Multifidi (bilaterally)*
Rotatores (bilaterally)*
Intertransversarii (bilaterally)*
Interspinalis*

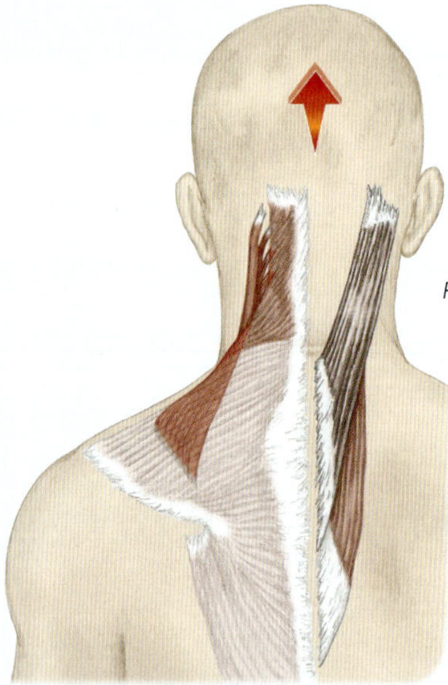

5.36 Extension of the cervical spine

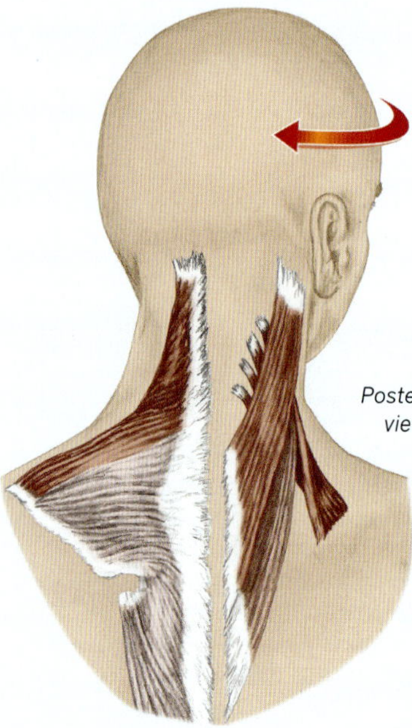

5.37 Rotation of the cervical spine

Rotation
(unilaterally to the same side)

Levator scapula
Splenius capitis
Splenius cervicis
Rectus capitis posterior major*
Oblique capitis inferior*
Longus colli*
Longus capitis*
Longissimus capitis (assists)*
Longissimus cervicis (assists)*
Iliocostalis cervicis (assists)*

Rotation
(unilaterally to the opposite side)

Trapezius (upper fibers)
Sternocleidomastoid
Anterior scalene
Middle scalene
Posterior scalene
Multifidi*
Rotatores*

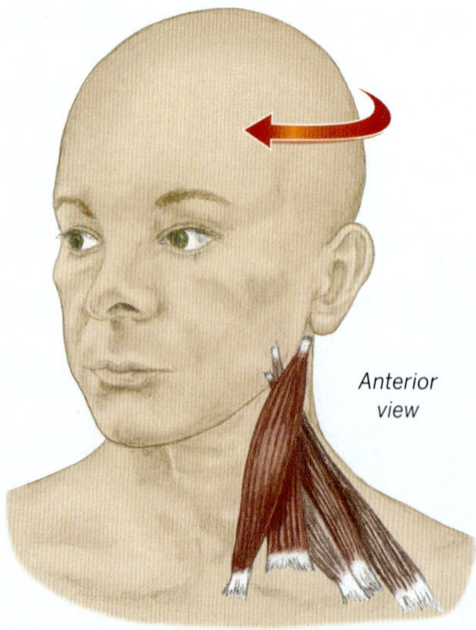

5.38 Rotation of the cervical spine

Cervical Spine

Lateral Flexion
(unilaterally to the same side)

- Trapezius (upper fibers)
- Levator scapula
- Sternocleidomastoid
- Anterior scalene (with ribs fixed)
- Middle scalene (with ribs fixed)
- Posterior scalene (with ribs fixed)
- Splenius capitis
- Splenius cervicis
- Longus capitis
- Longus colli
- Longissimus capitis (assists)*
- Longissimus cervicis (assists)*
- Iliocostalis cervicis (assists)*
- Oblique capitis superior*
- Intertransversarii*

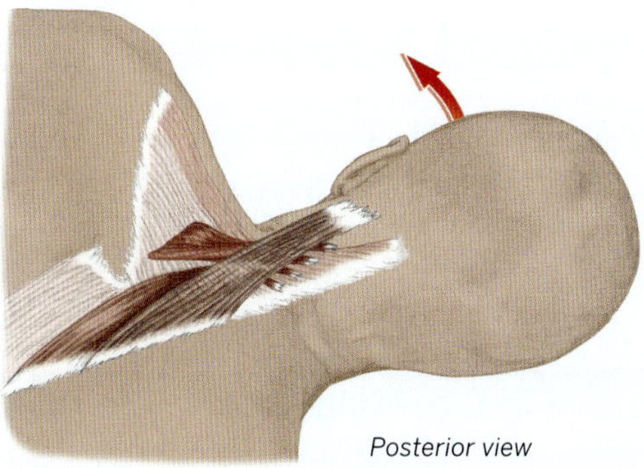

5.39 Lateral flexion of the cervical spine

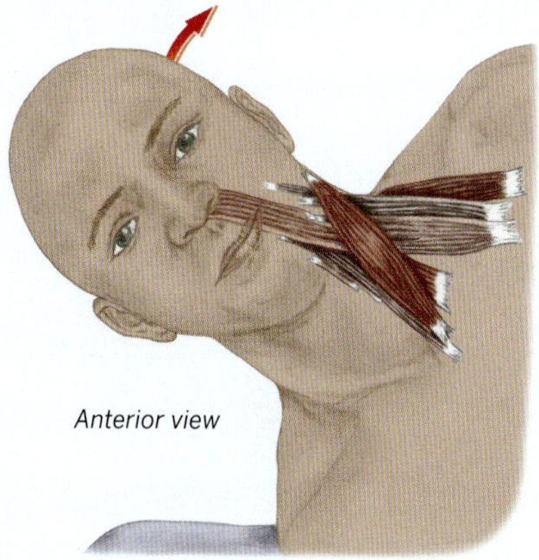

5.40 Lateral flexion of the cervical spine

Mandible
(temporomandibular joint)

Elevation
(antagonists on depression)

- Masseter
- Temporalis
- Medial pterygoid

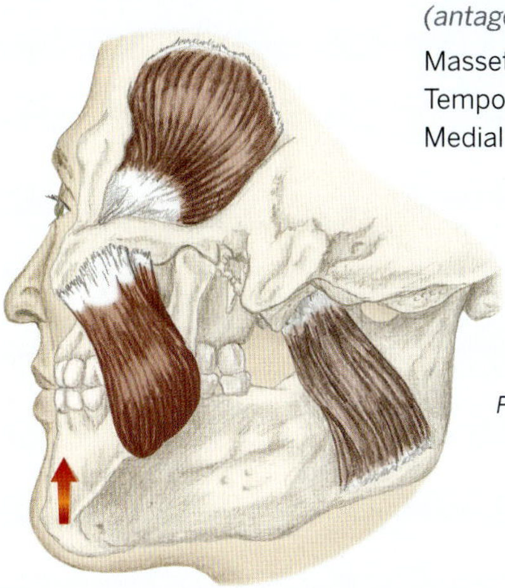

5.41 Elevation of the mandible

Depression
(antagonists on elevation)

- Geniohyoid*
- Mylohyoid*
- Stylohyoid
- Digastric (with hyoid bone fixed)
- Platysma (assists)

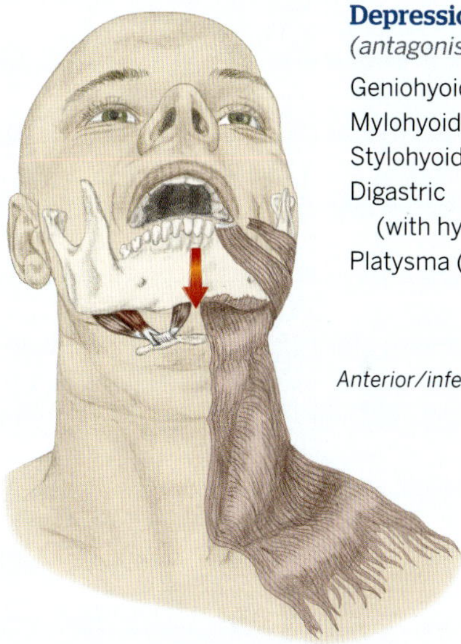

5.42 Depression of the mandible

Protraction
(antagonists on retraction)

- Lateral pterygoid (bilaterally)
- Medial pterygoid (bilaterally)
- Masseter (assists)*

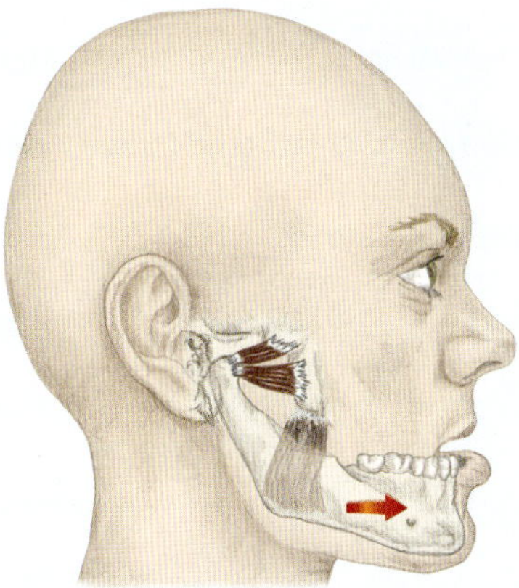

5.43 Protraction of the mandible

Retraction
(antagonists on protraction)

- Temporalis
- Digastric

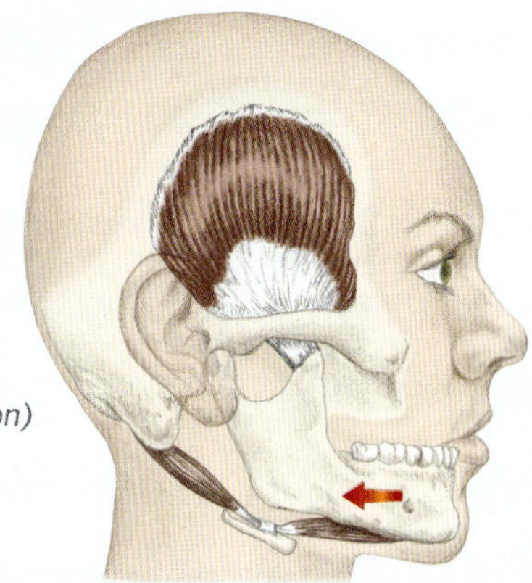

5.44 Retraction of the mandible

See p. 432 for synergists of lateral deviation of the mandible.

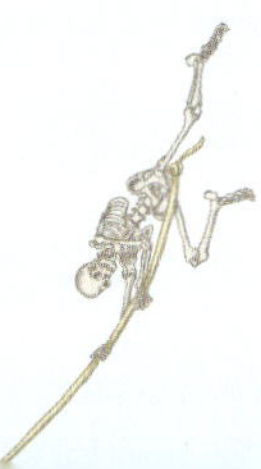

Muscles of the Head, Neck, and Face

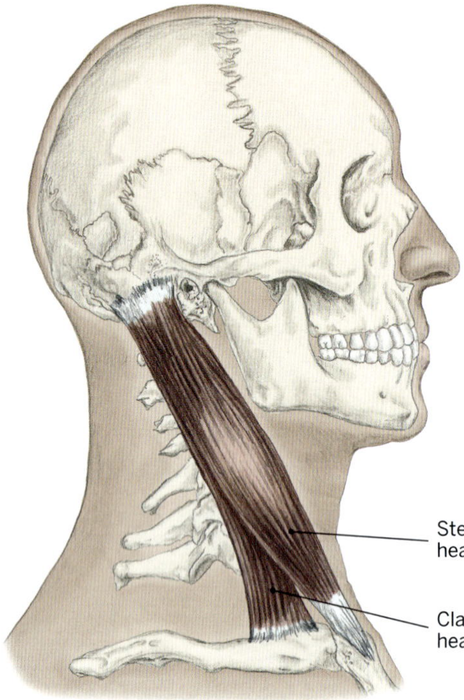

5.45 Lateral view of head and neck, showing sternocleidomastoid

Sternocleidomastoid ▶

The sternocleidomastoid (SCM) is located on the lateral and anterior aspects of the neck. It has a large belly with two heads: a flat, clavicular head and a slender, sternal head (**5.45**). Both heads merge to attach behind the ear at the mastoid process (**5.46**). The carotid artery (p. 271) passes deep and medial to the SCM; the external jugular vein lies superficial to it. The SCM is also superficial, completely accessible, and often visible when the head is turned to the side in Lord Byron–like fashion (**5.47**).

	STERNOCLEIDOMASTOID
A	*Unilaterally:* **Laterally flex** the head and neck to the same side **Rotate** the head and neck to the opposite side *Bilaterally:* **Flex** the neck Assist to **elevate** the rib cage during inhalation
O	***Sternal head:*** Top of manubrium ***Clavicular head:*** Medial one-third of the clavicle
I	Mastoid process of temporal bone and the lateral portion of superior nuchal line of occiput
N	Spinal accessory (XI) nerve, C**2**, 3

When Do You Use Your Sternocleidomastoid?

- Shaking your head "no" (opposite side rotation)
- Shaking your head "yes" (bilateral flexion)
- Stabilizing the head while riding a roller coaster
- Cocking your head to hear what someone is saying

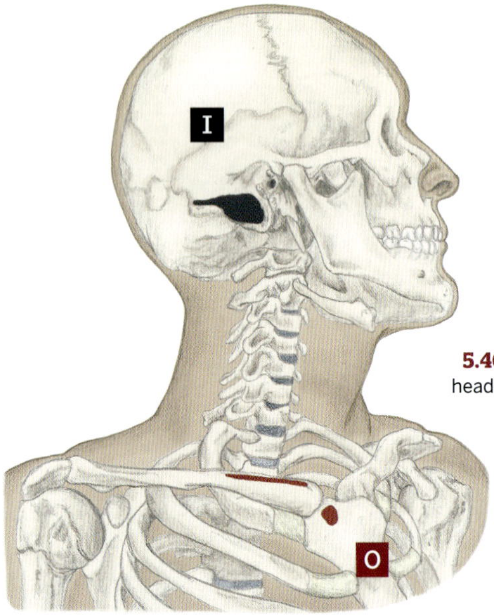

5.46 Lateral view of head and neck, with head rotated to the left, showing origin and insertion of sternocleidomastoid

The power of thought, the magic of the mind...

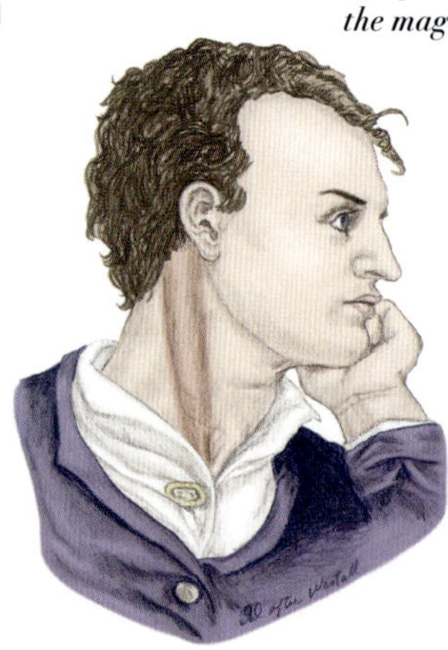

5.47 Lord Byron showing off the sternal head of his SCM

Discover More

The sternocleidomastoid and upper fibers of the trapezius (p. 64) begin as one muscle in the embryo and then split later on in development. The location of their attachments hints at their initial relationship: They form an almost continuous tendon along the superior nuchal line and mastoid process. Their other attachments are at either end of the clavicle.

sternocleidomastoid	***ster***-no-***kli***-do-***mas***-toyd	
jugular	***jug***-u-lar	L. throat

Sternocleidomastoid

1. Partner supine with practitioner at head of the table. Locate the mastoid process of the temporal bone, the medial clavicle, and the top of the sternum.
2. Draw an imaginary line between these landmarks to delineate the location of the SCM. Note how both SCMs form a V on the front of the neck.
3. Ask your partner to raise his head very slightly off the table as you palpate the SCM (**5.48**). It will usually protrude visibly. (To make the SCM more distinct, rotate the head slightly to the opposite side and then ask your partner to flex his neck.)
4. Palpate along the borders of the SCM, following it behind the earlobe and then down to the clavicle and sternum (**5.49**). Sculpt around the skinny sternal tendon and the wider clavicular tendon (**5.50**).

With your partner relaxed, can you grasp the SCM between your fingers and outline its thickness and shape? How much space is between the clavicular attachments of the SCM and trapezius? It should be roughly two to three inches.

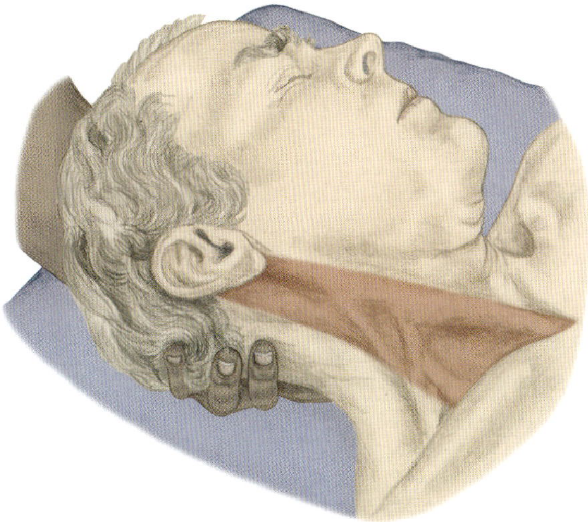

5.48 Partner supine, flexing his head slightly to engage the SCM while you palpate this muscle

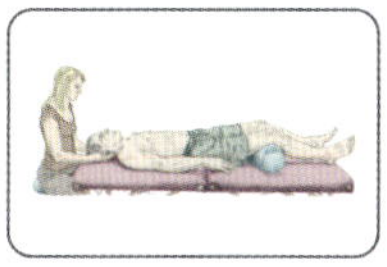

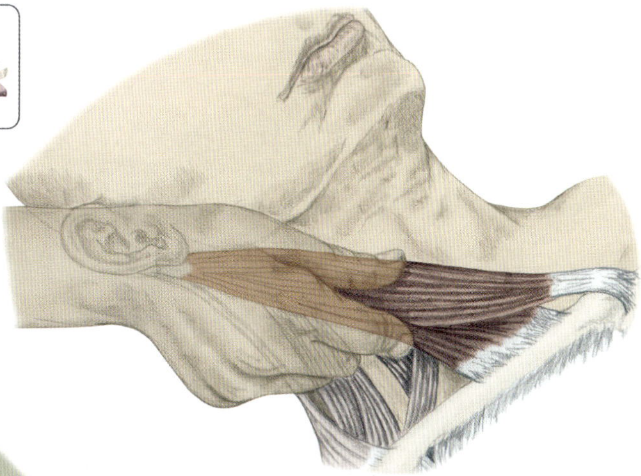

5.49 Partner supine, as you grasp the bellies of the SCM

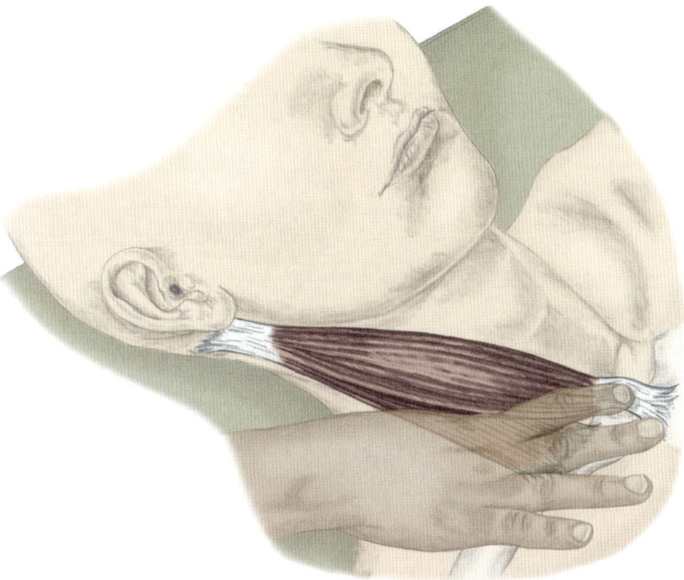

5.50 Partner supine, as you strum across the sternal tendon of the SCM

Since the carotid artery passes deep to the SCM, you might feel its strong pulse beneath (or between) your grasping fingers. If so, simply release and reposition your hand to ensure that the vessel is not impinged.

Scalenes ▶

Anterior
Middle
Posterior

The three scalenes are sandwiched between the sternocleidomastoid and the anterior flap of the trapezius on the anterior, lateral neck. Their fibers begin at the side of the cervical vertebrae, dive underneath the clavicle and attach to the first and second ribs (**5.51**, **5.52**; see also **5.57**). During normal inhalation, the scalenes perform the vital task of elevating the upper ribs.

The **anterior scalene** (**5.54**) lies partially tucked beneath the sternocleidomastoid. The **middle scalene** (**5.55**) is slightly larger and lies lateral to the anterior scalene. Both muscle bellies are directly accessible. The smaller **posterior scalene** (**5.56**) is located between the middle scalene and levator scapula. The posterior scalene is positioned deeper than the other scalenes. Due to its small size and buried location, the posterior scalene can be difficult to distinguish from the surrounding bellies.

The large branches of the brachial plexus and subclavian artery pass through a small gap between the anterior and middle scalenes. Individual nerves of the brachial plexus may penetrate through or in front of the anterior scalene (see **5.53**).

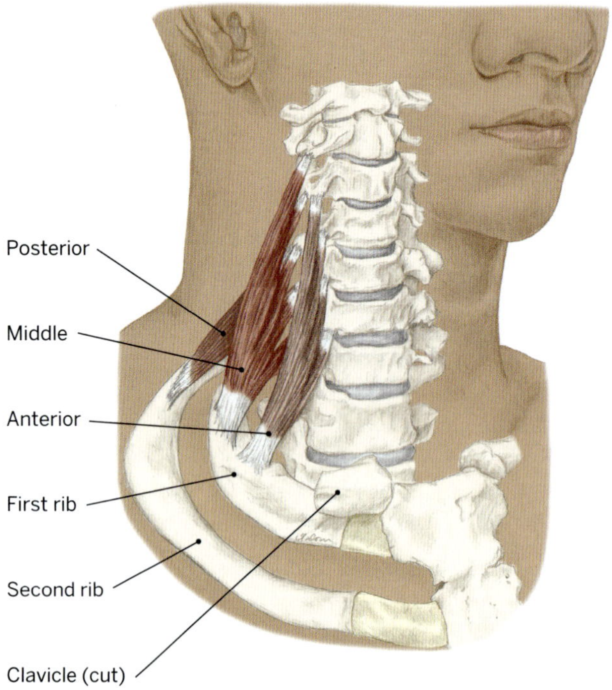

5.51 Anterior/lateral view of neck, showing scalenes

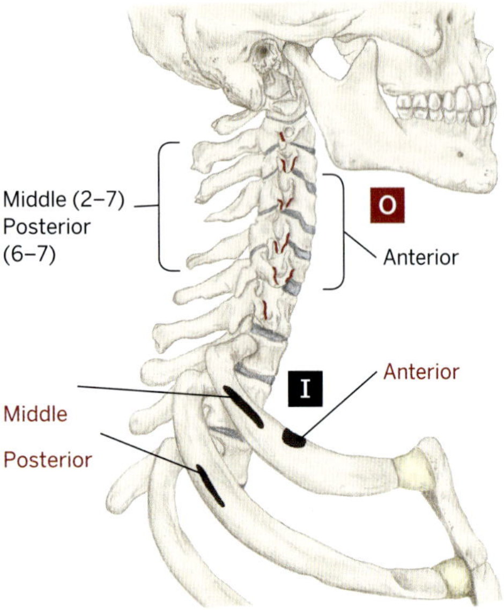

5.52 Lateral view of neck, showing origins insertions of scalenes

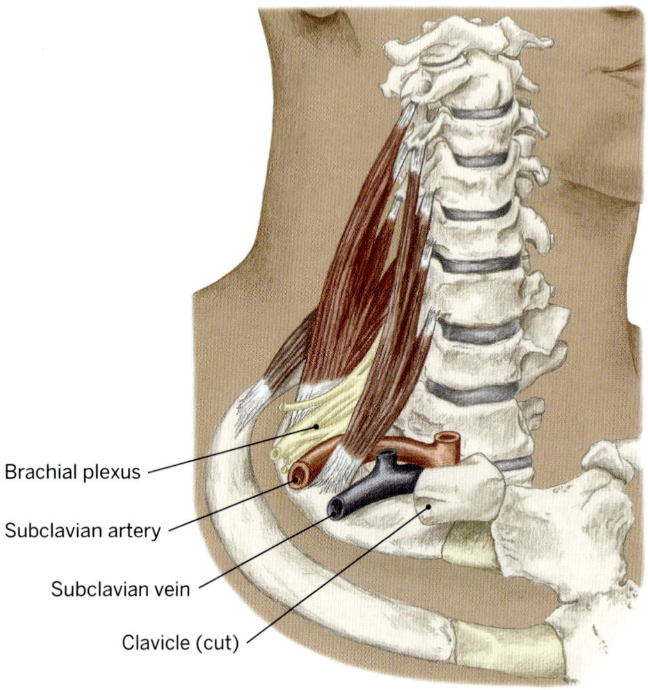

5.53 Anterior/lateral view of neck, showing brachial plexus and subclavian artery and vein

scalene *skay*-leen Grk. uneven

ALL SCALENES

A

Unilaterally:

With the ribs fixed, **laterally flex** the head and neck to the same side (all)

Rotate head and neck to the opposite side (all)

Bilaterally:

Elevate the ribs during inhalation (all)

Flex the head and neck (anterior)

When Do You Use Your Scalenes?

- Taking a deep breath into the upper chest
- Tipping your head to the side when trying to get water out of your ear
- Stabilizing your head when reading in a reclined position

ANTERIOR SCALENE

O Transverse processes of third through sixth cervical vertebrae (anterior tubercles)

I First rib

N C(3), **4–8**

MIDDLE SCALENE

O Transverse processes of second through seventh cervical vertebrae (posterior tubercles)

I First rib

N C(3), **4–8**

POSTERIOR SCALENE

O Transverse processes of sixth and seventh cervical vertebrae (posterior tubercles)

I Second rib

N C(3), **4–8**

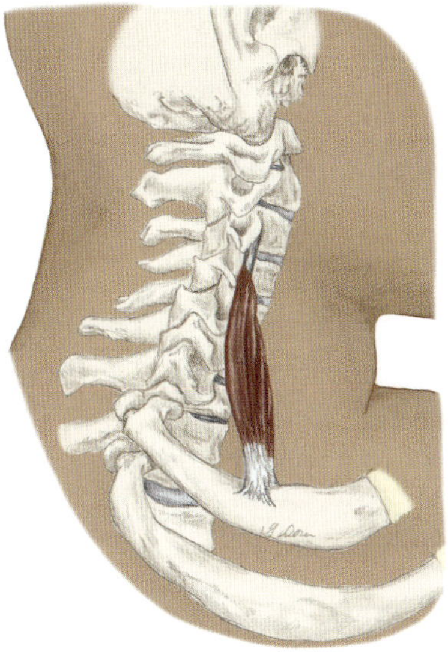

5.54 Lateral view of neck, showing anterior scalene

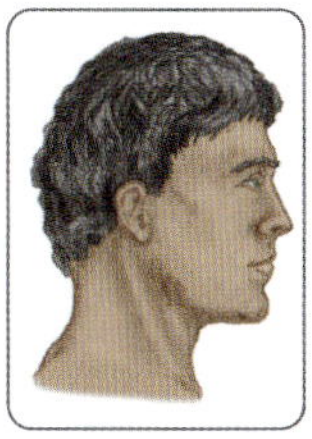

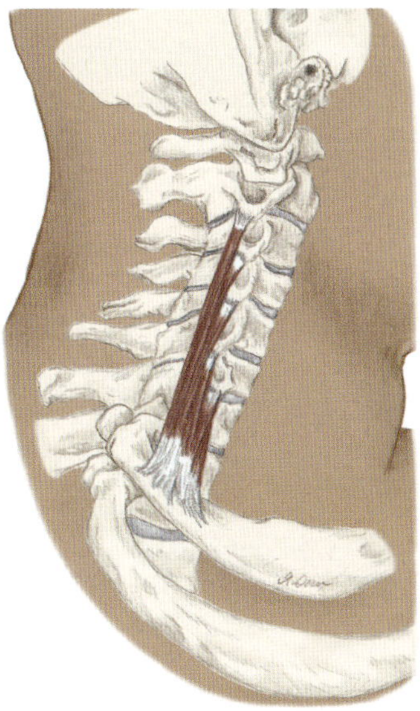

5.55 Lateral view of neck, showing middle scalene

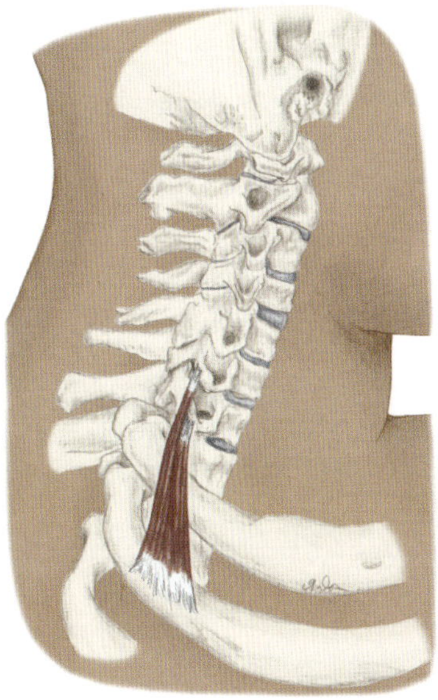

5.56 Lateral view of neck, showing posterior scalene

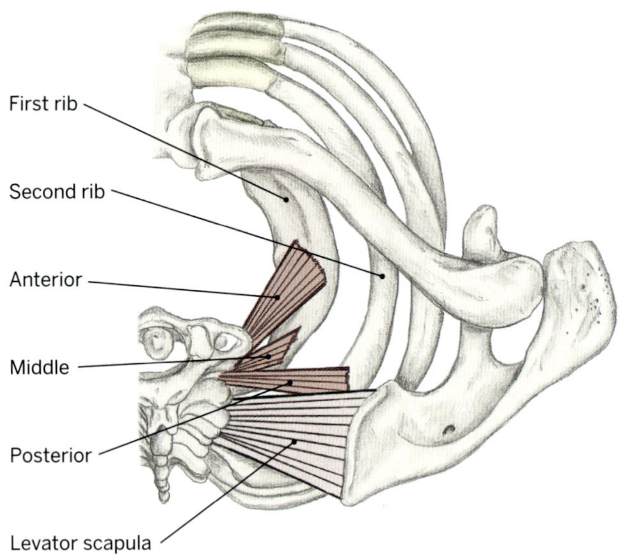

5.57 Superior view of thorax, showing the fiber direction of the scalenes and levator scapula. Muscles are not to scale.

Scalenes as a group

1. Partner supine, with practitioner at head of the table. Cradle the head (passively flexing it) to allow for easier palpation. Place your fingerpads along the anterior and lateral sides of the neck between the SCM and trapezius.
2. With the pads of your fingers, use gentle pressure to palpate the stringy, superficial muscle bellies in this triangle.

*Are you between the SCM and trapezius? Ask your partner to inhale deeply into her upper chest. As she fully inhales, do you feel the muscles in this triangle contract (**5.58**)?*

Anterior and middle scalenes

1. Partner supine. Because the anterior scalene lies partially deep to the lateral edge of the SCM, rotate the head slightly to the opposite side to better expose it. Gently palpate under the SCM's lateral edge and roll across the belly of the anterior scalene (**5.59**).
2. Follow it inferiorly as it tucks under the clavicle.
3. Move laterally to explore the middle scalene, noting its similarly shaped belly (**5.60**).

Do the muscles you feel have a slender, stringy texture? If you follow them inferiorly, do they sink beneath the clavicle (in the direction of the ribs)? Can you follow them superiorly to the transverse processes of the cervical vertebrae? Ask your partner to flex her head slightly. Can you feel the scalenes contract?

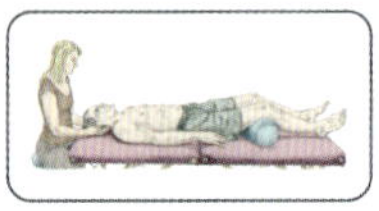

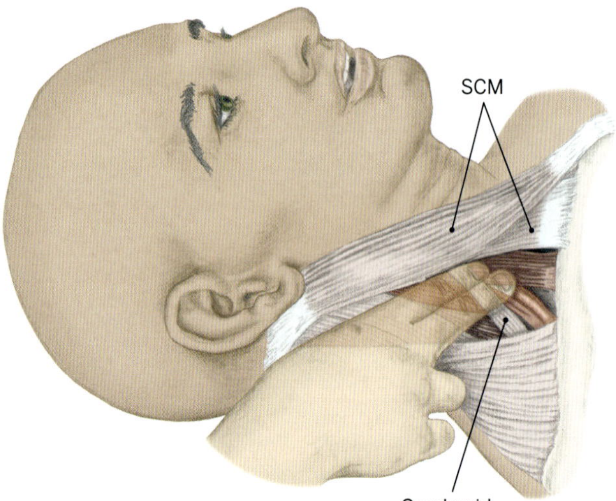

5.58 Partner supine, inhaling while you feel the scalenes contract

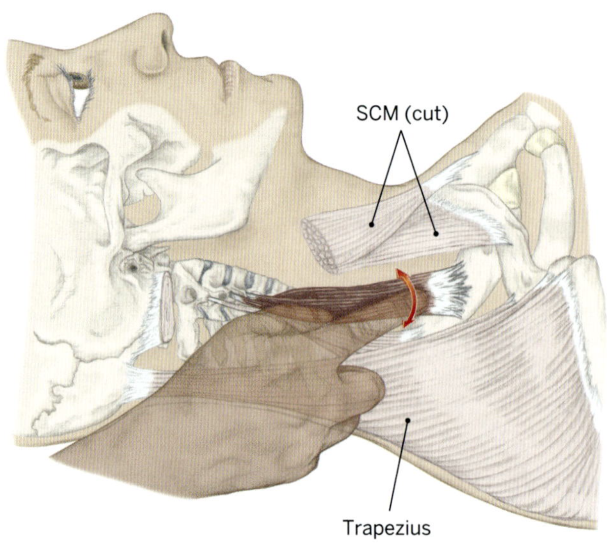

5.59 Partner supine, as you roll across the anterior scalene

Compression or impingement of the brachial plexus or one of its nerves can send a sharp, shooting sensation or numbness down the arm. If this should occur, immediately release and adjust your position posteriorly. Be sure to ask your partner for feedback while palpating the scalene muscles.

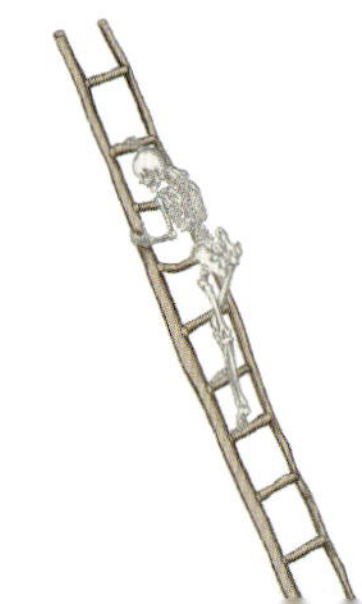

Posterior scalene

1. Partner supine. The posterior scalene extends laterally off the neck and is squeezed between the middle scalene and levator scapula (p. 79).
2. Locate the middle scalene and the levator scapula. Place a finger between these bellies and sink inferiorly (**5.61**).
3. Slowly strum across the thin band of tissue running laterally from the transverse processes to the second rib.

To distinguish between the posterior scalene and levator scapula, locate the posterior scalene and ask your partner to slowly elevate her scapula. Since the posterior scalene does not create this action, there should be no contraction of its fibers. However, if you ask your partner to slowly inhale into her upper chest, you should feel the posterior scalene contract.

All scalenes

Partner prone. Begin by isolating the edge of the upper fibers of the trapezius (p. 64). Then curl your fingers around the anterior edge of the trapezius into the tissue of the lateral neck (**5.62**). The levator scapula will be just anterior to the trapezius, followed by the posterior and middle scalenes.

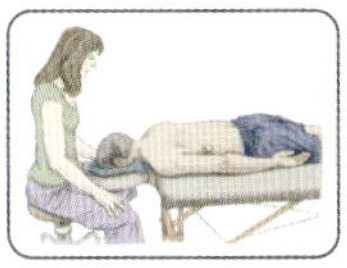

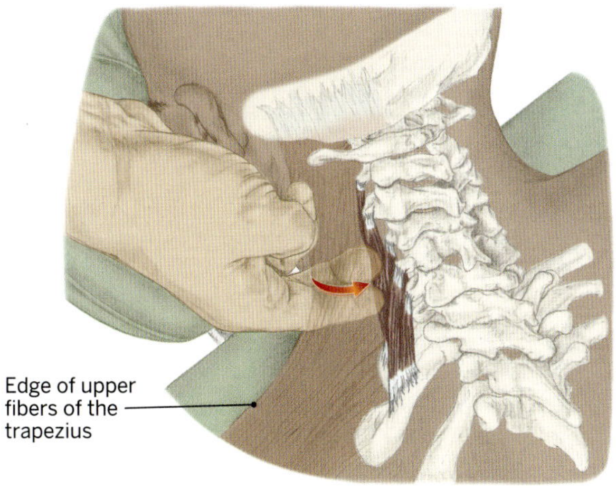

5.62 Partner prone, posterior/lateral view, as you palpate the middle and posterior scalenes

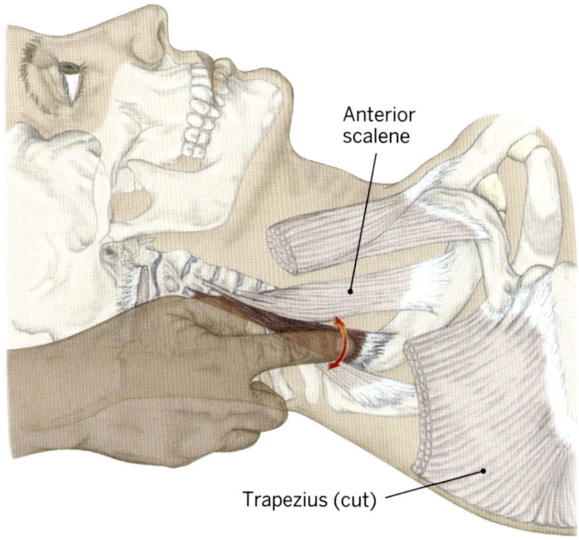

5.60 Partner supine, as you strum across the middle scalene

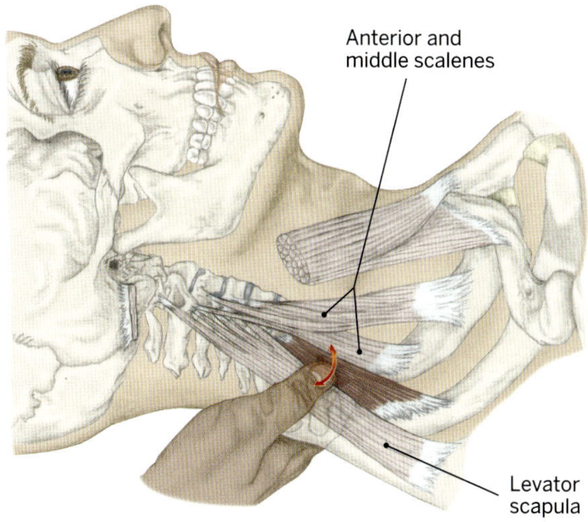

5.61 Partner supine, as you palpate the posterior scalene

Discover More

The existence of a fourth muscle, the scalene minimus, is one of several variations on the scalene muscle group. Present in roughly 40% of the population, the minimus often attaches from the sixth and seventh cervical vertebrae to the first rib or pleural dome of the lung. Lying inferior and deep to the anterior scalene, this muscle may nevertheless be quite strong.

Masseter ▶

The masseter is the strongest muscle in the body relative to its size. The two masseters together exert a biting force of nearly one hundred and fifty pounds of pressure—enough to bite off a finger! The masseter is the primary chewing muscle and is used in speaking and swallowing.

Located on the side of the mandible, the square-shaped masseter is composed of two overlapping bellies. The superficial belly can be accessed from the face (**5.63**); the deep belly is palpable from inside the mouth (**5.64**). The masseter is situated deep to the parotid gland (p. 272) yet is easily palpable.

	MASSETER
A	**Elevate** the mandible (temporomandibular joint) May assist to **protract** the mandible (TM joint)
O	Zygomatic arch
I	Angle and ramus of mandible
N	Trigeminal (V) nerve (mandibular division)

When Do You Use Your Masseter?

- Talking, gabbing, chin wagging, or chewing the fat
- Chomping down on a wad of gum
- Gnashing your teeth together during an argument

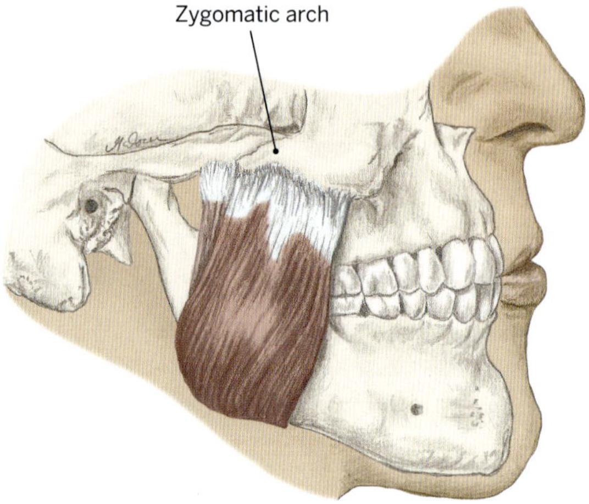

5.63 Lateral view of jaw, showing superficial head of masseter

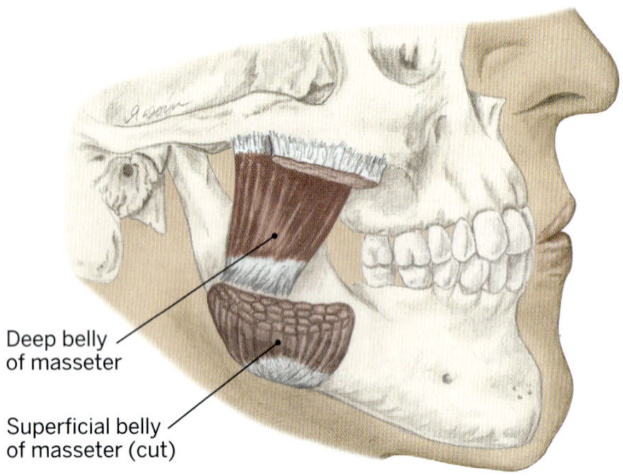

5.64 Lateral view of jaw, showing superficial and deep bellies of masseter

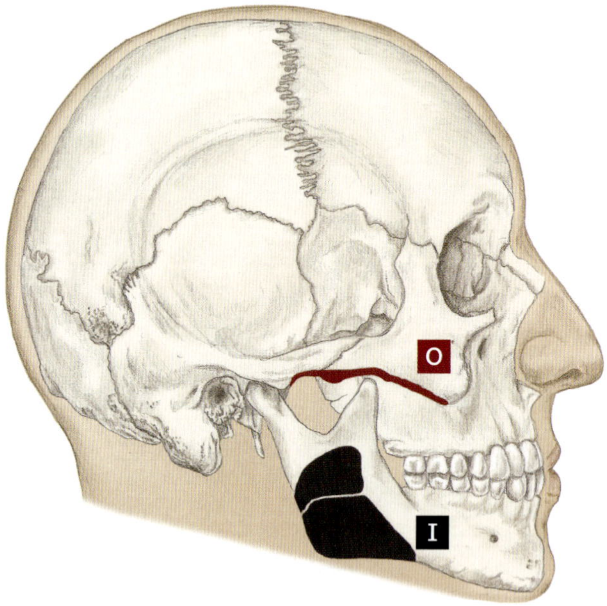

5.65 Lateral view of cranium, showing origin and insertion of masseter

masseter *mas*-se-ter Grk. chewer

Head, Neck & Face

Masseter

1. Partner supine. Locate the zygomatic arch and angle of the mandible. Place your fingers between these bony landmarks and palpate the surface of the masseter.
2. Ask your partner to alternately clench and relax her jaw as you sculpt out the square shape of the belly (**5.66**). Clarify the masseter's fiber direction by strumming your fingers horizontally across its muscle fibers.
3. Now ask your partner to relax and try grasping the chunky bellies of the masseter (**5.67**).

As your partner clenches her jaw, can you outline the anterior edge of the masseter? If your partner opens her jaw as wide as possible, can you feel the tissue lengthen?

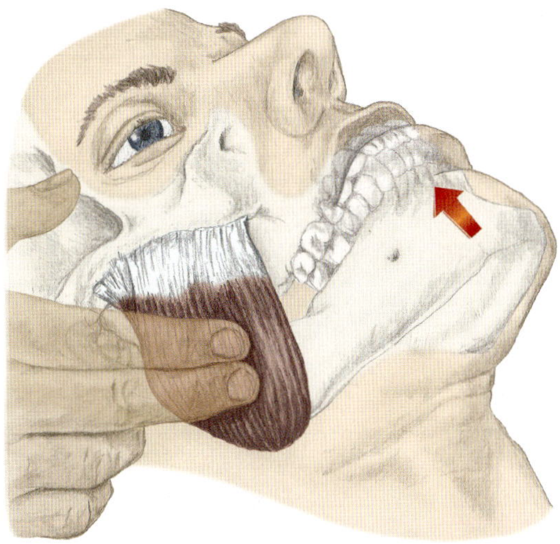

5.66 Partner supine, clenching her jaw while you palpate the masseter

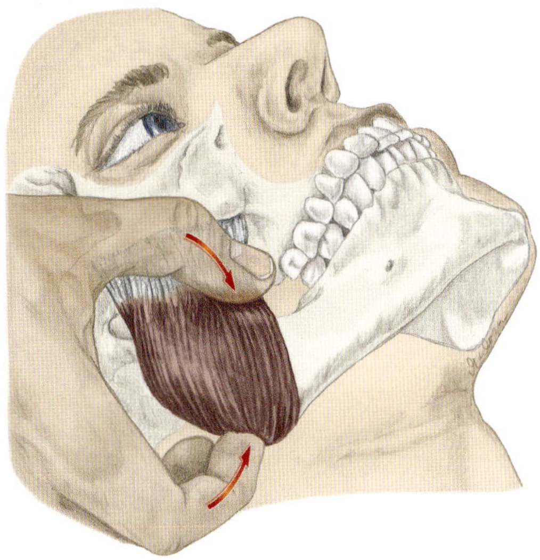

5.67 Partner supine, relaxing her jaw while you grasp the masseter

Temporalis ▶

The temporalis muscle is located on the temporal aspect of the cranium. Its broad origin attaches to the frontal, temporal, and parietal bones. Its fibers converge in a thick mass, reaching under the zygomatic arch to connect at the coronoid process (**5.68**, **5.69**). Though deep to the temporal fascia and artery, the temporalis is superficial and directly accessible.

	TEMPORALIS
A	**Elevate** the mandible (temporomandibular joint) **Retract** the mandible (TM joint)
O	Temporal fossa and fascia
I	Coronoid process and anterior edge of ramus of the mandible
N	Trigeminal (V) nerve (mandibular division)

When Do You Use Your Temporalis?

- Ripping off a piece of beef jerky with your teeth
- Chewing that beef jerky
- Grinding your teeth while you sleep, dreaming about beef jerky

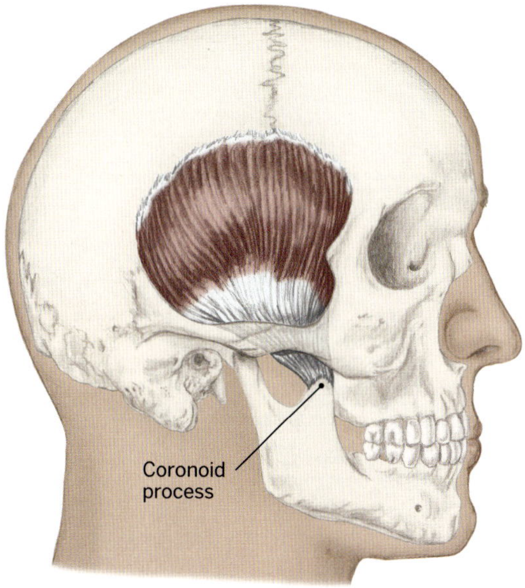

5.68 Lateral view of cranium, showing temporalis

temporalis *tem*-po-*ra*-lis L. time, seen by the graying of hairs in this region

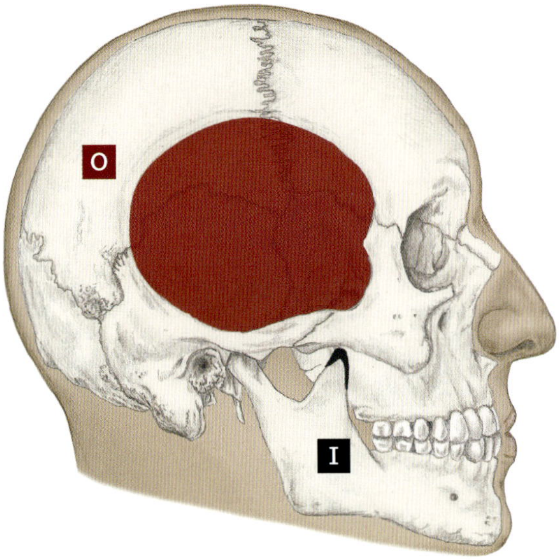

5.69 Lateral view of cranium, showing origin and insertion of temporalis

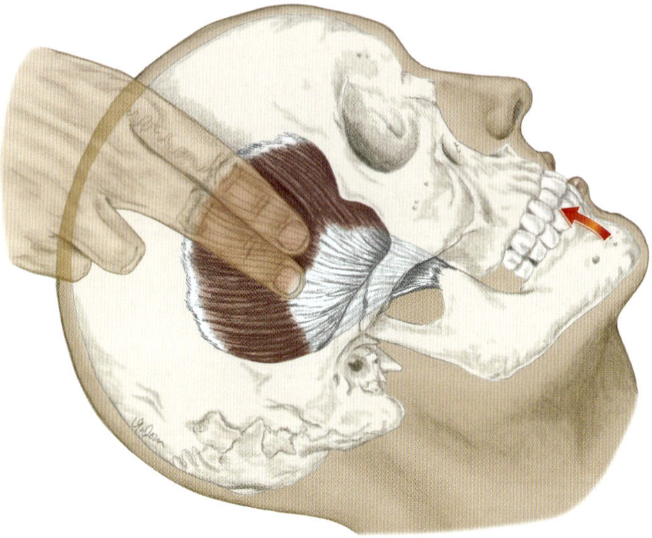

5.70 Partner supine, clenching her jaw while you feel the temporalis contract

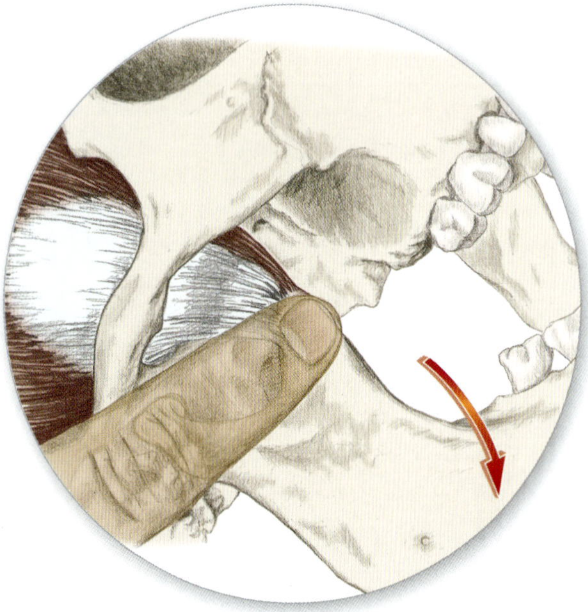

5.71 Partner supine with jaw open, lateral view, as you isolate the temporalis tendon at the coronoid process of the mandible

Temporalis

1. Partner supine with practitioner at head of the table. Locate the zygomatic arch.
2. Place your fingerpads one inch superior to the arch and ask your partner to alternately clench and relax her jaw. Do you feel the strong temporalis contracting beneath your fingers (**5.70**)?
3. To locate the insertion site of the temporalis tendon, ask your partner to open her mouth wide.
4. Locate and explore the coronoid process (**5.71**). Although the coronoid process is easily accessed, you may not be able to isolate the tendon of the temporalis.

When exploring the muscle belly, are you superior to the zygomatic arch on the side of the head? Can you discern the direction of the muscle fibers and feel them converge?

To outline the wide origin of the temporalis, place your fingers in various positions on the side of the head and ask your partner to alternately clench and relax her jaw. If your fingers are on the muscle, you will feel the temporalis fibers tighten and soften. If you are off the muscle, you will feel nothing.

Suprahyoids and Digastric ▶

The suprahyoids (**geniohyoid**, **mylohyoid**, and **stylohyoid**) form a wall of muscle along the underside of the jaw (**5.72**, **5.73**). Stretching from the edge of the mandible to the hyoid bone, they lie inferior to the glossus muscles (the muscles of the tongue).

Even though each of the three suprahyoids is quite small, collectively they affect the tongue and hyoid bone and are important in chewing, swallowing, and speaking. They are partially deep to the digastric muscle, yet are accessible. The suprahyoid bellies cannot be individually distinguished.

The long, round **digastric** muscle is composed of a posterior and an anterior belly. The posterior belly runs from the mastoid process to the hyoid bone (penetrating through the stylohyoid) and then loops through a tendinous sling on the hyoid's anterior surface. It continues on as the anterior belly to attach at the underside of the mandible (**5.74**). Both bellies are superficial, yet they are difficult to distinguish from the deeper suprahyoid muscles.

SUPRAHYOIDS

A	**Elevate** hyoid and tongue **Depress** mandible (temporomandibular joint)
O	***Geniohyoid, mylohyoid:*** Underside of mandible ***Stylohyoid:*** Styloid process
I	Hyoid bone
N	***Geniohyoid:*** C1, 2 ***Mylohyoid:*** Trigeminal (V) ***Stylohyoid:*** Facial (VII)

When Do You Use Your Suprahyoids?

- Chewing, swallowing, sucking on a straw
- Singing and speaking, since their actions affect the position of the larynx (voice box)

DIGASTRIC

A	With hyoid bone fixed, **depress** the mandible (temporomandibular joint) With mandible fixed, **elevate** the hyoid bone **Retract** the mandible (TM joint)
O	Mastoid process (deep to sternocleidomastoid and splenius capitis)
I	Inferior border of the mandible
N	***Anterior belly:*** Trigeminal (V) (mandibular division) ***Posterior belly:*** Facial (VII)

When Do You Use Your Digastric?

- Chewing, swallowing, sucking on a straw
- Singing and speaking, since their actions affect the position of the larynx (voice box)

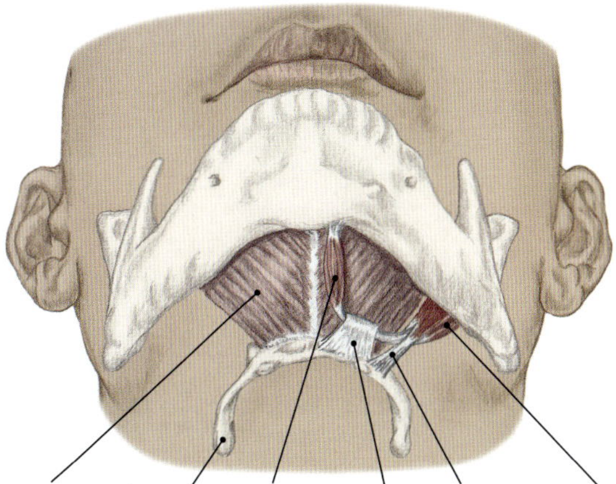

5.72 Anterior/inferior view of jaw, showing suprahyoids and digastric, with geniohyoid deep to mylohyoid

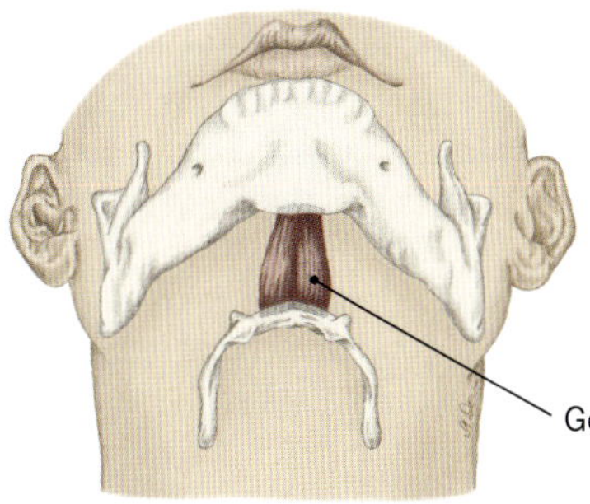

5.73 Anterior/inferior view of jaw, showing geniohyoid

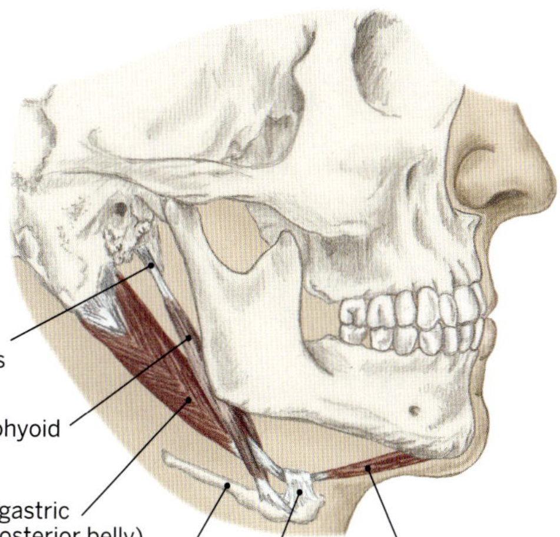

5.74 Lateral view of jaw, showing digastric (highlighted in dark red)

geniohyoid	*je*-ne-o-*hi*-oyd	Grk. *genion*, chin
glossus	*glah*-sis	Grk. tongue

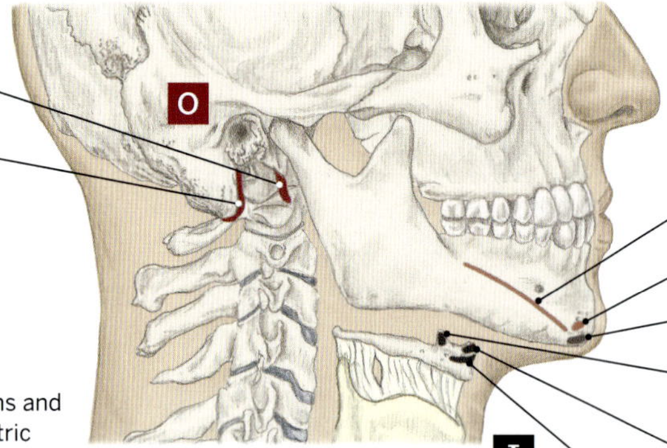

5.75 Lateral view of jaw, showing origins and insertions of suprahyoids and digastric

Suprahyoids

1. Partner supine. With your partner's jaw closed, place your finger along the underside of the mandible.
2. Contract the suprahyoids by asking your partner to press the tip of her tongue firmly against the roof of her mouth. Note how this action forms a wall of taut muscle along the base of the mandible (jawline). Follow it as it extends down to the hyoid bone (**5.76**).
3. With the tongue relaxed, palpate the flat surface of the suprahyoid tissues, distinguishing them from the lumpy texture of the submandibular gland (p. 272).

If you place a fingerpad underneath the tip of the chin and ask your partner to gently depress her mandible into your finger, do the suprahyoids contract? Also, ask your partner to swallow as you palpate the suprahyoids. Do these tissues contract?

Digastric

1. Partner supine with practitioner at head of table. Locate the mastoid process of the temporal bone and the hyoid bone.
2. Draw an imaginary line between these points. Using your index finger, palpate along this line for the skinny, posterior digastric (**5.77**).
3. Draw an imaginary line between the hyoid bone to the underside of the chin and palpate for its anterior belly.
4. To feel the digastric contract, place your finger under the chin and ask your partner to try to open her mouth against your gentle resistance. This contraction will sometimes allow both of the digastric bellies to be located more easily.

Is the muscle you are palpating superficial and pencil-width? Does it extend from the mastoid process to the hyoid bone to the chin?

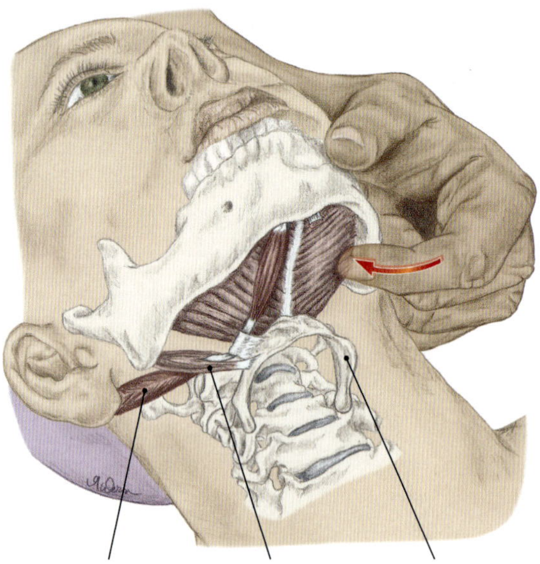

5.76 Partner supine, as you curl your finger around the mandible to palpate the mylohyoid

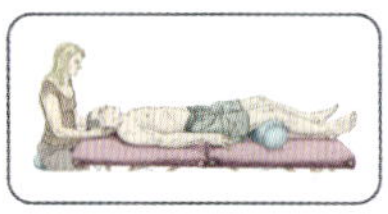

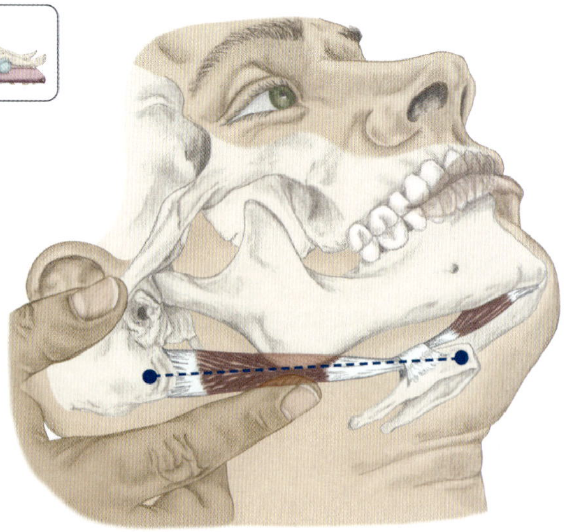

5.77 Partner supine, as you isolate the digastric between the mastoid process and the hyoid bone

digastric	di-***gas***-trik	Grk. double-bellied
mylohyoid	***my***-lo-***hi***-oyd	Grk. *myle*, mill
stylohyoid	***sti***-lo-***hi***-oyd	

Infrahyoids ▸

The infrahyoids are located on the anterior neck, superficial to the trachea (**5.78**). All four muscles are thin and delicate and function as antagonists to the suprahyoids. The superficial **sternohyoid** (**5.79**) and **sternothyroid** (**5.80**) are layered just to the side of the trachea and, although difficult to distinguish individually, are directly accessible. Deep to these two muscles is the **thyrohyoid** (**5.80**). As its name suggests, it spans from the thyroid cartilage to the hyoid bone.

The **omohyoid** (**5.81**) is perhaps the most bizarre muscle in the body. It has a skinny, ribbonlike belly running from the hyoid bone, passing underneath the SCM and scalenes, to the scapula. Aside from depressing the hyoid, the omohyoid tightens the fascia of the neck and dilates the internal jugular vein. Because of its depth and slender belly, the omohyoid is mostly inaccessible.

INFRAHYOIDS	
A	**Depress** the hyoid bone and thyroid cartilage
O	***Sternohyoid and sternothyroid:*** Top of manubrium ***Thyrohyoid:*** Thyroid cartilage ***Omohyoid:*** Superior border of the scapula
I	***Sternohyoid, thyrohyoid, and omohyoid:*** Hyoid bone ***Sternothyroid:*** Thyroid cartilage
N	***Sternohyoid, sternothyroid, and omohyoid:*** C1, 2, 3 ***Thyrohyoid:*** C1, 2

When Do You Use Your Infrahyoids?

- Drinking and swallowing
- Speaking (through their opposing action with the suprahyoids)
- Tightening the tissue of the anterior neck when threatened

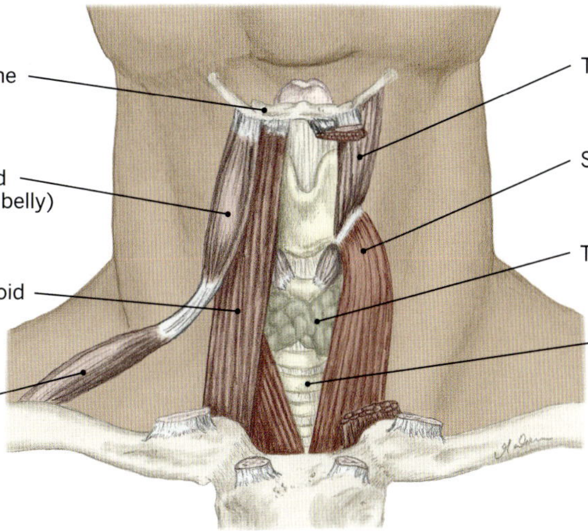

5.78 Anterior view of neck, SCM removed, showing infrahyoids

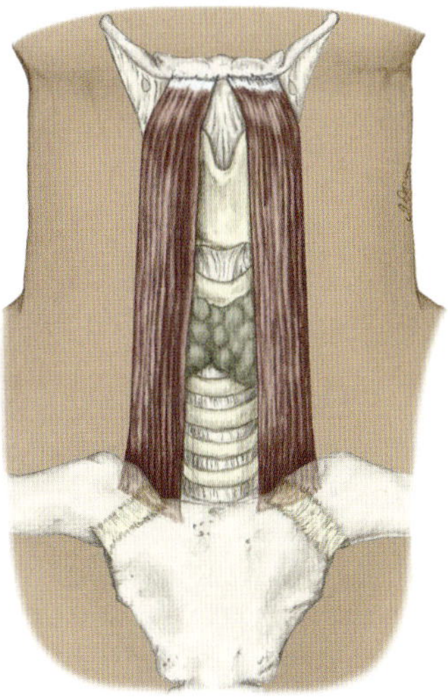

5.79 Anterior view of neck, showing sternohyoid

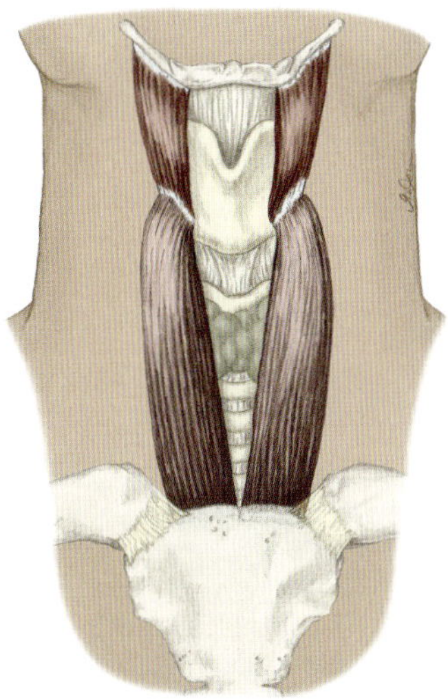

5.80 Anterior view of neck, showing thyrohyoid (top) and sternothyroid (below)

omohyoid	*o*-mo-***hi***-oyd	Grk. *omos*, shoulder
sternohyoid	*ster*-no-***hi***-oyd	
sternothyroid	*ster*-no-***thi***-royd	

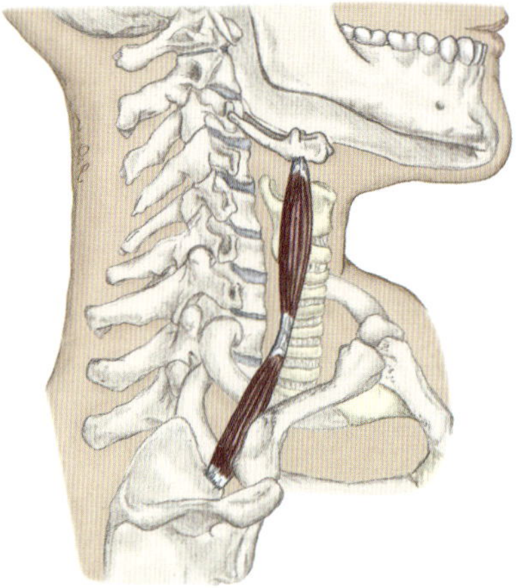

5.81 Lateral view of neck and right shoulder, showing omohyoid

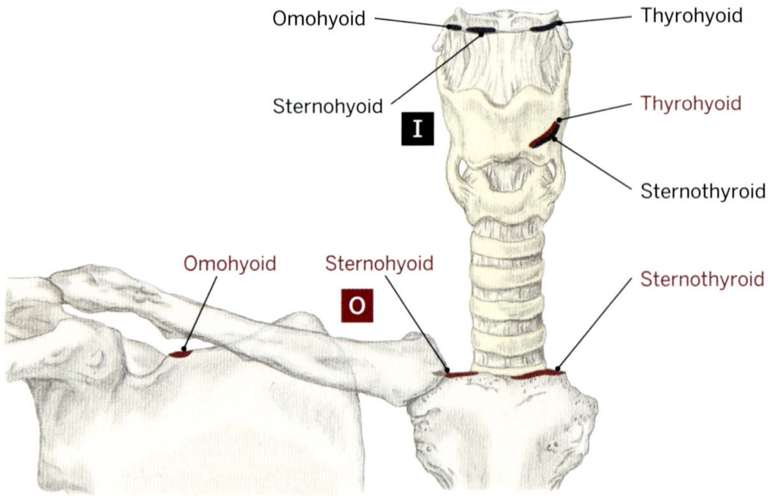

5.82 Anterior view of neck and right shoulder, showing origins (in **red**) and insertions (in **black**) of infrahyoids

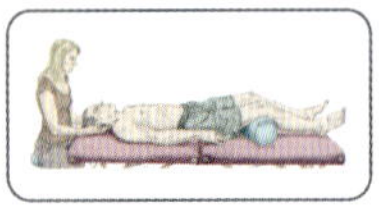

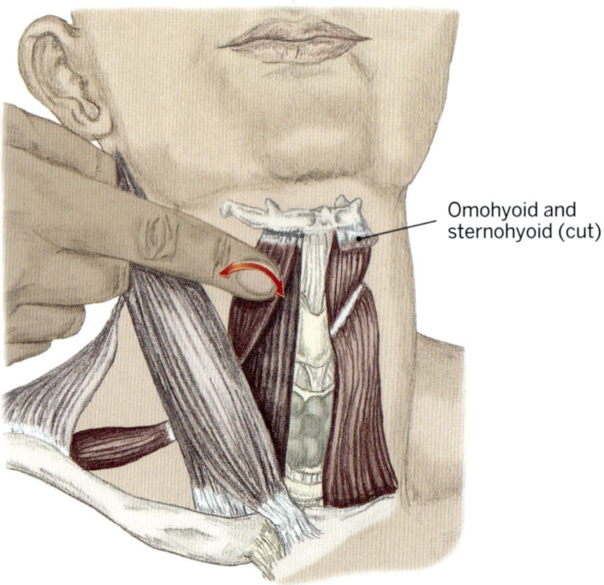

5.83 Partner supine, as you palpate the infrahyoids

Sternohyoid and sternothyroid

1. A hand (or two) on the front of the neck can be unnerving, so put your partner at ease by exploring with one hand at a time and then using only one fingerpad. Also, to avoid irritating the thyroid gland, explore only the superior half of these muscles.
2. Partner supine. Locate the surface of the trachea, just below the thyroid cartilage (Adam's apple). With one fingerpad, slide lateral to the trachea and gently explore the thin tissue lying superficial to the windpipe. Try to roll your finger across the thin bellies of the infrahyoids (**5.83**).
3. Ask your partner to tighten the muscles of the anterior neck. Sometimes this isometric contraction will make the infrahyoids quite solid and easily palpable.

Comparative Anatomy

A giraffe's trachea is formed by more than a hundred tracheal rings and is the cause of a unique breathing problem. Because of the windpipe's length, each inhalation includes nearly two gallons of air that never reach the lungs. (Comparatively, a resting human takes in two gallons of air every minute.) To counteract this anatomical dead space, a giraffe is equipped with a massive lung capacity of nearly twelve gallons. It has also been suggested that a giraffe's trachea might serve as a cooling device. As the trachea is filled with moist air, it cools the nearby blood vessels that travel up to the brain.

thyrohyoid ***thi***-ro-***hi***-oyd

Platysma

The platysma is a thin, superficial sheath spanning the anterior neck from the mandible to the chest (**5.84**). The platysma and other facial muscles are integumentary muscles. Instead of connecting to bones, these muscles are embedded in the superficial fascia and attach to the skin and overlying muscle. The platysma's claim to fame is its ability to create the infamous "Creature from the Black Lagoon" expression (**5.85**).

	PLATYSMA
A	Assist to **depress** the mandible (temporomandibular joint) **Tighten** the fascia of the neck **Draw down** corner of the mouth
O	Fascia covering superior part of pectoralis major
I	Base of mandible, skin of lower part of face
N	Facial (VII)

When Do You Use Your Platysma?

- Frowning or pouting
- Saying "ahh" at the dentist's office
- Forming an unequivocal expression of terror

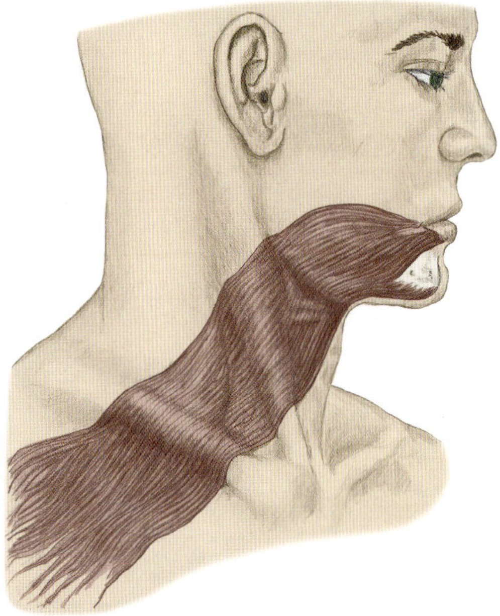

5.84 Anterior/lateral view of head and neck with head turned, showing platysma

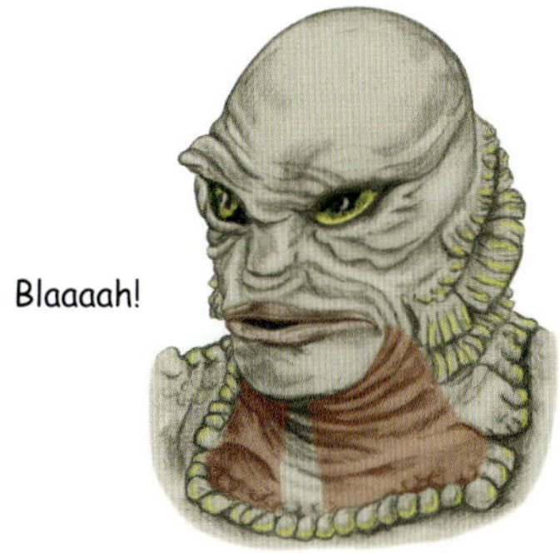

5.85 The Creature from the Black Lagoon, showing its platysma

Platysma

1. Partner supine. Ask your partner to jut his head anteriorly and protract his jaw (**5.86**). Then ask him to tighten the tissue on the front of his neck.
2. Explore this thin sheet of muscle from the mandible down to the upper chest. Note any "flaps" the platysma forms along the lateral side of the neck.

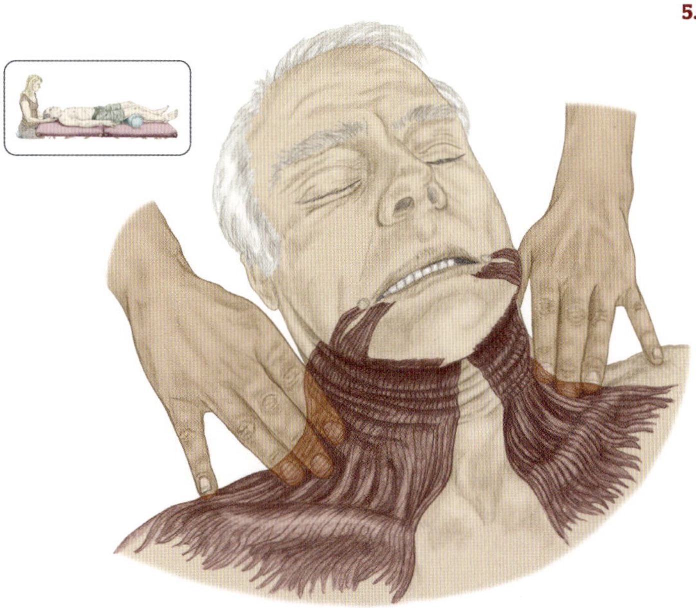

5.86 Partner supine, contracting the tissue of the anterior neck while you palpate the platysma

platysma pla-***tiz***-ma Grk. plate

Occipitofrontalis

(Frontalis and Occipitalis)

The occipitofrontalis is the muscle primarily responsible for raising the forehead into an expression of surprise. It is a unique muscle with four thin bellies—two **frontalis** bellies on the forehead and two **occipitalis** bellies located on the back of the head. The four bellies are joined by the galea aponeurotica, a broad sheath of connective tissue stretching across the top of the cranium (**5.87**). Although the occipitofrontalis is superficial, its thin fibers cannot be isolated.

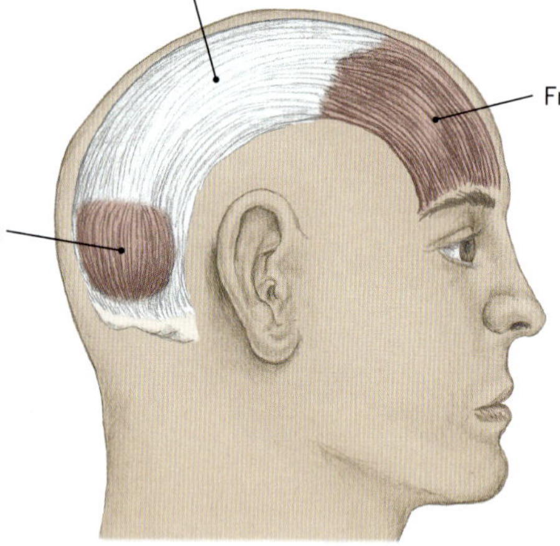

5.87 Lateral view of head, showing occipitofrontalis

OCCIPITOFRONTALIS	
A	*Frontalis:* **Raise** the eyebrows and wrinkle the forehead *Occipitalis:* **Anchor** and **retract** the galea posteriorly
O	*Both:* Galea aponeurotica
I	*Frontalis:* Skin superior to eyebrows *Occipitalis:* Superior nuchal line of the occiput
N	Facial (VII)

When Do You Use Your Occipitofrontalis?

- Raising your eyebrows in shock or surprise (frontalis)
- Smiling and yawning—according to a study of thirty volunteers who allowed electrodes to measure their muscle activity

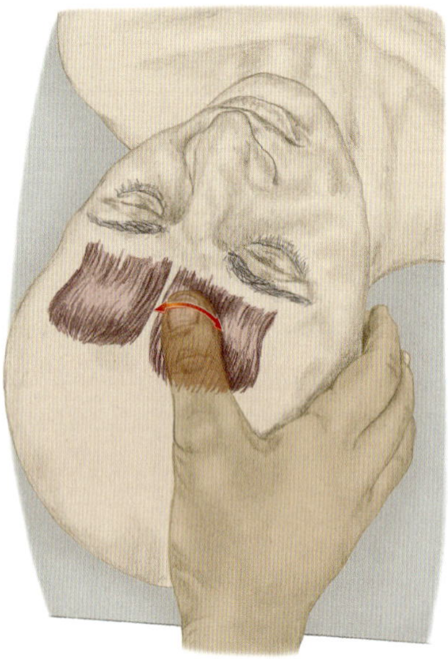

5.88 Partner supine, as you isolate the frontalis fibers

Frontalis fibers

Partner supine. Place your fingers on the forehead and ask your partner to raise his eyebrows (**5.88**). Do you feel the tissue of the forehead contract?

Occipitalis fibers

Partner supine or prone. Locate the superior nuchal line of the occiput (p. 232) and slide your fingers one inch superiorly to isolate the region of the oval occipitalis bellies (**5.89**).

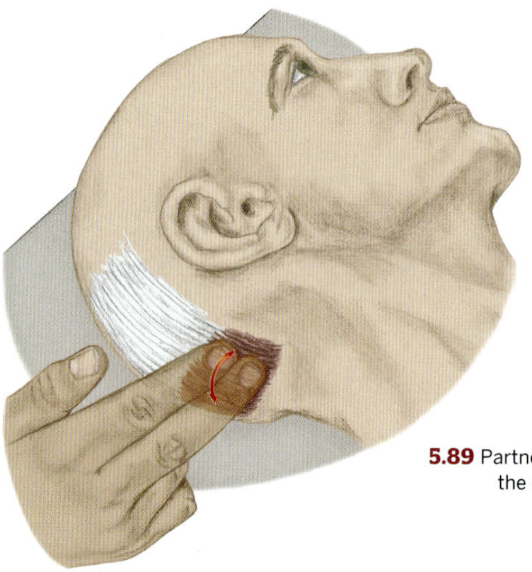

5.89 Partner supine, as you isolate the occipitalis fibers

occipitofrontalis ok-*sip*-i-to-fron-*ta*-lis

Medial and Lateral Pterygoids

The medial and lateral pterygoids assist the masseter and temporalis with movement of the mandible. The **medial pterygoid** helps to elevate the mandible, while the lateral pterygoid protracts it. The medial pterygoid is located on the *interior* side of the mandible (**5.90**, **5.91**) and its shape and position mirror the *exterior* masseter muscle (p. 250).

The **lateral pterygoid** has horizontal fibers that extend from the sphenoid bone to the joint capsule and articular disc of the temporomandibular joint (**5.92**, **5.93**). Portions of the pterygoids can be accessed from both inside and outside the mouth.

MEDIAL PTERYGOID

A *Unilaterally:*
Laterally deviate the mandible to the opposite side
Bilaterally:
Elevate the mandible
Protract the mandible

O Medial surface of lateral pterygoid plate of sphenoid bone and tuberosity of maxilla

I Medial surface of ramus of the mandible

N Trigeminal (V)

When Do You Use Your Medial Pterygoid?

- Chomping down on a wad of gum
- Grinding your teeth
- Ripping off a piece of beef jerky with your teeth

LATERAL PTERYGOID

A *Unilaterally:*
Laterally deviate the mandible to the opposite side
Bilaterally:
Protract the mandible

O *Superior head:*
Infratemporal surface and crest of greater wing of sphenoid bone
Inferior head:
Lateral surface of lateral pterygoid plate of sphenoid bone

I Articular disc and capsule of temporomandibular joint, neck of mandible

N Trigeminal (V)

When Do You Use Your Lateral Pterygoid?

- Chomping down on a wad of gum
- Grinding your teeth
- Ripping off a piece of beef jerky with your teeth

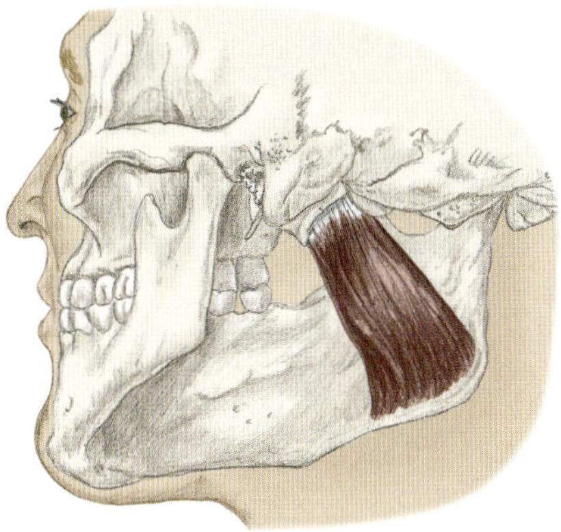

5.90 Posterior/lateral view of cranium, showing medial pterygoid

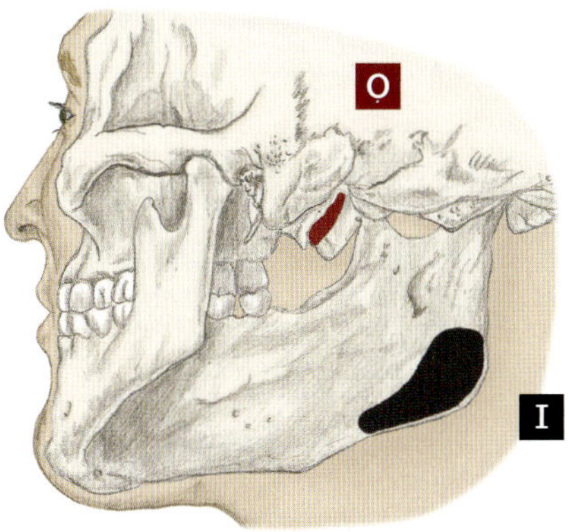

5.91 Posterior/lateral view of cranium, showing origin and insertion of medial pterygoid

pterygoid *ter-i-goyd* Grk. wing-shaped

Palpation Plus

While the pterygoids can be accessed safely and effectively through the mouth (and the longus muscles on p. 260 can be located on the anterior neck), these palpation techniques are best learned at a specific hands-on workshop in the presence of an experienced, patient instructor.

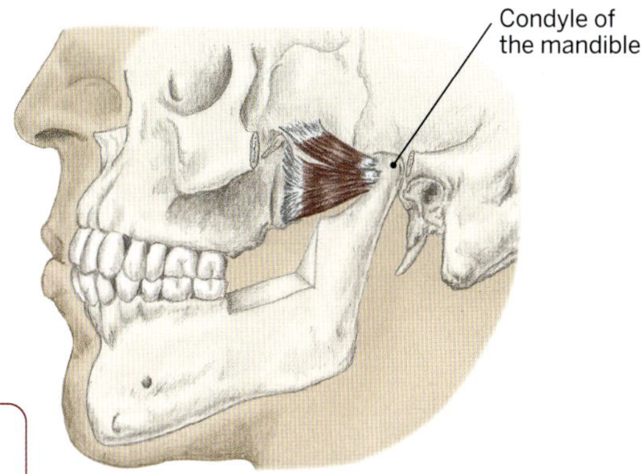

5.92 Lateral view of of cranium with zygomatic arch and mandible cut, showing lateral pterygoid

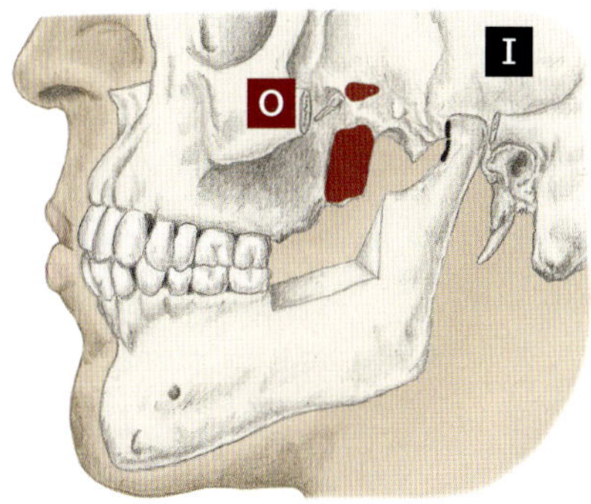

5.93 Lateral view of cranium with zygomatic arch and mandible cut, showing origin and insertion of lateral pterygoid

Longus Capitis and Longus Colli

Tucked between the trachea and the cervical vertebrae are two small muscles—**longus capitis** and **longus colli** (**5.94**, **5.95**). Attaching from the anterior surface of the cervical vertebrae to the occiput and atlas, they laterally flex, rotate, and flex the head and neck. They also help to reduce the lordotic curve of the cervical vertebrae. Each muscle has a multibranched design similar to that of the erector spinae muscles of the back.

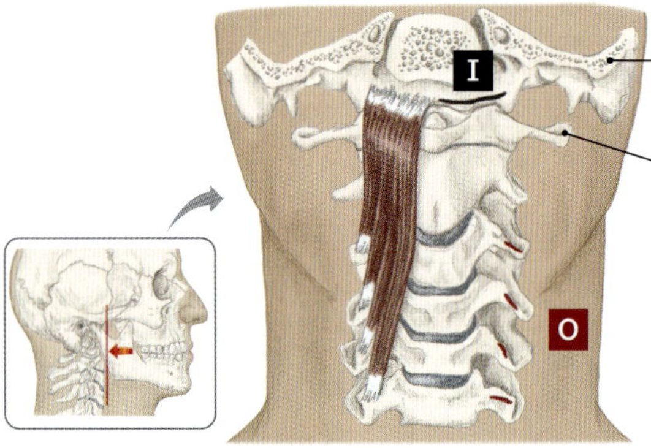

5.94 Anterior view of cervical vertebrae, showing longus capitis

LONGUS CAPITIS

A *Unilaterally:*

Laterally flex the head and neck to the same side

Rotate the head and neck to the same side

Bilaterally:

Flex the head and neck

O Transverse processes of C-3 through C-6

I Inferior surface of occiput

N C**1**, **2**, **3**, (4)

When Do You Use Your Longus Capitis?

- Looking to the left and right (same side rotation)
- Looking down toward your feet while lying on the couch (bilatera flexion)
- Stabilizing your head

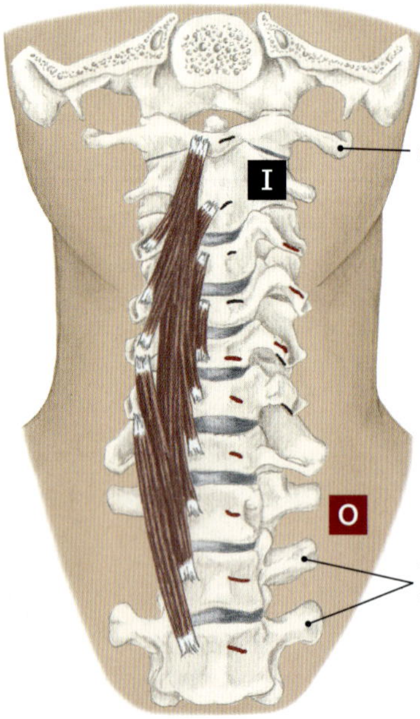

5.95 Anterior view of cervical vertebrae, showing longus colli

LONGUS COLLI

A *Unilaterally:*

Laterally flex the head and neck to the same side

Rotate the head and neck to the same side

Bilaterally:

Flex the head and neck

O Bodies of C-5 through T-3, transverse processes of C-3 through C-5

I Tubercle on anterior arch of the atlas; bodies of the axis, C-3, and C-4; transverse processes of C-5 and C-6

N C**2–6**, (7)

When Do You Use Your Longus Colli?

- Looking to the left and right (same side rotation)
- Looking down toward your feet while lying on the couch (bilateral flexion)
- Stabilizing your head

Discover More

There are two groups of muscles that coordinate the tongue: the glossus muscles and the intrinsic muscles. The three glossus muscles attach to the hyoid and other bones and move the tongue during chewing and swallowing. Three other intrinsic muscles of the tongue interweave with each other and are responsible for changing the tongue's shape during speech. As the tongue is basically a bag of fluid with a constant volume, these intrinsic muscles mold and twist it in the same way you might bend and shape a water balloon.

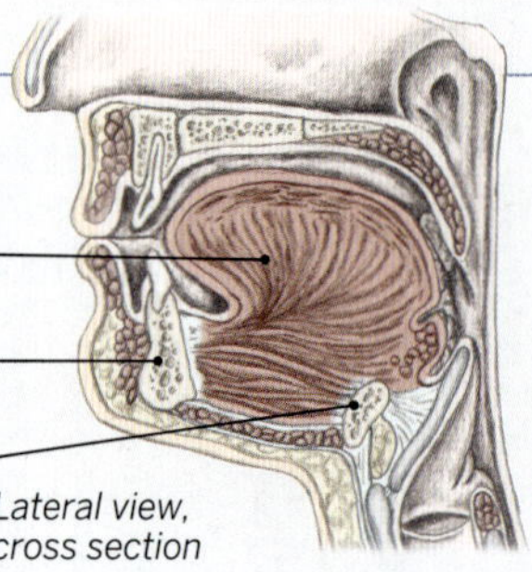

longus colli *long*-us ***ko***-li L. long (muscle) of the neck

Overview: Muscles of Facial Expression

The vast range of expressions the human face displays is created by thirty facial muscles—more than on any other animal (**5.96**, **5.97**). They can be divided into four groups: muscles of the mouth, nose, eyes, and scalp.

Unlike skeletal muscles that connect to bones, many of the muscles of facial expression are *integumentary* muscles, meaning they are embedded in the superficial fascia and attach to the skin and overlying muscle. They are also *mimetic* muscles, since they express emotion. Many of the facial muscles are structurally integumentary and functionally mimetic.

Collectively these muscles form expressions or actions such as crinkling the eyebrows in confusion, flaring the nostrils in anger, puckering the lips for a kiss, or raising the chin to pout. Smiling is generated by eight muscles, whereas frowning can require up to twenty.

5.96 Anterior view of head and neck, showing facial muscles

See p. 429 for the specific origins and insertions of the muscles of facial expression.

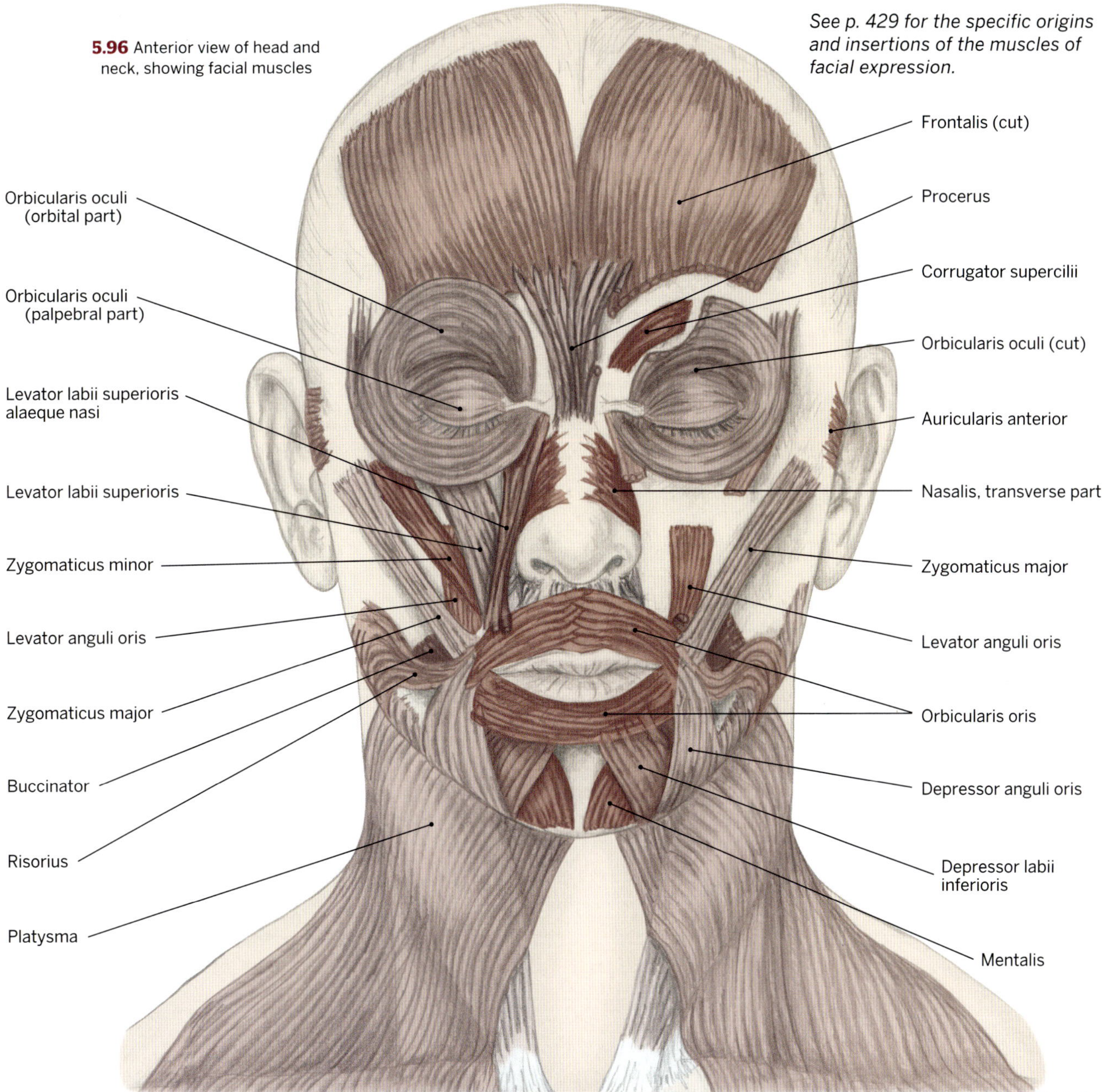

Discover More

Some muscles are identified with a certain expression. For example, a pout requires the mentalis. But, in reality, a clear facial message—doubt, fear, joy—is the result of several muscles. For that pout, the mentalis will push out the lower lip; for a more convincing sulk, one would also need both depressor anguli oris muscles to pull down the corners of the mouth and the corrugator supercilii to furrow the brow. Now *that's* an expression.

integumentary	in-***teg***-u-***ment***-ary	something that covers or encloses
mimetic	mi-***me***-tik	relating to, characterized by, or exhibiting mimicry

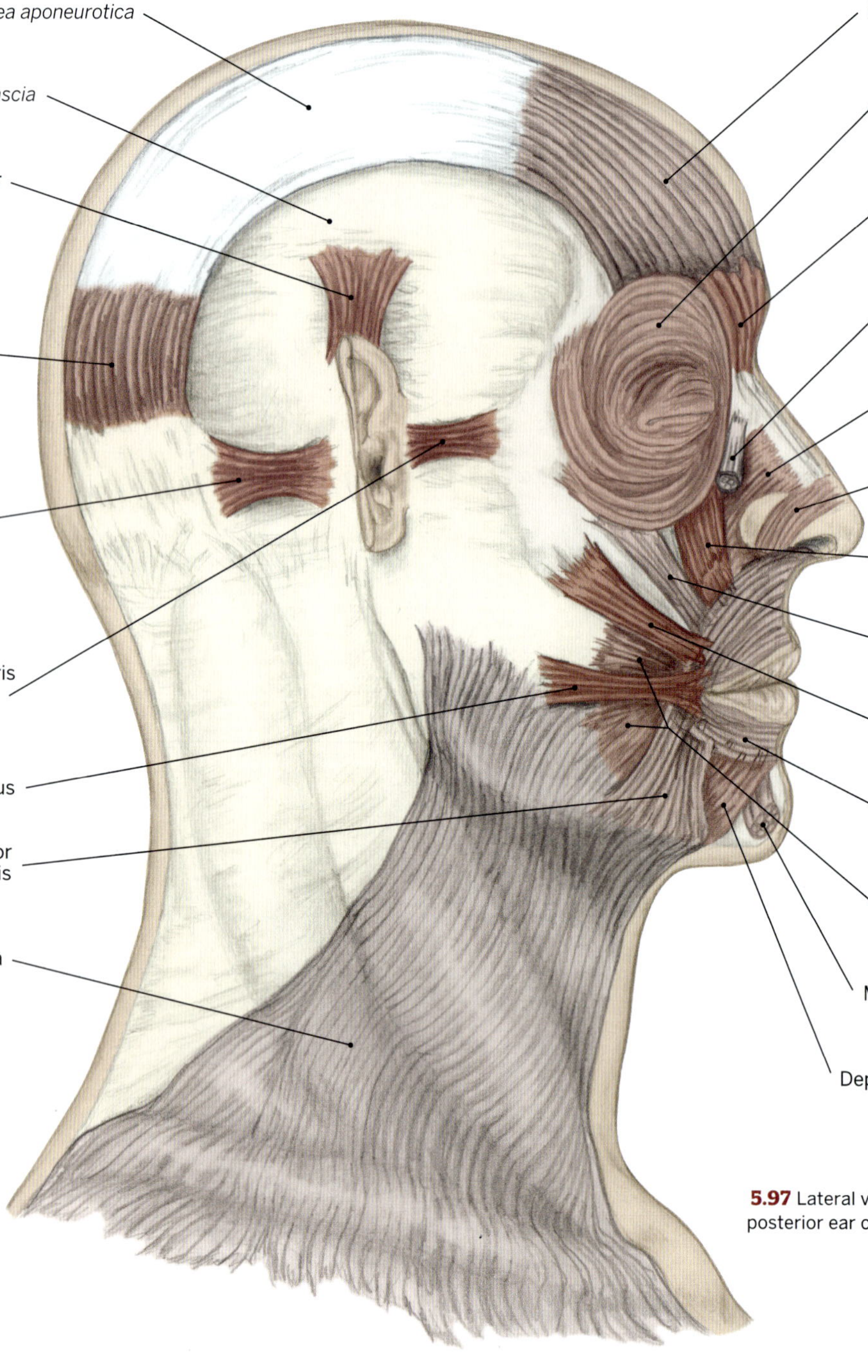

5.97 Lateral view of head and neck with posterior ear cut, showing facial muscles

Head, Neck & Face

Palpation Plus

Most of the facial muscles are superficial but, because of their ribbonlike thinness, can be difficult to isolate. Their locations, however, can be identified and the effects of their contractions can be seen.

Unlike other sections of *Trail Guide*, which are designed for you to palpate on a partner, this section is designed for you to palpate on your own face (optimally in front of a mirror). You may discover, while attempting to engage these muscles, that some of them only function on one side (or neither side) of your face. Do not be disheartened. This is not uncommon, and, with practice, muscles such as those that wiggle the ears can become active.

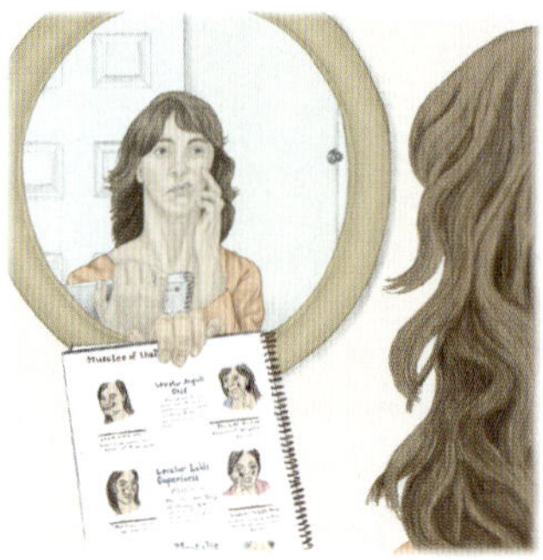

Curiously, when facial muscles are contracted involuntarily by emotion, they are more symmetrical, whereas deliberate or voluntary expressions often produce a more asymmetrical contraction.

Muscles of the Mouth

Eleven mimetic muscles form expressions of and around the mouth (twelve including the LLSAN, a muscle of the nose, p. 267). Except for the single orbicularis oris that encircles the mouth, all of these muscles are present bilaterally on the face. This brings the total number of muscles that create expressions of the mouth to twenty-three.

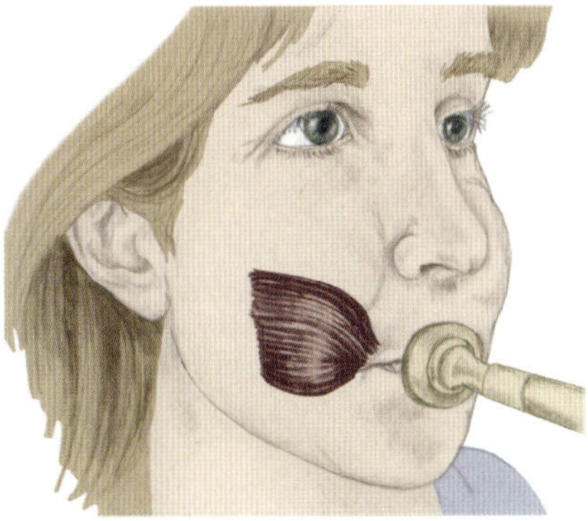

5.98 Engage the buccinators by blowing into a trumpet.

Buccinator

Located at the center of the cheek, this strong muscle tightens the corner of the lip and presses the cheek firmly against the teeth (**5.98**, **5.99**). Bilateral involvement will help to blow a trumpet, suck on a straw, or assist in mastication by keeping food between the molars.

Visually, it can produce a small dimple at the cheek's center and, with a unilateral contraction, generate a look of contempt. Blowing out the cheeks will stretch the buccinators.

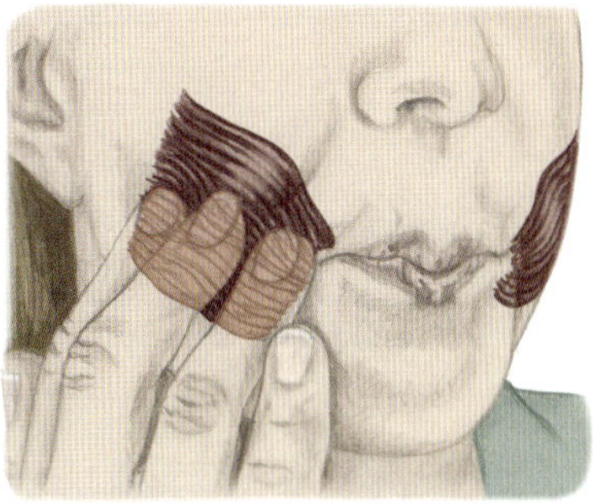

5.99 Purse the lips and press the cheeks against the teeth to feel the buccinator contract.

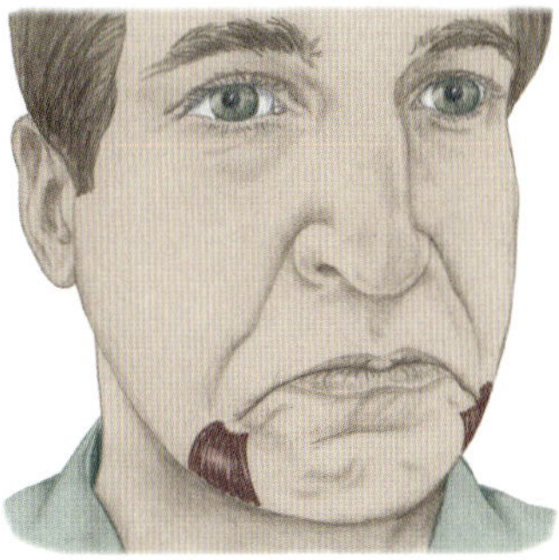

5.100 The DAO often works in conjunction with the mentalis (p. 264), creating expressions that range from a pout to a scowl.

Depressor Anguli Oris

The DAO pulls the corner of the mouth inferiorly and laterally (**5.100**, **5.101**). With a bilateral contraction, it forms an inverted "clown smile." Mild engagement of the DAOs is a common, involuntary signal of sadness, while a solid contraction is often associated with frowning. Look for it during both reprimands (upset parent to mischievous child) and apologies (contrite politician to skeptical public).

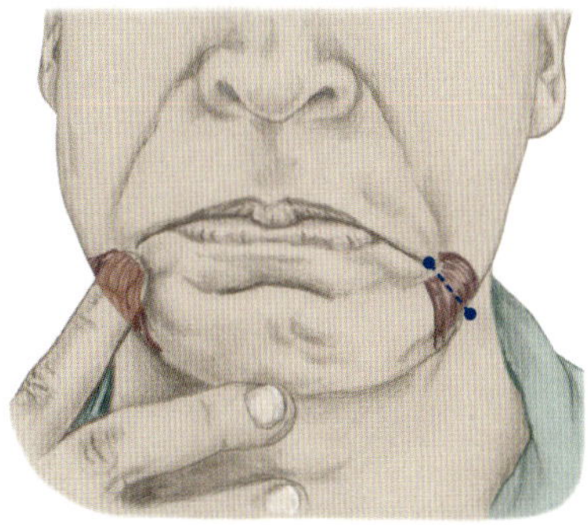

5.101 The DAO is located just inferior and lateral to the corner of the mouth, above the base of the mandible.

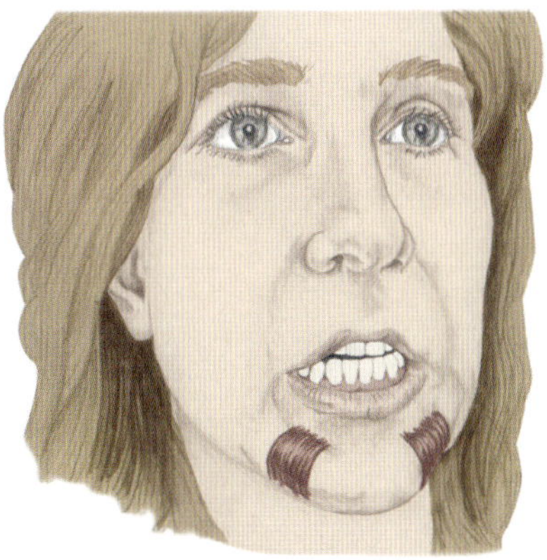

5.102 The DLI, along with orbicularis oris (p. 265), helps to shape the mouth during speech.

Depressor Labii Inferioris

Located just medial to DAO (above), the DLI depresses the corner of the mouth while protruding and drawing the lower lip laterally (**5.102**, **5.103**). By doing so, it bares the lower teeth, making it essential for brushing and flossing.

The DLI can be seen at sporting events both on the field and in the stands. An athlete's DLIs will engage to display determination (for example, a soccer player sprinting for the goal) while opposing fans will use their DLIs to express mock anger (especially if the player scores).

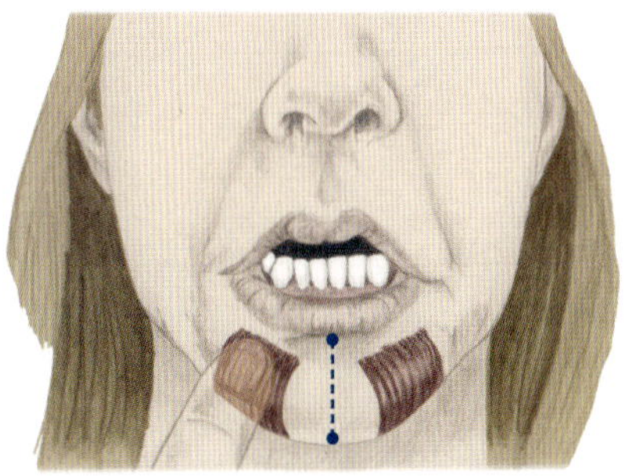

5.103 The DLI is located lateral to the center of the chin.

buccinator	*buk*-sin-*aye*-tor	L. trumpeter, proclaimer
labii	*lay*-bee-eye	L. pertaining to the lips

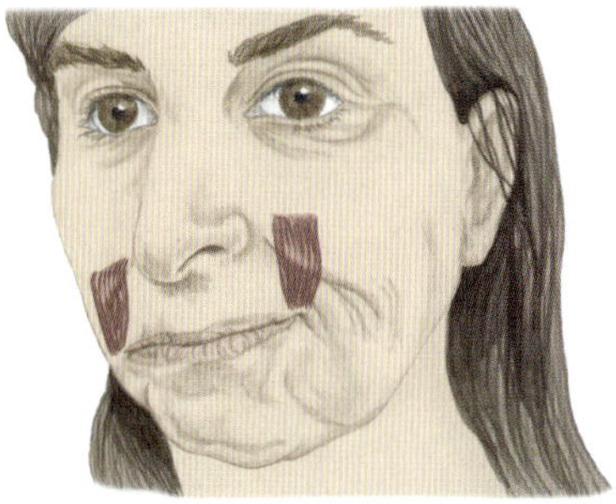

5.104 The LAO can create an ambiguous expression—is she being sardonic or just ticked off?

Levator Anguli Oris

This short muscle arises off the corner of the mouth and is located lateral to the levator labii superioris (below). *Bilateral* contraction of the LAOs will assist in smiling. A mild *unilateral* contraction of this muscle will elevate the corner of the mouth, giving the impression of self-confidence. A strong clench, however, will replace assuredness with a smirk (**5.104**, **5.105**).

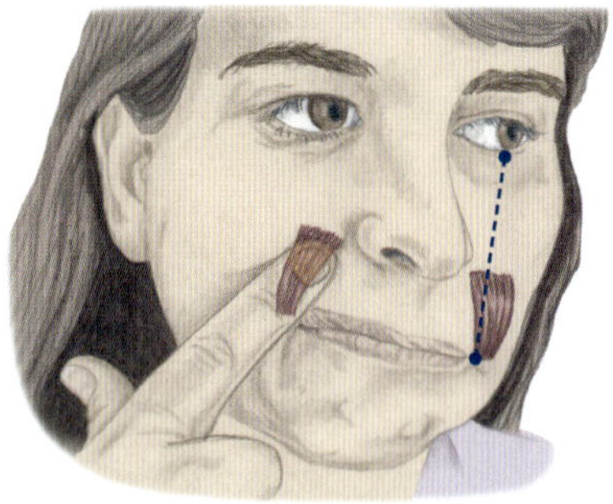

5.105 The LAO is located between the corner of the mouth and the center of the eye.

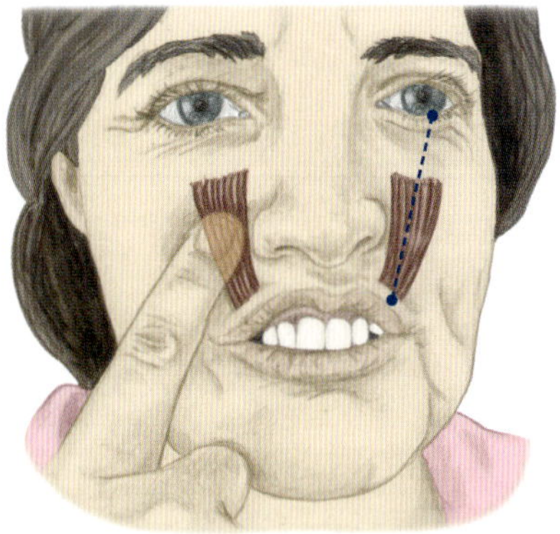

5.106 Locate the LLS between the upper lip and the center of the eye, passing next to the ala of the nose.

Levator Labii Superioris

The LLS is located medial to the levator anguli oris (above). *Bilateral* contraction will elevate and protrude the upper lip (**5.106**), such as when searching for food stuck between the teeth. A mild *unilateral* flex will produce an Elvis-like lip curl, while a strong contraction (**5.107**) manifests a contemptuous snarl that displays the canine tooth.

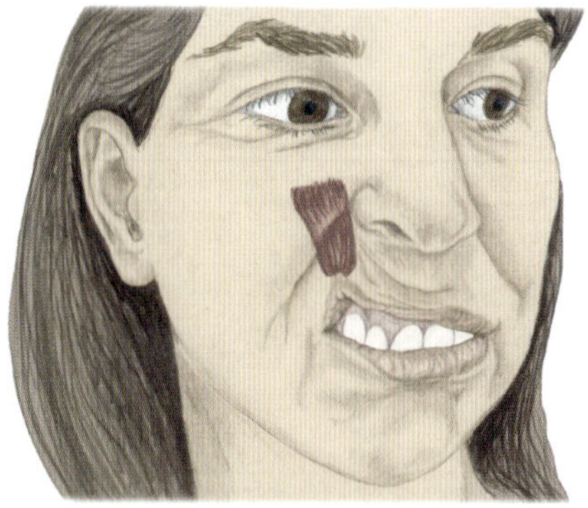

5.107 Grrr! A strong contraction of the LLS displays the canine tooth.

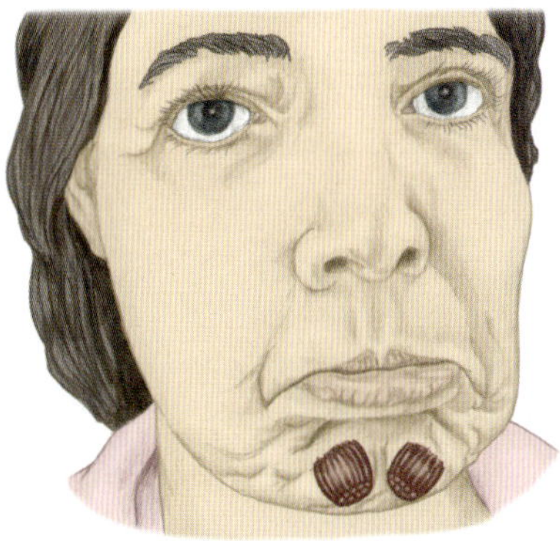

5.108 "Nobody wants to play with me." Contraction of the mentalis produces a pout.

Mentalis

The chin's most medial muscle is the mentalis (**5.108**, **5.109**). *Bilateral* contraction will elevate the skin of the chin and protrude the lower lip to form the universally understood signal of a pout. A *stronger* contraction will dimple the surface of the chin, forming a more sullen expression.

When you see this muscle's effects on the lower lip and chin, be well prepared for a cry of anguish or sadness in infants and some adults.

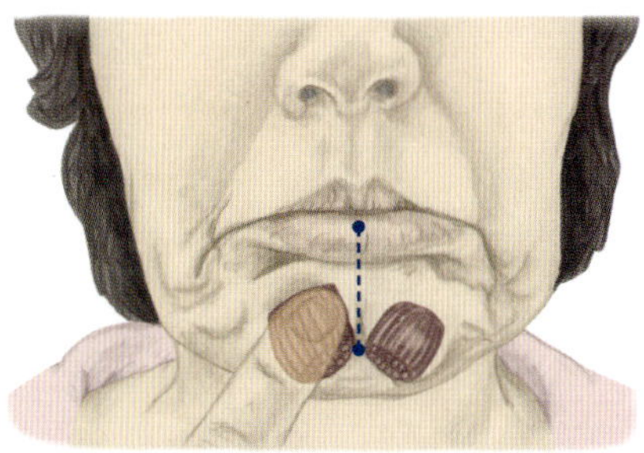

5.109 Locate the mentalis just off the centerline of the chin.

mentalis men-***tal***-is L. chin

Orbicularis Oris

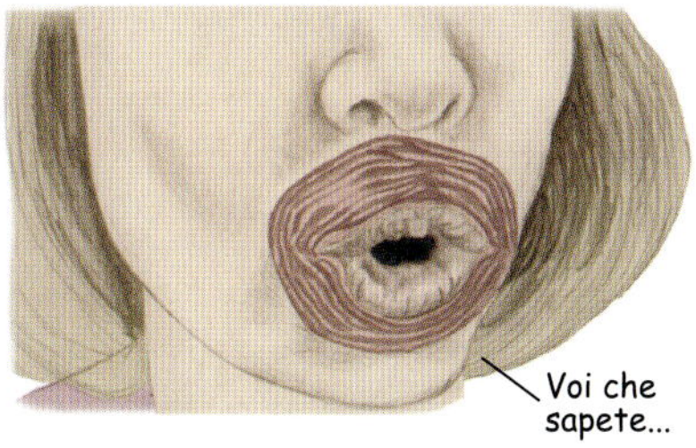

5.110 Look for a busy orbicularis oris during an opera recital.

This strong sphincter muscle encircles the mouth (**5.110**, **5.111**). It is responsible for closing the mouth and shaping the lips during speech and eating. The oris is indispensible to brass and woodwind players as well as to an anguished lover protruding his lips to deliver a long-distance kiss. Because its many strands can act separately, the oris can either narrow or protrude the lips, both signaling different states of anger.

See for yourself how necessary the orbicularis oris is for speech by enunciating the *Mary Poppins* phrase, "Supercalifragilisticexpialidocious."

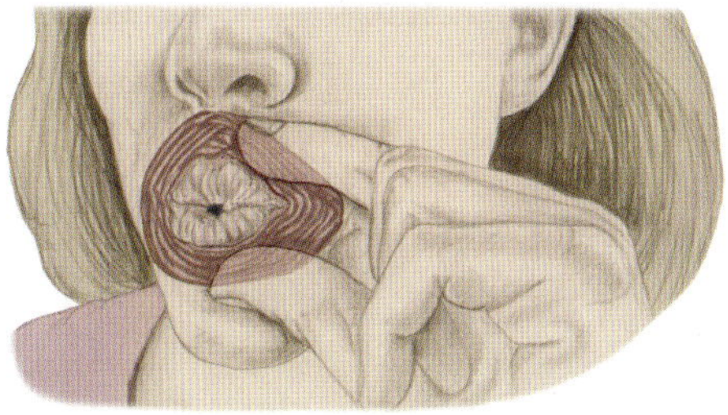

5.111 The orbicularis oris is located around the lips.

Discover More

There are seven primary facial expressions: anger, contempt, disgust, fear, happiness, sadness, and surprise—and few would confuse one with the other. But a miniscule shift of the face can transform these clear signals into something ambiguous. For example, (**a**) "happiness" raises the corners of the mouth, displays the upper teeth, and slightly narrows the eyes. Hold that expression, but now *raise the eyebrows* (**b**) and see how happiness becomes excitement. *Furrow the eyebrows* (**c**) and the face projects anxiety or confusion. Of course, if there are a hundred different expressions, there are a thousand different interpretations.

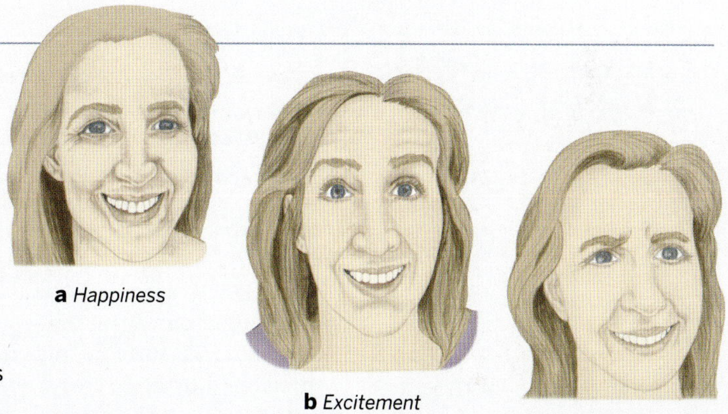

a *Happiness*

b *Excitement*

c *Anxious, confused, or both?*

Platysma

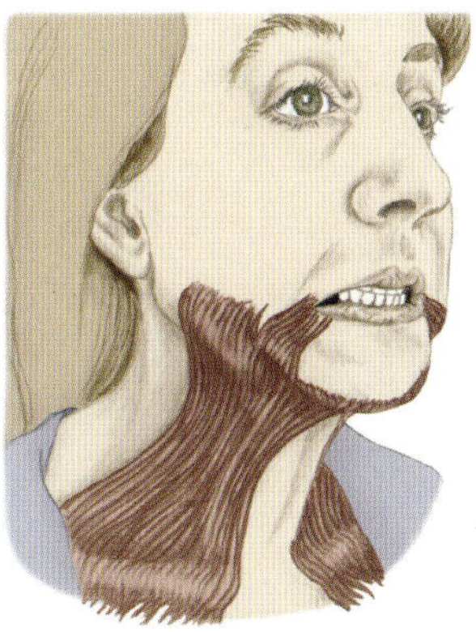

5.112 The platysma tightens the fascia of the neck and pulls down the corners of the mouth.

The platysma is a thin, superficial sheath spanning the anterior neck from the fascia of the superior part of the pectoralis major to the base of the mandible (**5.112**, **5.113**). It assists in depressing the jaw, drawing down the corners of the mouth and tightening the fascia of the neck. The platysma's claim to fame is its ability to create the infamous "Creature from the Black Lagoon" expression, but more commonly it is seen in moments of extreme fear, terror, or rage.

To palpate the playtsma on your partner, see p. 257.

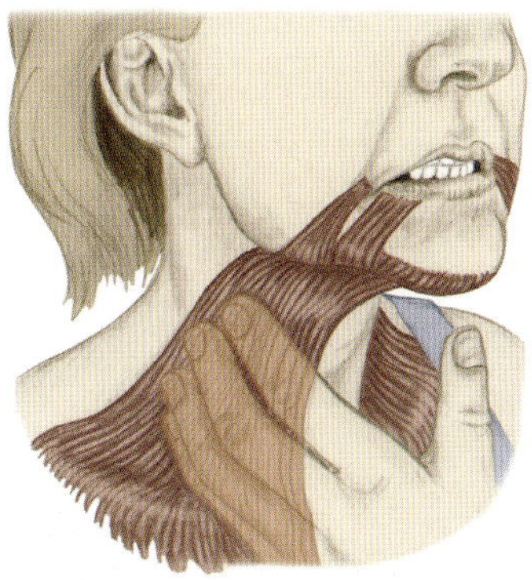

5.113 You can feel the platysma on the lateral neck.

orbicularis oris	or-***bik***-u-***la***-ris ***o***-ris	
platysma	pla-***tiz***-ma	Grk. plate
risorius	ri-***so***-re-us	L. to laugh

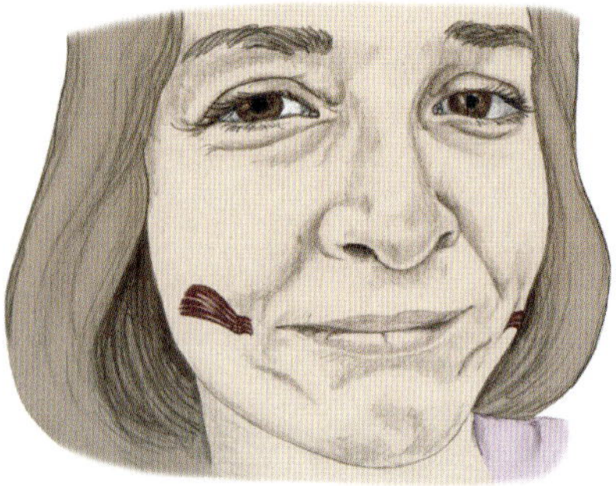

5.114 Yes, she's using the risorius to smile, but as her eyes and eyebrows are not involved, it's hard to believe she's sincere.

Risorius

Although it means "to laugh" in Latin, contraction of this muscle may indicate that there is nothing to laugh about. Positioned horizontally across the cheek, the risorius is superficial to the buccinator (p. 263). It retracts the corner of the mouth laterally and forms an insincere-looking smile (**5.114**, **5.115**). Look for it when someone is suffering through an unfunny joke.

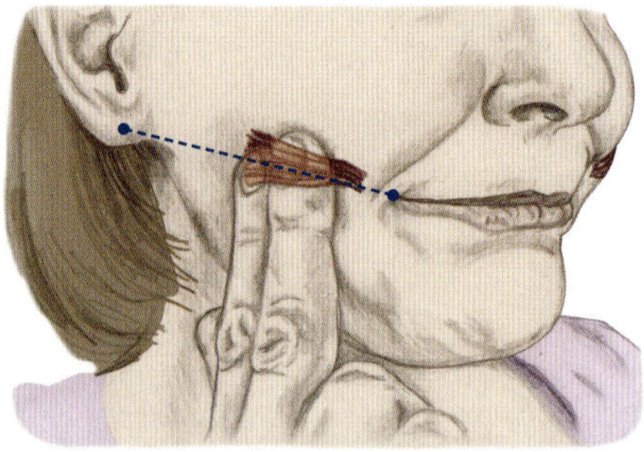

5.115 Locate the risorius by drawing an imaginary line between the corner of the mouth and the earlobe.

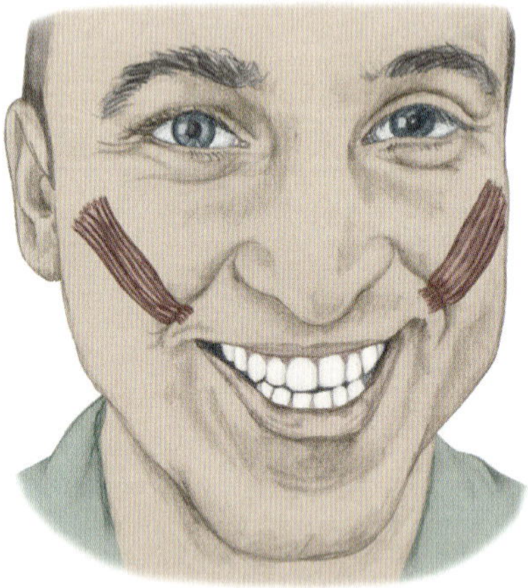

5.116 Now here's a genuine smile (note the alliance between the eyes and mouth), using the Z major.

Zygomaticus Major

This muscle draws the corner of the mouth upward and laterally with bilateral contraction, prominently displaying the upper row of teeth (**5.116**, **5.117**). It is the muscle often associated with joy, pleasure, and laughter.

When activated with the eye-squinting orbicularis oculi (p. 268), these muscles generate an authentic smile of enjoyment. However, without the oculi's participation, the zygomaticus's solo "smile" presents a *false* signal of enjoyment.

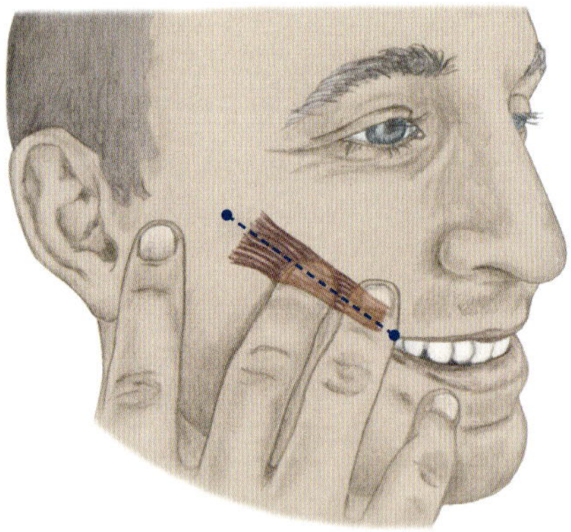

5.117 Locate the Z major by drawing an imaginary line between the corner of the mouth and the apex of the cheekbone.

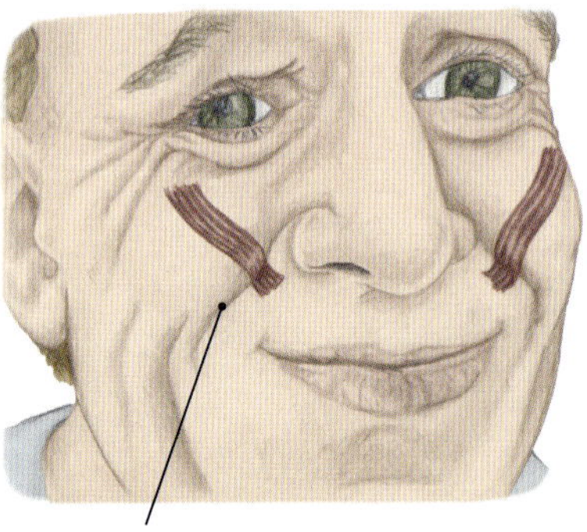

5.118 Unlike the joyous smile of the Z major (above), the Z minor forms a more understated and internal expression.

Zygomaticus Minor

Located medial to the zygomaticus major, the minor elevates and protrudes the upper lip. These actions deepen the nasolabial furrow and puff out the top of the cheek (**5.118**, **5.119**). Depending on the circumstances, this facial gesture can produce expressions ranging from a smile to a grimace.

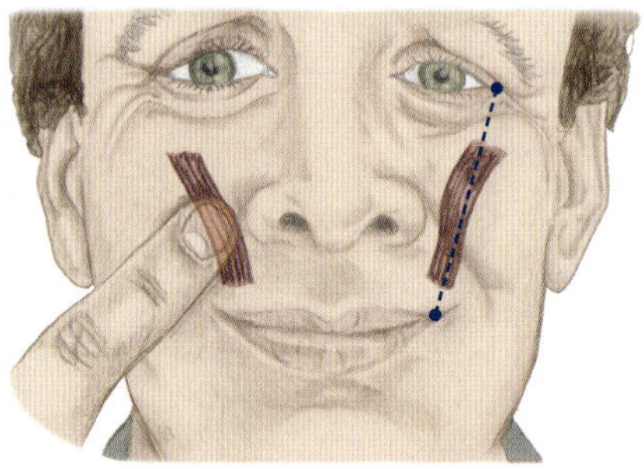

5.119 Locate the Z minor by drawing an imaginary line between the corner of the mouth and the corner of the eye.

nasalis	na-***sa***-lis	
zygomaticus	***zy***-go-***mat***-i-kus	Grk. cheekbone

Muscles of the Nasal Region

Three muscles are responsible for movement of the nose and its surrounding area. Unlike the mouth and eyes (where humans instinctively look for emotional signals), the movements and positions of the nose are somewhat secondary.

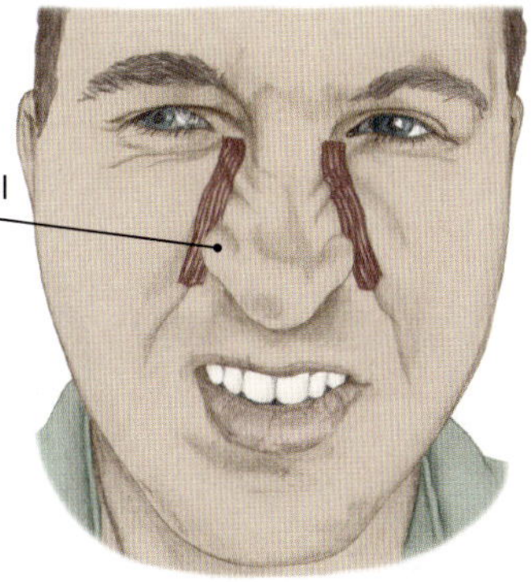

5.120 "What is that disgusting smell?" The LLSAN wrinkles the nose.

Levator Labii Superioris Alaeque Nasi

Aside from having the longest name of any muscle, the LLSAN is a vertical strip along the side of the nose that elevates the nasal ala (flaring the nostril). It also elevates and protrudes the upper lip. A strong, bilateral contraction deepens the nasolabial folds and forms diagonal wrinkles along the bridge of the nose, generating an expression of disgust (**5.120**, **5.121**). Look for it when a person hears an objectionable comment.

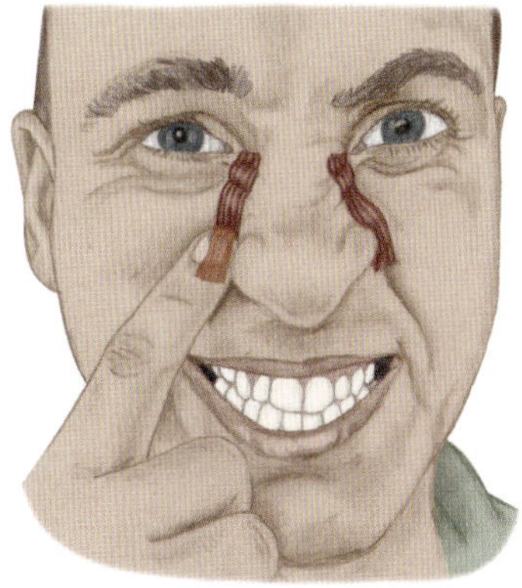

5.121 Locate the LLSAN alongside the nose.

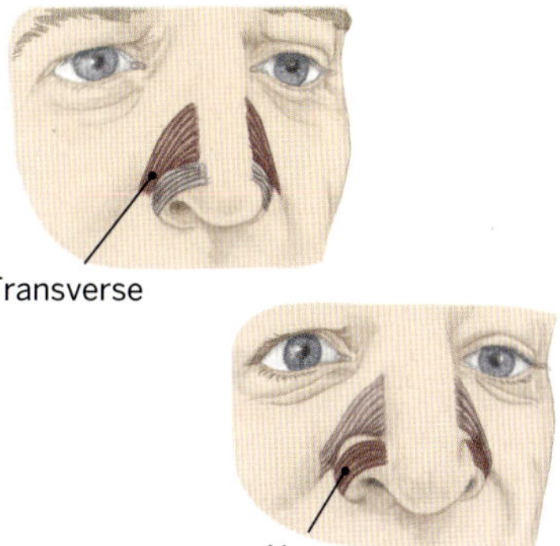

5.122 The transverse portion of the nasalis contracts at the smell of rotten food; the alar portion flares the nostril for a deep breath of fresh air.

Nasalis

The nasalis consists of two parts. The *transverse* portion, located on the side of the nose, constricts the nostril and draws down the tip of the nose. The *alar* portion wraps around the nasal ala and flares the nostril during forced respiration (**5.122**, **5.123**). Nostril expansion can also be useful when taunting an opponent or, in some cultures, as a discriminating tip-off of one's amorous intentions.

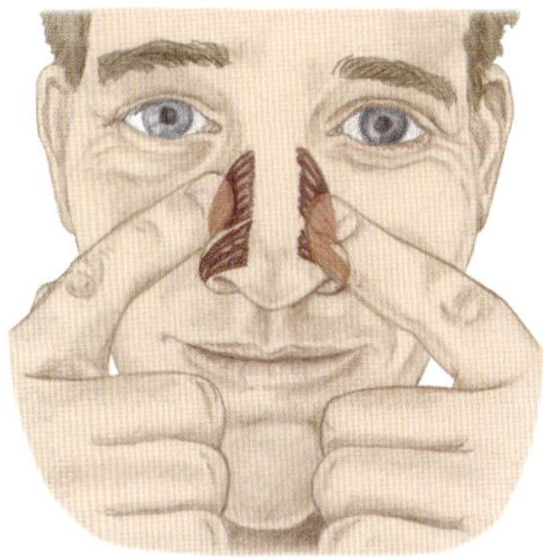

5.123 Access the transverse part of the nasalis on the sides of the nose.

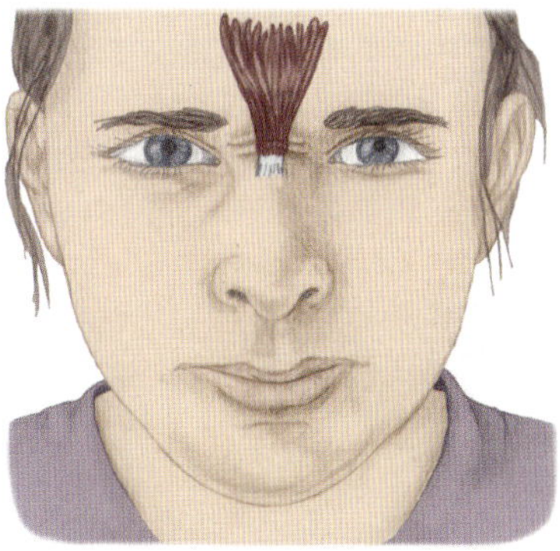

5.124 Contraction of the procerus can often appear as an expression of anger or concern.

Procerus

This small triangular muscle, located on the forehead, is often more involved with the eyebrows than with the nose (**5.124**, **5.125**). Along with the LLSAN, it wrinkles up the skin of the nose (such as when sneezing) and draws down the skin between the eyebrows (creating horizontal creases over the bridge of the nose). It often acts in conjunction with the corrugator supercilii (p. 268) to produce expressions of concentration or perplexity.

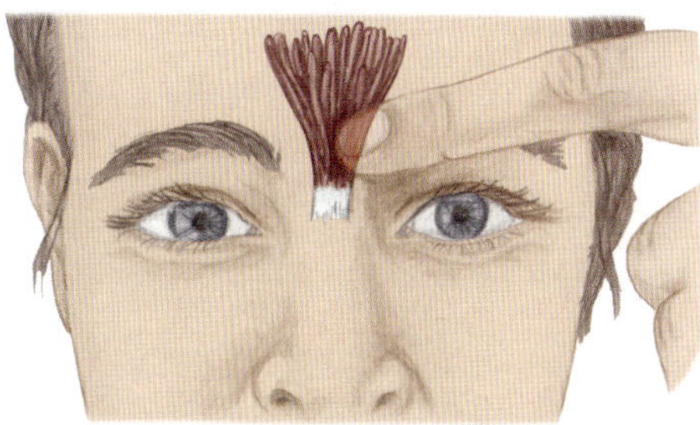

5.125 Locate the procerus between the eyebrows.

alaeque	a-***le***-kwe	L. wing (*ala* of nose)
levator labii superioris alaeque nasi		L. "lifter of the upper lip and of the wing of the nose"
procerus	pro-**se**-rus	L. slender, elongated

Head, Neck & Face

Muscles of the Eyes

These two muscles (as well as the procerus, p. 267) actually control the movement and position of the *eyebrows* and *eyelids*. Aside from protecting the eyeballs, they also convey visual signals about one's emotional state. This is an effective communication system because we instinctively glance at a person's eye region *first* for a hint of their underlying mood or intention.

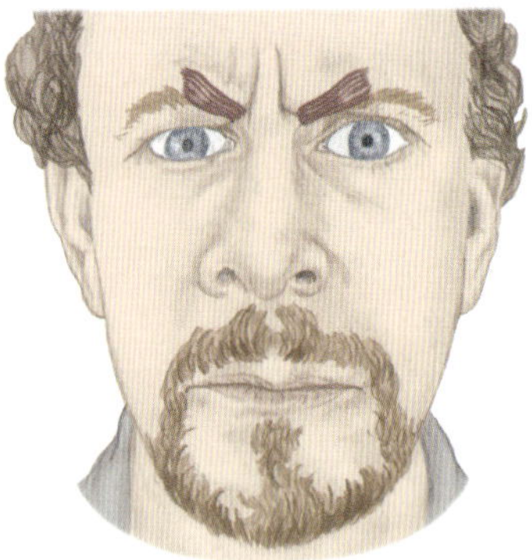

5.126 Chronic contraction of the CS can create permanent, vertical "frown lines" between the eyebrows.

Corrugator Supercilii

Charles Darwin called this the "muscle of difficulty" because of its involvement with anything demanding—emotional, mental, or physical. Located beneath the medial portion of the eyebrow, the corrugator draws the eyebrow medially and inferiorly (**5.126**, **5.127**). Bilateral contraction can form vertical wrinkles between the eyebrows, often creating a frown associated with anger, worry, or perplexion.

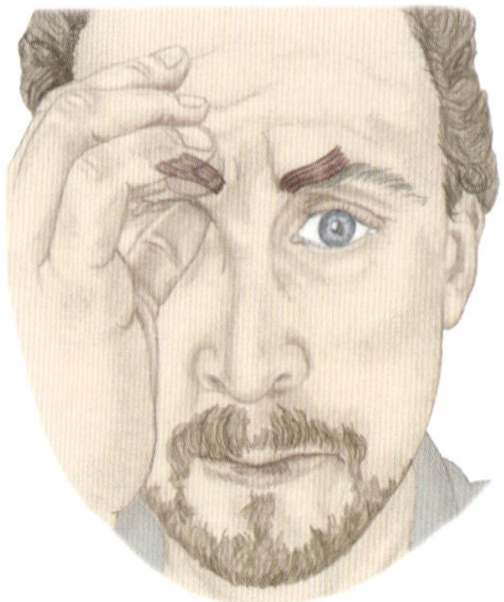

5.127 Locate the CS by squeezing the tissue under the medial eyebrow.

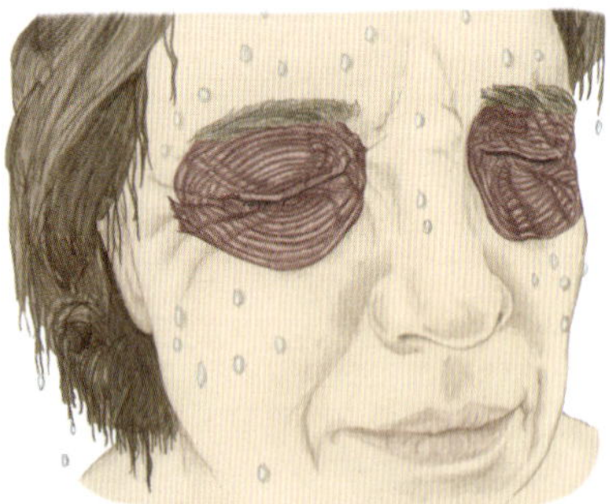

5.128 A glass of water in the face will activate the orbicularis oculi.

Orbicularis Oculi

This sphincter muscle encircles the eye and is responsible for closing the eyelid (**5.128**, **5.129**). The thicker, outer fibers form the *orbital* part of the muscle. They can squeeze the eyelid together or hold it in a partially closed position of a squint (creating an expression of distrust).

The inner fibers, the *palpebral* part of the muscle, involuntarily close the eyelid during blinking and sleeping.

"Smiling with your eyes" will engage the lateral portion of your oculi, but over time the chronic contraction of this muscle will form radiant creases of your skin called "crow's feet."

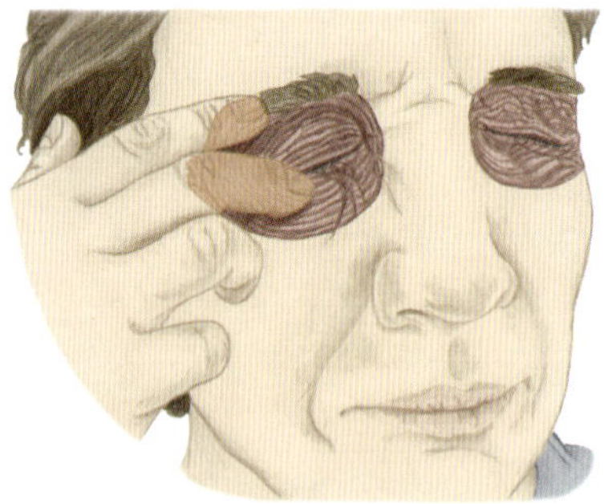

5.129 Palpate the tissue surrounding the eye to locate the orbicularis oculi.

Discover More

Moving Your Eyeball

The movements of the human eye are controlled by six muscles, four of which are the *superior, inferior, medial,* and *lateral rectus* muscles. Each rectus inserts on the corresponding side of the eyeball's anterior half. Depending on the position of the eye, the inserting tendon of a rectus muscle can be gently accessed. For example, rolling your eye downward will pull the superior rectus tendon out from under the eye socket and into a palpable position underneath the upper eyelid.

A seventh muscle, *levator palpebrae superioris*, attaches to the undersurface of the upper eyelid and is responsible for raising the eyelid.

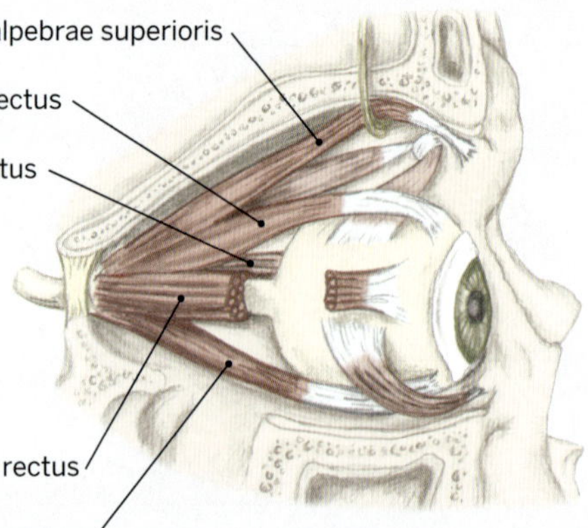

Lateral view of right eye

corrugator supercilii	***kor***-u-***ga***-tor su-per-***sil***-i-i	L. together + to wrinkle L. above eyelid

Head, Neck & Face

Muscles of the Scalp

The five muscles of the scalp are present bilaterally on the cranium. All of them are thin sheets that penetrate into the galea aponeurotica, a broad sheath of connective tissue that stretches across the top of the cranium.

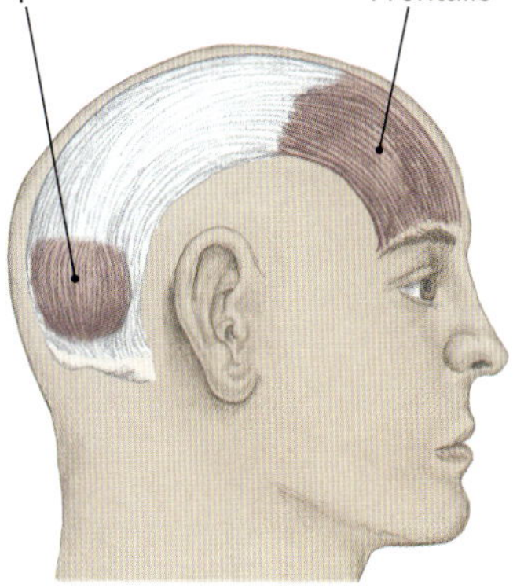

5.130 The occipitofrontalis has two parts, frontalis and occipitalis.

Occipitofrontalis (Frontalis and Occipitalis)

Each side of the cranium has an occipitofrontalis muscle consisting of two parts: a *frontalis* and an *occipitalis*. The frontalis is on the forehead, while the occipitalis is located on the back of the head (**5.130**). All four muscle bellies are joined by the galea aponeurotica.

The frontalis fibers are responsible for raising the eyebrows and wrinkling the forehead (**5.131–5.133**). Bilateral contraction of the frontalis's *medial* portion pulls up the inner eyebrows and produces an expression of sadness. A unilateral engagement of the *lateral* frontalis fibers can send a signal of skepticism or intimidation (**5.132**).

The occipitalis bellies anchor and retract the galea posteriorly. To palpate the occipitofrontalis on your partner, see p. 258.

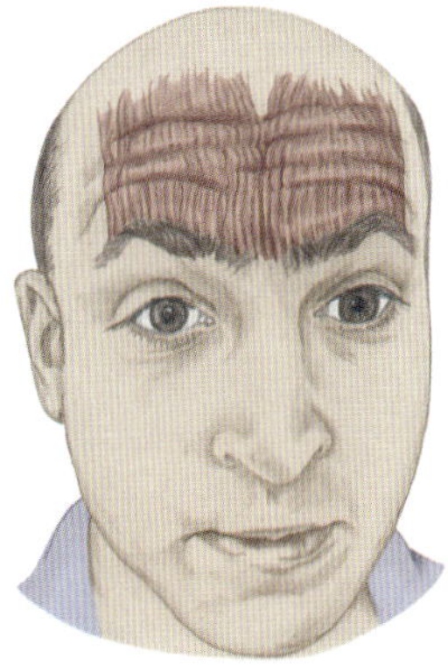

5.131 The frontalis muscles produce a look of surprise.

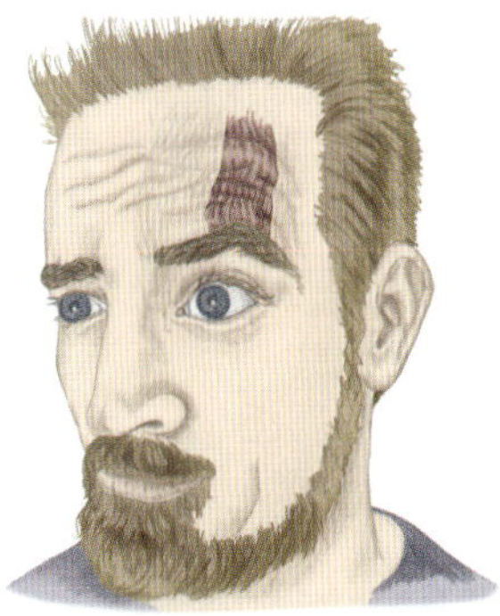

5.132 The classic raised-eyebrow expression is formed by the lateral portion of the frontalis.

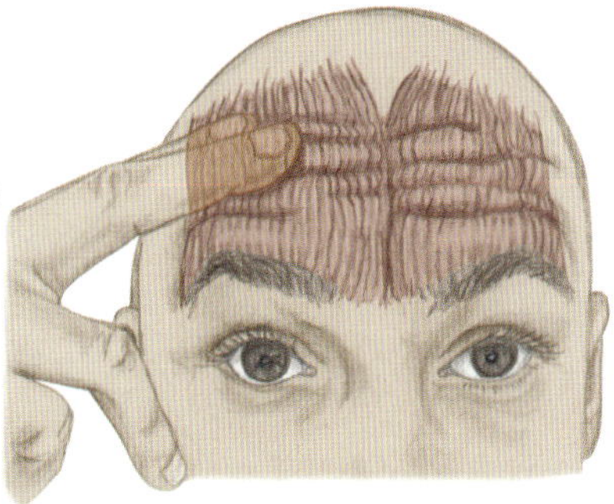

5.133 Locate the frontalis on the forehead.

Auricularis Muscles

The three auricularis muscles (*anterior, superior,* and *posterior*) are located above and alongside the ear on three sides (**5.134, 5.135**). They are thin, fan-shaped, and sheathed in the scalp. Theoretically, they have the capacity to move the ear.

The name of each muscle not only states where it is in respect to the ear, but also in which direction it will pull the ear. For example, the *auricularis posterior* is located posterior to the ear and, if you are coordinated, will move it posteriorly. Strong, alternating contractions of the *anterior* and *posterior* muscles can produce an impressive wiggling of the ear.

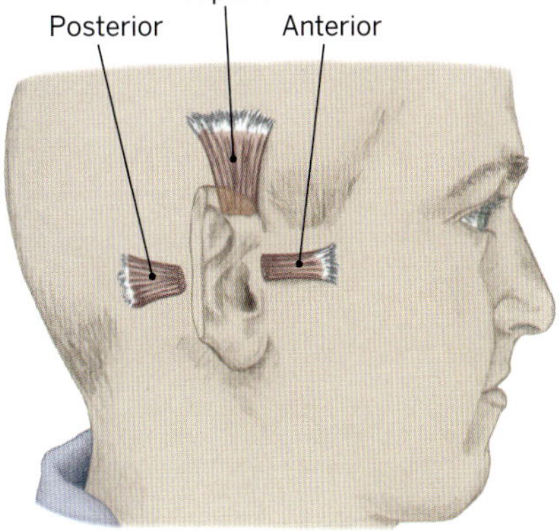

5.134 The three auricularis muscles are positioned around the ear (cut).

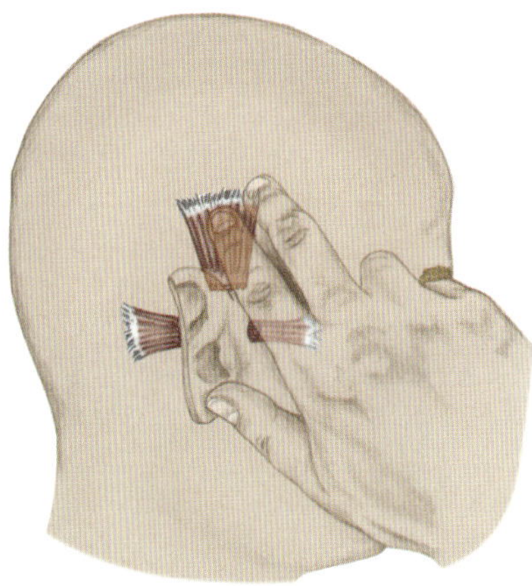

5.135 The location of the auricularis superior is just above and in front of the ear (cut).

auricularis	aw-***rik***-u-***la***-ris	L. little ear
occipitofrontalis	ok-***sip***-i-to-fron-***ta***-lis	

Other Structures of the Head, Neck, and Face

There are several accessible arteries, glands, and nerves in the head, neck, and face (**5.136**). Many are superficial and delicate and should therefore be palpated gently. It is advisable to locate and explore these structures on yourself before palpating them on a partner.

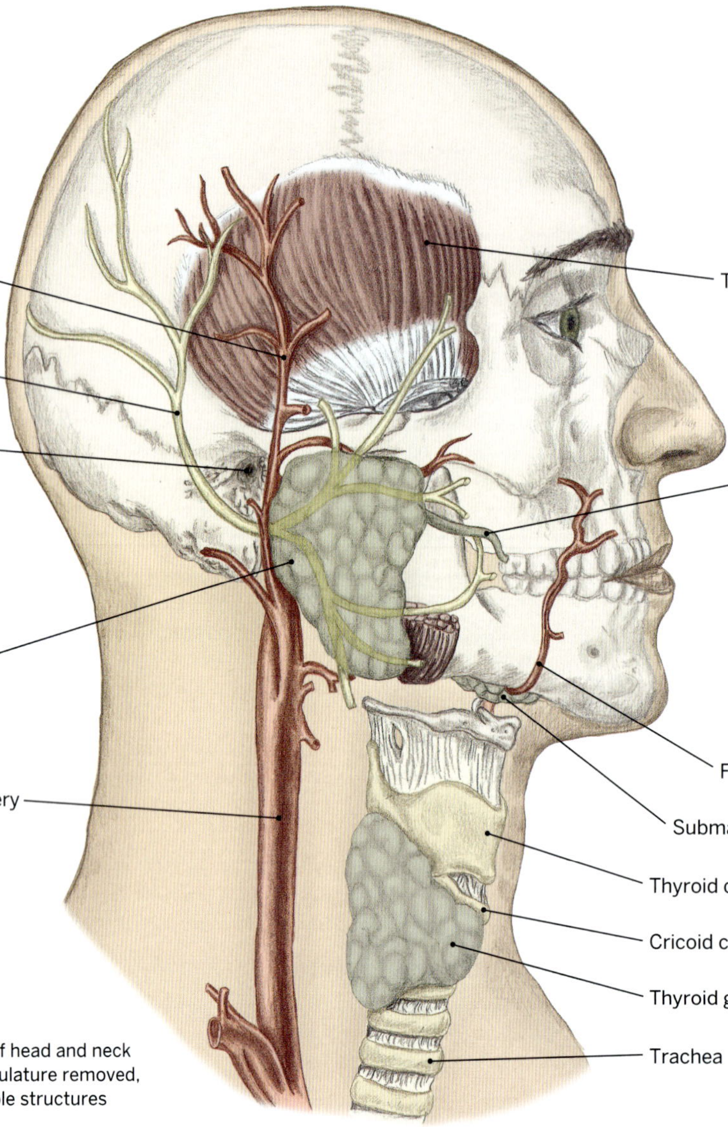

5.136 Lateral view of head and neck with superficial musculature removed, showing accessible structures

Comparative Anatomy

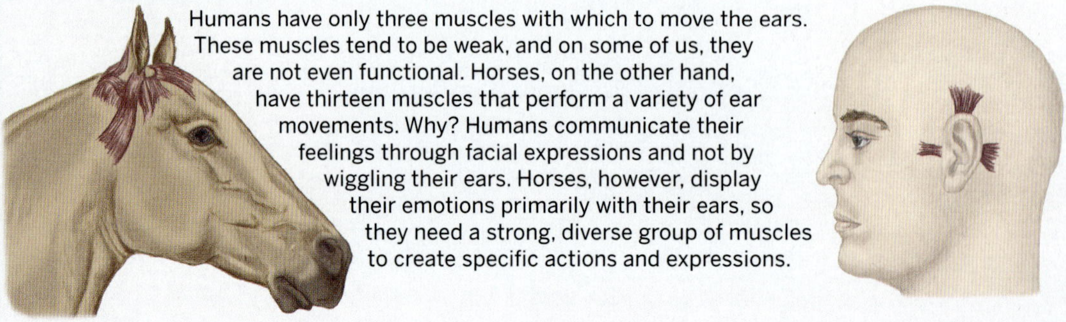

Humans have only three muscles with which to move the ears. These muscles tend to be weak, and on some of us, they are not even functional. Horses, on the other hand, have thirteen muscles that perform a variety of ear movements. Why? Humans communicate their feelings through facial expressions and not by wiggling their ears. Horses, however, display their emotions primarily with their ears, so they need a strong, diverse group of muscles to create specific actions and expressions.

Common Carotid Artery

The carotid artery is the primary supplier of blood to the head and neck. It ascends the anterior and lateral sides of the neck and lies deep to the sternocleidomastoid (SCM) and infrahyoid muscles. Its strong pulse can be felt medial to the SCM at the level of the hyoid bone.

Common carotid artery

1. Partner supine or seated. Place two fingerpads at the angle of the mandible.
2. Slide off the angle in an inferior and medial direction and press gently into the neck (**5.137**). The strong pulse of the carotid artery should be quite noticeable.

Are you medial to the SCM? Are you under the mandible at the level of the hyoid bone?

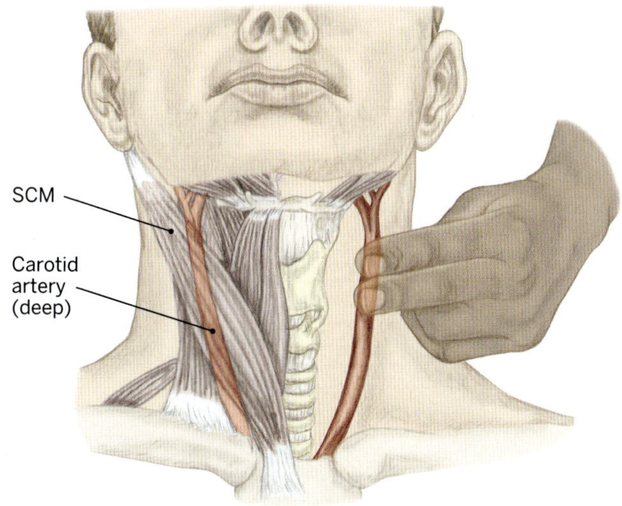

5.137 Partner supine, as you feel the pulse of the carotid artery

Superficial Temporal Artery

The superficial temporal artery branches off the external carotid artery and crosses over the top of the zygomatic arch. It continues superiorly along the side of the cranium, lying superficial to the temporalis muscle. The pulse of the superficial temporal artery can be detected in front of the ear along the zygomatic arch.

Superficial temporal artery

1. Partner supine or seated. Place your fingerpad in front of the ear at the zygomatic arch (**5.138**).
2. Gently explore and palpate for the artery's pulse. If you do not feel it, adjust your finger position and make sure your pressure is not too deep.

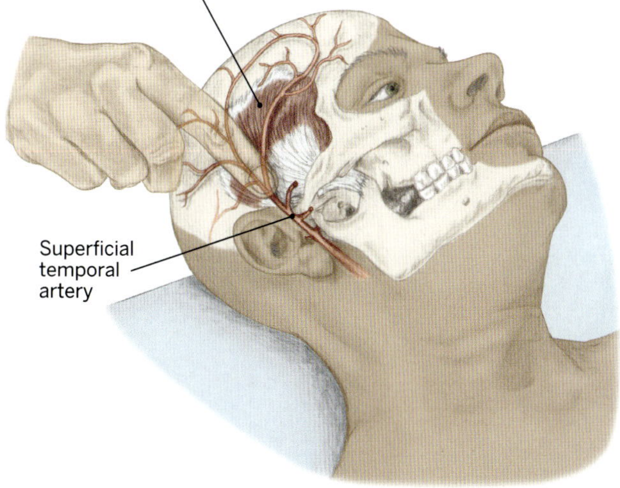

5.138 Partner supine, as you access the superficial temporal artery

Facial Artery

The facial artery is a small, superficial vessel that branches off from the external carotid artery and curves around the base of the mandible (jawline) toward the mouth and nose. Its pulse may be difficult to detect but can be felt along the base of the mandible at the anterior edge of the masseter.

Facial artery

1. Partner supine. With your partner clenching her jaw, locate the masseter's anterior edge.
2. Position your finger next to the base of the mandible and gently palpate for the pulse of the artery (**5.139**).

Are you at the base of the mandible, along the anterior edge of the masseter?

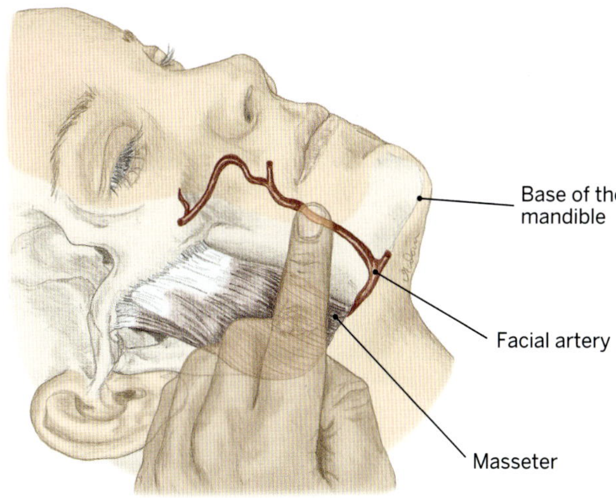

5.139 Partner supine, as you gently palpate the facial artery

carotid ka-*rot*-id Grk. causing deep sleep

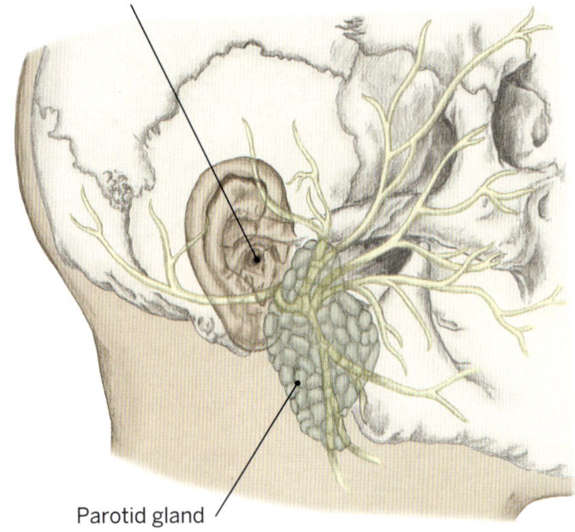

5.140 Lateral view of head, showing branches of the facial nerve

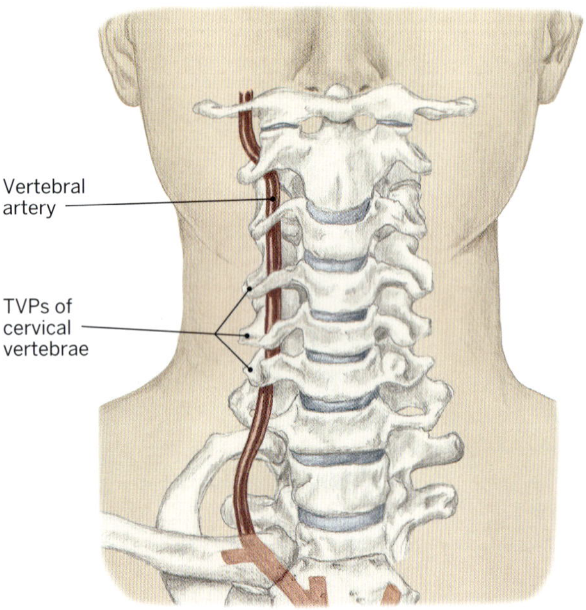

5.141 Anterior view of head and neck, showing vertebral artery

Facial Nerve

The facial nerve is not a structure you will want to palpate specifically, but, because of its proximity to other palpable structures on the side of the face, you will need to be aware of its location.

The facial nerve (cranial nerve VII) exits from the cranium and emerges superficially just anterior to the mastoid process. As it passes beneath the parotid gland, the nerve branches off and spreads across the face, scalp, and neck (**5.140**). Often two or more branches of the facial nerve cross superficially over the zygomatic arch.

When exploring the parotid gland, masseter, or zygomatic arch, be mindful of the facial nerve's presence. Static pressure on the nerve can cause irritation or inflammation, or even induce nausea in your partner.

Vertebral Artery

The vertebral artery branches off the subclavian artery and supplies blood to the brain and spinal cord. It ascends the neck through the transverse foramen of C-6 to C-1 before passing through the foramen magnum of the occiput (**5.141**). It is inaccessible, of course, but a vital structure to be aware of when palpating and/or passively moving the head and neck.

Parotid Gland and Duct, Submandibular Gland

There are three salivary glands in the neck and face: the parotid, submandibular, and sublingual. All are accessible, but be aware that palpation of the salivary glands can stimulate the production of saliva.

The **parotid gland** is located in front of the earlobe, superficial to the masseter muscle (p. 250). It has a soft, lumpy surface and is penetrated by branches of the facial nerve. The **parotid duct** is a spaghetti-sized tube extending anteriorly from the parotid gland. It tucks around the anterior edge of the masseter to funnel saliva to the mouth.

True to its name, the **submandibular gland** is tucked underneath the base of the mandible. Its round shape can be located anterior to the angle of the mandible.

Discover More

The flap of tissue that hangs from the roof of the mouth (soft palate) is called the uvula. It is designed to cover the nasal passages during swallowing. When a person sleeps on her back with her mouth open, air passes the uvula and palate, causing these and other tissues to vibrate. This, of course, produces a snore. The loudest snore ever recorded was 69 decibels—frightening when you consider that a pneumatic drill produces 70 to 90 decibels!

parotid	pa-***rot***-id	Grk. beside the ear
uvula	***uv***-u-la	L. a little grape

Parotid gland

1. Partner supine. Place your fingerpads in front of the earlobe on the masseter muscle.
2. Using gentle pressure along the superficial tissue, palpate between the angle of the mandible and the zygomatic arch for the gland's gelatinous texture (**5.142**).
3. Press deep to the gland in order to feel the striated fibers of the masseter muscle. Compare the different textures of these structures.

Parotid duct

1. Ask your partner to clench her jaw.
2. Place your fingerpads below the zygomatic arch, along the anterior edge of the masseter. Roll your finger back and forth (in a superior/inferior direction) and palpate for the mobile, horizontal tube.

Are you along the anterior edge of the masseter? Is the duct the diameter of a strand of spaghetti, and does it run horizontally?

Submandibular gland

1. Place a finger along the base of the mandible.
2. Move your fingers medially, underneath the base, to palpate the superficial, marble-sized gland (**5.143**).

Can you roll your finger along the surface of the gland, outlining its shape?

Thyroid Gland

The left and right lobes of the thyroid gland are located on the anterior surface of the trachea. The gland lies deep to the infrahyoid muscles and has a soft, spongy texture that can be difficult to distinguish from the surrounding tissues.

Thyroid gland

1. Partner supine or seated. Using one fingerpad, locate the surface of the trachea between the jugular notch and cricoid cartilage.
2. Palpate for the soft texture of the thyroid gland lying on top of the trachea (**5.144**). Respecting the gland's delicacy, explore gently and briefly.

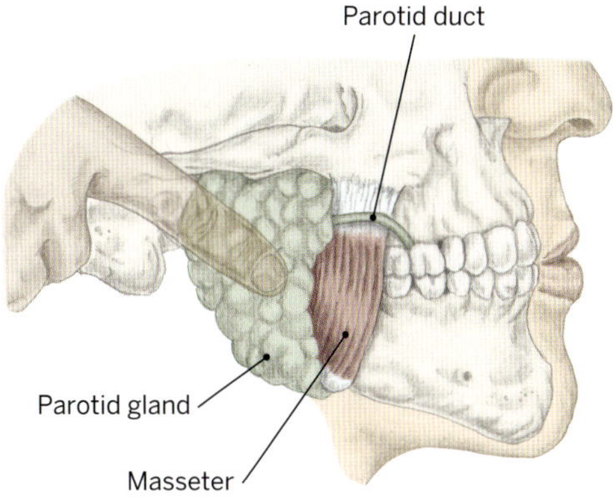

5.142 Lateral view of jaw, as you palpate the parotid gland

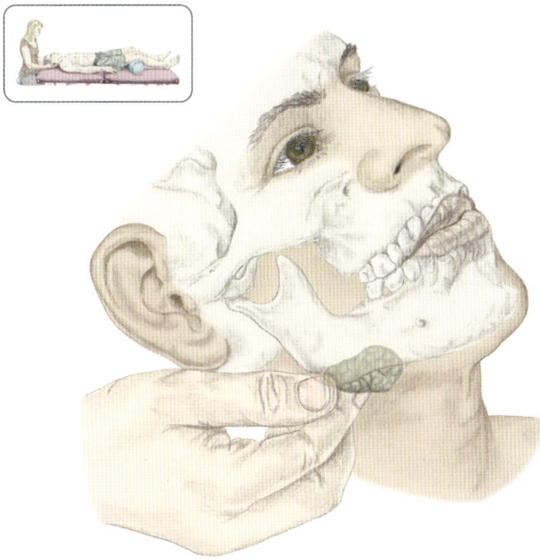

5.143 Anterior/lateral view of head, as you access under the base of the mandible for the submandibular gland

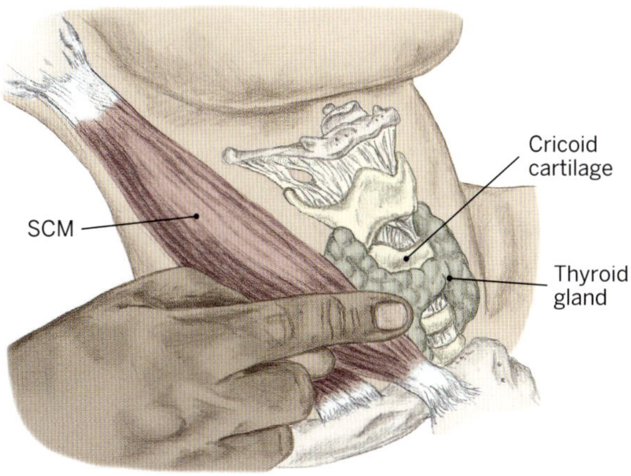

5.144 Anterior/lateral view of neck, as you palpate the thyroid gland

thyroid *thi*-royd Grk. shield

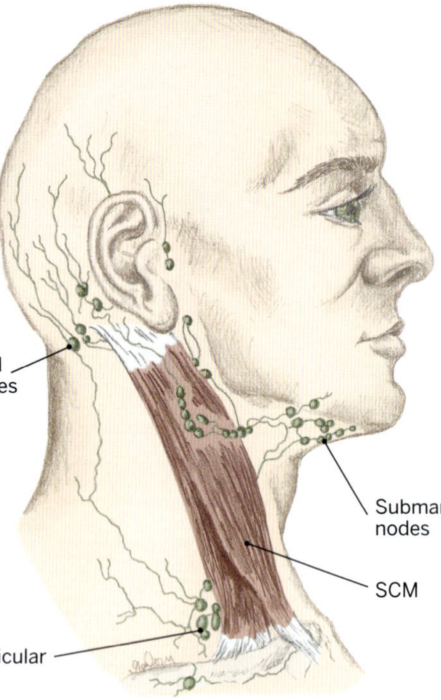

5.145 Lateral view of head and neck, showing cervical lymph nodes

Cervical Lymph Nodes

The numerous bundles of lymph nodes in the cervical region are divided into two groups: superficial and deep. The superficial cervical nodes (**5.145**) are located primarily along the underside of the mandible, posterior and inferior to the earlobe, and in the posterior triangle (p. 226) between the platysma and the deep fascia. The deep cervical nodes are larger and lie beside several large vessels and glands. Both the superficial and deep lymph nodes are slightly movable and have the size and texture of soft lentils or moist raisins. They are often tender on palpation.

Cervical lymph nodes

1. Partner supine or seated. Place your fingers on the lateral side of the neck. Using your broad fingerpads, gently palpate under the skin for the superficial cervical nodes.
2. Explore along the underside of the mandible and in the posterior triangle. Once you have located a node, carefully outline its size and shape.

Are they slightly movable and the size and texture of soft lentils?

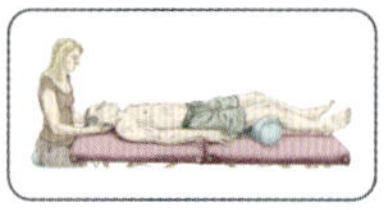

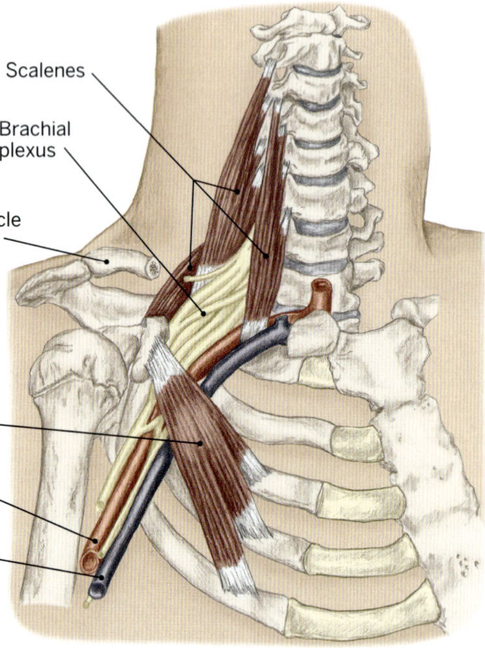

5.146 Anterior/lateral view of right shoulder and cervical spine, showing brachial plexus

Brachial Plexus

The brachial plexus is a large bundle of nerves that innervates the shoulder and upper extremity. After exiting from the transverse processes of C-5 to T-1, it squeezes between the anterior and middle scalenes, continues inferiorly and laterally, and ducks underneath the clavicle to the axillary region (**5.146**).

Although the brachial plexus can be accessed, it is best avoided. Compressing or impinging one of its nerves can create a sharp, shooting sensation down the arm.

Comparative Anatomy

Most mammals have a broad, thin sheet of muscle called the panniculus carnosus. It is an integumentary muscle that attaches to the underside of the skin and, in some species, covers the entire thorax. It enables a horse to shake off flies, an armadillo to roll into a ball, and a cat to raise the hair on its back (left). For humans, the platysma (p. 257) is believed to be all that remains of the panniculus carnosus.

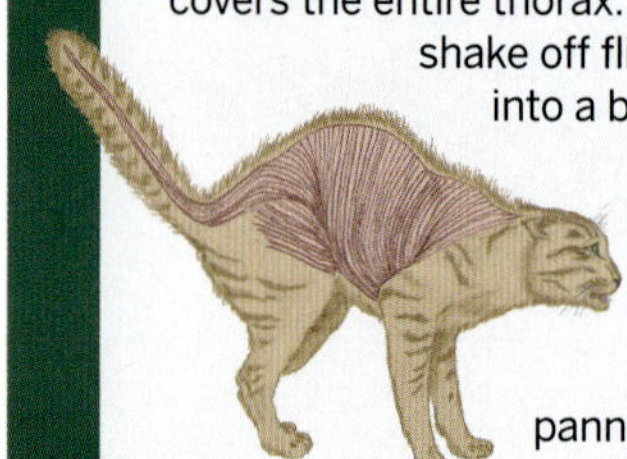

panniculus carnosus	pan-***ik***-u-lus car-***no***-sis	L. small, fleshy garment
plexus	***plek***-sus	L. interwoven

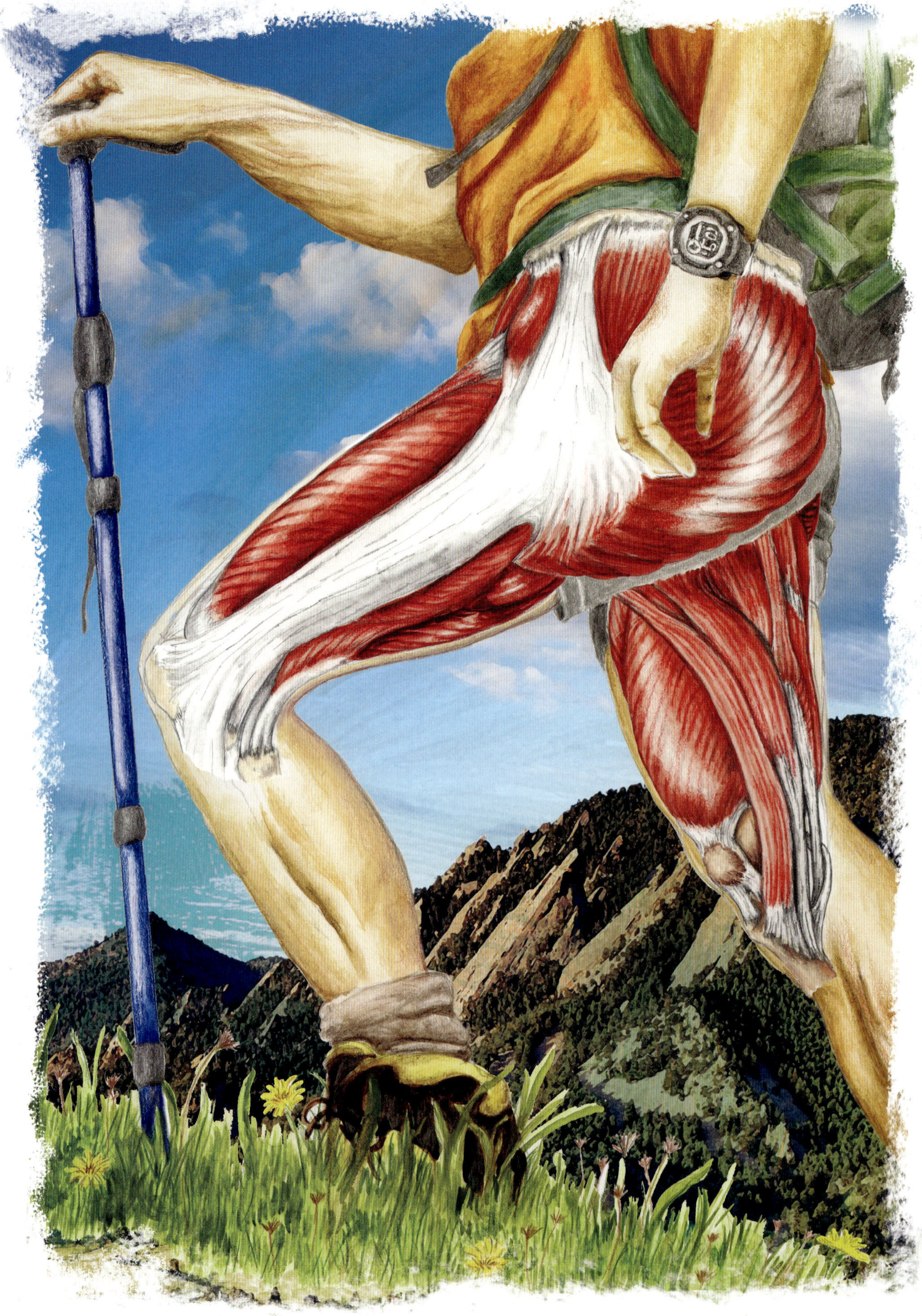

6

Pelvis & Thigh

Sitting, climbing stairs, squatting, lifting your leg to get into a car— many everyday movements depend on structures in the pelvis and thigh region. Because some of these structures are close to intimate areas, learning how to palpate in this region calls for careful, respectful practice and touch.

Please remember that therapeutic touch is a unique privilege given to health care professionals. Take some to time to consider the style of communication you would want to receive as a client. What would you need to hear and understand from your practitioner to feel safe? How could nonverbal elements—facial expressions, tone, gestures, and draping techniques—increase your comfort?

Knowledge is key, and this chapter will help you. Just like the hiker in this picture, we will go one step at a time. Your future clients will appreciate your ability to provide trustworthy and professional palpation in this region.

See for yourself:

- Look at the picture of the hiker on the previous page. Which of the shown muscle bellies and borders can you feel on your own hips and legs?
- What might be different about palpation techniques for these large muscles compared to smaller structures in the face and hands? Think about pressure, depth, and access to bony landmarks.
- Sit down and put your hands along the top of your pelvis. Feel the bony ridge that starts in the front and trails all the way around to the posterior side of the hips. Locate the two bony knobs that contact the chair underneath you. Are they bones of the thigh or hip?

Topographical Views

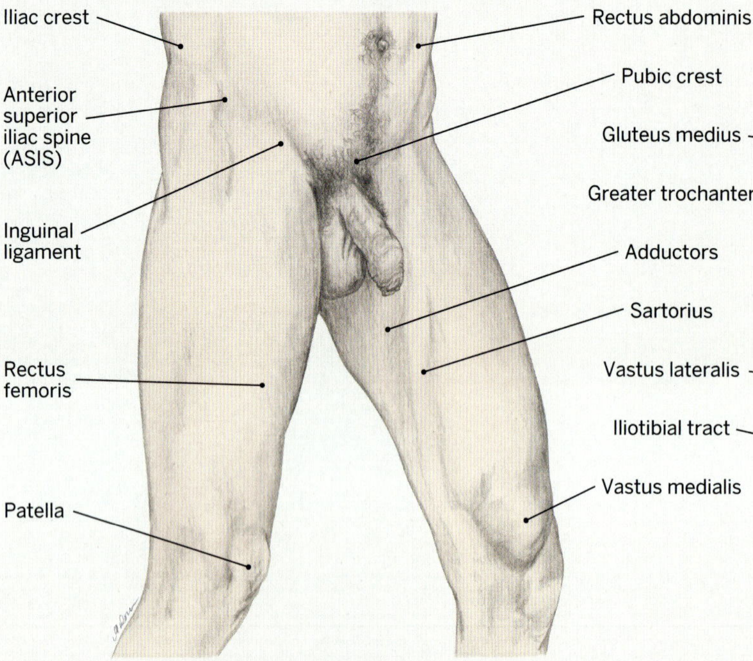

6.1 Anterior/lateral view of right thigh and anterior/medial view of the left thigh

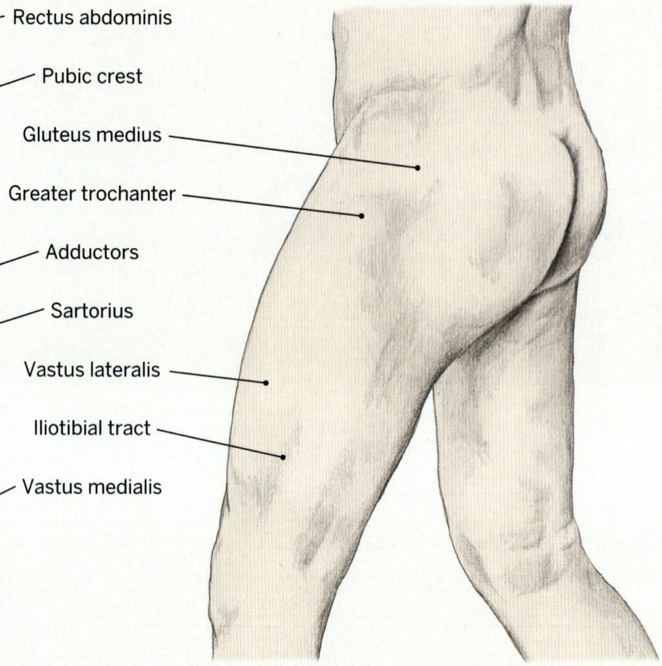

6.2 Posterior/lateral view of the left thigh and posterior/medial view of the right thigh

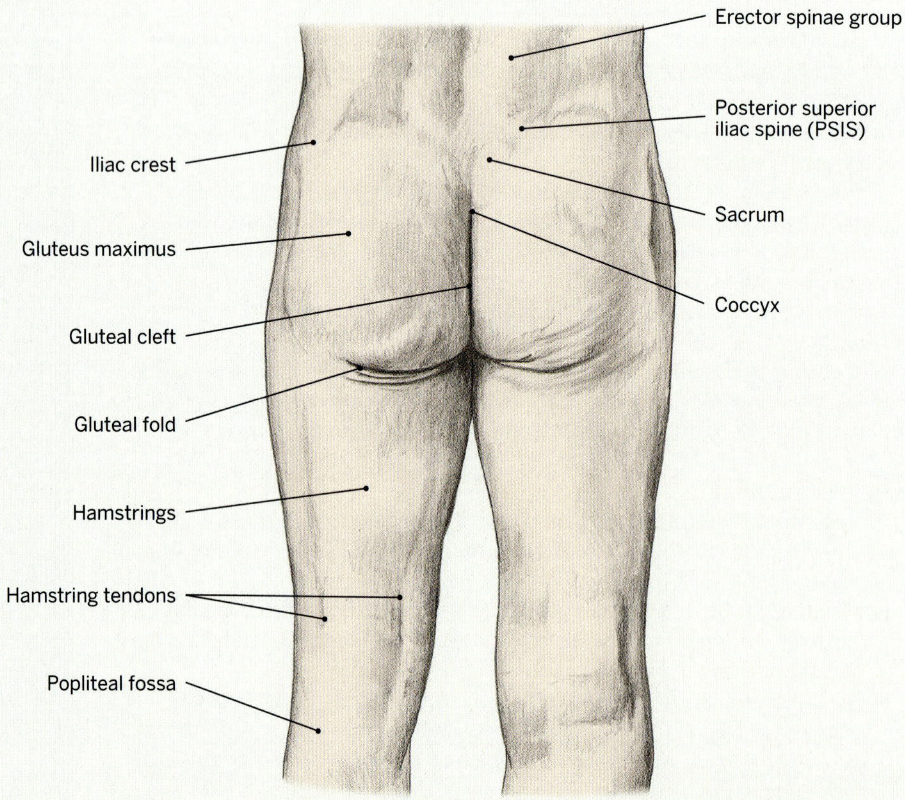

6.3 Posterior view of hips, buttocks, and thighs

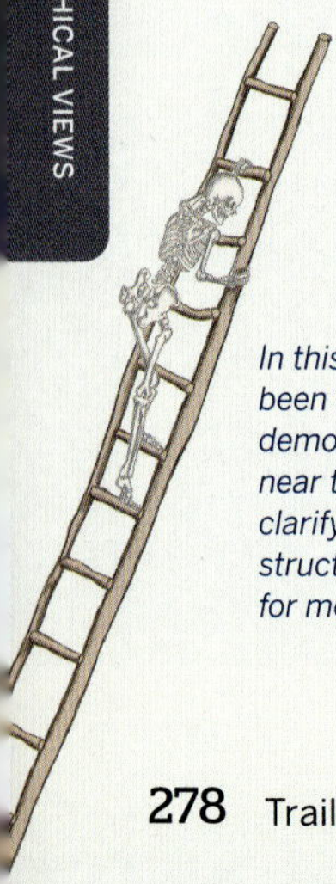

In this chapter, the male genitals have been included in the illustrations that demonstrate palpatory techniques near the base of the pelvis. This is to clarify their location with respect to the structure you are palpating. *See p. 297 for more information.*

Pelvis & Thigh

TOPOGRAPHICAL VIEWS

Exploring the Skin and Fascia

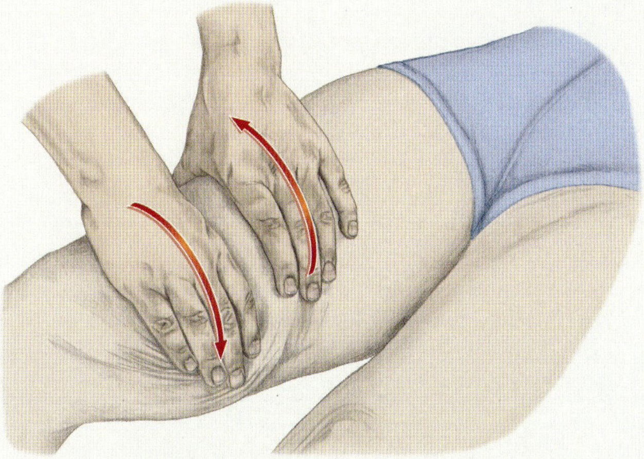

6.4 Partner supine, medial view of right thigh, as you palpate the thigh tissue

Thigh

1. Partner supine. Begin by placing your hands on your partner's thigh. Explore from the pelvis to the knee, sensing the temperature of the tissue. Be sure to access the thigh's medial and lateral sides as well.
2. Sink your hands into the thigh and gently twist the tissue in opposite directions (**6.4**). Take particular note of its thickness and elasticity. For example, the skin and fascia just proximal to the knee may be thinner than the tissue near the pelvis.

Posterior knee

1. Partner prone. Holding the ankle, passively flex the knee. Use your other hand to gently grasp the skin and fascia proximal to the posterior knee. As you roll it between your fingers, note the tissue's pliability and texture.
2. Compare what you have felt to the thicker tissue of the medial thigh and the denser fascia of the lateral thigh.
3. Still grasping the skin and fascia, passively flex and extend the knee (**6.5**). Feel the tissue stretch as the knee extends. Continue this same movement while grasping the sides of the thigh. If the tissue is difficult to grasp, you may want to use the flat of your hand to sense the changes in the tissue.

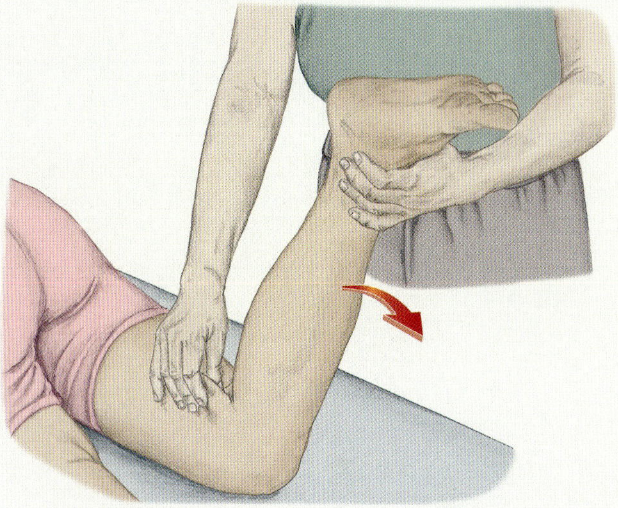

6.5 Partner prone, posterior/medial view of right thigh, as you passively flex and extend the knee

Buttocks

1. Partner prone. Using the back of your hand, explore the temperature of the posterior and lateral buttocks. It is not uncommon for the tissue to be cooler here than it is on the posterior thigh or low back.
2. Since the buttocks are composed of both large muscles and large quantities of adipose, they are a good area for exploring tissue differences. Setting your thumb on the gluteal fold (see **6.3**), gently but firmly grasp the tissue of the buttock.
3. Try grasping just the superficial skin and fascia, sensing its gelatinous quality. Then grasp a bit deeper and feel the thick, striated mass of the gluteal muscles (**6.6**).

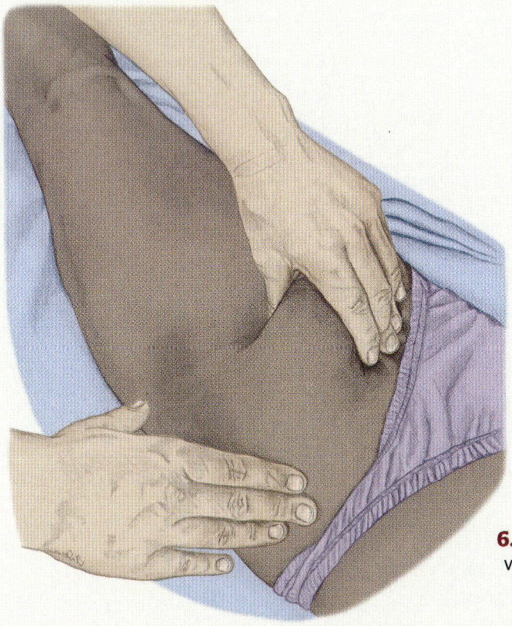

6.6 Partner prone, superior/lateral view of right thigh, as you palpate the gluteal muscles

Bones of the Pelvis and Thigh

The **pelvis** (pelvic girdle) consists of the sacrum, the coccyx, and the two hip bones (**6.7**). Each **hip** (coxal) bone is formed by the fusion of three smaller bones: the **ilium**, **ischium**, and **pubis** (**6.8**). Although the pelvis is deep to surrounding muscles, organs, and adipose tissue, aspects of it are easily palpable.

The superficial **sacrum** lies posteriorly between the hip bones. The small **coccyx** extends inferiorly from the sacrum. The sacrum and coccyx, both made up of fused vertebrae, are considered part of the vertebral column.

The **femur** is the longest, heaviest, and strongest bone in the body. Its proximal end articulates with the hip at the acetabulum to form the ball-and-socket-shaped coxal (hip) joint. Portions of the proximal femur are partially accessible. The femoral shaft is surrounded by the thick muscles of the thigh, while the distal end of the femur is superficial.

The distal femur articulates with the proximal tibia to form the tibiofemoral (knee) joint. The tibiofemoral joint is a modified hinge joint, which means it can flex and extend and, when in a flexed position, can medially and laterally rotate the knee.

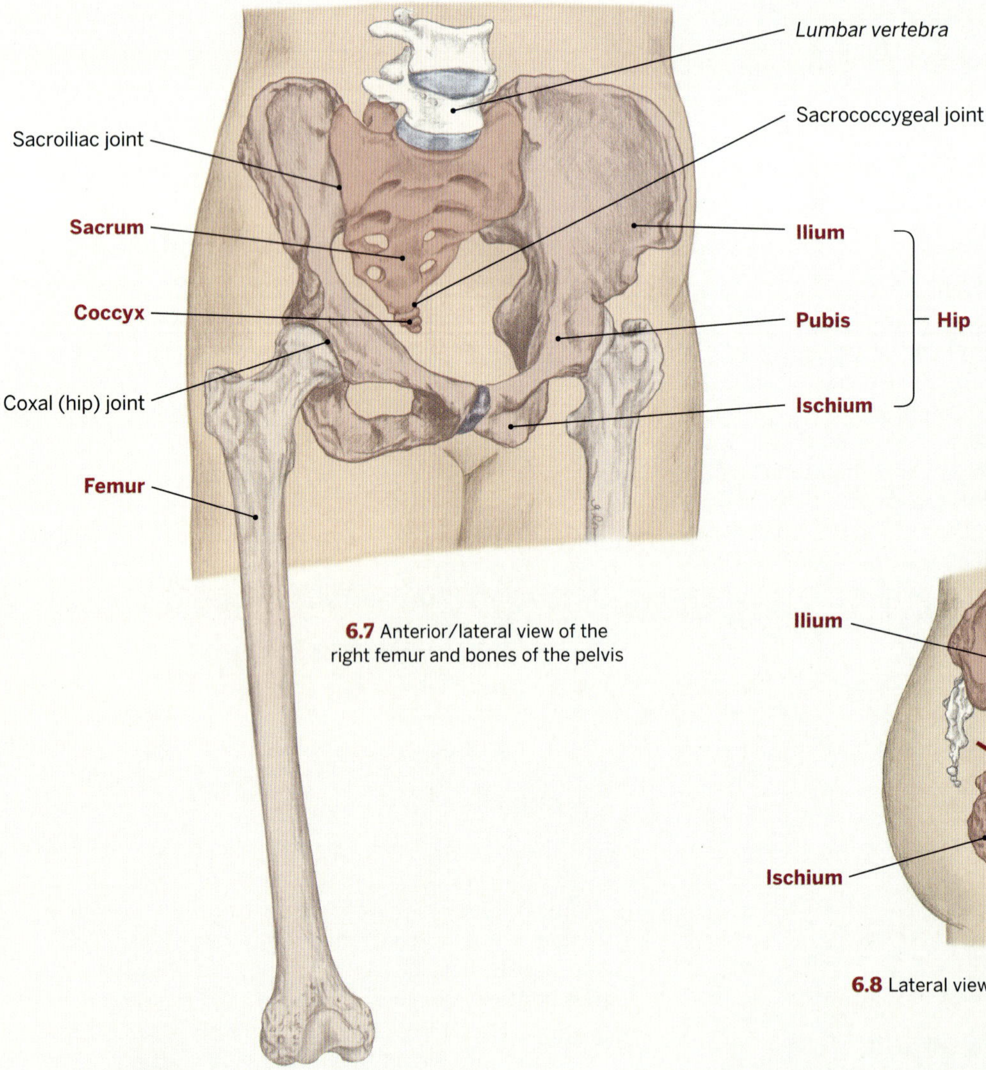

6.7 Anterior/lateral view of the right femur and bones of the pelvis

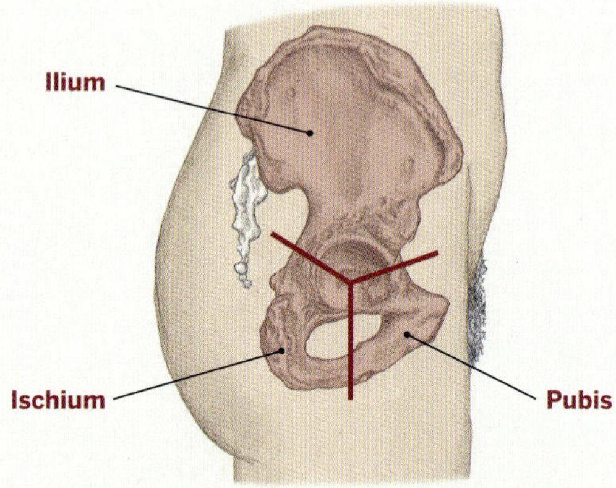

6.8 Lateral view of bones of the right hip

Discover More

The shape of the pelvis is different in females and males. The female pelvis is broader, for carrying and delivering a child. It has a wider iliac crest, a larger pelvic "bowl," and a greater distance between ischial tuberosities.

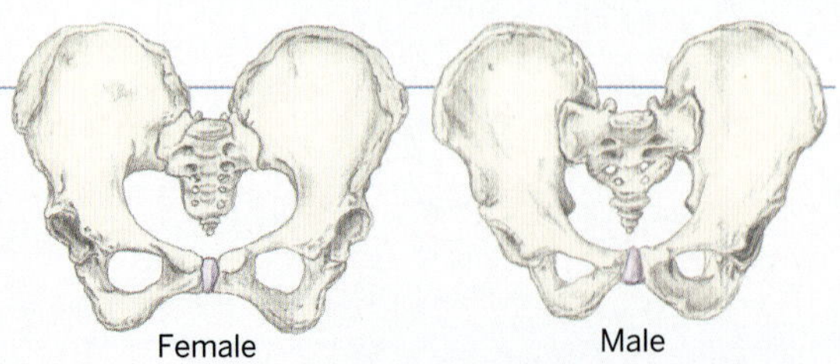

acetabulum	***as***-e-***tab***-u-lum	L. a little saucer for vinegar
femur	***fee***-mur	L. thigh
pelvis	***pel***-vis	L. basin

Bony Landmarks of the Pelvis and Thigh

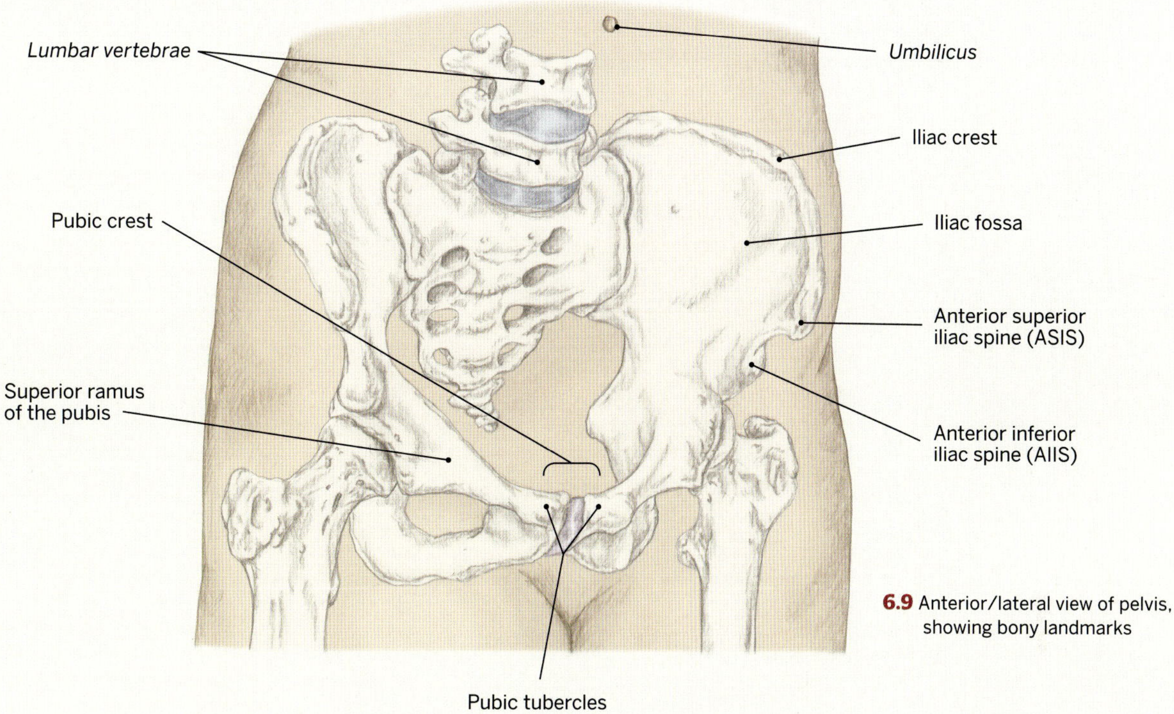

6.9 Anterior/lateral view of pelvis, showing bony landmarks

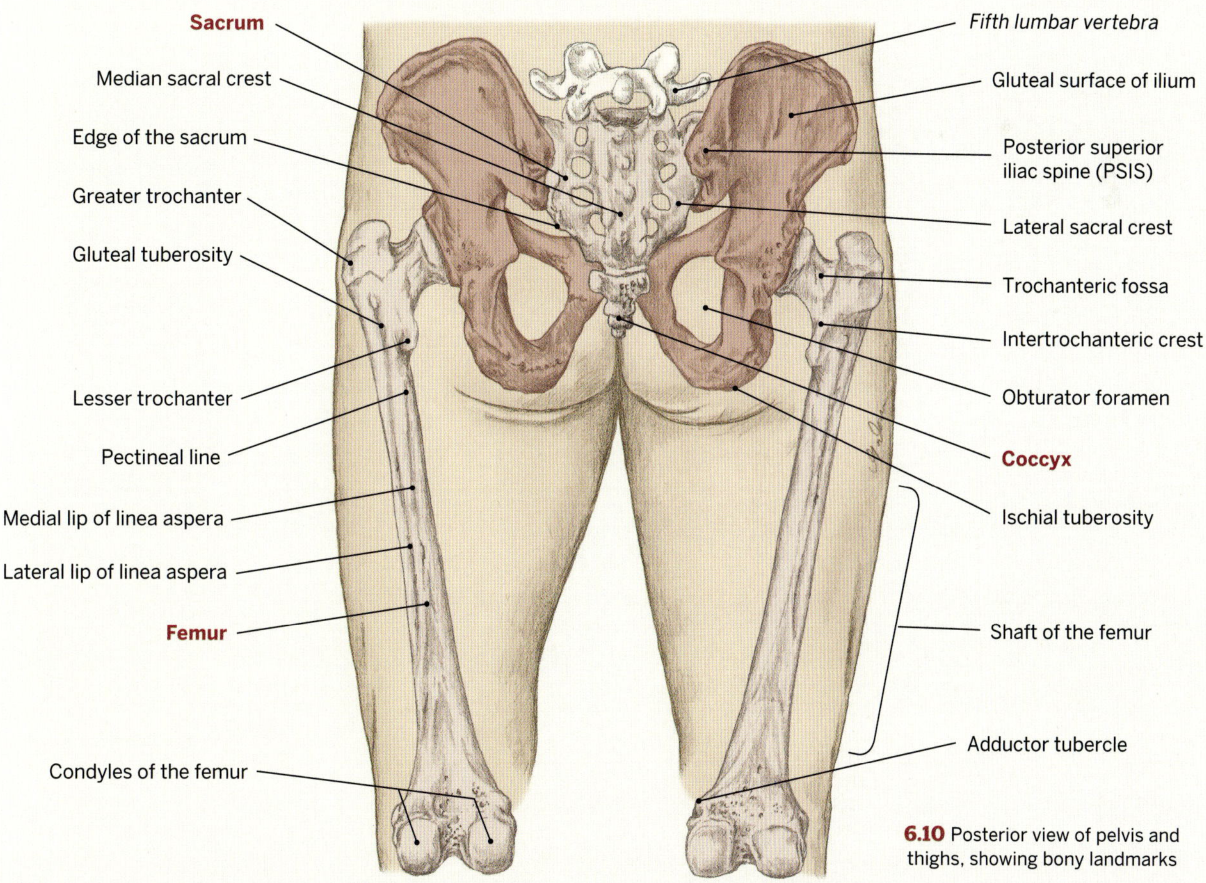

6.10 Posterior view of pelvis and thighs, showing bony landmarks

ischium	***ish**-ee-um*	Grk. hip	**linea aspera**	***lin**-e-a **as**-per-a*	L. rough line
ilium	***il**-ee-um*	L. groin, flank	**pubis**	***pu**-bis*	NL. bone of the groin

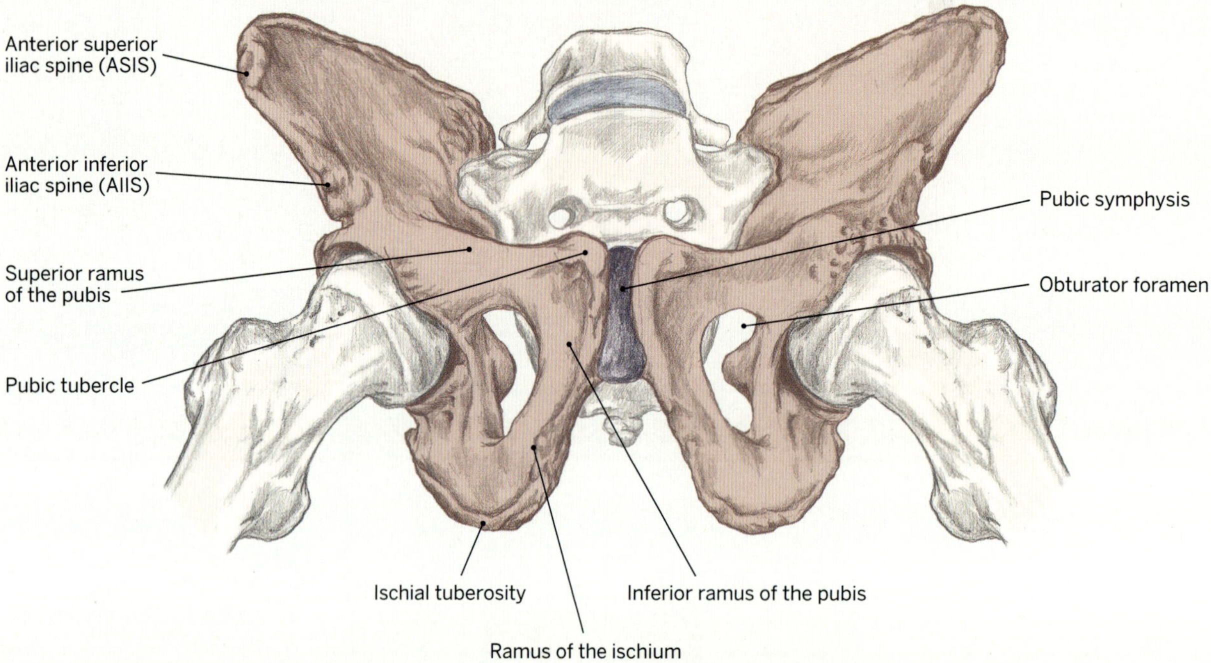

6.11 Inferior view of pelvis, with femurs abducted and externally rotated, showing bony landmarks

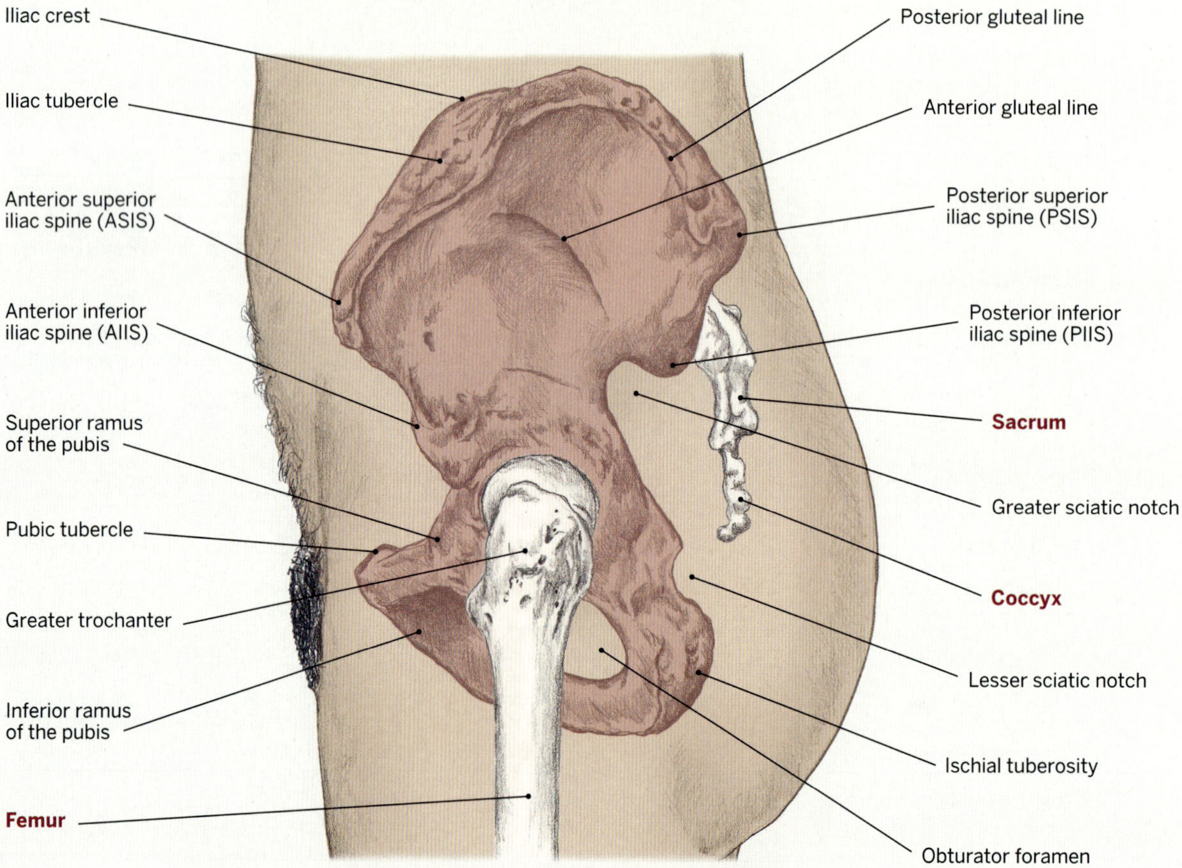

6.12 Lateral view of pelvis and left thigh, showing bony landmarks

foramen for-***aye***-men L. a passage or opening

The Hip

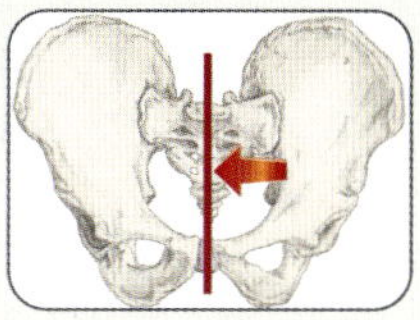

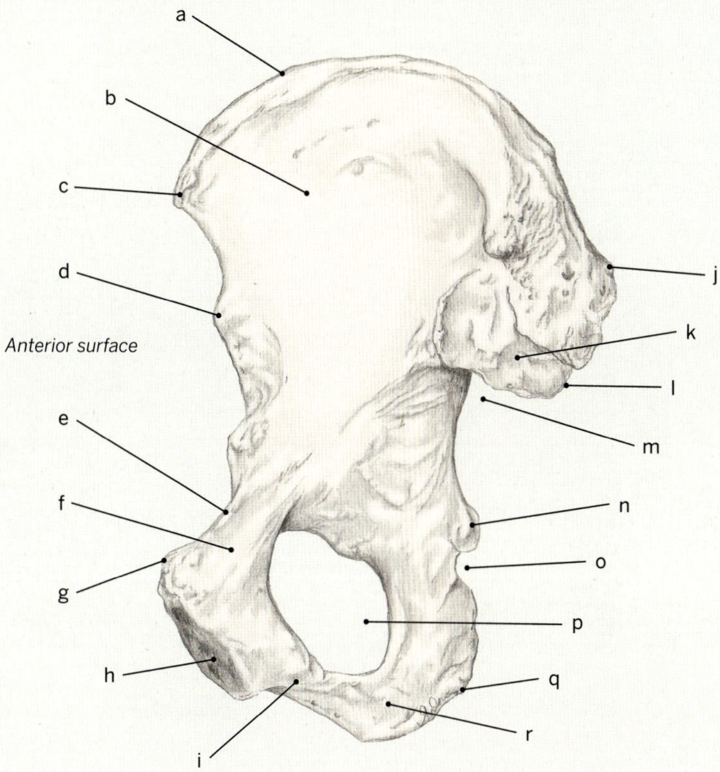

- **a.** Iliac crest
- **b.** Iliac fossa
- **c.** Anterior superior iliac spine (ASIS)
- **d.** Anterior inferior iliac spine (AIIS)
- **e.** Pectineal line
- **f.** Superior ramus of the pubis
- **g.** Pubic tubercle
- **h.** Symphyseal surface
- **i.** Inferior ramus of the pubis
- **j.** Posterior superior iliac spine (PSIS)
- **k.** Articular surface for sacrum
- **l.** Posterior inferior iliac spine (PIIS)
- **m.** Greater sciatic notch
- **n.** Ischial spine
- **o.** Lesser sciatic notch
- **p.** Obturator foramen
- **q.** Ischial tuberosity
- **r.** Ramus of the ischium

6.13 Medial view of right hip

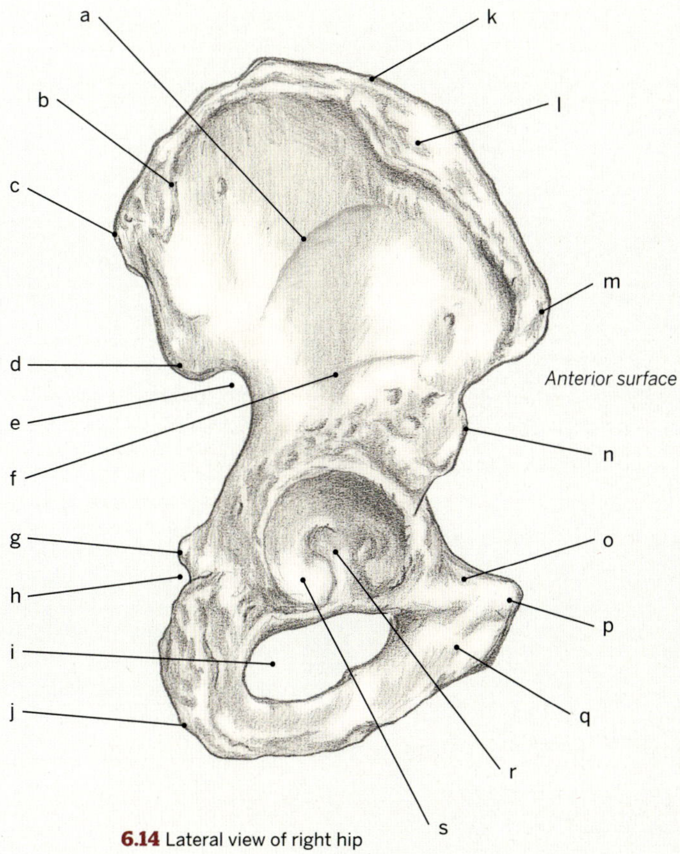

6.14 Lateral view of right hip

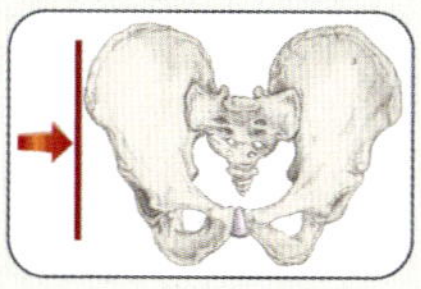

- **a.** Anterior gluteal line
- **b.** Posterior gluteal line
- **c.** Posterior superior iliac spine (PSIS)
- **d.** Posterior inferior iliac spine (PIIS)
- **e.** Greater sciatic notch
- **f.** Inferior gluteal line
- **g.** Ischial spine
- **h.** Lesser sciatic notch
- **i.** Obturator foramen
- **j.** Ischial tuberosity
- **k.** Iliac crest
- **l.** Iliac tubercle
- **m.** Anterior superior iliac spine (ASIS)
- **n.** Anterior inferior iliac spine (AIIS)
- **o.** Superior ramus of the pubis
- **p.** Pubic tubercle
- **q.** Inferior ramus of the pubis
- **r.** Acetabulum
- **s.** Lunate surface of acetabulum

The Sacrum and Coccyx

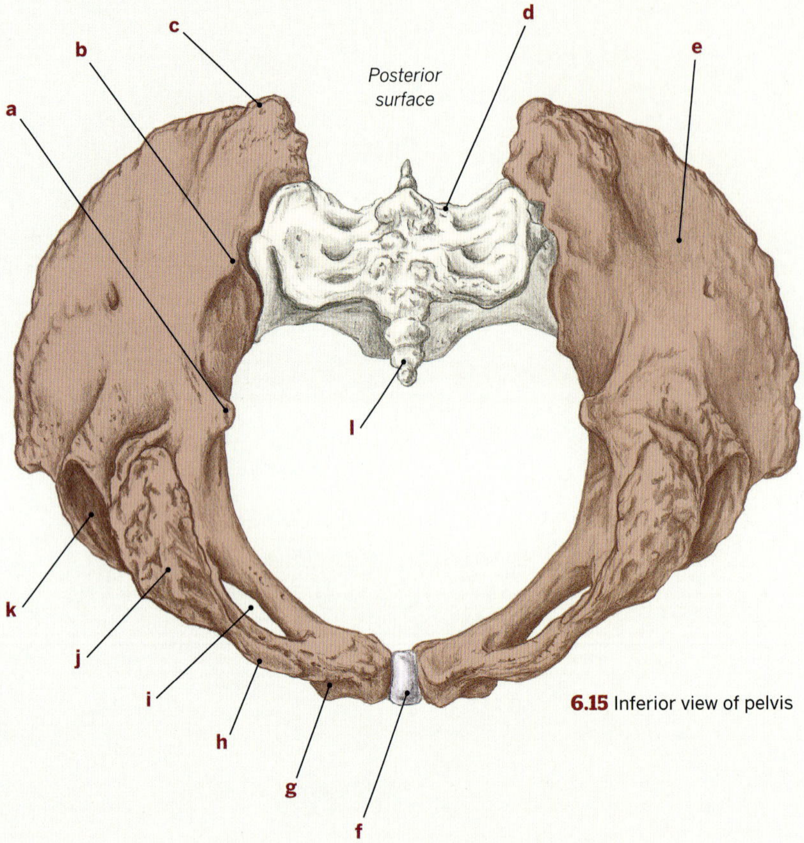

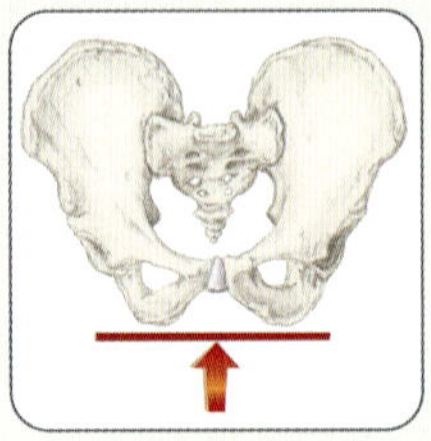

a. Ischial spine
b. Posterior inferior iliac spine (PIIS)
c. Posterior superior iliac spine (PSIS)
d. **Sacrum**
e. Gluteal surface of ilium
f. Pubic symphysis
g. Inferior ramus of the pubis
h. Ramus of ischium
i. Obturator foramen
j. Ischial tuberosity
k. Acetabulum
l. **Coccyx**

6.15 Inferior view of pelvis

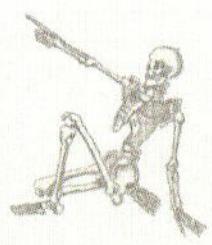

Black letters indicate bones; **red** letters indicate bony landmarks or other structures.

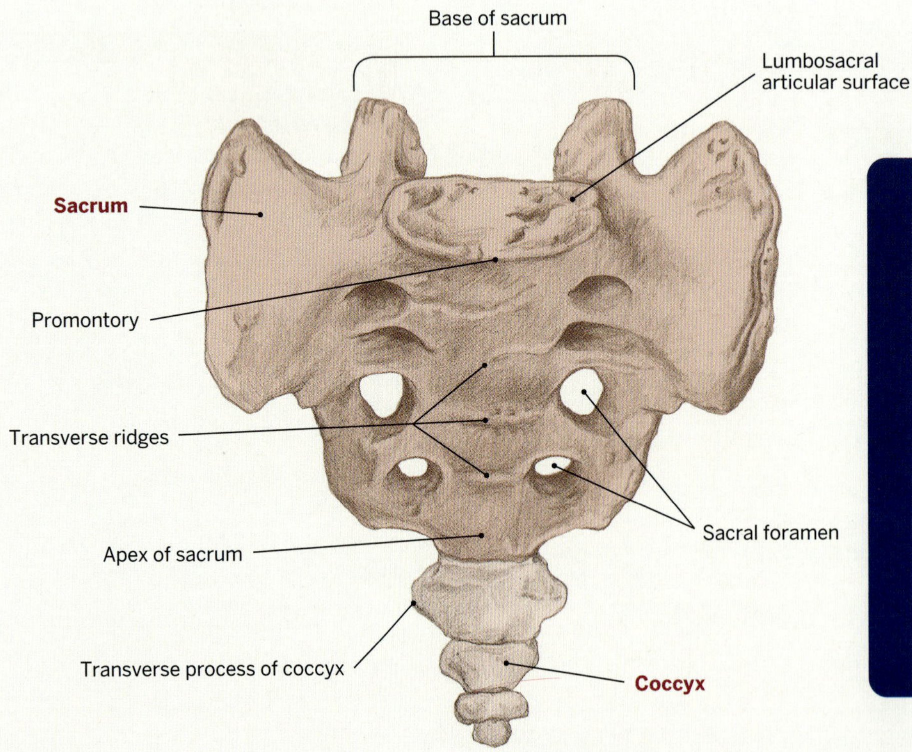

6.16 Anterior view of sacrum and coccyx

Discover More

Why is there a big hole in the hip? The **obturator foramen** (**6.14**, i) is located along the inferior part of the pelvis, surrounded by the pubis and ischium. It began quite small—as seen in the skeletal remains of early reptiles. On humans, the foramen is situated between weight-bearing lines, and, since bone is heavy and (in a sense) costly to maintain, the foramen evolved into a larger hole covered with a membrane.

symphysis *sim*-fi-sis Grk. growing together

The Femur

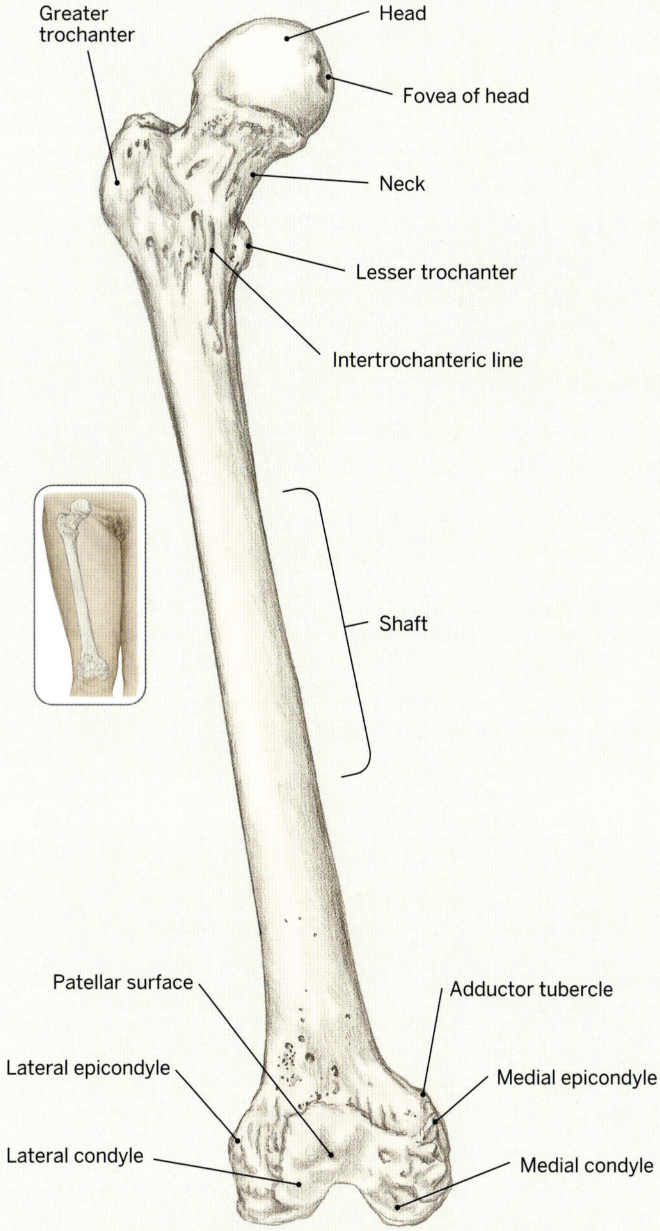

6.17 Anterior view of right femur

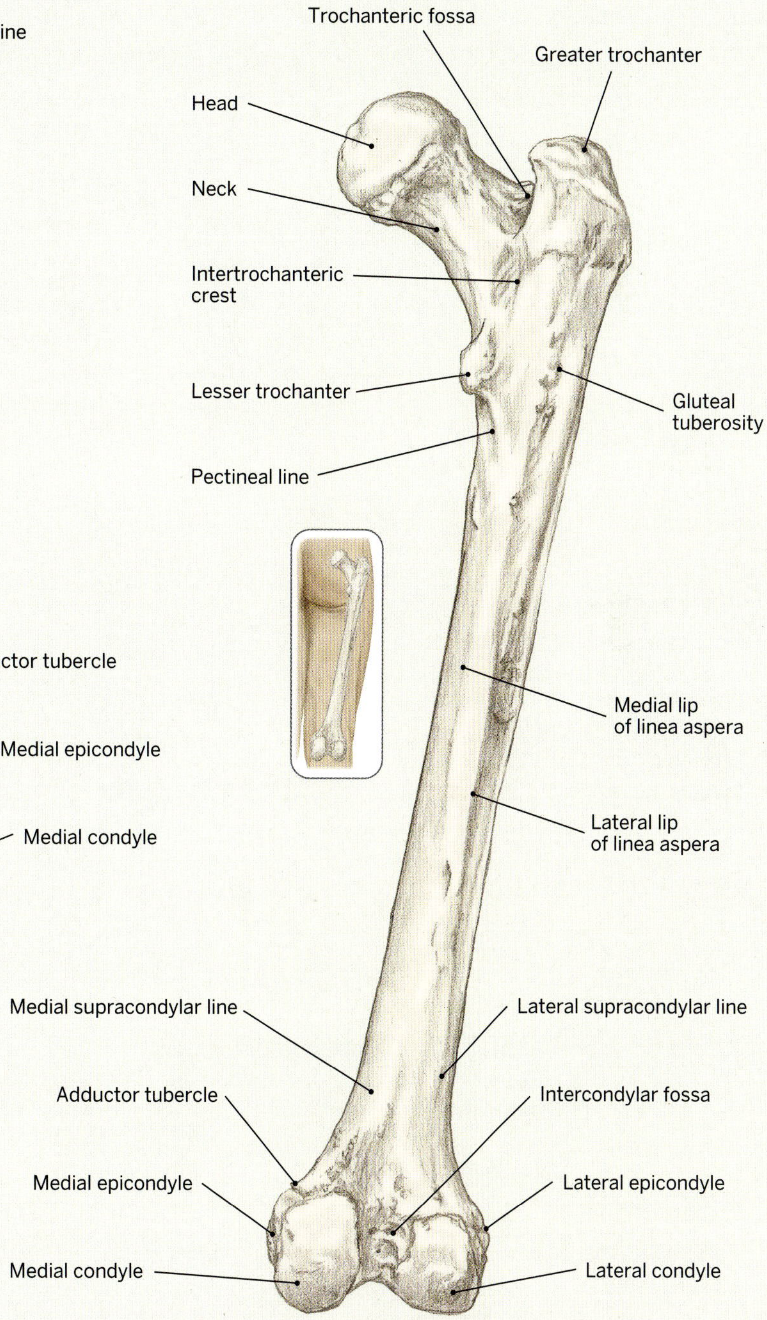

6.18 Posterior view of right femur

Overview: **Bony Landmark Trails**

Trail 1 Solo Pass

Due to the pelvis's multifaceted shape and proximity to sensitive areas, palpating your partner's pelvic region may challenge you initially. **Trail 1** is designed to give you an opportunity to access your own pelvic region first. This will generate the confidence needed to palpate effectively on your partner over the next four trails. These six landmarks can be seen as your "base camps"—they are clearly accessible and will lead you to the other landmarks of the pelvis.

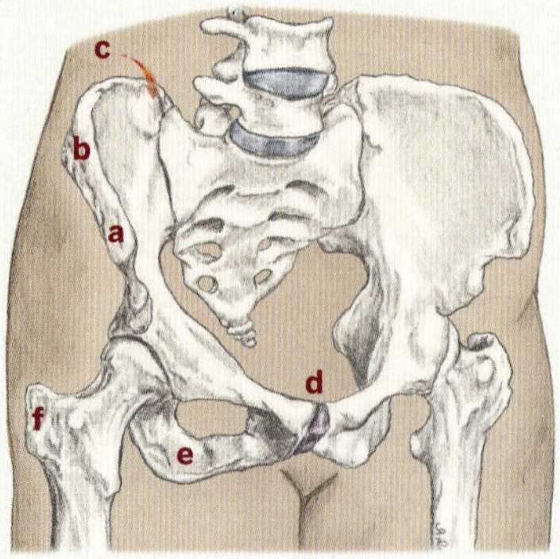

Trail 1

- **a** Anterior superior iliac spine (ASIS)
- **b** Iliac crest
- **c** Posterior superior iliac spine (PSIS)
- **d** Pubic crest
- **e** Ischial tuberosity
- **f** Greater trochanter of the femur

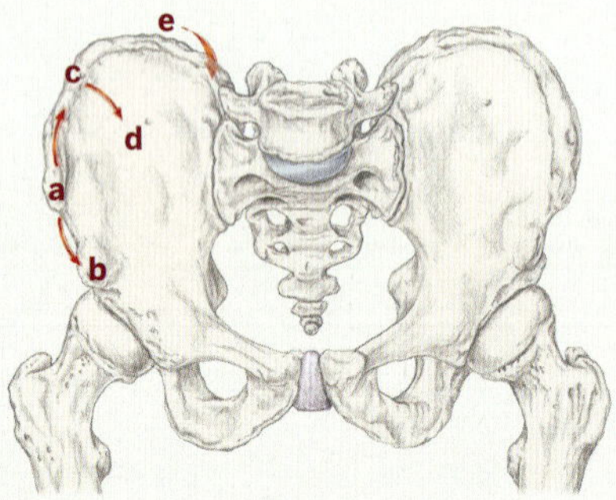

Trail 2

Trail 2 Iliac Avenue travels along the superior aspect of the pelvis on the ilium.

- **a** Anterior superior iliac spine (ASIS)
- **b** Anterior inferior iliac spine (AIIS)
- **c** Iliac crest
- **d** Iliac fossa
- **e** Posterior superior iliac spine (PSIS)

Trail 3 Tailbone Trail accesses the bones at the base of the spine.

- **a** Posterior superior iliac spine (PSIS)
- **b** Sacrum
- **c** Median sacral crest
- **d** Edge of the sacrum
- **e** Coccyx
- **f** Sacroiliac joint

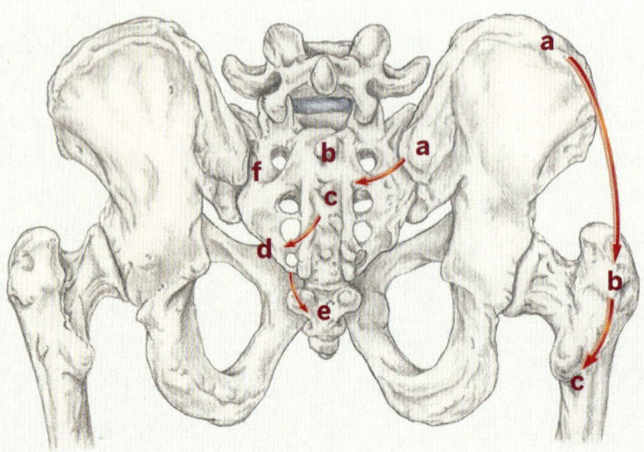

Trail 3

Trail 4

Trail 4 Hip Hike explores the lateral hip and landmarks of the proximal femur.

- **a** Iliac crest
- **b** Greater trochanter
- **c** Gluteal tuberosity

Trail 5 The Underpass follows around the pubic region to access the landmarks of the medial thigh.

- **a** Umbilicus
- **b** Pubic crest and tubercles
- **c** Superior ramus of the pubis
- **d** Inferior ramus of the pubis and ramus of the ischium
- **e** Ischial tuberosity

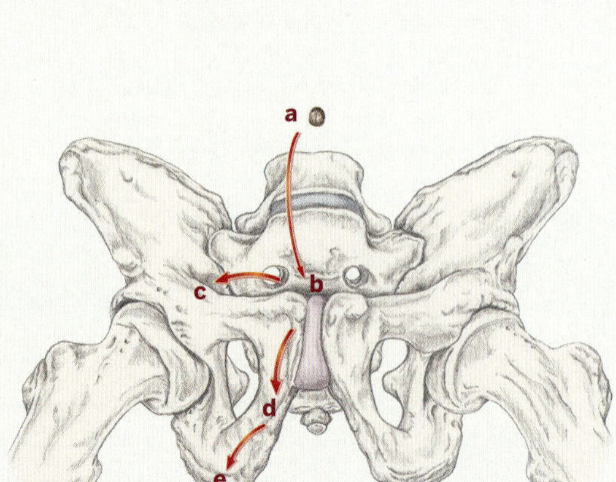

Trail 5

Anterior Superior Iliac Spine (ASIS)

As the name suggests, the ASIS is located on the anterior and superior aspect of the ilium. Both ASISs are the superficial tips located below the waistline. The ASIS serves as the attachment site for the sartorius muscle and the inguinal ligament.

(Note: Prior to the mid-1990s, when pants were designed and worn in a manner that fit the pelvic region, the ASISs were located "underneath the front pants pockets." Nowadays, with the waistbands of both young men and women rarely seen "north" of the mid-gluteal cleft, this helpful hint no longer applies.)

ASIS

1. Locate both anterior superior iliac spines by placing your hands on your hips with fingers in front, thumbs behind. Feel for the tip of the pelvis that sticks out anteriorly (**6.19**).
2. Explore these points and the surrounding structures of the ilium. Try palpating them on yourself from a seated position so that the overlying tissue will be soft.

Are the bones you feel just beneath the surface of the skin? Are you inferior to the level of the umbilicus?

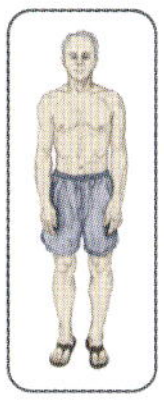

Palpate on yourself first.

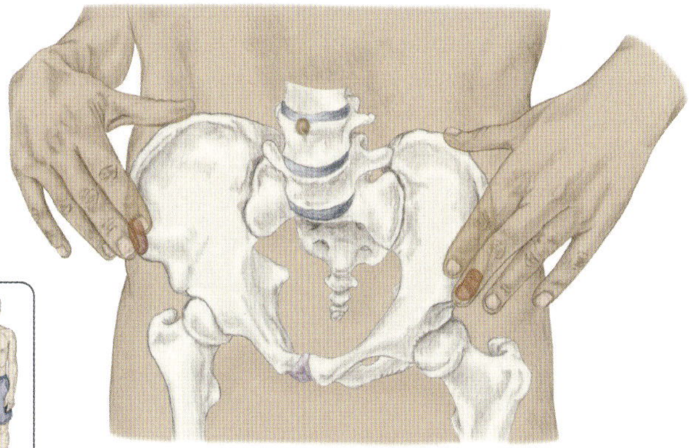

6.19 Anterior view of pelvis, as you palpate your ASISs

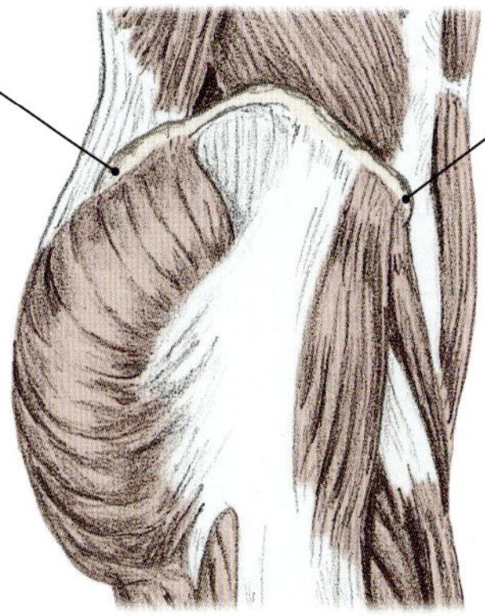

6.20 Lateral view of pelvis, showing the muscles that surround the iliac crest

Iliac Crest

The iliac crest is the long, superior edge of the ilium. It begins at the ASIS and extends around the side of the torso to end at the posterior superior iliac spine (PSIS). Besides helping to keep your pants up, the iliac crests serve as attachment sites for the quadratus lumborum (p. 207) and abdominal muscles. Each crest is superficial and easily palpable, as the muscles that attach to it do not cross over its edge (**6.20**).

Iliac crest

1. Locate the ASIS. Slowly walk your fingers around the side of your hip, pressing into the wide edge of the crest. Note how the crest rises from the ASIS and soon after may widen laterally (**6.21**).
2. Follow the crest as it continues around to the posterior side of the body and ends at the PSIS.

Can you sink your fingers into the flesh of the abdomen just above the iliac crest?

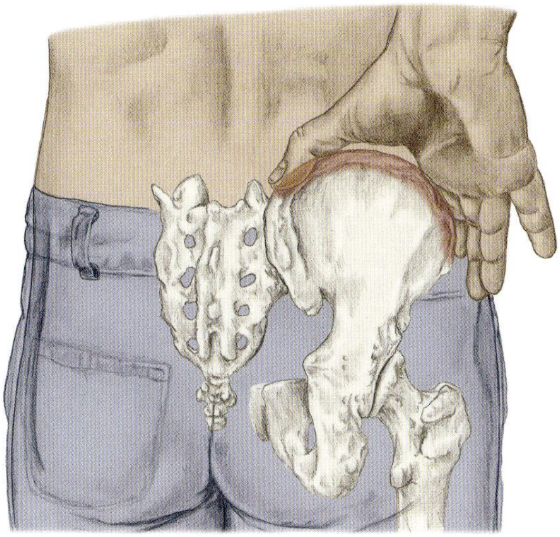

6.21 Posterior view of pelvis, as you slide your fingers along your iliac crest

Pelvis & Thigh

Posterior Superior Iliac Spine (PSIS)

The superficial PSIS is located at the posterior end of the iliac crest. In most people, both PSISs can be visibly identified by the two small dimples found at the base of the low back. Without the help of a mirror, you might have trouble seeing your own PSISs, but you can still palpate them.

PSIS

1. Standing. Place your thumbs on your iliac crests. Follow the crests around the posterior hip. Note how they descend as you move medially.
2. The PSISs might feel like small humps surrounded by thicker tissues and are not as pronounced as the ASISs (**6.22**).

Are you at the posterior end of the iliac crests? Are the points you feel three to four inches apart from each other?

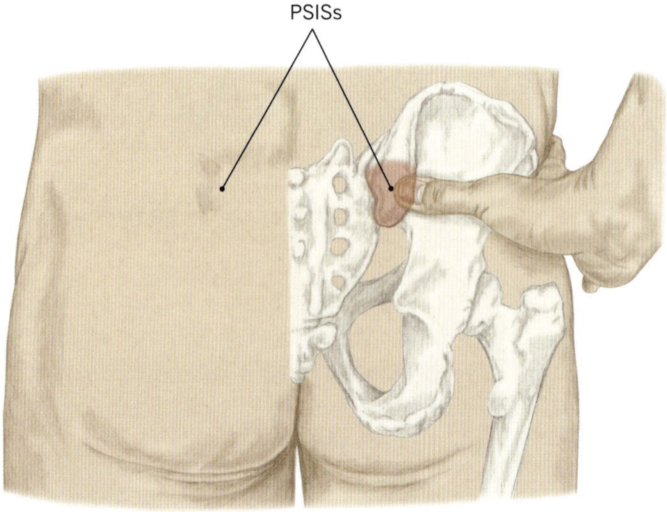

6.22 Posterior view of pelvis, as you locate your PSIS

Pubic Crest

The pubic crest is located directly inferior to the navel and superior to the genitals. Formed by the superior, medial edge of both pubic bones, the horizontal crest is roughly two inches wide and clearly palpable. It is an attachment site for the rectus abdominis muscle (p. 209) and the rectus sheath.

Pubic crest

1. Position your fingers at your navel.
2. Slowly slide your fingers down the midline of the body toward the pubic region (**6.23**). You might travel five to eight inches before you feel the firm ridge of the pubic crest. You will be one to two inches superior to the genitals.

Are you at the midline of the body? Are you inferior to the level of the ASISs? Do you feel a solid, horizontal ridge of bone just above the genital region?

Locate the ASIS. Follow the inguinal ligament (p. 341) inferiorly 45° to the midline of the body until you reach the crest.

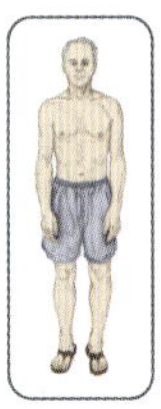

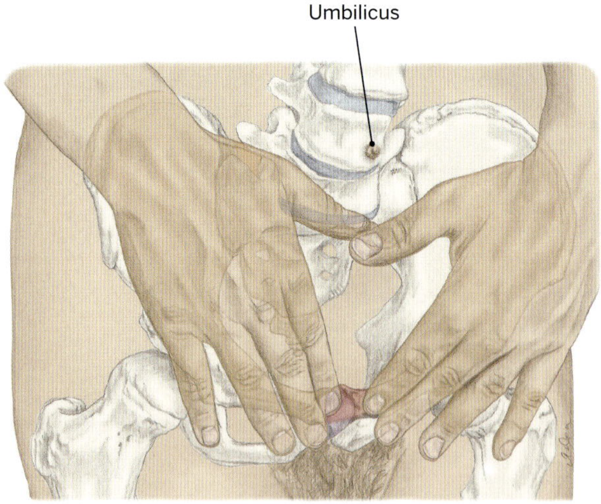

6.23 Anterior view of pelvis, as you access your pubic crest

Pelvis & Thigh

Ischial Tuberosity

If you have ever sat through a long musical or sporting event on a metal folding chair, then your ischial tuberosities are no strangers to you. The "sits bones" are located on the most inferior aspect of the pelvis at the level of the gluteal fold (the horizontal crease between the buttocks and thigh). The ischial tuberosity serves as an attachment site for the hamstrings, adductor magnus, and the sacrotuberous ligament.

Ischial tuberosity

1. Have a seat on a hard chair or surface and rock side-to-side, feeling your "sits bones."
2. Stand up and palpate the bone you were sitting on—your ischial tuberosity (**6.24**). Explore in all directions the large surface of the tuberosity.

Do you feel an identical structure between the other buttock and thigh?

Greater Trochanter of the Femur

Located distal to the iliac crest, the greater trochanter is the large, superficial mass located on the side of the hip. It is easily palpable and serves as an attachment site for the gluteus medius, gluteus minimus, and lateral rotators of the hip.

Greater trochanter

1. Locate the middle of the iliac crest.
2. Slide your fingerpads inferiorly four to six inches along the lateral side of the thigh until you reach the superficial mass of the greater trochanter. Explore and sculpt around all sides of its wide hump.

*Medially and laterally rotate your hip as you palpate the trochanter. Do you feel its wide, knobby surface swivel back and forth under your fingers (**6.25**)?*

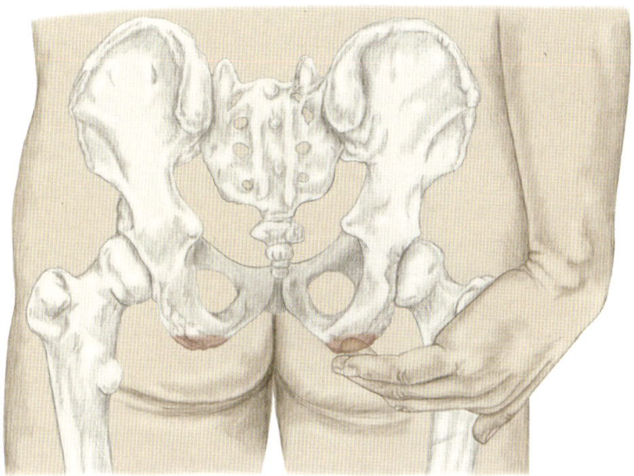

6.24 Posterior view of pelvis, as you palpate your ischial tuberosity

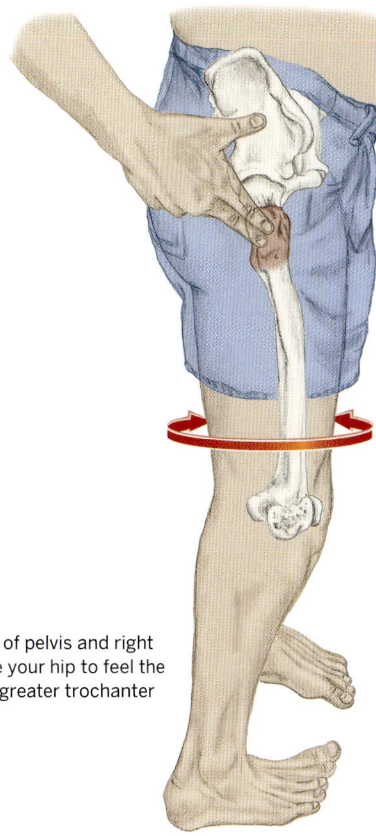

6.25 Lateral view of pelvis and right thigh, as you rotate your hip to feel the movement of the greater trochanter

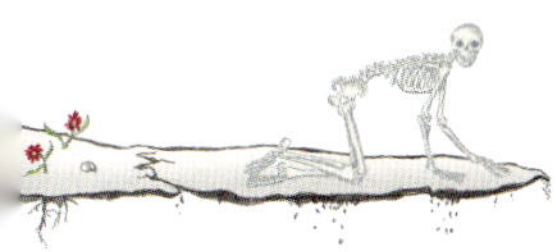

When exploring the area around the sacrum and posterior iliac crest, it is not uncommon to locate small nodules of fibrofatty tissue. Embedded in the superficial fascia, they may vary in size from a pea to a large marble.

trochanter tro-***kan***-ter Grk. to run

Trail 2 Iliac Avenue ▸

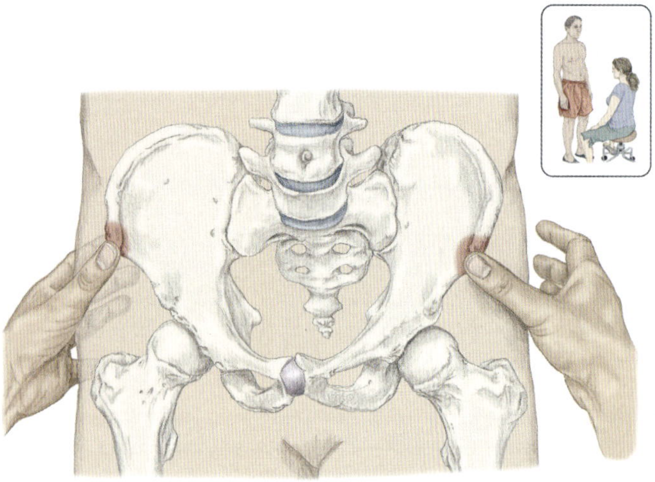

6.26 Partner standing, anterior view of pelvis, as you locate both ASISs

Anterior Superior Iliac Spine (ASIS)

(Refer to p. 287 for more information.)

ASIS

1. Partner standing. Place your hand on the side of the abdomen, below the level of the umbilicus.
2. Gently compress inferiorly until you feel the superficial tip of the ASIS (**6.26**). Palpate and observe the distance between the two ASISs and their relationship to each other.

Is the bony tip you feel superficial? Are you inferior to the level of the navel? Are you superior to the genital region?

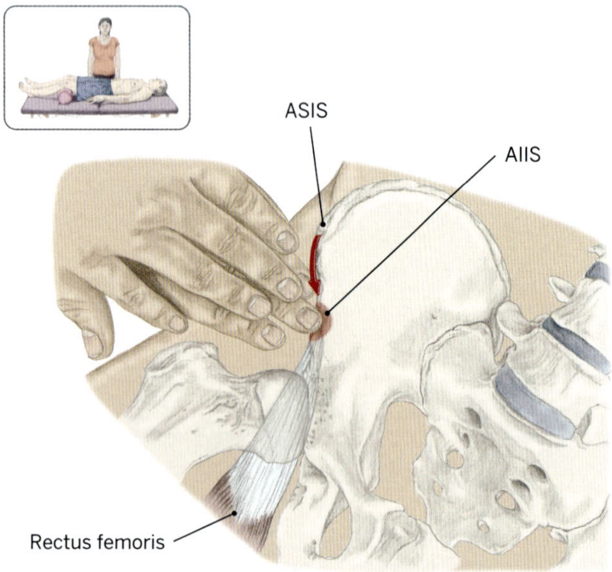

6.27 Partner supine, anterior/medial view of pelvis, as you access the AIIS

Anterior Inferior Iliac Spine (AIIS)

The AIIS is located inferior and medial to the ASIS and is the attachment site for the rectus femoris muscle (p. 308). Smaller and flatter than the ASIS, the AIIS is deep to the sartorius muscle and inguinal ligament. Because of its subtle shape and its depth to the sartorius, the AIIS can be difficult to distinguish.

AIIS

1. Partner supine. Flex the hip by bolstering under your partner's knee to shorten and soften the overlying tissue.
2. Locate the ASIS. Slide inferiorly and medially approximately one inch.
3. Palpate deep to the overlying tendons and explore for the small mound of the AIIS (**6.27**).

Are you medial and inferior to the ASIS? If your partner flexes his hip slightly, can you feel the tendon of the rectus femoris tighten under your fingers? (The overlying sartorius tendon will also become taut with this action.)

Palpation Plus

Along the lateral edge of the iliac crest, there is a subtle widening called the iliac tubercle. It designates the boundary between the origins of the tensor fasciae latae and gluteus medius muscles.

1. Locate the ASIS.
2. Slide posteriorly along the iliac crest approximately two inches. Explore the lateral edge of the iliac crest where it swells slightly. This is the iliac tubercle.

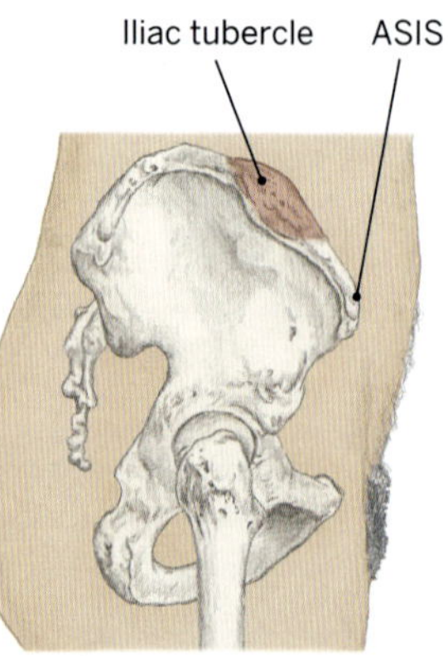

Iliac Crest

(*Refer to p. 287 for more information.*)

Iliac crest

1. Partner side lying. Locate the ASIS.
2. Slide posteriorly along the iliac crest, observing how it widens and rises up along its path.
3. Follow the crest as it continues around the posterior side of the body to the PSIS (**6.28**).

Can you spread the webbing between your finger and thumb along the length of the crest?

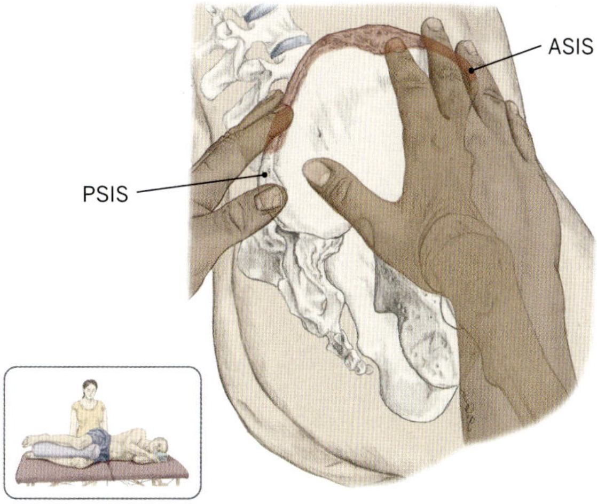

6.28 Partner side lying, as you sculpt out the iliac crest

Iliac Fossa

The bowl-shaped iliac fossa is located on the medial surface of the ilium and is an attachment site for the iliacus muscle. The presence of the iliacus and the abdominal contents makes the majority of the fossa inaccessible; however, you can sink your fingers slowly over the iliac crest and into the fossa to palpate it.

Iliac fossa

1. Partner supine. Flex the hip by bolstering under your partner's knee to shorten and soften the overlying tissue.
2. Lay the fingertips of one hand along the iliac crest just posterior and superior to the ASIS.
3. Moving slowly and patiently, curl your fingertips over the lip of the iliac crest into the iliac fossa (**6.29**). Depending on the firmness of the tissue, you might sink in only a small distance.

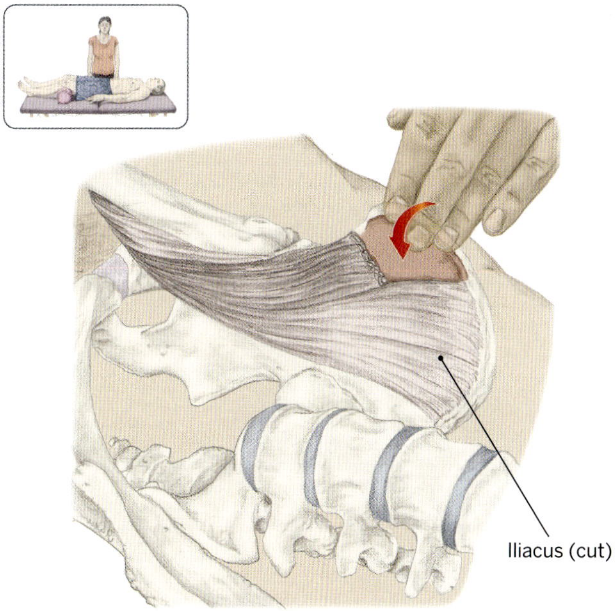

6.29 Partner supine, as you curl your fingers into the iliac fossa

Posterior Superior Iliac Spine (PSIS)

(*Refer to p. 288 for more information.*)

PSIS

1. Partner standing. Follow both iliac crests posteriorly around the waist.
2. Follow the crests as they descend toward the sacrum and end at each PSIS (**6.30**). The PSIS will feel like a shallow hump surrounded by thicker tissues. It is not as pronounced as the ASIS but is nevertheless accessible.
3. If possible, visibly locate the dimples of the low back and explore the surrounding region.

Are you at the posterior end of the iliac crest? Are both landmarks roughly horizontal to each other and three to four inches apart?

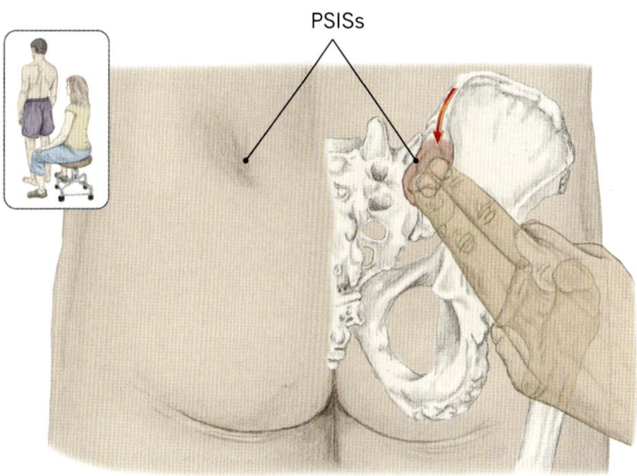

6.30 Partner standing, posterior view of pelvis, as you isolate the PSIS

fossa *fos*-a L. a shallow depression

Trail 3 Tailbone Trail ▸

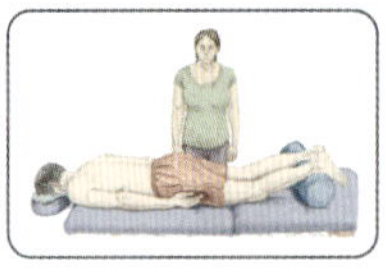

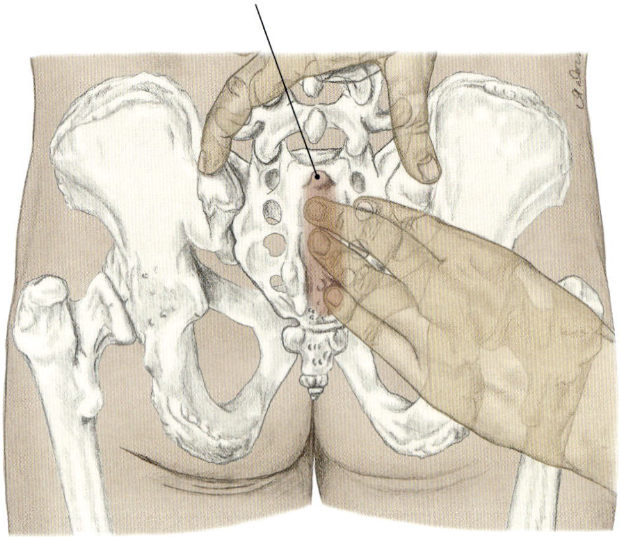

6.31 Partner prone, posterior view of pelvis, as you use the PSISs as guides to locate the median sacral crest of the sacrum

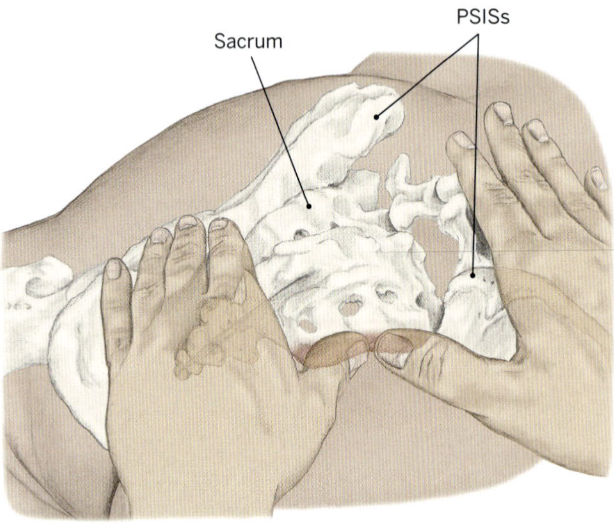

6.32 Partner prone, posterior/lateral view of pelvis, as you explore the edge of the sacrum

Sacrum

Median Sacral Crest
Lateral Sacral Crest
Edge of the Sacrum

The **sacrum** is a large, triangular bone at the inferior end of the vertebral column. Situated between the overhanging sides of the pelvis, the sacrum is made up of a series of four or five vertebrae that are fused together.

Running down the center of the sacrum and composed of three to four points is the **median sacral crest**. On either side of the median sacral crest is the **lateral sacral crest**—a smaller series of bony knobs. The **edge of the sacrum** is part of the attachment site for the gluteus maximus and the sacrotuberous ligament. Although the sacrum's bumpy surface lies deep to the thoracolumbar fascia and sacroiliac ligaments, it is easily accessible.

Sacrum

1. Partner prone. Place a thumb and finger on each PSIS and explore between and below these points for the surface of the sacrum.
2. Locate the midline of the sacrum and explore the points of the sacral crest (**6.31**). Palpate superiorly to the level of the PSIS and just above the coccyx.
3. Slide your fingers laterally off the side of the sacrum, pressing your fingertips into its solid edge (**6.32**). Follow the lateral edge up toward the PSIS and down to the coccyx.

How many small tips can you feel along the sacral crest? Can you follow both lateral edges inferiorly to where they converge at the coccyx? If you move laterally from the outer edge of the sacrum, can you feel the mass of the gluteus maximus (p. 317)?

Comparative Anatomy

Reptiles and most birds have two sacral vertebrae, whereas mammals have between three and five. Humans in particular have more because, as upright creatures, the entire weight of the upper body is transferred through the sacrum to the pelvis and legs. All that remains of the spinous processes of the sacrum's vertebrae are the time-worn tips of the median sacral crest.

sacrum *sa*-krum L. sacred or holy thing, from the use of the sacrum in Roman animal sacrifice

Coccyx

The coccyx is located at the top of the gluteal cleft and attaches to the end of the sacrum. Composed of three or four fused bones, it has a segmented, bumpy contour and can be an inch or more in length. Its tip may curve in toward the body or veer slightly to the left or right.

Because of its proximity to the gluteal cleft, palpating the coccyx may be challenging initially for both you and your partner, so palpate your own coccyx before palpating your partner's.

Coccyx

1. Partner prone. Walk your fingers down the median sacral crest toward the gluteal cleft. At the top of the cleft, you will feel the bumpy surface of the coccyx.
2. Explore the surface and sides of the coccyx, noting how the wide upper part narrows to a tip (**6.33**). The tip of the coccyx might not be accessible since it curves into the body.

Are you palpating the most inferior aspect of bone in this region? Can you sculpt out the edges of the coccyx and its shape?

Sacroiliac Joint

The sacroiliac joint is the junction between the sacrum and the ilium. It is located medial to the PSIS and is deep to the thoracolumbar fascia and posterior sacroiliac ligaments (p. 342). The ilium overhangs the sacroiliac joint, leaving only the edge of the joint accessible.

Sacroiliac joint

1. Partner prone. Locate the PSIS. Move slightly inferior and medial to locate the sacroiliac joint.
2. Create a small widening at the joint by keeping one hand on it while the other hand flexes the knee to 90°. Then passively rotate the hip medially, feeling for a small opening at the joint space (**6.34**). Also try to laterally rotate the hip.

Are you just medial and distal to the PSIS? Can you sculpt out the edge of the ilium as it overlaps the sacrum?

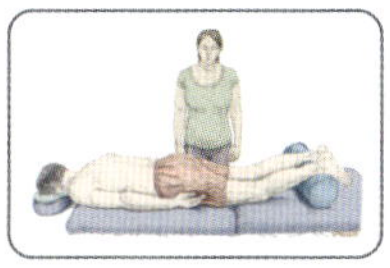

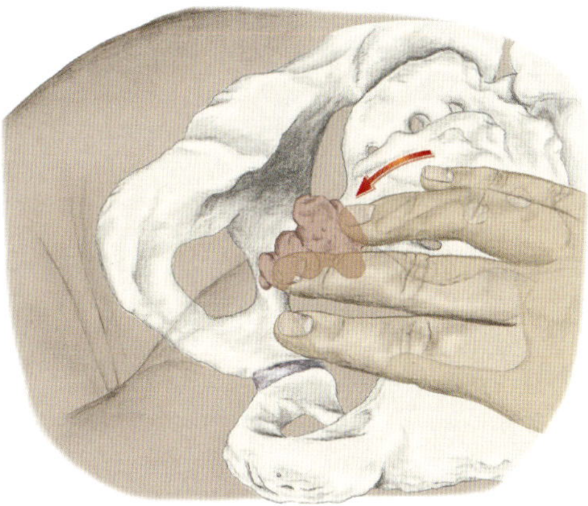

6.33 Partner prone, posterior/lateral view of pelvis, as you palpate the coccyx

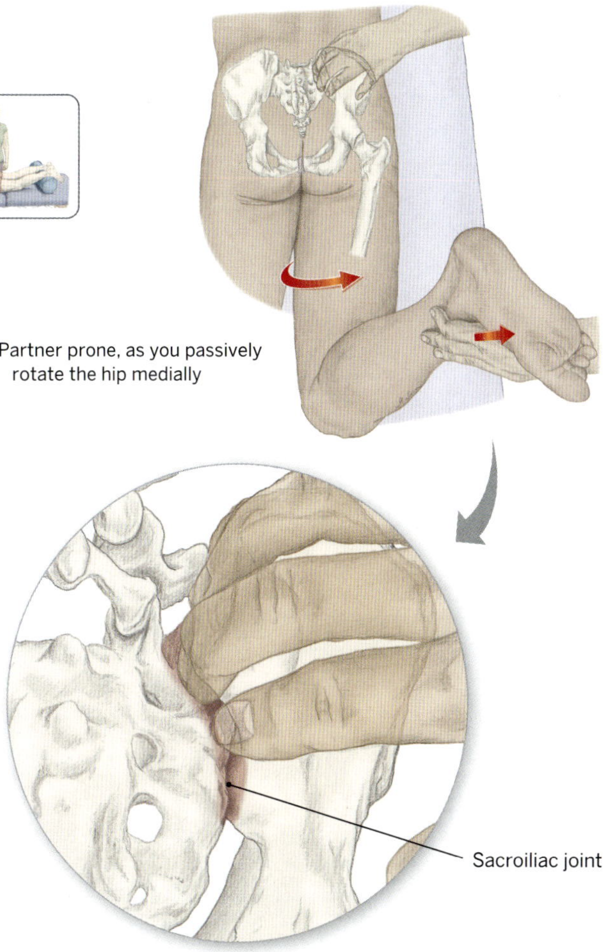

6.34 Partner prone, as you passively rotate the hip medially

Discover More

The Greek philosopher Herophilus named the last segments of the vertebral column the "kokkyx" since it resembled a cuckoo's beak. However, during the Renaissance, the French anatomist Jean Riolan thought the term referred to the release of gas from the anus that can sound like the cry of a cuckoo. The coccyx is also called the "tailbone"—an appropriate term when referring to the human fetus. During early development a small, distinct tail extends off the sacrum, but by the eighth week it disappears, leaving just what is recognizable as the coccyx.

coccyx *kok*-siks Grk. cuckoo

Trail 4 Hip Hike ▸

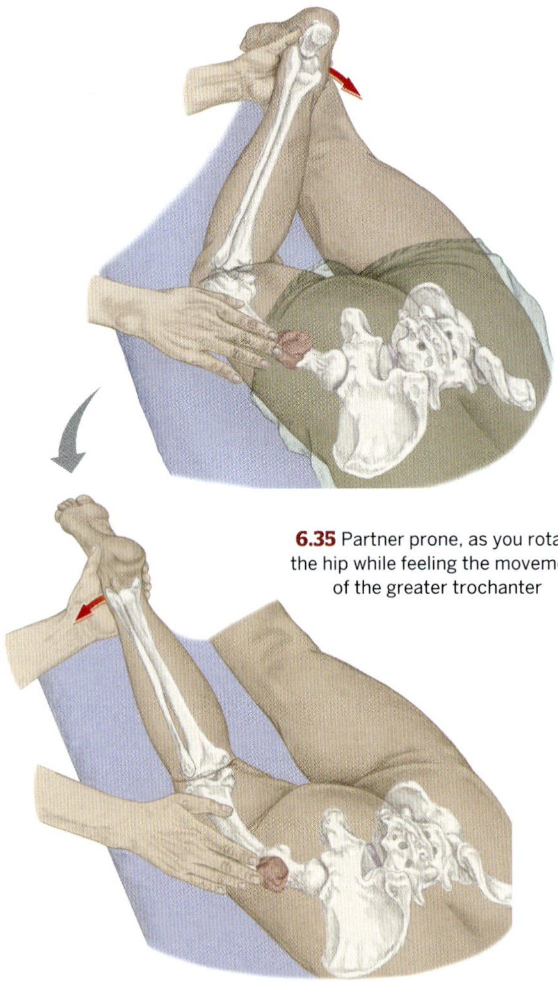

6.35 Partner prone, as you rotate the hip while feeling the movement of the greater trochanter

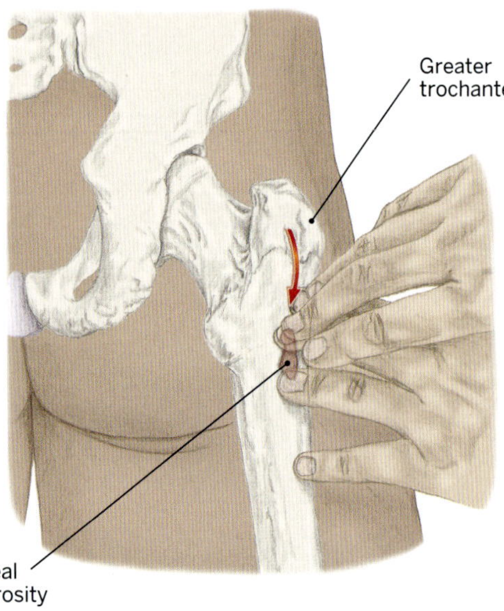

6.37 Posterior view of right hip, as you locate the gluteal tuberosity

Greater Trochanter

(Refer to p. 289 for more information.)

Greater trochanter

1. Partner prone. Locate the middle of the iliac crest.
2. Slide your fingerpads distally four or five inches along the side of the thigh. There you will feel the superficial hump of the greater trochanter.
3. Sculpt around its two-inch-wide surface and explore all of its sides.

*Holding the ankle, flex the knee to 90°. As your proximal hand palpates the greater trochanter, use the other hand to medially and laterally rotate the hip (**6.35**). Do you feel the trochanter swivel back and forth under your fingers?*

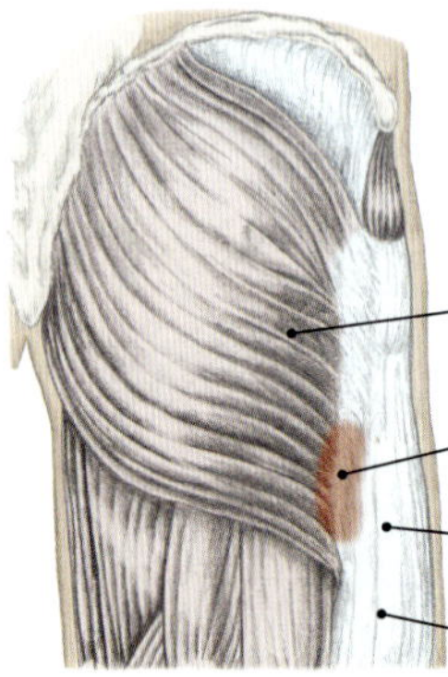

6.36 Posterior view of pelvis, showing the gluteal tuberosity's relationship to the surrounding muscles

Gluteal Tuberosity

The gluteal tuberosity is located distal to the posterior surface of the greater trochanter. It is a small ridge serving as an attachment site for the lower fibers of the gluteus maximus muscle. Although it is surrounded by the gluteus maximus tendon and the upper fibers of the vastus lateralis muscles (**6.36**), the gluteal tuberosity is relatively superficial and accessible.

Gluteal tuberosity

1. Partner prone. Locate the posterior surface of the greater trochanter.
2. Slide one or two inches distally along the posterior shaft of the femur until you feel the solid surface of the tuberosity (**6.37**). It might feel not like a ridge but more like a flat, superficial portion of bone.

Can you press into the area you are palpating and feel the superficial surface of the femur? Are you directly lateral to the ischial tuberosity (p. 289)?

Pelvis & Thigh

Umbilicus

The umbilicus (or navel) will, of course, be visible when the abdomen is undraped. When not exposed, the umbilicus can be felt at the midline of the body, superior to the level of the ASISs.

Pubic Crest and Tubercles

(Refer to p. 288 for more information.)

The pubic tubercles are located on the superior aspect of the pubic crest. Each tubercle is shaped like a small horn and serves as an attachment site for the adductor longus muscle and the inguinal ligament. The tubercles might be one to two inches apart and are not always easy to palpate.

Pubic crest and tubercles

1. Face your partner as he lies supine on the table. Set your fingertips on his umbilicus, allowing your palm to rest on the abdomen. The heel of your hand will be on (or just superior to) the pubic crest.
2. Turn your hand and relocate the crest with your fingers (**6.38**). Explore its horizontal ridge. Remember that the pubic crest is the only horizontal stretch of bone in this vicinity.
3. Move laterally and explore for the tips of the pubic tubercles. Palpate both tubercles, noting the distance between them.

Do you feel a firm, bony prominence inferior and medial to the level of the ASIS? With respect to the pubic tubercles, are the bony prominences you feel on the superior part of the pubic crest? Are the tubercles on the same level as the greater trochanters?

Begin at the ASIS and follow the inguinal ligament (p. 341) inferiorly and medially 45° to the pubic tubercle.

Trail 5 The Underpass ▸

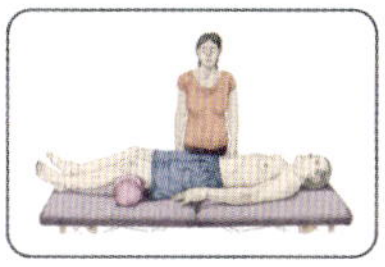

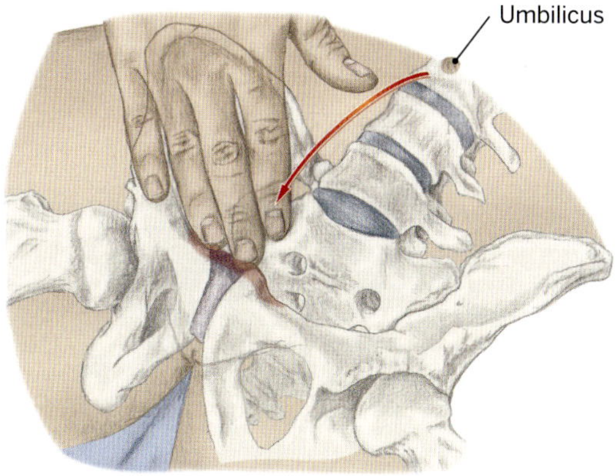

6.38 Partner supine, anterior/lateral view of pelvis, as you locate the pubic crest

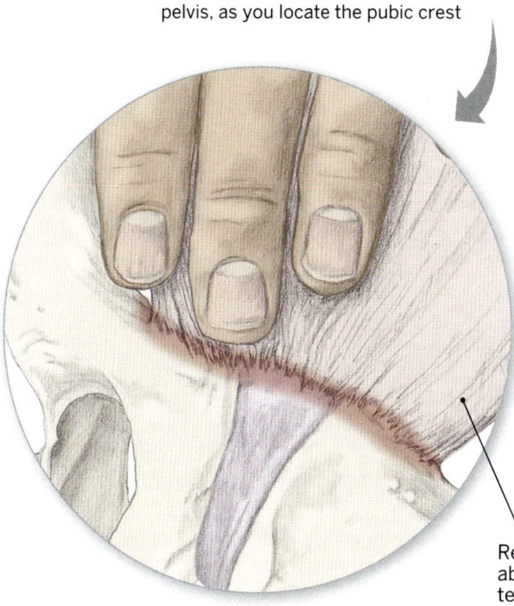

Palpation Plus

Here are two suggestions to make sure this route is comfortable for you and your partner: (**a**) Explain to your partner what you will be doing and obtain permission to proceed. (**b**) If your partner would be more comfortable, use their hand to palpate with your hand guiding on top (right).

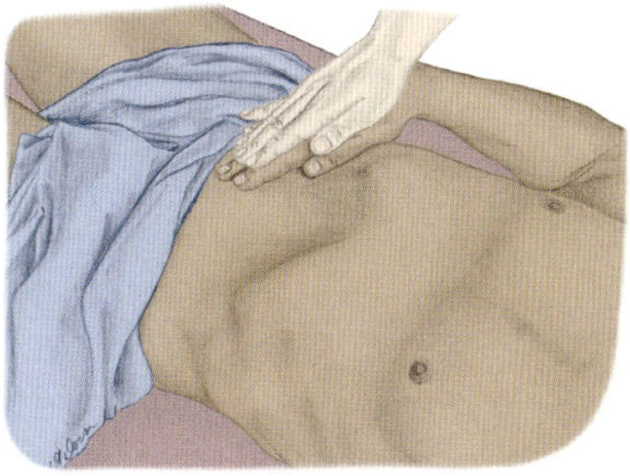

Partner supine

umbilicus um-***bil***-i-kus L. navel, center

When palpating the superior ramus, be mindful of the pulse of the femoral artery (p. 341).

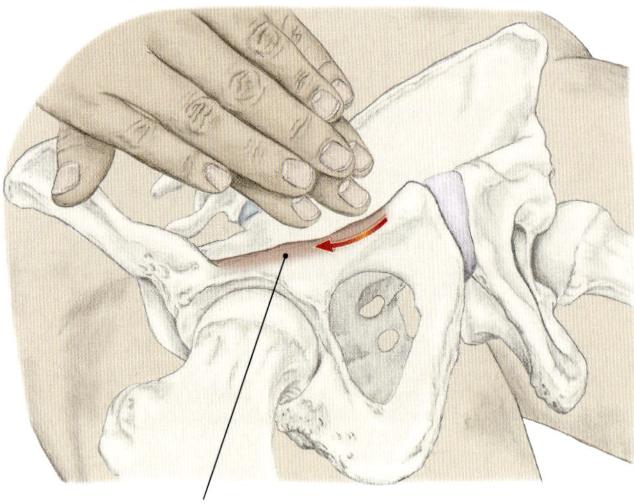

6.39 Partner supine, as you palpate the superior ramus of the pubis

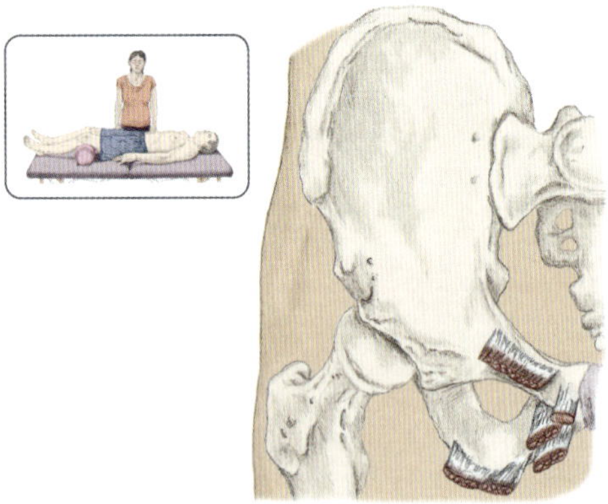

6.40 Anterior view of right hip and pelvis, showing adductor muscle attachment sites along the rami

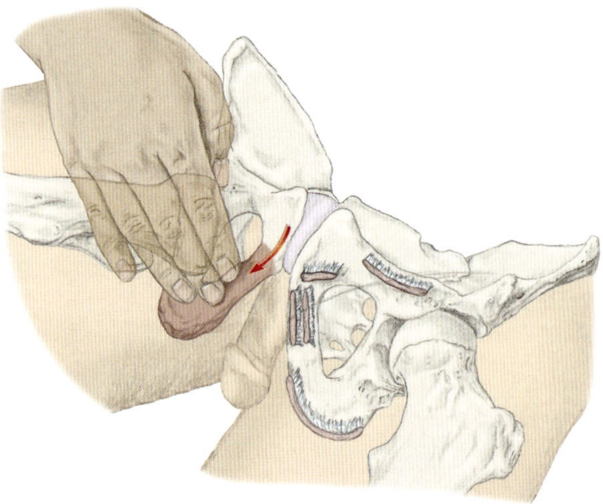

6.41 Partner supine, as you palpate from the rami to the ischial tuberosity

Superior Ramus of the Pubis

The superior ramus of the pubis spans 45° from the pubic tubercle toward the AIIS. It forms a ridge that serves as an attachment site for the pectineus muscle (p. 321). Because it is deep to the inguinal ligament and a neurovascular bundle, the superior ramus can be challenging to palpate.

Superior ramus

1. Partner supine. Place your flexed knee under your partner's knee. This position will flex and laterally rotate the hip, allowing for easier palpation.
2. Locate the pubic crest. Slide laterally off the crest toward the AIIS. Sink into the tissue, feeling for the buried ridge of the superior ramus (**6.39**).

Are you lateral and slightly superior to the pubic tubercle? If you cannot feel the edge of the ramus, can you sense its density beneath the superficial tissue?

Inferior Ramus of the Pubis and Ramus of the Ischium

The two rami are located along the inferior aspect of the pelvis and together form a bridge between the pubic crest and the ischial tuberosity. The ramus of the pubis, the anterior half of the bridge, serves as an attachment site for the gracilis and adductor brevis muscles; both rami are attachment sites for the adductor magnus muscle (**6.40**). When palpating the rami, use your fingertips, keeping them close to the medial thigh. The angle formed by the rami will be wider on females than males.

Inferior ramus

1. Partner supine. Place your flexed knee under your partner's knee.
2. Locate the pubic crest. Then move to the lateral edge of the pubic crest and slide posteriorly around the medial thigh (**6.41**). Using slow but firm pressure, palpate for the hard ridge of the rami. This "bridge of bone" is the only bony mass in the area, so if you are pressing on a solid line of bone, you have found it.
3. Continue around the thigh until you reach the large ischial tuberosity.

As you follow the rami, do they lead you posteriorly around the inside of the thigh? As you move around the thigh, do you feel the rami widen laterally? Can you feel where any of the adductor tendons (p. 321) attach to the rami?

ramus *ray*-mus L. branch

Ischial Tuberosity

(Refer to p. 289 for more information.)

Ischial tuberosity

1. Partner prone. Locate the gluteal fold, the horizontal line between the buttock and thigh. Place your fingers at the center of the gluteal fold and press superiorly and medially until your fingertips bump into the large surface of the ischial tuberosity (**6.42**).
2. Explore all sides of its large mass and note its relationship to the greater trochanter.

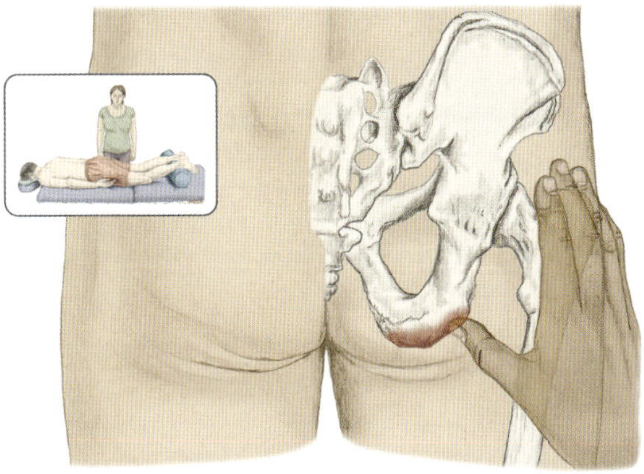

6.42 Posterior view of right hip and pelvis, as you locate the ischial tuberosity

Are you palpating between the inferior buttock and proximal thigh? Can you feel the large hamstring tendons attach to the ischial tuberosity?

Partner side lying, with the top hip flexed. Place your hand on the medial thigh. Slide proximally to the gluteal fold and ischial tuberosity (**6.43**).

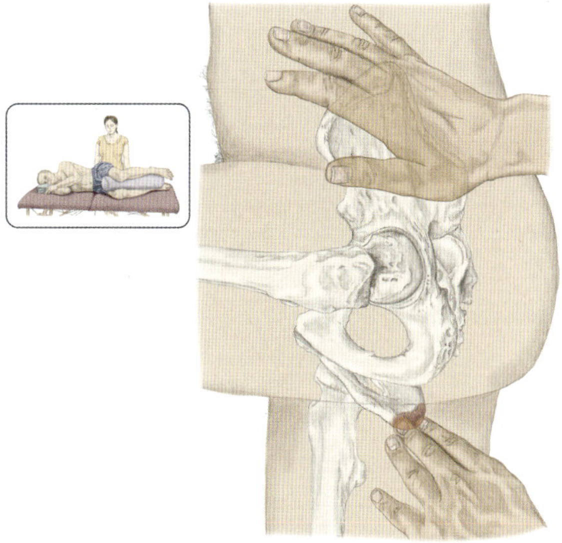

6.43 Partner side lying, as you locate your partner's right ischial tuberosity

Palpation Plus ▶

How do you access bones and muscles that are close to the genitals? Actually, all of the bony landmarks, tendons, and blood vessels in this region can be easily palpated without contacting the genitals (below). If you follow the instructions given, you will maintain your and your partner's comfort.

With that said, it should be obvious that palpation on males is complicated by the position of the penis and testicles. In a supine position, flexion and lateral rotation of the thigh will bring it away from the pelvis and allow for easier palpation. (See p. 324, for example.)

The side lying position allows the genitals to shift away from the base of the pelvis. To make sure your partner's genitals are away from the area you are trying to access, ask him to shift and hold his genitals away from the side you will be contacting (above).

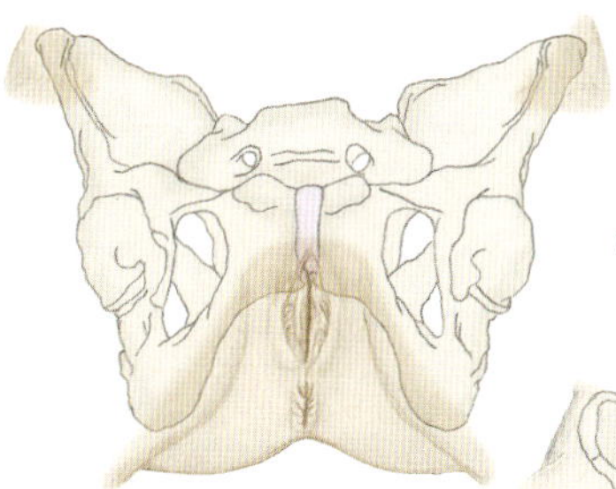

Inferior view of female genitals

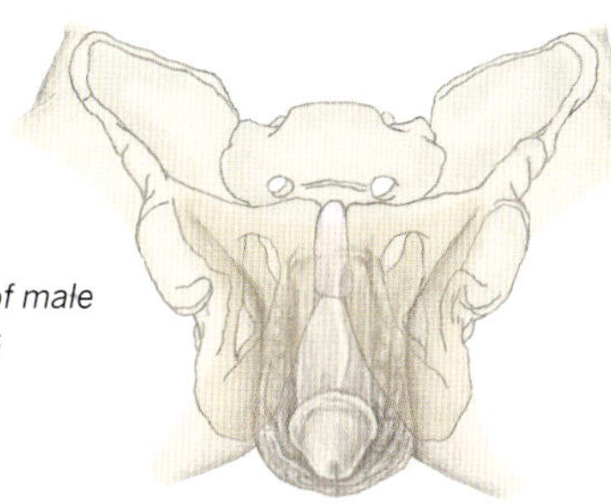

Inferior view of male genitals

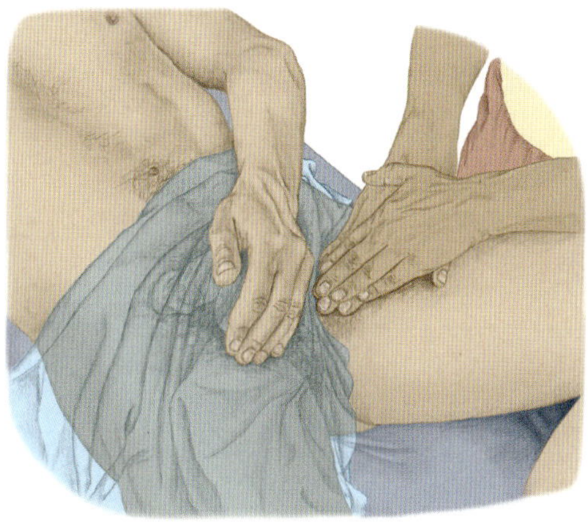

Partner supine

Overview: **Muscles of the Pelvis and Thigh**

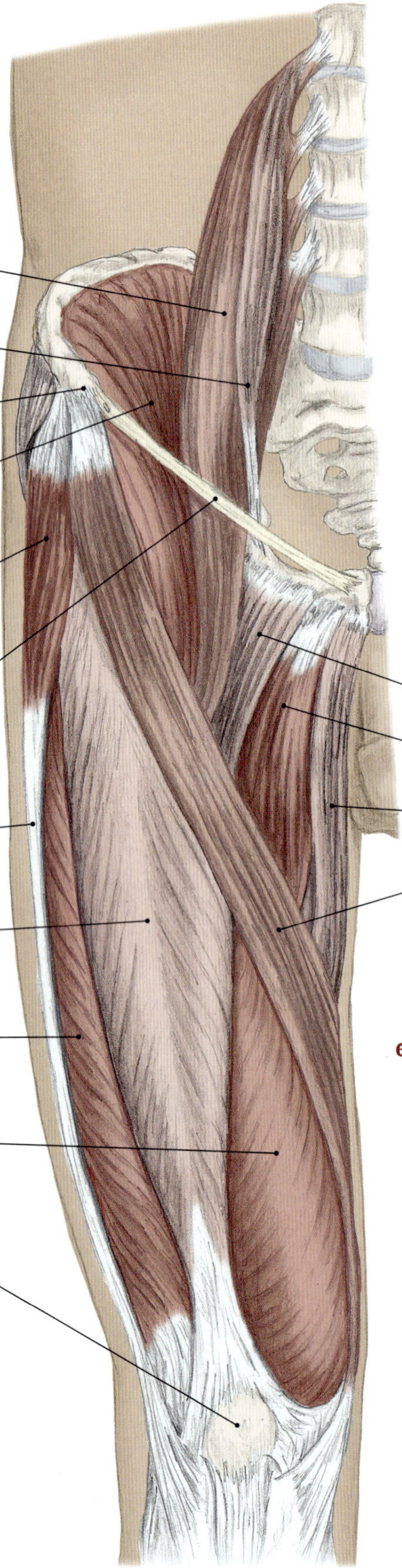

The muscles of the pelvis and thigh create movement primarily at the coxal (hip) and tibiofemoral (knee) joints. Most of the hip and thigh muscles can be divided into five groups. There are two groups in the buttock region while three make up the mass of the thigh:

1. Three **gluteal** muscles give shape to the buttock and lateral hip.
2. Six small **lateral rotators** are deep to the large gluteals.
3. Four **quadriceps** are located on the thigh's anterior and lateral surfaces.
4. Three long **hamstrings** lie along the posterior thigh.
5. Five **adductors** are tucked between the quadriceps and hamstrings along the medial thigh.

Additional muscles include the iliopsoas, sartorius, and tensor fasciae latae.

6.44 Anterior view of muscles of right hip and thigh

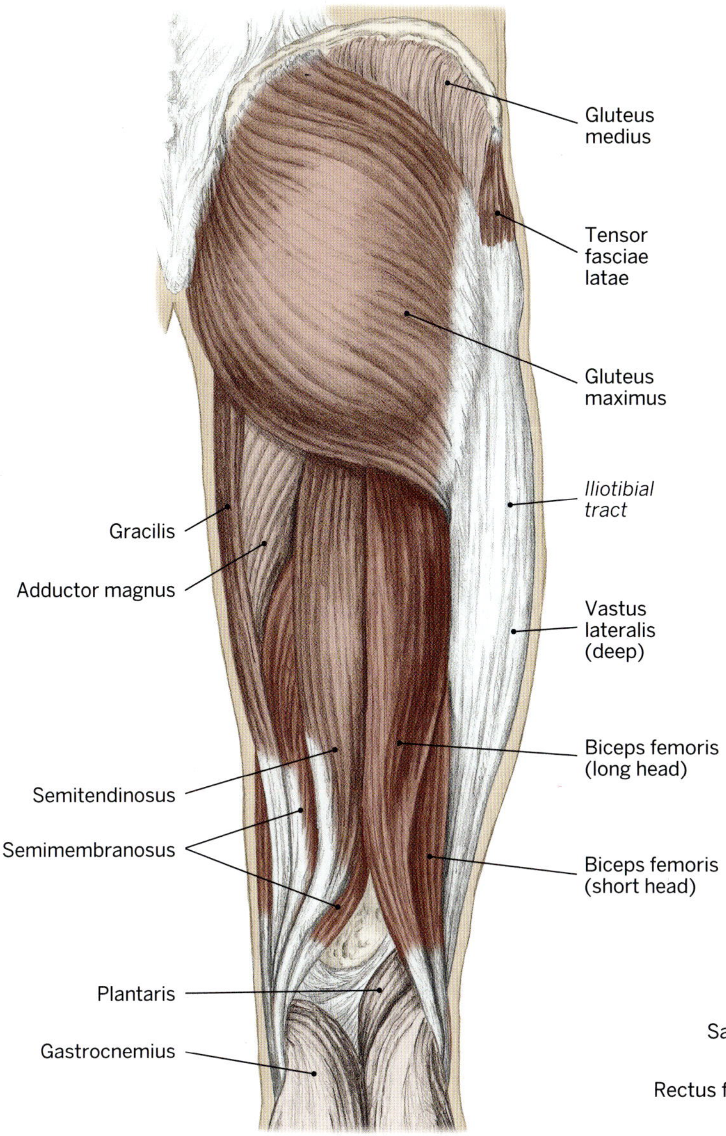

6.45 Posterior view of muscles of right hip and thigh

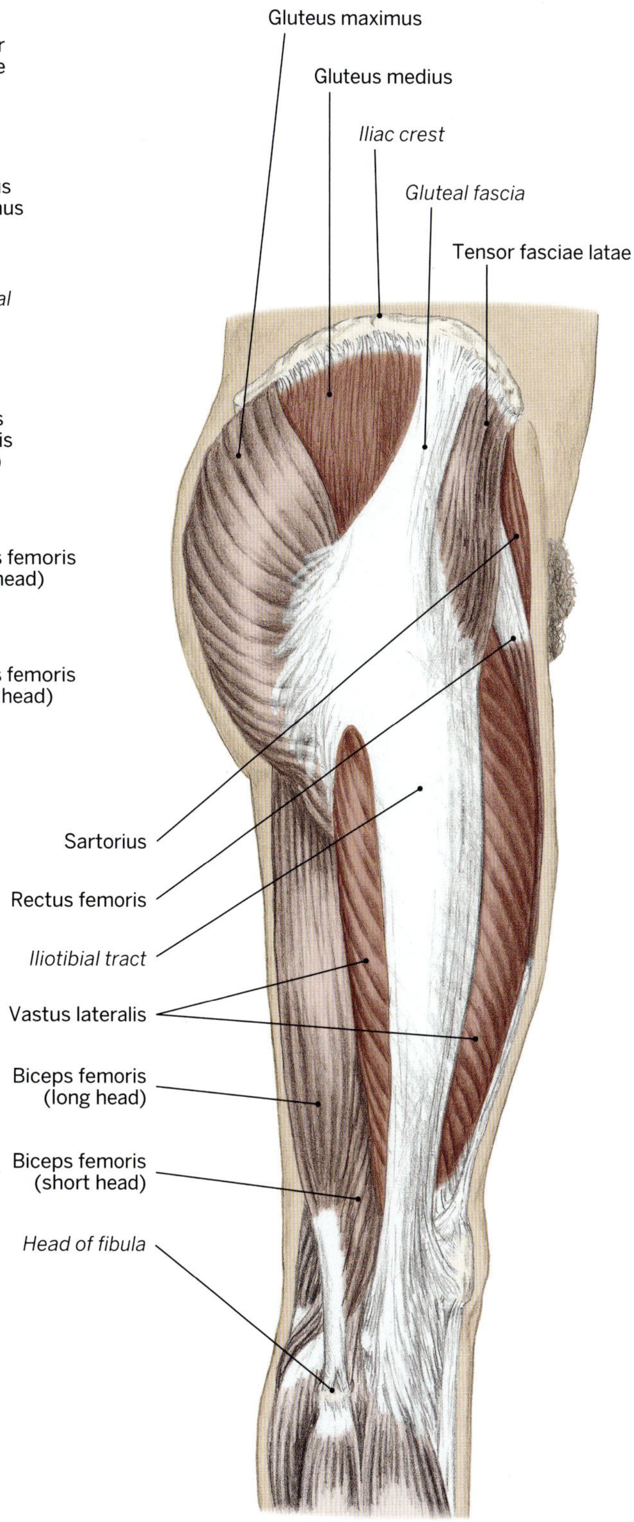

6.46 Lateral view of muscles of right hip and thigh

Pelvis & Thigh

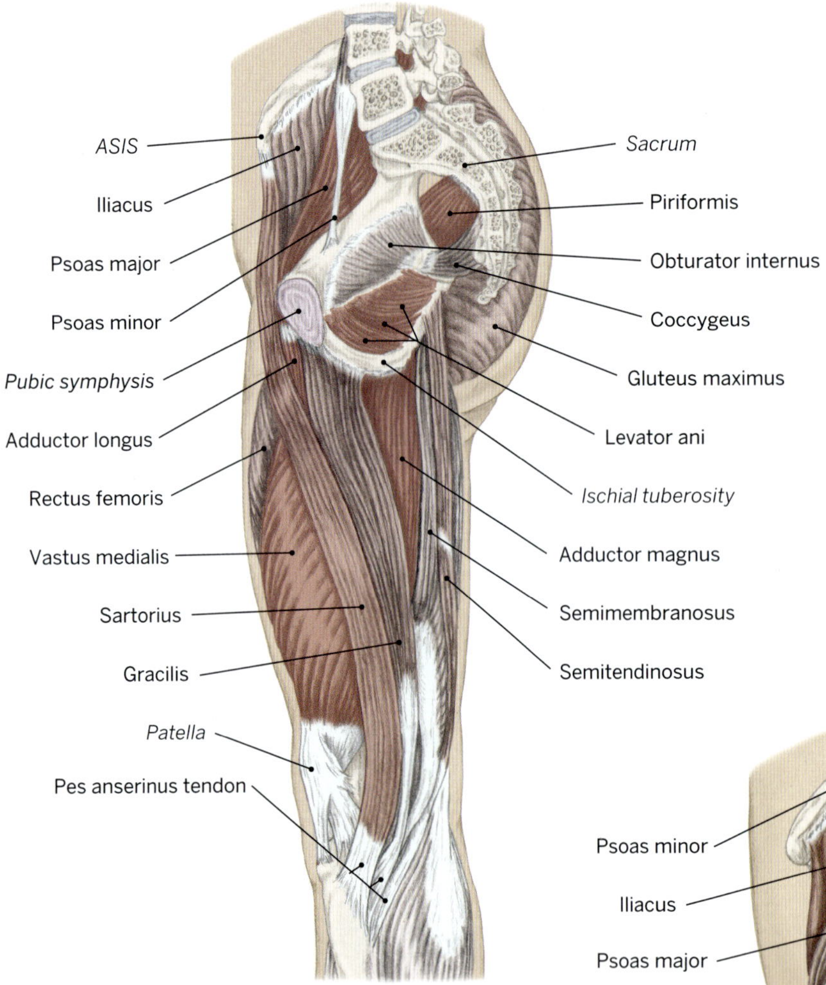

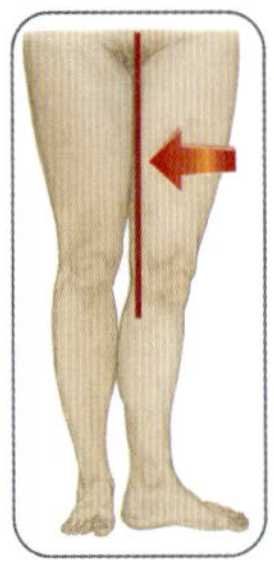

6.47 Medial view of muscles of right hip and thigh, superficial layer

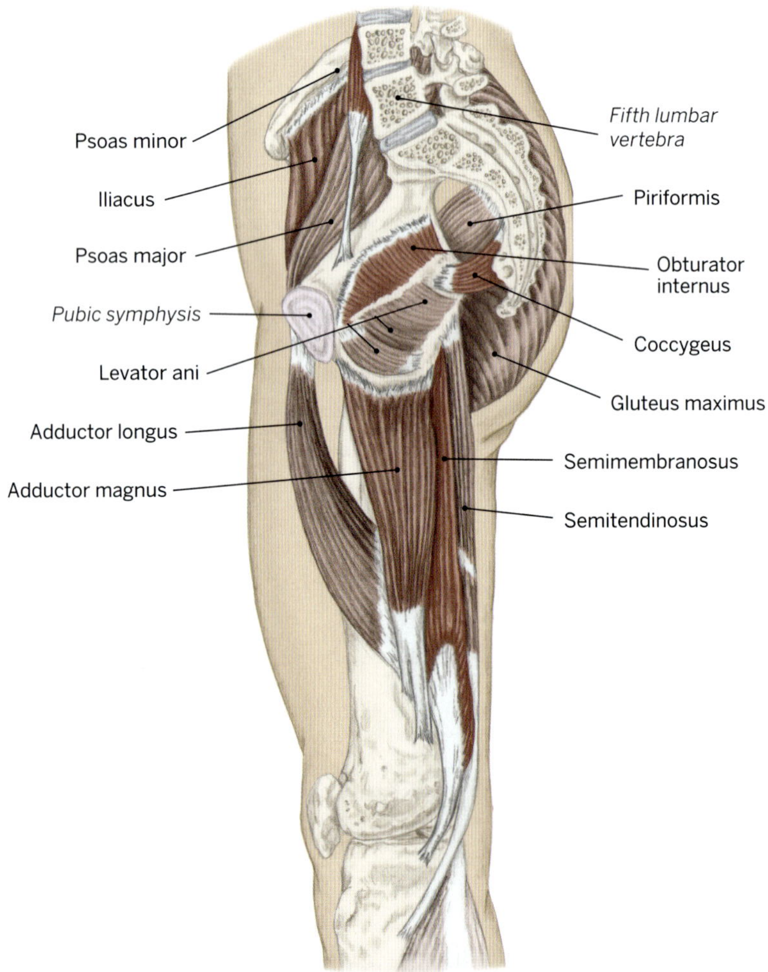

6.48 Medial view of muscles of right hip and thigh, deeper layer

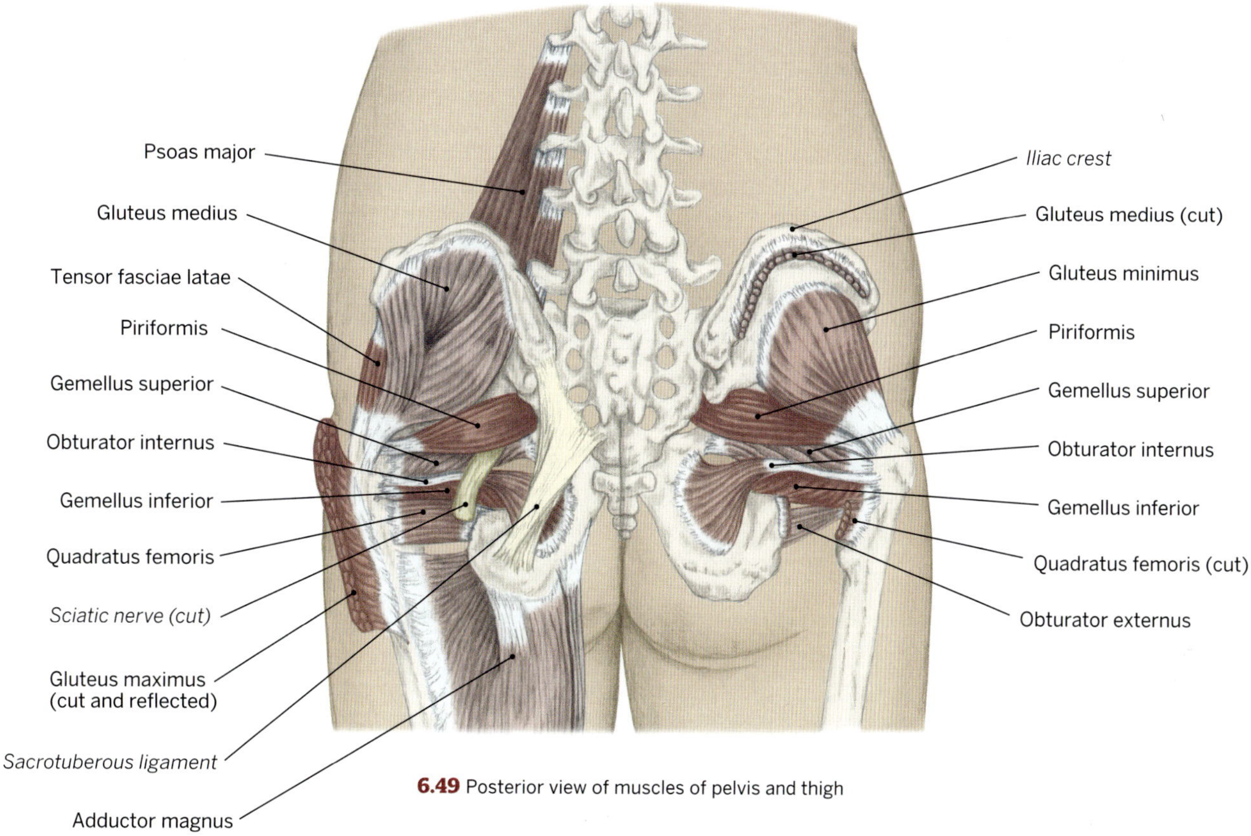

6.49 Posterior view of muscles of pelvis and thigh

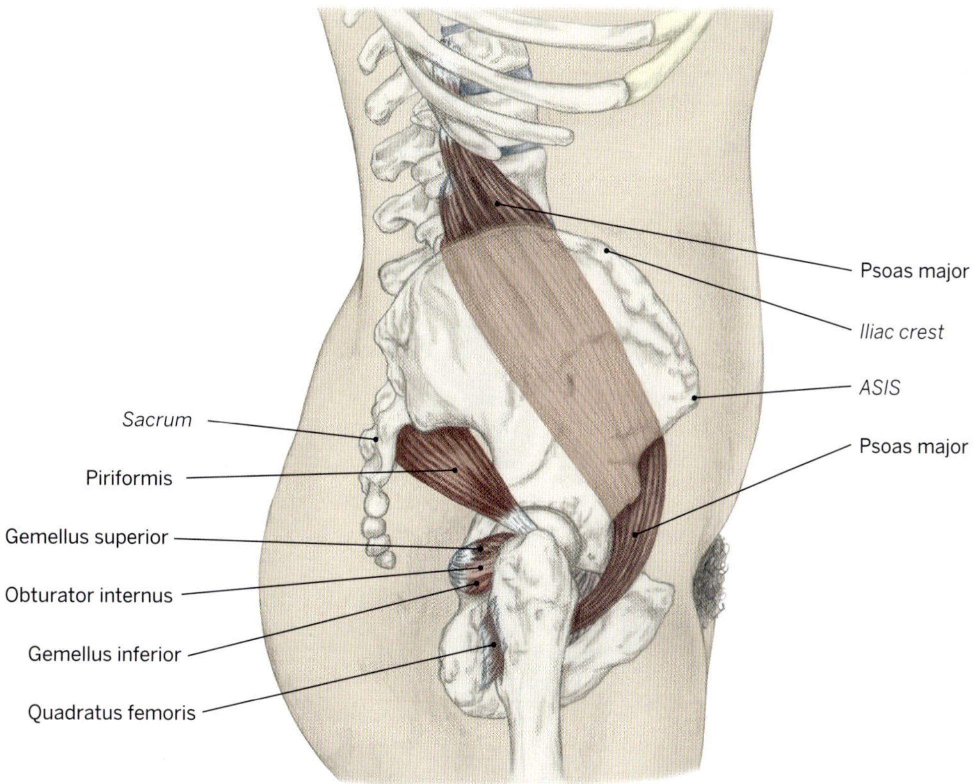

6.50 Lateral view of muscles of right hip

Perineum and Pelvic Floor

The **perineum** is the diamond-shaped area at the *inferior* aspect of the pelvis (**6.51**). It is framed by the pubic symphysis, the ischial tuberosities, and the coccyx. A line drawn between the ischial tuberosities divides the perineum into two triangles. The anterior (**a**) *urogenital triangle* contains the external genitals, and the posterior (**b**) *anal triangle* contains the anus.

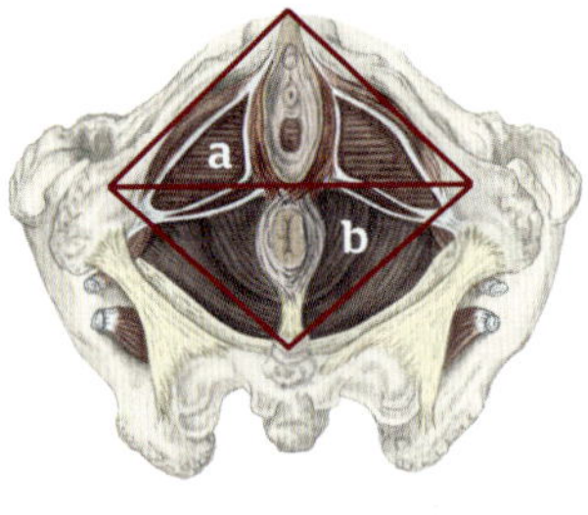

6.51 Inferior view of pelvis, showing perineum

The **pelvic floor** is formed primarily by the two levator ani and two coccygeus muscles (**6.52–6.55**). Together with their surrounding fascia, they form the funnel-shaped pelvic diaphragm, which spans the inside floor of the pelvis. The pelvic floor supports the abdominal and pelvic viscera, such as the sigmoid colon and rectum.

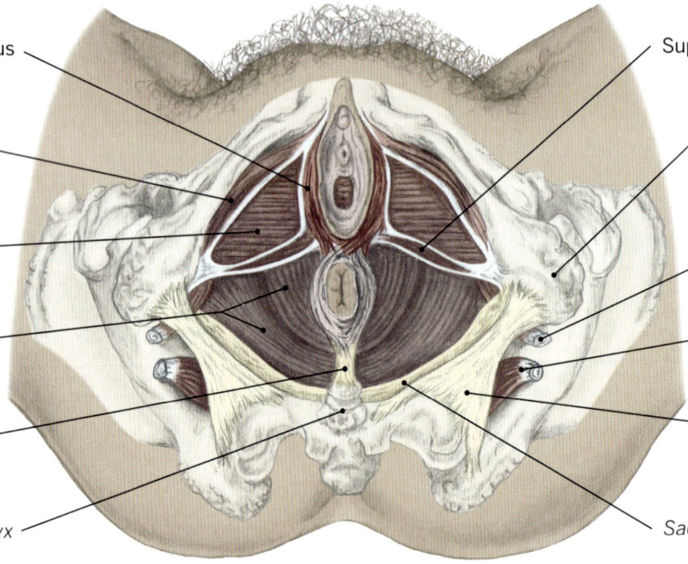

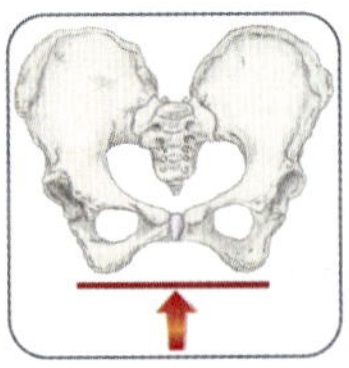

6.52 Inferior view of pelvis, showing superficial layer of female pelvic floor (hips abducted)

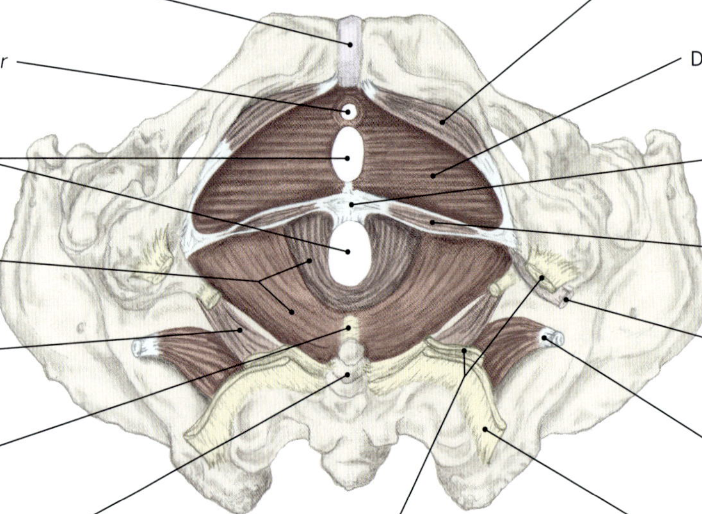

6.53 Inferior view of pelvis, showing intermediate layer of female pelvic floor

perineum	***per***-i-***nee***-um	Gr. space between anus and scrotum
pubococcygeus	***pu***-bo-kok-***si***-je-us	
puborectalis	***pu***-bo-rek-***tal***-is	

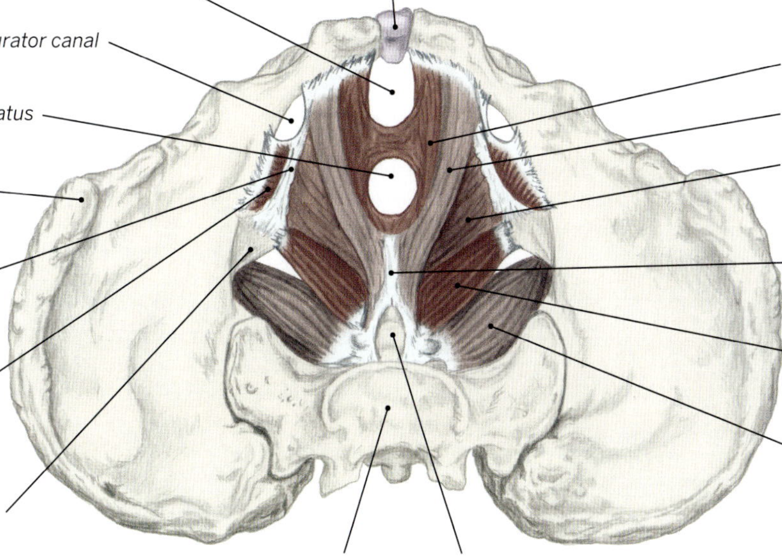

6.54 Superior view of pelvis, showing superficial layer of female pelvic floor

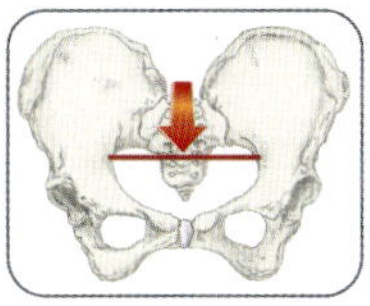

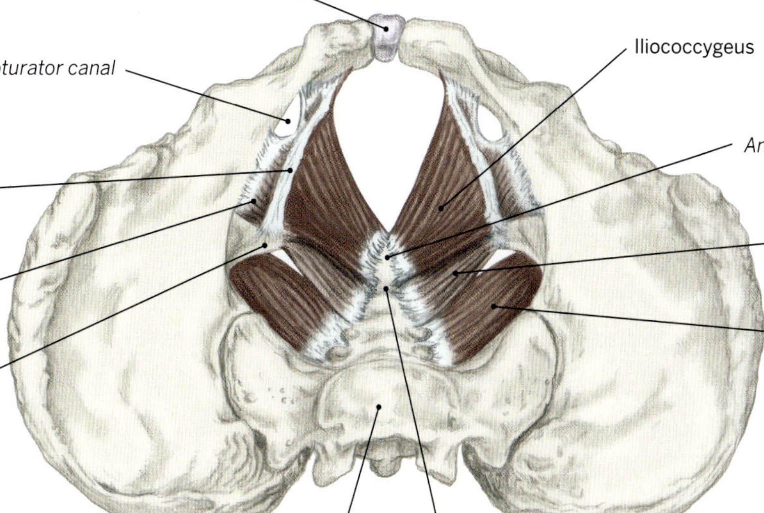

6.55 Superior view of pelvis, showing deep layer of female pelvic floor

Palpation Plus

"Why no palpation instructions for the perineal region?" The perineum—as well as other challenging areas such as the mouth, nose, and ear cavities—are best learned not in a text such as *Trail Guide*, but at a specific hands-on workshop in the presence of an experienced instructor.

In the meantime, consider exploring the landmarks and muscles of your own perineum and pelvic floor. Initially, you may snicker and be intimidated, but this often-avoided region of the body is as much a part of you as your fingers and toes.

anococcygeal	***a***-no-kok-***si***-je-al	L. *anus*, anus + Grk. *kokkyx*, coccyx
bulbospongiosus	***bul***-bo-***spon***-je-***o***-sus	L. *bulbus*, bulbous root + Gr. *spongos*, sponge
iliococcygeus	***il***-ee-o-kok-***si***-je-us	

Synergists—Muscles Working Together

Muscles are listed in the order of their ability to create the movement. Asterisk indicates muscles not shown.

Coxal

(hip joint)

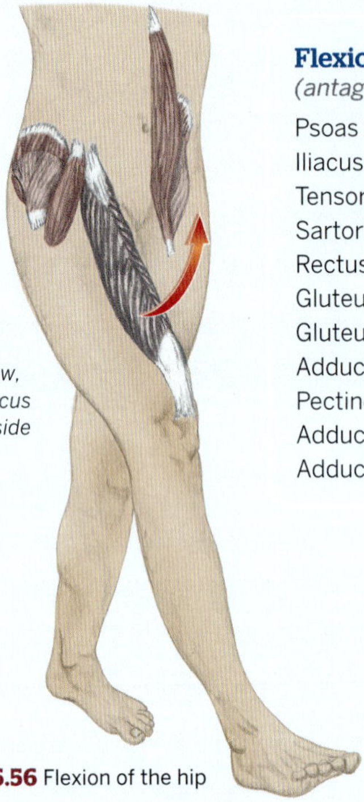

Anterior/lateral view, psoas major and iliacus shown on opposite side

6.56 Flexion of the hip

Flexion

(antagonists on extension)

Psoas major
Iliacus
Tensor fasciae latae
Sartorius
Rectus femoris
Gluteus medius (anterior fibers)
Gluteus minimus
Adductor longus (assists)
Pectineus (assists)
Adductor brevis (assists)
Adductor magnus (assists)

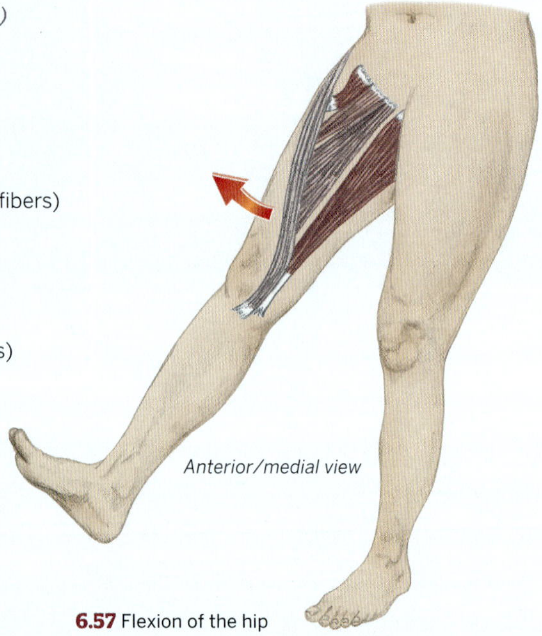

Anterior/medial view

6.57 Flexion of the hip

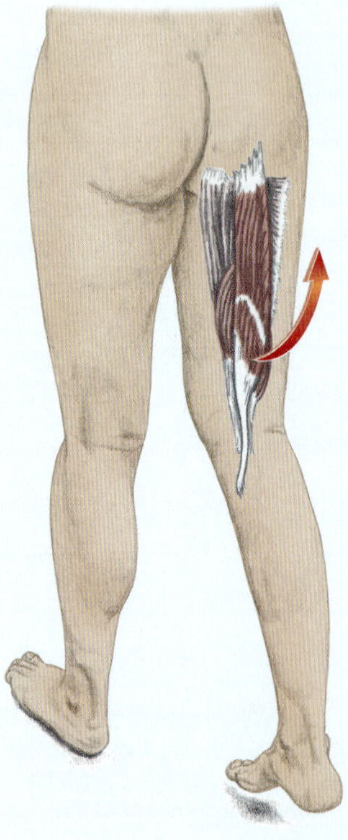

Posterior/medial view

6.58 Extension of the hip

Extension

(antagonists on flexion)

Gluteus maximus (all fibers)
Biceps femoris (long head)
Semitendinosus
Semimembranosus
Adductor magnus (posterior fibers)
Gluteus medius (posterior fibers)

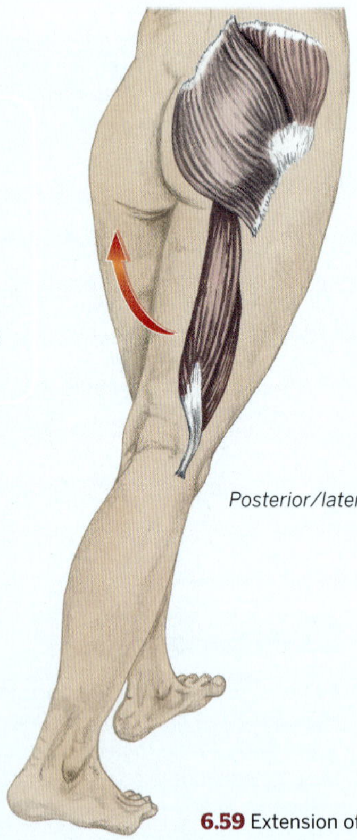

Posterior/lateral view

6.59 Extension of the hip

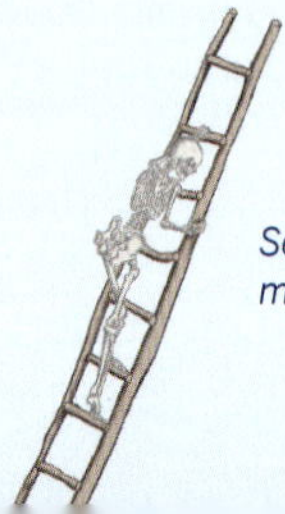

See p. 432 for a complete list of muscles that tilt the pelvis.

Coxal

(hip joint)

Medial Rotation (internal rotation)

(antagonists on lateral rotation)

- Gluteus medius (anterior fibers)
- Gluteus minimus
- Tensor fasciae latae
- Adductor magnus
- Adductor longus
- Adductor brevis
- Pectineus
- Gracilis
- Semitendinosus (assists)
- Semimembranosus (assists)

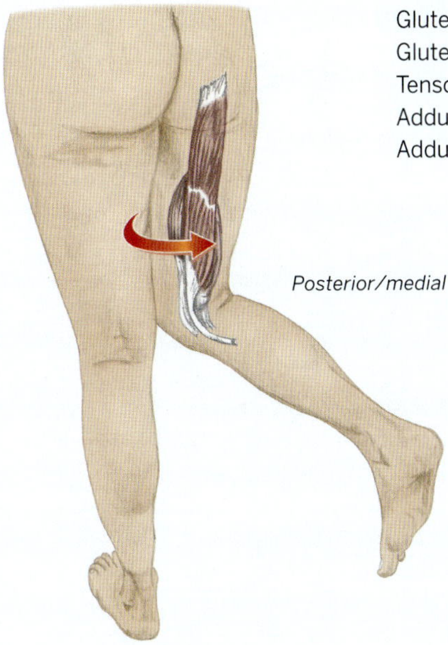

6.60 Medial rotation (internal rotation) of the hip

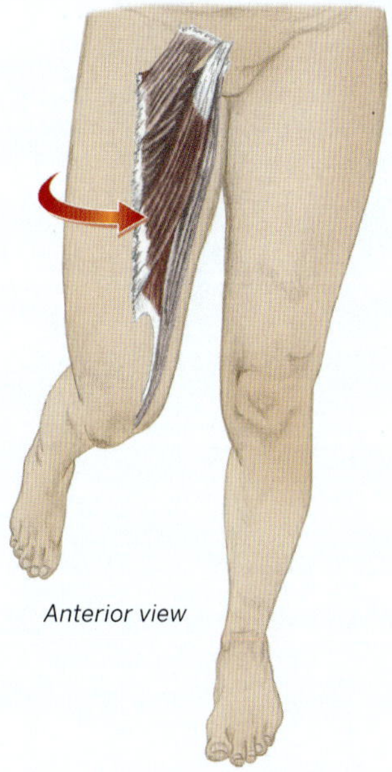

6.61 Medial rotation (internal rotation) of the hip

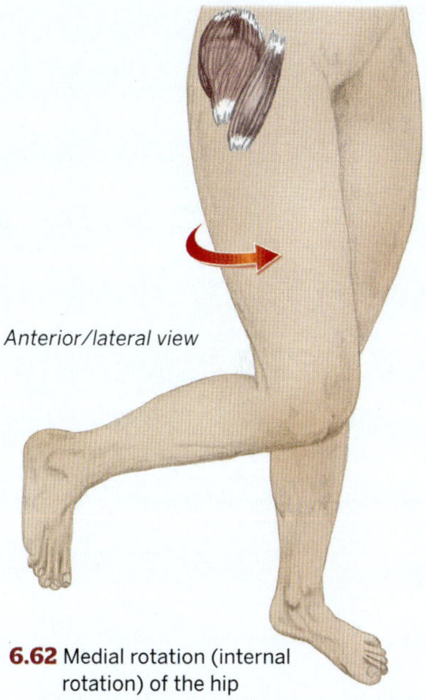

6.62 Medial rotation (internal rotation) of the hip

Lateral Rotation (external rotation)

(antagonists on medial rotation)

- Gluteus maximus (all fibers)
- Piriformis
- Quadratus femoris
- Obturator internus
- Obturator externus
- Gemellus superior
- Gemellus inferior
- Gluteus medius (posterior fibers)
- Psoas major
- Iliacus
- Sartorius
- Biceps femoris (assists, long head)

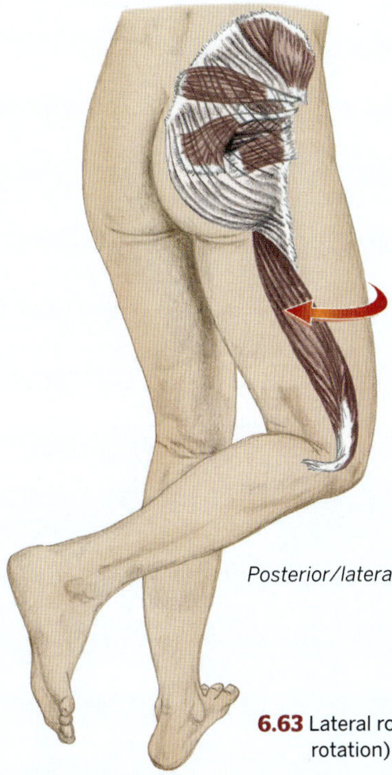

6.63 Lateral rotation (external rotation) of the hip

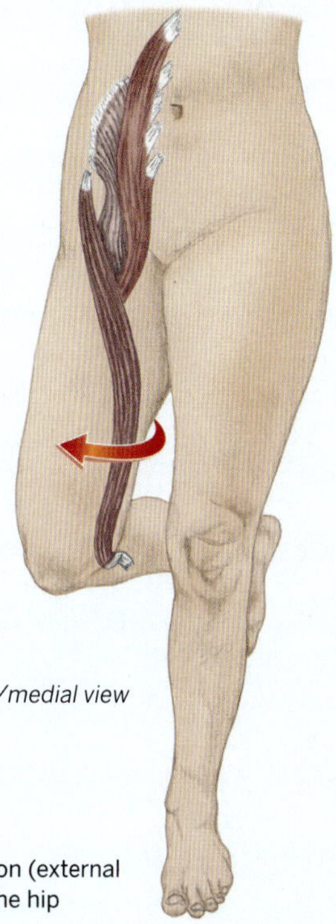

6.64 Lateral rotation (external rotation) of the hip

Coxal

(hip joint)

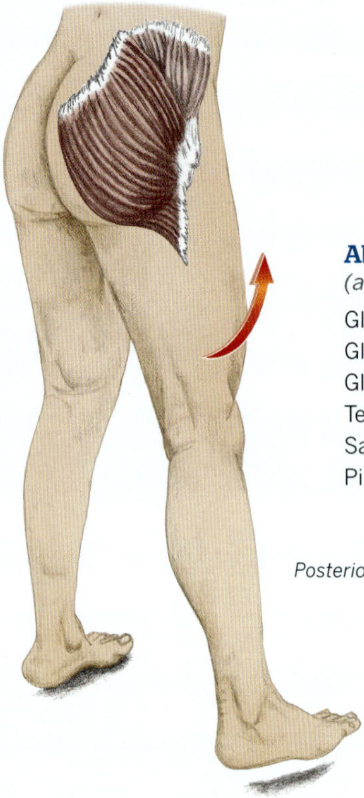

6.65 Abduction of the hip

Abduction

(antagonists on adduction)

Gluteus maximus (all fibers)
Gluteus medius (all fibers)
Gluteus minimus
Tensor fasciae latae
Sartorius
Piriformis (when the hip is flexed)*

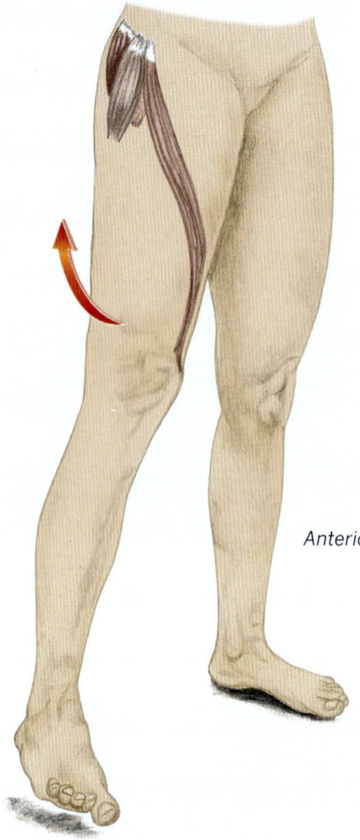

6.66 Abduction of the hip

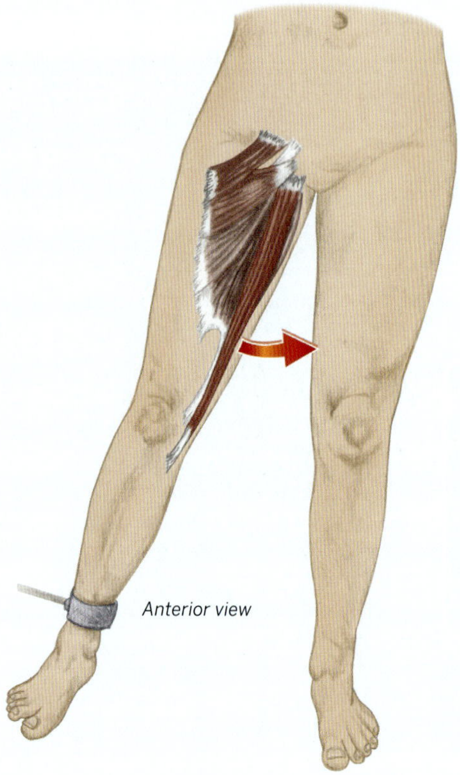

6.67 Adduction of the hip

Adduction

(antagonists on abduction)

Adductor magnus
Adductor longus
Adductor brevis
Pectineus
Gracilis
Gluteus maximus (lower fibers)

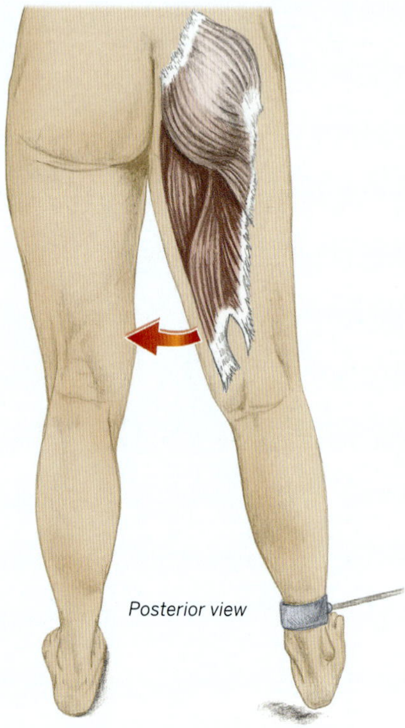

6.68 Adduction of the hip

Knee

(tibiofemoral joint)

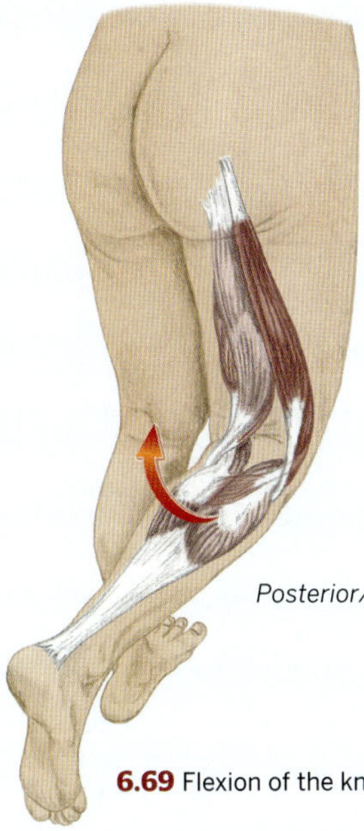

6.69 Flexion of the knee

Flexion

(antagonists on extension)

Biceps femoris
Semitendinosus
Semimembranosus
Gracilis
Sartorius
Gastrocnemius
Popliteus
Plantaris (weak)*

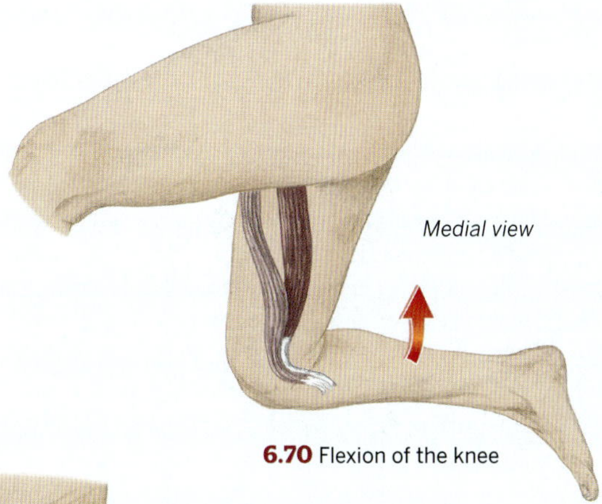

6.70 Flexion of the knee

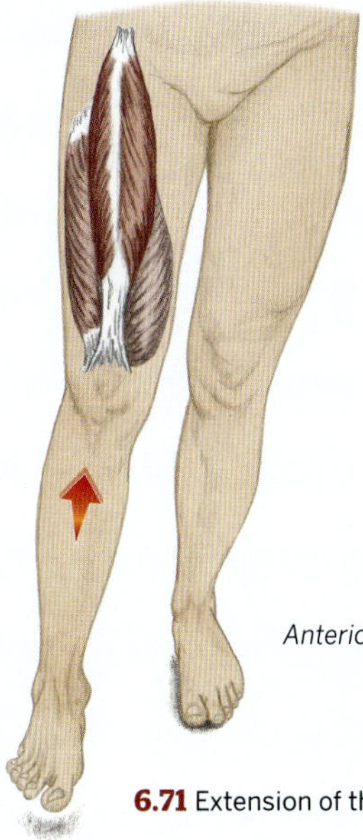

6.71 Extension of the knee

Extension

(antagonists on flexion)

Rectus femoris
Vastus lateralis
Vastus medialis
Vastus intermedius*

Medial Rotation of Flexed Knee

(antagonists on lateral rotation)

Semitendinosus
Semimembranosus
Gracilis
Sartorius
Popliteus*

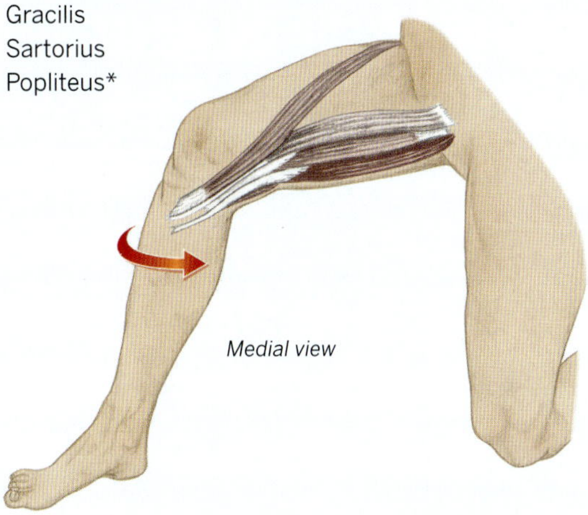

6.72 Medial rotation of flexed knee

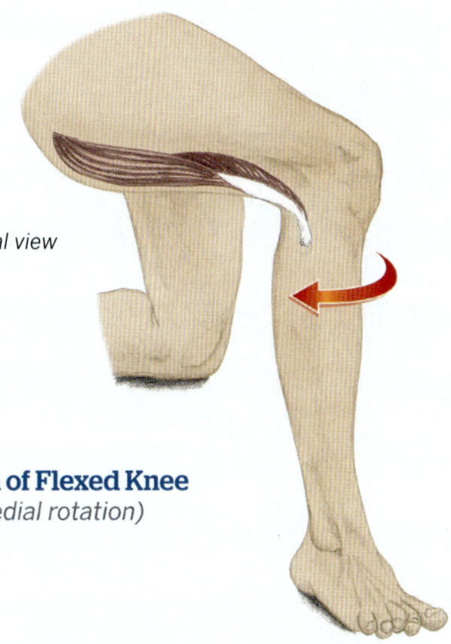

Lateral Rotation of Flexed Knee

(antagonist on medial rotation)

Biceps femoris

6.73 Lateral rotation of flexed knee

Muscles of the Pelvis and Thigh

Quadriceps Femoris Group ▶

Rectus Femoris
Vastus Medialis
Vastus Lateralis
Vastus Intermedius

The four large quadriceps muscles primarily extend the knee. The cylindrical, superficial **rectus femoris** is located on the anterior thigh and is the only quadriceps that crosses two joints—the hip and knee (**6.74**). **Vastus intermedius** is deep to the rectus femoris; however, its edges can be accessed if the rectus femoris is shifted to the side (**6.75**).

The palpable aspect of **vastus medialis** forms a teardrop shape at the distal portion of the medial thigh (**6.76**) while the **vastus lateralis** is the sole muscle of the lateral thigh. The posterior edge of the lateralis lies next to the biceps femoris, one of the hamstrings. Although vastus lateralis is deep to the iliotibial tract (p. 326), its fibers are easily accessible (**6.77**, **6.78**).

All four quadriceps muscles converge into a single tendon above the knee. The tendon connects to the top and sides of the patella before attaching—via the patellar ligament—to the tibial tuberosity (**6.79**, **6.80**).

QUADRICEPS FEMORIS GROUP

A
All:
Extend the knee (tibiofemoral joint)
Rectus femoris:
Flex the hip (coxal joint)

O
Rectus femoris: Anterior inferior iliac spine (AIIS)
Vastus medialis: Medial lip of linea aspera
Vastus lateralis: Lateral lip of linea aspera, gluteal tuberosity, and greater trochanter
Vastus intermedius: Anterior and lateral shaft of the femur

I
Tibial tuberosity (via the patella and patellar ligament)

N
Femoral L**2**, **3**, **4**

When Do You Use Your Quadriceps Femoris Group?

- Kicking a soccer ball
- Stabilizing yourself in a stationary squat position
- Raising your knee quickly into a bad guy's cojones (rectus femoris)

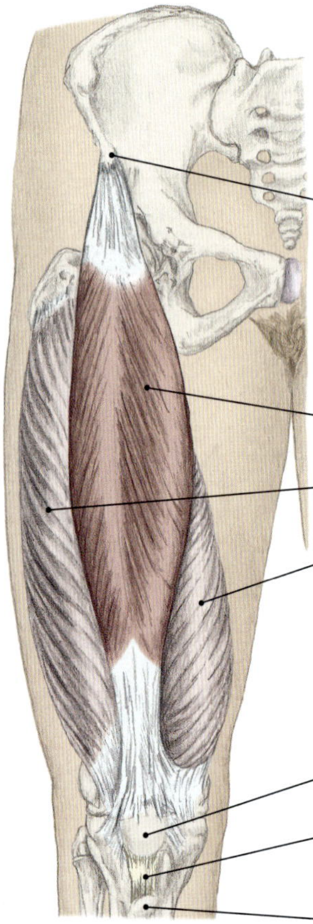

6.74 Anterior view of right hip and thigh, showing rectus femoris (highlighted in dark red)

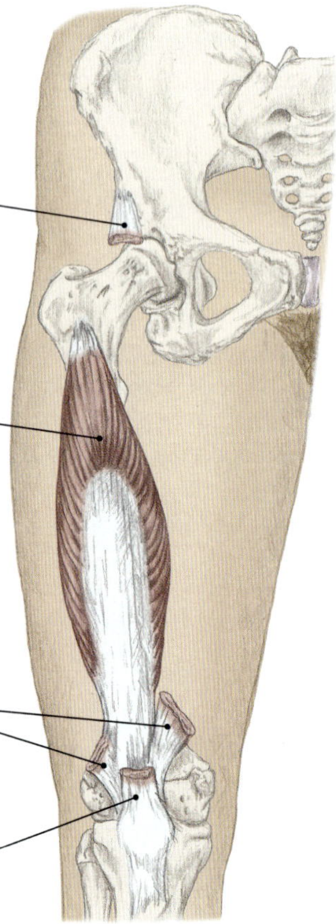

6.75 Anterior view of right hip and thigh, showing vastus intermedius

quadriceps	***kwod***-ri-seps	L. four-headed
rectus	***rek***-tus	L. straight

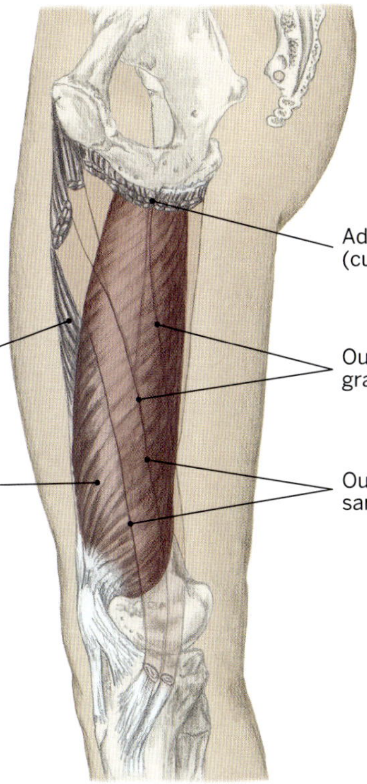

6.76 Medial view of right thigh, showing vastus medialis

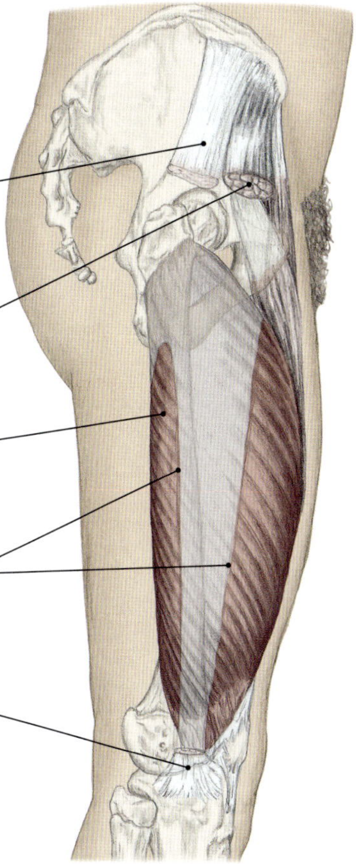

6.77 Lateral view of right hip and thigh, showing vastus lateralis

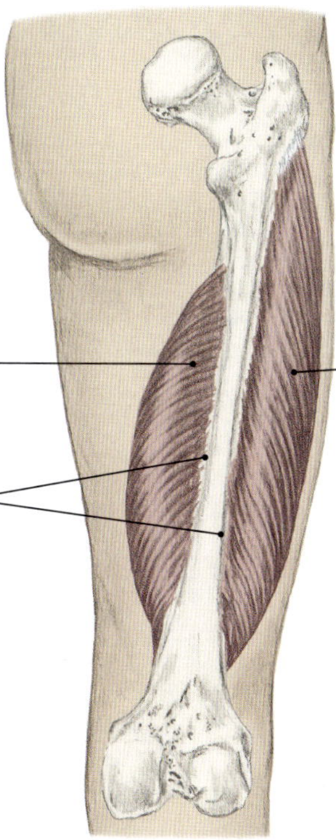

6.78 Posterior view of right femur, showing vastus medialis and vastus lateralis

Discover More

The distal tendon of the quadriceps and the patellar ligament are one and the same structure (see **6.74**). Because the tendon attaches one bone to another (the patella to the tibia), it is actually considered a ligament.

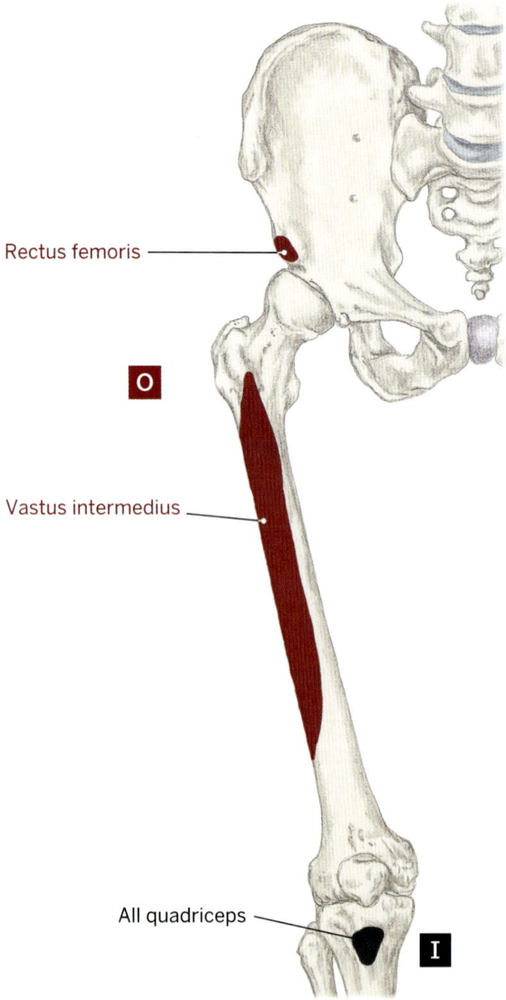

6.79 Anterior view of right hip and thigh, showing origins of rectus femoris and vastus intermedius and insertions of quadriceps

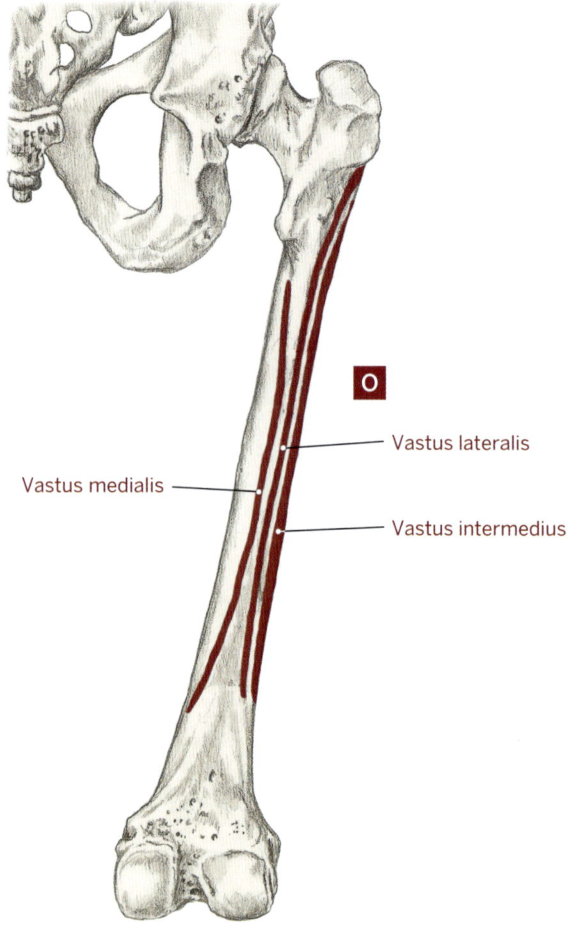

6.80 Posterior view of right hip and femur, showing origins of vastus medialis, vastus lateralis, and vastus intermedius

Palpation Plus

Ask your supine partner to extend his knee by fully contracting his quadriceps. Observe and palpate the distal ends of the vastus medialis and vastus lateralis. Do you notice that the vastus medialis extends farther distally than the vastus lateralis? The reason for this variance concerns the tracking (or movement) of the patella. The angle of the femur, combined with the pull of the quadriceps, causes the patella to track laterally. This is prevented, however, in two ways: first, the edge of the lateral condyle of the femur (p. 356) is elevated, forming a lateral wall; and second, the distal fibers of vastus medialis are set at an angle, pulling the patella medially..

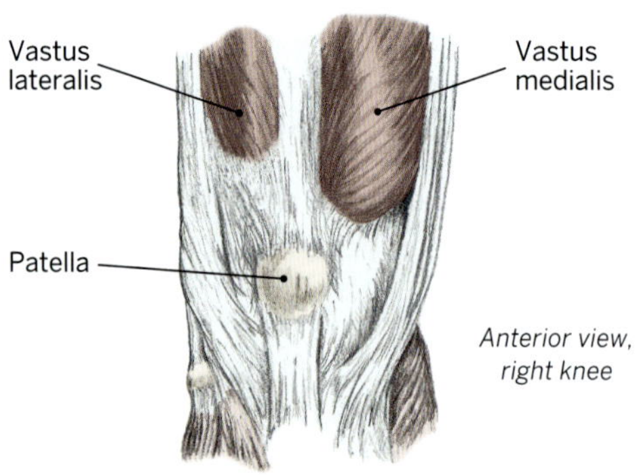

Quadriceps as a group

1. Partner seated. Lay the flat of your hands on the anterior surface of the thigh.
2. Ask your partner to alternately extend and relax his knee slowly. Explore the lateral and medial sides of the thigh (**6.81**). Do you feel the quadriceps tighten as the knee extends? For greater contraction, provide a little resistance below the knee as your partner tries to raise it.

Rectus femoris

1. Partner supine with knee bolstered. Locate the AIIS (p. 290) and the patella (p. 354).
2. Draw an imaginary line between these two points and follow the path of the rectus femoris (**6.82**).
3. Palpate along this line and strum across the rectus fibers. (It will be two to three fingers wide.)
4. Ask your partner to flex his hip and hold his foot up off the table (**6.83**). This position contracts the rectus femoris, making it more pronounced.

Are you on the anterior surface of the thigh? Can you follow the muscle belly to the patella and toward the AIIS? Can you shift it to the side and feel the density of vastus intermedius beneath it?

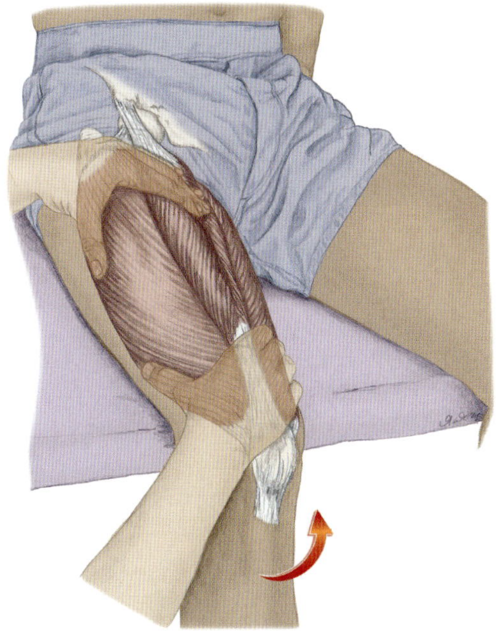

6.81 Partner seated, palpating the quadriceps as a group

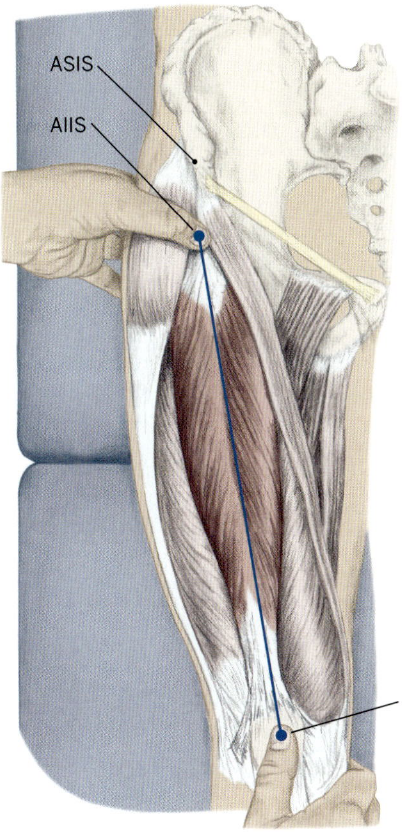

6.82 Partner supine, anterior view of thigh, as you draw an imaginary line between the AIIS and patella to isolate the rectus femoris

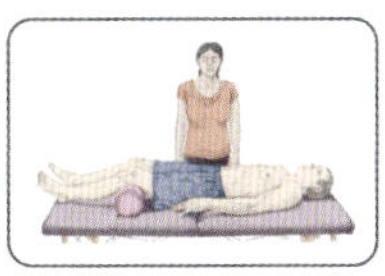

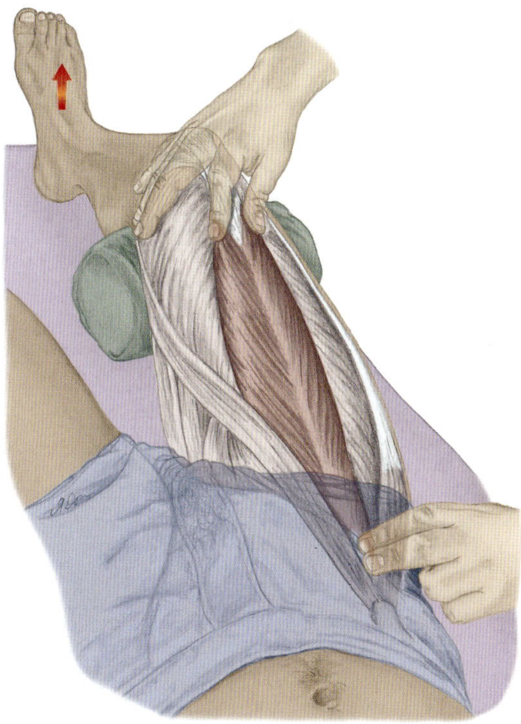

6.83 Partner supine, flexing his hip and holding his foot off the table while you locate the rectus femoris

Vastus medialis

1. Supine with the knee bolstered. Ask your partner to fully contract his quadriceps by extending his knee. Palpate just medial and proximal to the patella for the bulbous shape of the medialis.
2. Locate the rectus femoris and sartorius (p. 328), noting how these muscles surround the medialis to form its long teardrop shape (**6.84**).

Are you medial to the rectus femoris? Can you make out the round shape of the vastus medialis and follow its fibers to the patella?

Vastus lateralis

1. Partner side lying. Place the flat of your hand on the lateral side of the thigh while your partner slowly extends and relaxes his knee (**6.85**). Notice the vastus lateralis contracting and relaxing.
2. Palpate its entire belly—posteriorly to the biceps femoris (p. 313) and proximally to the greater trochanter. With the thigh relaxed, identify the direction and depth of the lateralis fibers and the superficial iliotibial tract (p. 326).

*Can you follow its fibers to the patella? Can you differentiate between the vertical fibers of the iliotibial tract and the deeper, oblique fibers of the lateralis (**6.86**)?*

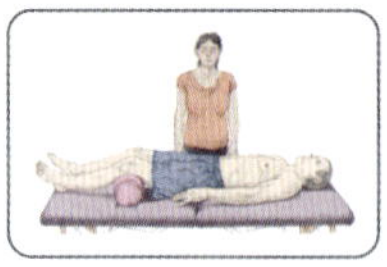

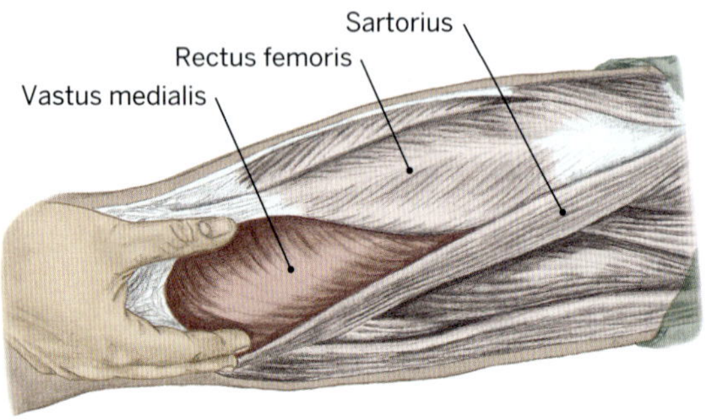

6.84 Partner supine, anterior/medial view of right thigh, as you explore vastus medialis

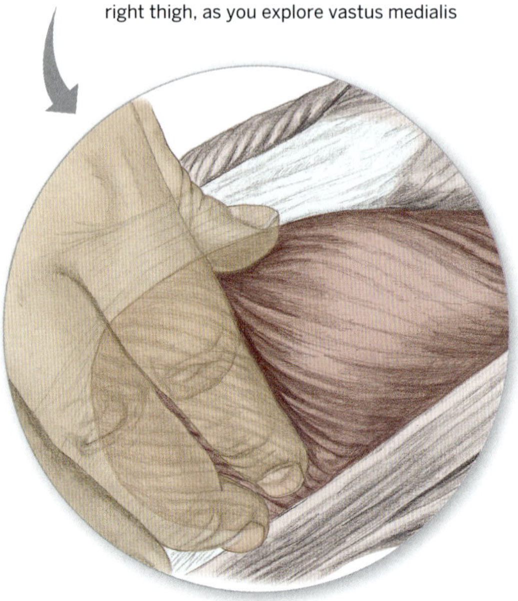

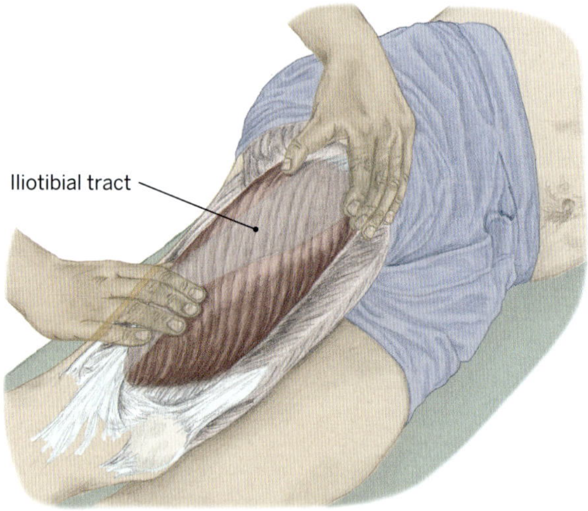

6.85 Partner side lying, as you palpate the vastus lateralis deep to the iliotibial tract

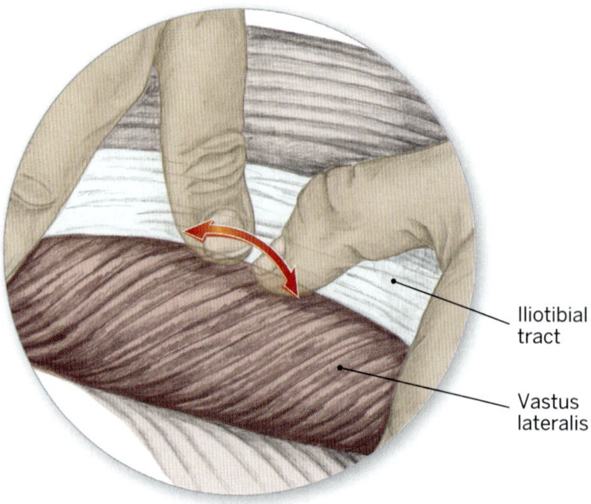

6.86 Partner side lying, lateral view, as you roll your fingers across the fibers of the vastus lateralis

Hamstrings ▶

Biceps Femoris
Semitendinosus
Semimembranosus

The hamstrings are located along the posterior thigh between the vastus lateralis and adductor magnus (**6.87**). Comparatively, the hamstrings are not as massive as the quadriceps femoris group, but they are nonetheless strong hip extensors and knee flexors. All three hamstrings have a common origin at the ischial tuberosity (see **6.92**). Their tubular bellies extend superficially down the thigh before becoming long, thin tendons that stretch across the posterior knee. As a group, the hamstrings and their distal tendons are easily palpable.

Biceps femoris is the lateral hamstring. It has two heads—a superficial long head and a deeper, indiscernible short head (**6.88**, **6.89**). The medial hamstrings include the two "semi" muscles. The **semitendinosus** lies superficial to the wider and deeper **semimembranosus** (**6.90**, **6.91**).

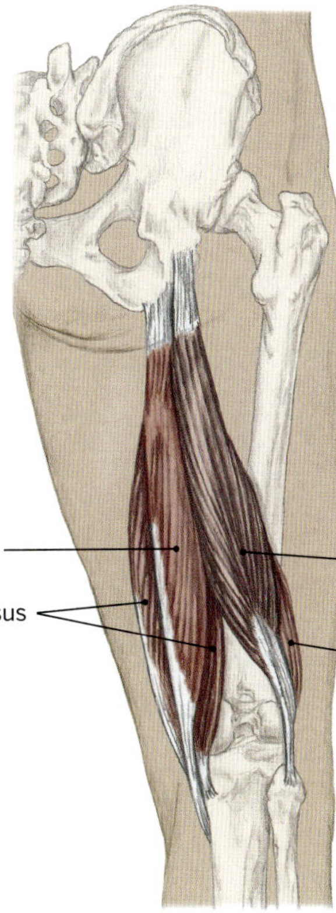

6.87 Posterior view of right thigh, showing superficial hamstrings

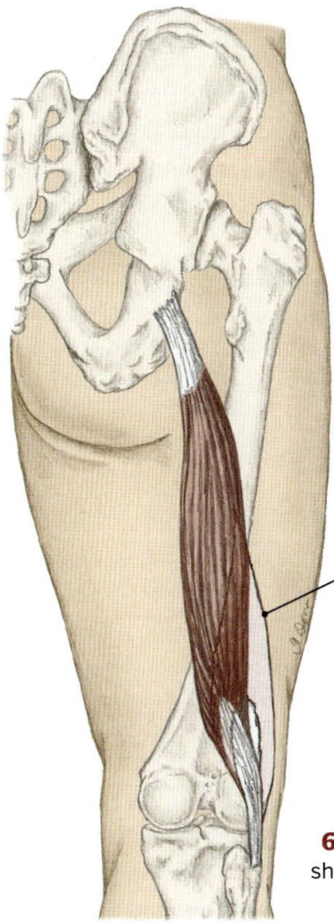

6.88 Posterior view of right thigh, showing long head of biceps femoris

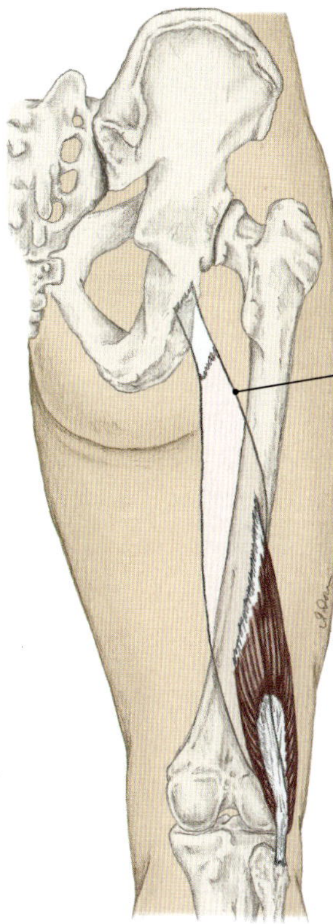

6.89 Posterior view of right thigh, showing short head of biceps femoris

Discover More

The term "hamstring" originated in 18th-century England. Back then, butchers would display pig carcasses in their shop windows by hanging them from the long tendons at the back of the knee.

semimembranosus	*sem*-eye-*mem*-bra-*no*-sus	L. half membranous
semitendinosus	*sem*-eye-*ten*-di-*no*-sus	L. half tendinous

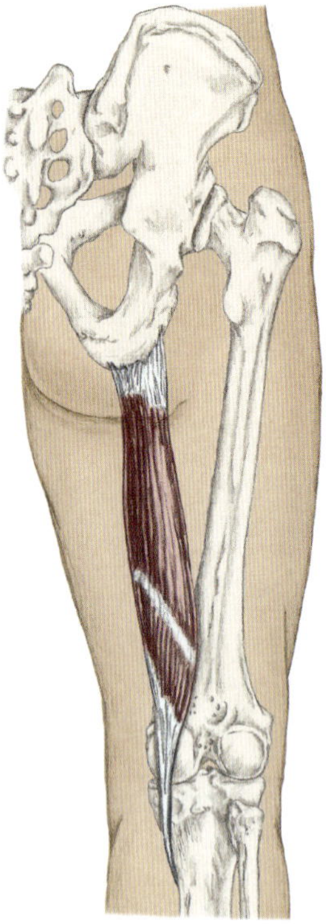

6.90 Posterior view of right thigh, showing semitendinosus

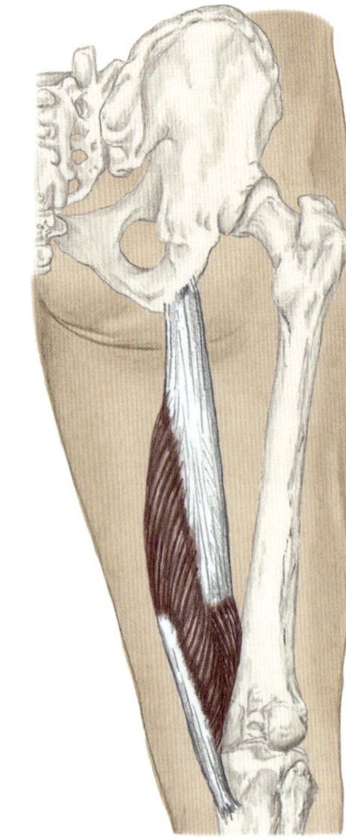

6.91 Posterior view of right thigh, showing semimembranosus

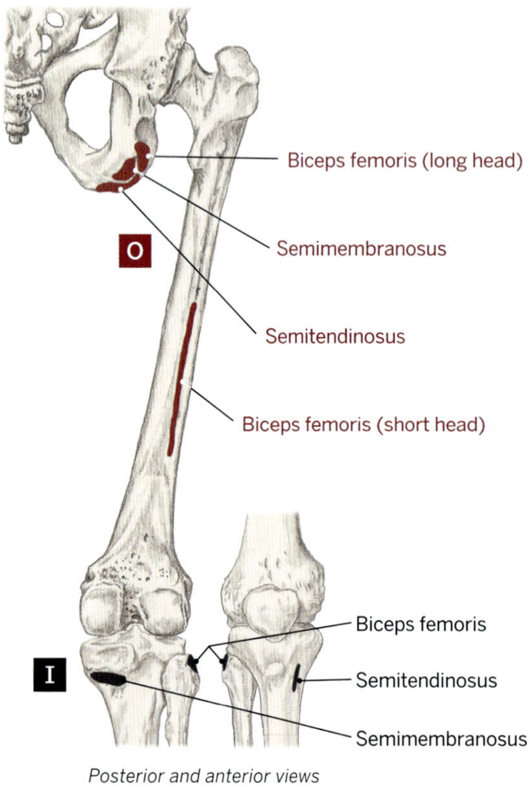

6.92 Posterior view of right thigh (left) and anterior view of right knee (right), showing origins and insertions of hamstrings

BICEPS FEMORIS

A
Flex the knee (tibiofemoral joint)
Laterally rotate the flexed knee (T/F joint)
Long head:
Extend the hip (coxal joint)
Long head:
Assist to **laterally rotate** the hip (coxal joint)
Tilt the pelvis posteriorly

O
Long head: Ischial tuberosity
Short head: Lateral lip of linea aspera

I
Head of the fibula

N
Long head: Sciatic (tibial branch) L5, S**1**, **2**, 3
Short head: Sciatic (fibular branch) L**5**, S**1**, **2**

When Do You Use Your Biceps Femoris?

- Running, cycling, swimming, climbing stairs
- Stabilizing your hip while bending over to tie your shoes
- Scraping mud off your boots (extension of the hip)

SEMITENDINOSUS

A
Flex the knee (tibiofemoral joint)
Medially rotate the flexed knee (T/F joint)
Extend the hip (coxal joint)
Assist to **medially rotate** the hip (coxal joint)
Tilt the pelvis posteriorly

O
Ischial tuberosity

I
Proximal, medial shaft of the tibia at pes anserinus tendon

N
Sciatic (tibial branch) L4, **5**, S**1**, **2**

When Do You Use Your Semitendinosus?

- Running, cycling, swimming, climbing stairs
- Stabilizing your hip while bending over to tie your shoes
- Scraping mud off your boots (extension of the hip)

SEMIMEMBRANOSUS

A
Flex the knee (tibiofemoral joint)
Medially rotate the flexed knee (T/F joint)
Extend the hip (coxal joint)
Assist to **medially rotate** the hip (coxal joint)
Tilt the pelvis posteriorly

O
Ischial tuberosity

I
Posterior aspect of medial condyle of tibia

N
Sciatic (tibial branch) L4, **5**, S**1**, 2

When Do You Use Your Semimembranosus?

- Running, cycling, swimming, climbing stairs
- Stabilizing your hip while bending over to tie your shoes
- Scraping mud off your boots (extension of the hip)

Hamstrings as a group

1. Partner prone. Place a hand on the posterior thigh between the buttocks and knee. Ask your partner to flex his knee, holding his foot off the table. As the hamstrings contract, explore their mass and width (**6.93**).
2. Locate the ischial tuberosity. Slide your fingertips distally one inch and strum across the large, solid tendon of the hamstrings (**6.94**).
3. Follow the tendon distally as it spreads out into the separate bellies of the hamstrings (**6.95**).

Follow the bellies proximally. Do they attach to the ischial tuberosity? Follow the bellies distally. Do you feel their skinny tendons along the posterior knee?

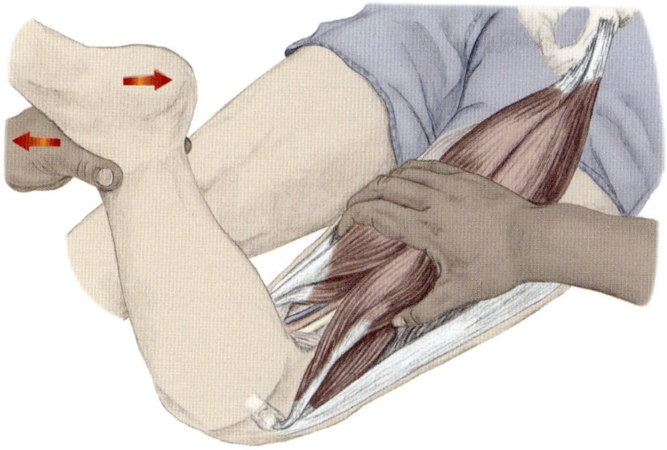

6.93 Partner prone, flexing his knee while you grasp the hamstrings group

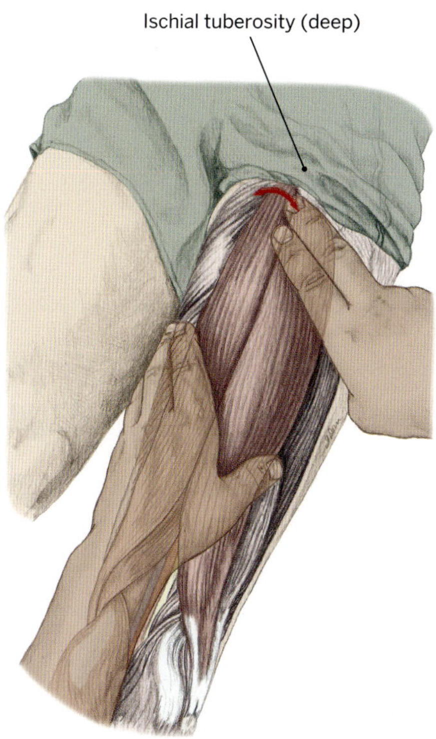

6.94 Partner prone, as you isolate the hamstrings tendon at the ischial tuberosity

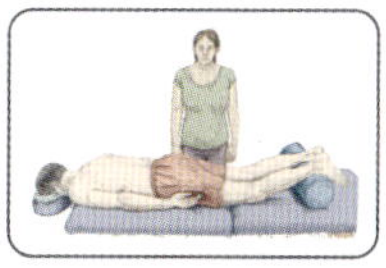

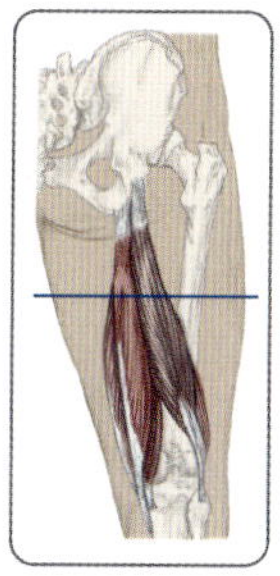

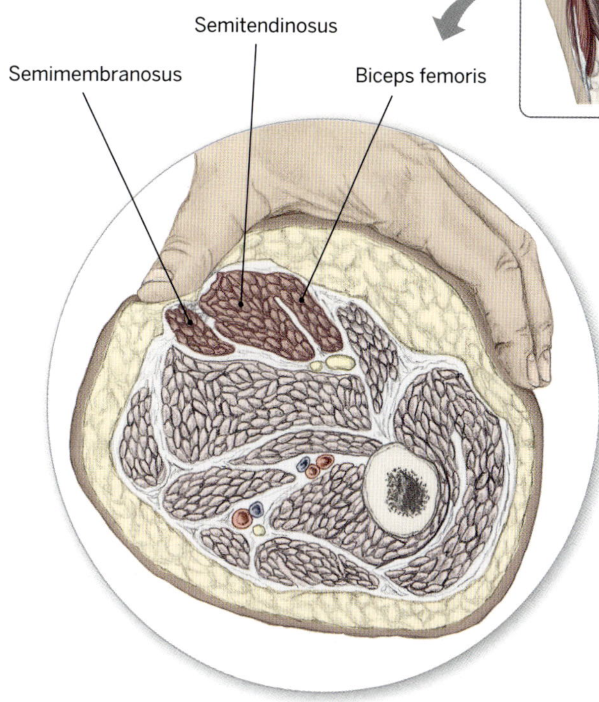

6.95 Superior view, cross section of right thigh, as you sink your thumb into the medial edge of the hamstrings

biceps femoris	***bi***-seps fe-***mor***-is	Grk. the two-headed (muscle) of the thigh
pes anserinus	pes ***an***-ser-***i***-nus	L. *pedis*, foot; *anserinus*, goose-like

Individual bellies and distal tendons

1. Partner prone. Ask him to hold his knee in a flexed position. Again, explore the bellies of the hamstrings.
2. The lateral half of the hamstring belly is the biceps femoris. Its belly will lead toward the head of the fibula. Palpate on the lateral side of the knee for the long, prominent tendon of the biceps femoris and follow it toward the head of the fibula (**6.96**).
3. The medial half of the hamstrings consists of the layered bellies of the semitendinosus and semimembranosus. Move to the medial side of the knee and palpate for the tendons of these muscles (**6.97**).
4. The most superficial tendon will be the semitendinosus. Turn your partner supine and follow it distally as it merges with the pes anserinus tendon. The semimembranosus is tucked deep to the semitendinosus and is often difficult to isolate.

Are the tendons along the back of the knee slender and superficial? Does the biceps femoris tendon lead to the head of the fibula? Can you follow the "semis" as they seem to disappear into the medial knee?

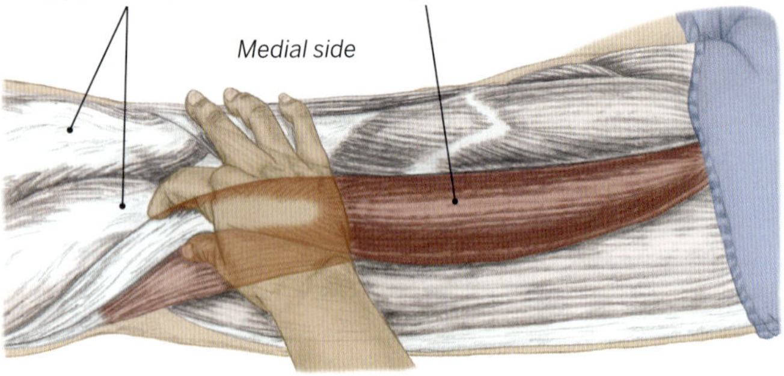

6.96 Partner prone, posterior/lateral view of right knee, as you palpate biceps femoris

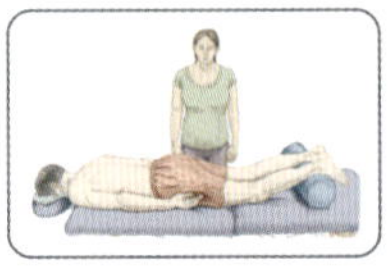

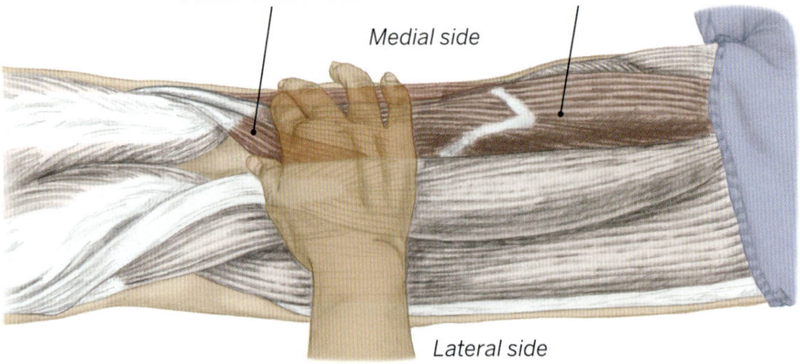

6.97 Partner prone, posterior/lateral view of right knee, as you palpate semimembranosus and semitendinosus

Palpation Plus

How do you differentiate the vastus lateralis from the biceps femoris on the posterior, lateral thigh? Have these muscles do what comes naturally— be antagonists.

1. Partner side lying. Bend the top knee to 90° and clasp the ankle. Lay your other hand on the lateral thigh.
2. Ask your partner to alternate between flexing and extending his knee ever so slightly against your resistance. Sense how the vastus lateralis contracts upon extension while the biceps femoris remains lax. The opposite will happen when flexing the knee.
3. Often there will be a palpable dividing line or depression between the edges of these muscles.

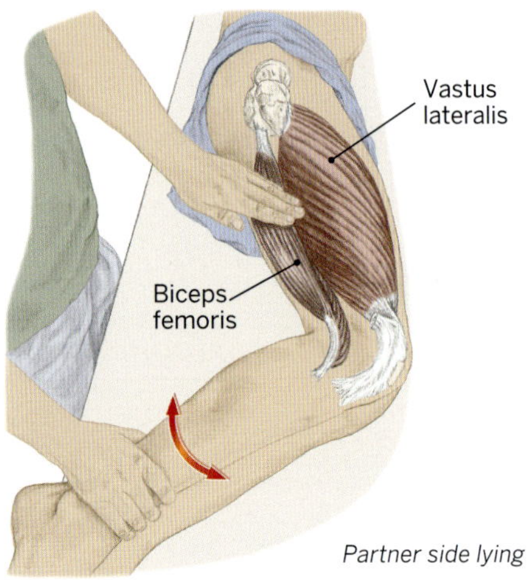

Gluteals ▶

Gluteus Maximus, Medius, and Minimus

The three gluteal muscles are located in the buttock region, deep to the surrounding adipose tissue. The large, superficial **gluteus maximus** is the most posterior of the group and has fibers that run diagonally across the buttock (**6.98**).

The **gluteus medius** is located on the lateral side of the hip and is also superficial, except for the posterior portion which is deep to the maximus (**6.99**). Both the gluteus maximus and medius are strong extensors and abductors of the hip. With its convergent fibers that pull the femur in multiple directions, the gluteus medius could be thought of as the "deltoid muscle of the coxal joint."

The **gluteus minimus** lies deep to the gluteus medius and is inaccessible; however, its dense fibers can be felt beneath the medius (**6.100**). Because it attaches to the anterior surface of the greater trochanter, the gluteus minimus flexes and medially rotates the hip, thus performing the opposite actions of the gluteus maximus (**6.101, 6.102**).

GLUTEUS MAXIMUS

A
All fibers:
Extend the hip (coxal joint)
Laterally rotate the hip (coxal joint)
Abduct the hip (coxal joint)
Lower fibers:
Adduct the hip (coxal joint)

O Coccyx, edge of sacrum, posterior iliac crest, sacrotuberous and sacroiliac ligaments

I Iliotibial tract (upper fibers) and gluteal tuberosity (lower fibers)

N Inferior gluteal L**5**, S**1**, **2**

When Do You Use Your Gluteus Maximus?

- Climbing stairs
- Running, cycling, swimming, skating
- Latin dancing (lots of lateral rotation of the hip)

GLUTEUS MEDIUS

A
All fibers:
Abduct the hip (coxal joint)
Anterior fibers:
Flex the hip (coxal joint)
Medially rotate the hip (coxal joint)
Posterior fibers:
Extend the hip (coxal joint)
Laterally rotate the hip (coxal joint)

O Gluteal surface of ilium, between posterior and anterior gluteal lines, just below the iliac crest

I Lateral aspect of greater trochanter

N Superior gluteal L**4**, **5**, S**1**

When Do You Use Your Gluteus Medius?

- Climbing stairs
- Running, cycling, swimming, skating
- Latin dancing (lots of lateral rotation of the hip)

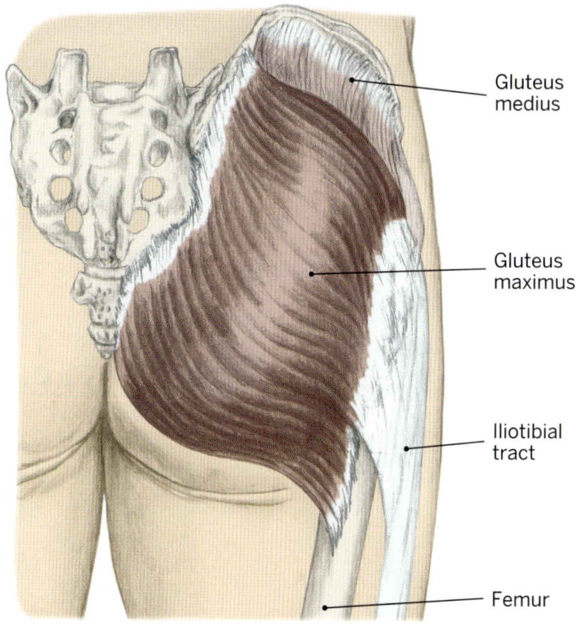

6.98 Posterior view of right buttock, showing gluteus maximus

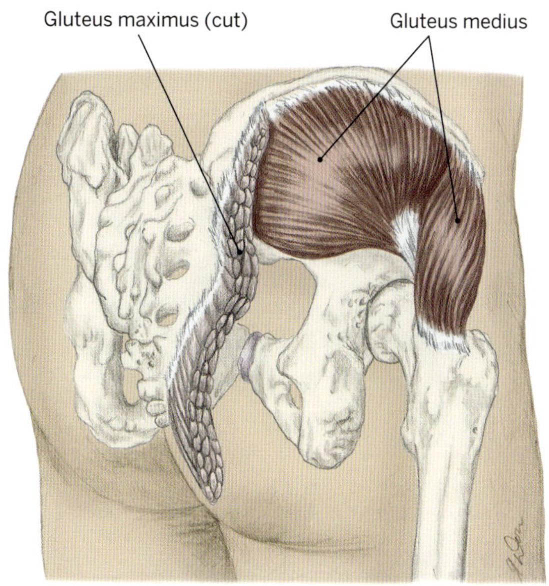

6.99 Posterior/lateral view of right buttock, showing gluteus medius

gluteus *gloo*-te-us Grk. *gloutos*, buttocks, which in turn is Anglo-Saxon for *buttuc*, meaning end

Pelvis & Thigh

GLUTEUS MINIMUS

A **Abduct** the hip (coxal joint)
Medially rotate the hip (coxal joint)
Flex the hip (coxal joint)

O Gluteal surface of the ilium between the anterior and inferior gluteal lines

I Anterior aspect of greater trochanter

N Superior gluteal L**4**, **5**, S**1**

When Do You Use Your Gluteus Minimus?

- Climbing stairs
- Running, cycling, swimming, skating
- Latin dancing (lots of lateral rotation of the hip)

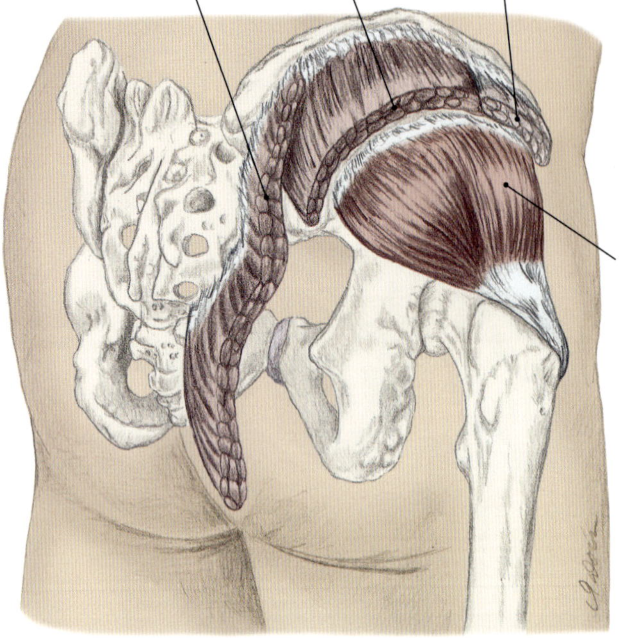

6.100 Posterior/lateral view of right buttock, showing gluteus minimus

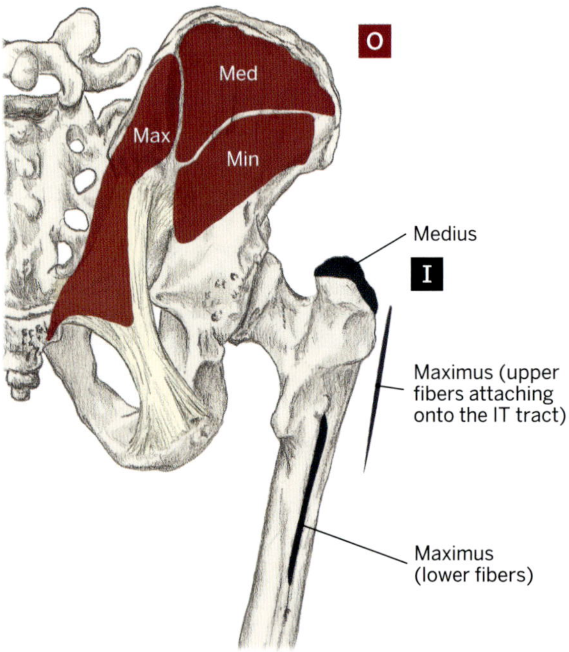

6.101 Posterior view of right hip and femur, showing origins and insertions of gluteal muscles

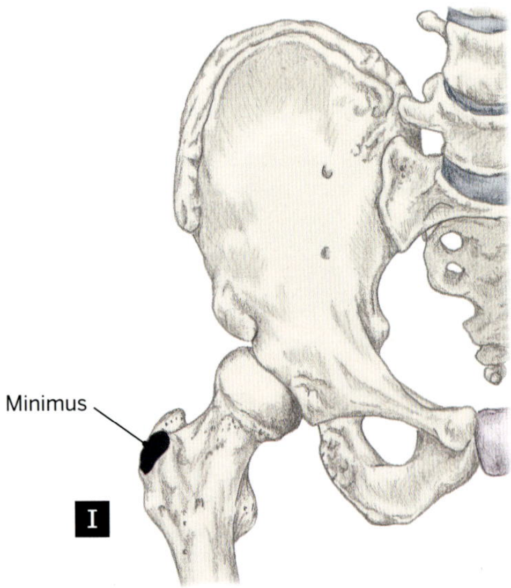

6.102 Anterior view of right hip and femur, showing insertion of gluteus minimus

Gluteus maximus

1. Partner prone. Locate the coccyx, the edge of the sacrum, the PSIS, and the posterior two inches of the iliac crest to isolate the landmarks that form the origin of the maximus (**6.103**).
2. Locate the insertion of the maximus at the gluteal tuberosity.
3. Connect its origin to its insertion by drawing the fiber direction on your partner. Then palpate its thick, superficial fibers. Also notice differences in texture and depth between the adipose tissue of the buttock and the muscle fibers of the maximus. The adipose is superficial to the maximus and often has a soft, gel-like consistency.

*Ask your partner to extend his hip (**6.104**). Palpate the bulging fibers that lead to the gluteal tuberosity. If this is difficult with the knee extended for your partner while prone, try palpating with the knee flexed or with your partner standing.*

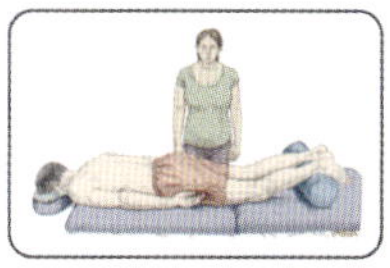

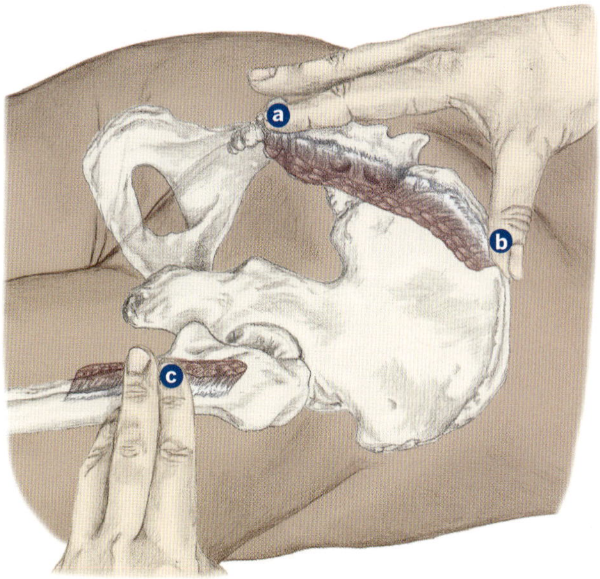

6.103 Partner prone, as you isolate the borders of the gluteus maximus: (**a**) coccyx, (**b**) posterior iliac crest, (**c**) gluteal tuberosity

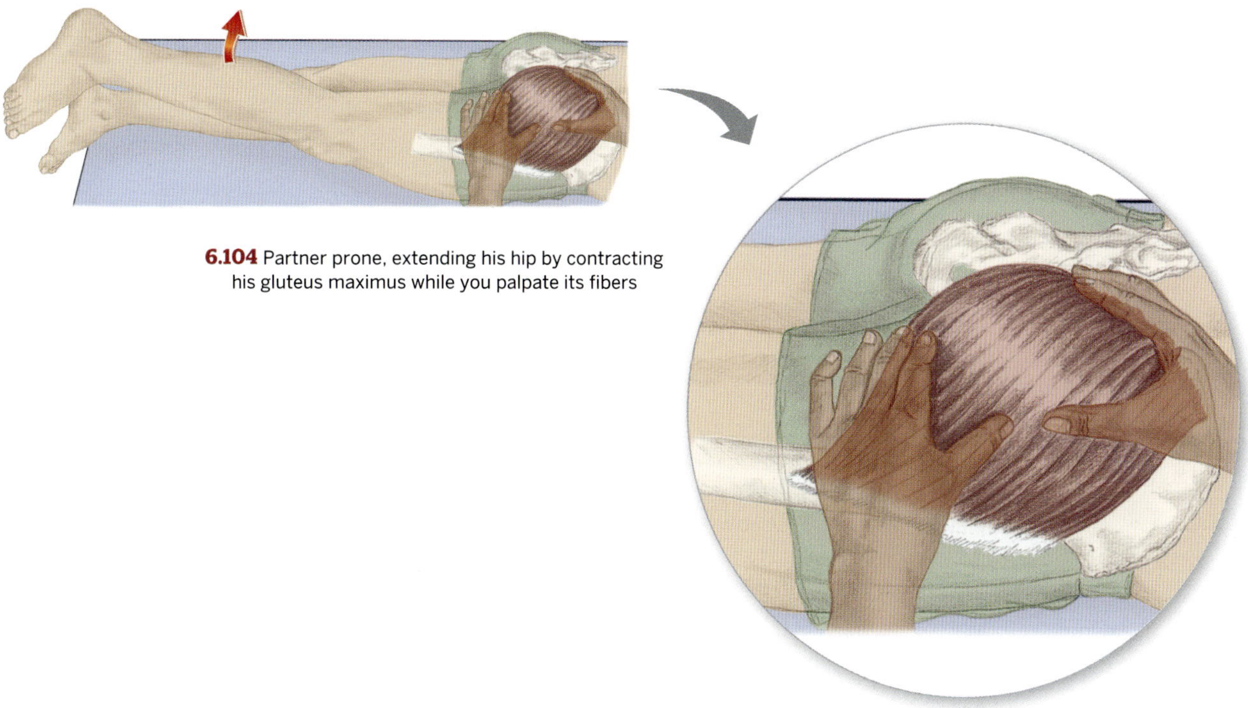

6.104 Partner prone, extending his hip by contracting his gluteus maximus while you palpate its fibers

Pelvis & Thigh

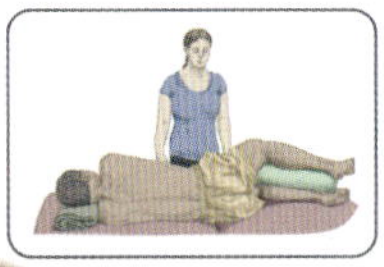

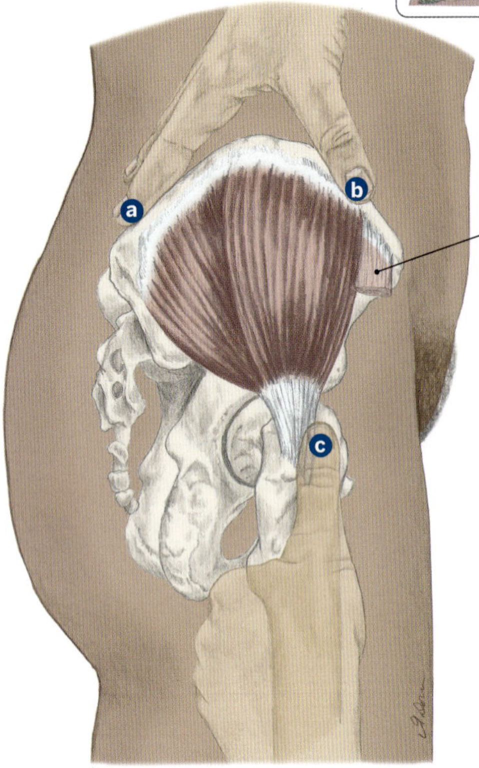

6.105 Partner side lying, as you isolate the borders of the gluteus medius: (**a**) PSIS, (**b**) iliac crest, (**c**) greater trochanter

Gluteus medius and minimus

1. Partner side lying. Isolate the shape of the gluteus medius by placing the webbing of one hand along the iliac crest (from PSIS to nearly the ASIS) while the other hand locates the greater trochanter.
2. Your hands will form a shape that looks like a slice of pie. This is the outline of the gluteus medius (**6.105**).
3. Palpate in this area from just below the iliac crest to the greater trochanter for the dense fibers of the gluteus medius.
4. Sink your fingers deep to the gluteus medius to explore for the density and mass of the gluteus minimus.

*Ask your partner to abduct his hip slightly (**6.106**). Do you feel the medius contract?*

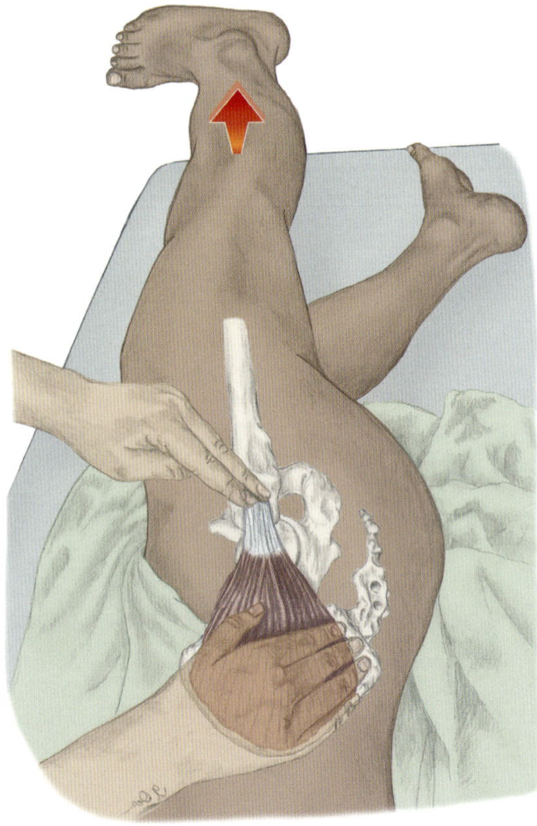

6.106 Partner side lying, abducting the hip while you isolate the gluteus medius

Discover More

Humans are unique among mammals not only with respect to their extra-large brains, but also because of their well-padded buttocks. No other mammal has such deposits of adipose tissue in the gluteal region, and no one seems to know *why* we have them. It was thought that the buttocks gave us something to sit upon, but we really sit upon our ischial tuberosities. And for good reason: if we did not, the gluteus maximus and gluteal fascia would be compressed beneath us. Since women typically have larger buttocks than men, it was conjectured that the buttocks served as fat-storage sites during pregnancy. Not so.

One thing is known: The gluteal fold—the crease between the buttock and thigh—helps localize the subcutaneous adipose at the top of the thigh. Biomechanically, it is easier to swing the thigh back and forth when walking with the tissue situated proximally rather than dispersed down the thigh.

Adductor Group ▶

Adductor Magnus
Adductor Longus
Adductor Brevis
Pectineus
Gracilis

The five adductors are located along the medial thigh between the hamstrings and quadriceps femoris muscles (**6.107**, **6.108**). Their proximal tendons attach at specific locations along the base of the pelvis (see **6.113–6.115**). Together these tendons form a connective tissue drape that extends from the superior ramus of the pubis to the ischial tuberosity.

When the thigh is viewed anteriorly, the muscle bellies of the adductors lie in three layers. The **pectineus** and **adductor longus** are most anterior (**6.109**). Behind them is the **adductor brevis** (**6.110**), and most posterior is the **adductor magnus** (**6.111**, **6.112**). The broad span of adductor magnus, known as the "floor of the adductors," lies anterior to the hamstrings. These four muscles tuck posteriorly to the quadriceps femoris group and insert on the posterior femur. The fifth adductor, **gracilis**, lies superficially on the medial thigh. It is the only adductor that crosses the knee (see **6.110**).

Although their individual bellies can be challenging to isolate, as a group, the adductors are easy to locate. When palpating the adductor tendons near the pubic bone, you will find a prominent tendon that extends off of or near the pubic tubercle. The source of this superficial tendon is either the gracilis or adductor longus; in some cases, it is a merging of both tendons.

In either case, the tendon can serve as an important guidepost for locating not only gracilis and adductor longus, but also pectineus and adductor magnus. The pectineus will be located on the anterior side of this tendon while the adductor magnus will be located posterior to it.

ADDUCTOR GROUP

A

All: **Adduct** the hip (coxal joint)
Medially rotate the hip (coxal joint)
All except gracilis: Assist to **flex** the hip (coxal joint)
Gracilis: **Flex** the knee (tibiofemoral joint)
Medially rotate the flexed knee (T/F joint)
Posterior fibers of adductor magnus: **Extend** the hip (coxal joint)

When Do You Use Your Adductors?

- Ice skating (doing a crossover step when turning)
- Gripping a horse with your thighs when riding
- Stabilizing your pelvis when walking

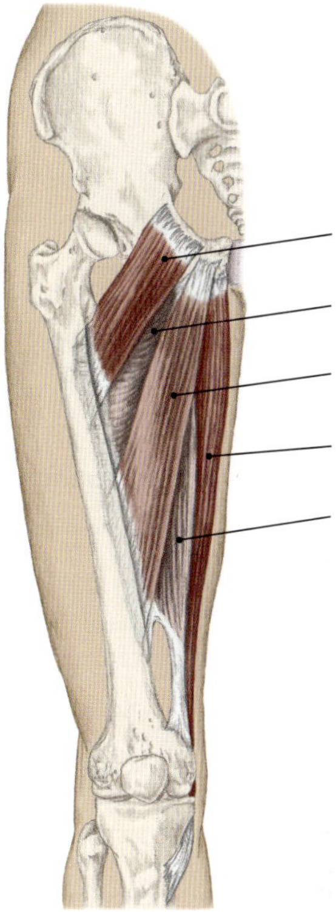

6.107 Anterior view of right hip and thigh, showing adductors

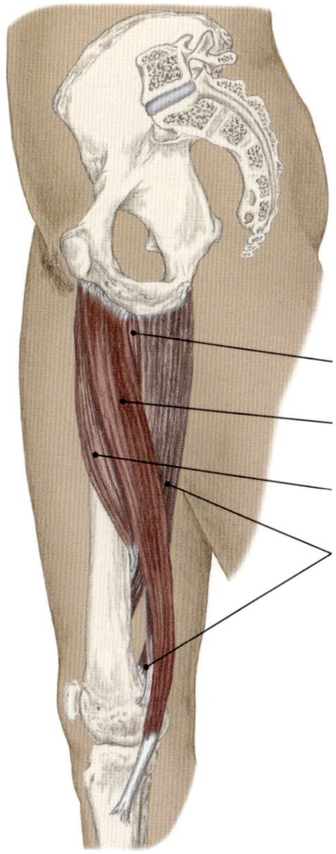

6.108 Medial view of right hip and thigh, showing adductors

brevis	***breh***-vis	L. short
gracilis	gra-***cil***-is	L. slender, graceful
pectineus	pek-***tin***-e-us	L. comblike

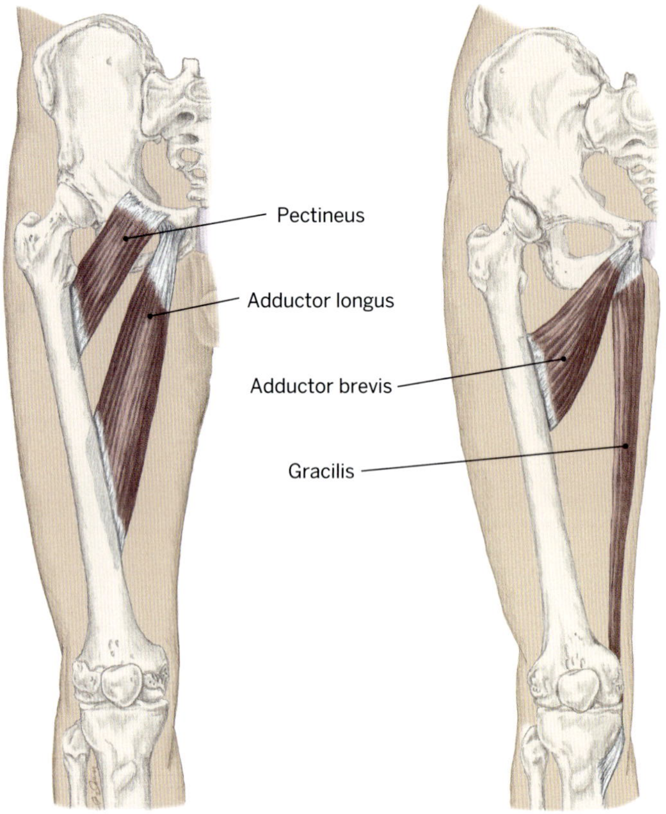

6.109 Anterior view of right hip and thigh, showing pectineus and adductor longus

6.110 Anterior view of right hip and thigh, showing adductor brevis and gracilis

ADDUCTOR MAGNUS

O	Inferior ramus of the pubis, ramus of ischium, and ischial tuberosity
I	Medial lip of linea aspera and adductor tubercle
N	Obturator L2, **3**, **4** and sciatic L**4**, 5, S1

ADDUCTOR LONGUS

O	Pubic tubercle
I	Medial lip of linea aspera
N	Obturator L**2**, **3**, 4

ADDUCTOR BREVIS

O	Inferior ramus of pubis
I	Pectineal line and medial lip of linea aspera
N	Obturator L**2**, **3**, **4**

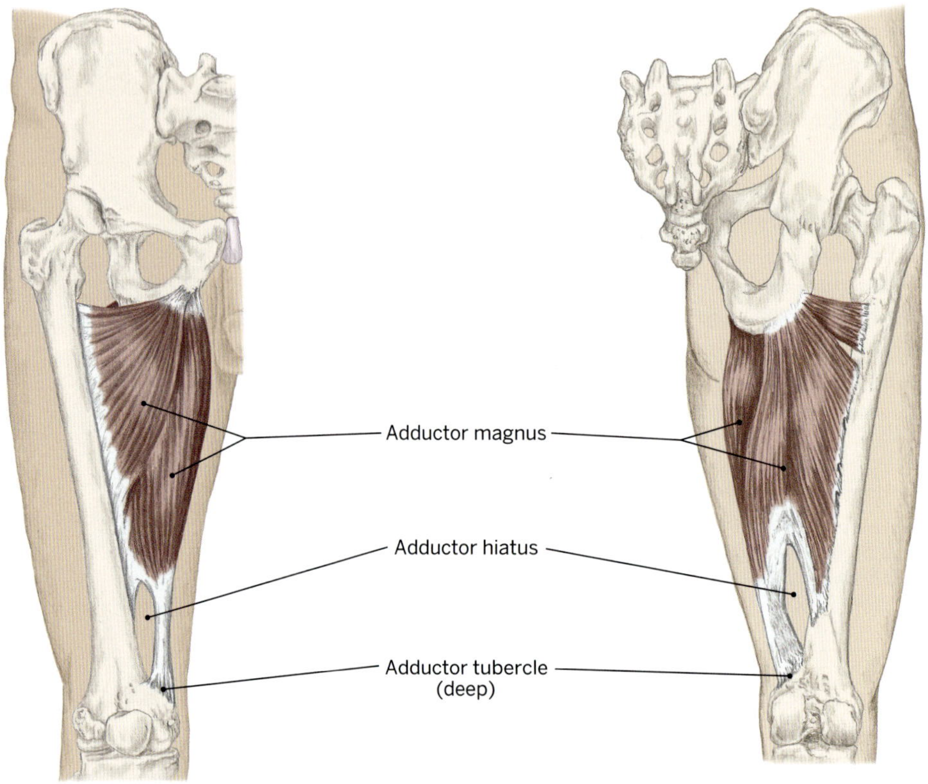

6.111 Anterior view of right hip and thigh, showing adductor magnus

6.112 Posterior view of right hip and thigh, showing adductor magnus

Pelvis & Thigh

PECTINEUS

O	Superior ramus of pubis
I	Pectineal line of femur
N	Femoral and obturator L**2**, **3**, 4

GRACILIS

O	Inferior ramus of pubis
I	Proximal, medial shaft of tibia at pes anserinus tendon
N	Obturator L**2**, **3**, **4**

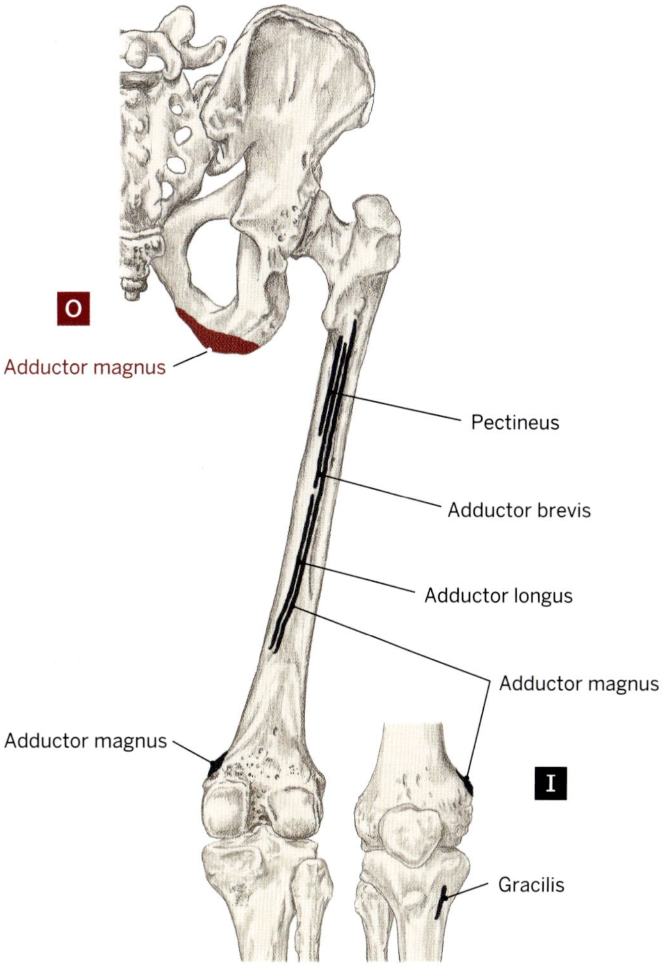

Posterior and anterior views

6.113 Posterior view of right hip and thigh (left) and anterior view of right knee (right), showing origin of adductor magnus and insertions of adductors

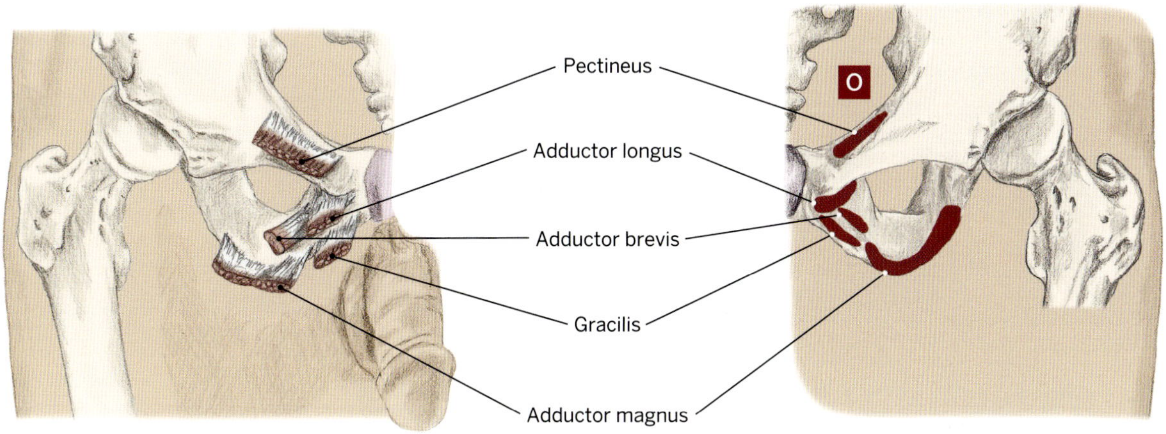

Right thigh and hip

6.114 Anterior view of right hip and thigh, showing origins of adductors

Left thigh and hip

6.115 Anterior view of left hip and thigh, showing origins of adductors

Pelvis & Thigh

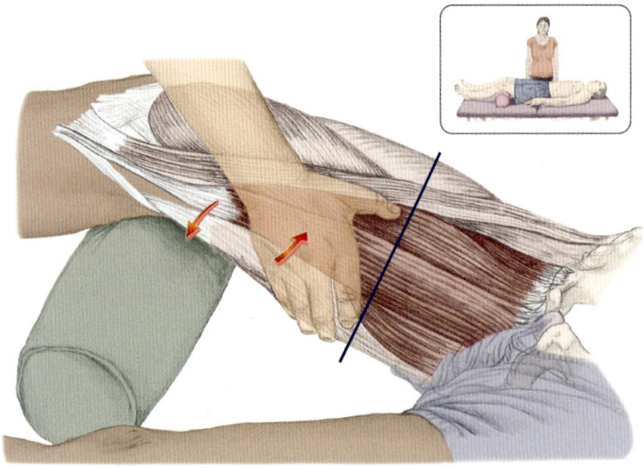

6.116 Partner supine, as you palpate the adductors as a group. The line indicates the cross section shown in 6.117.

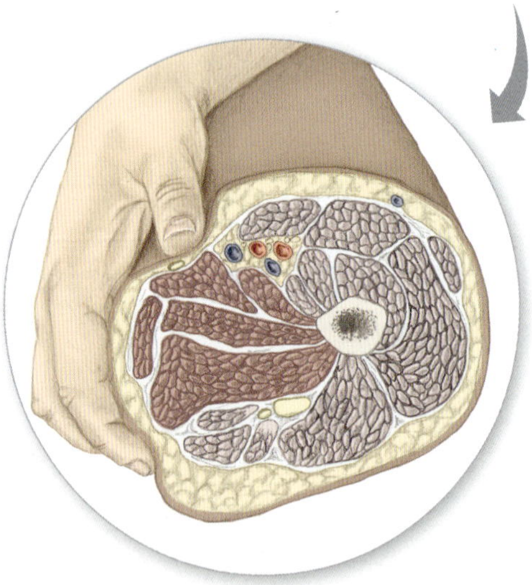

6.117 Inferior view, cross section of right thigh, as you grasp the highlighted adductors

Adductors as a group

1. Partner supine with the hip slightly flexed and laterally rotated. Place your hand along the medial thigh and ask your partner to adduct his hip against your resistance (**6.116**). Do you feel the adductors tighten?
2. Ask your partner to alternately adduct and relax as you palpate proximally to the adductor tendons. Then move distally, exploring anterior and posterior to the edges of the adductor bellies.

*Are you on the medial side of the thigh? Explore either side of the adductors to determine if you are between the hamstrings and quadriceps femoris group (**6.117**). You should be.*

Gracilis and adductor longus

1. Partner supine with the hip slightly flexed and laterally rotated. Place the flat of your hand at the middle of the medial thigh. Ask your partner to adduct his hip slightly.
2. While your partner contracts, slide your fingers proximally to the pubic bone and locate the taut, prominent tendon(s) of the gracilis and adductor longus extending off of (or near) the pubic tubercle.
3. Strum your fingertip across this tendon and follow it distally as it develops into muscle tissue (**6.118**). If the muscle belly slowly angles into the medial thigh, you are palpating adductor longus. If the belly is slender and continues down the medial thigh toward the knee, you are accessing gracilis.

The shape and location of the sartorius (p. 328) are similar to the shape and location of the gracilis. Distinguish between the two by simply following the muscle you are palpating proximally. If it leads toward the ASIS, it is the sartorius; if toward the pubis, the muscle is the gracilis.

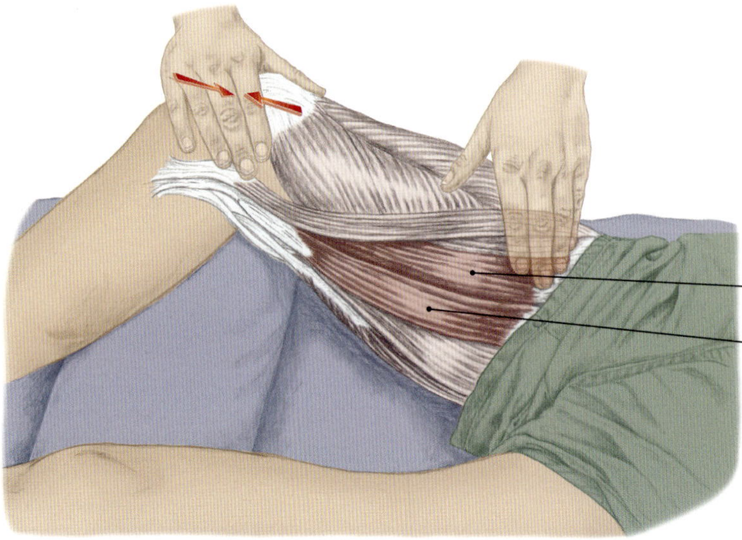

6.118 Partner supine, as you locate the prominent tendon(s) of the adductors

Pectineus

1. Partner supine with the hip slightly flexed and laterally rotated. Place the flat of your hand on the middle of the medial thigh and ask your partner to adduct his hip slightly.
2. Locate the prominent tendon of the adductor longus or gracilis. Slide off the tendon laterally toward the ASIS. Slowly sink into the belly of pectineus (**6.119**). You should be inferior to the superior ramus of the pubis (p. 296).
3. Ask your partner to alternately adduct and relax his hip and feel the fibers of pectineus contract.

Are you just anterior to the prominent adductor tendon? Do the fibers you are palpating contract upon adduction?

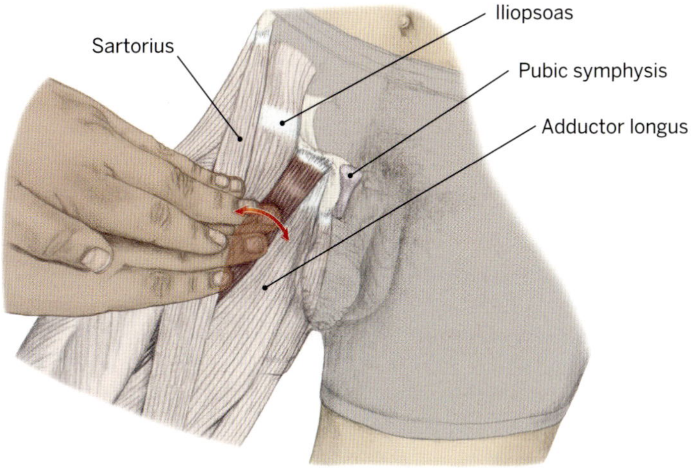

6.119 Partner supine, as you roll your fingers across the pectineus

Adductor magnus

1. Partner side lying with his top hip flexed. Begin by locating the ischial tuberosity.
2. Ask your partner to adduct his hip slightly. Shifting anteriorly, locate the prominent tendon of adductor longus or gracilis. Then slide off the tendon posteriorly. Palpate the wide tendon of adductor magnus as it stretches to the ischial tuberosity (**6.120**).
3. Follow the fibers of adductor magnus distally by strumming your fingers across its belly. It is difficult to differentiate magnus fibers from semimembranosus fibers. Nevertheless, the thin, distal tendon of the magnus is distinguishable and can be accessed where it attaches to the adductor tubercle (p. 357).

Be alert to the pulse of the femoral artery (p. 341). If you feel it under your fingers, remove your pressure and shift to one side.

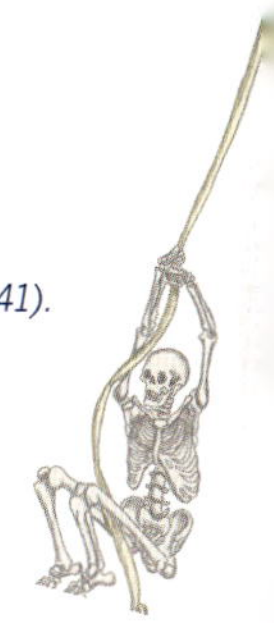

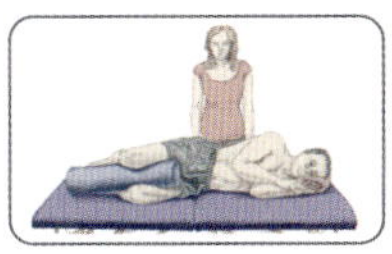

Top hip flexed

Palpation Plus

Because the adductors attach on the posterior femur, you might assume that they would rotate the coxal joint *laterally* rather than *medially*. In anatomical position, however, the adductors will medially rotate the femur. With that said, if the femur is in a laterally rotated position, some of the adductors will produce lateral rotation.

Partner supine. Lay your hand on the adductors. Ask your partner to alternately rotate his hip medially and laterally. Grasping the ankle to create a little resistance will verify this movement. Do you feel the adductors contract on medial rotation? What do they do when the hip is laterally rotated?

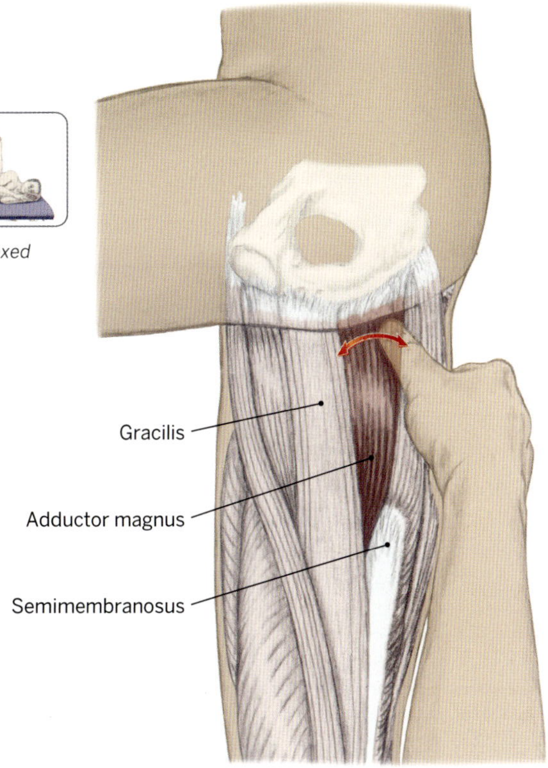

6.120 Partner side lying, as you access the adductor magnus

Tensor Fasciae Latae and Iliotibial Tract ▶

The **tensor fasciae latae** (TFL) is a small, superficial muscle located on the lateral side of the upper thigh (**6.121**, **6.122**). Approximately three fingers wide, the TFL is easily accessible between the upper fibers of the rectus femoris and the gluteus medius. The TFL attaches to the iliotibial tract along with the gluteus maximus.

The **iliotibial tract** (sometimes known as the iliotibial band) is a superficial sheet of fascia with vertical fibers that run along the lateral thigh. It emerges from the gluteal fascia, is wide and dense over the vastus lateralis muscle (p. 308), and funnels into a strong cable along the side of the knee before inserting at the tibial tubercle (see box, p. 355).

The fibers of tensor fasciae latae and some fibers of gluteus maximus (p. 317) attach to the proximal aspect of the iliotibial tract. The iliotibial tract has a thick, matted texture (similar to packing tape) that makes it a strong, stabilizing component of the hip and knee.

The iliotibial tract is entirely accessible. The distal cable portion, anterior to the biceps femoris tendon, is the easiest part of the iliotibial tract to isolate.

	TENSOR FASCIAE LATAE AND ILIOTIBIAL TRACT
A	**Flex** the hip (coxal joint) **Medially rotate** the hip (coxal joint) **Abduct** the hip (coxal joint)
O	Iliac crest, posterior to the ASIS
I	Iliotibial tract
N	Superior gluteal L**4**, **5**, S**1**

When Do You Use Your TFL?

- Running, bicycling, squatting at the hips
- Raising your leg to climb into a car (flex, medially rotate, and abduct the hip)
- The windup for a karate kick to the side—again, all three movements (see *Fist of Fury* with Bruce Lee for examples)

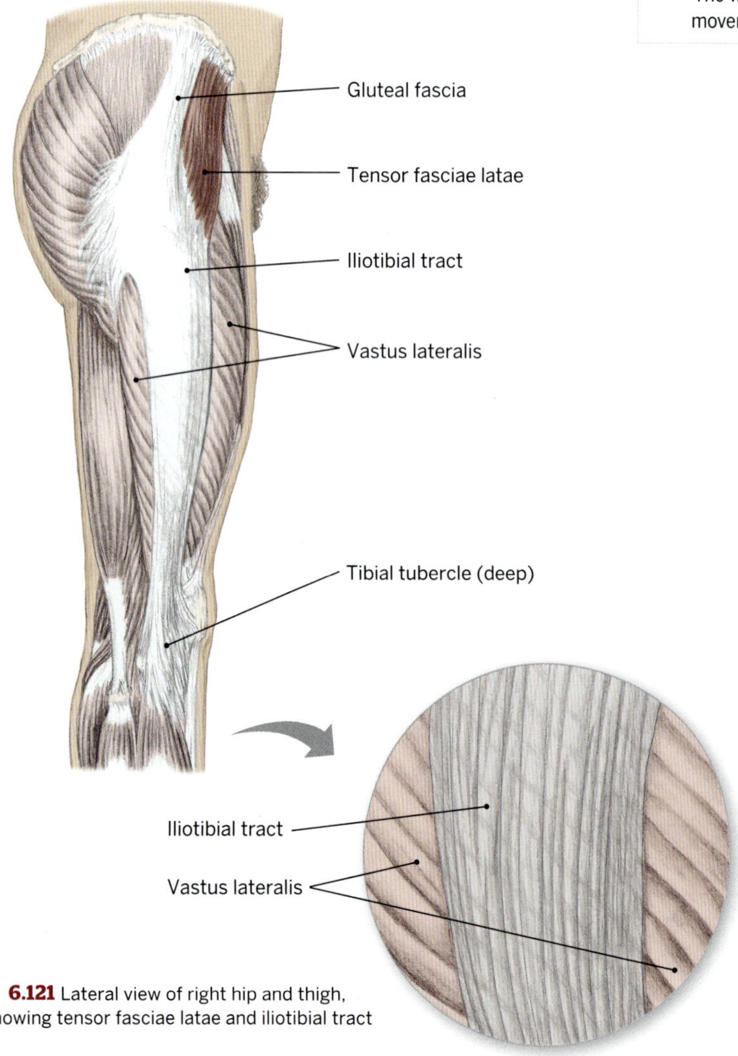

6.121 Lateral view of right hip and thigh, showing tensor fasciae latae and iliotibial tract

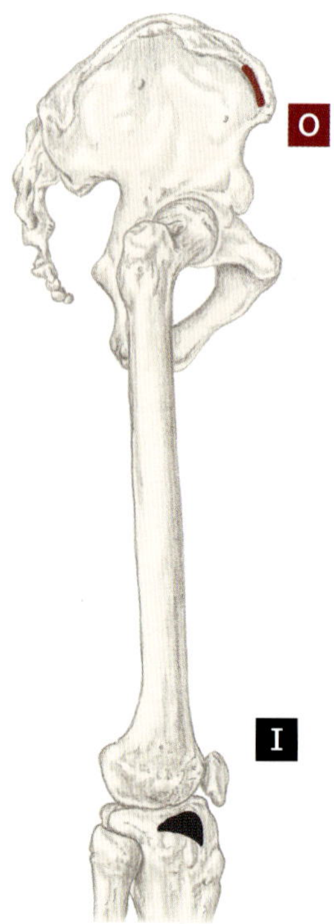

6.122 Lateral view of right hip and femur, showing origin of TFL and insertion of iliotibial tract

latae	*la*-ta	L. broad
tensor	*ten*-sor	L. a stretcher
tract		L. extent, drawn out

Tensor fasciae latae

1. Partner supine. Locate the ASIS. Place the flat of your hand posterior and distal to the ASIS and iliac crest.
2. Ask your partner to alternate medial rotation with relaxation of the hip. Upon medial rotation, the TFL will contract into a solid, oval mound beneath your hand (**6.123**).
3. Palpate its vertical fibers, outline its width, and follow it distally until the TFL blends into the iliotibial tract.

Are you posterior and distal to the anterior iliac crest? If you ask your partner to rotate the hip laterally, does the TFL contract? It should not.

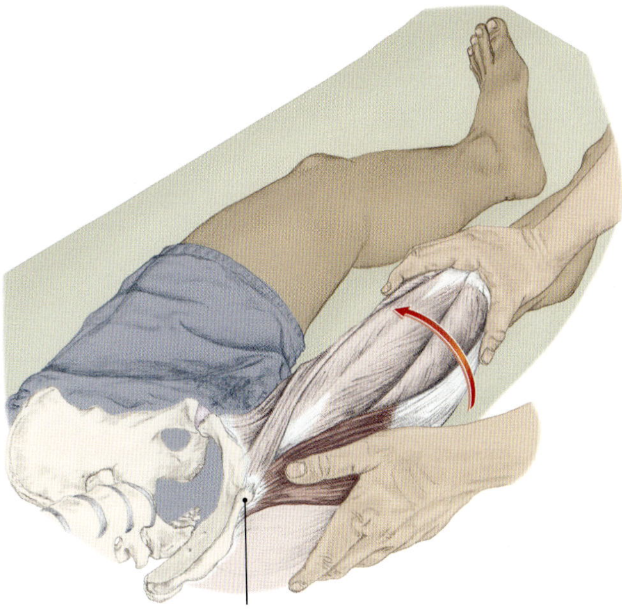

6.123 Partner supine, medially rotating his hip while you feel the TFL contract

Distal end of the iliotibial tract

1. Partner side lying. Locate the biceps femoris tendon (p. 313) just proximal to the back of the knee.
2. Slide anteriorly from the biceps femoris tendon to the lateral thigh. Roll your fingers horizontally across the fibers of the iliotibial tract and explore for its tough, superficial quality. Its most distal aspect may feel similar in size and shape to the biceps femoris tendon.
3. Follow it distally as it disappears toward the tibial tubercle. Explore proximally and note how it becomes broader and thinner as it progresses up the thigh. Feel the tension of the iliotibial tract change by asking your partner to alternately abduct and relax his hip (**6.124**).

Are the fibers you feel superficial and stringy compared to the deeper, fleshier vastus lateralis fibers? Do the fibers run vertically down the thigh and converge into a thin, cable-like tendon at the tibial tubercle?

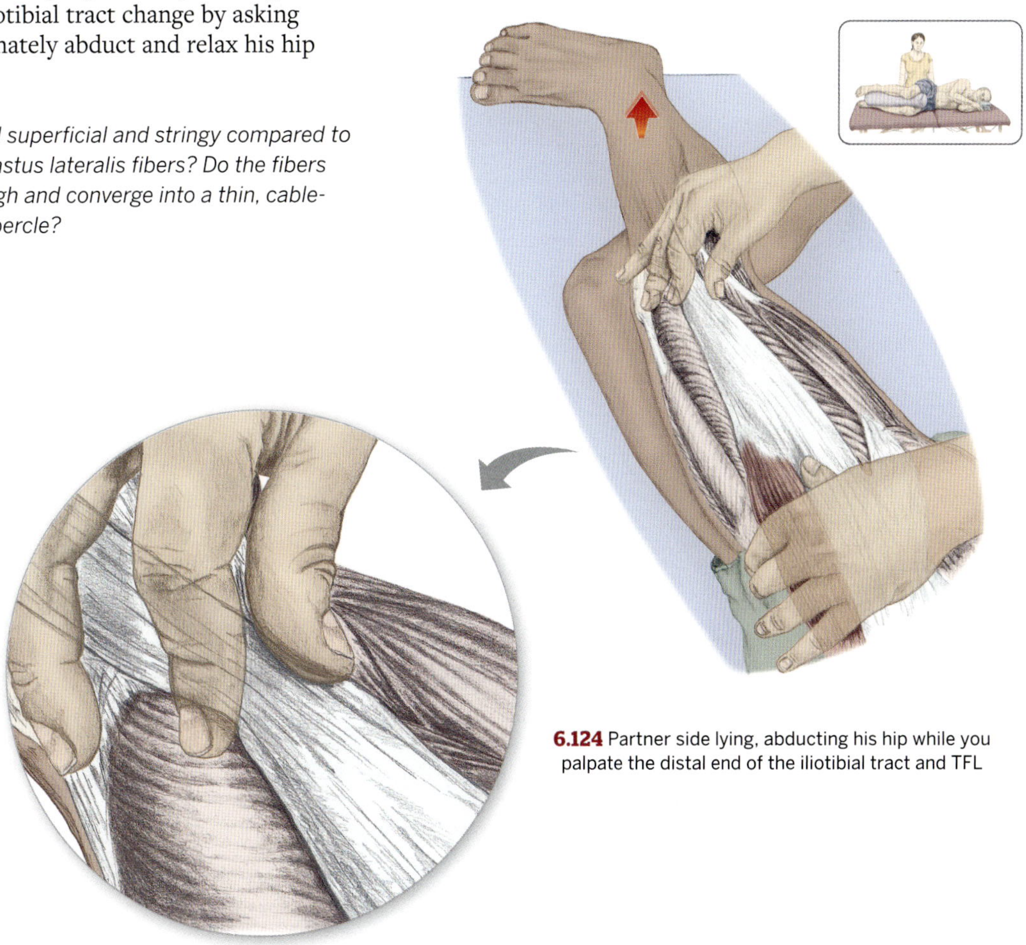

6.124 Partner side lying, abducting his hip while you palpate the distal end of the iliotibial tract and TFL

Sartorius ▶

The sartorius is the longest muscle in the body, stretching from the anterior superior iliac spine (ASIS), across the thigh, to the medial knee (**6.125**, **6.126**). Though it is entirely superficial, the slender belly of the sartorius, roughly two fingers wide, can be difficult to isolate. Its proximal fibers are lateral to the femoral artery (p. 341). Its name (L. *sartor*, tailor) refers to its ability to bring the thigh and leg into the position a tailor would use when sewing (**6.127**).

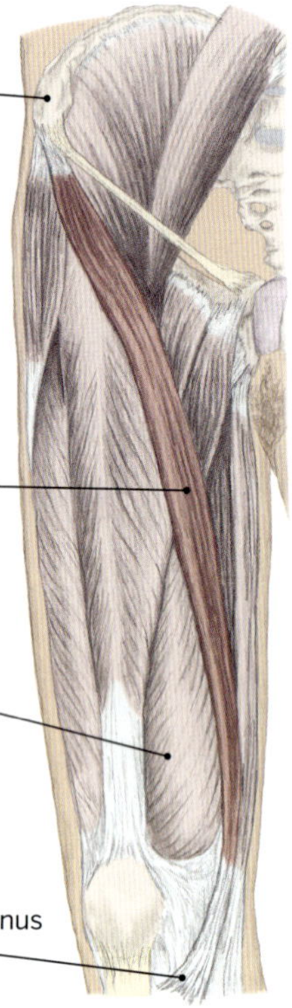

6.125 Anterior/medial view of right hip and thigh, showing sartorius

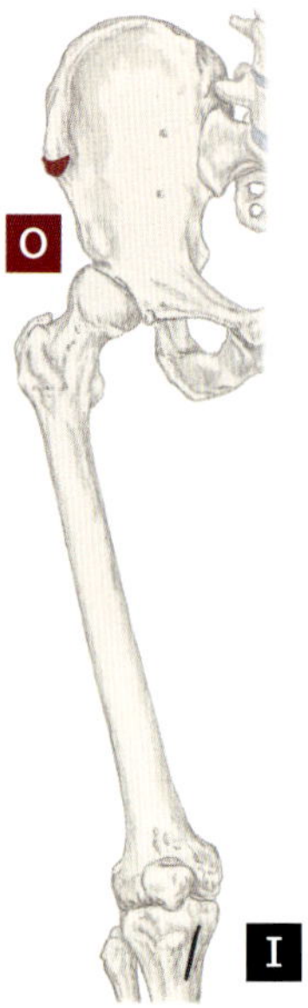

6.126 Anterior view of right hip and thigh, showing origin and insertion of sartorius

SARTORIUS	
A	**Flex** the hip (coxal joint) **Laterally rotate** the hip (coxal joint) **Abduct** the hip (coxal joint) **Flex** the knee (tibiofemoral joint) **Medially rotate** the flexed knee (T/F joint)
O	Anterior superior iliac spine (ASIS)
I	Proximal, medial shaft of the tibia at pes anserinus tendon
N	Femoral L**2**, **3**, (4)

When Do You Use Your Sartorius?

- Folding your hips into a lotus position for meditation
- Sitting in a tailor position (common among men)
- Crossing and uncrossing your legs (common among all genders)

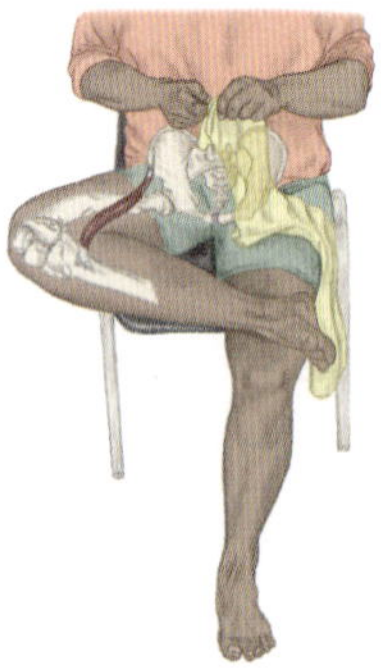

6.127 Anterior view of right thigh and leg in a tailor's position

Sartorius

1. Partner supine. Ask your partner to position his foot so it is resting on his opposite knee. The hip will be flexed and laterally rotated.
2. Place your hand along the middle of the medial thigh. Ask your partner to raise his knee toward the ceiling (contracting the sartorius).
3. Strum your fingers across the slender sartorius, following it proximally to the ASIS and distally to the medial tibia (**6.128**).
4. Maintain your hand placement and ask your partner to relax his hip. Continue to palpate, noticing how the sartorius curves from the ASIS to the medial side of the thigh.

Is the muscle belly you feel roughly two fingers wide and superficial? When distal to the ASIS, can you strum across its tendon? Are you medial to the vastus medialis belly? The sartorius and gracilis are slender, superficial muscles along the medial thigh. Differentiate between them by following their respective bellies proximally: the sartorius will lead toward the ASIS, the gracilis toward the pubic tubercle.

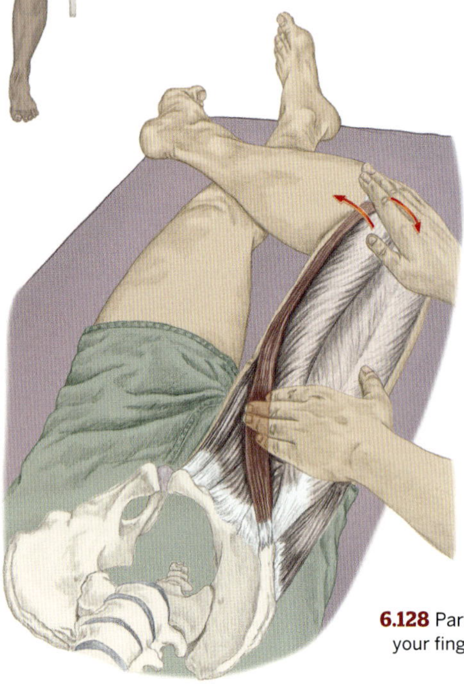

6.128 Partner supine, as you strum your fingers across the sartorius

sartorius sar-***tor***-ee-us L. *sartor*, tailor

Tendons of the Posterior Knee

Five distinct tendons are located on the posterior aspect of the knee (**6.129**). Biceps femoris and the iliotibial tract are located on the lateral/posterior knee; sartorius, gracilis, and semitendinosus are bundled together on the medial/posterior knee. These three tendons merge distally at the proximal, medial shaft of the tibia to become the pes anserinus tendon.

Where is the semimembranosus tendon? Its distal tendon is very short and deep to the semitendinosus and gracilis. The distal aspect of semimembranosus can be accessed by palpating between the tendons of semitendinosus and gracilis.

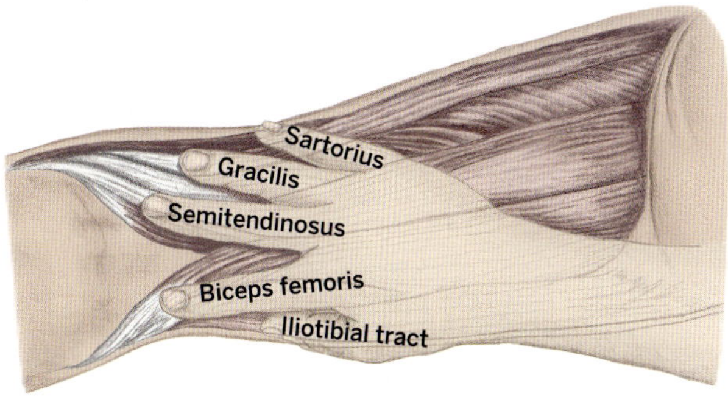

6.129 Posterior view of right thigh with your fingers on the posterior knee, showing location of distal tendons

Lateral tendons

1. Partner side lying. Ask your partner to flex and hold his knee at 45°. The tendons will become taut in this position. For greater clarity, place your hand on the ankle and give your partner some resistance.
2. The most prominent tendons will be biceps femoris and semitendinosus. Follow the slender biceps femoris tendon as it extends down to the head of the fibula (**6.130**).
3. Move laterally approximately one inch from the biceps tendon and palpate the iliotibial tract. Unlike the biceps femoris, the iliotibial tract is broad and located on the lateral side of the thigh.

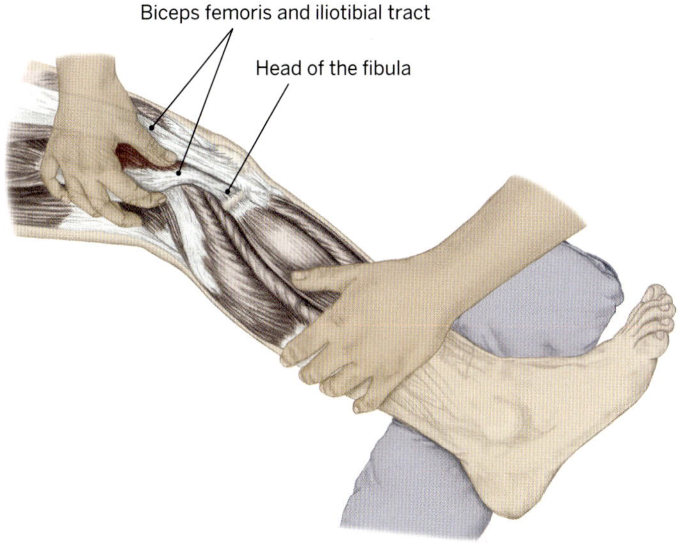

6.130 Partner side lying, lateral view of right knee, as you isolate the biceps femoris and iliotibial tract

Medial tendons

1. Partner supine. Move to the medial side of the knee and palpate the thin, prominent tendon of the semitendinosus.
2. Slide off semitendinosus anteriorly and palpate the equally slender tendon of gracilis.
3. Situated anterior to gracilis will be sartorius. Compared to the long, skinny tendons of semitendinosus and gracilis, the sartorius tendon is wider (**6.131**). For this reason, it may be challenging to isolate.
4. Follow the three tendons distally as they blend together to become the pes anserinus tendon, which attaches on the proximal, medial shaft of the tibia.

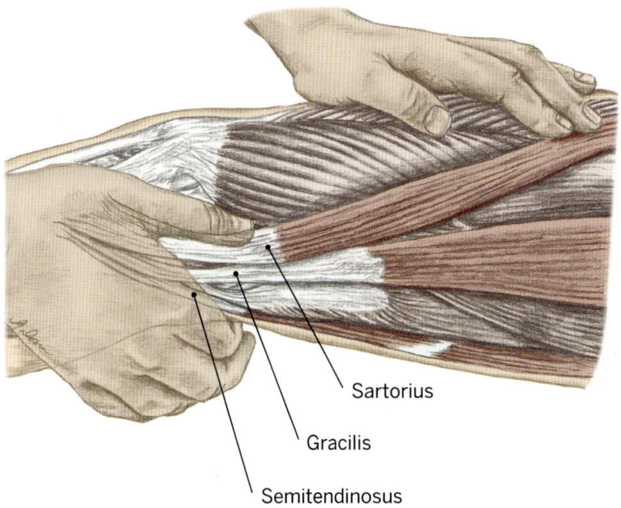

6.131 Partner supine, medial view of right knee, as you isolate the medial tendons

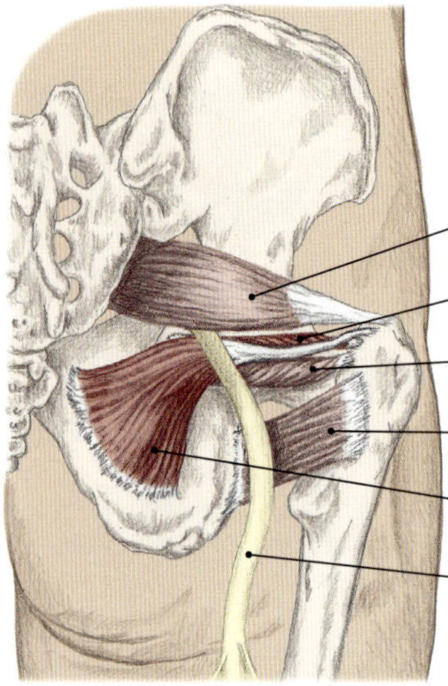

6.132 Posterior view of right hip with gluteals removed, showing lateral rotators

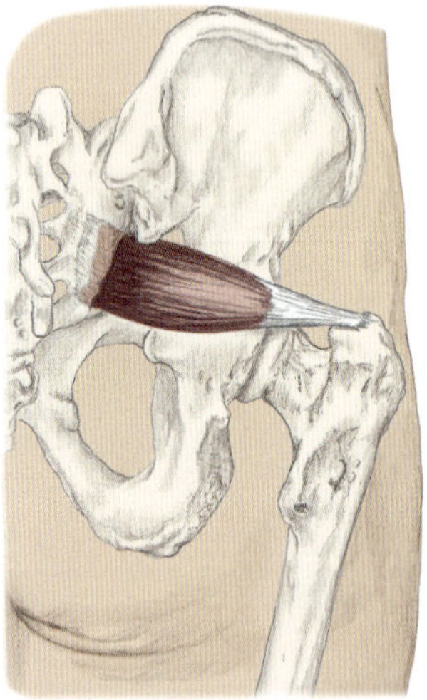

6.133 Posterior view of right hip, showing piriformis

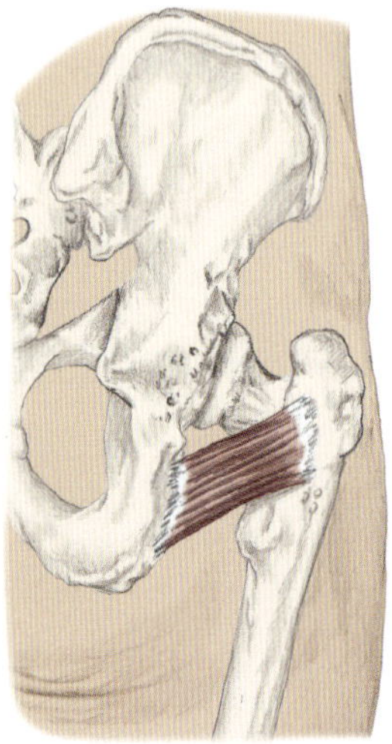

6.134 Posterior view of right hip, showing quadratus femoris

Lateral Rotators of the Hip ▶

Piriformis and Quadratus Femoris
Obturator Internus and Obturator Externus
Gemellus Superior and Gemellus Inferior

Sometimes known as the "deep six," these small muscles are located deep to the gluteus maximus and create lateral rotation of the hip. All attach to aspects of the greater trochanter and fan medially to attach to the sacrum and pelvis (**6.132–6.140**).

All of the lateral rotators are deep to the large sciatic nerve (p. 343) except for the piriformis. The piriformis lies superficial to the sciatic nerve and, if overcontracted, can compress it. Nevertheless, the lateral rotators are accessible as a group, with the piriformis and quadratus femoris being the most discernible.

PIRIFORMIS	
A	**Laterally rotate** the hip (coxal joint) **Abduct** the hip when the hip is flexed
O	Anterior surface of sacrum
I	Superior aspect of greater trochanter
N	Sacral plexus L(5), S**1**, **2**

QUADRATUS FEMORIS	
A	**Laterally rotate** the hip (coxal joint)
O	Lateral border of ischial tuberosity
I	Intertrochanteric crest, between the greater and lesser trochanters
N	Sacral plexus L**4**, **5**, S**1**, (2)

OBTURATOR INTERNUS	
A	**Laterally rotate** the hip (coxal joint)
O	Obturator membrane and inferior surface of obturator foramen
I	Medial surface of greater trochanter
N	Sacral plexus L**5**, S**1**, **2**

Discover More

The obturator membrane, one of the origins of the obturator internus, is a fibrous wall of connective tissue that forms a partial covering of the obturator foramen.

gemellus	jem-*el*-us	L. twin
obturator	*ob*-tu-*ra*-tor	L. obstructor

OBTURATOR EXTERNUS

A	**Laterally rotate** the hip (coxal joint)
O	Rami of pubis and ischium, obturator membrane
I	Trochanteric fossa of femur
N	Obturator L**3**, **4**

GEMELLUS SUPERIOR

A	**Laterally rotate** the hip (coxal joint)
O	Ischial spine
I	Medial surface of greater trochanter
N	Sacral plexus L**5**, S**1**, **2**

GEMELLUS INFERIOR

A	**Laterally rotate** the hip (coxal joint)
O	Ischial tuberosity
I	Medial surface of greater trochanter
N	Sacral plexus L**4**, **5**, S**1**, (2)

When Do You Use Your Lateral Rotators?

- Stabilizing the pelvis while standing
- Walking, running, hiking, climbing, biking
- Piriformis: Controlling rapid medial rotation of the hip during the early phase of walking and running

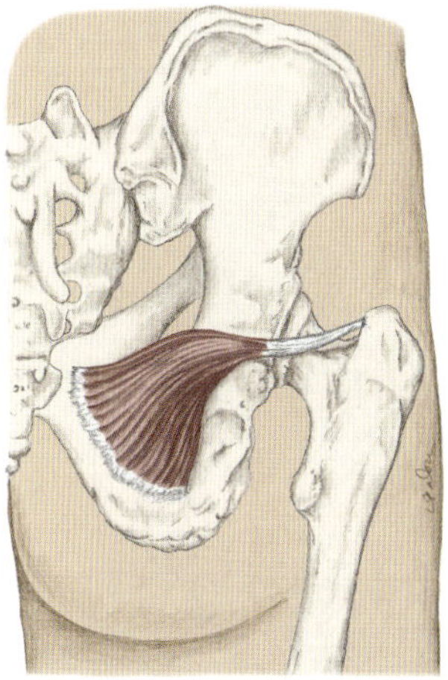

6.135 Posterior view of right hip, showing obturator internus

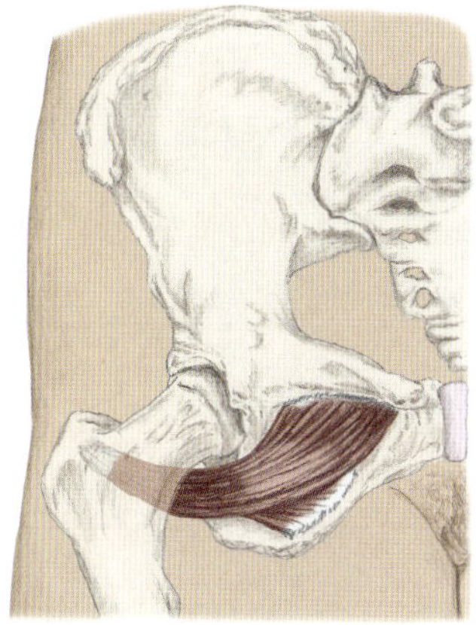

6.136 Anterior view of right hip, showing obturator externus

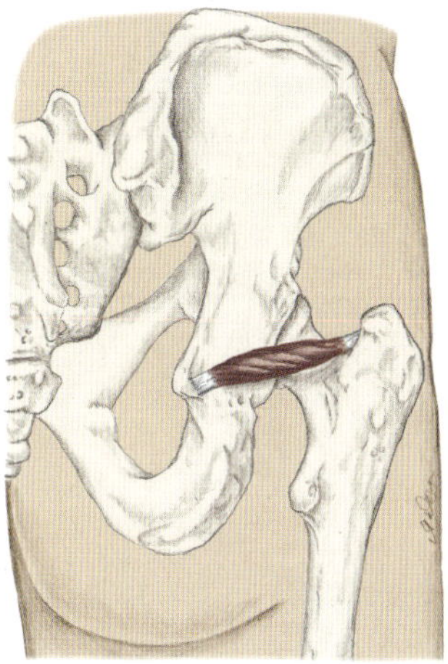

6.137 Posterior view of right hip, showing gemellus superior

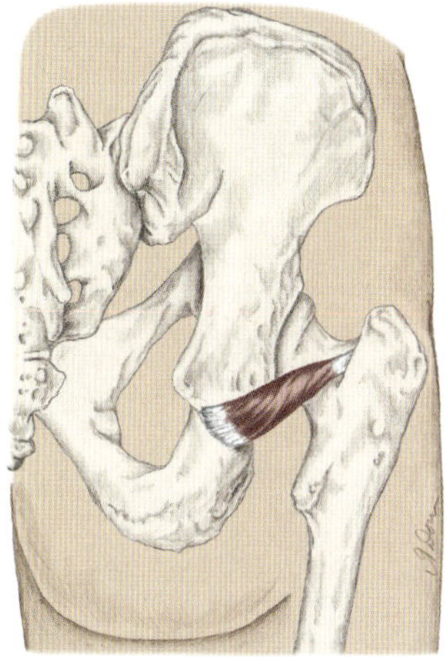

6.138 Posterior view of right hip, showing gemellus inferior

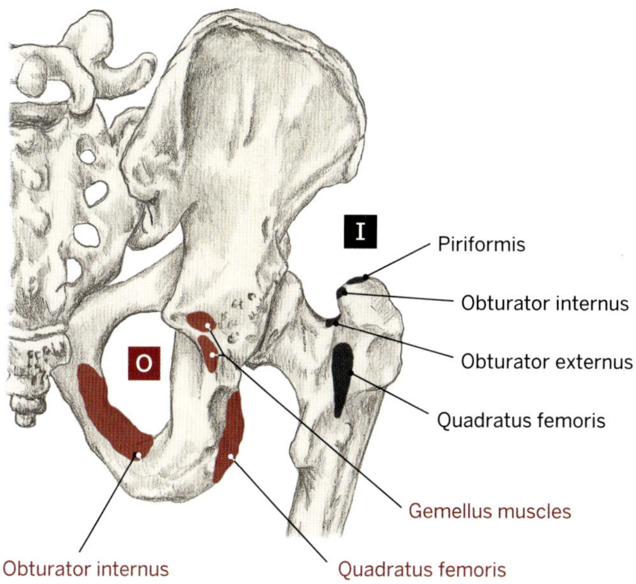

6.139 Posterior view of right hip, showing origins and insertions of lateral rotators

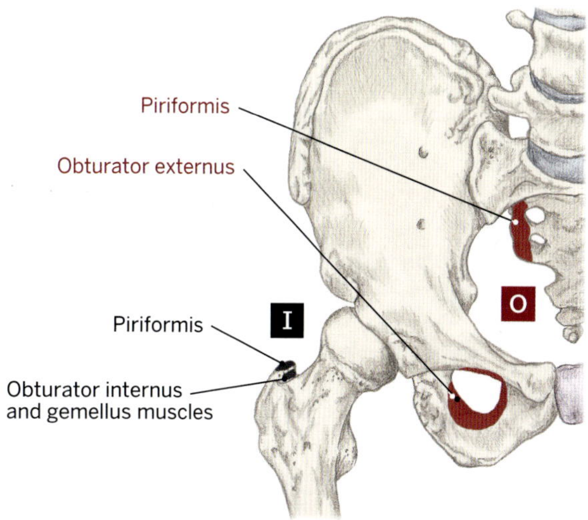

6.140 Anterior view of right hip, showing origins and insertions of lateral rotators

Piriformis

1. Partner prone. Locate the coccyx, PSIS, and greater trochanter. Together, these landmarks form a T. The piriformis is located along the base of the T (**6.141**).
2. Place your fingers along this line. Working through the thick gluteus maximus, roll your fingers across the belly of the slender piriformis.
3. Strum across the belly to clarify its location, staying mindful of the deeper sciatic nerve (**6.142**).

*Are you compressing through the thick gluteus maximus fibers? With your fingers on the piriformis, bend the knee to 90° and ask your partner to rotate his hip laterally against your gentle resistance (**6.143**). You may feel gluteus maximus contract, but can you feel piriformis contract beneath it?*

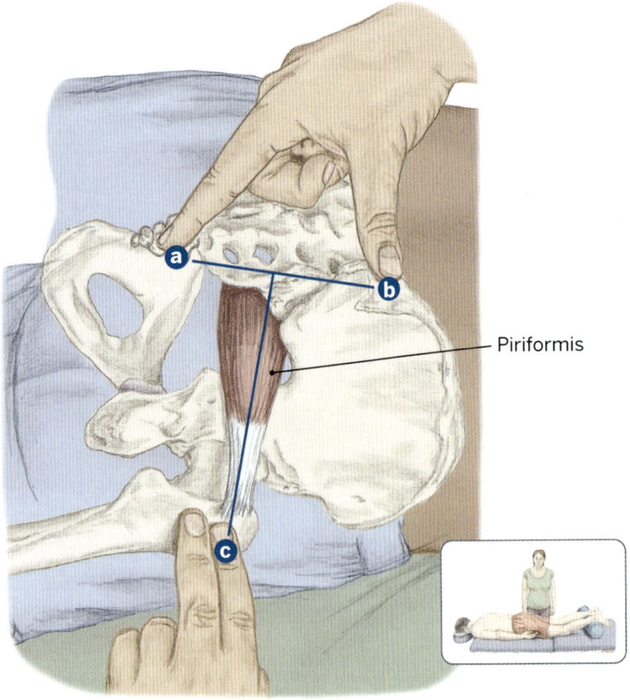

6.141 Partner prone, posterior/lateral view, as you isolate the piriformis by forming a T: (**a**) coccyx, (**b**) PSIS, (**c**) greater trochanter

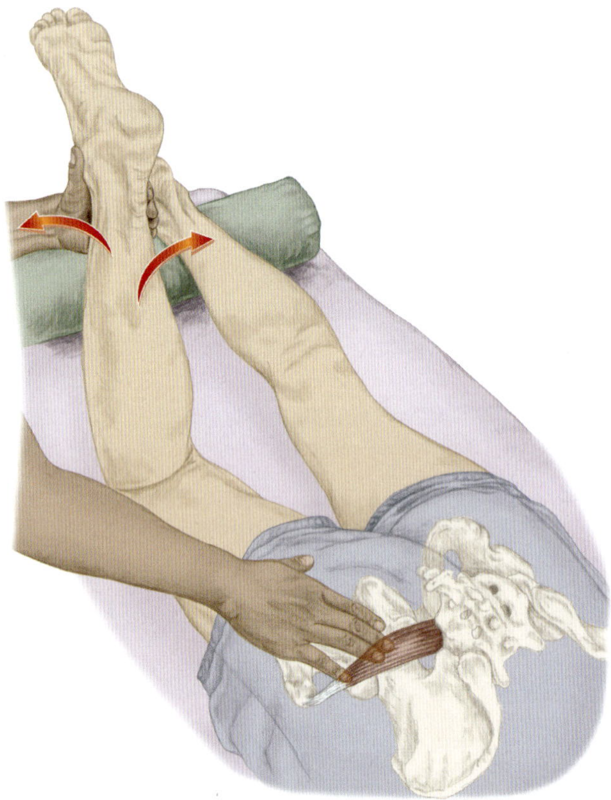

6.143 Partner prone, laterally rotating his hip against your resistance while you feel the piriformis contract

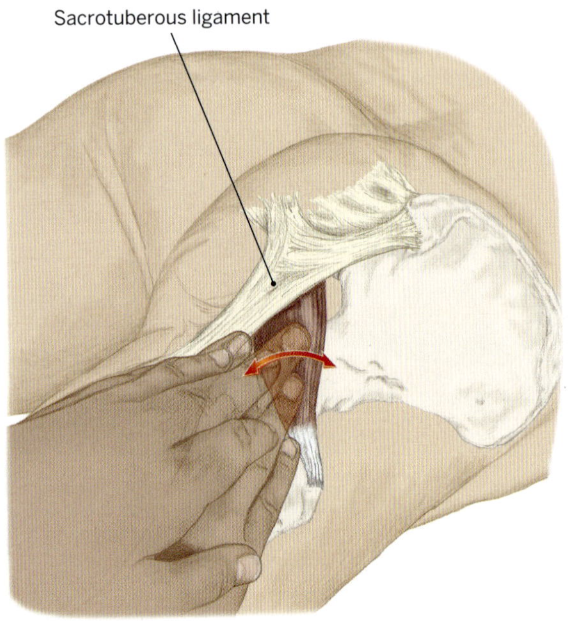

6.142 Partner prone, posterior/lateral view, as you roll your fingers over piriformis

piriformis	*pir*-i-*form*-is	L. pear-shaped
quadratus	kwod-*rait*-us	L. squared, four-sided

Quadratus femoris

1. Partner prone. Locate the distal, posterior aspect of the greater trochanter and the ischial tuberosity. Place your fingerpads between these two landmarks.
2. Pressing firmly through the gluteus maximus fibers, strum vertically across the fibers of the rectangle-shaped quadratus femoris.

*Does the belly stretch between the ischial tuberosity and the distal trochanter? Rolling your fingers over the belly, can you feel its horizontal fibers (**6.144**)? Flex the knee to 90° and passively rotate the hip medially and laterally. Can you sense changes in the muscle's tension as it shortens and lengthens?*

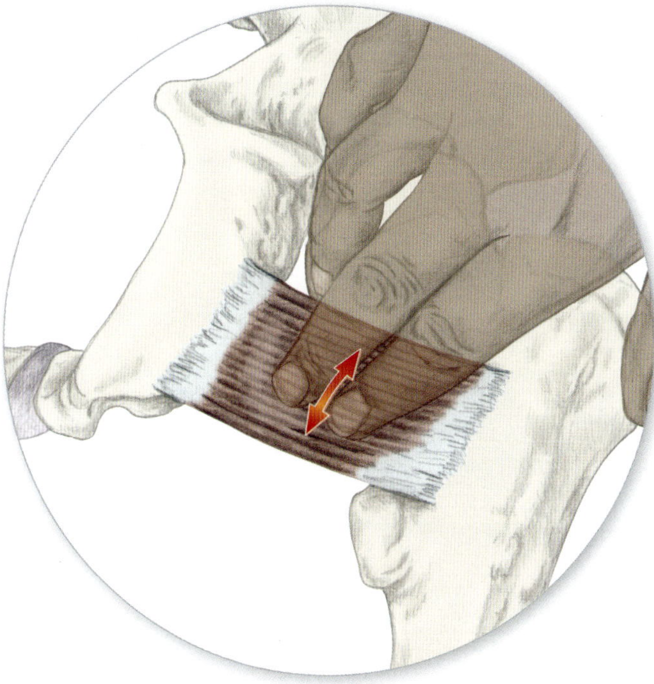

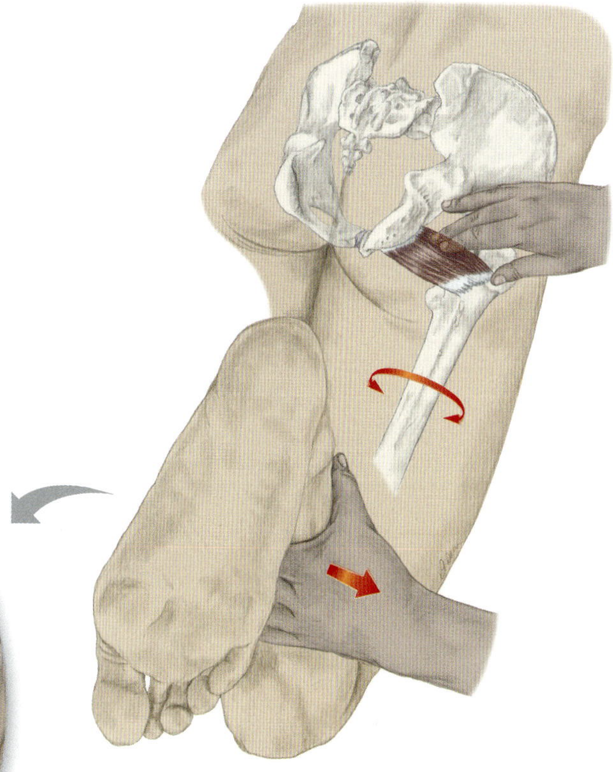

6.144 Partner prone, laterally rotating his hip against your resistance while you sense the quadratus femoris contract

Comparative Anatomy

Compared to its evolutionary precursors, the piriformis is a remnant of its former glory. It is a descendant of the great caudofemoral elevator muscles that can still be seen today extending from a reptile's femur to its tail. These large muscles provide reptiles with the tremendous thrusting force needed to extend the femur while running.

Pelvis & Thigh

Iliopsoas ▶

Psoas Major and Iliacus

The iliacus and psoas major, together called the iliopsoas, are important hip flexors and low back stabilizers (**6.145**). Best known to your local butcher as "tenderloin" or "filet mignon," the long, slender **psoas major** is located deep to the abdominal contents (**6.146**). It stretches from the lumbar vertebrae, underneath the inguinal ligament, to the lesser trochanter.

The stockier **iliacus** is located deep to the abdomen in the iliac fossa (**6.147**). Because of their respective locations, these muscles are only partially accessible and may be challenging to palpate (**6.148**, **6.149**).

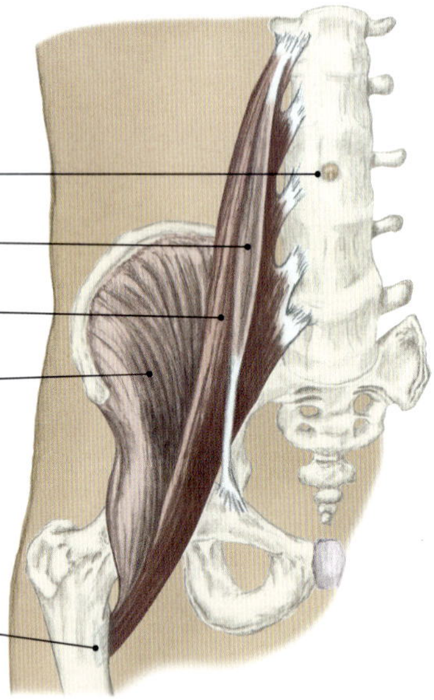

6.145 Anterior view of spine and right hip, showing iliopsoas

PSOAS MAJOR

A *With the origin fixed:*
Flex the hip (coxal joint)
May **laterally rotate** the hip (coxal joint)
With the insertion fixed:
Flex the trunk toward the thigh
Tilt pelvis anteriorly
Unilaterally:
Assist to **laterally flex** the lumbar spine

O Bodies and transverse processes of lumbar vertebrae

I Lesser trochanter

N Lumbar plexus L1, **2**, **3**, 4

When Do You Use Your Psoas Major?

- Hiking, climbing, or walking up an incline
- Getting up from a reclined position (the movement of a small sit-up)

ILIACUS

A *With the origin fixed:*
Flex the hip (coxal joint)
May **laterally rotate** the hip (coxal joint)
With the insertion fixed:
Flex the trunk toward the thigh
Tilt pelvis anteriorly

O Iliac fossa

I Lesser trochanter

N Femoral L(1), **2**, **3**, 4

When Do You Use Your Iliacus?

- Reaching up, against gravity, to untie the ropes around your ankles that suspend you upside down from a tree limb (It could happen!)

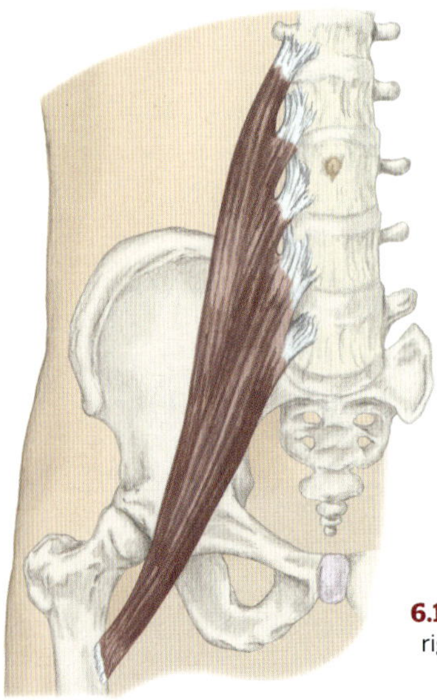

6.146 Anterior view of spine and right hip, showing psoas major

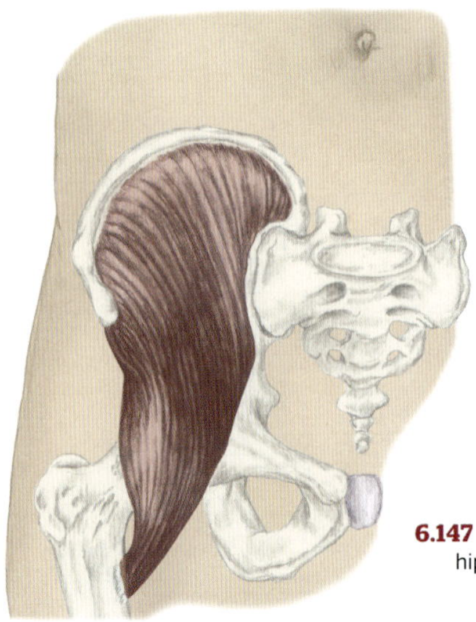

6.147 Anterior view of right hip, showing iliacus

iliacus	i-*lee*-a-cus	L. pertaining to the loin
psoas	*so*-as	Grk. muscle of the loin

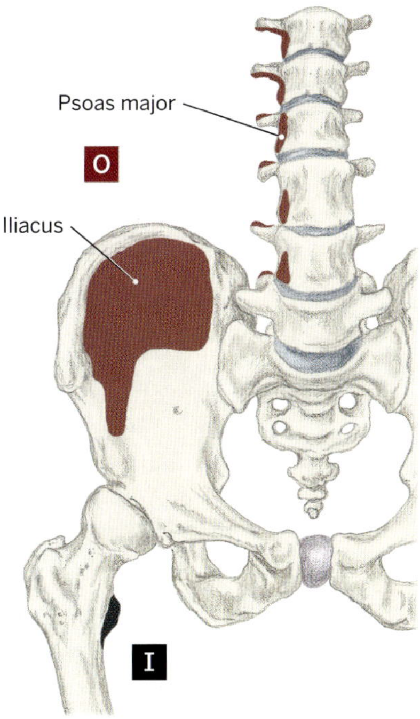

6.148 Anterior view of spine and right hip, showing origins and insertions of psoas major and iliacus

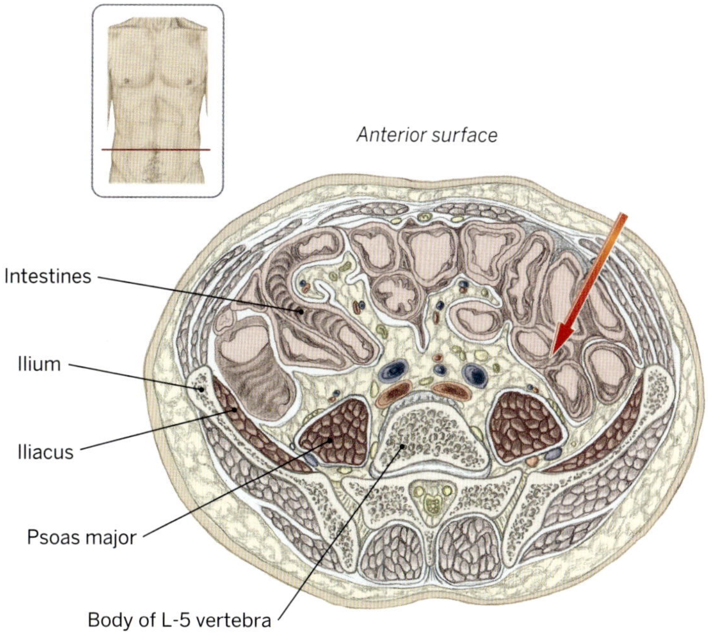

6.149 Cross section of the trunk at the level of L-5, arrow showing direction of fingers when accessing the psoas major

Discover More

Psoas Minor

Roughly 40% of the population has a psoas minor. It is a small muscle that extends from the lumbar vertebrae to the superior ramus of the pubis. When present, the psoas minor assists in posterior tilt (upward rotation) of the pelvis—the opposite action of the psoas major (see box, p. 336). Interestingly, the psoas minor is an important muscle of locomotion on a dog or cat because of the relationship of the pelvis to the vertebrae in quadrupeds. In a human biped, however, the psoas minor is a relatively insignificant muscle.

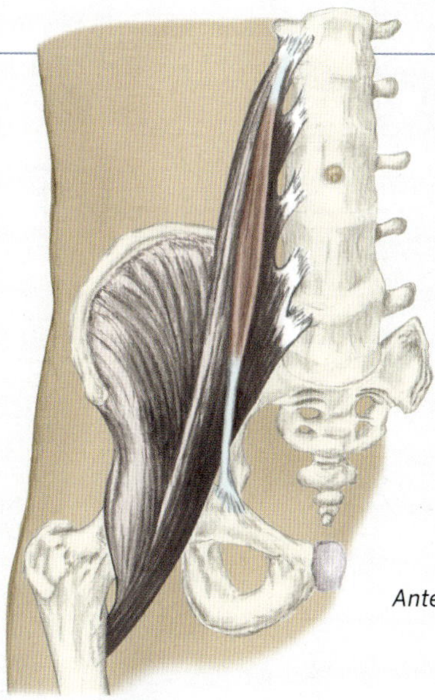

Anterior view of right hip

A	Assist to **create** lordotic curvature in the lumbar spine **Tilt** pelvis posteriorly
O	Body and transverse process of first lumbar vertebra
I	Superior ramus of pubis
N	Lumbar plexus L**1**, **2**

Pelvis & Thigh

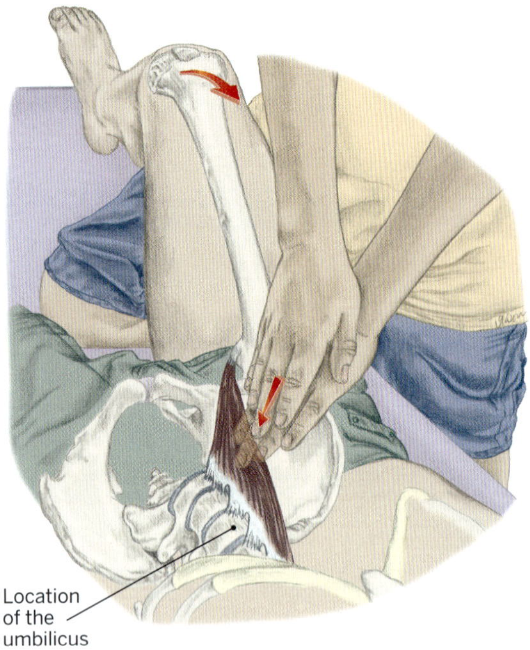

6.150 Partner supine, flexing his hip while you access the psoas major

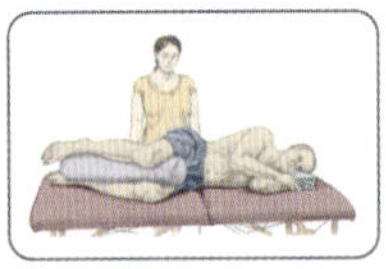

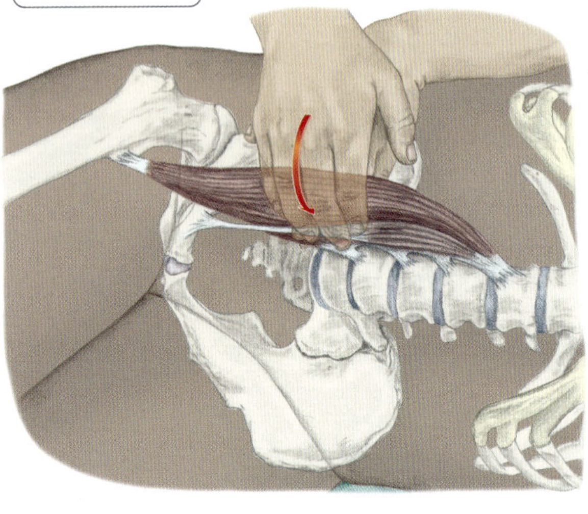

6.151 Partner side lying with hips flexed, as you curl your fingers into the abdomen

Psoas major

When accessing either the psoas or iliacus, palpate slowly and communicate with your partner. If at any point he does not feel comfortable or safe, slowly remove your hands. The psoas major lies just lateral to the abdominal aorta (p. 219). If you feel a strong pulse directly beneath your fingers when accessing the muscle, realign them more laterally.

1. Partner supine, with the hip slightly flexed and laterally rotated. Support your partner's thigh by placing your thigh underneath it. Locate the navel and ASIS, placing your fingerpads hand-on-hand between these points.
2. Slowly compress your fingerpads into the abdomen, moving only when your partner exhales. (Compressing in small circles upon your partner's initial exhalations will assist in moving the abdominal contents to the side.) As you compress further, keep your fingerpads stationary and direct your fingers downward toward the table.
3. Check that you are palpating the psoas, not the surrounding tissues, by asking your partner to flex his hip ever so slightly. If your fingers are accessing the psoas, you will feel a definite, solid contraction (**6.150**).

Are you between the ASIS and navel? Is the direction of your fingers at a slight angle toward the spine? Have you compressed slowly, allowing the overlying tissue to relax? If you did not feel the muscle contract, try again with the fingers repositioned farther inferiorly.

Side lying position allows the abdominal contents to shift away from the psoas and, oftentimes, offers a less invasive position for your partner.

1. With the hips in a flexed position, place a bolster between your partner's knees. Locate the navel and ASIS, placing your fingerpads hand-on-hand between these points (**6.151**).
2. Following your partner's breath, curl your fingers into the abdomen and onto the surface of the psoas. Ask your partner to flex his hip slightly so you can feel for the psoas's contraction.

Discover More

Psoas major primarily flexes the hip. But when the femur is stabilized, the psoas, in conjunction with iliacus, can increase the lordotic curvature in the lumbar spine and create anterior tilt (downward rotation) of the pelvis. It has also been theorized that only the superficial fibers of the psoas increase the lordotic curve, whereas the deeper fibers may decrease it.

Pelvis & Thigh

Iliacus

1. Partner supine, with the hip slightly flexed and laterally rotated. Support your partner's thigh by placing your thigh underneath it.
2. Locate the anterior portion of the iliac crest and place your fingerpads hand-on-hand an inch medial to its ridge. (Beginning medially will allow you to penetrate more easily through the abdominal muscles.)
3. Slowly curl your fingers into the iliac fossa, moving only when your partner exhales (**6.152**). Your fingers might sink only a short distance into the tissue. Here's a hint: The intention of your touch needs to go beyond the superficial abdominal muscles and be directed toward the anterior surface of the ilium.
4. Ask your partner to flex his hip slightly, with your fingers in place. You will feel the strong iliacus contract.

Are you in the iliac fossa? Have you compressed slowly, allowing the overlying tissue to relax?

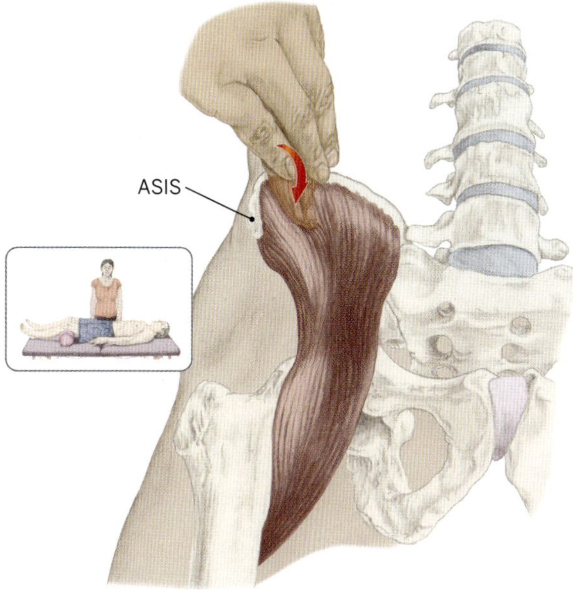

6.152 Partner supine, anterior/inferior view, as you curl your fingers around the iliac crest to access the iliacus

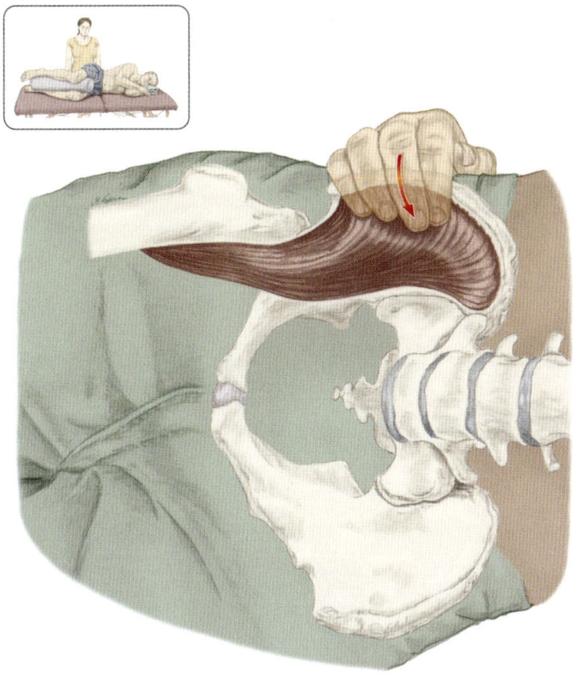

6.153 Partner side lying with hips flexed, as you curl your fingers into the abdomen to access the iliacus

As with the psoas, side lying position allows the abdominal contents to fall away from the iliacus and can be a more comfortable position for your partner. With the hips in a flexed position, place a bolster between your partner's knees and follow the instructions above (**6.153**).

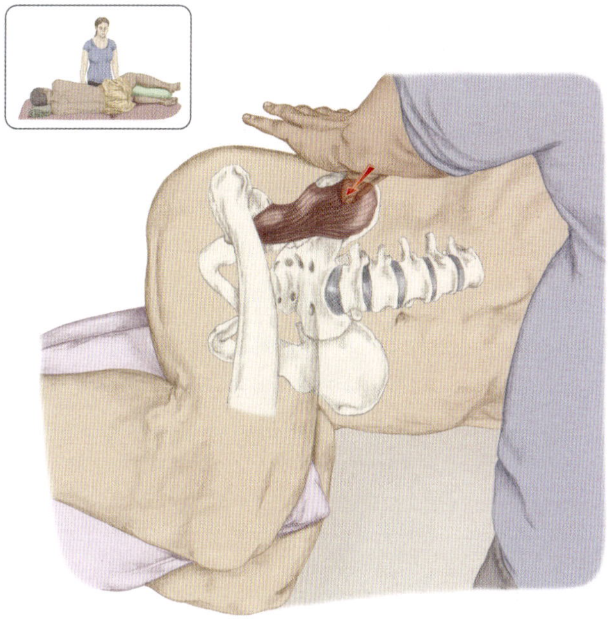

6.154 Partner side lying, as you palpate the iliacus

Following the above procedure, access the iliacus from the opposite side of the table. Try curling into the iliac fossa with your thumbs (**6.154**).

Ligaments and Other Structures of the Pelvis and Thigh

The femoral triangle is located on the anterior, medial surface of the thigh (**6.155**). It is formed by the inguinal ligament, adductor longus, and sartorius. Several important vessels, including the femoral artery, nerve, and vein, pass superficially through the femoral triangle (**6.156**).

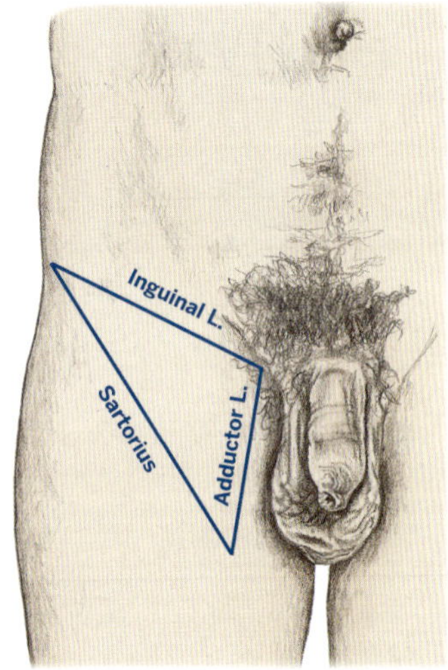

6.155 Anterior view of right hip, showing the three borders of the femoral triangle

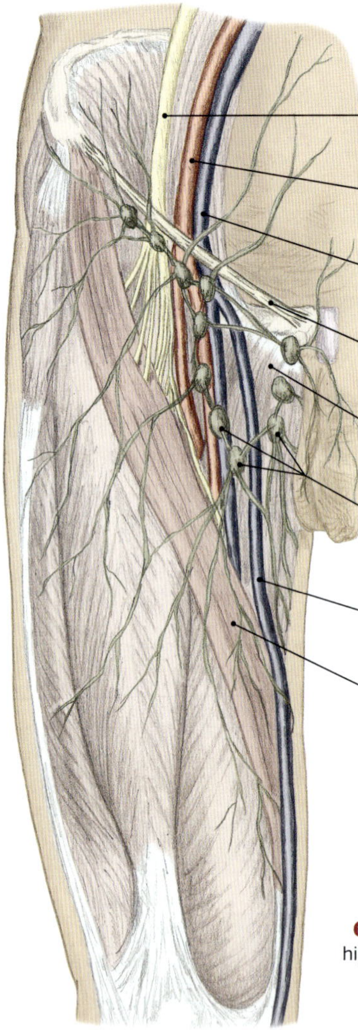

6.156 Anterior view of right hip and thigh, showing vessels and structures

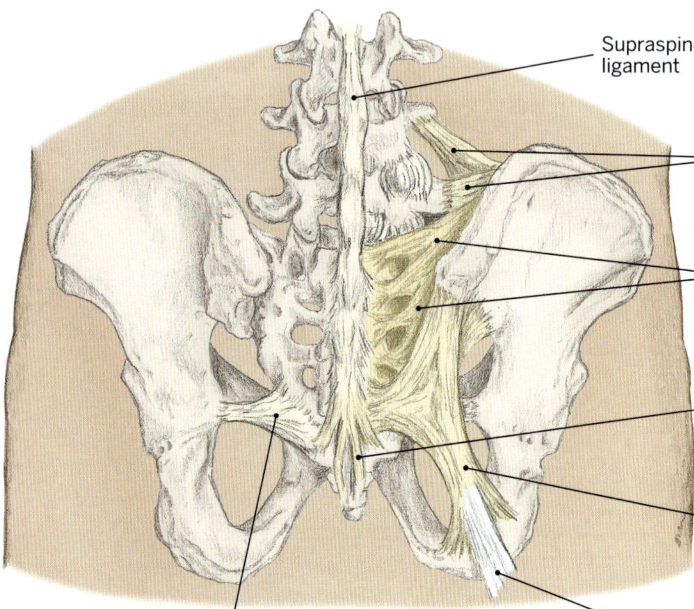

6.157 Posterior view of pelvis, showing ligaments

Discover More

The great saphenous vein is a superficial vessel traveling the length of the lower extremity. Often visible, it begins near the ankle, passes along the medial aspect of the tibia and follows the sartorius up the thigh to empty into the femoral vein at the femoral triangle. Since it is long and easily accessible, the saphenous vein is often used for grafts in coronary bypass surgery.

sacrococcygeal *sa*-kro-kok-*sij*-e-al
saphenous *sa*-fe-nus origin unclear, perhaps Arabic *saphin*, standing; or Greek *saphen*, clearly visible

Pelvis & Thigh

Ligaments of the Pelvis

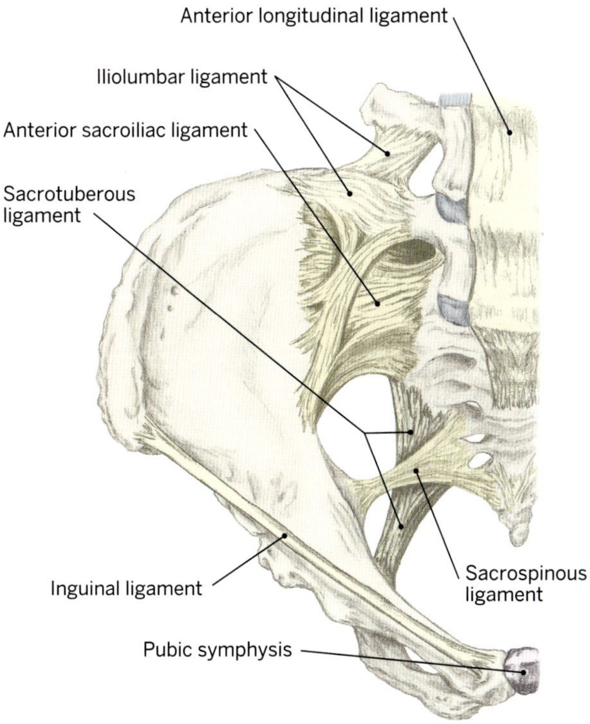

6.158 Anterior view of right hip and pelvis, showing ligaments

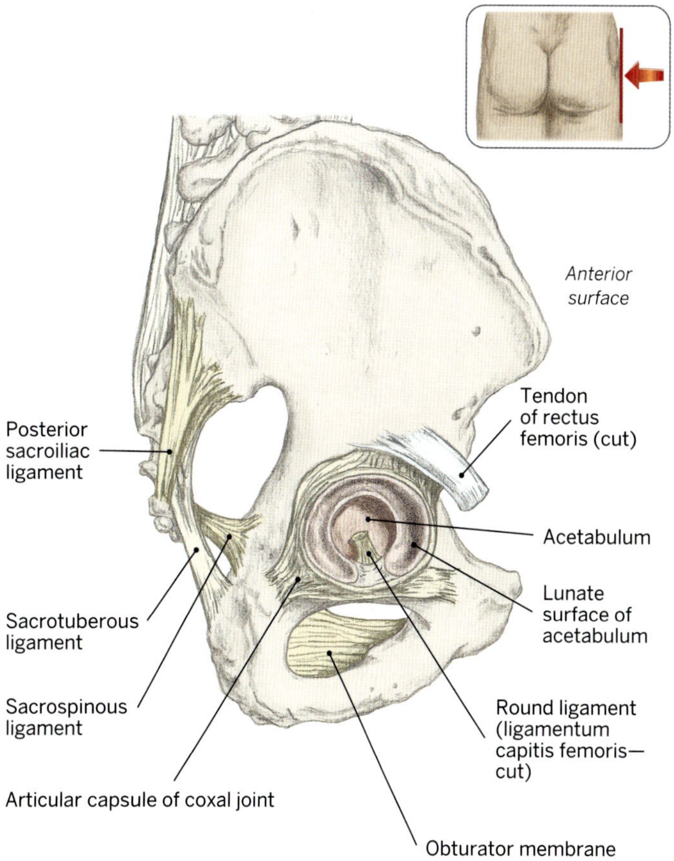

6.159 Lateral view of right hip and pelvis, showing ligaments

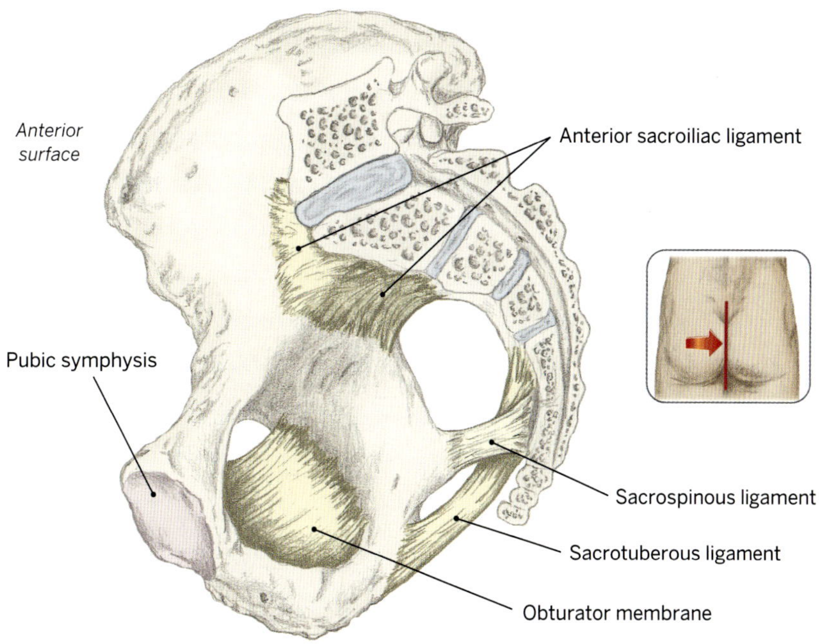

6.160 Cross section of pelvis, medial view from midline, showing ligaments

sacrotuberous ***sa***-kro-***tu***-ber-us

Ligaments of the Coxal Joint

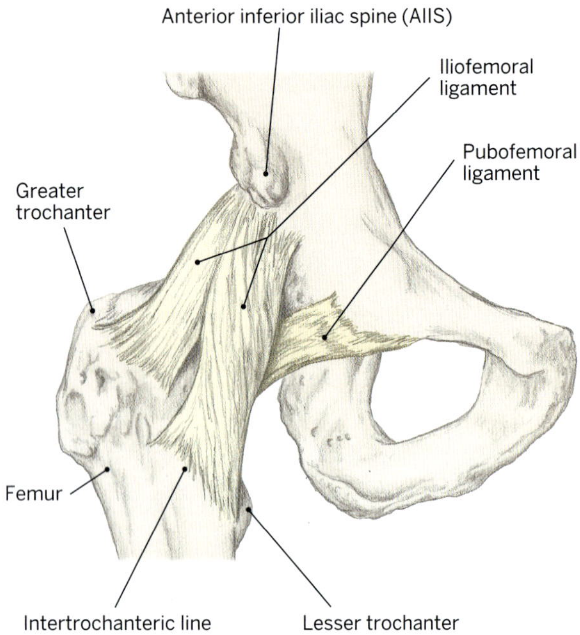

6.161 Anterior view of right coxal joint, showing ligaments

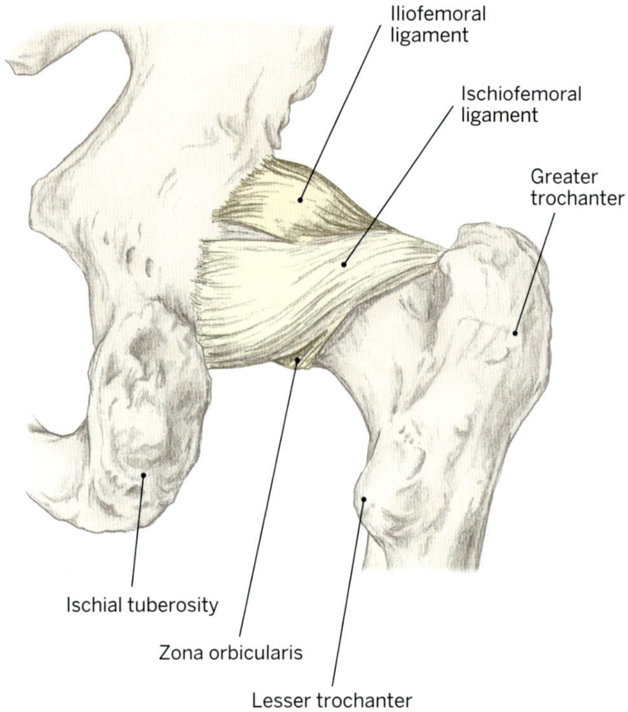

6.162 Posterior view of right coxal joint, showing ligaments

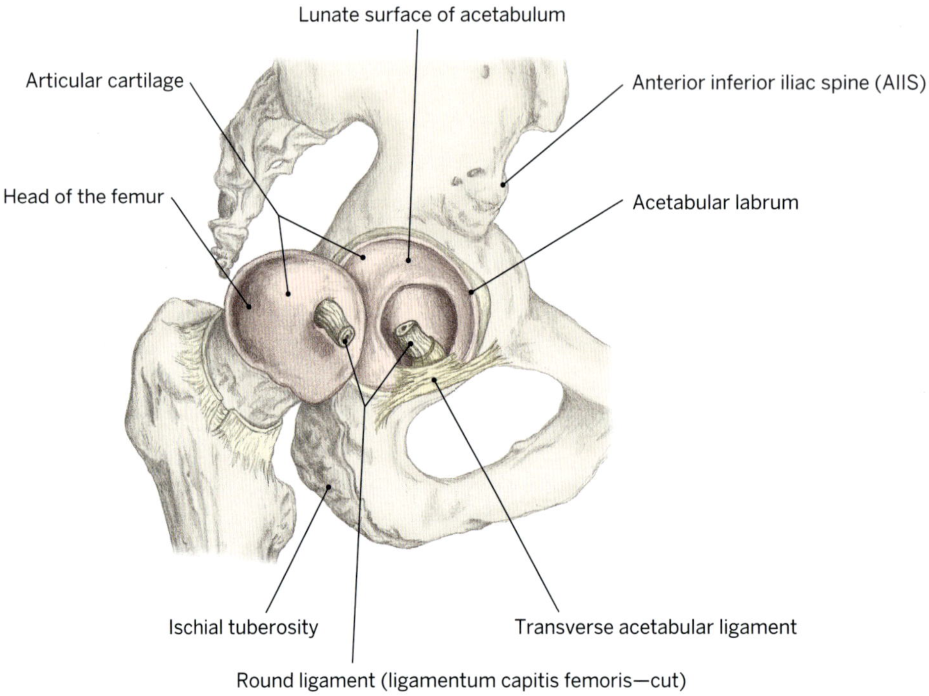

6.163 Lateral view of right coxal joint, femur reflected, showing ligaments

zona orbicularis	***zo***-na or-***bik***-u-***lar***-is	L. girdle + little circle

Inguinal Ligament

The inguinal ligament is a superficial band stretching between the ASIS and the pubic tubercle. It forms the superior border of the femoral triangle and the lower edge of the rectus sheath. It is an attachment site for the lower portion of the external oblique muscle.

Inguinal ligament

1. Partner supine. Soften the surrounding tissue of the ligament by bolstering your partner's knee.
2. Locate the ASIS and slide diagonally in the direction of the pubic tubercle (**6.164**).
3. Strum gently across the slender ligament, feeling its cord-like quality.

Can you feel a thin, superficial band just beneath the skin? Does the band stretch from the ASIS and extend to the pubic tubercle?

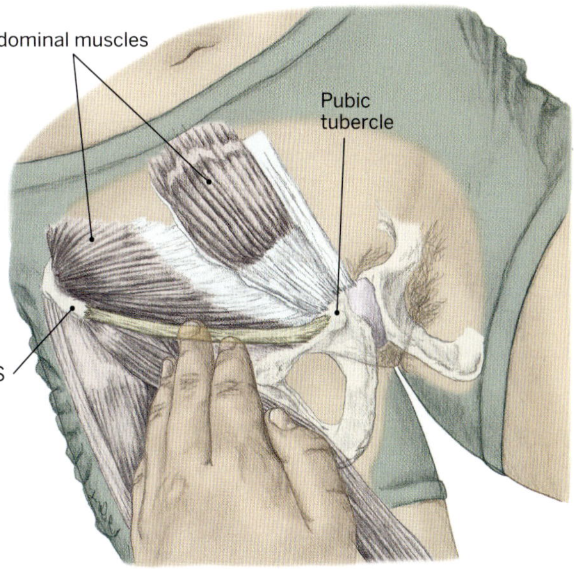

6.164 Partner supine, as you locate the inguinal ligament

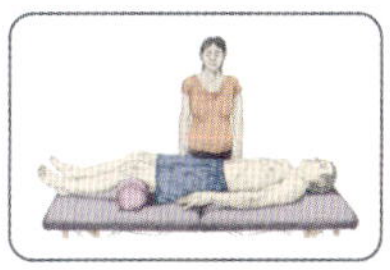

Femoral Artery, Nerve, and Vein

The femoral artery, nerve, and vein form a neurovascular bundle that courses through the femoral triangle. These vessels lie beneath the inguinal ligament and extend distally into the tissue of the thigh. The bundle is relatively superficial; the pulse of the femoral artery can be easily felt.

Pulse of the femoral artery

1. Partner supine. Slide your flexed knee behind your partner's knee. This position will flex and laterally rotate the hip, allowing for easier palpation.
2. Place the flat of your fingerpads halfway between the ASIS and the pubic tubercle just distal to the inguinal ligament. Feel for the strong pulse of the femoral artery (**6.165**).

Are you distal to the inguinal ligament? Are you between the ASIS and the pubic tubercle?

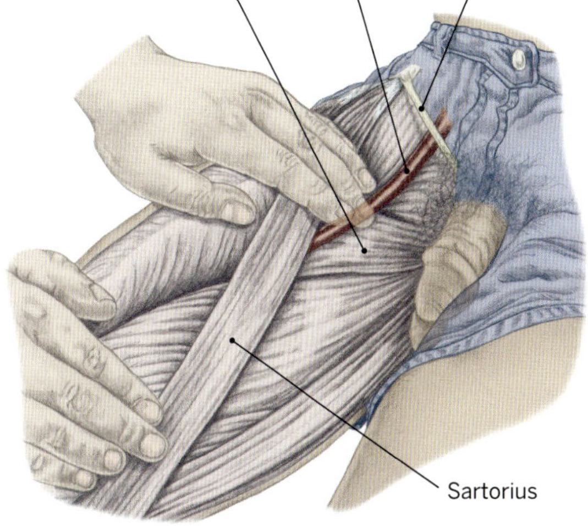

6.165 Partner supine, as you locate the femoral artery

Discover More

The penis contains no muscle tissue. During sexual arousal, the arteries of the penis dilate and a small muscle (ischiocavernosus) at the base of the penis helps to maintain an erection. The testicles are enwrapped by the cremaster muscle. It protects the sperm inside by lowering the testes when they become too warm and pulling them up closer to the body when they become too cold.

inguinal	*ing*-gwi-nal	L. of the groin
penis		L. tail

Pelvis & Thigh

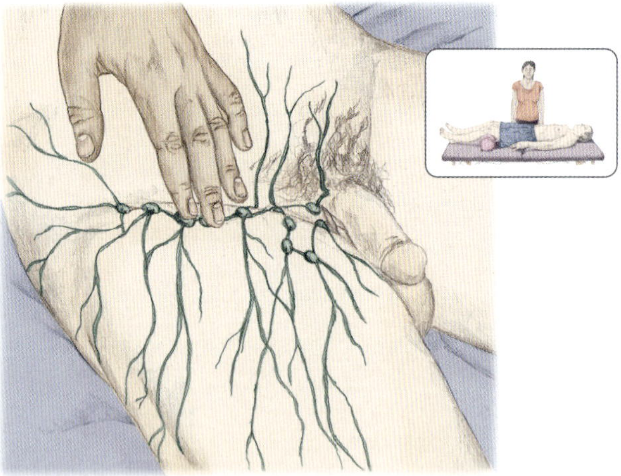

6.166 Partner supine, as you palpate the inguinal lymph nodes

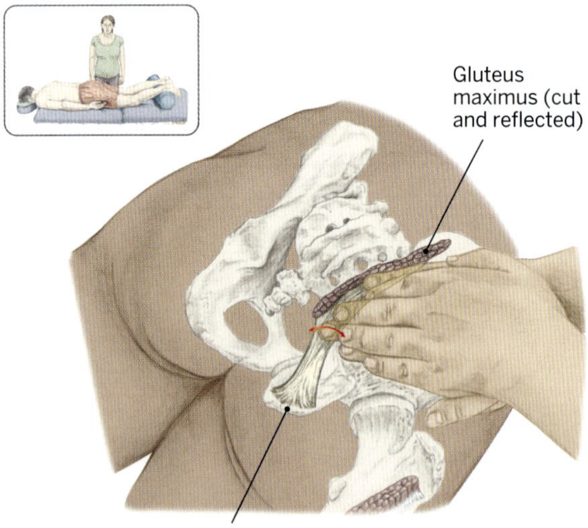

6.167 Partner prone, as you roll your fingertips across the sacrotuberous ligament

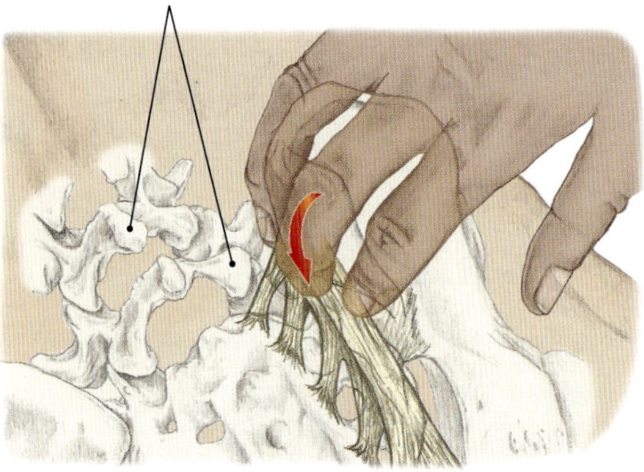

6.168 Partner prone, as you locate the sacroiliac ligaments

Inguinal Lymph Nodes

Distal to the inguinal ligament, the superficial inguinal lymph nodes are easily palpable. They number between eight and ten and vary in size from a small lentil to a raisin.

Inguinal lymph nodes

1. Partner supine, with the knee bolstered. This position will flex and laterally rotate the hip, allowing for easier palpation.
2. Locate the inguinal ligament. Slide inferiorly and explore for the superficial nodes (**6.166**).

Sacrotuberous Ligament

This broad, solid ligament stretches between the ischial tuberosity and the edge of the sacrum. Although it is deep to the gluteus maximus muscle, it is distinctly palpable and might feel like a span of bone.

Sacrotuberous ligament

1. Partner prone. Locate the ischial tuberosity. Locate the edge of the sacrum (p. 292).
2. Slide your fingertips off the tuberosity toward the edge of the sacrum. Using firm pressure, palpate through the gluteus maximus belly and strum broadly across the ligament (**6.167**).

Are you deep to the gluteus maximus fibers? Is the structure you are rolling over roughly an inch wide and inflexible? Does it stretch from the ischial tuberosity toward the sacrum?

Posterior Sacroiliac Ligaments

Superficial to the sacroiliac joint, the dense sacroiliac ligaments support the union of the posterior sacrum and the ilium. There are several segments, which attach from the sacrum to the area around the PSIS. The ligaments are deep to the thoracolumbar fascia, and their oblique fibers may be difficult to distinguish.

Posterior sacroiliac ligaments

1. Partner prone. Locate the surface of the sacrum.
2. Using firm pressure, strum your fingertips across the dense fibers of the sacroiliac ligaments (**6.168**).

Are you medial to the PSIS, on top of the sacroiliac joint space (p. 293)?

Iliolumbar Ligament

The iliolumbar ligament is located between the transverse processes of the fourth and fifth lumbar vertebrae and the posterior iliac crest. The strong, horizontal fibers of the ligament are important in stabilizing L-4 and L-5. The ligament is difficult to palpate, being deep to the thoracolumbar fascia, the thick multifidi (p. 200), and the quadratus lumborum (p. 207). However, its location and density can be determined.

Iliolumbar ligament

1. Partner prone. Locate the PSIS.
2. Slide your thumb straight superior from the PSIS to the level of L-4 and L-5. Your thumb should be between the iliac crest and the transverse processes of the lumbar vertebrae.
3. Using firm pressure, sink into the dense muscles of the low back and attempt to roll vertically across the ligament's taut fibers (**6.169**).

Can you palpate its dense, horizontal fibers?

Sciatic Nerve

The sciatic nerve is the largest nerve in the body—sometimes measuring three-quarters of an inch in diameter. It is formed by the spinal nerves of L-4 through S-3. The nerve passes through the greater sciatic notch, between the ischial tuberosity and greater trochanter, and extends down the posterior thigh. Distally, it branches into the tibial and fibular nerves.

Because the sciatic nerve runs deep to the piriformis (p. 330), there is considerable potential for the piriformis to compress or entrap the nerve. In general, the sciatic nerve is difficult to isolate in the gluteal region and, of course, is best avoided.

Sciatic nerve

1. First, *outline* the placement of the sciatic nerve. With your partner prone, locate the edge of the sacrum.
2. Draw an imaginary line down the buttock between the ischial tuberosity and greater trochanter. Continue down the middle of the posterior thigh. This is the location of the nerve.
3. To *access* the sciatic nerve, turn your partner side lying and flex the hip. Locate the ischial tuberosity and greater trochanter.
4. Palpate between these landmarks for the pathway of the sciatic nerve (**6.170**). You can avoid pinching the nerve by palpating with the pad of your thumb.

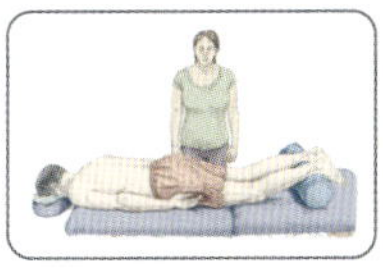

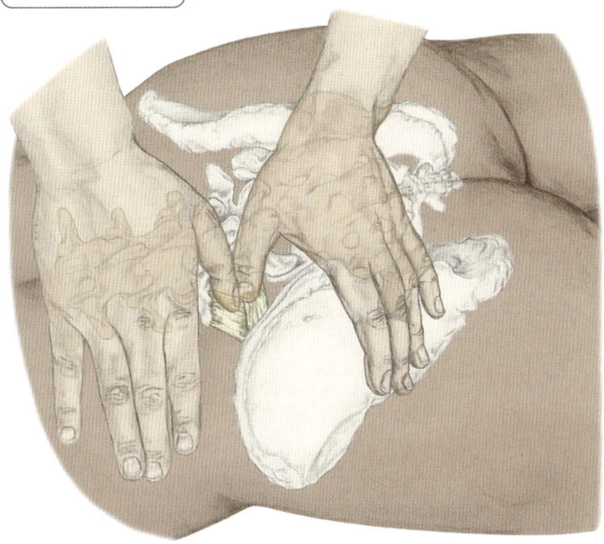

6.169 Partner prone, posterior/lateral view, as you sink your thumb onto the iliolumbar ligament

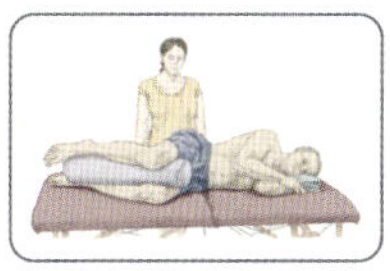

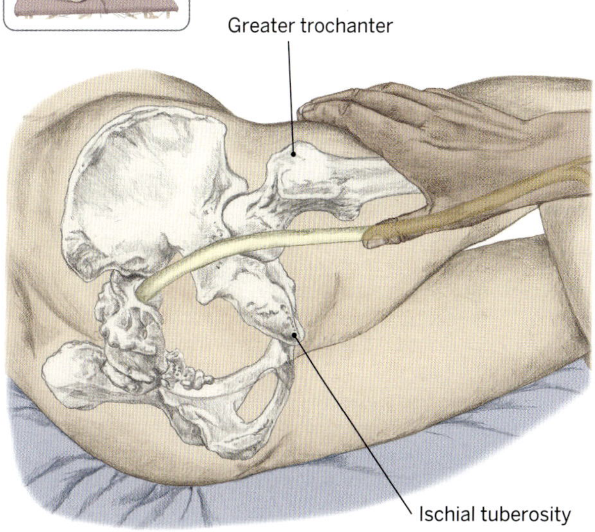

6.170 Partner side lying, as you locate the sciatic nerve

sciatic si-***at***-ik Grk. *ischion*, hip joint

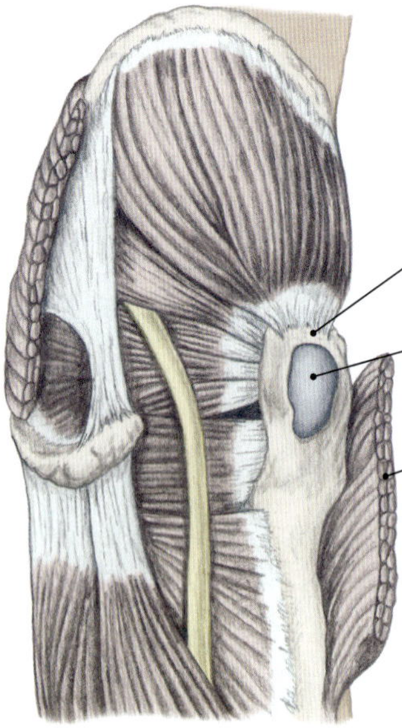

6.171 Posterior view of right hip, showing trochanteric bursa

Trochanteric Bursa

Positioned along the posterior/lateral aspect of the greater trochanter, this large bursa reduces friction between the trochanter and the gluteus maximus (**6.171**). Other bursae are located along the lateral and anterior sides of the trochanter and separate it from the gluteus medius and minimus. Unless they are inflamed or distended, the bursae will be impalpable.

Palpation Plus

Ligaments, tendons, fasciae, and retinacula are all forms of connective tissue. They are composed of virtually the same ingredients (collagen, elastin, and ground substance), differing only in the proportions of these materials. For anatomical purposes, these bands and sheaths have been categorized individually, although they are not separate structures. Collectively they form an incredible matrix that spreads throughout the entire body and supports it.

Now that you have explored the location of several connective tissue structures, here is an exercise to help you get a feel for how some of them connect together.

1. Partner prone. Locate the proximal hamstrings tendon (p. 313) as it attaches to the ischial tuberosity.
2. Follow the tendon superiorly as it melds into the sacrotuberous ligament and then to the posterior sacroiliac ligaments (p. 342) and iliolumbar ligaments (p. 343) on the sacrum.
3. Continue superiorly as the sacroiliac ligaments blend into the thoracolumbar fascia (p. 220) and the supraspinous ligament (p. 219) between the spinous processes of the vertebrae.
4. Ultimately, follow the supraspinous ligament all the way up the spine to the ligamentum nuchae (p. 218) and, finally, to the galea aponeurotica (p. 262) surrounding the cranium.

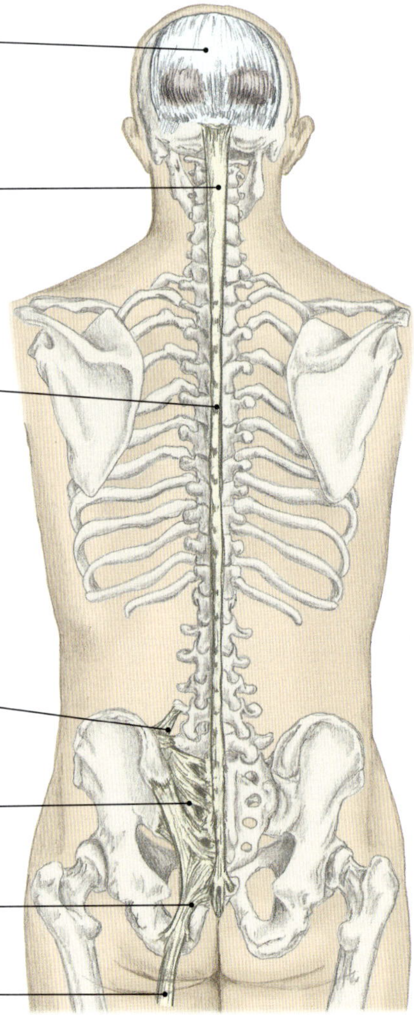

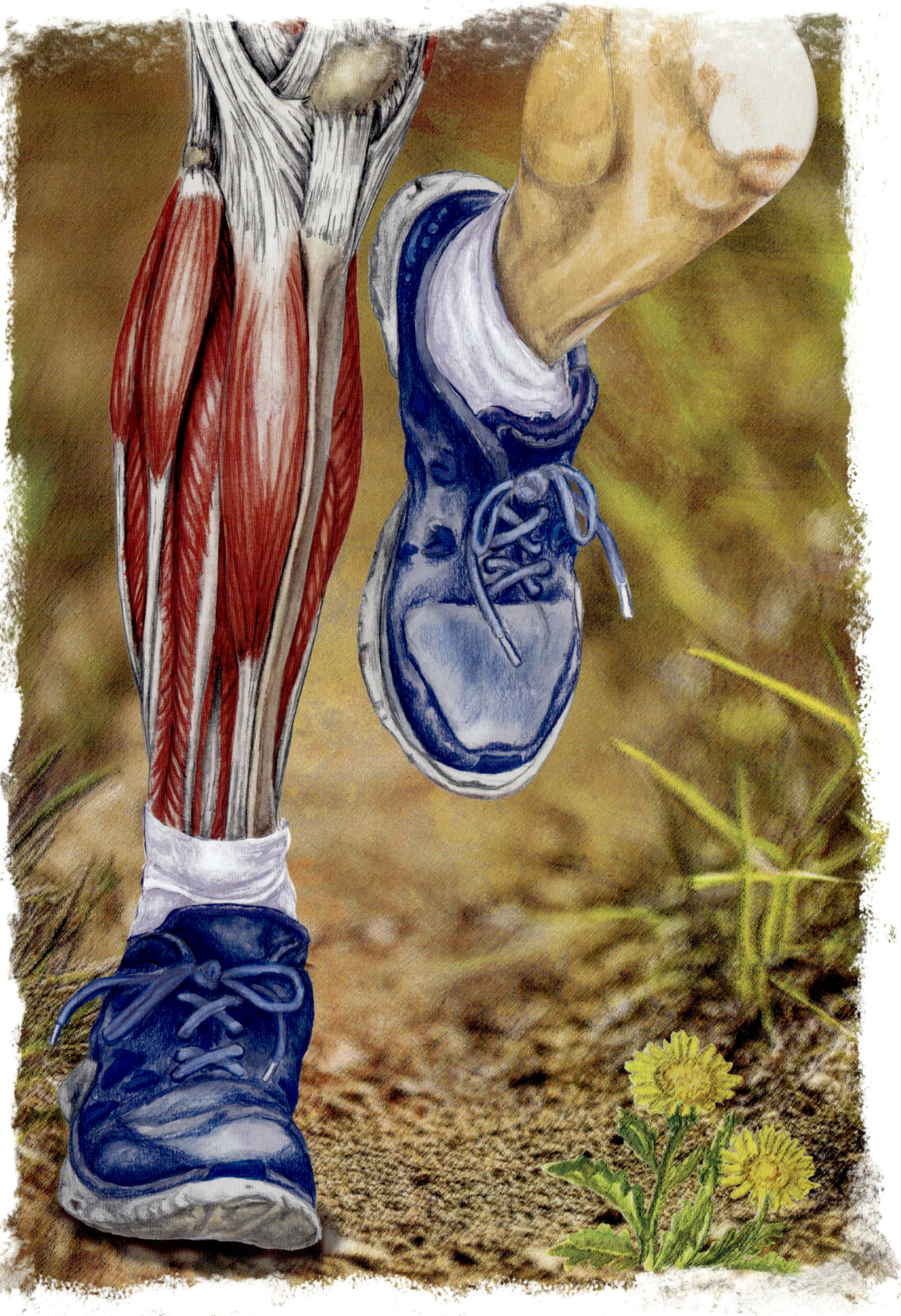

7

Leg & Foot

As you read this chapter, how is your body positioned? Are you sitting, standing, or lying down? Are your feet planted on the ground, moving, or raised up in the air? Are your knees flexed or extended? Perhaps you're wiggling your toes or forming circles with your ankles.

Consider the types and quantities of bones, muscles, joints, ligaments, and other structures that might be at work as you move your legs and feet. The foot alone has twenty-six bones! Look at the picture of the runner on the previous page. How many muscles can you see shown in the leg?

The muscles of the leg and foot are especially busy when the body is moving—walking, hiking, running, pedaling a bicycle, and more. They not only play a part in producing movement but also have critical roles in maintaining stability and balance.

See for yourself:

- Look at your leg—that's the portion between your knee and ankle. Dorsiflex and plantar flex your ankle. Where can you see different sets of muscles contracting as you move?
- If you invert (turn in) and evert (turn out) your foot, are the muscles used for dorsiflexion and plantar flexion of the ankle the same or different during these movements?
- Standing with bare feet, try to balance on one foot. What do you feel in the balancing foot? How about in the ankle? If you flex your toes to "grab" the ground, how does that affect your balance?

Topographical Views

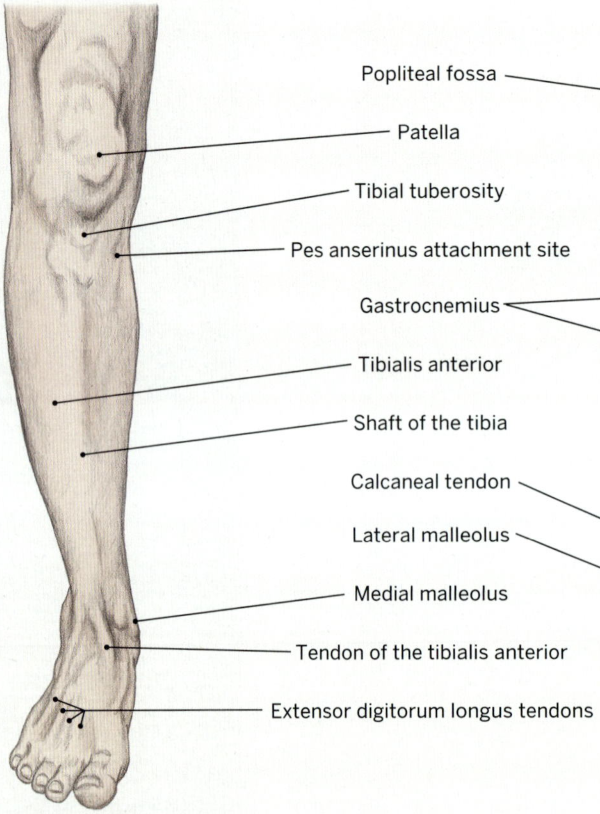

7.1 Anterior view of right leg

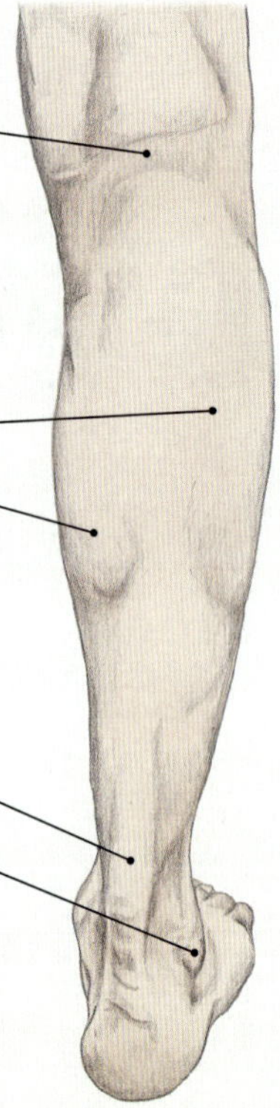

7.2 Posterior view of right leg

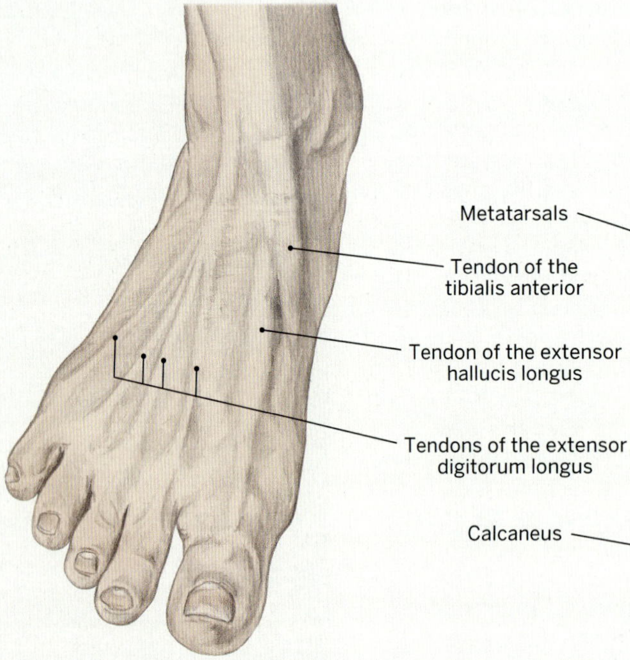

7.3 Dorsal view of right foot

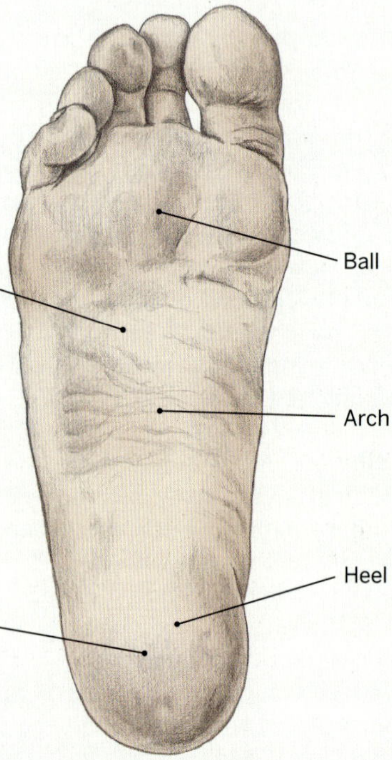

7.4 Plantar view of right foot

Leg & Foot

TOPOGRAPHICAL VIEWS

Exploring the Skin and Fascia

Leg

1. Partner seated. Using one hand to stabilize the leg, use your other hand to gently twist the skin and fascia around the leg's shaft (**7.5**). Note the tissue's mobility or resistance as you pull it in opposite directions.
2. Now try to tug the skin superiorly and inferiorly. Often the tissue has less mobility when moving in the vertical direction than in the horizontal direction.

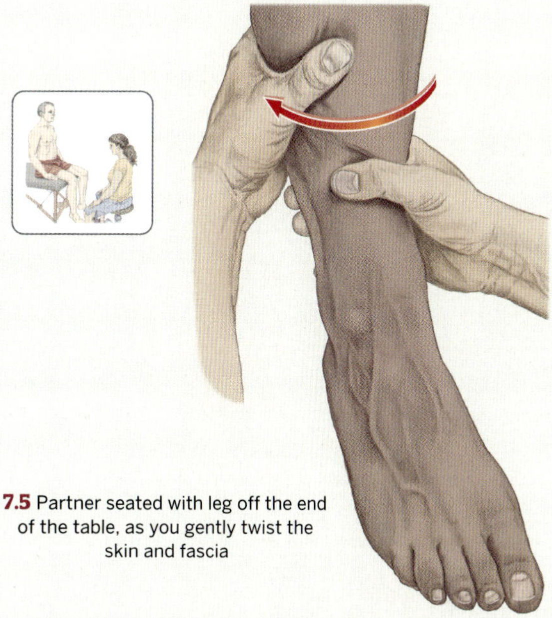

7.5 Partner seated with leg off the end of the table, as you gently twist the skin and fascia

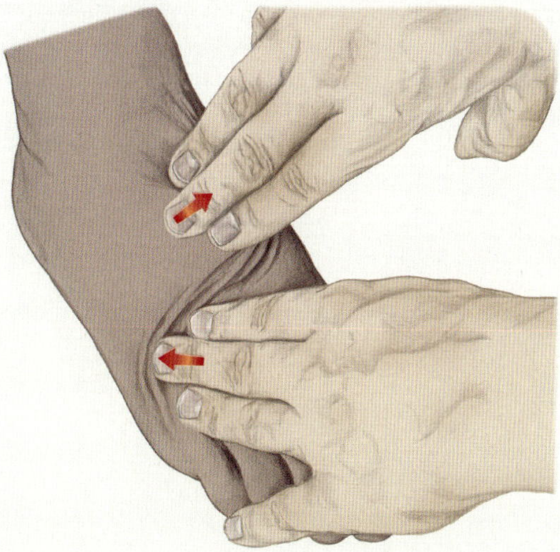

7.6 Partner seated, as you explore the dorsal surface of the foot

Foot

1. Partner seated. Place your hands on the foot's dorsal and plantar surfaces and sense their respective temperatures. Is one side warmer than the other?
2. Explore the dorsal surface by shifting the skin from side to side (**7.6**). Note the thin, delicate quality of its skin and fascia. Now palpate the plantar surface and note the tissue's thick, tough quality.

Ankle

1. Partner prone. Here is an opportunity to feel the skin and fascia stretch upon passive movement. Grasp the tissue of the posterior ankle and passively plantar flex and dorsiflex the ankle (**7.7**). Feel how supple the tissue is when the ankle is plantar flexed. When you dorsiflex the ankle, however, the skin might be pulled out from between your fingers.
2. Continue to move the ankle while grasping the tissue on all sides of the leg. Now ask your partner to actively move his ankle and toes while you grasp the skin and fascia. Encourage him to move slowly. Play with isolating specific actions—such as plantar flexion of the ankle versus flexion of the toes—to feel how the tissue shifts upon different movements.

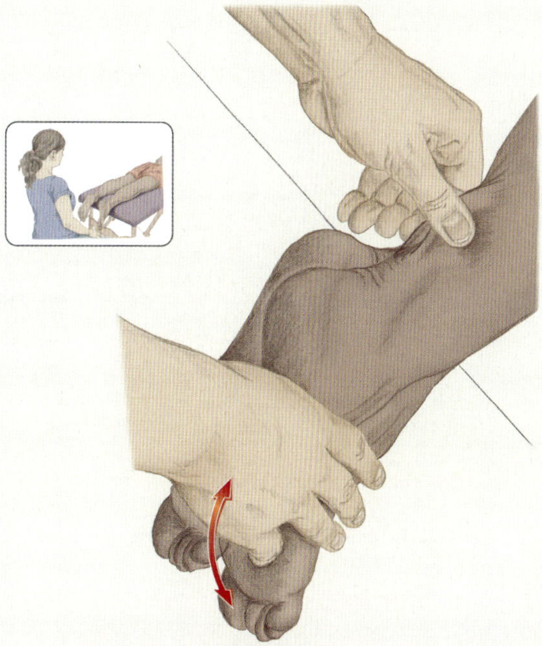

7.7 Partner prone with foot off the end of the table, as you passively plantar flex and dorsiflex the ankle

Bones of the Knee, Leg, and Foot

The knee is formed by the articulation of the distal femur and proximal tibia (**7.8**). The tibiofemoral (knee) joint, the largest synovial joint in the body, is a modified hinge joint. It is capable of flexion and extension; and when the knee is in a flexed position, it can medially and laterally rotate the knee (see box, p. 352).

The region of the knee also includes the small **patella** (kneecap) and the proximal fibula. The bony surfaces of the knee are superficial and easily accessible.

The **tibia** and **fibula** are the bones of the leg. The tibia (shinbone) runs superficially from the knee to the ankle just as the ulna runs superficially from the elbow to the wrist. The fibula's relationship to the tibia is also similar to the radius's relationship to the ulna: it is lateral to the tibia and virtually deep to the surrounding muscles. The fibula bears only 10% of the body's weight and rightfully so: it is the thinnest bone in the body in proportion to its length.

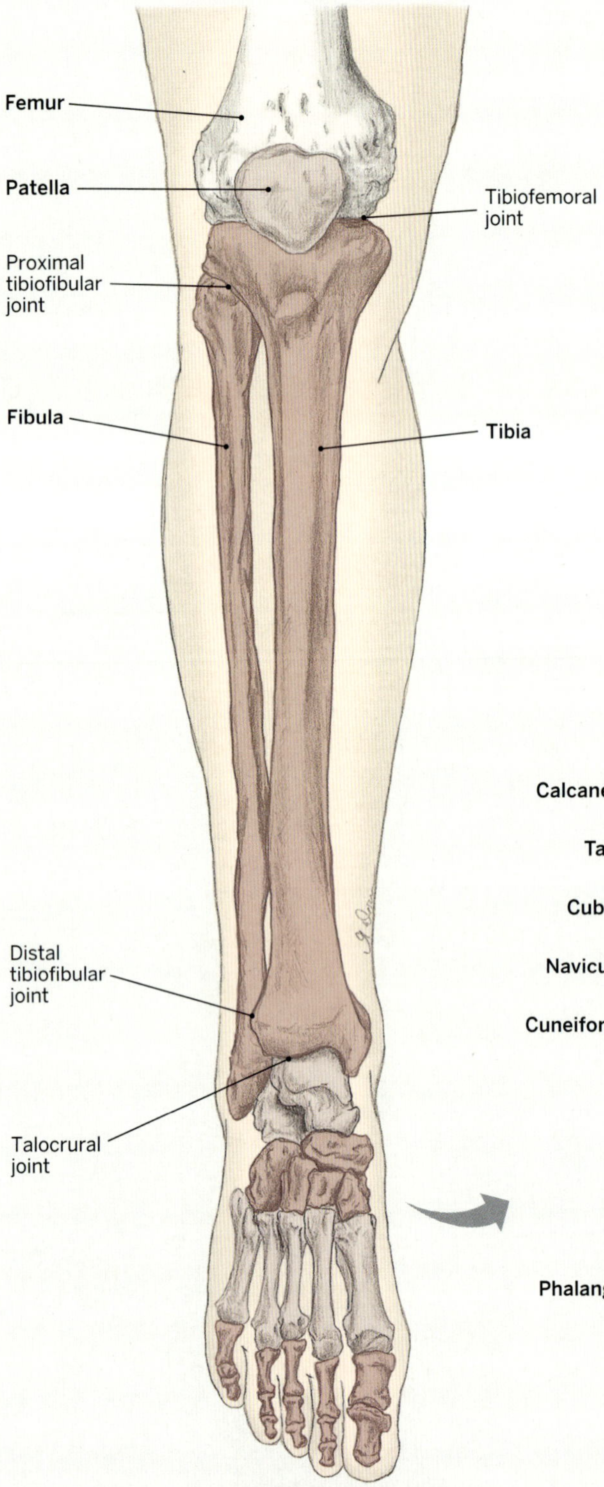

7.8 Anterior view of bones of right leg and foot, foot plantar flexed

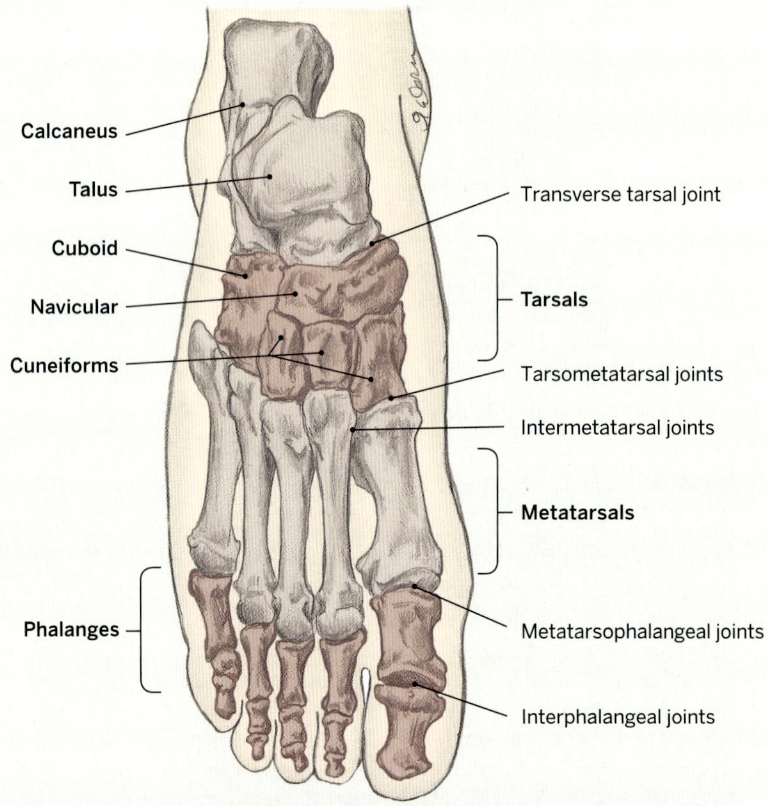

7.9 Dorsal view of bones of right foot

fibula	***fib***-u-la	L. pin or buckle
patella	pa-***tel***-a	L. small pan

The Tibia, Fibula, and Patella

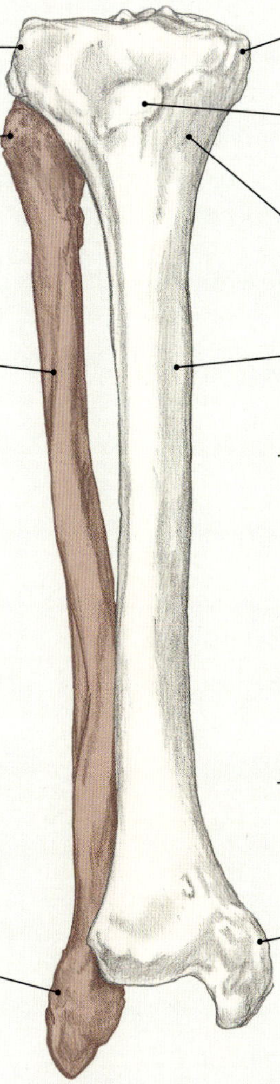

7.10 Anterior view of right tibia and fibula

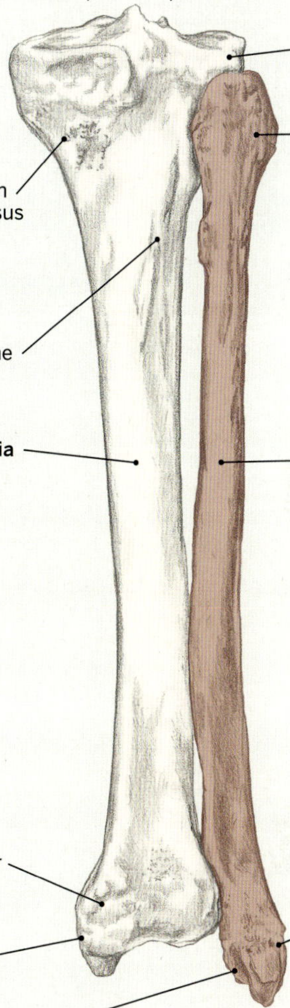

7.11 Posterior view of right tibia and fibula

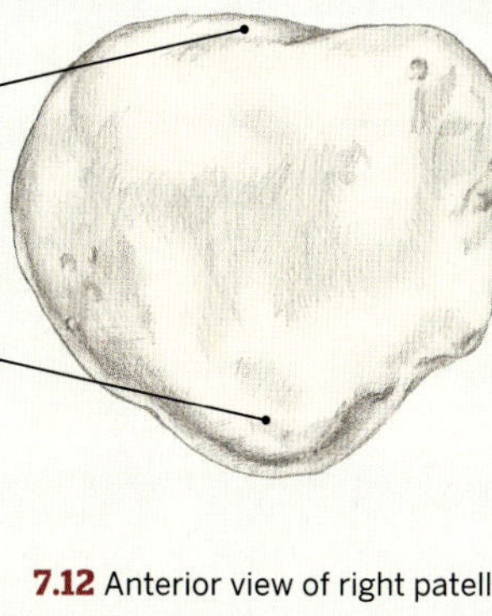

7.12 Anterior view of right patella

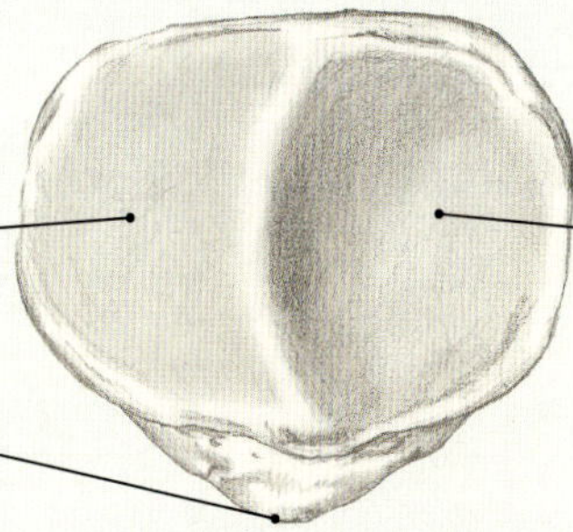

7.13 Posterior view of right patella

Leg & Foot

BONES

talocrural *ta*-lo-***kroo***-ral L. ankle + *crus*, leg

Bony Landmarks of the Knee and Leg

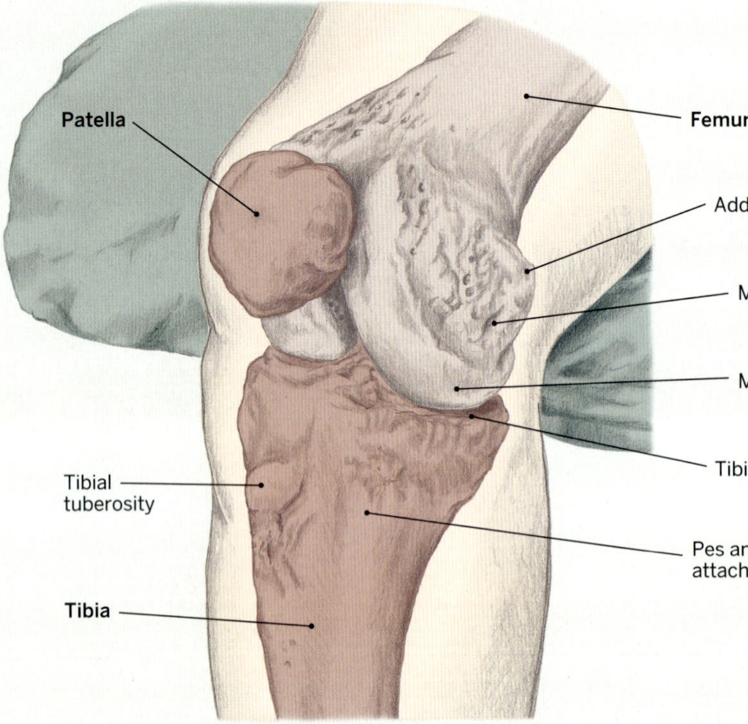

7.14 Anterior/medial view of right knee, showing tibiofemoral joint and bony landmarks

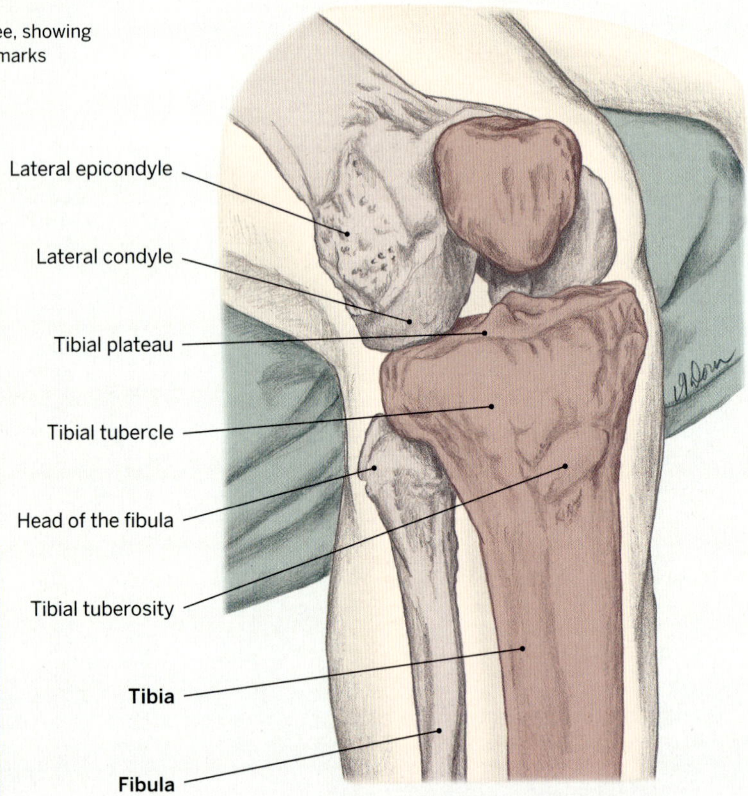

7.15 Anterior/lateral view of right knee, showing tibiofemoral joint and bony landmarks

Discover More

When the knee is in a flexed position, the tibia can rotate medially and laterally.

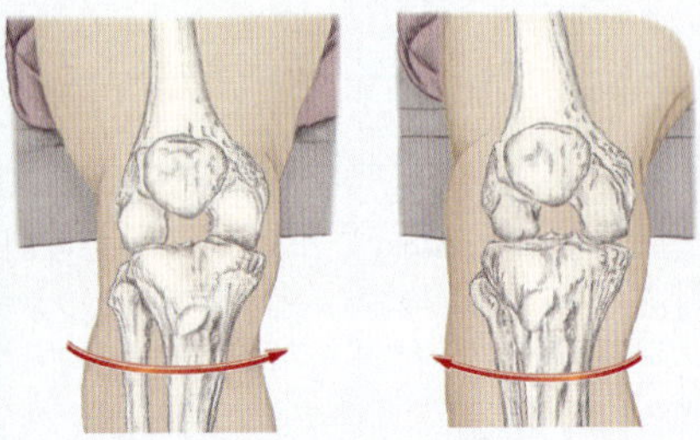

tibia	***tib*-e-a**	L. shinbone

Leg & Foot

BONY LANDMARKS

Overview: **Bony Landmark Trails**

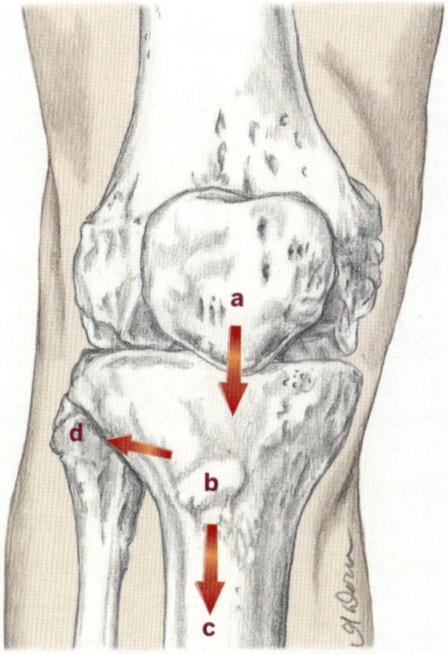

Trail 1 Landmark Trail links together the most prominent landmarks of the knee.

a Patella
b Tibial tuberosity
c Shaft of the tibia
d Head of the fibula

Trail 2 Waddle Walk has two paths exploring the medial and lateral aspects of the proximal tibia. It ends at the pes anserinus ("goose foot" in Latin) attachment site.

a Patella
b Medial and lateral tibial plateaus
c Pes anserinus attachment site

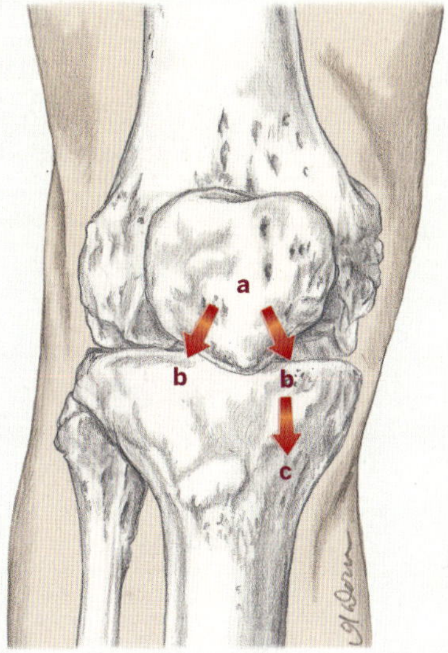

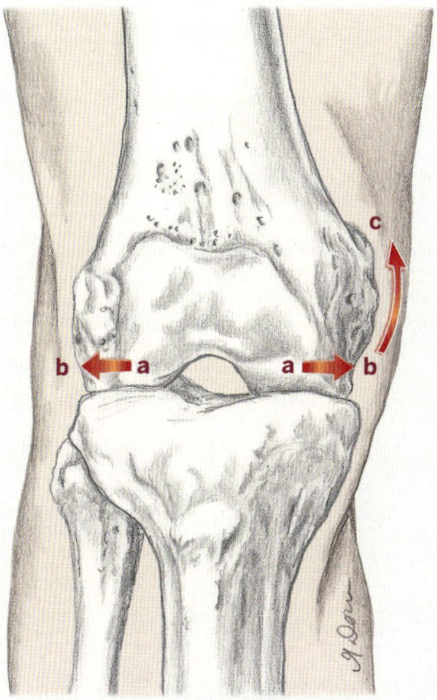

Patella removed

Trail 3 Hills on Both Sides explores the bumps of the distal end of the femur.

a Edges of the medial and lateral femoral condyles
b Medial and lateral epicondyles of the femur
c Adductor tubercle

Discover More

The thickest layering of cartilage in the body can be found on the posterior surface of the patella. This eighth-of-an-inch-thick coating protects the patella from the incredible pressure applied by the quadriceps when the knee is flexed. Simply walking up or down stairs can place as much as six hundred pounds of pressure on the patella.

tuberosity *tu*-ber-*os*-i-tee L. a swelling

Trail 1 Landmark Trail ▸

Patella

The patella is located on the anterior surface of the knee. It is superficial and round with an apex that points distally. The largest sesamoid bone in the body, the patella is an attachment site and junction point for the quadriceps femoris tendon (p. 308) and patellar ligament. When the knee is flexed, the patella seems to disappear, sinking into the space between the proximal tibia and femoral condyles.

Patella

1. Partner supine with the knee extended. In this position the quadriceps tendon is shortened and the patella is more mobile and easier to access.
2. Locate the patella on the anterior knee and palpate its round surface and edges. Try gently shifting it from side to side (**7.16**). Note any bumps or crevices along its edges.
3. Have your partner sit with his legs hanging off the table. Passively flex and extend the knee as you explore the patella's movements and its relationship to the rectus femoris tendon (**7.17**).

Tibial Tuberosity and Shaft of the Tibia

The **tibial tuberosity** is a superficial knob located distal to the patella on the shaft of the tibia. It is roughly half an inch in diameter and serves as an attachment site for the patellar ligament. It sometimes protrudes visibly. The **shaft of the tibia** runs superficially along the anterior leg. From the tibial tuberosity to the medial malleolus (p. 361), its edges and flat surface are easily palpable.

Tibial tuberosity and shaft of the tibia

1. Partner seated with the knee flexed. Locate the patella. Slide your fingers three or four inches inferior from the patella and, using your thumbpad, explore for the tuberosity (**7.18**).
2. Continue to palpate inferiorly along the shaft of the tibia. Determine the width of the shaft by palpating along its edges. Follow it down to the medial malleolus.

With your fingers at the tibial tuberosity, ask your partner to extend his knee slightly. With this action, the patellar ligament will tighten, and you will be able to feel where it attaches to the tibial tuberosity. When palpating the tibial shaft, can you feel its distinct edges leading toward the medial ankle?

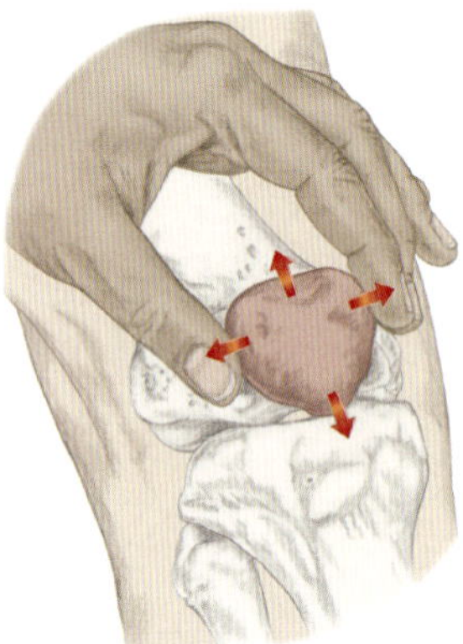

7.16 Partner supine, anterior/lateral view of extended right knee, as you palpate the patella

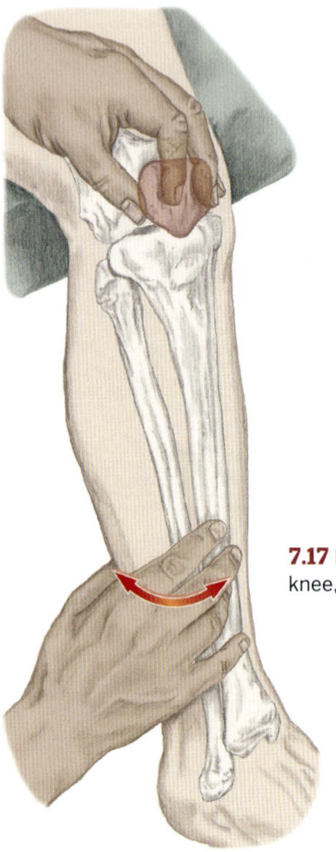

7.17 Partner seated, anterior view of right knee, as you passively flex and extend the knee to feel the patella shift

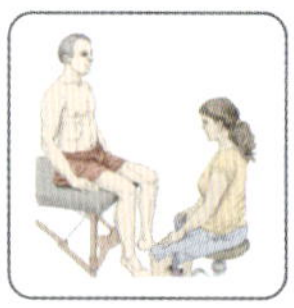

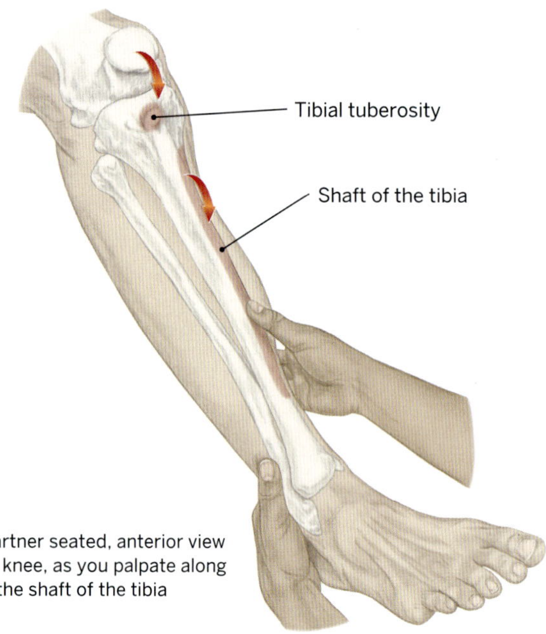

7.18 Partner seated, anterior view of right knee, as you palpate along the shaft of the tibia

Leg & Foot

sesamoid	***ses***-a-moyd	L. resembling a sesame seed

Head of the Fibula

The head of the fibula is located on the lateral side of the leg and sometimes protrudes visibly. It is the attachment site for the biceps femoris muscle and a portion of the soleus muscle as well as the fibular collateral ligament.

Be aware of the common fibular nerve (p. 401), which lies along the posterior aspect of the head of the fibula.

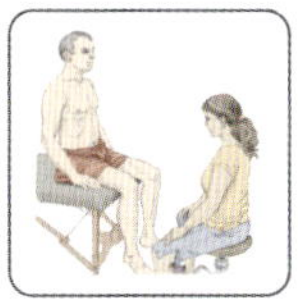

Head of the fibula

1. Partner seated with the knee flexed. Locate the tibial tuberosity.
2. Slide your fingers laterally three to four inches toward the outside of the leg. Palpate for the head of the fibula (**7.19**). Explore its inch-wide tip.

Is the knob you are palpating lateral to the tibial tuberosity? Can you sculpt a circle around it, outlining its shape? Does the biceps femoris tendon lead to the head of the fibula?

With your partner prone, bend the knee to 90° and follow the biceps femoris tendon (p. 313) distally to where it inserts at the head of the fibula.

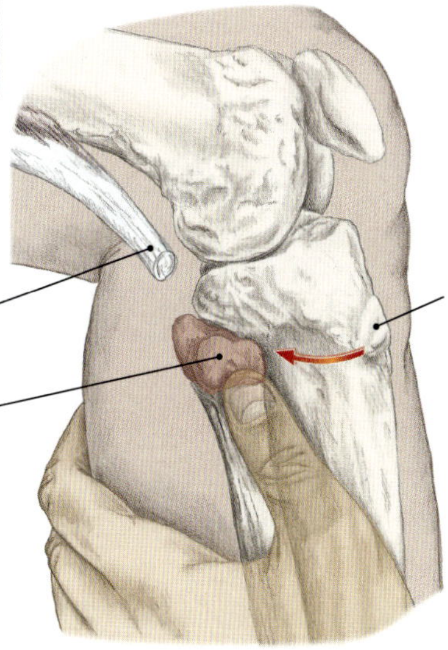

7.19 Lateral view of flexed right knee, as you locate the head of the fibula

Trail 2 Waddle Walk ▸

Tibial Plateaus

The medial and lateral plateaus are located on the proximal end of the tibia. Situated inside the knee joint, the plateaus cannot be palpated, but their edges, located superficially on either side of the patellar ligament, are easily accessible.

Tibial plateaus

1. Partner seated with the knee flexed. Place your thumbs on either side of the patella.
2. Slide inferiorly, compressing into the tissue. You will feel a softening in the knee as your thumbs sink into the joint space between the femur and tibia.
3. Continue inferiorly until you feel the plateau edges (**7.20**). Palpate both edges and follow them in either direction.

Can you follow the edges of both plateaus horizontally to the sides of the knee? Can you feel the soft joint space superior to them? If you passively extend the knee with one hand while palpating the edges with the other, can you feel the edges move closer to the patella?

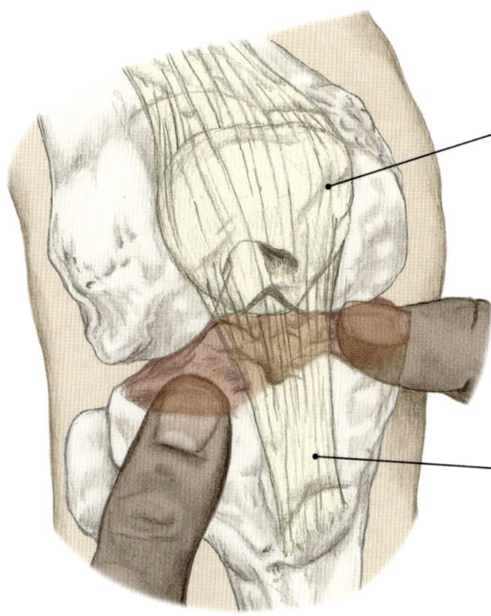

7.20 Anterior view of flexed right knee, as you access the tibial plateaus

Palpation Plus

Distal to the lateral plateau is a swelling of bone called the tibial tubercle (see **7.15**), which is the attachment site for the iliotibial tract (p. 326). Slide distally off the lateral plateau and explore the tubercle's girth. When the knee is extended, the tubercle usually lies between the patella and the head of the fibula.

Pes Anserinus Attachment Site

Three tendons of the thigh—the sartorius, gracilis, and semitendinosus—converge at the medial knee to form the larger pes anserinus tendon, which attaches to the proximal, medial shaft of the tibia (**7.21**). More generally, the pes anserinus is the flat area medial to the tibial tuberosity.

Pes anserinus attachment site

1. Partner seated with the knee flexed. Locate the tibial tuberosity.
2. Slide medially one inch and explore its flat surface and any palpable tendons (**7.22**).

Is the region you are isolating medial to the tibial tuberosity? Is it on the anterior/medial shaft of the tibia?

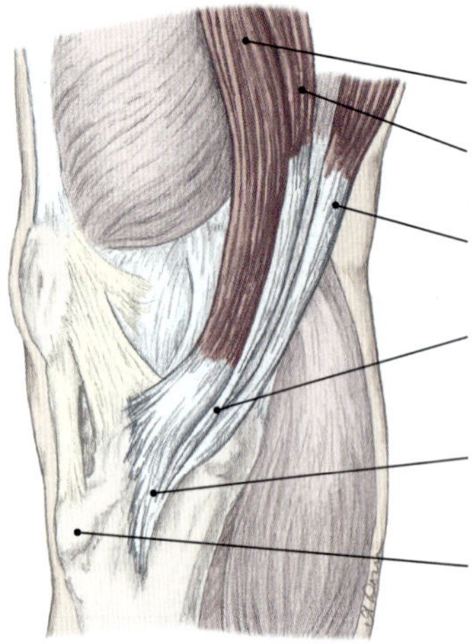

7.21 Medial view of right knee, showing pes anserinus attachment site

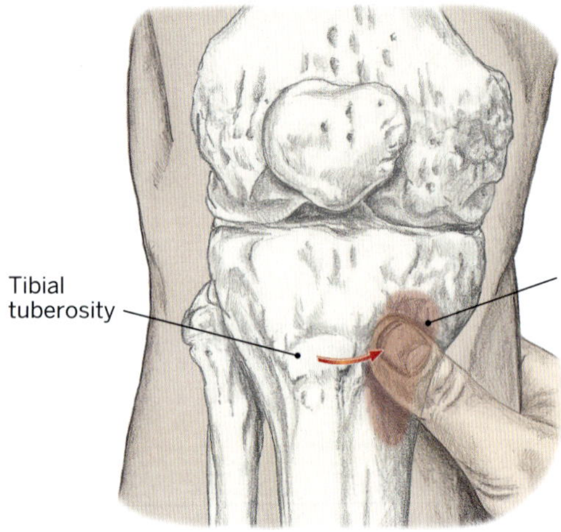

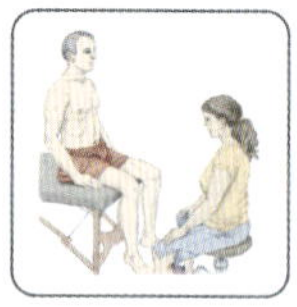

7.22 Anterior view of right knee, as you palpate around the pes anserinus attachment site

Trail 3 Hills on Both Sides ▸

Edges of Femoral Condyles

The two large, round femoral condyles are mostly inaccessible; however, their edges, located on either side of the patella, are easily accessible. The edges of the femoral condyles play an important role in the tracking of the patella when the knee is flexed and extended.

Edges of femoral condyles

1. Partner supine with the knee fully extended. Locate the sides of the patella.
2. Shift the patella medially and slide off of it onto the lateral condyle. Explore the condyle's distinct edge (**7.23**) and follow it distally as it continues toward the joint space.
3. Palpate the edge of the medial condyle in the same manner. Compare the size and height of the two edges and the relationship of both to the patella.

Are the edges slightly underneath the patella? Can you follow them distally toward the joint space of the knee?

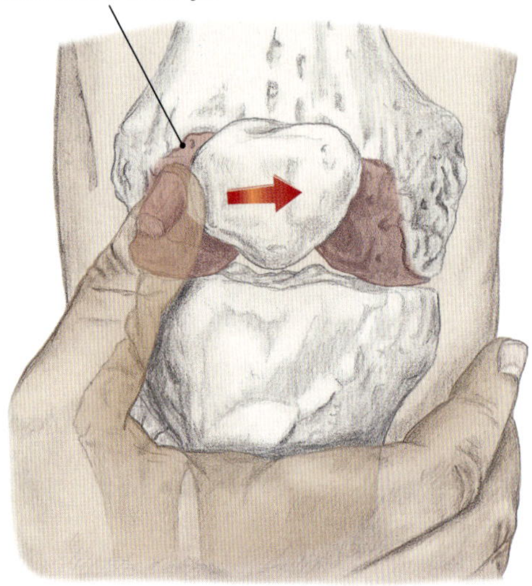

7.23 Anterior view of right knee, as you explore the femoral condyles

pes anserinus pes ***an***-ser-***i***-nus L. *pedis*, foot; *anserinus*, goose-like

Leg & Foot

Epicondyles of the Femur

The lateral epicondyle is a bald, knobby area located on the lateral surface of the knee. It serves as an attachment site for the fibular collateral ligament. It is deep to the iliotibial tract and anterior to the biceps femoris tendon.

The medial epicondyle is deep to the tendon of the sartorius, distal to the vastus medialis muscle, and serves as an attachment site for the tibial collateral ligament.

Epicondyles of the femur

1. Partner seated with the knee flexed. Locate the patella.
2. Slide directly lateral from the patella to the outside of the knee. Explore this region, noting the lateral epicondyle's location proximal to the head of the fibula (**7.24**).
3. Return to the patella and slide to the medial epicondyle on the inside of the knee. Note the epicondyle's superficial quality and round surface, as well as its location superior to the tibiofemoral joint.

Is the head of the fibula distal to the lateral epicondyle? Can you palpate the vastus medialis (p. 308) proximal to the medial epicondyle?

Adductor Tubercle

The adductor tubercle is located proximal to the medial epicondyle, between the belly of the vastus medialis and the hamstring tendons. Its small tip sticks out from the top of the medial epicondyle and is an attachment site for the adductor magnus tendon (p. 321). It is often tender to the touch.

Adductor tubercle

1. Partner seated with the knee flexed. Locate the medial epicondyle of the femur.
2. Slide superiorly along the medial side of the femur. As the outline of the femur drops off into the soft tissue, explore for the small point of the tubercle (**7.25**).
3. Strum across the adductor magnus tendon by rubbing your thumbpad anteriorly and posteriorly.

Are you directly proximal to the medial epicondyle? With your thumb on the proximal aspect of the tubercle (on the adductor magnus tendon), have your partner gently adduct his hip. Does the tendon of the magnus become taut and press into your finger?

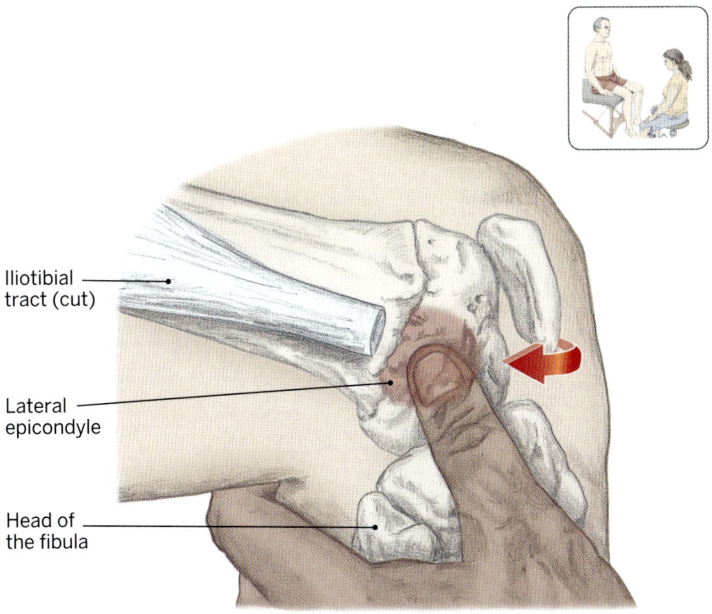

7.24 Lateral view of right knee, as you palpate the lateral epicondyle of the femur

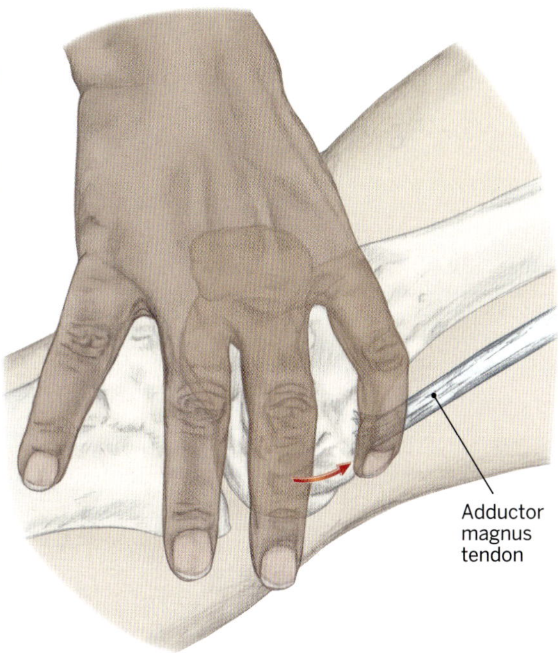

7.25 Anterior/medial view of right knee, as you explore for the adductor tubercle

Bones of the Ankle and Foot

The foot contains twenty-six bones (**7.26–7.30**). The hindfoot is the union of the talus and calcaneus. The **talus** articulates with the tibia and fibula to form the talocrural, or ankle, joint. The large, chunky **calcaneus** is the bone at the heel of the foot.

The midfoot is composed of five tarsals. Small and uniquely shaped, like the carpal bones of the wrist, the **tarsals** are tightly wedged together. They are most accessible along the dorsal surface of the foot.

The forefoot is formed by the long, superficial metatarsals and phalanges. Similar to a metacarpal, each **metatarsal** consists of a proximal base, a shaft, and a distal head. The first toe is formed by two sizable **phalanges**; the remaining toes have three phalanges each. The phalanges are accessible on all sides.

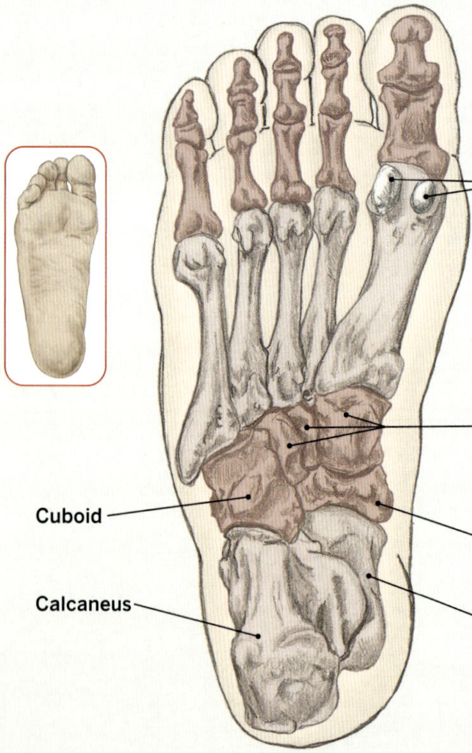

7.26 Plantar view of bones of right foot

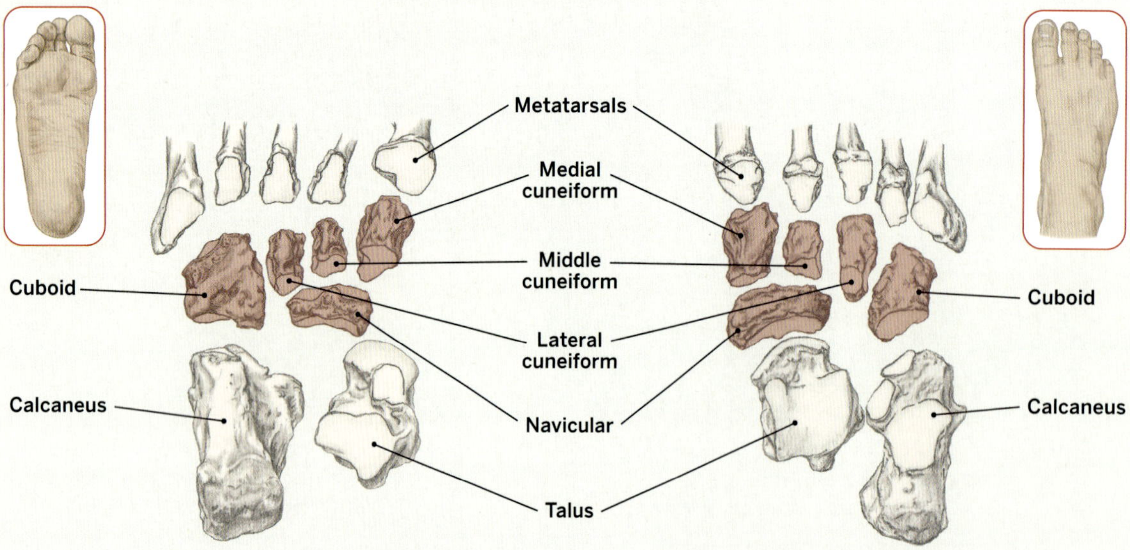

7.27 Plantar view of right foot, bones separated

7.28 Dorsal view of right foot, bones separated

metatarsophalangeal ***met***-a-***tar***-so-***fa***-lan-***jee***-al

Bony Landmarks of the Ankle and Foot

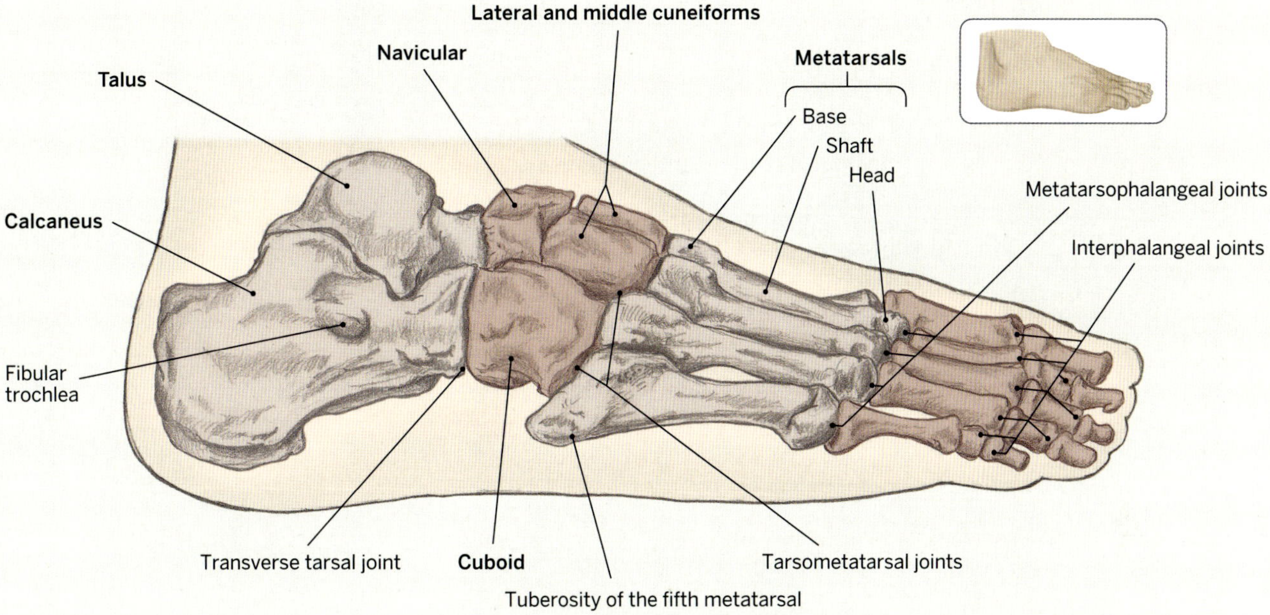

7.29 Lateral view of bones of right foot

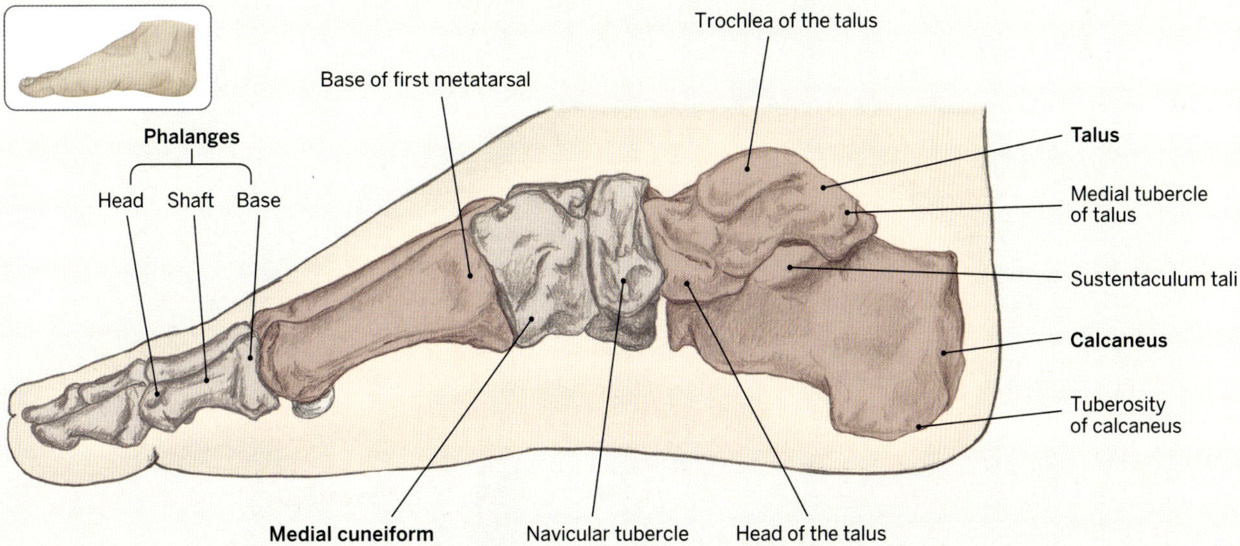

7.30 Medial view of bones of right foot

Leg & Foot

BONY LANDMARKS

phalanges fa-***lan***-jeez Grk. closely knit row, line of battle

Overview: **Bony Landmark Trails**

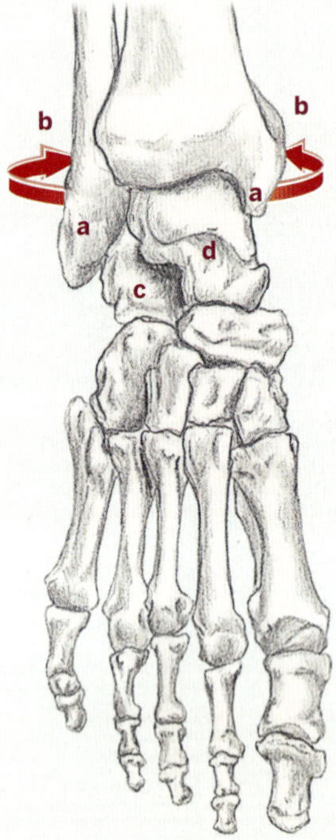

Trail 1 The Back Road locates the bones and landmarks of the hindfoot and ankle.

a Lateral and medial malleoli
b Malleolar grooves
c Calcaneus
  Tuberosity of calcaneus
  Sustentaculum tali
  Fibular trochlea
d Talus
  Head
  Trochlea
  Medial tubercle

Discover More

The bony landmark trails of the foot present the hindfoot and forefoot first, followed by the more challenging structures of the midfoot.

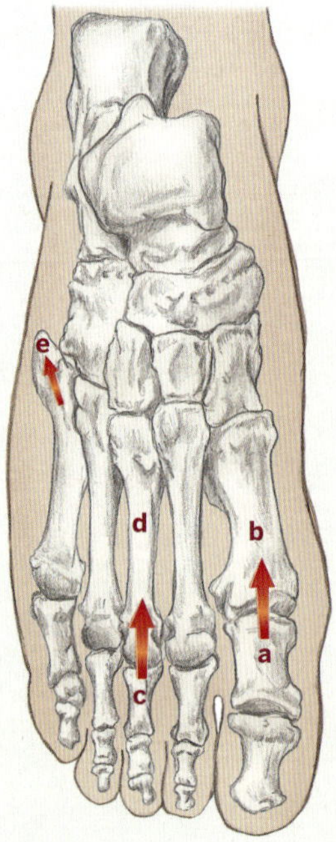

Trail 2 This route, Little Piggies, palpates the bones and joints of the toes and forefoot.

a Hallux
b First metatarsal
c Second through fifth digits (toes)
d Second through fifth metatarsals
e Tuberosity of fifth metatarsal

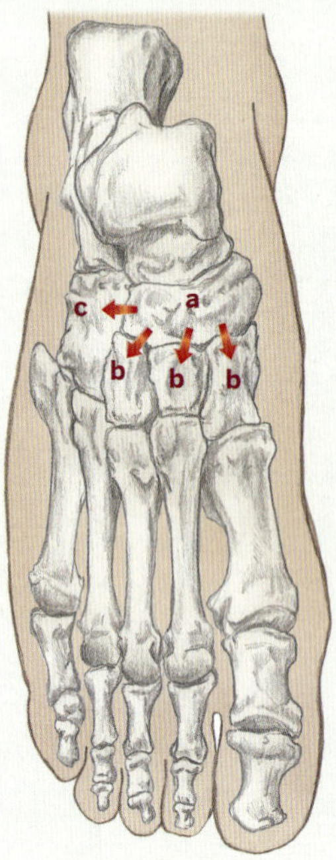

Trail 3 The Archway explores the bones of the midfoot located at the arch of the foot.

a Navicular and navicular tuberosity
b Medial, middle, and lateral cuneiforms
c Cuboid

Discover More

As with the carpals of the wrist, the names of the tarsals speak for themselves:

cuboid	L. cube-shaped
cuneiform	L. wedge-shaped
navicular	L. boat-shaped

metatarsal	***met**-a-**tar**-sal*	Grk. *meta*, after or beyond
tarsal	***tar**-sul*	Grk. wicker basket

Lateral and Medial Malleoli

The lateral and medial malleoli are the large, conspicuous knobs on either side of the ankle. The broader medial malleolus is located at the distal end of the tibia, while the more slender lateral malleolus protrudes from the distal fibula.

Lateral and medial malleoli

Partner seated or supine. Explore and compare the shapes and sizes of the two malleoli. Palpating all sides of their surfaces, note how the lateral malleolus extends further distally than its medial counterpart (**7.31**).

Sliding proximally, can you connect the medial malleolus to the shaft of the tibia and then to the tibial tuberosity? Is the medial malleolus more proximal than the lateral?

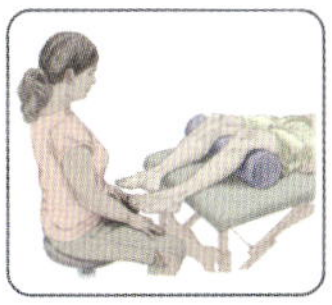

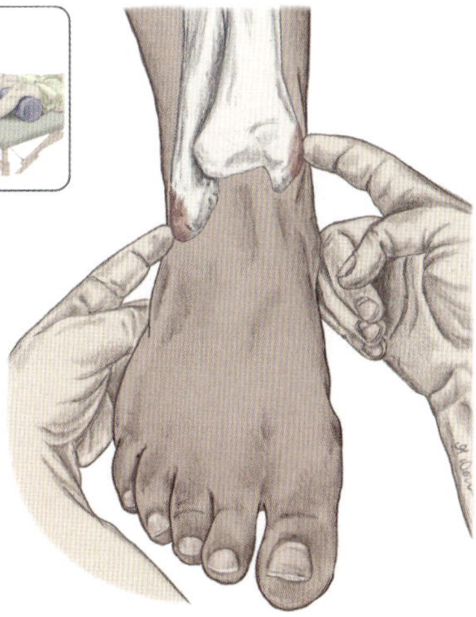

7.31 Dorsal view of right foot, as you palpate the level of each malleolus

Malleolar Grooves

Both the medial and lateral malleoli have small vertical grooves carved into their posterior surfaces. These grooves are designed to offer stability and leverage to tendons that bend around the ankle. Because these tendons lie either inside the groove or beside it, it can be difficult to feel the actual depression of the groove.

Malleolar grooves

1. Partner supine or seated. Locate the medial malleolus.
2. Slide roughly half an inch posteriorly to palpate the posterior aspect of the malleolus for a slender, vertical groove (**7.32**).
3. Shorten the surrounding tissue by passively inverting the foot and explore the length of the medial groove and the superficial tendons.
4. Try this same method along the lateral malleolus, only now, passively evert the foot to shorten the surrounding tissue and locate the lateral groove (**7.33**).

Because each groove runs vertically, can you roll your finger horizontally across each vertical groove to determine its location and shape?

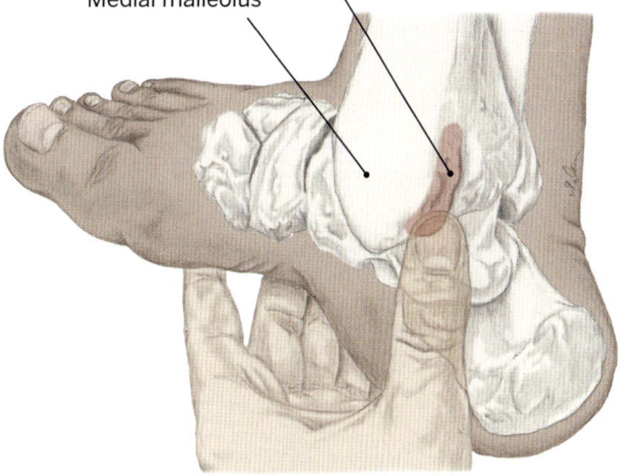

7.32 Posterior/medial view of right foot, as you palpate the medial malleolar groove

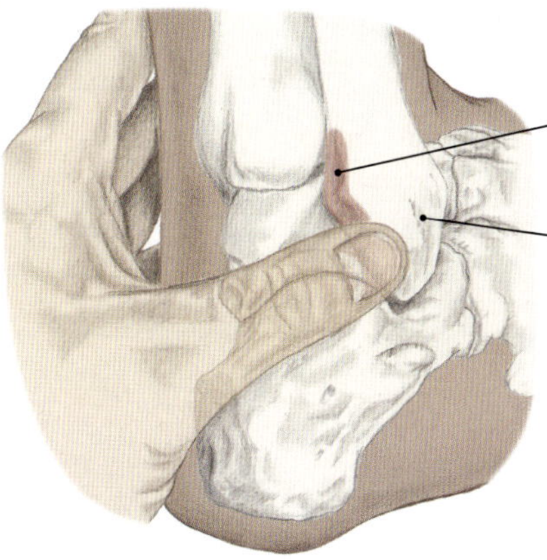

7.33 Posterior/lateral view of right foot, as you locate the lateral malleolar groove

calcaneus	kal-***kay***-nee-us	L. heel
malleolus	***mal***-e-**o**-lus	L. little hammer

Calcaneus

Tuberosity, Sustentaculum Tali, and Fibular Trochlea

The large, solid **calcaneus** forms the heel of the foot (**7.34**). It is situated beneath the talus and projects two inches posteriorly from the malleoli. The medial and lateral sides of the calcaneus are deep to tendons, yet easily palpable. The **tuberosity** of the calcaneus is a rounded region located along its posterior surface. The calcaneal tendon attaches to the superior aspect of the tuberosity.

The **sustentaculum tali** is located on the medial side of the calcaneus, roughly one inch distal to the medial malleolus (**7.35**). Shaped like a plank, the sustentaculum supports the talus on the calcaneus. It is also an attachment site for the deltoid ligament (p. 405) and is deep to the flexor tendons. Only its small tip is accessible.

The **fibular trochlea** is located on the lateral side of the foot (see 7.34). Roughly an inch distal to the lateral malleolus, the trochlea is a small, superficial prominence that protrudes from the calcaneal surface to help stabilize the fibularis muscles (p. 380).

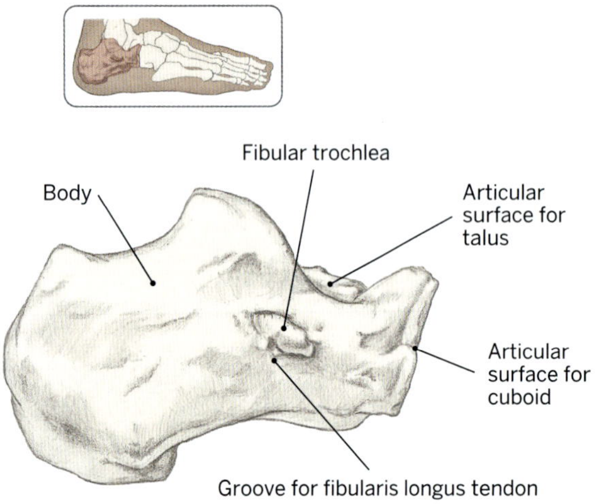

7.34 Lateral view of right calcaneus

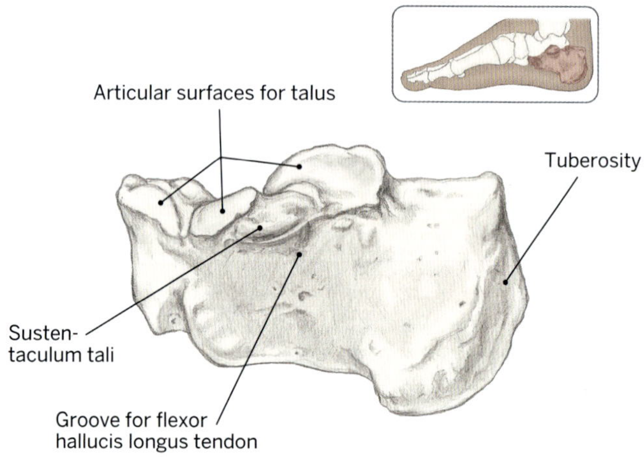

7.35 Medial view of right calcaneus

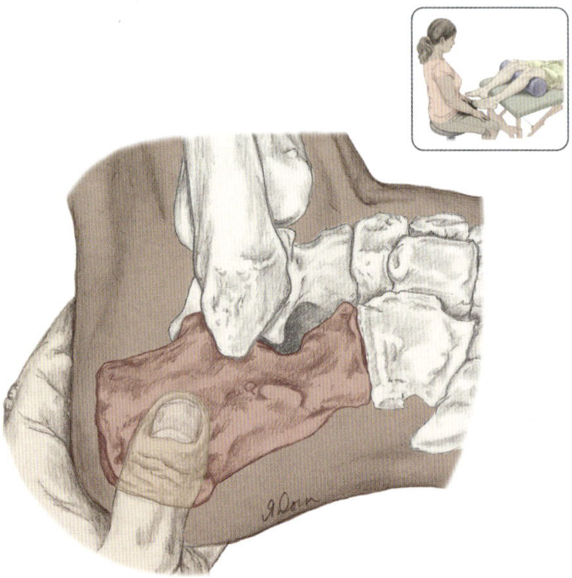

7.36 Lateral view of right foot, as you explore the calcaneus

Tuberosity of calcaneus

1. Partner supine or seated. Walk your fingers distally from the malleoli down to the heel. Palpate and explore the shape and girth of the posterior calcaneus.
2. Move to the plantar surface to isolate the tuberosity at the base of the heel (**7.36**). The tuberosity will feel more like a flat region than a distinct bump.

Place one hand at the malleoli and the other at the tuberosity. Note how far the calcaneus extends posteriorly.

sustentaculum *sus*-ten-*tak*-u-lum L. support

Sustentaculum tali

1. Partner supine or seated. Place the ankle in a neutral position and locate the medial malleolus.
2. Slide approximately one inch distal to the small tip of the sustentaculum (**7.37**). Passively inverting the foot will soften the surrounding tissues.
3. Sculpt around its sides, noting the soft tissues just distal to it.

Are you distal to the medial malleolus? If you slide distally off the sustentaculum tali, do you feel the thick tissues at the sole of the foot?

Fibular trochlea

1. Partner supine or seated. With the ankle in a dorsiflexed position, locate the lateral malleolus.
2. Slide roughly an inch inferiorly and explore for the small, superficial trochlea. It may feel like a short ridge on the surface of the calcaneus (**7.38**). Passively everting the foot will soften the surrounding tissues.
3. Sculpt around its edges, noting the soft tissues just distal to the trochlea.

Are you distal to the lateral malleolus? If you slide off the trochlea distally, do you feel the thick tissues of the foot? Ask your partner to alternately evert and relax her foot. Do the fibularis tendons pass along either side of the trochlea?

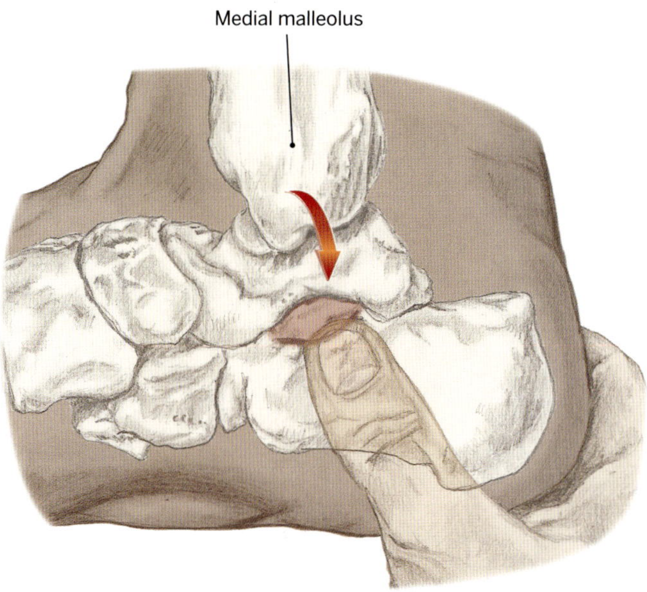

7.37 Medial view of right ankle, as you locate the sustentaculum tali

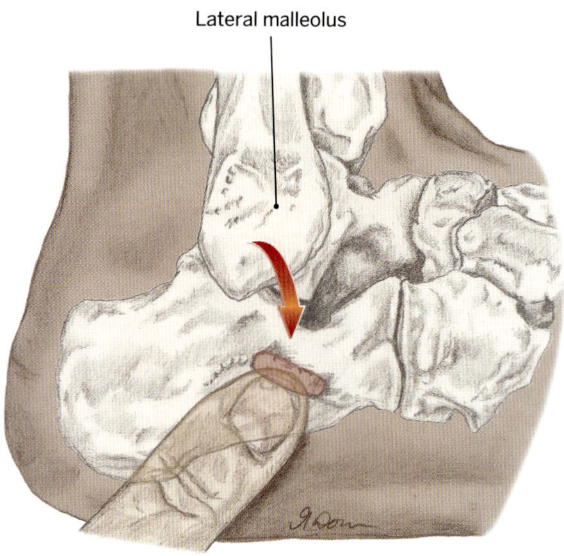

7.38 Lateral view of right ankle, as you isolate the fibular trochlea

Comparative Anatomy

Of the two hundred different kinds of primates in the world, humans are the only ones with a nongrasping first toe. Since we are no longer tree climbers, our foot has lost its handlike capabilities in order to become a platform for an upright body.

This does not mean, however, that the toes were designed to be inactive. An infant's foot has twenty times the toe-grasping capacity of a shoe-wearing adult. And in shoeless cultures, people retain the prehensile abilities of their feet throughout adulthood, using them for sewing and even threading needles.

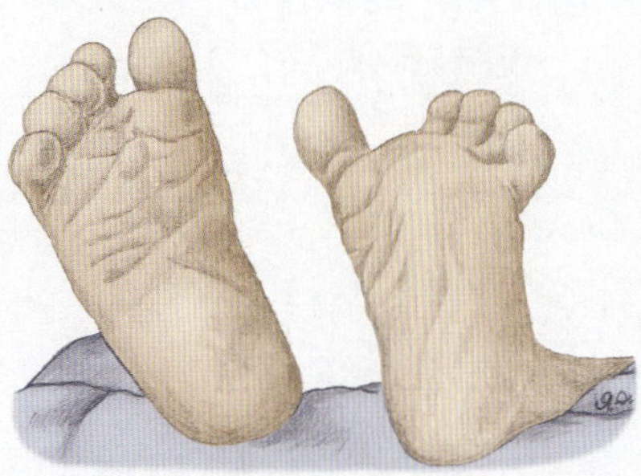

Talus

Head, Trochlea, and Medial Tubercle

The **talus** has three accessible landmarks (**7.39**, **7.40**). The **head** is the round, anterior portion that articulates with the navicular. The medial aspect of the head is accessible posterior to the navicular tubercle (p. 369). The **trochlea**, the large, superior prominence of the body of the talus, is wedged between the distal ends of the fibula and tibia. The anterior part of the trochlea is located between the malleoli. Finally, the small **medial tubercle** of the talus is posterior to the medial malleolus and serves as an attachment site for the deltoid ligament (p. 405).

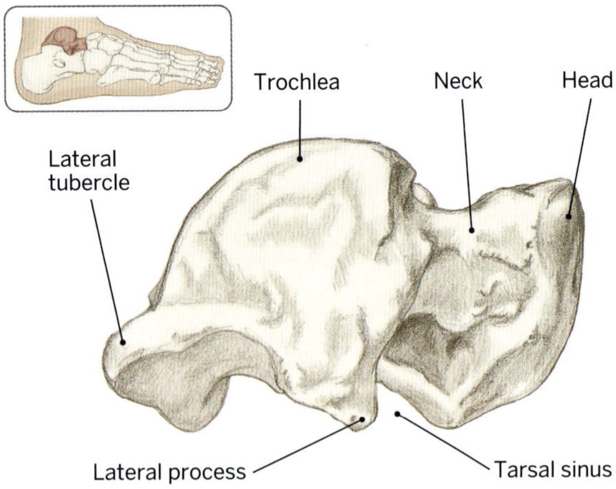

7.39 Lateral view of right talus

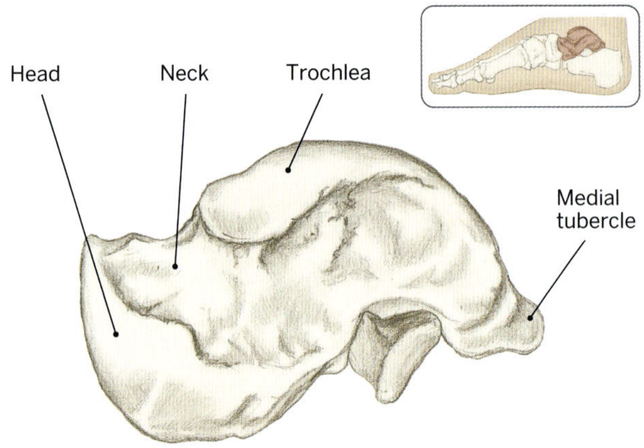

7.40 Medial view of right talus

Discover More

The calcaneus, talus, and cuboid bones are all roughly cube-shaped. The soldiers of ancient Rome used these bones (probably from horses) to carve out playing dice. For this reason, the talus is sometimes called the astragalus, which in Latin means *die*, the singular form of the plural *dice*.

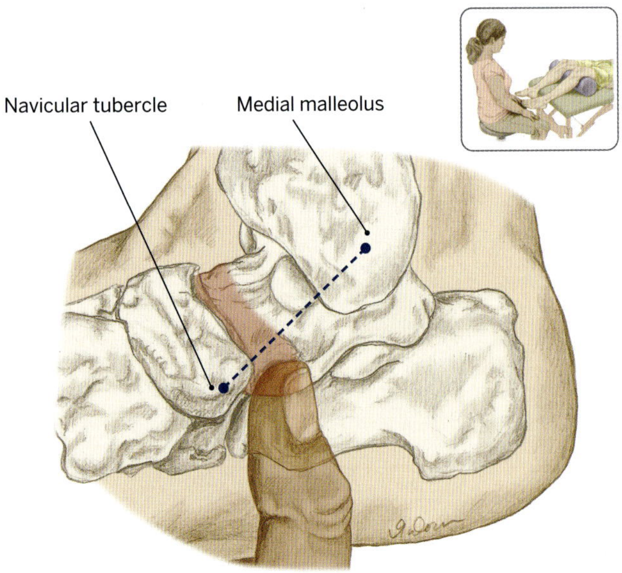

7.41 Medial view of right ankle, as you draw a line between the navicular tubercle and medial malleolus to access the head of the talus

Head of the talus

1. Partner supine or seated, with the ankle in a neutral position. Locate the navicular tubercle (p. 369).
2. Slide proximally off the tubercle to the head of the talus. The head may feel like a depression in comparison to the tubercle.
3. Passively invert and evert the foot to distinguish clearly between these two landmarks. When the foot is inverted, the navicular tubercle will become more prominent; when the foot is everted, the talar head will be more pronounced.

*If you draw a line between the medial malleolus and navicular tubercle, the head of the talus will be located along that line (**7.41**).*

talus	***ta**-lus*	L. ankle
trochlea	***trok**-lee-ah*	Grk. pulley

Trochlea of the talus

1. Partner supine. Passively invert and plantar flex the foot.
2. Draw a horizontal line connecting the malleoli and drop inferiorly off the center of the line, looking for a bony prominence. The trochlea will be deep to the overlying tendons and more prominent near the lateral malleolus (**7.42**).

Is the tissue you are palpating hard and immovable like bone, or firm and mobile like tendon? If you passively move the foot back to neutral, does the bony mound you are palpating seem to disappear into the ankle?

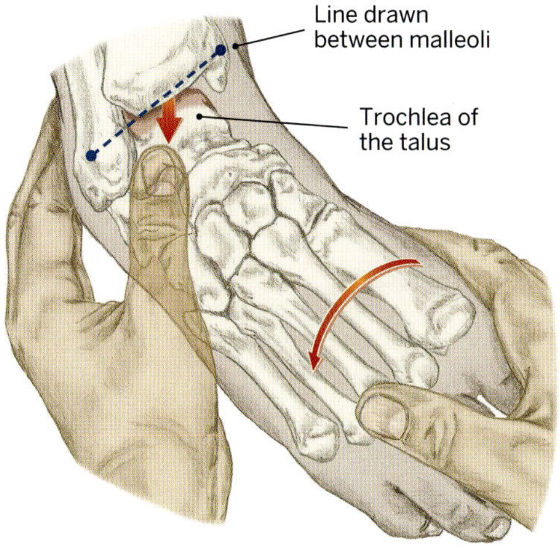

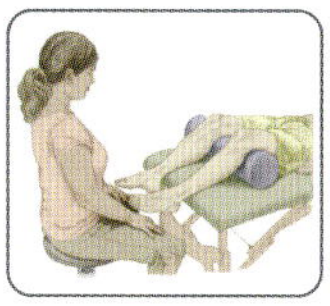

7.42 Dorsal/lateral view of right foot, with foot inverted and plantar flexed, as you locate the trochlea

Medial tubercle

1. Partner supine. Locate the medial malleolus. Instead of sliding straight distally for the sustentaculum tali (see **7.37**), slide posteriorly just off the malleolus at a 45° angle to locate the medial tubercle (**7.43**).
2. Passively dorsiflex and plantar flex the ankle, noting how the tubercle seems to slide around the malleolus.

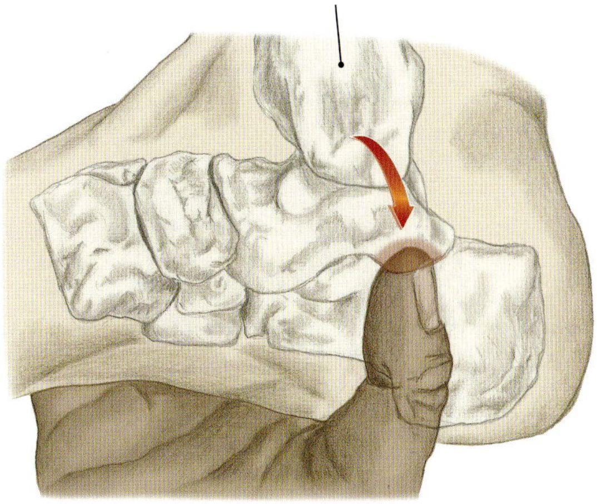

7.43 Medial view of right foot, as you contact the medial tubercle

Trail 2 Little Piggies

Hallux

The hallux (big toe) is composed of two phalanges. The joint between the phalanges, the interphalangeal, is a hinge joint wrapped in supportive ligaments. The first metatarsophalangeal joint is located at the ball of the foot. It is an ellipsoid joint with a large, bulbous shape.

Hallux

1. Partner seated or supine. Palpate the entire surface of the first toe, noting the differences in thickness and texture between its dorsal and plantar surfaces (**7.44**).
2. Explore the surface of each joint by passively moving it through its range of motion.

Is the proximal phalanx nearly twice as long as its distal counterpart?

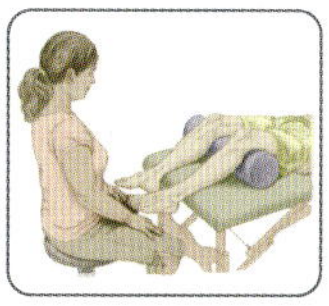

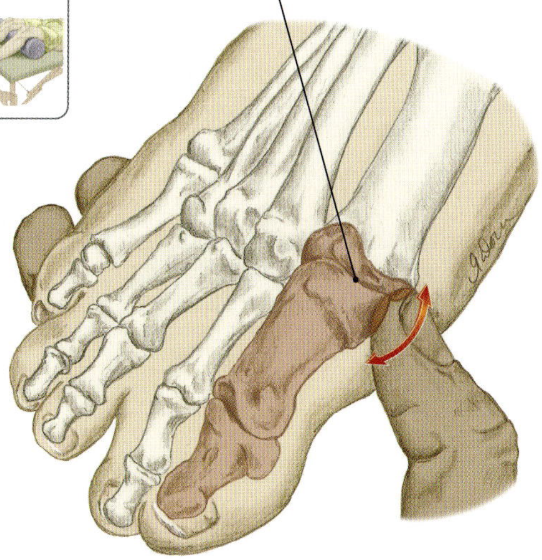

7.44 Dorsal/medial view of right foot, as you palpate the hallux

Leg & Foot

First Metatarsal

Unlike the long, slender metatarsals of toes two through five, the first metatarsal is short and stocky. Its dorsal and medial sides are superficial and easily accessible; its plantar surface is deep to several thick muscles (**7.45**). The proximal end of the first metatarsal flares to articulate with the medial cuneiform. This articulation often forms a visible crest on the top of the foot that can be irritated by wearing tight shoes.

First metatarsal

1. Partner seated or supine. Locate the metatarsal shaft along the medial side of the foot.
2. Explore the shaft's size and length by sliding across its entire surface. Palpate the junction and crest at the metatarsal head and medial cuneiform (**7.46**).

Are the head and base broader than the shaft of the metatarsal? Can you feel the cylindrical shape of the shaft?

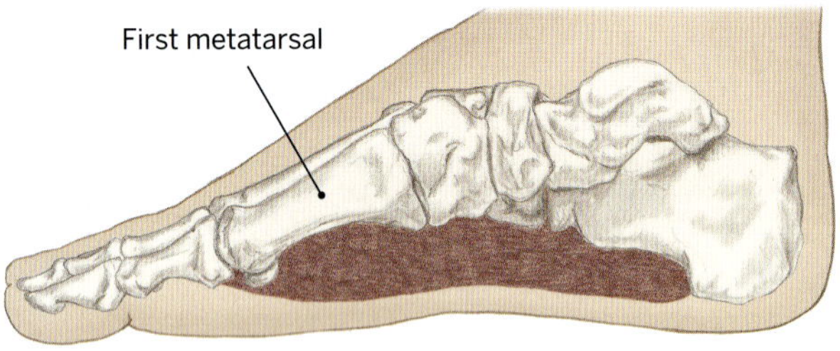

7.45 Medial view of right foot, shaded area indicating muscle mass along the foot's plantar surface

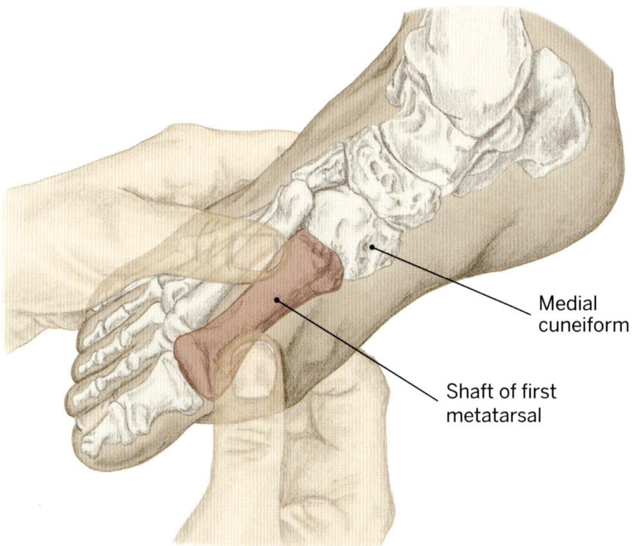

7.46 Dorsal/medial view of right foot, as you explore the first metatarsal

Second through Fifth Digits (Toes)

Unlike the hallux, the second through fifth toes contain three phalanges each. In each toe there are two articulations, the **p**roximal **i**nter**p**halangeal (or "**pip**" joint) and the **d**istal **i**nter**p**halangeal (or "**dip**" joint).

Toes

Partner seated or supine. Palpate along all surfaces of the toes, noting the thin tissue along their inner sides. Explore one toe at a time, slowly moving each one through its range of motion (**7.47**).

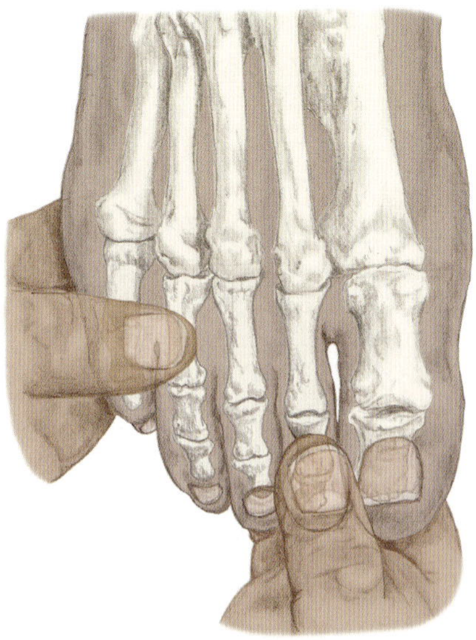

7.47 Dorsal view of right foot, as you explore the phalanges

hallux	***hal**-uks*	L. first toe
hallucis	***hal**-ah-sis*	

Second through Fifth Metatarsals

Each of the long, slender bones of the second through fifth metatarsals has an enlarged base and head. The bases are set close together in articulation with the tarsals. The spaces between the metatarsals are filled with the small intrinsic muscles of the toes and are easily palpated on the dorsal surface of the foot.

The tuberosity of the fifth metatarsal is a superficial knob that extends laterally off the base of the metatarsal and is the attachment site for the fibularis brevis (p. 380).

Metatarsals

1. Partner seated or supine. Grasp the foot with both hands and palpate the head of each metatarsal on the dorsal side of the foot.
2. Use both thumb tips to explore the length of each bone and its surrounding spaces. Follow the shaft of each metatarsal proximally (**7.48**). Note how it widens to form the base of the metatarsal.

Tuberosity of the fifth metatarsal

1. Partner seated or supine. Locate the shaft of the fifth metatarsal.
2. Follow the shaft proximally to where the base bulges laterally (**7.49**). Explore the superficial shape of the tuberosity and its surrounding landmarks as it projects from the side of the foot.

When the ankle is dorsiflexed, are you roughly two inches distal (anterior) to the lateral malleolus? Is the tip you are palpating connected to the fifth metatarsal?

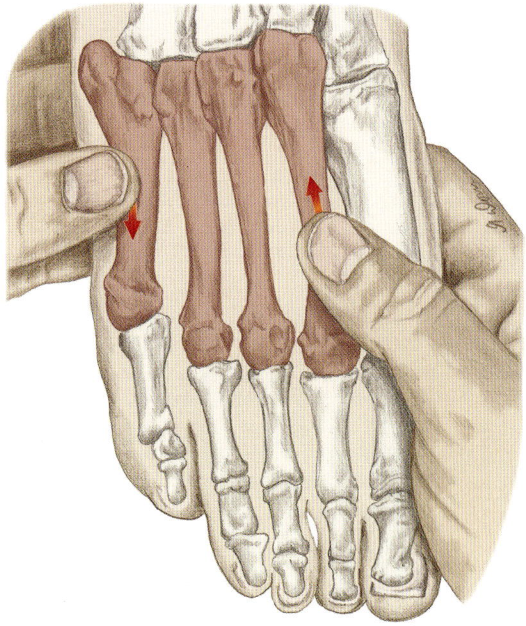

7.48 Dorsal view of right foot, as you explore the second through fifth metatarsals

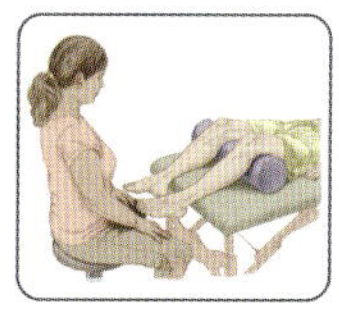

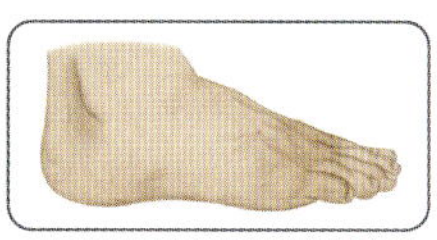

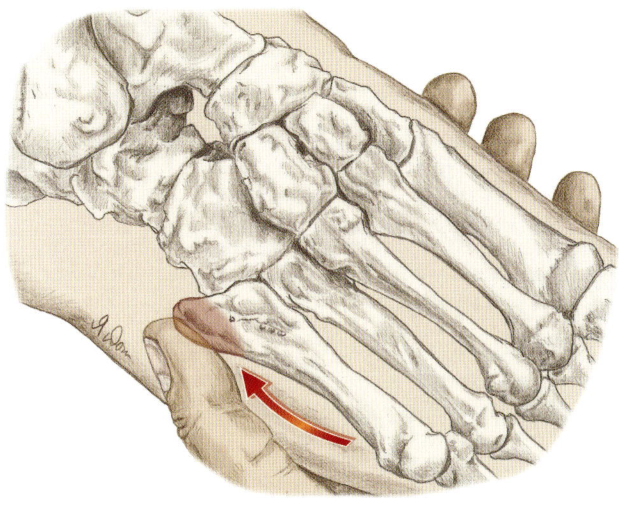

7.49 Dorsal/lateral view of right foot, as you access the tuberosity of the fifth metatarsal

Discover More

While strapping on shoes has certainly protected our feet and reduced the number of sprained ankles, it has also wreaked havoc on our arches. With the external support of shoes, our arches no longer need to adapt to varying terrain, and so the normally supportive musculature weakens. Eventually, the arch on the medial side of the foot collapses, resulting in a condition commonly known as flat foot.

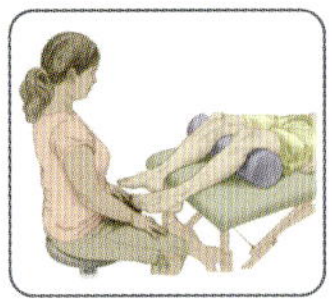

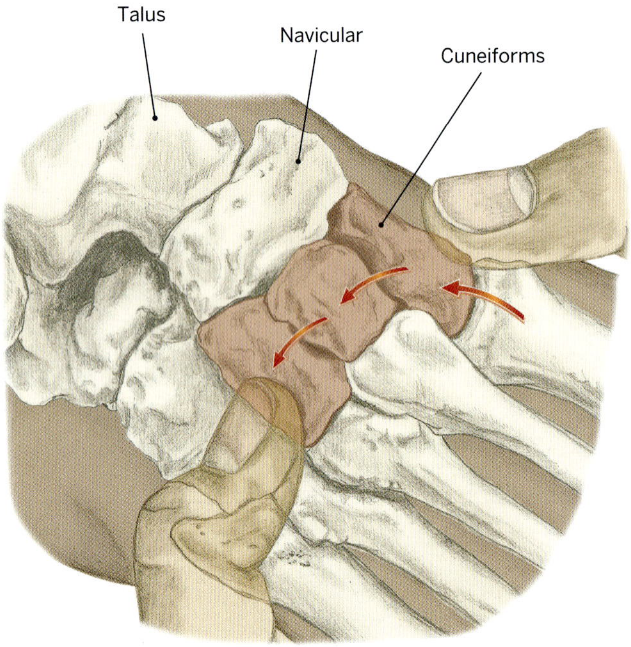

7.50 Dorsal/lateral view of right foot, as you explore the cuneiforms

Medial, Middle, and Lateral Cuneiforms

The three cuneiforms lie in a row between the navicular and metatarsals. The medial cuneiform serves as an attachment for the tibialis anterior and tibialis posterior muscles. It can be isolated along its dorsal and medial surfaces. The middle and lateral cuneiforms, sandwiched between the medial cuneiform and the cuboid, are accessible on their dorsal surfaces.

Cuneiforms

1. Partner seated or supine. Locate the base of the first metatarsal.
2. Glide proximally to the skinny ditch of the first tarsometatarsal joint. Continue proximally onto the surface of the medial cuneiform.
3. Slide laterally from the medial cuneiform along the dorsal surface of the foot and explore the surfaces of the middle and lateral cuneiforms (**7.50**).

Are you proximal to the base of the first metatarsal and can you isolate the joint between these two bones? If you follow the tibialis anterior tendon, does it lead to the same location at which you were palpating the medial cuneiform?

The tibialis anterior tendon (p. 382) runs superficially down the dorsal surface of the ankle and leads directly to the medial side of the medial cuneiform. Have your partner dorsiflex his foot, and follow the tendon distally as it blends into the medial cuneiform.

Comparative Anatomy

Mammals such as cats and dogs are called digitigrades, meaning they walk on their toes (digits). When digitigrades are standing, their tarsals and metatarsals are off the ground, forming what appears to be the leg. For this reason, the ankle of a dog or cat is often mistaken for the knee, while the actual knee appears to be hyperextended.

Digitigrades are raised up on their toes this way for additional height. The extra height enhances sensory perception and increases stride length.

Hooved animals, call unguligrades, go a step further than digitigrades in lifting themselves up on all their phalanges except the distal one. With this wide, four-point stance, these animals literally walk on the tips of their toes all the time.

Walking "tippy-toe" will quickly tell you that neither of these designs work for humans. We are plantigrades, meaning we walk on the soles of our feet. As we are also bipeds, we must spread our feet out, pressing all of our foot bones firmly on the ground in order to keep our balance.

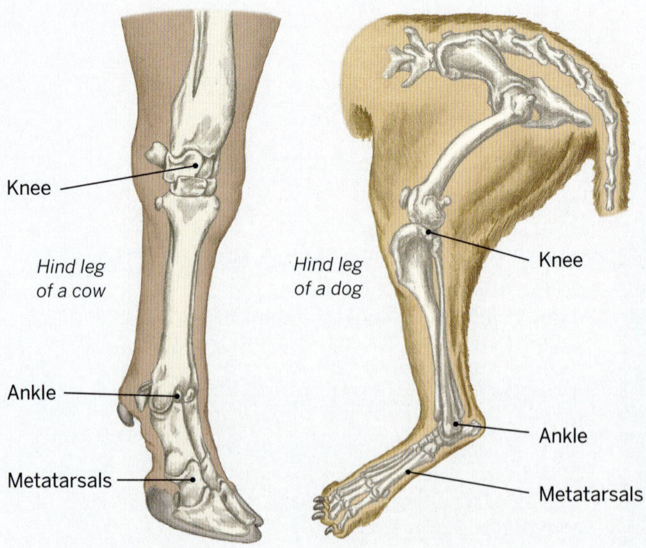

cuneiform ku-*ne*-i-form L. *cuneus*, wedge-shaped

Navicular

The bean-shaped navicular is sandwiched between the medial and middle cuneiforms and the talus. Its dorsal and medial surfaces are superficial and palpable. The superficial tuberosity bulges out of the medial side of the foot and is an attachment site for the tibialis posterior muscle (p. 385) and the spring ligament (p. 405).

Navicular

1. Partner seated or supine. Locate the base of the first metatarsal.
2. Sliding along the foot's medial side, move proximally across the surface of the medial cuneiform and the slender joint between the medial cuneiform and the navicular.
3. As you move onto the surface of the navicular, explore the shape and size of the navicular tuberosity (**7.51**). The tuberosity will lie approximately one to two inches distal to the medial malleolus.

Does the bone you are palpating project more medially than the surfaces of the other bones on the medial foot? If you place a finger on the tuberosity of the fifth metatarsal and the navicular tuberosity simultaneously, does the metatarsal tuberosity lie slightly distal to the navicular tuberosity? (See box to the right.)

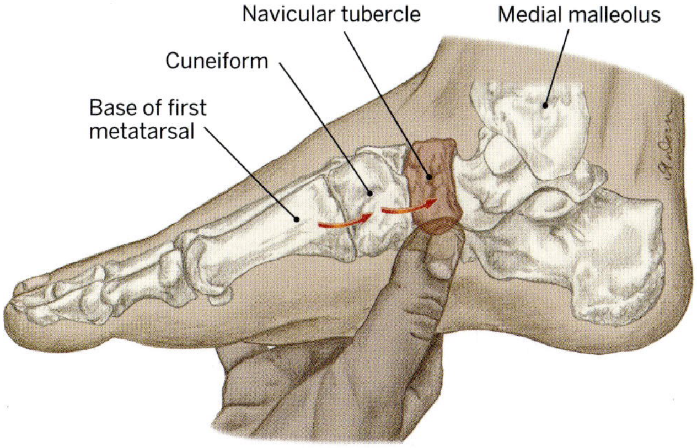

7.51 Medial view of right foot, as you locate the navicular tuberosity

Palpation Plus

The tuberosity of the fifth metatarsal (**a**) and the navicular tubercle (**b**) can be helpful landmarks. Palpate both structures and notice how the tuberosity of the fifth metatarsal is further distal than the navicular.

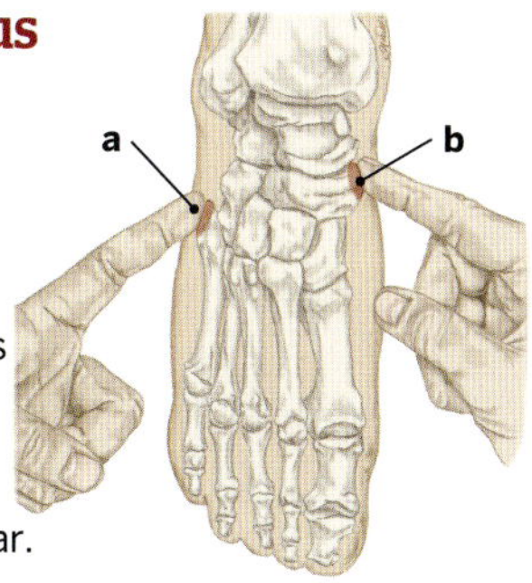

Cuboid

As the translation of its name suggests, the cuboid is cube-shaped. It is surrounded on three of its four sides by the fourth and fifth metatarsals, the lateral cuneiform, and the calcaneus. The cuboid's dorsal surface is partially covered by the belly of the extensor digitorum brevis (p. 391). Because of its cramped location and the covering of the brevis, the cuboid is only partially accessible.

Cuboid

1. Partner seated or supine. Draw an imaginary line from the tuberosity of the fifth metatarsal to the lateral malleolus.
2. Following this line, the cuboid is roughly half an inch from the tuberosity (**7.52**).

Are you proximal to the tuberosity of the fifth metatarsal? With the foot dorsiflexed, are you roughly an inch dorsal/distal to the lateral malleolus?

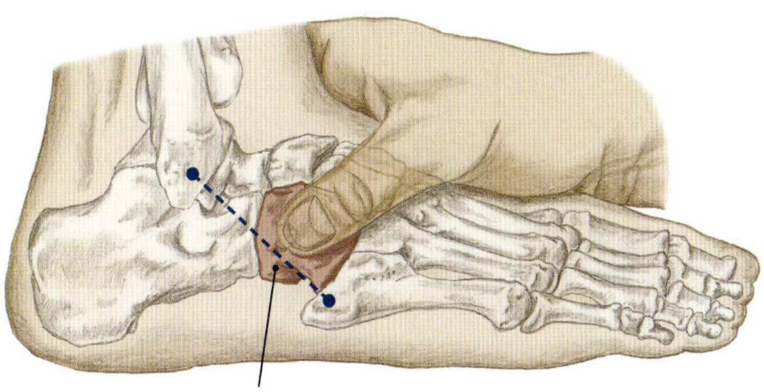

7.52 Lateral view of right foot, as you draw a line between the lateral malleolus and tuberosity of fifth metatarsal to access the cuboid

navicular	na-***vik***-u-lar	L. boat-shaped
cuboid	***ku***-boyd	Grk. cube-shaped

Overview: **Muscles of the Leg and Foot**

Like the forearm and hand, the leg and foot feature numerous muscles (**7.53–7.59**). Most are directly or partially accessible, and their names reveal a great deal about their actions. Most of the muscles of the leg can be divided into four groups:

a. The large **gastrocnemius** and **soleus** form the calf muscles of the posterior leg.
b. The **fibularis longus and brevis** are slender muscles located along the lateral side of the leg.
c. The **extensors** of the ankle and toes (tibialis anterior, extensor digitorum longus, and extensor hallucis longus) are layered together on the anterior leg and the dorsum of the foot.
d. The small **flexors** of the ankle and toes include tibialis posterior, flexor digitorum longus, and flexor hallucis longus. They are deep to the gastrocnemius and soleus on the posterior leg.

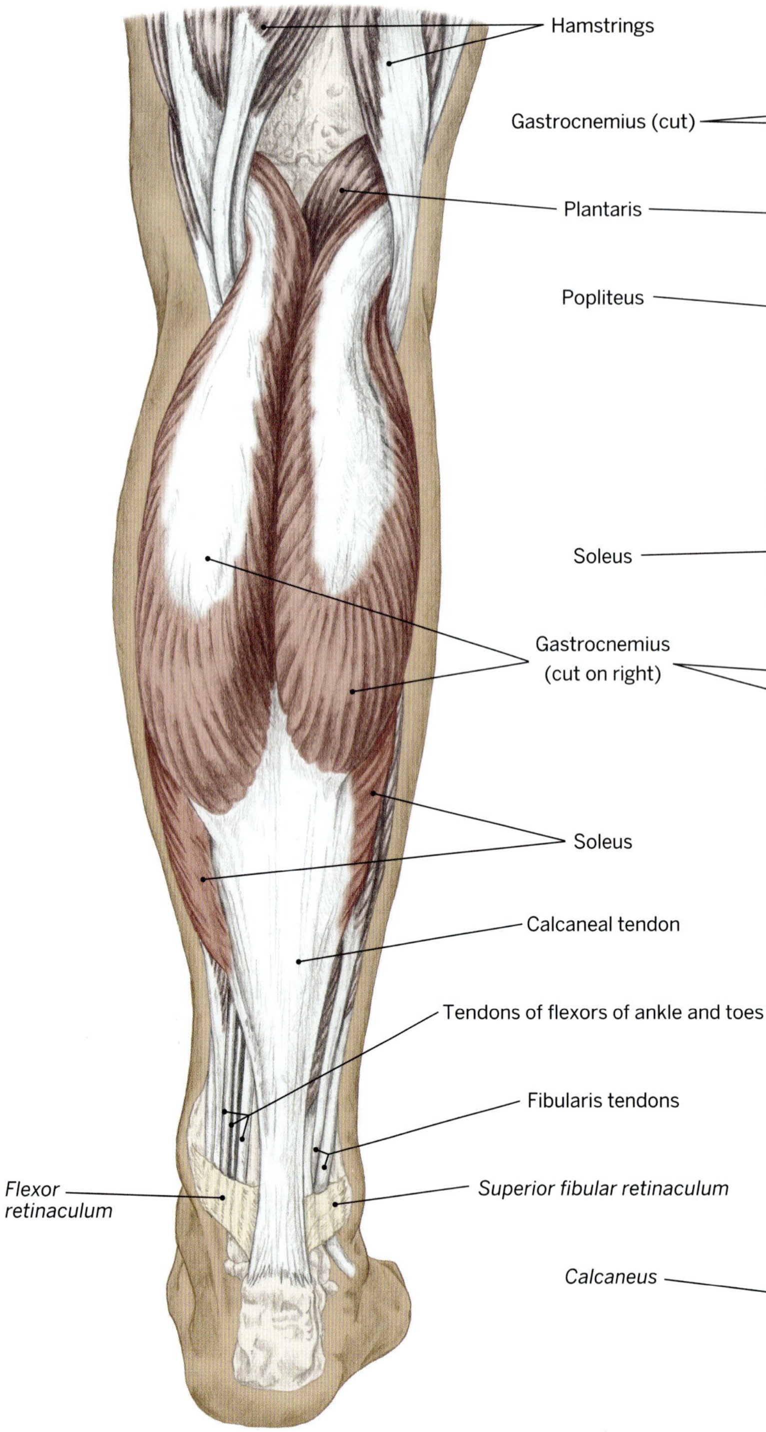

7.53 Posterior view of right leg, showing superficial muscles

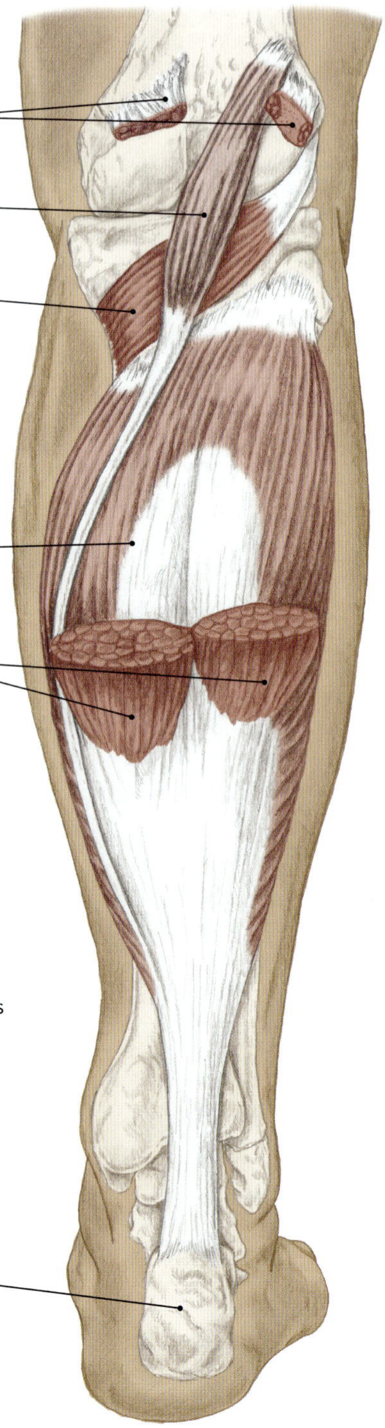

7.54 Posterior view of right leg, showing deeper muscles

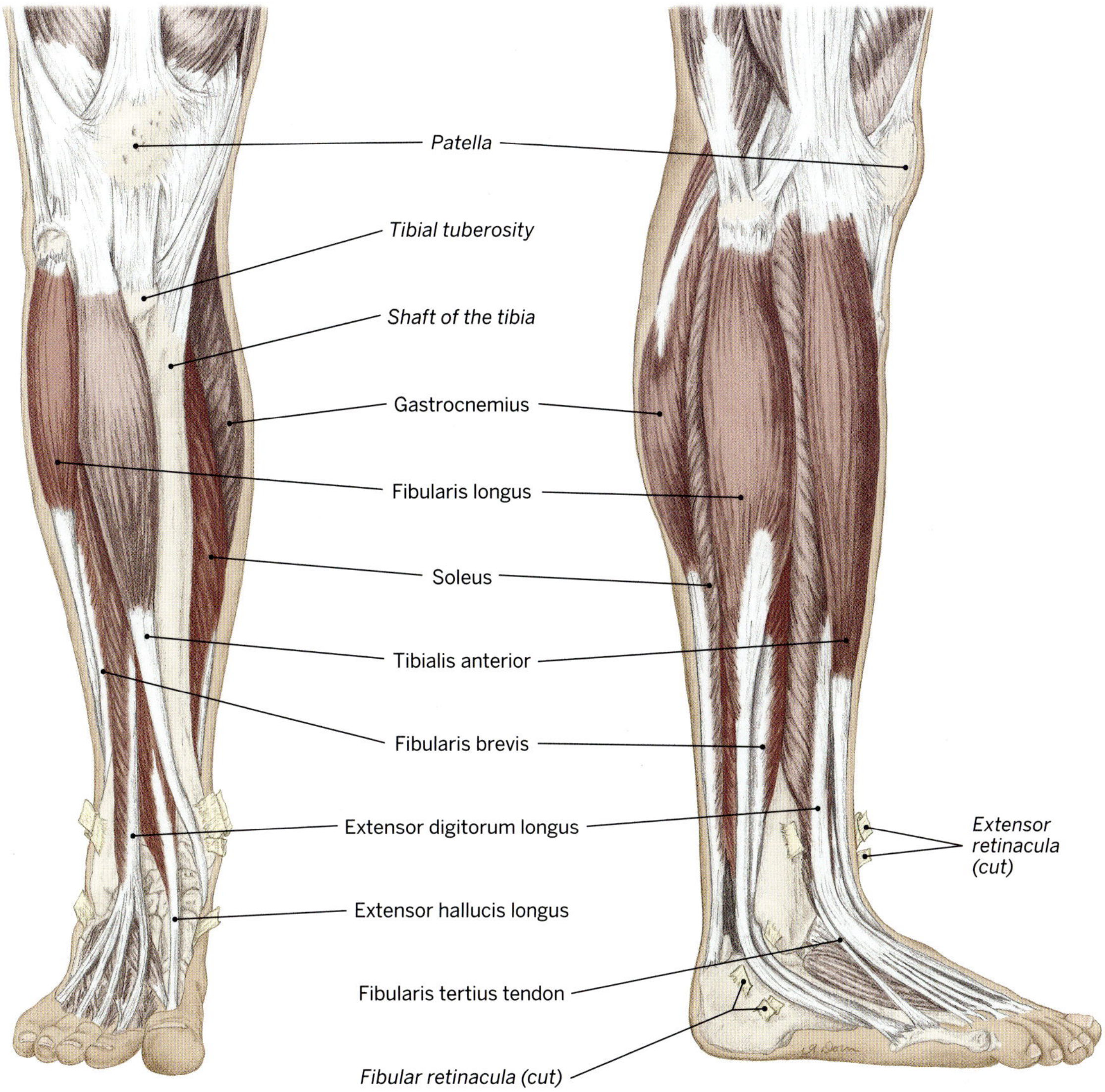

7.55 Anterior view of muscles of right leg and foot

7.56 Lateral view of muscles of right leg and foot

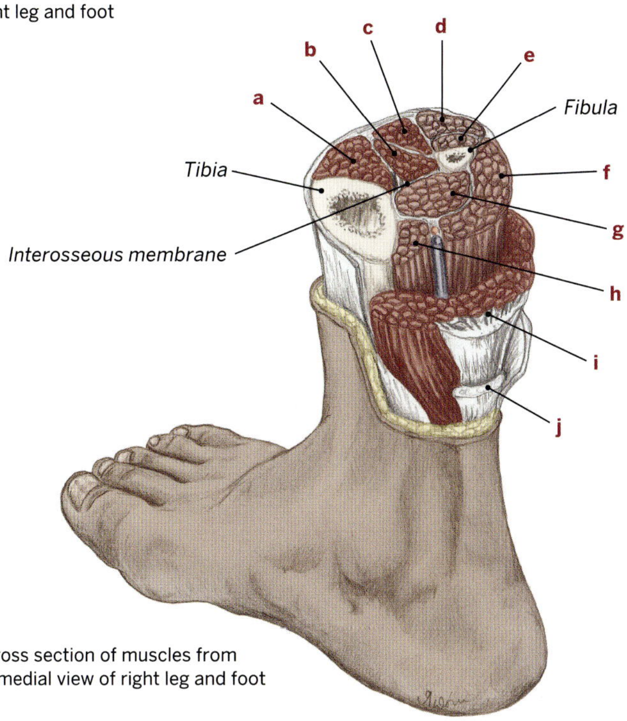

- **a.** Tibialis anterior
- **b.** Extensor hallucis longus
- **c.** Extensor digitorum longus
- **d.** Fibularis longus
- **e.** Fibularis brevis
- **f.** Flexor hallucis longus
- **g.** Tibialis posterior
- **h.** Flexor digitorum longus
- **i.** Soleus
- **j.** Calcaneal tendon

7.57 Cross section of muscles from posterior/medial view of right leg and foot

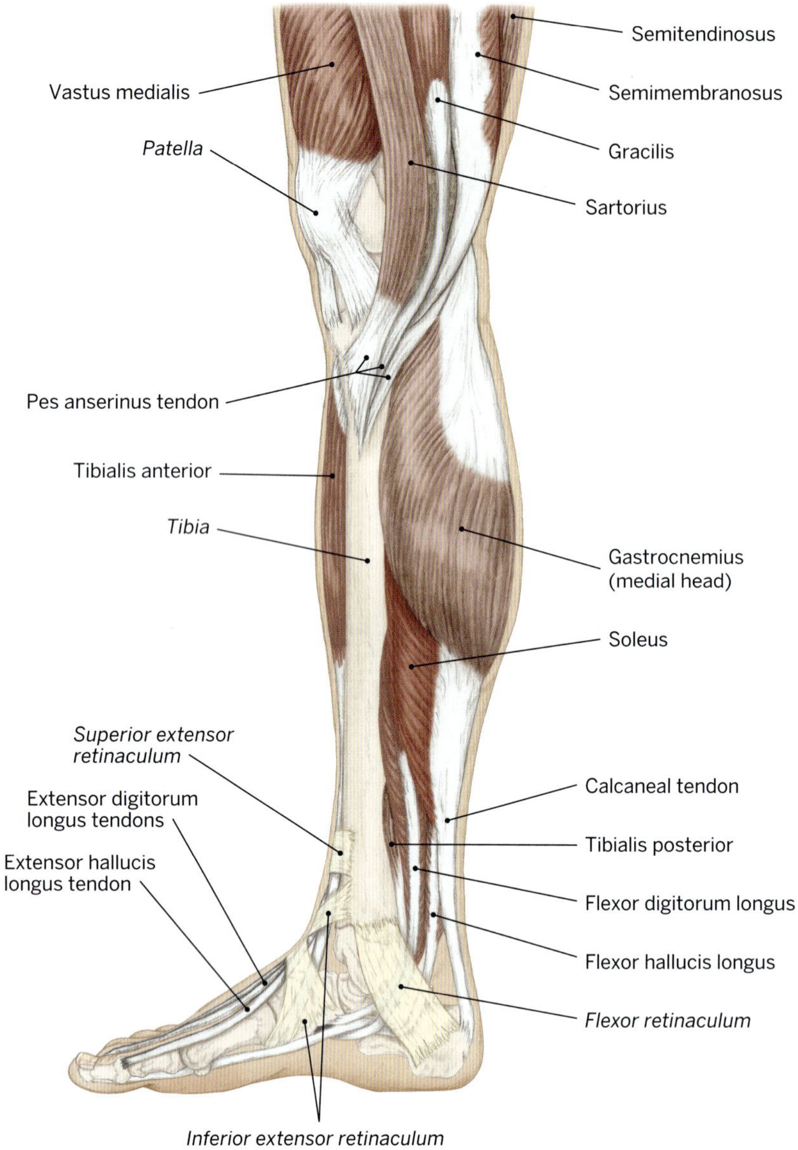

7.58 Medial view of right knee, leg, and foot, showing superficial layer of muscles and tendons

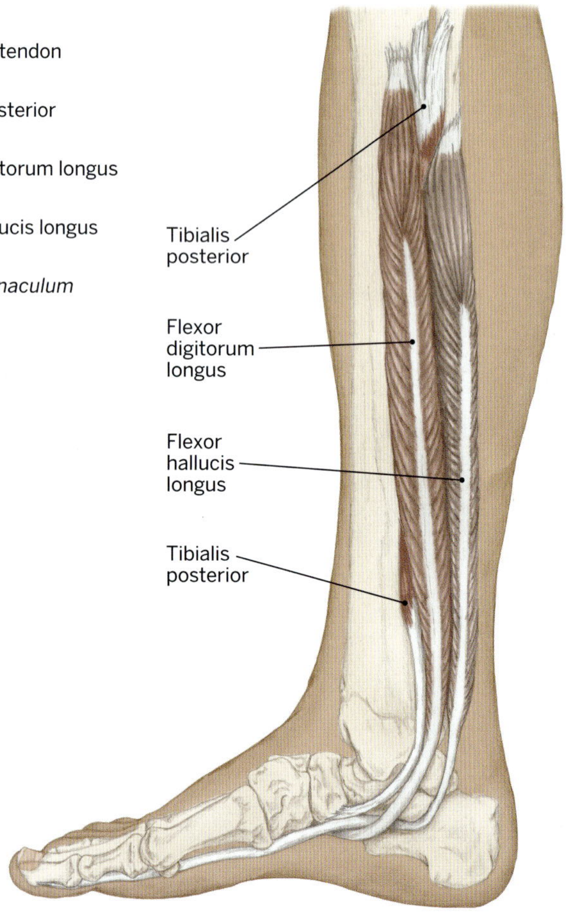

7.59 Medial view of right leg and foot, showing deep layer of muscles

Synergists—Muscles Working Together

Muscles are listed in the order of their ability to create the movement. Asterisk indicates muscles not shown.

Ankle

(talocrural joint)

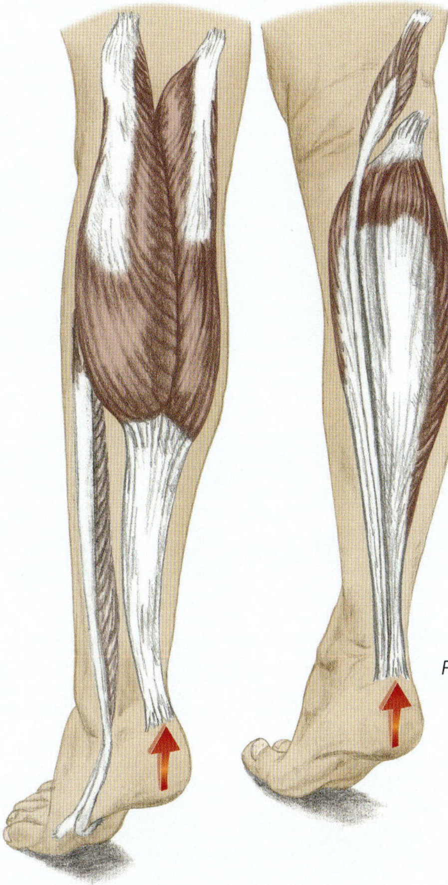

7.60 Plantar flexion of the ankles

Plantar Flexion

(antagonists on dorsiflexion)

Gastrocnemius
Soleus
Tibialis posterior
Fibularis longus (assists)
Fibularis brevis (assists)
Flexor digitorum longus (weak)
Flexor hallucis longus (weak)
Plantaris (weak)

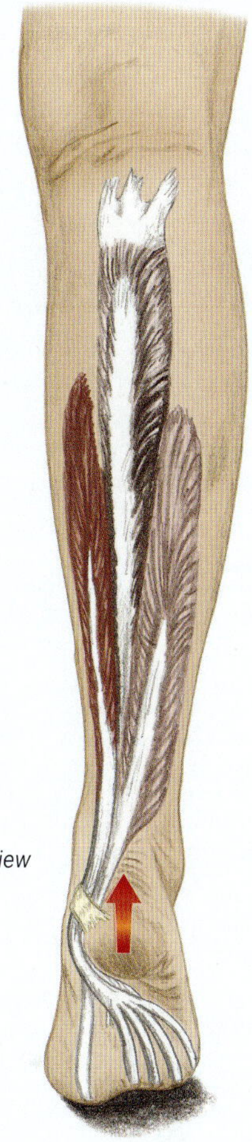

7.61 Plantar flexion of the ankle

Dorsiflexion

(antagonists on plantar flexion)

Tibialis anterior
Extensor digitorum longus
Extensor hallucis longus

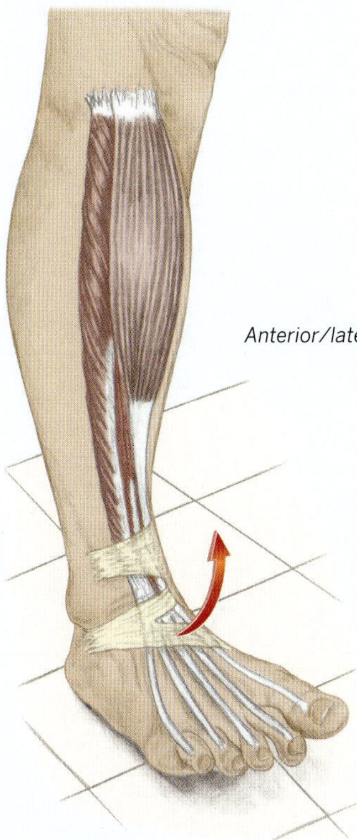

7.62 Dorsiflexion of the ankle

Foot and Toes

(talotarsal, midtarsal, tarsometatarsal,metatarsophalangeal, proximal and distal interphalangeal joints)

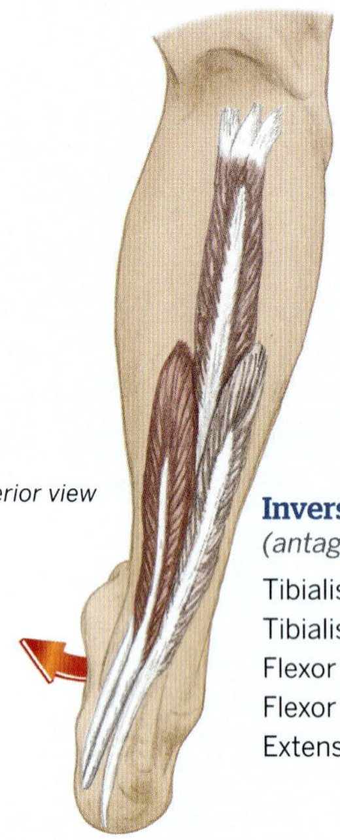

Inversion
(antagonists on eversion)

Tibialis anterior
Tibialis posterior
Flexor digitorum longus
Flexor hallucis longus
Extensor hallucis longus

7.63 Inversion of the foot

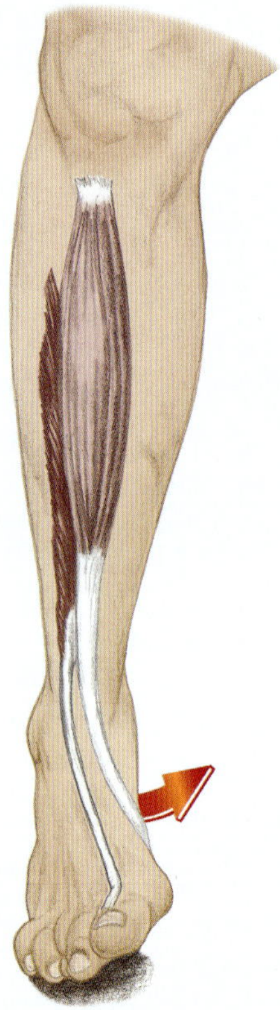

7.64 Inversion of the foot

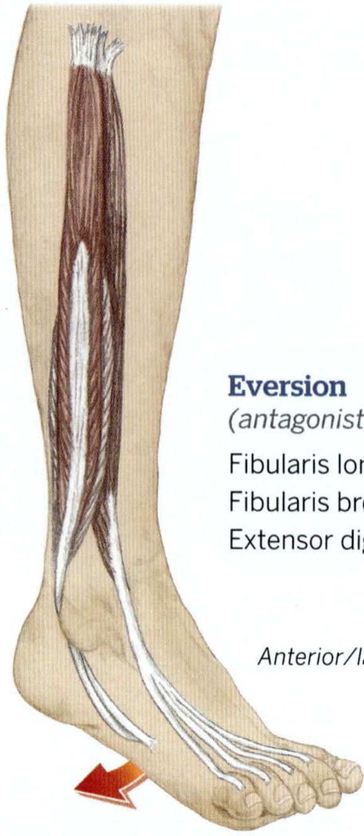

Eversion
(antagonists on inversion)

Fibularis longus
Fibularis brevis
Extensor digitorum longus

7.65 Eversion of the foot

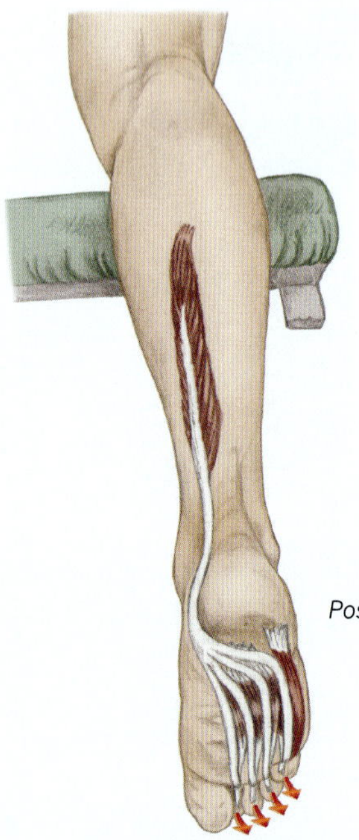

Flexion of Second through Fifth Toes
(antagonists on extension of toes)

Flexor digitorum longus
Flexor digitorum brevis
Lumbricals*
Quadratus plantae (assists)*
Dorsal interossei (2nd–4th)*
Plantar interossei (3rd–5th)*
Abductor digiti minimi (5th)
Flexor digiti minimi brevis (5th)*

7.66 Flexion of second through fifth toes

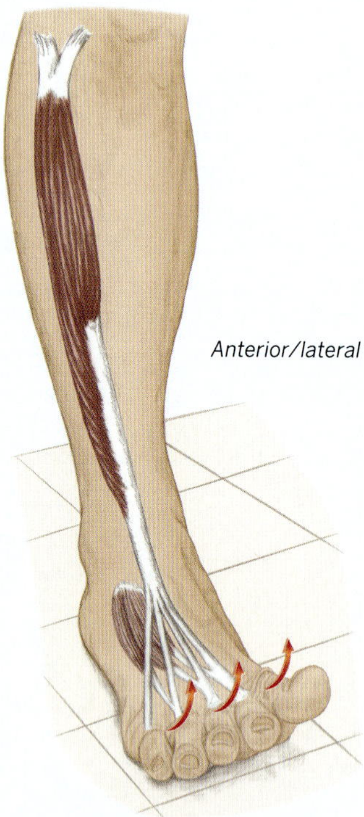

Extension of Second through Fifth Toes
(antagonists on flexion of toes)

Extensor digitorum longus
Extensor digitorum brevis (2nd–4th)
Lumbricals*

7.67 Extension of second through fifth toes

See p. 433 for a list of muscles performing flexion, extension, abduction, and adduction of the toes.

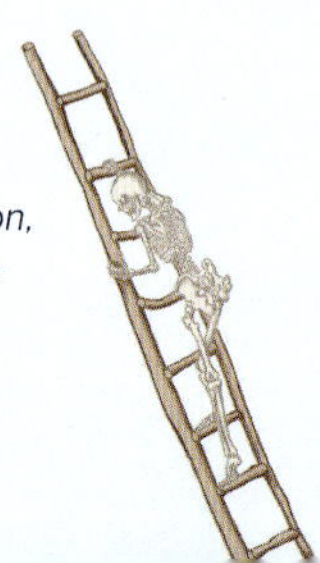

Leg & Foot
SYNERGISTS

Muscles of the Leg and Foot

Gastrocnemius and Soleus ▶

The large muscle mass of the posterior leg is composed of the gastrocnemius and the soleus muscles. Together they form what is known as the triceps surae, which attaches to the strong calcaneal (Achilles) tendon. Both the gastrocnemius and soleus are easily accessible.

The superficial **gastrocnemius** has two heads and crosses two joints—the knee and ankle (**7.68**, **7.69**). Emerging from between the hamstring tendons, the short gastrocnemius heads extend halfway down the leg before blending into the calcaneal tendon. Although its name (Greek for "belly of the leg") suggests that the gastrocnemius is rotund, it is actually quite thin when compared to the thick soleus.

The **soleus** is deep to the gastrocnemius, yet its medial and lateral fibers bulge from the sides of the leg and extend further distal than the gastrocnemius heads (**7.69**, **7.70**). The soleus is sometimes called the "second heart" because of the important role its strong contractions play in returning blood from the leg to the heart.

GASTROCNEMIUS

A	**Flex** the knee (tibiofemoral joint) **Plantar flex** the ankle (talocrural joint)
O	Condyles of the femur, posterior surfaces
I	Calcaneus via calcaneal tendon
N	Tibial S**1**, **2**

When Do You Use Your Gastrocnemius?

- Peeking over a fence (standing on your toes)
- Walking, running, climbing—virtually all forms of ambulation

SOLEUS

A	**Plantar flex** the ankle (talocrural joint)
O	Soleal line; proximal, posterior surface of tibia; and posterior aspect of head of fibula
I	Calcaneus via calcaneal tendon
N	Tibial L5, S**1**, **2**

When Do You Use Your Soleus?

- Carrying a heavy backpack up a steep hill (plantar flexion with strength and balance)
- Pedaling your bike up the grueling hairpin turns of L'Alpe d'Huez in France

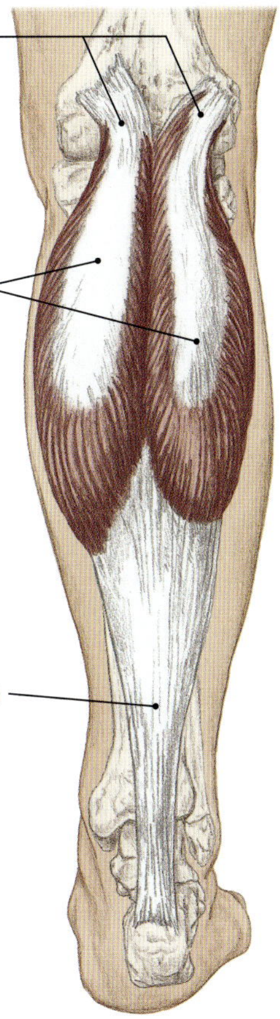

7.68 Posterior view of right leg, showing gastrocnemius

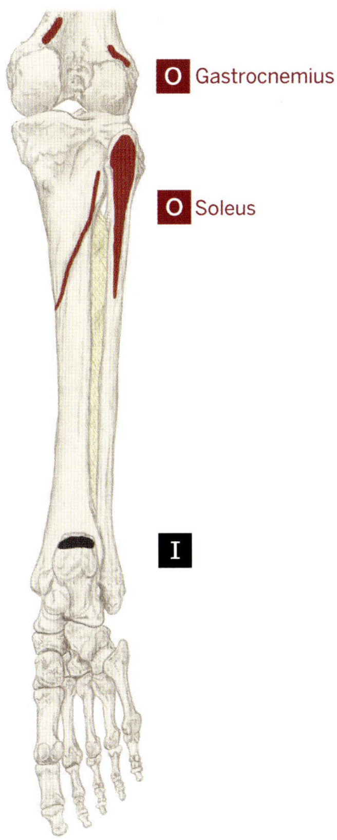

7.69 Posterior view of right leg with foot plantar flexed, showing origins and insertions of gastrocnemius and soleus

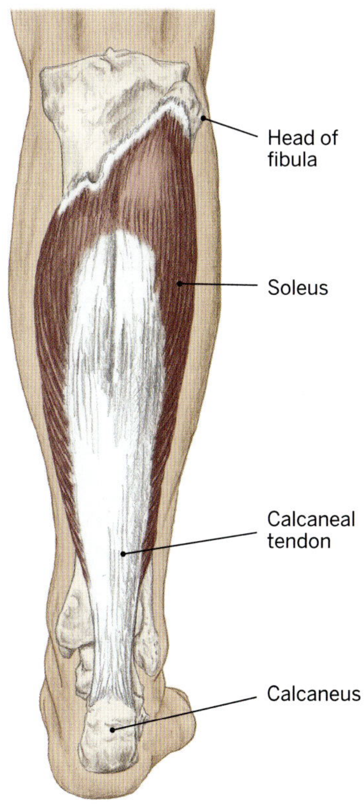

7.70 Posterior view of right leg with gastrocnemius removed, showing soleus

gastrocnemius	***gas***-trok-***ne***-me-us	Grk. *gaster*, stomach + *kneme*, leg
soleus	so-***lay***-us	L. *solea*, as in a sole fish (right)

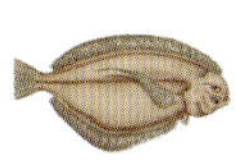

Gastrocnemius and soleus - standing #1

1. Ask your partner, supported by a chair, to stand on her toes.
2. Palpate the posterior leg, sculpting out the gastrocnemius's oval heads. Follow both heads proximally to the back of the knee. Then follow them distally, noting how the medial head extends further distal than the lateral head (**7.71**, **7.72**).
3. Move distal to the gastrocnemius and palpate the distal portion of the soleus. Also explore the medial and lateral sides of the soleus that bulge out from the gastrocnemius.
4. Follow both muscles distally as they blend into the calcaneal tendon.

Can you follow the gastrocnemius heads proximally between the hamstring tendons? Is the medial gastrocnemius head slightly longer than the lateral? Can you feel the difference in texture between the fleshy muscle bellies and the tough, dense calcaneal tendon?

Discover More

Why was the calcaneal tendon originally called the Achilles tendon? As a baby, the Greek mythological warrior Achilles was dipped in the River Styx by his mother to make him invulnerable. He was completely immersed except for the ankle by which she held him. After fighting in the Trojan War, Achilles was mortally wounded when an arrow penetrated his heel. Hence, "Achilles' heel" refers to a small but fatal weakness.

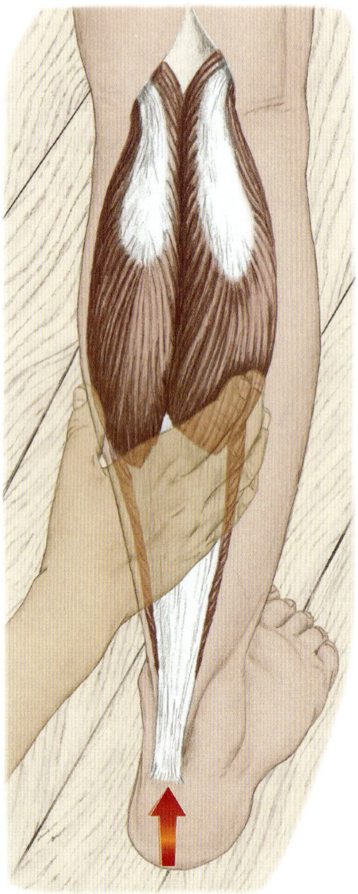

7.71 Partner raising her heel to stand up on her toes, as you sculpt out gastrocnemius

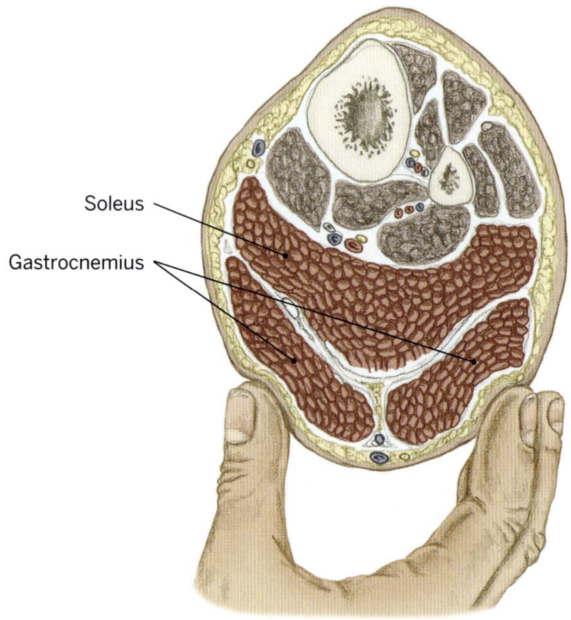

7.72 Superior view, cross section of right leg, as you palpate gastrocnemius

Gastrocnemius and soleus - standing #2

1. Although these muscles are located on the posterior leg, they are also accessible from an *anterior* direction. With your partner standing on her toes, locate the tibial shaft.
2. Slide medially off the shaft of the tibia and feel the wad of muscle that bulges along the medial side of the leg (**7.73**). This tissue is the triceps surae.
3. Ask your partner to lie supine and, with the tissue relaxed, note how your thumb can sink around the medial edge of the tibial shaft to specifically locate the soleus.

Gastrocnemius and soleus - prone

1. Partner prone. Bend the knee to 90° and investigate the soft, massive bellies of the gastrocnemius and soleus and the thick calcaneal tendon.
2. When the knee is flexed, the gastrocnemius muscle is shortened and ineffectual as a plantar flexor. Isolate the soleus by asking your partner to gently plantar flex against your resistance. Notice how the thick soleus contracts while the thin, superficial bellies of the gastrocnemius remain flaccid (**7.74**).

*Can you feel the difference in texture between the fleshy muscle bellies and the tough, dense calcaneal tendon (**7.75**)?*

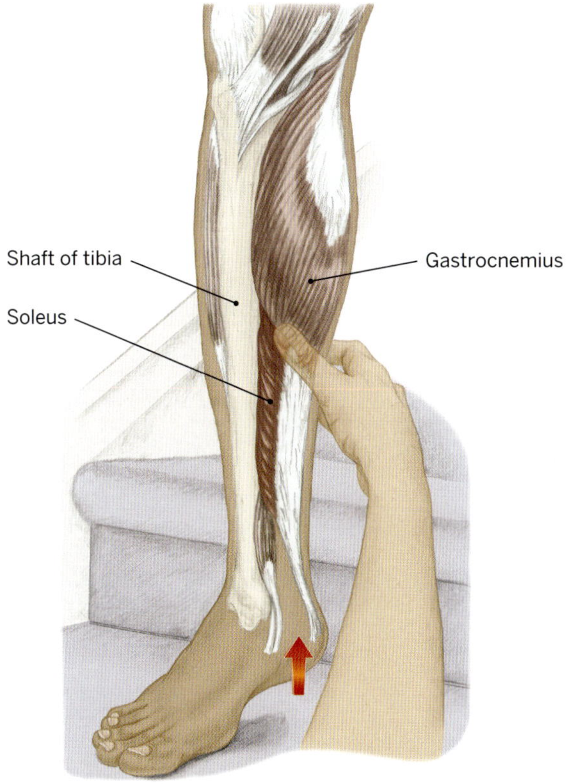

7.73 Partner raising her right heel, anterior/medial view of right leg, as you access gastrocnemius and soleus

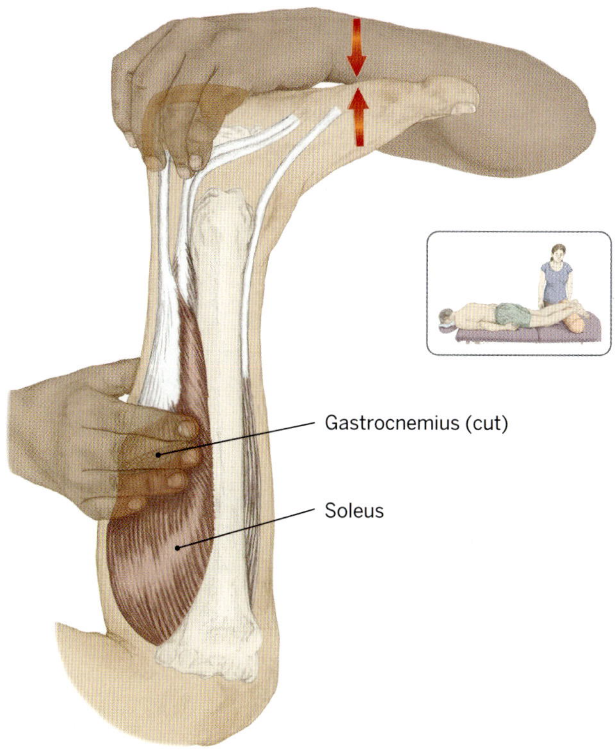

7.74 Partner prone with right knee flexed, medial view of right leg, as you isolate the soleus

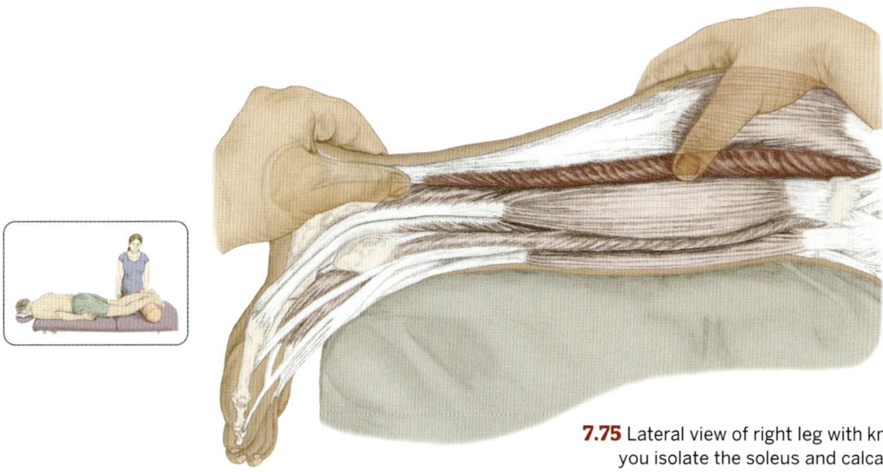

7.75 Lateral view of right leg with knee extended, as you isolate the soleus and calcaneal tendon

triceps surae *tri*-seps *sir*-eye L. three-headed muscle of the calf

Plantaris ▶

The plantaris has a short muscle belly but the longest tendon in the body. Its belly lies at an oblique angle along the popliteal space of the posterior knee between the gastrocnemius heads; its tendon extends down the length of the leg and attaches to the calcaneus (**7.76**). Although the plantaris belly is situated in a small, cramped area, it can be readily accessed.

From the standpoint of evolution, the plantaris is thought to be what remains of a larger plantar flexor of the foot. The plantaris of reptiles, which serves as an important muscle of propulsion, still retains much of the basic character of this older, larger flexor.

PLANTARIS	
A	Weak **plantar flexion** of the ankle (talocrural joint) Weak **flexion** of the knee (tibiofemoral joint)
O	Lateral supracondylar line of femur
I	Calcaneus via calcaneal tendon
N	Tibial L4, **5**, S**1**, (2)

When Do You Use Your Plantaris?

- Assists with actions of the gastrocnemius, such as bending your knee

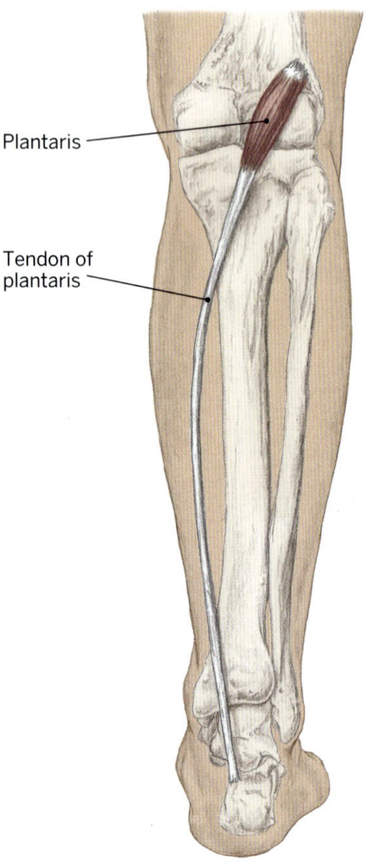

7.76 Posterior view of right leg, showing plantaris

Plantaris

1. Partner prone with the knee flexed. Locate the head of the fibula.
2. Move your thumb medial into the popliteal space between the gastrocnemius heads. (Sliding your thumb a little more proximally in the popliteal space will position it off the gastrocnemius heads.)
3. With your thumb between the gastrocnemius heads, slowly sink into the tissue of the posterior knee (**7.77**). Explore for an inch-wide belly that runs at an oblique angle from lateral to medial. When you believe you have located the plantaris, outline its shape by strumming your thumb across its belly.

Are you medial and proximal to the head of the fibula?
Are you accessing between the gastrocnemius heads?
Is the belly you are palpating one to two fingers wide with oblique fibers?

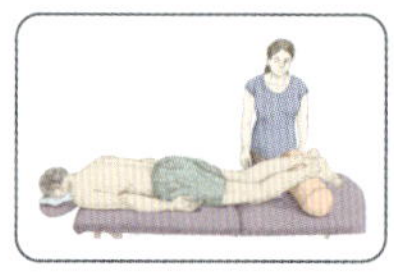

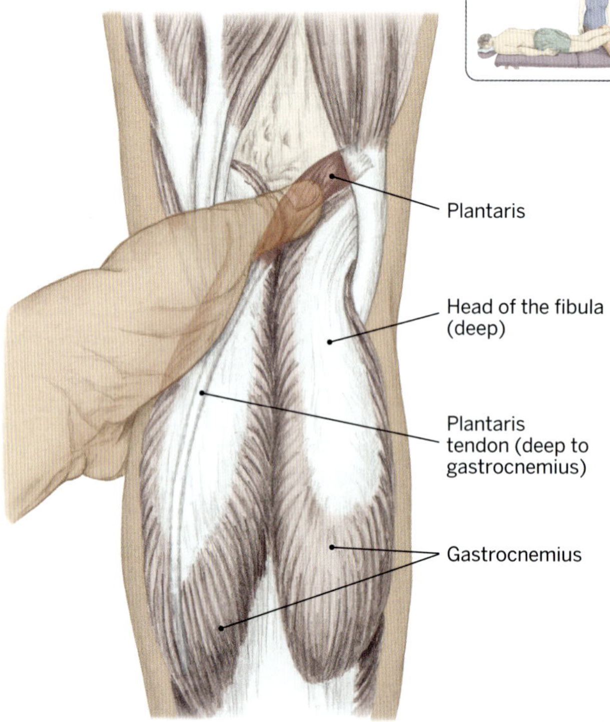

7.77 Posterior view of right knee, as you locate plantaris

Discover More

It is no mere coincidence that the plantaris of the leg bears a marked resemblance to the palmaris longus (p. 138) in the forearm: the two muscles have short bellies followed by long tendons, feature limited capabilities, and are absent in nearly 10% of the population.

plantaris plan-***tar***-is Fr. the sole of the foot

Popliteus ▶

As its name suggests, the popliteus is located in the popliteal space. This muscle has a small, short belly with diagonal fibers (**7.78**, **7.79**). Lying beneath the upper fibers of the gastrocnemius and plantaris, it is the deepest muscle of the posterior knee. Because of its depth, the popliteus is inaccessible; nevertheless, its tendinous insertion on the posterior tibia (**7.80**) can be palpated. Although the popliteus is a weak flexor of the knee, it is vital in "unlocking" the joint from an extended position; hence its nickname, "the key which unlocks the knee."

	POPLITEUS
A	**Medially rotate** the flexed knee (tibiofemoral joint) **Flex** the knee (T/F joint)
O	Lateral condyle of the femur
I	Proximal, posterior aspect of tibia
N	Tibial L4, **5**, S**1**

When Do You Use Your Popliteus?

- Walking, running, climbing

Popliteus

1. Partner prone with the knee flexed. Access a portion of the popliteus by locating the tibial tuberosity and sliding medially around the tibia to the posterior surface of its shaft.
2. Explore the posterior surface of the tibia for the popliteus tendon by pushing the overlying edge of the soleus and gastrocnemius muscles to the side (**7.81**).
3. Although the popliteus will not readily present itself as a palpable structure, if you are accessing the posterior region of the tibial shaft, you will be on its tendinous attachment.

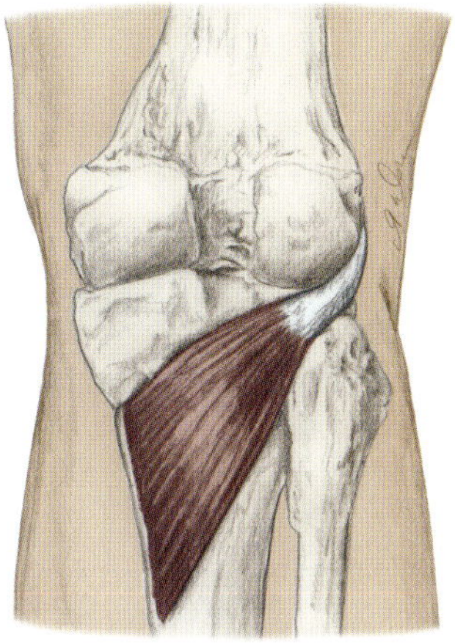

7.78 Posterior view of right knee, showing popliteus

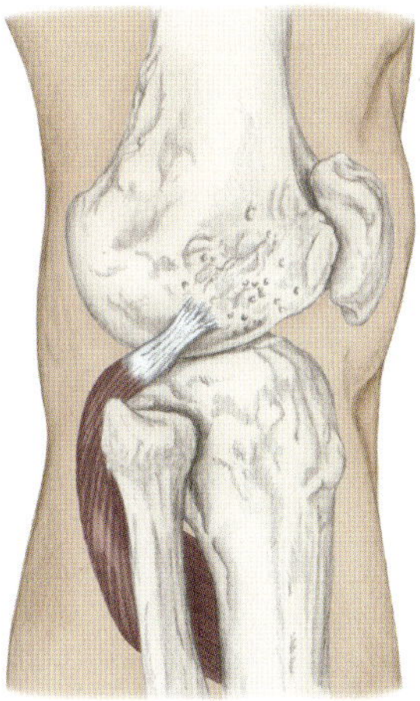

7.79 Lateral view of right knee, showing popliteus

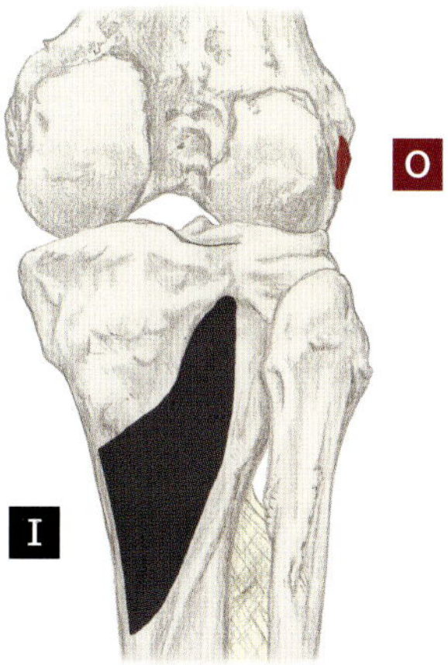

7.80 Posterior view of right knee, showing origin and insertion of popliteus

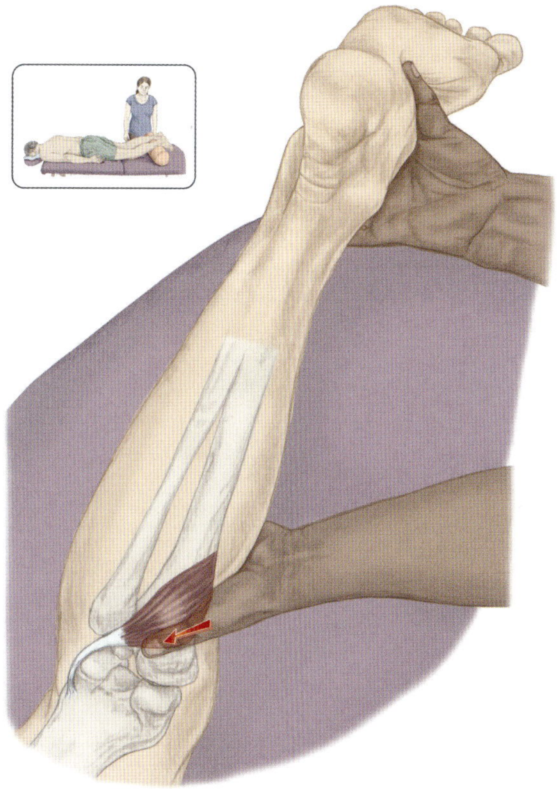

7.81 Posterior view of right knee, as you explore deep to gastrocnemius and soleus for the popliteus

popliteus pop-***lit***-e-us L. *poples*, ham of the knee

Fibularis Longus and Brevis ▶

Known also as the *peroneus longus* and *brevis*, the slender fibularis muscles are located on the lateral side of the fibula (**7.82–7.85**). More specifically, they lie between the extensor digitorum longus and the soleus. A portion of the fibularis brevis lies deep to the fibularis longus, yet both are accessible. Their distal tendons are superficial and palpable behind the lateral malleolus and along the side of the heel.

	FIBULARIS LONGUS
A	**Evert** the foot Assist to **plantar flex** the ankle (talocrural joint)
O	Head of fibula and proximal two-thirds of lateral fibula
I	Base of the first metatarsal and medial cuneiform
N	Superficial fibular L4, **5**, S**1**

When Do You Use Your Fibularis Longus?

- Scraping mud off the inside edge of your boot (eversion of the ankle)
- Hiking on a rocky trail (small, specific stabilizing movements of the foot)

	FIBULARIS BREVIS
A	**Evert** the foot Assist to **plantar flex** the ankle (talocrural joint)
O	Distal two-thirds of lateral fibula
I	Tuberosity of fifth metatarsal
N	Superficial fibular L4, **5**, S**1**

When Do You Use Your Fibularis Brevis?

- Hiking on a rocky trail (small, specific stabilizing movements of the foot)
- Ice skating or skate skiing (eversion occurring at the end of a stroke)

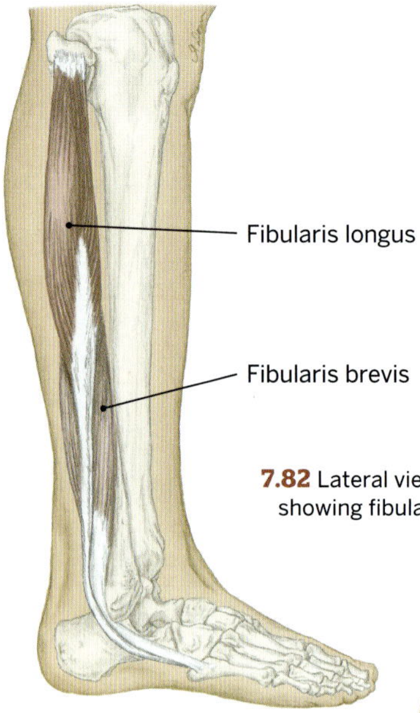

7.82 Lateral view of right leg and foot, showing fibularis longus and brevis

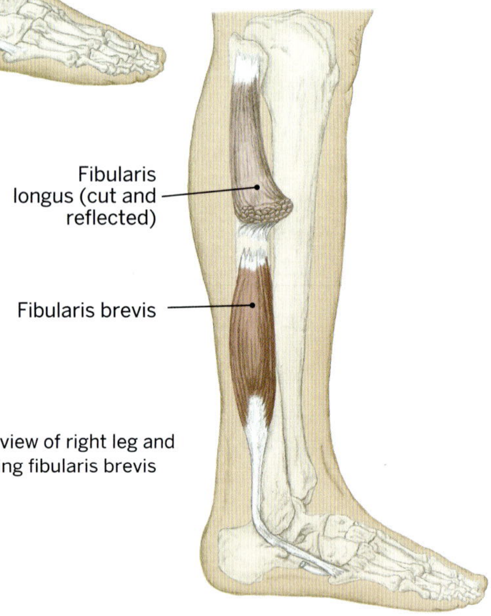

7.83 Lateral view of right leg and foot, showing fibularis brevis

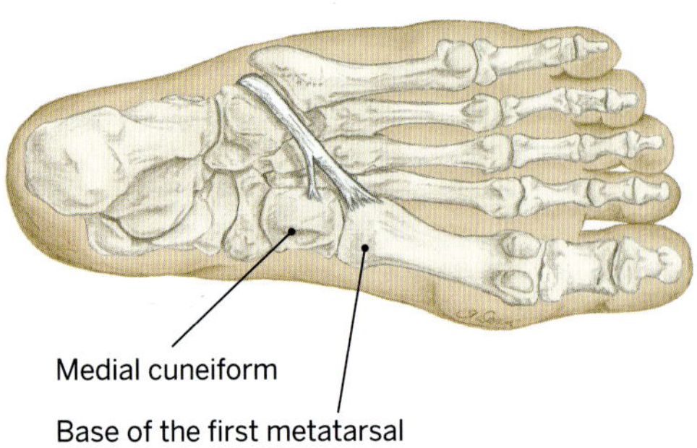

7.84 Plantar view of right foot, showing fibularis longus tendon

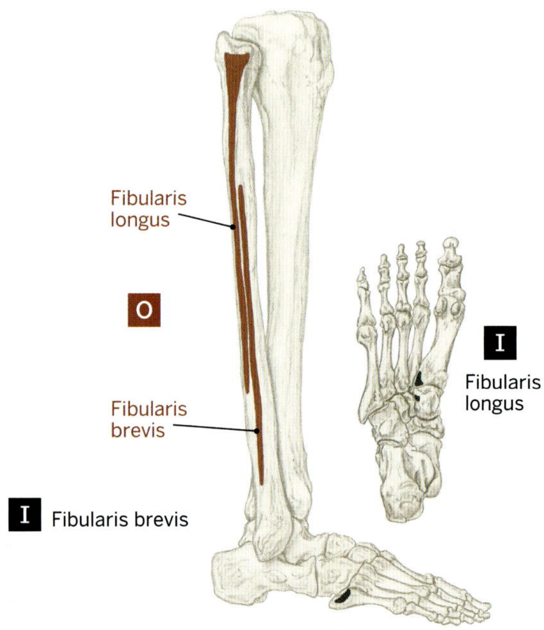

7.85 Lateral view of right leg and foot, showing origins and insertions of fibularis longus and brevis

fibularis ***fib***-u-***lar***-is L. pin or buckle

Leg & Foot

Fibulares

1. Partner side lying. Place a finger at the head of the fibula and the lateral malleolus. The fibularis bellies are located between these two landmarks (**7.86**).
2. Lay your fingers between these landmarks and ask your partner to alternately evert and relax her foot. Feel the fibulares tighten upon eversion. This action will sometimes create a visible dimple or depression along the side of the leg (**7.87**).
3. As your partner continues to evert and relax her foot, follow the fibularis longus proximally toward the head of the fibula. Now follow both muscles distally to where their tendons wrap around the back of the lateral malleolus.
4. Follow the fibularis brevis tendon to the base of the fifth metatarsal (**7.88**).

Are you on the lateral side of the leg between the head of the fibula and the lateral malleolus? Can you differentiate the slender fibulares from the lateral edge of the larger gastrocnemius and soleus? Can you feel the tendon of the fibularis brevis attach to the base of the fifth metatarsal?

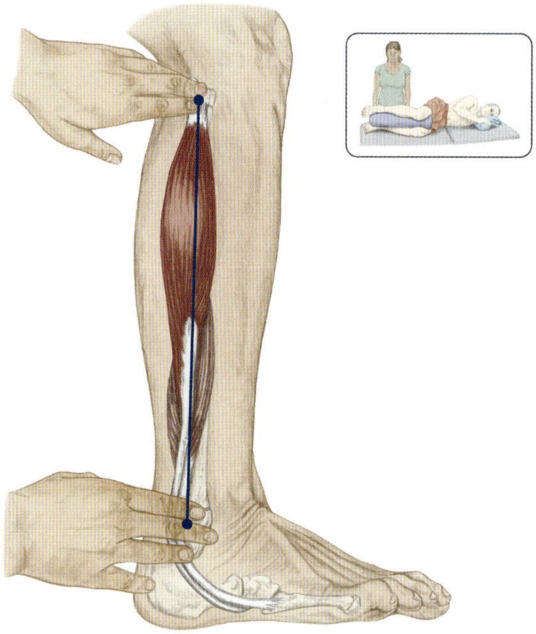

7.86 Lateral view of right leg, as you draw a line between the head of the fibula and the lateral malleolus

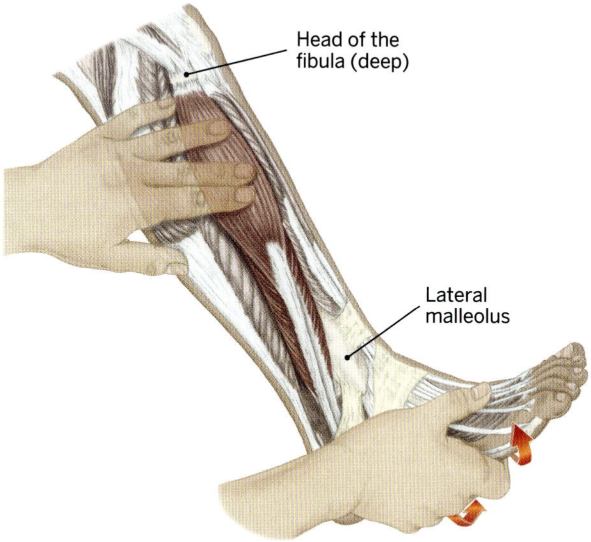

7.87 Partner side lying, everting her right foot while you explore fibularis longus

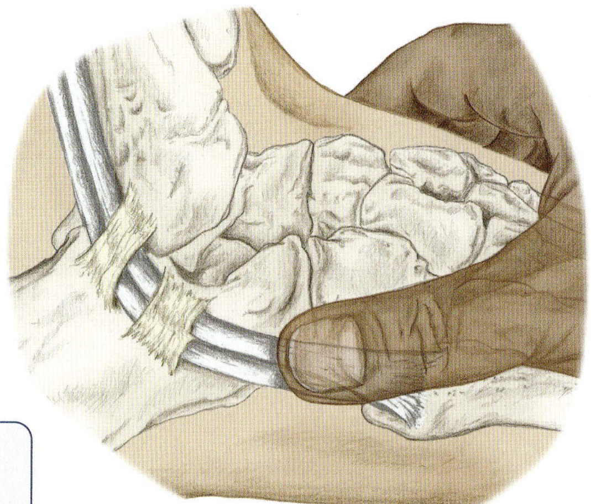

7.88 Lateral view of right ankle, as you access the fibularis tendons

Discover More

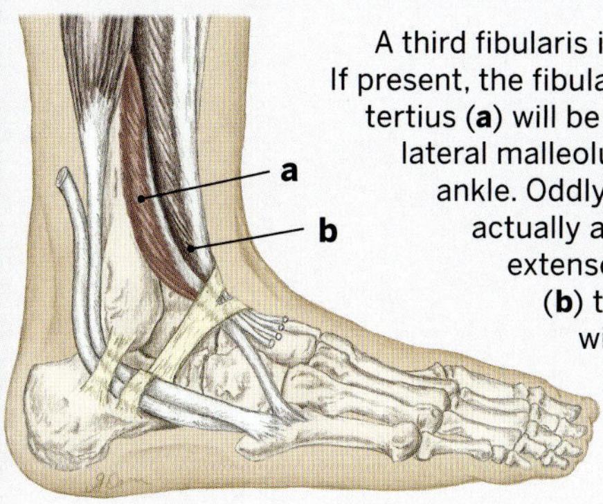

A third fibularis is not uncommon. If present, the fibularis (or peroneus) tertius (**a**) will be found anterior to the lateral malleolus on the front of the ankle. Oddly enough, the tertius is actually a short branch of the extensor digitorum longus (**b**) that attaches, along with fibularis brevis, at the tuberosity of the fifth metatarsal.

tertius *ter*-she-us L. third

Extensors of the Ankle and Toes ▸

Tibialis Anterior
Extensor Digitorum Longus
Extensor Hallucis Longus

These extrinsic muscles are located on the anterior aspect of the leg between the shaft of the tibia and the fibularis muscles (see **7.93**). The tendons of all three muscles cross beneath the extensor retinacula at the ankle (p. 407). The **tibialis anterior** is large, superficial, and the most clearly isolated of the group. It lies directly lateral to the tibial shaft (**7.89**).

Squeezed between the tibialis anterior and the fibularis muscles, the **extensor digitorum longus** is partially superficial. Its four tendons are clearly palpable on the dorsal surface of the foot (**7.90**, **7.91**).

The muscle belly of the **extensor hallucis longus** lies deep to the other two muscles and can be accessed only indirectly; however, like the extensor digitorum, its distal tendon is easily found on the dorsal surface of the foot as it leads toward the first toe (**7.91**, **7.92**).

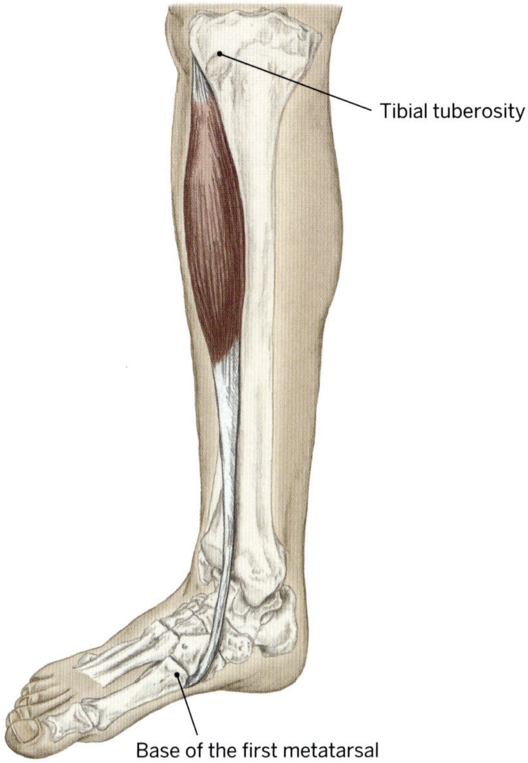

7.89 Anterior/medial view of right leg and foot, showing tibialis anterior

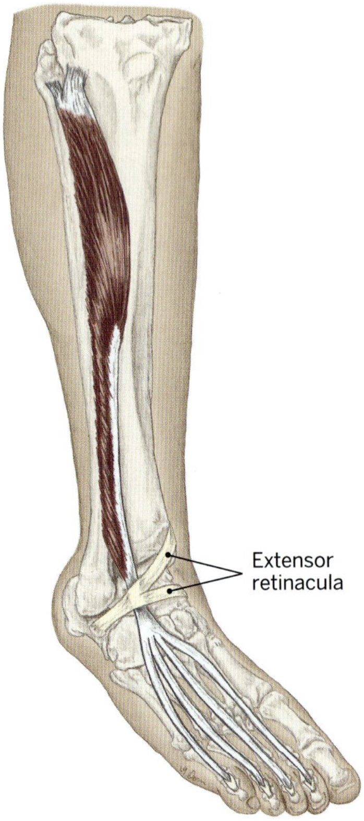

7.90 Anterior/lateral view of right leg and foot, showing extensor digitorum longus

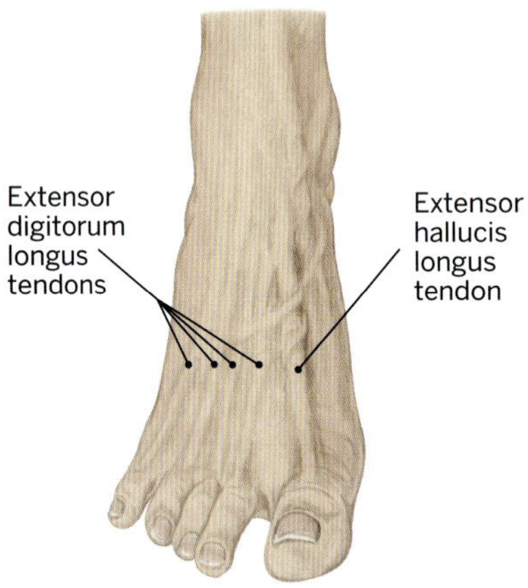

7.91 Dorsal view of right foot, showing tendons of extensor digitorum longus and extensor hallucis longus

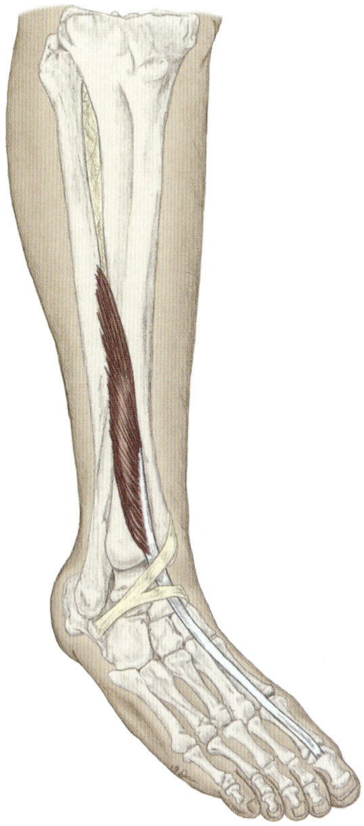

7.92 Anterior/lateral view of right leg and foot, showing extensor hallucis longus

TIBIALIS ANTERIOR

A **Invert** the foot
Dorsiflex the ankle (talocrural joint)

O Lateral condyle of tibia; proximal, lateral surface of tibia; and interosseous membrane

I Medial cuneiform and base of the first metatarsal

N Deep fibular L**4**, **5**, S1

When Do You Use Your Tibialis Anterior?

- Balancing on one foot

EXTENSOR DIGITORUM LONGUS

A **Extend** the second through fifth toes (metatarsophalangeal and interphalangeal joints)
Dorsiflex the ankle (talocrural joint)
Evert the foot

O Lateral condyle of tibia; proximal, anterior shaft of fibula; and interosseous membrane

I Middle and distal phalanges of second through fifth toes

N Deep fibular L**4**, **5**, S**1**

When Do You Use Your Extensor Digitorum Longus?

- Putting on and taking off your socks and shoes

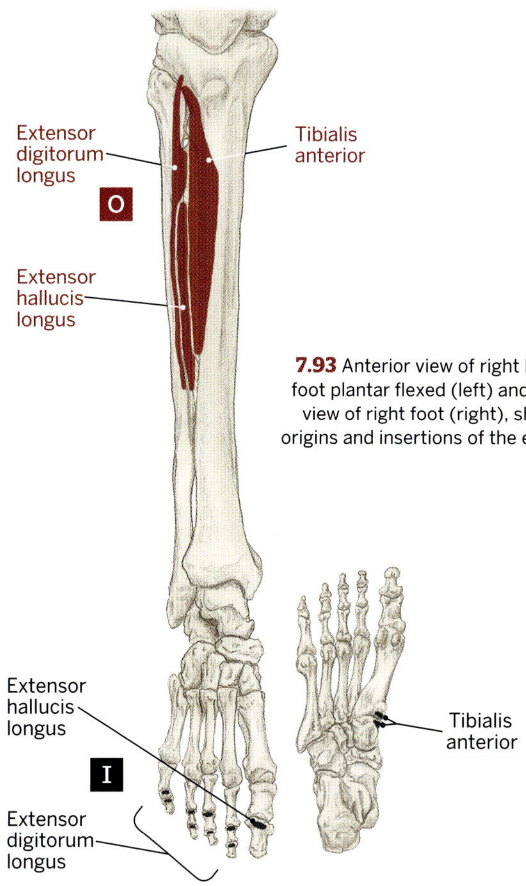

7.93 Anterior view of right leg with foot plantar flexed (left) and plantar view of right foot (right), showing origins and insertions of the extensors

EXTENSOR HALLUCIS LONGUS

A **Extend** the first toe (metatarsophalangeal and interphalangeal joints)
Dorsiflex the ankle (talocrural joint)
Invert the foot

O Middle, anterior surface of fibula and interosseous membrane

I Distal phalanx of first toe

N Deep fibular L4, **5**, S**1**

When Do You Use Your Extensor Hallucis Longus?

- During the swing phase of your gait (lifting the foot after toe-off so that your foot clears the ground)

Tibialis anterior

1. Partner supine. Locate the shaft of the tibia and slide off it laterally onto the tibialis anterior.
2. Ask your partner to dorsiflex his ankle and palpate its long, inch-wide belly (**7.94**).
3. With the ankle dorsiflexed, palpate the muscle distally as it becomes a thick, tendinous cord. Follow it to the medial side of the foot as it disappears at the medial cuneiform.

As your partner alternately dorsiflexes and relaxes his ankle, can you feel and see the tendon that crosses the top of the ankle? Ask your partner to invert his foot and note whether the tibialis anterior is involved. Can you feel where the tendon passes under the extensor retinacula?

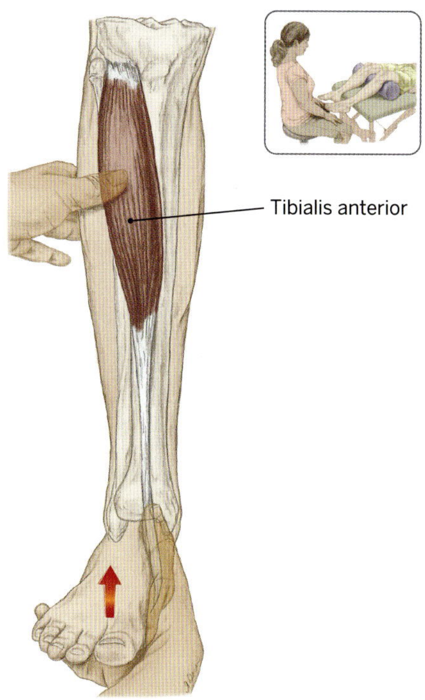

7.94 Anterior view of right leg, as you palpate tibialis anterior

Extensor digitorum longus

1. Partner supine. The easiest way to begin is by palpating the digitorum's distal tendons. Ask your partner to extend his toes. Visibly identify and palpate the four tendons of the digitorum on the top of the foot.
2. With the toes still extended, follow the tendons toward the ankle. Notice how they converge into a single tendinous bundle that loops underneath the extensor retinacula (**7.95**).
3. Follow this tendon proximally as it merges into its muscle belly. Explore the slender belly of the digitorum as it squeezes between the tibialis anterior and the fibularis muscles.

Locate the digitorum and tibialis anterior tendons on the top of the ankle. With the ankle dorsiflexed, ask your partner to slowly invert and evert his foot. Do you feel the tibialis tighten upon inversion and the digitorum tighten upon eversion?

Extensor hallucis longus

1. Partner supine. Ask your partner to extend his first toe. Visibly identify and palpate the solid tendon running along the dorsal surface of the foot to the first toe (**7.96**).
2. With the toe still extended, follow the tendon toward the ankle. Note how it snuggles between and underneath the extensor digitorum and tibialis anterior tendons.

Can you follow the tendon from the first toe to the dorsal surface of the ankle? Can you distinguish the three separate tendons of the extensors (hallucis, digitorum, and tibialis anterior) along the dorsal surface of the ankle?

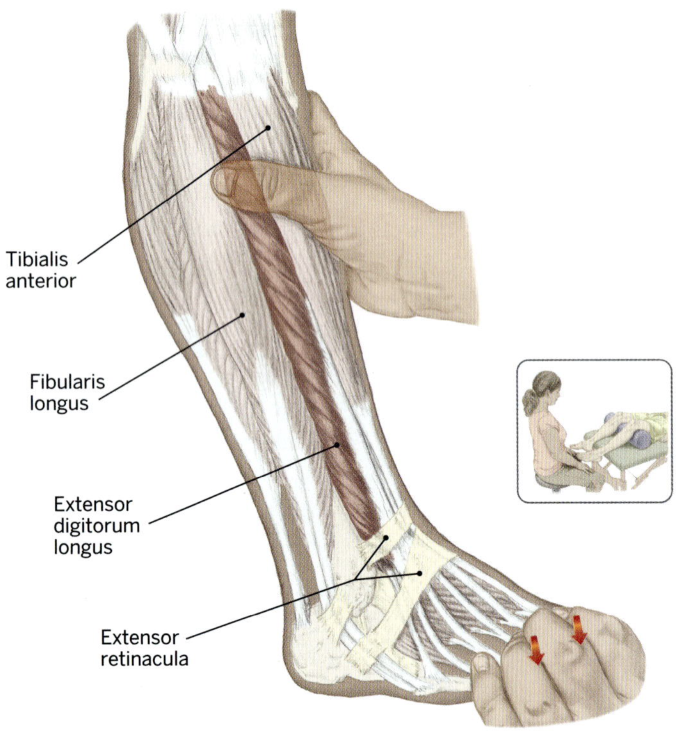

7.95 Lateral view of right leg, partner extending the toes of right foot against your resistance while you palpate extensor digitorum longus

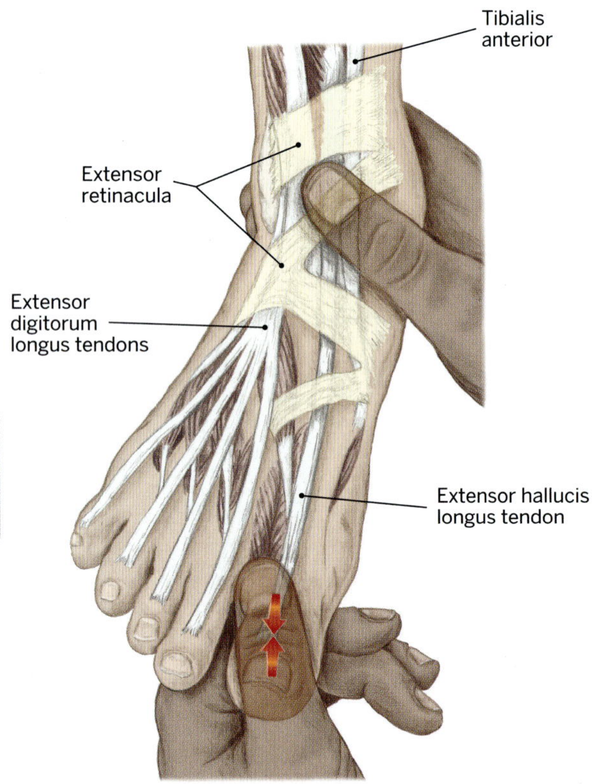

7.96 Partner extending the first toe of right foot against your resistance while you palpate extensor hallucis longus

Leg & Foot

Flexors of the Ankle and Toes ▶

Tibialis Posterior
Flexor Digitorum Longus
Flexor Hallucis Longus

Buried deep to the gastrocnemius and soleus on the posterior leg are three slender muscles primarily responsible for inverting the foot and flexing the toes (**7.97–7.102**). All three muscles are virtually inaccessible except at the small region on the medial side of the leg. This small gap between the tibial shaft and the edge of the calcaneal tendon is where the most distal fibers and tendons of the flexors can be palpated directly (**7.101**). The tendons of these three muscles curve around the medial malleolus and pass deep to the flexor retinaculum. The tibial artery and tibial nerve (pp. 387, 408) are situated between the tendons at the medial ankle.

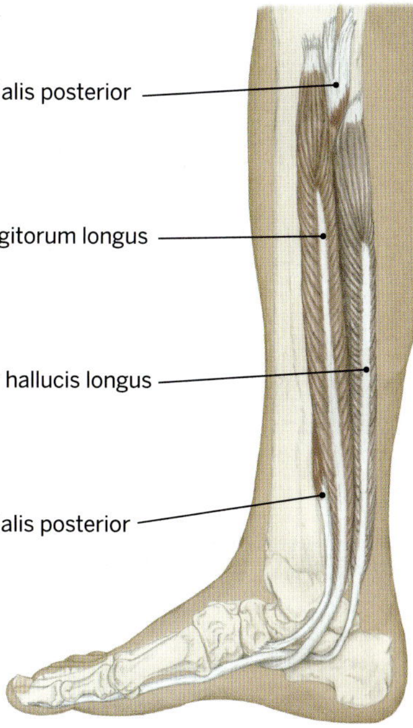

7.97 Medial view of right leg and foot, showing flexors of the ankle and toes

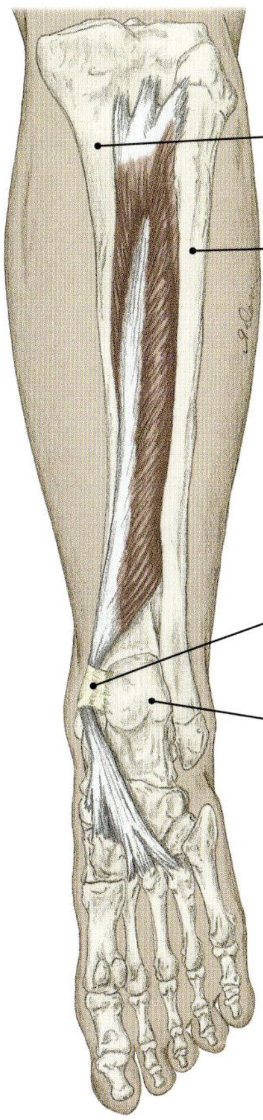

7.98 Posterior view of right leg with foot plantar flexed, showing tibialis posterior

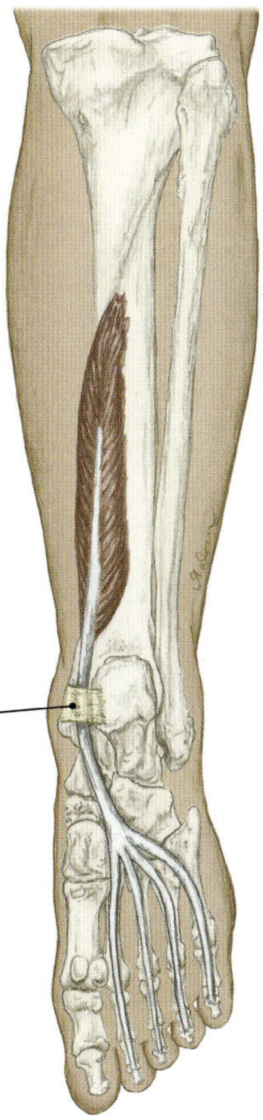

7.99 Posterior view of right leg with foot plantar flexed, showing flexor digitorum longus

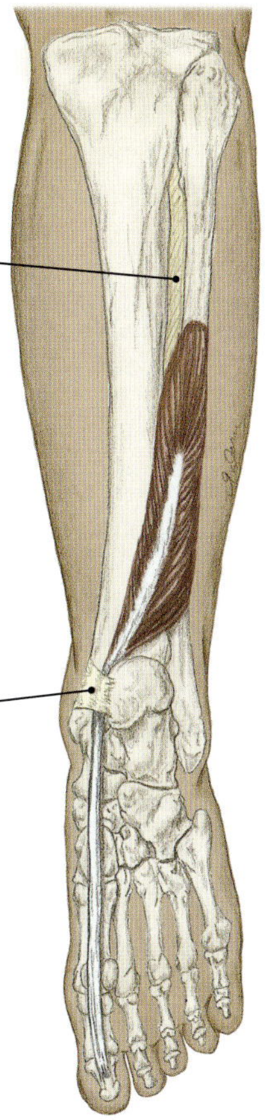

7.100 Posterior view of right leg with foot plantar flexed, showing flexor hallucis longus

Leg & Foot

TIBIALIS POSTERIOR

A **Invert** the foot
Plantar flex the ankle (talocrural joint)

O Proximal, posterior shafts of tibia and fibula; and interosseous membrane

I All five tarsal bones and bases of second through fourth metatarsals

N Tibial L(4), **5**, S**1**

When Do You Use Your Tibialis Posterior?

- Walking on your tiptoes
- Hiking on a rocky trail (small, specific stabilizing movements of the foot and ankle)

FLEXOR DIGITORUM LONGUS

A **Flex** the second through fifth toes (metatarsophalangeal and interphalangeal joints)
Weak **plantar flexion** of ankle (talocrural joint)
Invert the foot

O Middle, posterior surface of tibia

I Distal phalanges of second through fifth toes

N Tibial L**5**, S**1**, (2)

When Do You Use Your Flexor Digitorum Longus?

- Walking on your tiptoes
- Hiking on a rocky trail (small, specific stabilizing movements of the foot and ankle)

FLEXOR HALLUCIS LONGUS

A **Flex** the first toe (metatarsophalangeal and interphalangeal joints)
Weak **plantar flexion** of ankle (talocrural joint)
Invert the foot

O Middle half of posterior fibula

I Distal phalanx of first toe

N Tibial L**5**, S**1**, **2**

When Do You Use Your Flexor Hallucis Longus?

- Turning the water tap with your toes when lying in the bathtub (flexion of the toes with subtle movements of the foot and ankle)

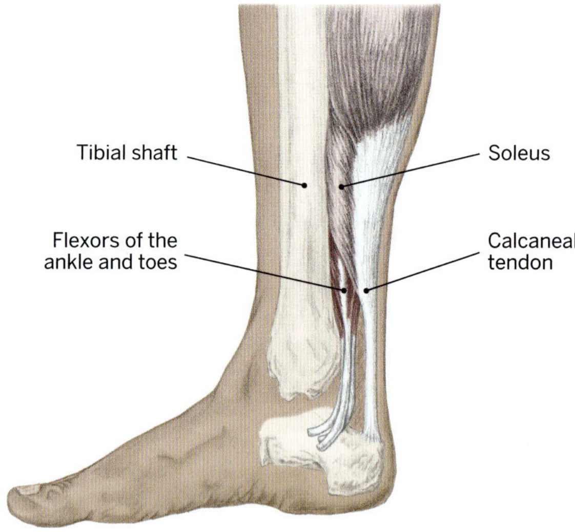

7.101 Medial view of right leg and foot, showing calcaneal tendon and flexors

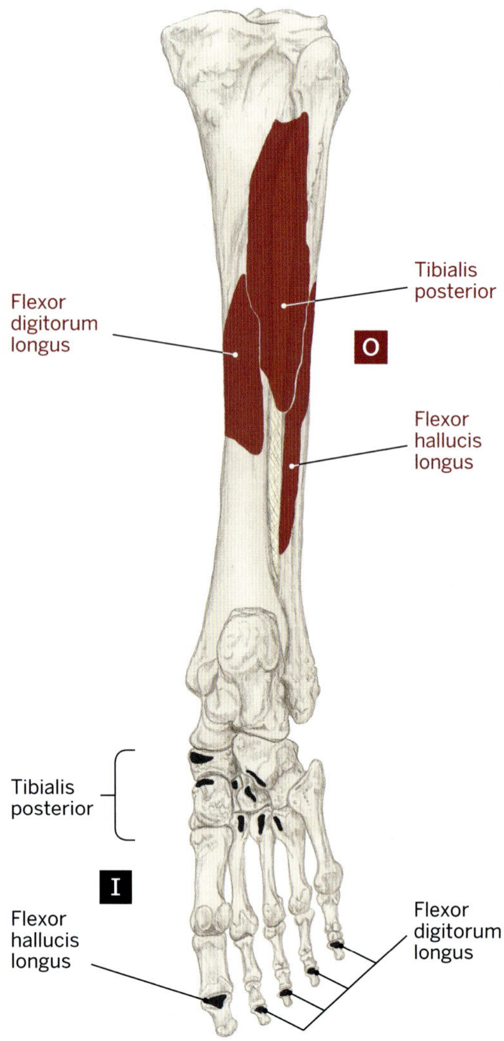

7.102 Posterior view of right leg with foot plantar flexed, showing origins and insertions of flexors

All flexors

1. Partner supine, prone, or side lying. Locate the medial malleolus. Slide off the malleolus posteriorly and proximally into the space between the posterior shaft of the tibia and the calcaneal tendon.
2. Explore this region for the distal bellies and tendons of these muscles. Follow the tendons distally around the back of the medial malleolus.
3. It is difficult to isolate specific tendons; however, tibialis posterior will be the most anterior. Have your partner invert his foot as you follow this tendon around the ankle to the underside of the foot.

*Place your fingers on the distal bellies and ask your partner to slowly wiggle all his toes (**7.103**). Can you feel the muscles or tendons shift? Can you locate the medial malleolar groove (p. 361) and feel the tendons in and posterior to it? Can you locate the pulse of the tibial artery?*

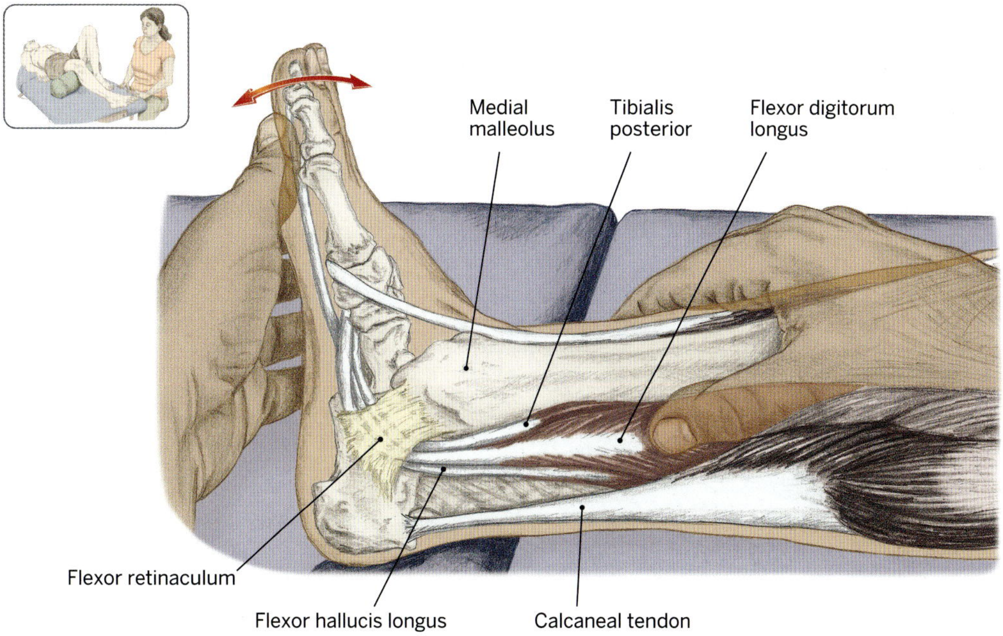

7.103 Medial view of right leg and foot, as your partner wiggles his toes while you palpate the flexors

Discover More

"Tom, Dick, AN' Harry" is a mnemonic device that corresponds to the initials of the tendons and vessels in the order that they pass by the medial malleolus. **T**ibialis posterior is the most anterior, followed by flexor **D**igitorum, the tibial **A**rtery, tibial **N**erve, and then flexor **H**allucis.

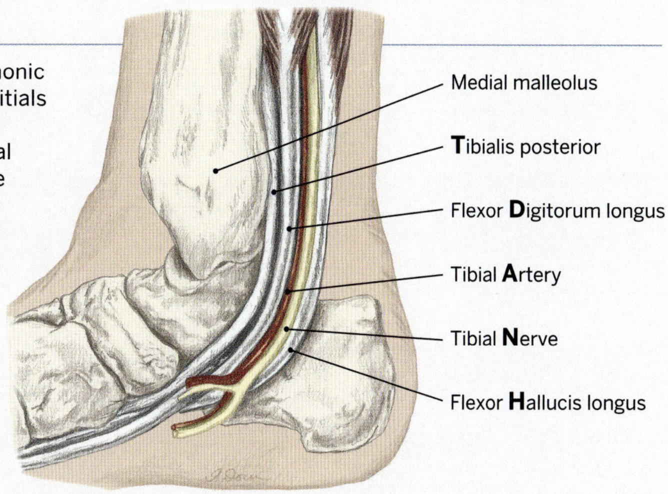

Medial view of right ankle

Overview: **Muscles of the Foot**

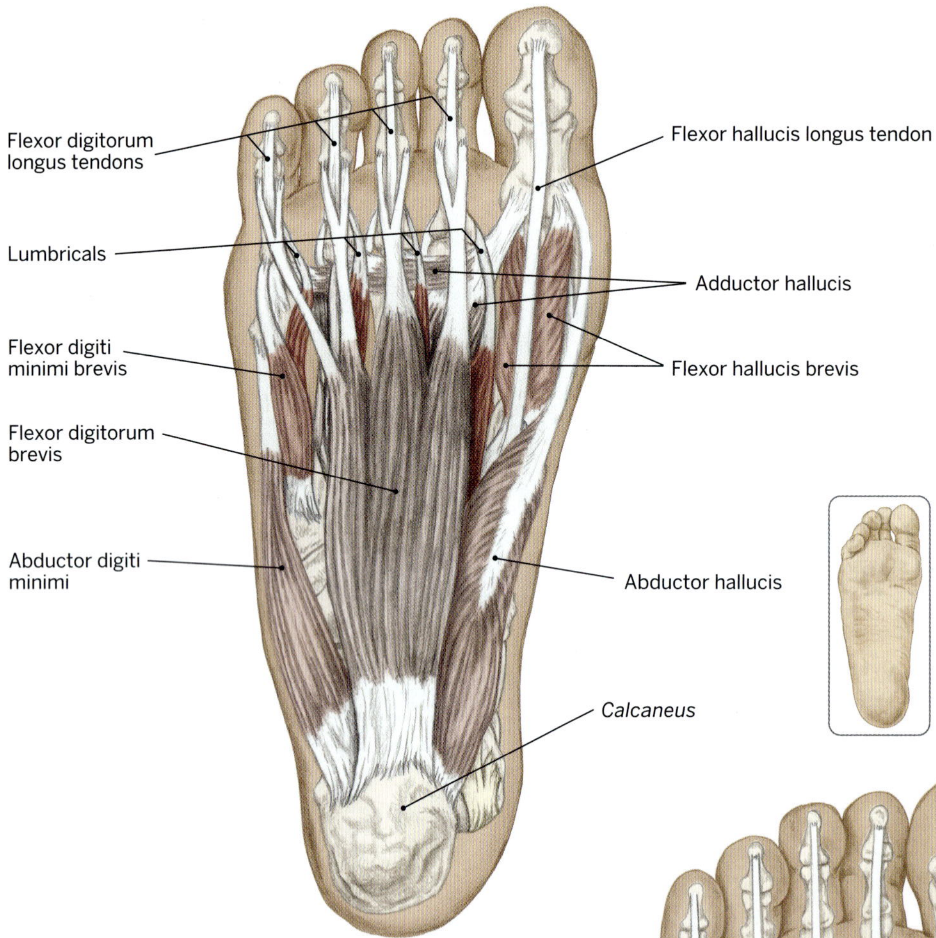

7.104 Plantar view of muscles of right foot, superficial layer

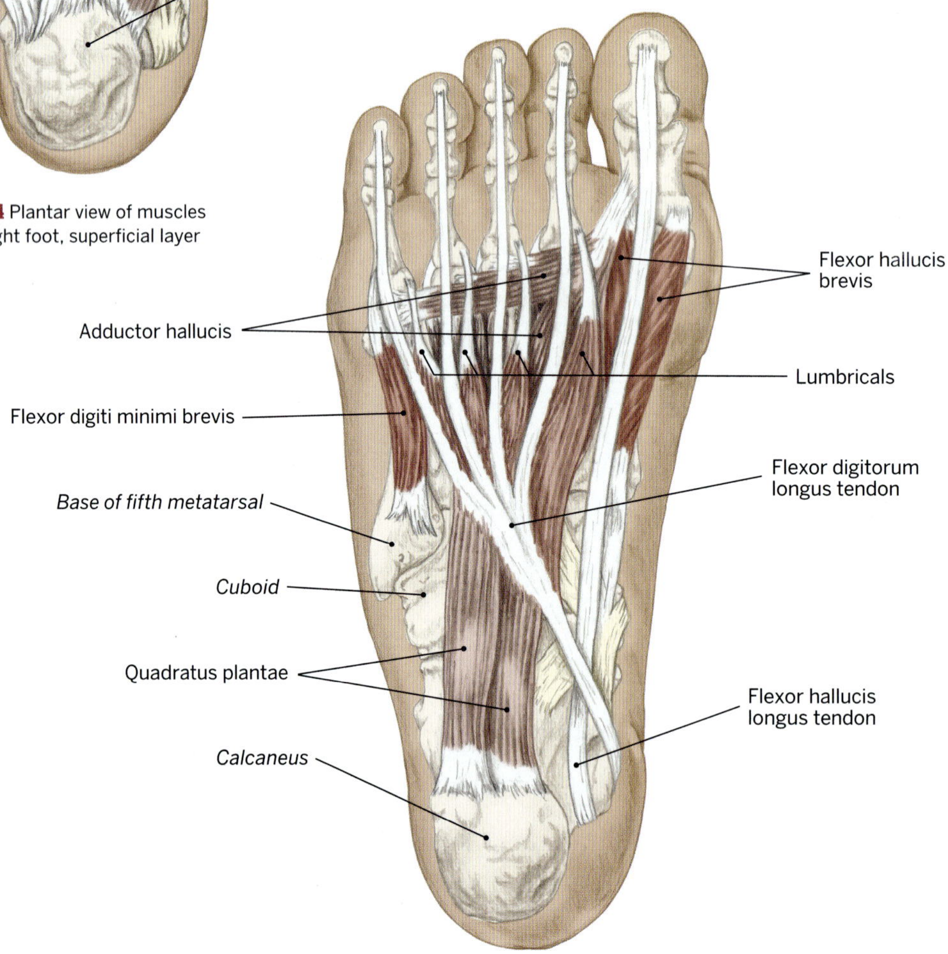

7.105 Plantar view of muscles of right foot, intermediate layer

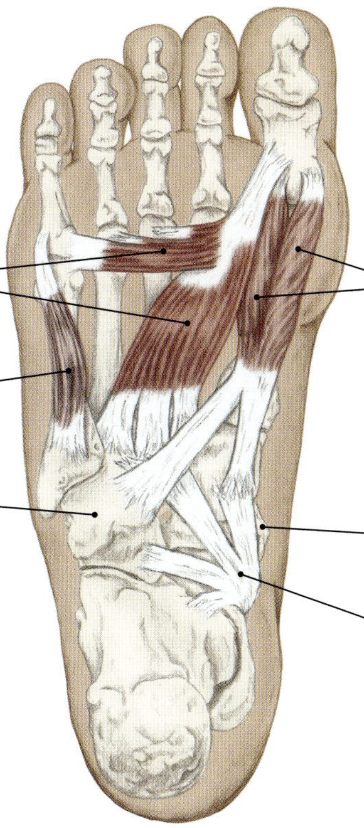

7.106 Plantar view of muscles of right foot, deep layer

Discover More

Because they bear the weight of the body when standing, walking, and running, the feet are sometimes known as the "little soldiers." In comparison to standing, walking increases the pressure on the feet twofold, while running increases it fourfold.

These stresses demand that the foot be designed for more than lying flat and idle on the ground. Thus the bones and ligaments of the foot are arranged to form three arches—the medial longitudinal, lateral longitudinal, and transverse. These arches connect with three points of contact—the calcaneus and the heads of the first and fifth metatarsals.

The three arches together raise the center of the foot, creating a structure that is ideally shaped to distribute and absorb the weight of the body. The arches also help the plantar surface of the foot adapt to uneven terrain while hiking or climbing.

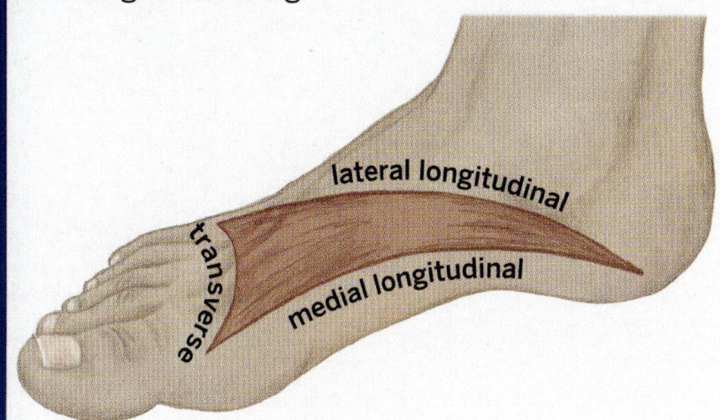

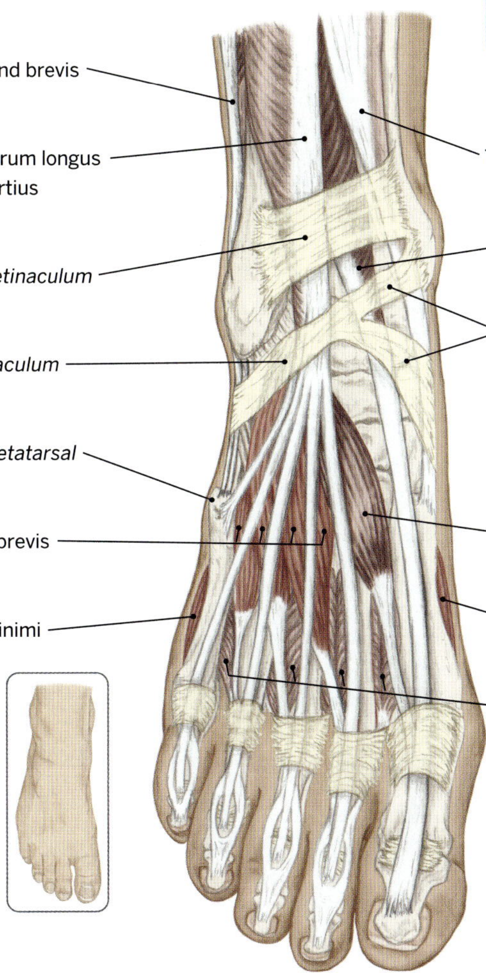

7.107 Dorsal view of muscles of right foot

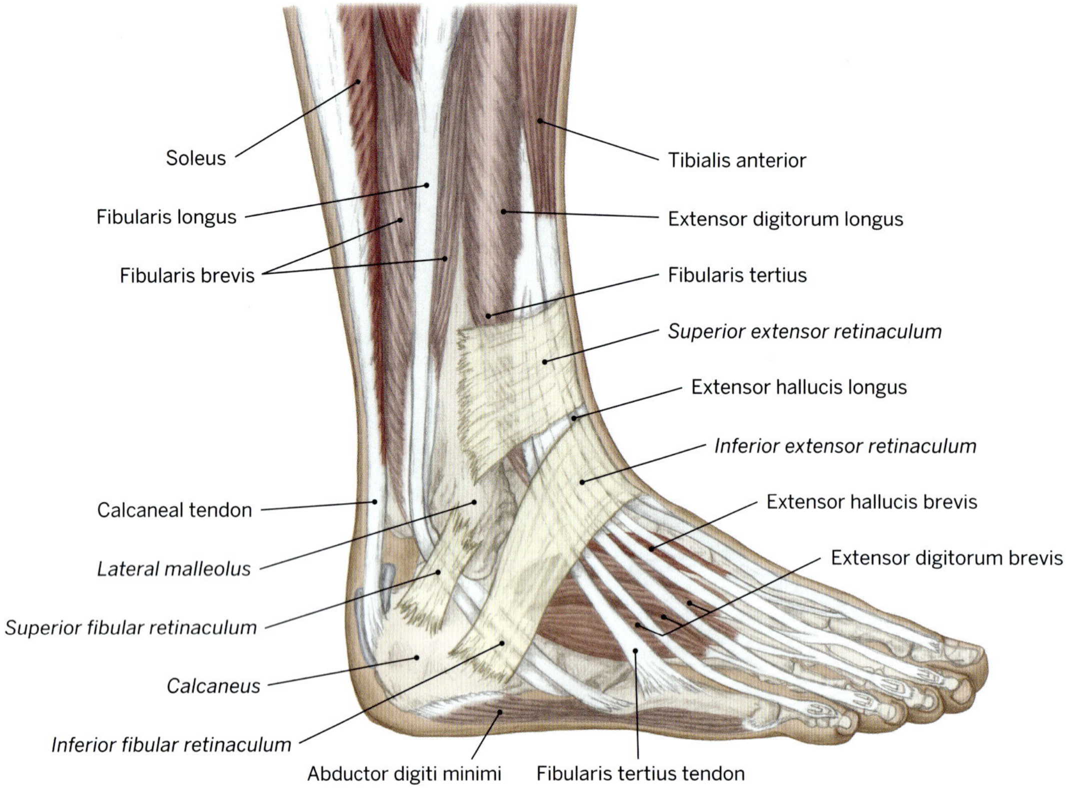

7.108 Lateral view of muscles of ankle and foot

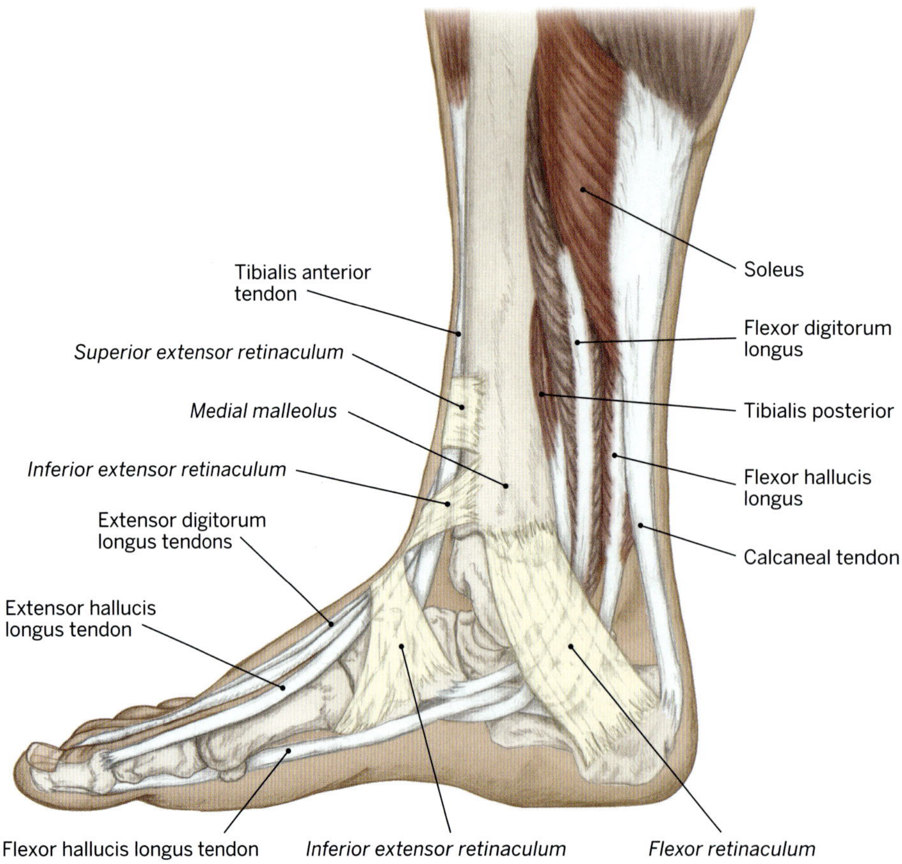

7.109 Medial view of muscles of ankle and foot

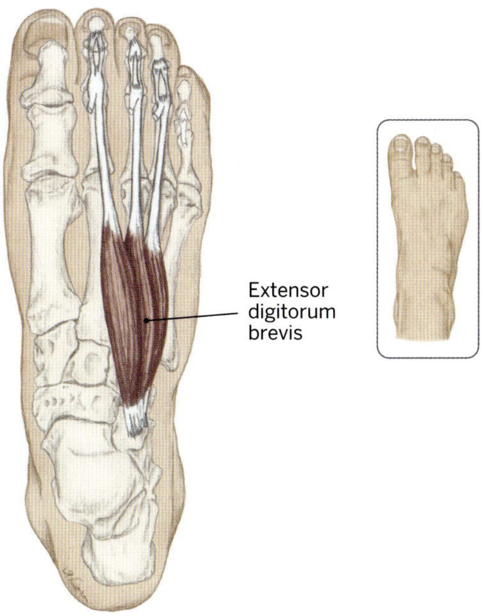

7.110 Dorsal view of right foot, showing extensor digitorum brevis

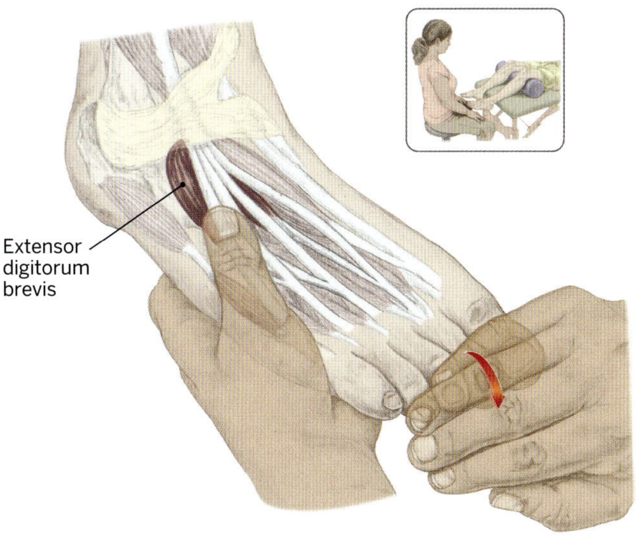

7.111 Dorsal/lateral view of right foot, partner extending the toes against your resistance while you palpate extensor digitorum brevis

Discover More

If the discomfort of wearing high-heeled shoes were not enough, try this on for size: The point of a spike heel worn by the average-sized woman is subjected to nearly 2,000 pounds of pressure per square inch with every step she takes. This force is shot into the heel and reverberates up the entire body. When air travel was in its infancy, women wearing high heels were actually prohibited from boarding airplanes because the heels of their shoes might pierce the thin metal floors.

minimi *min*-i-mee L. smallest

Muscles of the Foot ▶

Extensor Digitorum Brevis
Flexor Digitorum Brevis
Abductor Hallucis
Abductor Digiti Minimi

The dorsal surface of the foot is home to the **extensor digitorum brevis** (**7.110**). Its small belly lies deep to the extensor digitorum longus tendons but is still palpable (**7.111**).

Unlike the minimally muscled dorsal surface, the foot's plantar surface is made up of several layers of muscle. The first layer, located deep to the plantar aponeurosis, (p. 408), is formed by three muscles that lie side by side. The center muscle is the **flexor digitorum brevis** (**7.112**). It extends down the center of the foot from the calcaneus to the phalanges. Medial to the flexor digitorum brevis is the thick, superficial **abductor hallucis**; lateral to it is the superficial **abductor digiti minimi** (**7.113**). Both abductors are easily accessible and often visible along the sides of the foot. Although deep to the plantar aponeurosis, all three muscles are relatively superficial on the sole of the foot and are thus palpable (**7.114**).

	EXTENSOR DIGITORUM BREVIS
A	**Extend** the second through fourth toes (metatarsophalangeal and interphalangeal joints)
O	Dorsal surface of calcaneus
I	Second through fourth toes via the extensor digitorum longus tendons
N	Deep fibular L4, **5**, S**1**

When Do You Use Your Extensor Digitorum Brevis?

- Stabilization when you are balancing on one foot
- Rock climbing (serious work on behalf of all of the toes)
- Walking on a patch of ice (Notice how your toes suddenly "grab.")
- Picking up a pencil off the floor with your toes

Extensor digitorum brevis

1. Partner supine, with the feet off the end of the table. Locate the lateral malleolus. Slide two inches off the malleolus toward the fifth toe. Palpate beneath and lateral to the extensor digitorum longus tendons to locate the small belly of extensor digitorum brevis.
2. Ask your partner to extend her toes against your resistance to feel the muscles contract (see **7.111**). Note how the belly forms a dense mound over the cuboid and lateral cuneiform upon contraction.

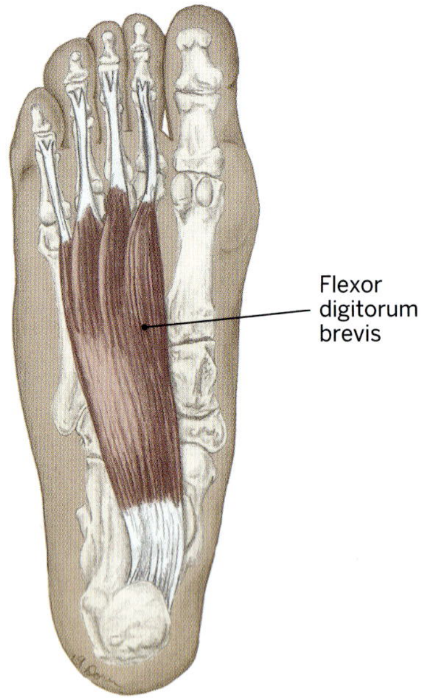

7.112 Plantar view of right foot, showing flexor digitorum brevis

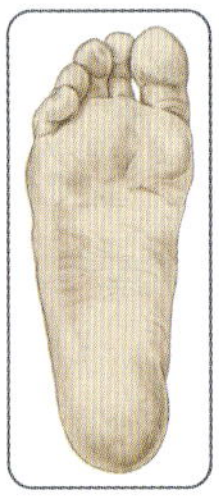

FLEXOR DIGITORUM BREVIS

A **Flex** middle phalanges of the second through fifth toes (proximal interphalangeal joints)

O Medial process of calcaneus and plantar aponeurosis

I Middle phalanges of second through fifth toes

N Tibial L4, **5**, S**1**

When Do You Use Your Flexor Digitorum Brevis?

- Stabilization when you are balancing on one foot
- Rock climbing (serious work on behalf of all of the toes)

ABDUCTOR HALLUCIS

A **Abduct** the first toe (metatarsophalangeal joint)
Assist to **flex** the first toe (metatarsophalangeal joint)

O Medial process of calcaneus and plantar aponeurosis

I Proximal phalanx of first toe (medial surface) and medial sesamoid bone

N Tibial L4, **5**, S**1**

When Do You Use Your Abductor Hallucis?

- Stabilization when you are balancing on one foot
- Walking on a patch of ice (Notice how your toes suddenly "grab.")

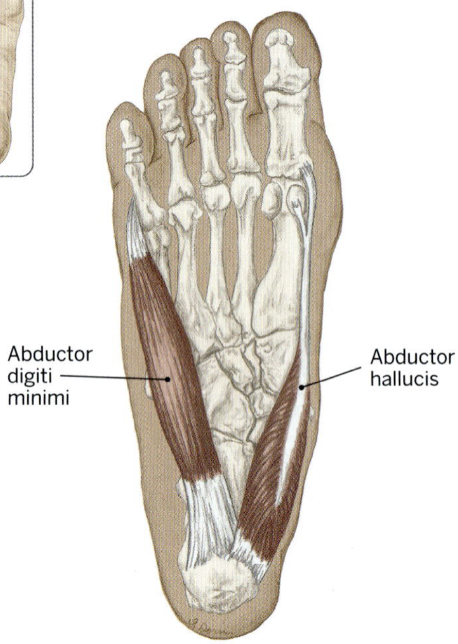

7.113 Plantar view of right foot, showing abductor hallucis and abductor digiti minimi

ABDUCTOR DIGITI MINIMI

A **Flex** the fifth toe
Assist to **abduct** the fifth toe (metatarsophalangeal joint)

O Lateral process of calcaneus and plantar aponeurosis

I Proximal phalanx of fifth toe (lateral surface)

N Tibial S**1**, **2**

When Do You Use Your Abductor Digiti Minimi?

- Stabilization when you are balancing on one foot
- Picking up a pencil off the floor with your toes

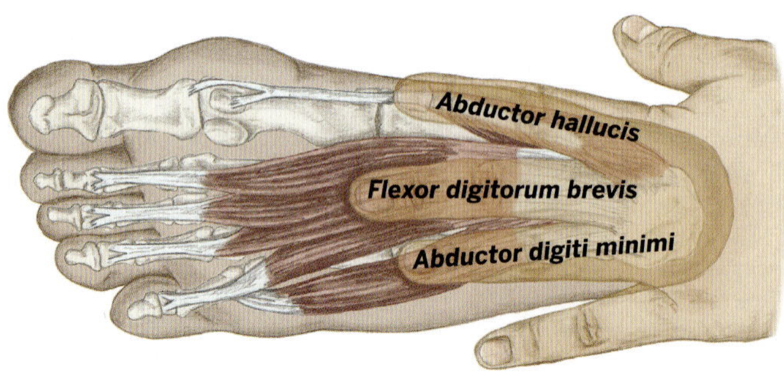

7.114 Plantar surface of right foot with fingers showing order of muscles

Flexor digitorum brevis

1. Partner supine, with the feet off the end of the table. Locate the plantar surface of the heel and the second through fifth toes. Visualize this muscle's location by drawing imaginary lines between these points.
2. Palpating along the arch of the foot, sink your thumbs along these lines and roll across the muscle fibers (**7.115**). Ask your partner to alternately flex and relax her toes. It may be challenging to isolate the flexor digitorum brevis belly, but have faith that you are in the correct location.

Abductor hallucis

1. Partner supine, with the feet off the end of the table. Locate the medial surface of the heel and the medial side of the first toe.
2. Palpate between these points and note the thick, superficial tissue running alongside the medial/plantar surface of the foot (**7.116**).
3. Ask your partner to flex his first toe against your resistance and note the strength and density of the abductor hallucis belly.

Abductor digiti minimi

1. Partner supine, with the feet off the end of the table. Locate the plantar surface of the heel and the lateral surface of the fifth toe.
2. Palpate between these points for the thick, superficial tissue running alongside the lateral/plantar surface of the foot (**7.117**).
3. Ask your partner to abduct or flex his fifth toe against your resistance in order to feel the fibers contract.

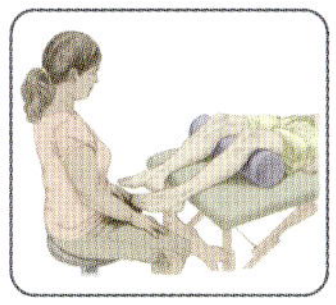

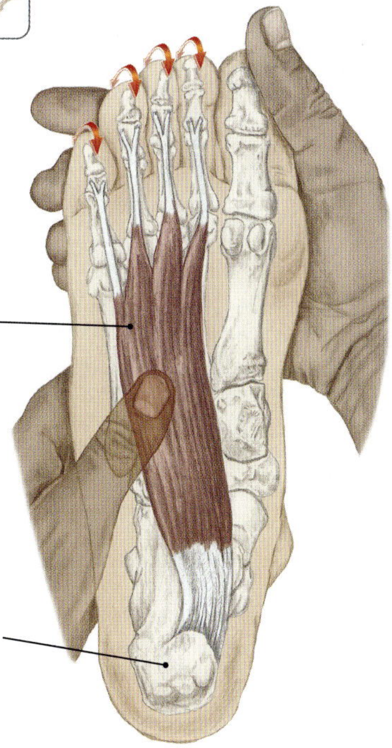

7.115 Plantar view of right foot, partner flexing her toes while you palpate flexor digitorum brevis

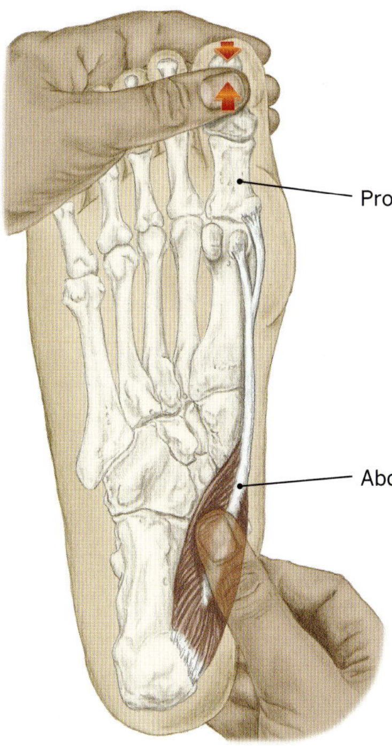

7.116 Plantar view of right foot, partner flexing the first toe against your resistance while you palpate abductor hallucis

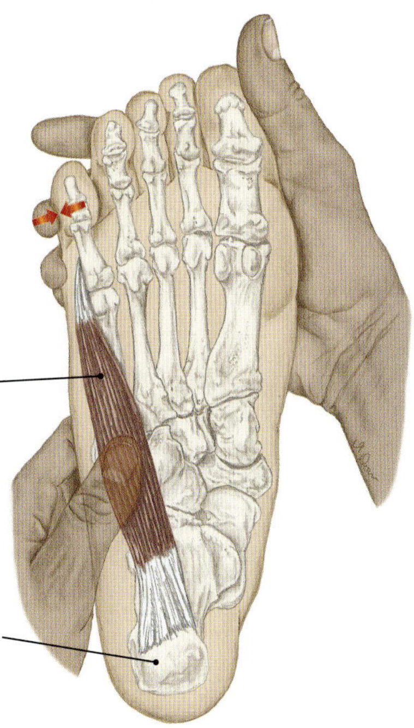

7.117 Plantar view of right foot, partner abducting the fifth toe against your resistance while you palpate abductor digiti minimi

Other Muscles of the Foot

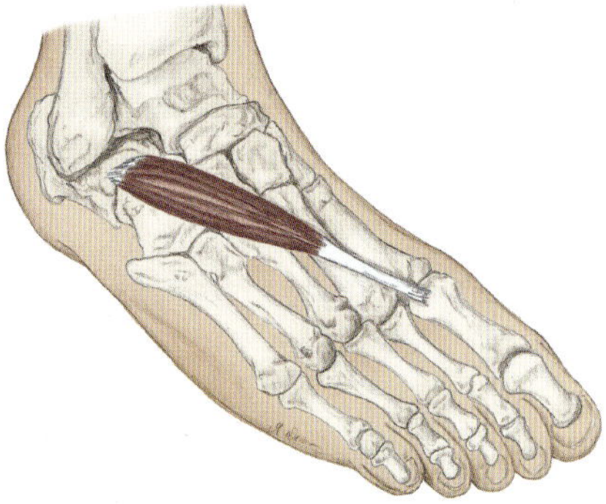

7.118 Dorsal/lateral view of right foot, showing extensor hallucis brevis

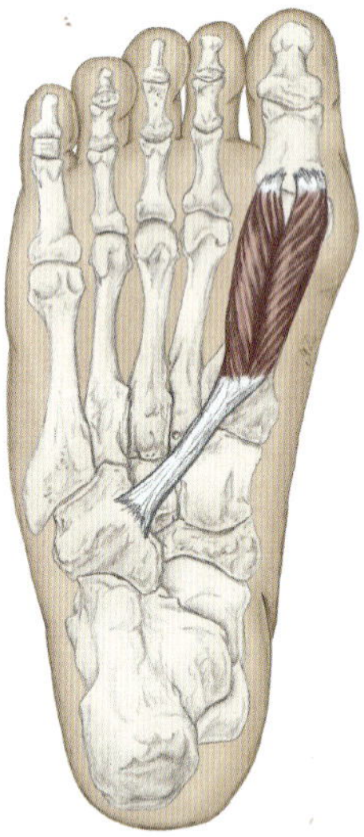

7.119 Plantar view of right foot, showing flexor hallucis brevis

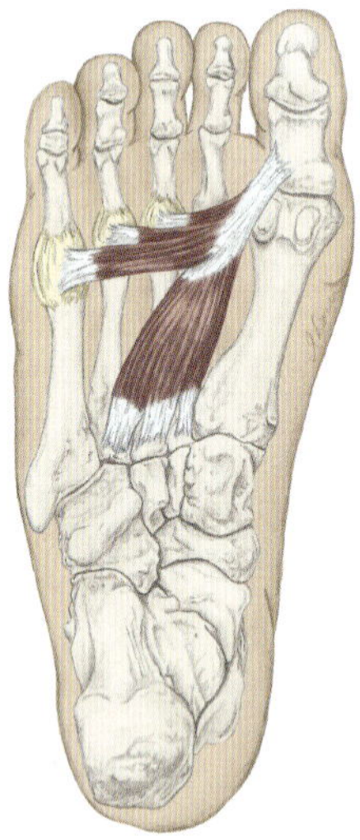

7.120 Plantar view of right foot, showing adductor hallucis

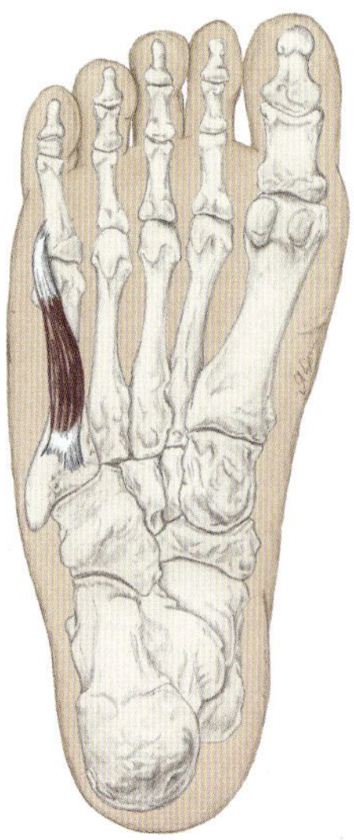

7.121 Plantar view of right foot, showing flexor digiti minimi brevis

EXTENSOR HALLUCIS BREVIS

A **Extend** the first toe (metatarsophalangeal joint)

O Dorsal surface of calcaneus

I Proximal phalanx of first toe

N Deep fibular L4, **5**, S**1**

When Do You Use Your Extensor Hallucis Brevis?

- Maintaining your balance while walking barefoot along a beach

FLEXOR HALLUCIS BREVIS

A **Flex** the first toe (metatarsophalangeal joint)

O Plantar surfaces of cuboid and lateral cuneiform

I Medial and lateral surfaces of base of proximal phalanx of first toe

N Tibial L4, **5**, S**1**

When Do You Use Your Flexor Hallucis Brevis?

- Maintaining your balance while walking barefoot along a beach

ADDUCTOR HALLUCIS

A **Adduct** the first toe
Assist to **maintain** transverse arch of foot
Assist to **flex** the first toe

O *Oblique head:*
Bases of second through fourth metatarsals
Transverse head:
Plantar ligament of third through fifth metatarsophalangeal joints

I Lateral surface of base of proximal phalanx of first toe

N Tibial S**1**, **2**

When Do You Use Your Adductor Hallucis?

- Maintaining your balance while walking barefoot along a beach

FLEXOR DIGITI MINIMI BREVIS

A **Flex** the fifth toe (metatarsophalangeal joint)

O Base of fifth metatarsal

I Base of proximal phalanx of fifth toe

N Tibial S**1**, **2**

When Do You Use Your Flexor Digiti Minimi Brevis?

- Maintaining your balance while walking barefoot along a beach

QUADRATUS PLANTAE

A Assist flexor digitorum longus to **flex** 2nd–5th toes

O Medial and lateral sides of plantar surface of calcaneus

I Posterior, lateral aspect of flexor digitorum longus tendon

N Tibial S**1**, **2**

When Do You Use Your Quadratus Plantae?

- Maintaining your balance while walking barefoot along a beach

PLANTAR INTEROSSEI

A **Adduct** 3rd–5th toes (metatarsophalangeal joints)
Flex 3rd–5th toes (metatarsophalangeal joints)

O Medial surfaces of 3rd–5th metatarsals

I Medial surfaces of proximal phalanges of 3rd–5th toes

N Tibial S**1**, **2**

When Do You Use Your Plantar Interossei?

- Maintaining your balance while walking barefoot along a beach

DORSAL INTEROSSEI

A **Abduct** 2nd–4th toes (metatarsophalangeal joints)
Flex 2nd–4th toes (metatarsophalangeal joints)

O Adjacent surfaces of all metatarsals

I ***First:*** Medial surface of proximal phalanx of 2nd toe
Second through fourth: Lateral surfaces of proximal phalanges of 2nd–4th toes

N Tibial S**1**, **2**

When Do You Use Your Dorsal Interossei?

- Maintaining your balance while walking barefoot along a beach

LUMBRICALS OF THE FOOT

A **Flex** the proximal phalanges of the 2nd–5th toes at the metatarsophalangeal joints
Extend the middle and distal phalanges of the 2nd–5th toes at the interphalangeal joints

O Tendons of flexor digitorum longus

I Bases of proximal phalanges of 2nd–5th toes and extensor digitorum longus tendons (on dorsal surface of the toes)

N ***First:*** Tibial L4, **5**, S**1**
Second through fourth: Tibial L(4), (5), S**1**, **2**

When Do You Use Your Lumbricals of the Foot?

- Maintaining your balance while walking barefoot along a beach

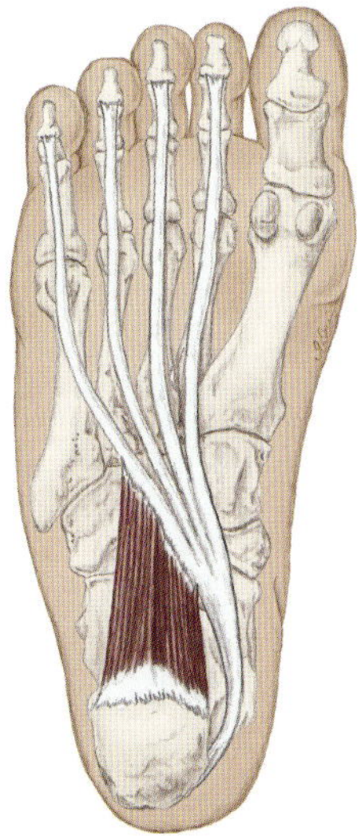

7.122 Plantar view of right foot, showing quadratus plantae

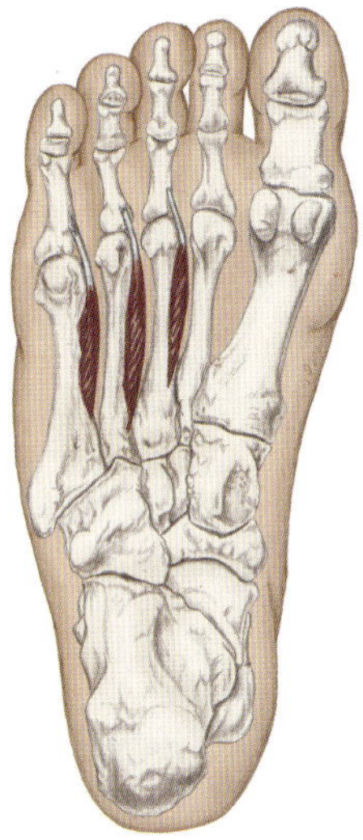

7.123 Plantar view of right foot, showing plantar interossei

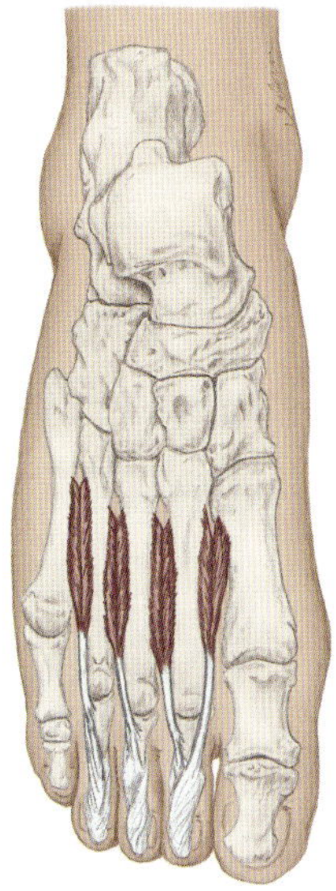

7.124 Dorsal view of right foot, showing dorsal interossei

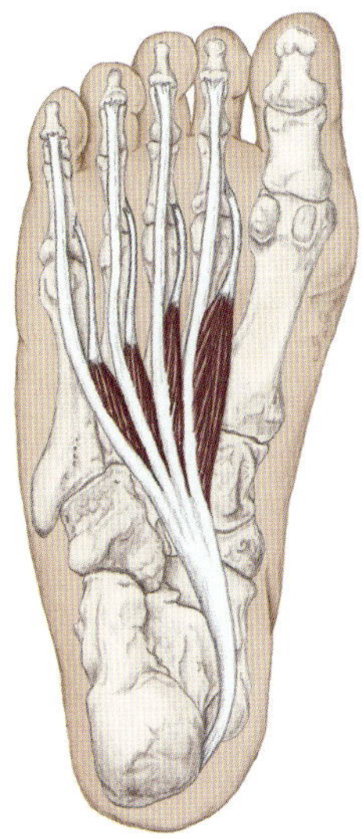

7.125 Plantar view of right foot, showing lumbricals

Leg & Foot

Ligaments and Other Structures of the Knee and Leg

Tibiofemoral Joint

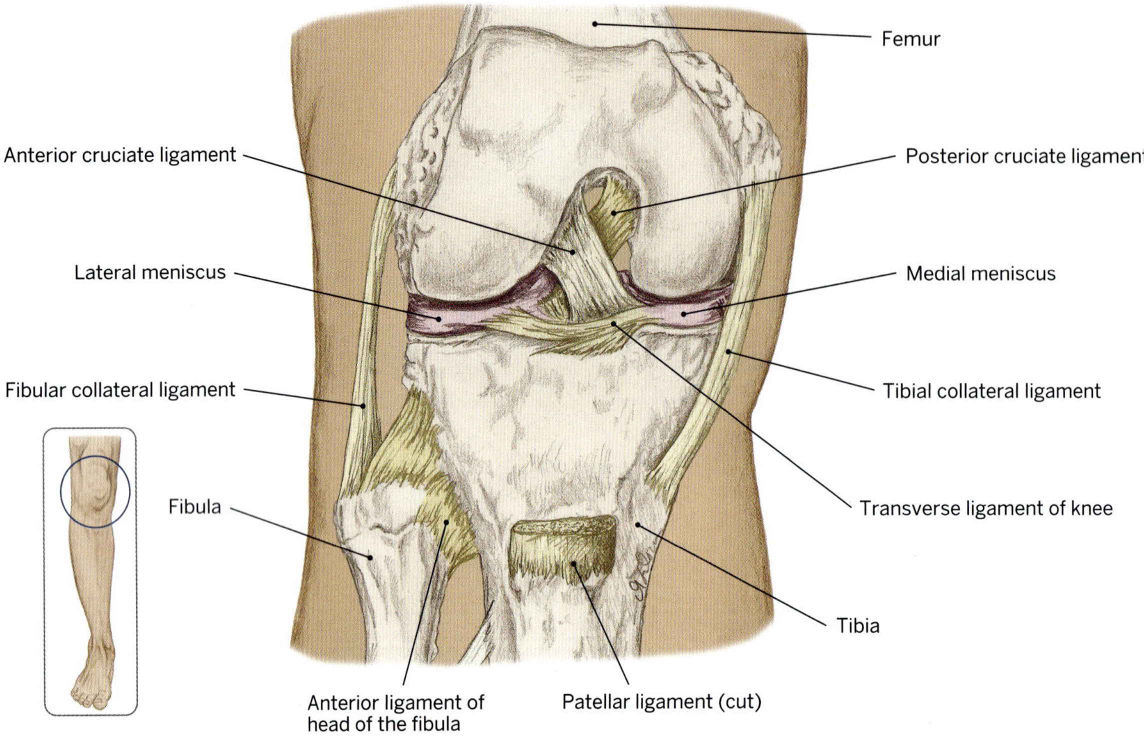

7.126 Anterior view of right knee with patella removed, showing menisci and ligaments of tibiofemoral joint

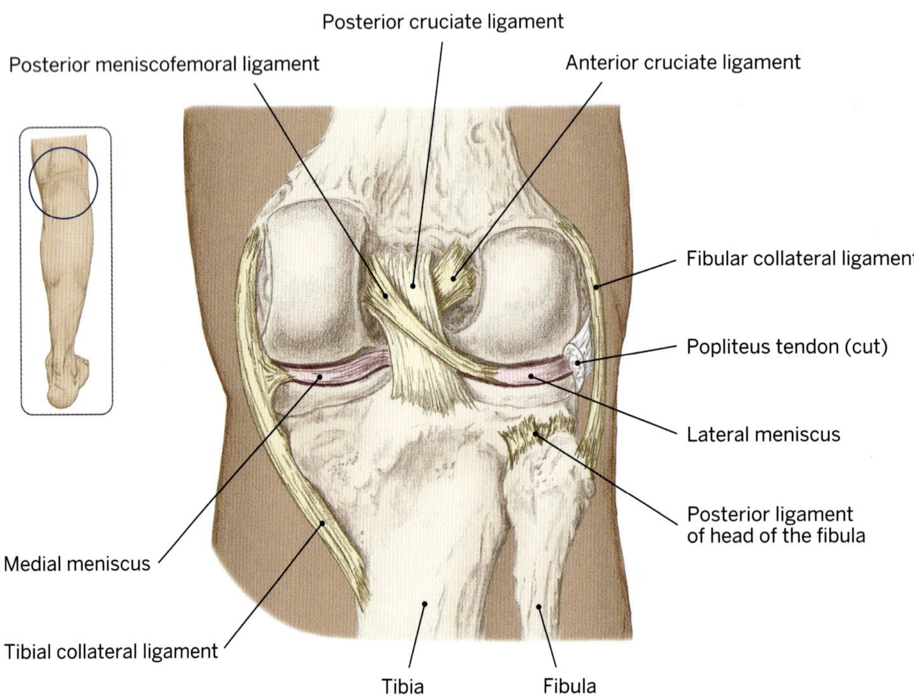

7.127 Posterior view of right knee, showing menisci and ligaments of tibiofemoral joint

cruciate	***kroo***-she-at	L. cross-shaped
meniscofemoral	men-***is***-ko-fem-***or***-al	

Tibiofemoral and Tibiofibular Joints

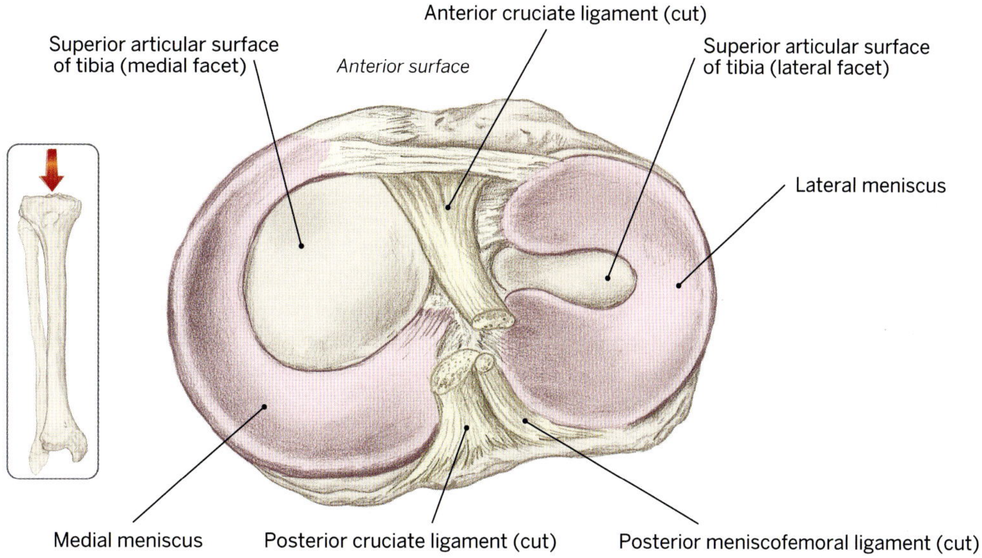

7.128 Superior view of right tibia, showing menisci and ligaments of tibiofemoral joint

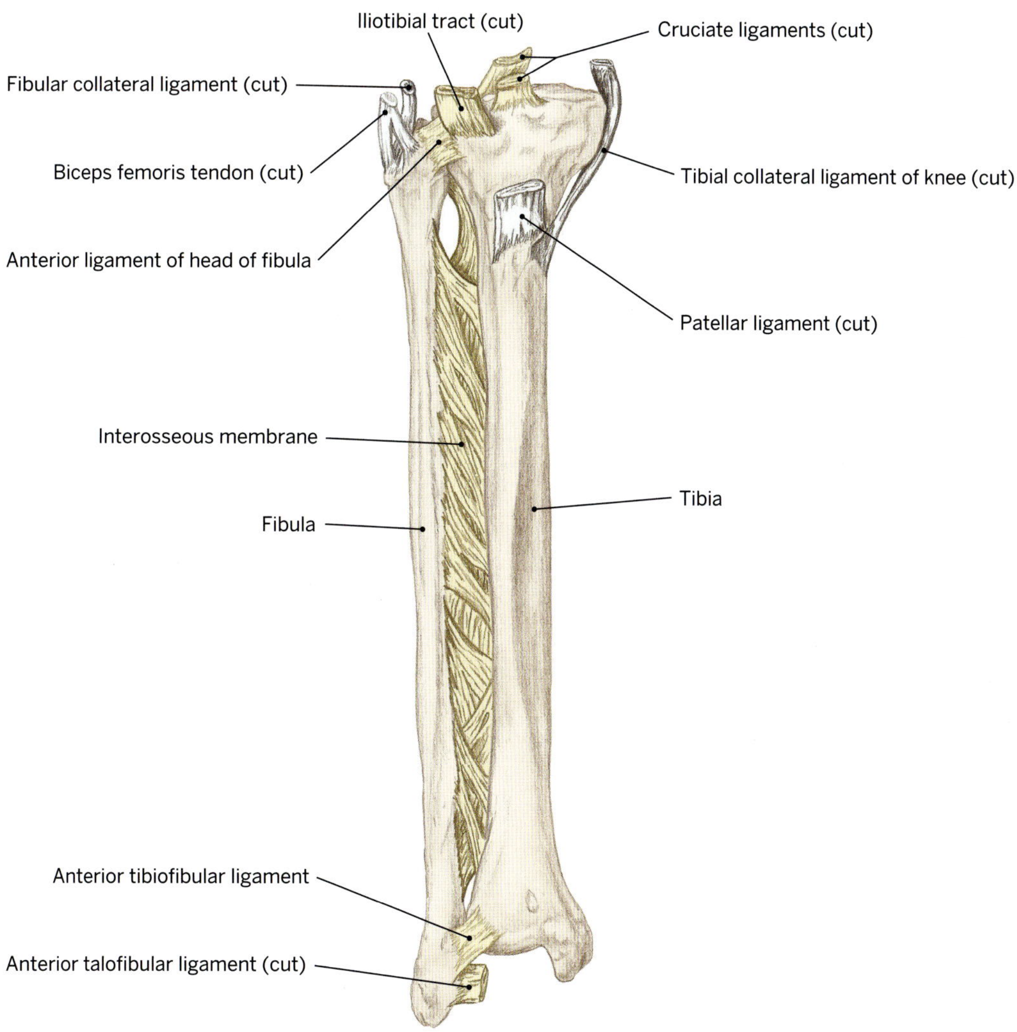

7.129 Anterior view of right tibia and fibula, showing ligaments of tibiofibular joints

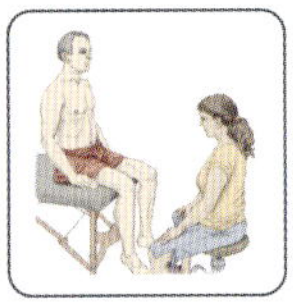

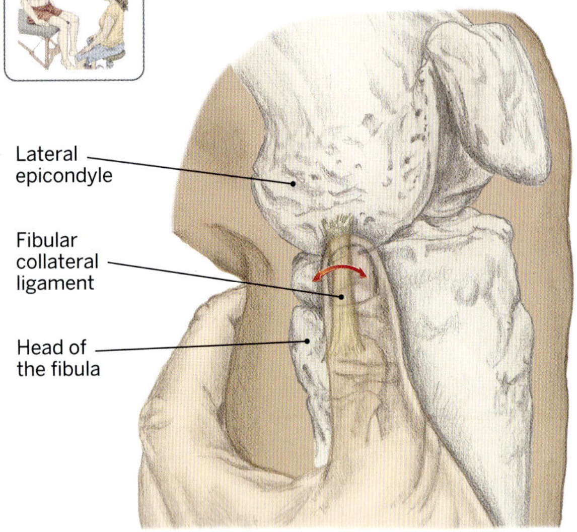

7.130 Lateral view of right knee, as you locate the fibular collateral ligament

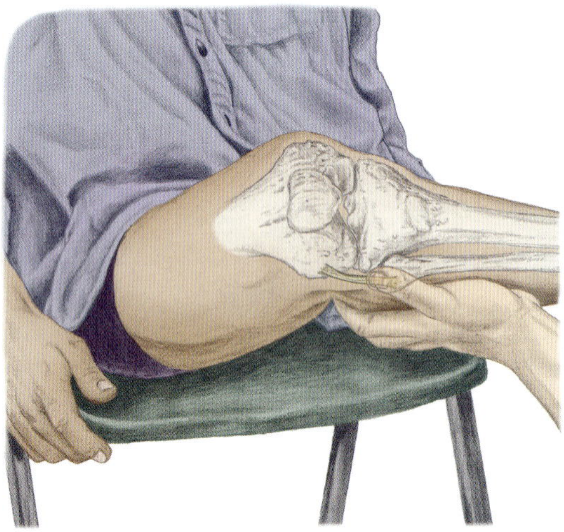

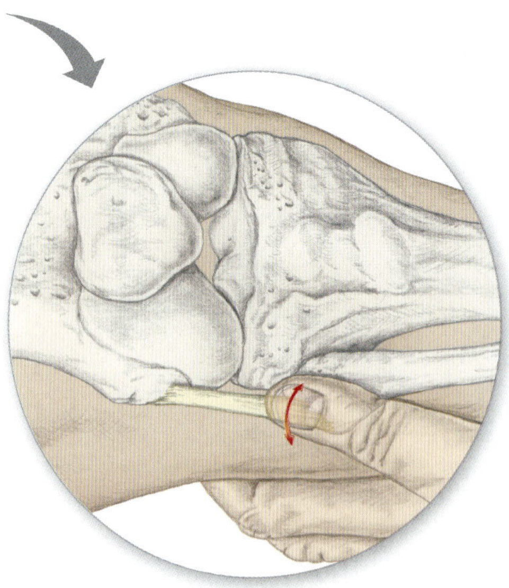

7.131 Anterior/lateral view of right knee, showing an alternate method for locating the fibular collateral ligament

Fibular and Tibial Collateral Ligaments

The **fibular collateral ligament** is a strong, thin strap that crosses the knee joint running from the lateral epicondyle of the femur to the head of the fibula. It is superficial and located between the biceps femoris tendon and the iliotibial tract.

The broad **tibial collateral ligament** lies superficial to the joint capsule of the knee, but may not be as easy to isolate as its lateral counterpart. Stretching nearly two inches distal to the knee joint, it is deep to the pes anserinus tendon.

Both collateral ligaments resist medial rotation of the knee. The fibular collateral also stabilizes the knee against genu varum stresses (often seen in bowlegged cowboys) while the tibial collateral protects against genu valgum (knock-knee) stresses. An example would be a blow from a football helmet to the lateral side of the knee joint.

Fibular collateral ligament

1. Partner seated with knee flexed. Locate the head of the fibula and the lateral epicondyle (**7.130**).
2. Slide your finger between these points and gently strum in a horizontal direction across this superficial ligament.

Is the band of tissue you feel the width of a pencil? Does it run from the epicondyle to the fibular head? Is it anterior to the biceps femoris tendon?

Ask your partner to cross his leg so the ankle is resting on top of the opposite knee. This position will allow the fibular collateral ligament to be easily accessed. Roll your finger between the epicondyle and the head of the fibula and palpate the ligament (**7.131**).

collateral	ko-***lat***-er-al	L. of both sides
genu valgum	***je***-noo ***val***-gum	
genu varum	***je***-noo ***va***-rum	

Tibial collateral ligament

1. Partner seated with the knee flexed. Locate the medial epicondyle of the femur. Slide distally to the joint space, the thin crevice between the tibia and femur.
2. Strum your fingertip horizontally across this space, exploring for the broad fibers of the ligament (**7.132**).

Are you on the medial side of the knee, just distal to the medial epicondyle of the femur?

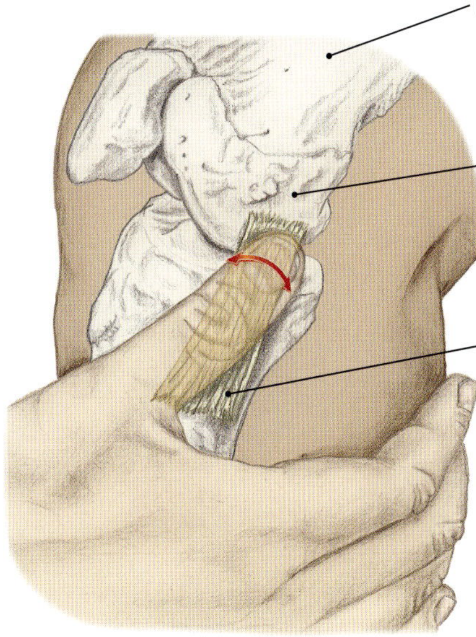

7.132 Medial view of right knee, as you strum your fingertip across the tibial collateral ligament

Menisci of the Knee

The menisci are fibrocartilaginous discs attached to the tibial condyles (see **7.128**). They not only are important for weight distribution and friction reduction, but also help the round femoral condyles sit comfortably upon the flat tibial plateaus. The edge of the medial meniscus can be palpated just above the edge of the medial tibial plateau. The smaller, more mobile lateral meniscus is difficult to access.

Medial meniscus

1. Partner seated with the knee flexed. Place your thumb superior to the medial tibial plateau in the joint space between the femur and tibia.
2. Grasp the leg with your other hand and slowly rotate the knee medially (**7.133**).
3. As the medial side of the tibia rotates posteriorly, the edge of the medial meniscus will be pushed anteriorly into your thumb. The sensation may be quite subtle—a gentle pressure against your thumbpad.

Is your thumb in the knee joint space? If you slowly switch from lateral to medial rotation of the knee, do you feel a difference under your thumb?

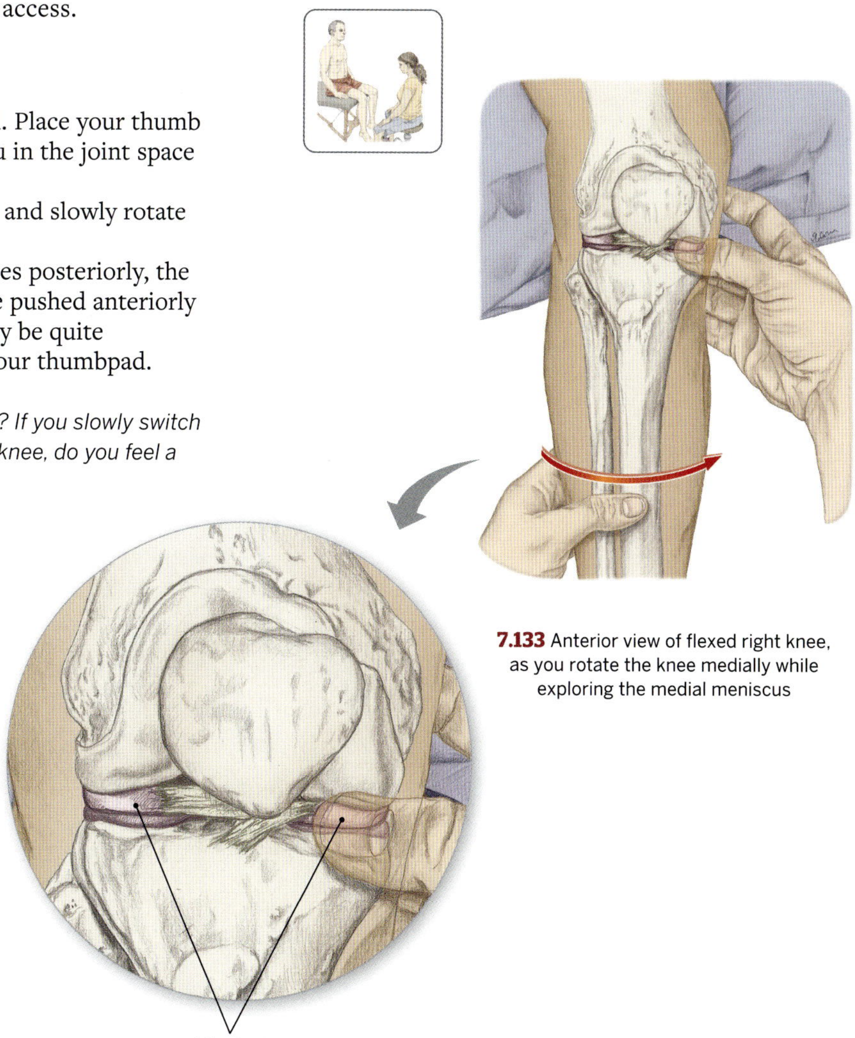

7.133 Anterior view of flexed right knee, as you rotate the knee medially while exploring the medial meniscus

meniscus	men-*is*-kus	Grk. crescent-shaped
menisci	men-*is*-ki	plural for meniscus

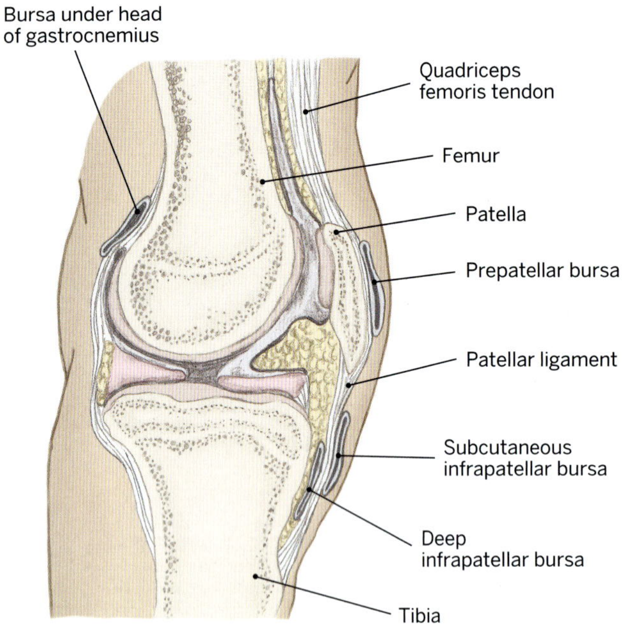

7.134 Midline cut, lateral view of knee, showing bursae (pes anserine bursa not shown)

Bursae of the Knee

Tremendous pressures, repetitive movements, and chafing tendons constantly challenge the knee joint. Nearly a dozen bursae help to protect the joint and its surrounding structures. The primary bursae are included here (**7.134**).

Lying superficial to the patella, the **prepatellar bursa** helps the skin to move freely over the patella, even with the knee flexed. Excessive kneeling and squatting can inflame the vulnerable bursa, a condition called "housemaid's knee" (or "carpenter's knee," depending on your vocation).

The **subcutaneous infrapatellar bursa** and the **deep infrapatellar bursa** are located on either side of the patellar ligament. The deep bursa reduces friction between the tendon and the surface of the tibia. The superficial bursa can become irritated with prolonged kneeling, sometimes called "parson's knee" (or "Buddhist's knee," depending on your faith).

The **pes anserine bursa** serves as a buffer between the pes anserinus tendons (those of the gracilis, sartorius, and semitendinosus) and the tibia.

When inflamed, the superficial bursae of the knee are palpable and sometimes visible; under normal conditions, however, they are impalpable.

Popliteal Artery

The popliteal artery branches from the femoral artery to pass through the popliteal fossa at the back of the knee. It is situated deep in the fossa and, for this reason, its pulse can be difficult to detect.

Popliteal artery

1. Partner supine. Flex your partner's knee in order to soften the overlying tissues. Hold the knee so that the fingertips of both hands are at the midline of the posterior knee.
2. Sink your fingerpads deep into the popliteal fossa and explore for the subtle pulse (**7.135**).

If the pulse is undetectable, follow the same instructions with your partner prone.

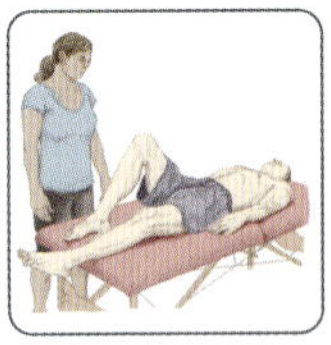

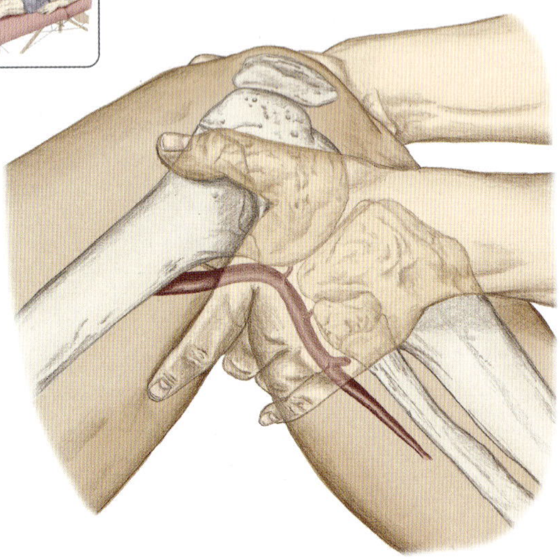

7.135 Lateral view of right knee, as you feel the pulse of the popliteal artery

Leg & Foot

Common Fibular Nerve

Branching off from the sciatic nerve, the fibular nerve courses superficially along the posterior/lateral side of the knee. Roughly the diameter of a thick piece of spaghetti, it lies medial to the biceps femoris tendon and lateral to the gastrocnemius belly. It becomes particularly accessible (and vulnerable) along the posterior surface of the head of the fibula (**7.136**).

Common fibular nerve

1. Partner prone. Passively flex the knee and locate the biceps femoris tendon and head of the fibula.
2. Gently roll your thumb from side to side, exploring the region just distal to the biceps tendon on the posterior surface of the fibular head.
3. Distinguish between the slender, slightly mobile nerve and the gastrocnemius fibers by asking your partner to gently flex her knee against your resistance. The nerve, of course, will remain soft and mobile, while the muscle fibers will become taut (**7.137**).

Locate the biceps femoris tendon by asking your partner to flex her knee against your resistance. Follow the tendon to the head of the fibula, noting the nerve pathway that runs alongside it. If you follow the nerve past the head of the fibula, does it continue down the lateral side of the leg?

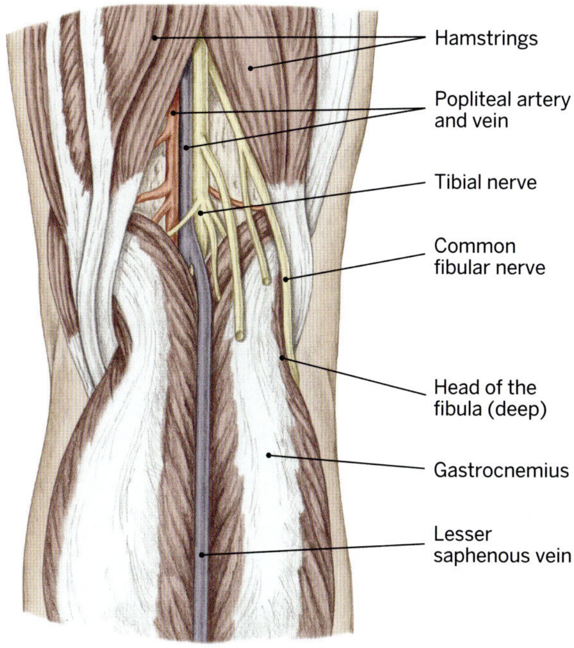

7.136 Posterior view of right knee, showing the common fibular nerve and surrounding structures

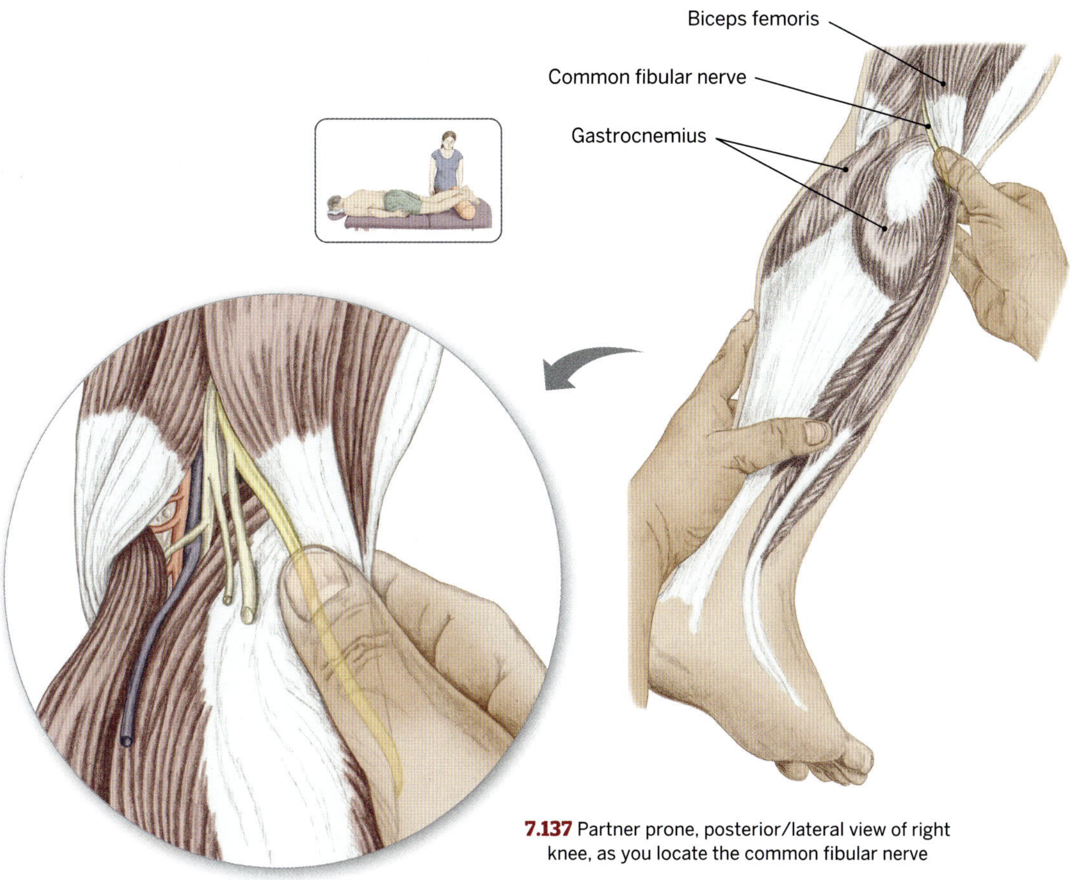

7.137 Partner prone, posterior/lateral view of right knee, as you locate the common fibular nerve

Ligaments and Other Structures of the Ankle and Foot

Talocrural Joint

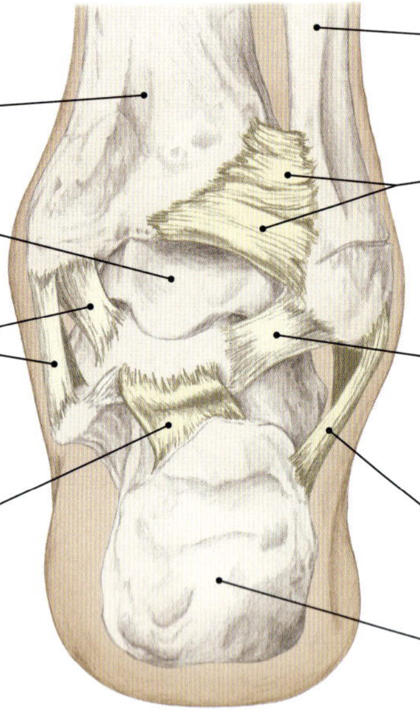

7.138 Posterior view of right ankle, showing ligaments of talocrural joint

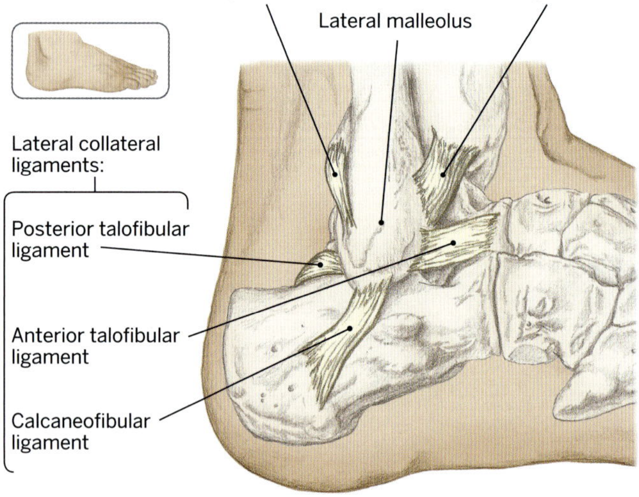

7.139 Lateral view of right ankle, showing ligaments of talocrural joint

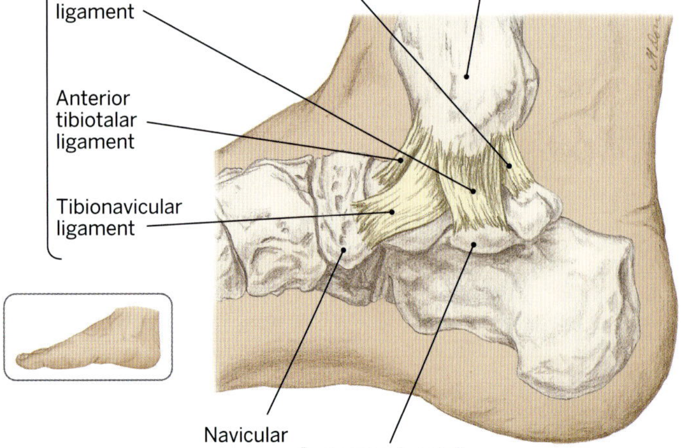

7.140 Medial view of right ankle, showing ligaments of talocrural joint

calcaneofibular	kal-***ka***-ne-o-***fib***-u-lar
talocalcaneal	***ta***-lo-kal-***ka***-ne-al
talofibular	***ta***-lo-***fib***-u-lar

Talotarsal Joints and Ligaments of the Foot

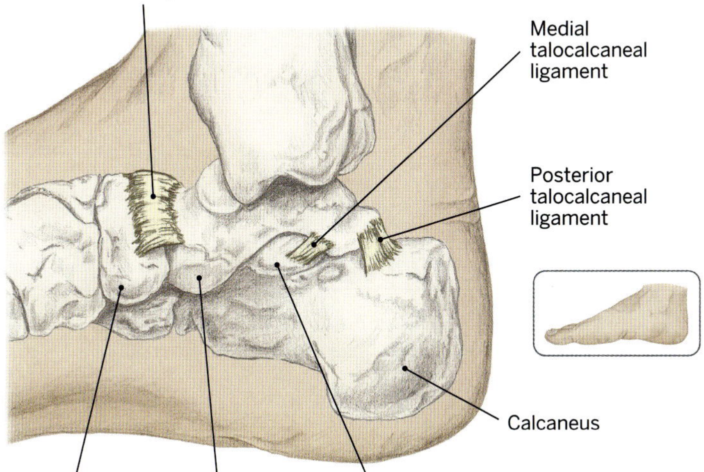

7.141 Medial view of right ankle, showing ligaments of talotarsal joints

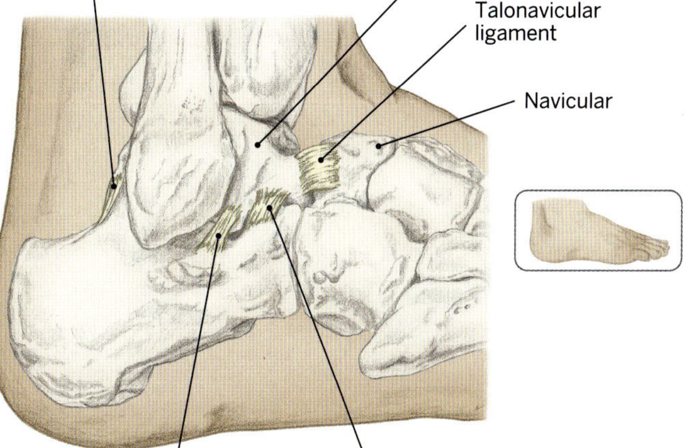

7.142 Lateral view of right ankle, showing ligaments of talotarsal joints

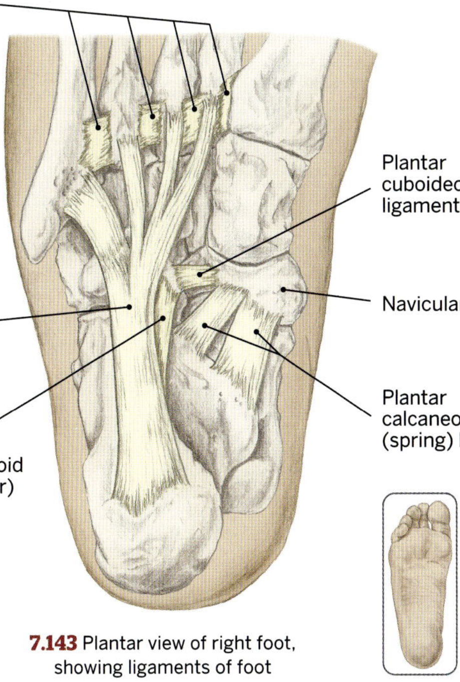

7.143 Plantar view of right foot, showing ligaments of foot

calcaneocuboid kal-***ka***-ne-o-***ku***-boyd
cuboideonavicular ku-***boyd***-e-o-na-***vik***-u-lar
talonavicular ***ta***-lo-na-***vik***-u-lar

Leg & Foot

Ligaments of the Foot

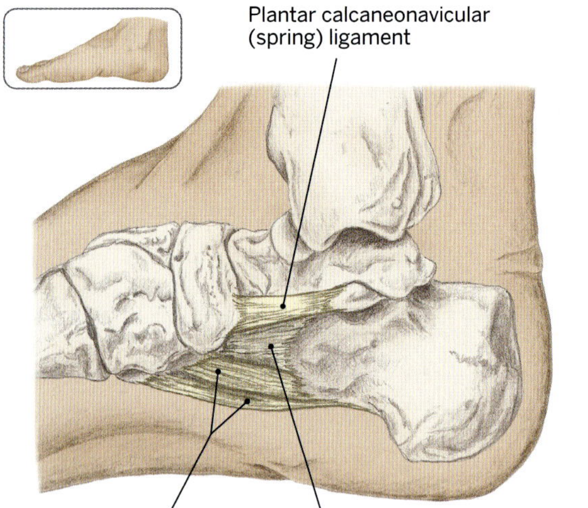

7.144 Medial view of right ankle, showing ligaments of subtalar joints

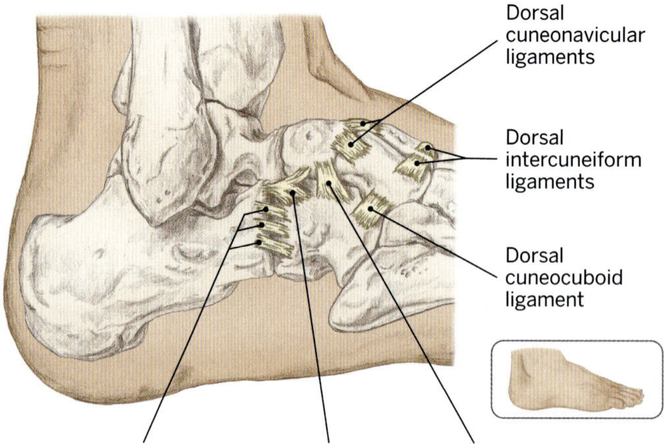

7.145 Lateral view of right ankle, showing ligaments of intertarsal joints

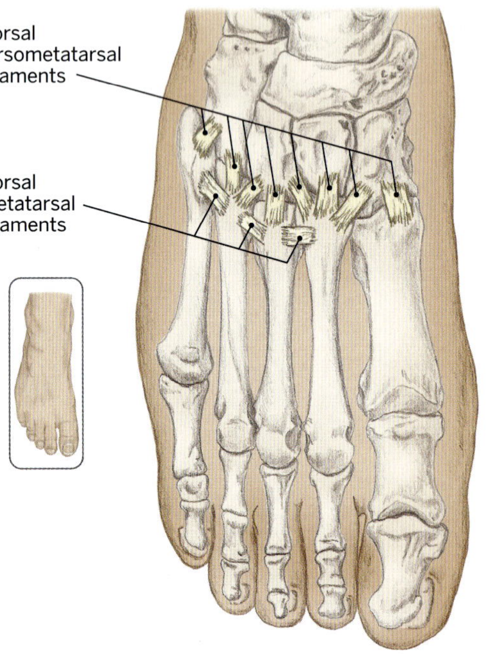

7.146 Dorsal view of right foot, showing ligaments of tarsometatarsal and intermetatarsal joints

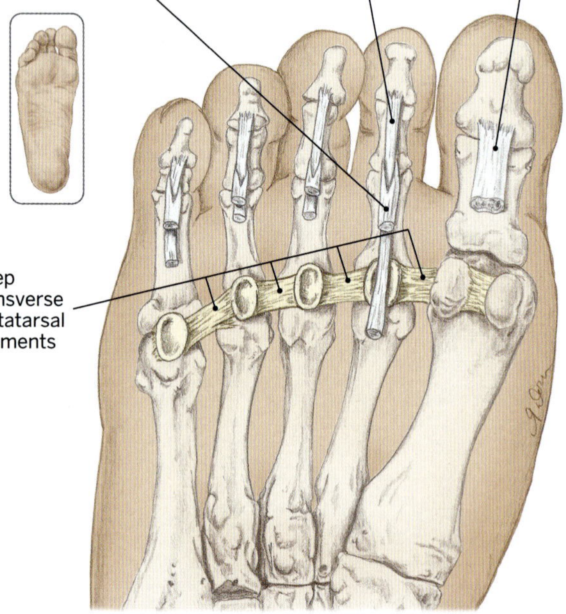

7.147 Plantar view of right foot, showing ligaments of metatarsophalangeal and interphalangeal joints

Deltoid Ligament

The deltoid ligament is composed of several ligaments that originate at the medial malleolus and fan distally to attach at the talus, sustentaculum tali, and navicular (**7.148**). It is designed to protect against medial stress of the talocrural joint. The deltoid ligament is deep to the flexor retinaculum and flexor tendons (p. 385), yet is palpable.

Deltoid ligament

1. Partner supine or seated. Locate the medial malleolus and sustentaculum tali.
2. Place your finger between these points and strum horizontally to isolate the fibers of the ligaments.
3. Slide distally from the medial malleolus at a 45° angle and palpate its angled fibers to define the anterior and posterior aspects of the deltoid ligament (**7.149**).

Are you palpating in the space between the medial malleolus and sustentaculum tali? Do the fibers you feel fan out from the medial malleolus and have a firm, dense texture?

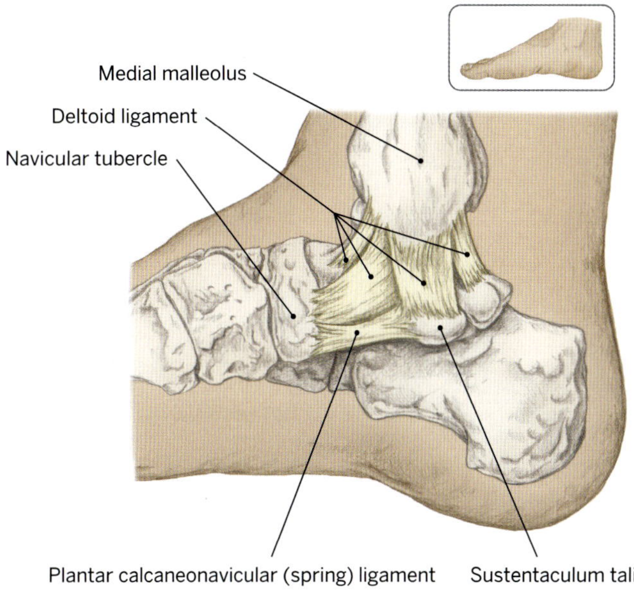

7.148 Medial view of right ankle, showing deltoid and spring ligaments

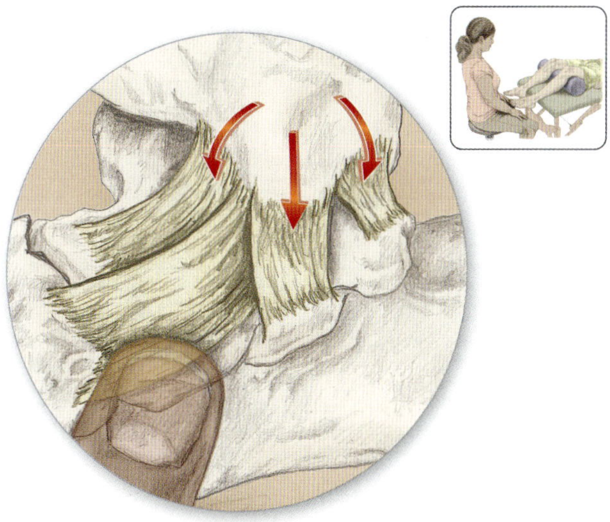

7.149 Medial view of right ankle, as you palpate the deltoid ligament

Plantar Calcaneonavicular (Spring) Ligament

The spring ligament is a small, tough band of tissue that plays an important role in stabilizing the medial longitudinal arch of the foot (see **7.148**). Located along the medial side of the foot, the ligament stretches from the sustentaculum tali to the navicular tubercle and might be positioned deep to the tibialis posterior tendon. The spring ligament might be extremely tender and should be accessed slowly. Be sure to communicate with your partner.

Spring ligament

1. Partner supine or seated. Passively invert the foot to soften any surrounding tissue and locate the sustentaculum tali and navicular tubercle.
2. Palpating between these bony landmarks, use a fingertip to slowly explore the taut surface of the spring ligament (**7.150**).

Are you between the sustentaculum tali and navicular tubercle? Can you roll your fingertip slowly across the surface of the ligament?

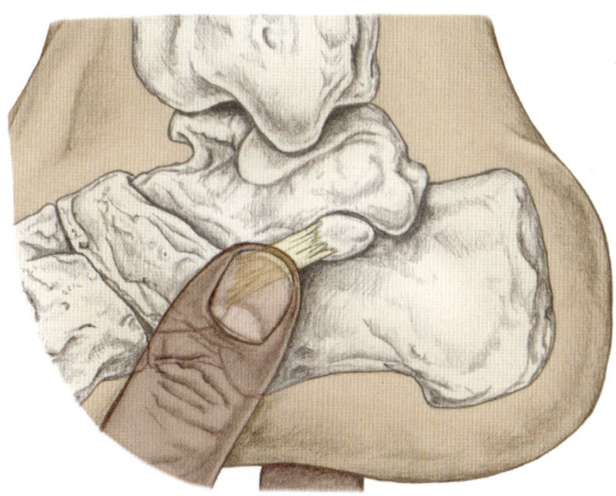

7.150 Medial view of right ankle, as you palpate the spring ligament

Leg & Foot

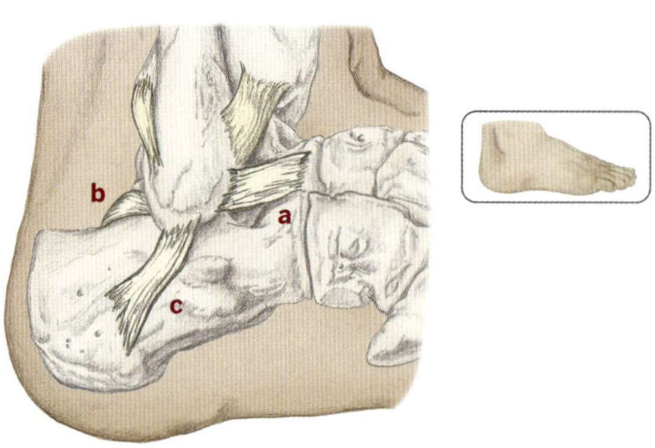

7.151 Lateral view of right ankle, showing lateral collateral ligaments: (**a**) anterior talofibular ligament, (**b**) posterior talofibular ligament, and (**c**) calcaneofibular ligament

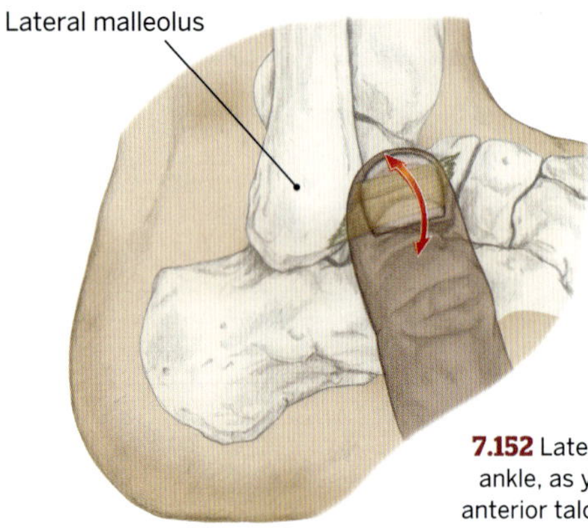

7.152 Lateral view of right ankle, as you palpate the anterior talofibular ligament

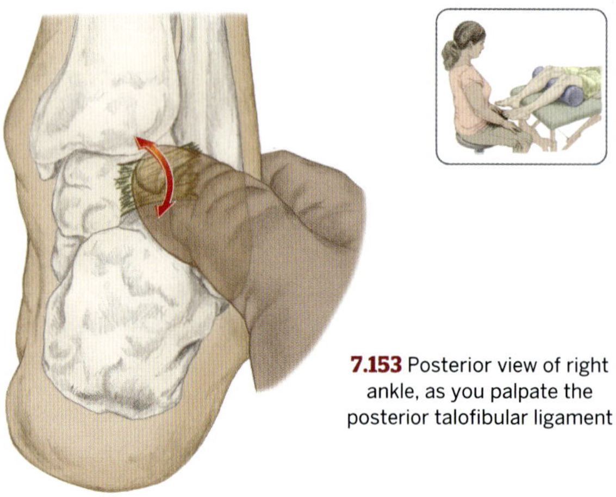

7.153 Posterior view of right ankle, as you palpate the posterior talofibular ligament

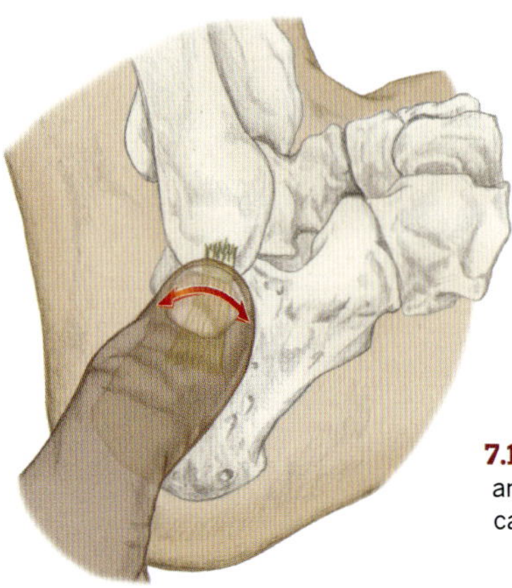

7.154 Lateral view of right ankle, as you palpate the calcaneofibular ligament

Lateral Collateral Ligaments of the Ankle

To understand why the ankle is the most frequently injured articulation in the body, you might begin with the ankle's lateral collateral ligaments (**7.151**). Designed to stabilize the distal end of the fibula to the calcaneus and talus, these three bands are the most often torn ligaments during ankle sprains. They are nowhere near as strong as the deltoid ligament on the ankle's medial side and are most vulnerable when the foot is inverted and plantar flexed.

The **anterior talofibular ligament** (**a**) spans from the anterior surface of the lateral malleolus to the lateral side of the talus's neck. When the foot is weight-bearing and excessively inverted, this ligament is often the first to be torn.

The **posterior talofibular ligament** (**b**) is much stronger than its anterior counterpart and only damaged in the most severe of ankle injuries, such as dislocations. It attaches to the posterior side of the lateral malleolus and the talus's lateral tubercle.

Between these two ligaments is the **calcaneofibular ligament** (**c**). It spans from the lateral malleolus down to the lateral surface of the calcaneus, deep to the fibularis tendons. Only during severe ankle sprains, after the anterior talofibular has ripped, will this ligament be torn as well.

Lateral collateral ligaments of the ankle

1. Partner supine or seated.
2. **Anterior talofibular** (**7.152**): This ligament is not very distinguishable, but its position can be isolated by first locating the anterior aspect of the lateral malleolus. Slide your thumb toward the head of the talus (p. 364), roughly an inch. The ligament passes just medial to the extensor digitorum brevis belly (p. 391).
3. **Posterior talofibular** (**7.153**): Set your finger on the posterior side of the lateral malleolus. Continue around the mallelous to the surface of the talus's lateral tubercle. (If you reach the calcaneal tendon, you have gone too far.) Between these landmarks will be the ligament. Also, use gentle pressure here since this region can often be tender.
4. **Calcaneofibular** (**7.154**): Locate the distal end of the lateral malleolus and the lateral aspect of the calcaneus. This ligament runs at a slight oblique angle and passes posterior to the fibular tubercle.

Retinacula of the Ankle

The tendons of the extensor muscles (p. 382) are supported by the superior and inferior extensor retinacula. The **superior extensor retinaculum** is broad and crosses the front of the ankle just proximal to the malleoli. The **inferior extensor retinaculum** is Y-shaped and begins distal to the lateral malleolus on the calcaneus. It spans the ankle and then divides, with one fork attaching at the medial malleolus and the other connecting to the navicular (**7.155**).

The fibularis muscles are stabilized by the superior and inferior fibular retinacula. The **superior fibular retinaculum** stretches from the lateral malleolus to the calcaneus, and the **inferior fibular retinaculum** pins the fibularis tendons down at the fibular tubercle.

The **flexor retinaculum** is a broad strap extending from the medial calcaneus to the medial malleolus. It is designed to hold in place the tendons of the flexor muscles and the tibial artery and nerve (see **7.158**).

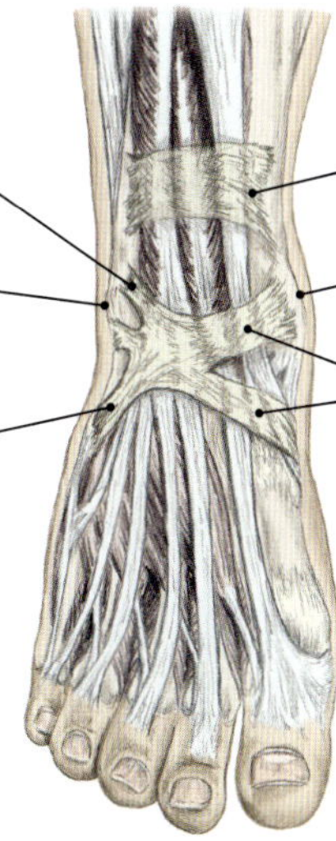

7.155 Dorsal view of right foot and ankle, showing retinacula

Extensor retinacula

1. Partner supine. Ask your partner to dorsiflex her ankle and extend her toes. The pressure from the bulging tendons will make the retinacula more pronounced.
2. Palpate an inch proximal to the medial malleolus for the broad fibers of the superior extensor retinaculum.
3. Locate the inferior extensor retinaculum by moving distally to the level of the malleolus (**7.156**). Explore either side of the large tibialis anterior tendon for easy access to this retinaculum.

Are the fibers you are accessing superficial and perpendicular to the extensor tendons? Ask your partner to relax her ankle and notice how the retinacula soften.

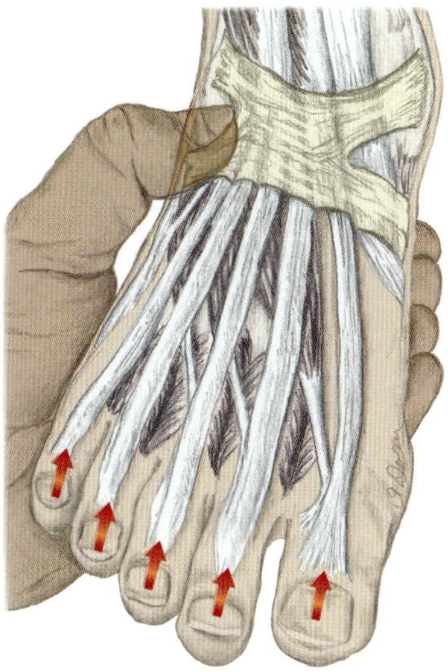

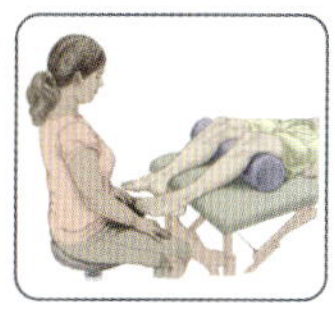

7.156 Dorsal view of right foot, partner extending her toes while you locate the inferior extensor retinaculum

Fibular retinacula

1. Ask your partner to evert her foot. The tension from the fibularis tendons will make the retinacula more pronounced.
2. Locate the fibularis tendons between the lateral malleolus and lateral calcaneus (**7.157**). Roll your fingers along either side of the fibularis tendons to feel the small, short fibers of the retinacula.

For the superior retinaculum, does the tissue you feel strap across the fibularis tendons from the lateral calcaneus to the lateral malleolus? For the inferior retinaculum, do you feel a short band crossing over the fibular tubercle?

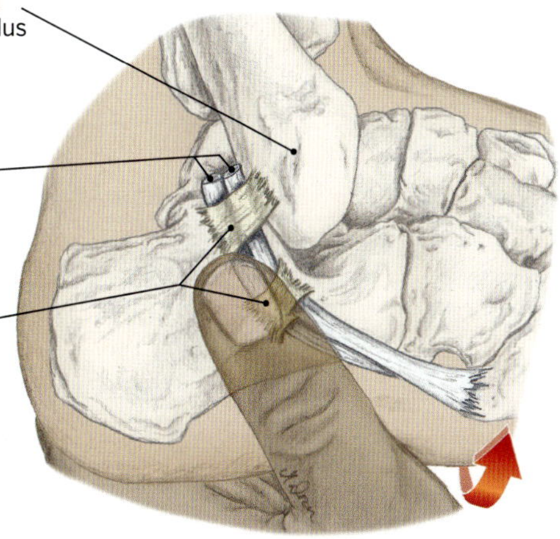

7.157 Lateral view of right ankle, partner everting foot while you locate the fibular retinacula

retinaculum	*ret*-i-***nak***-u-lum	L. halter, band, rope
retinacula	*ret*-i-***nak***-u-la	plural for retinaculum

Flexor retinaculum

1. Ask your partner to dorsiflex and invert her foot. The tension from the flexor tendons will elevate the retinaculum closer to the surface.
2. Locate the medial malleolus and the medial side of the calcaneus.
3. Palpate between these landmarks, strumming across the broad, superficial fibers of the flexor retinaculum (**7.158**).

Are you between the medial calcaneus and medial malleolus? Continue to explore the retinaculum with the foot relaxed.

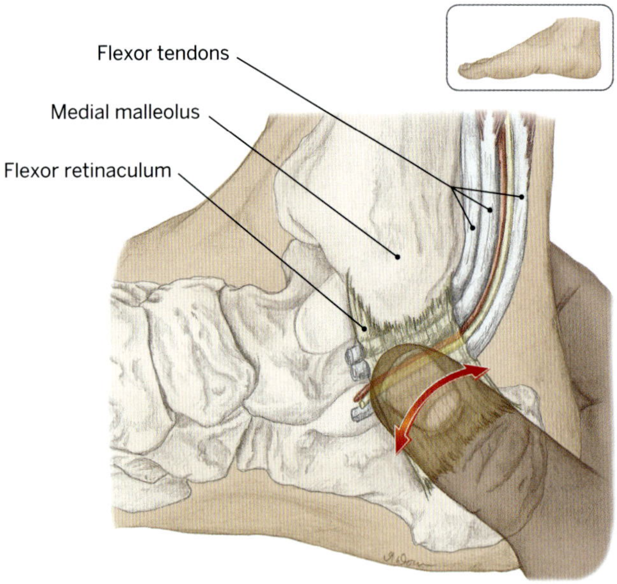

7.158 Medial view of right ankle, as you palpate flexor retinaculum

Plantar Aponeurosis

The plantar aponeurosis is a thick, superficial band of fascia stretching from the heel to the ball of the foot (**7.159**). Originating from the tuberosity of the calcaneus and expanding toward the metatarsal heads, it is important for supporting the longitudinal arch of the foot. Because the aponeurosis is located between the skin and muscles of the foot, it can be difficult to isolate from the surrounding tissues.

Plantar aponeurosis

1. Partner seated or supine. Crossing the ball of the foot, draw an imaginary triangle extending down to the heel.
2. Within this triangle explore the superficial layers of tissue along the sole of the foot. Passively flex and extend the toes, noting how this movement affects the tension of the plantar aponeurosis.

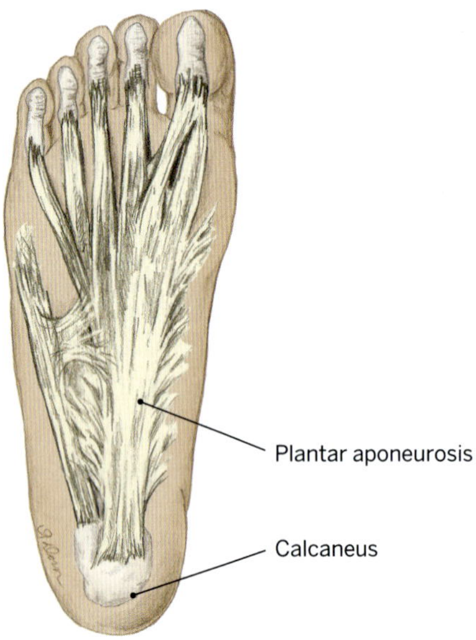

7.159 Plantar view of right foot, showing plantar aponeurosis

Posterior Tibial Artery

The posterior tibial artery extends from the popliteal artery. It is superficial and its pulse can be felt just inferior and posterior to the medial malleolus.

Posterior tibial artery

Partner supine. Locate the medial malleolus. Using two fingerpads, slide posterior to the malleolus and feel for the pulse of the artery (**7.160**).

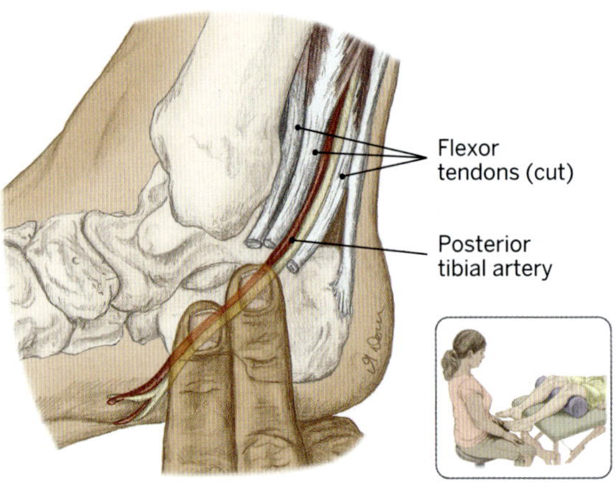

7.160 Medial view of right ankle, as you locate the posterior tibial artery

dorsalis pedis	*dor*-sal-is ***peh***-dis	L. *dorsum*, back; *pedis*, foot
aponeurosis	*ap*-o-nu-***ro***-sis	Grk. *apo*, from + *neuron*, nerve or tendon

Dorsalis Pedis Artery

Located between the first and second metatarsal bones, the dorsalis pedis artery lies superficial along the dorsal side of the foot.

Dorsalis pedis artery

Partner supine. Locate the first and second metatarsals. Place two fingerpads between the two bones and, using gentle pressure, explore for the pulse of the dorsalis pedis artery (**7.161**).

Are you lateral to the extensor hallucis longus tendon? If the pulse is undetectable, move slightly lateral.

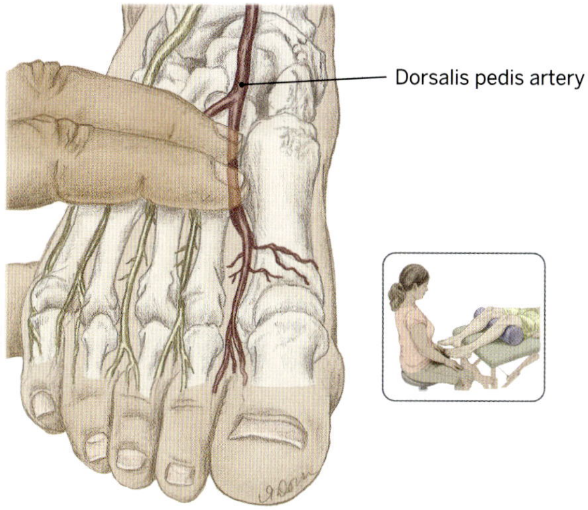

7.161 Dorsal view of right foot, as you locate the dorsalis pedis artery

Sesamoid Bones of First Metatarsal

The sesamoid bones of the first metatarsal are located along the plantar surface of the first metatarsal head. Usually there are two of these bones, but sometimes more are present. The sesamoids are spherical and imbedded in the tendon of the flexor hallucis brevis. Often only their location and density, not their specific shapes, are palpable.

Sesamoid bones of first metatarsal

1. Partner seated or supine. Locate the head of the first metatarsal. Slide around to its plantar surface at the ball of the foot.
2. Using your thumbpad, explore this surface for the small sesamoid bones. Passively flex and extend the first toe to soften the surrounding tissues (**7.162**).

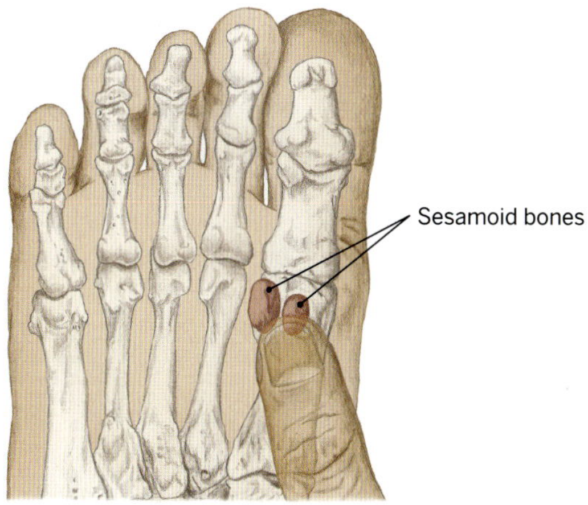

7.162 Plantar view of right foot, as you explore the sesamoid bones

Calcaneal Bursae

The **calcaneal bursa** (**7.163, a**) is located between the attachment of the calcaneal tendon and the overlying skin. The **retrocalcaneal bursa** (**b**) is positioned on the opposite side of the calcaneal tendon. It serves to cushion the tendon against the calcaneus.

Both bursae are impalpable; however, they can become thick or inflamed from tight shoes and, especially, from high heels.

Calcaneal bursae

1. Partner seated or supine. With the ankle in a neutral position, locate the calcaneal tendon.
2. Follow it distally until it merges into the calcaneus. Gently squeeze the skin posterior to the tendon. This is where the calcaneal bursa is located (**7.163**).
3. Shift your fingers between the tendon and calcaneus. If the bursae are healthy, they will not be palpable.

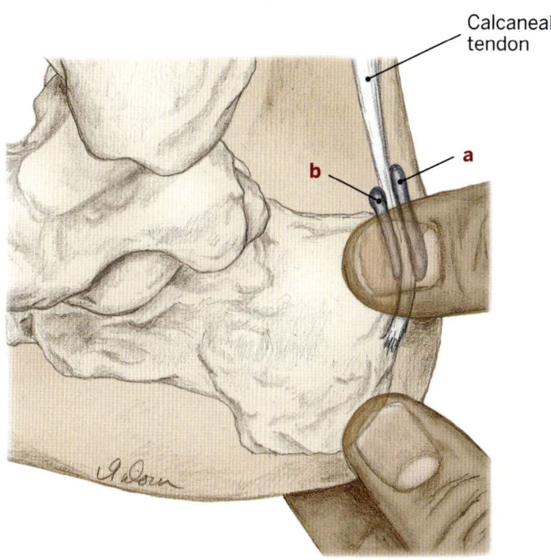

7.163 Medial view of right foot, as you locate (**a**) the calcaneal bursa and (**b**) the retrocalcaneal bursa

Leg & Foot

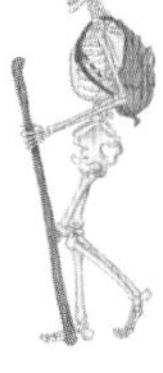

. . . to arrive where we started
and know the place for the first time . . .

A Day in the Life of Your Nervous System

Trail Guide to the Body focuses on the anatomical and palpatory aspects of the musculoskeletal system, including details to locate (or avoid) nerves. This appendix is designed to help you further explore some of the fascinating features of the nervous system (**A.1**). To make it fun, we'll experience it over the course of one day. And it might look a bit like *your* day.

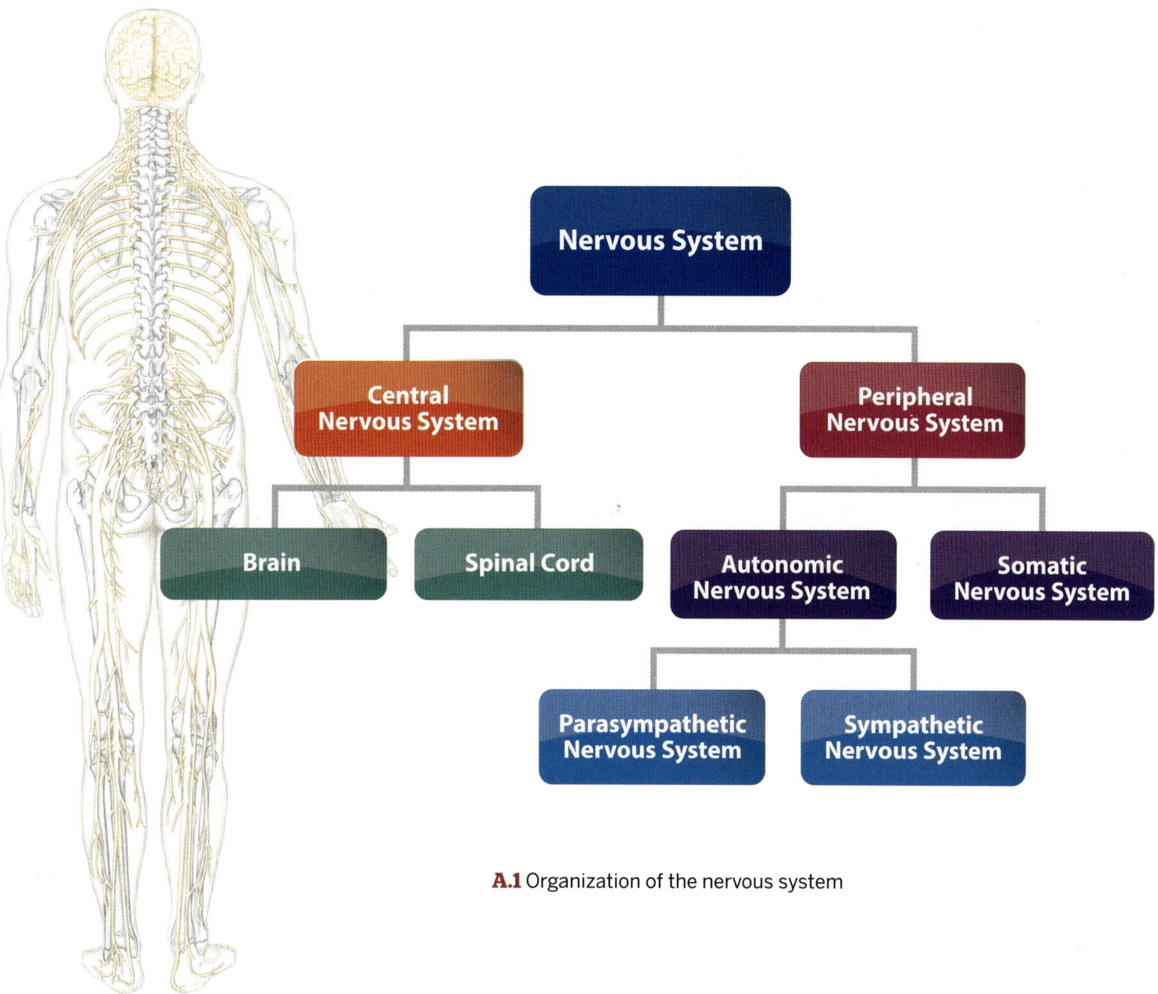

A.1 Organization of the nervous system

An Introduction

It's early. Still dark outside. You roll over, flip on the light next to your bed, and (being a good student) open Trail Guide to the Body *to this very page. You blink a few times until these words come into focus. Unbeknownst to you, your nervous system was busy all night regulating hundreds of processes throughout your body—even producing dreams. But now it must perform an astonishingly intricate task—reading.*

First, your nervous system needs to recognize squiggly symbols and comprehend their groupings. Then it needs to interpret those figures with previously formed understandings and memories. Finally, it must formulate new thoughts and images based on those interpretations. How you do all this instantaneously is courtesy of a vast network of neural tissues that comprise your brain, your spinal cord, and thousands of miles of neural pathways.

The nervous system—with your brain serving as the command center—uses electrochemical signals to *send, receive,* and *relay* messages throughout your body. Doing so, it *coordinates and controls* your thoughts, movements, and automatic responses to everyday life.

Working both consciously and unconsciously, the nervous system affects virtually every aspect of life, from sleeping to standing to climbing stairs; regulating your heart rate, breathing, emotions, and digestion; even recalling yesterday's lunch. The list is long.

It performs these functions through an extensive network of nerve tissue that sends electrical signals back and forth between cells, muscles, and glands throughout your body. And while the nervous system is managing your internal environment, it simultaneously receives, integrates, and processes information from the world around you.

For instance, you stop reading, look on your nightstand, and spy an apple. You gather this information via your senses. This data is then processed by your brain (*I see an apple*) (**A.2**) and then integrated with information from your digestive system (*I'm hungry*) (**A.3**). Then a set of commands is sent back to your body, prompting the desired response (*I grab the apple*) (**A.4**).

Let's take that apple into the kitchen, prepare a hearty breakfast, and lay out a general picture of this complex and beautiful system.

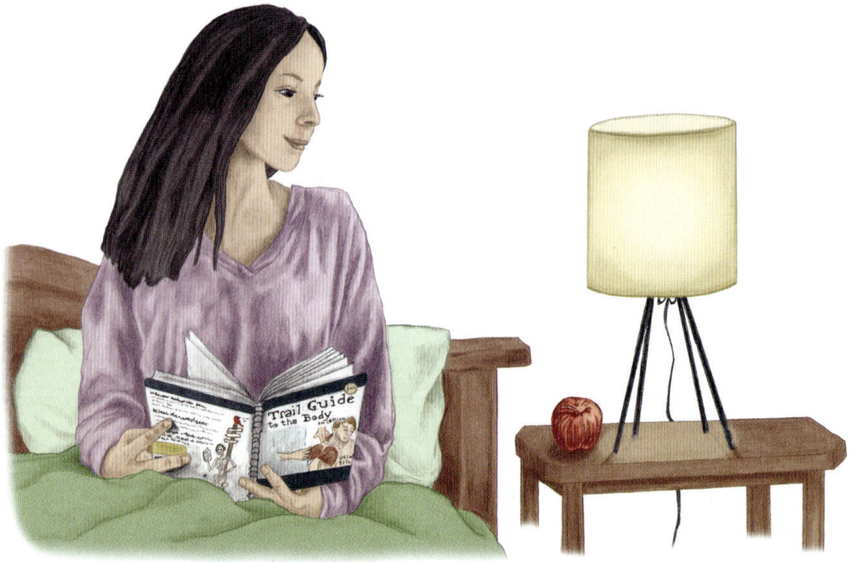

A.2 Seeing an apple

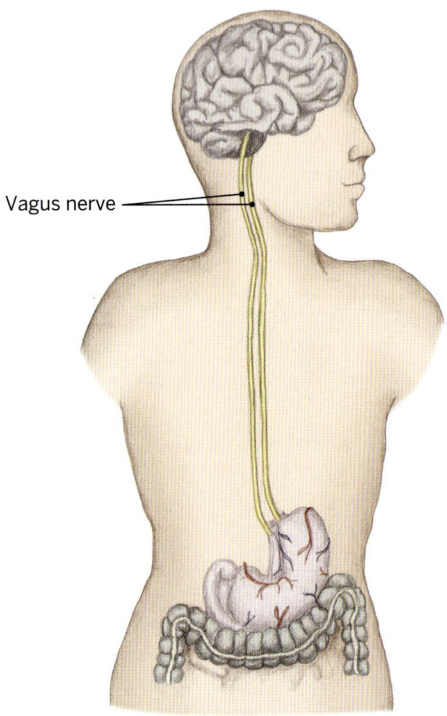

A.3 Hearing your stomach rumble

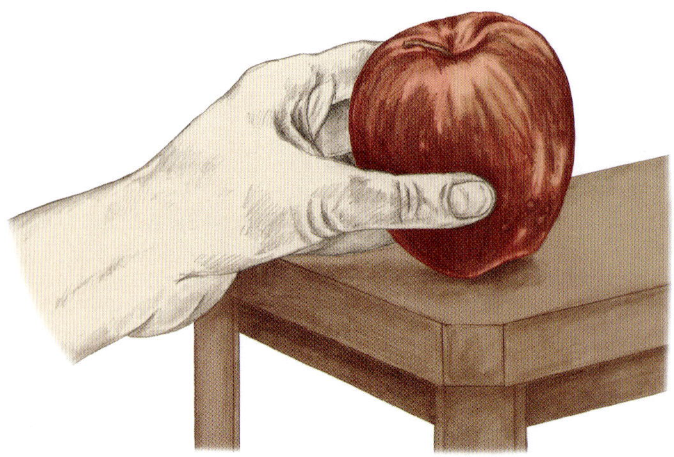

A.4 Reaching for the apple

The Nervous System in General

As you cut up the apple and inhale the aroma of cooked bacon, your **central nervous system (CNS)** is fully engaged. Composed of the brain and spinal cord, the CNS regulates all bodily functions (knife handling, for example) and responds to external stimuli (bacon, *yum*).

The vast network of nerves distributed throughout your body forms the **peripheral nervous system (PNS)**. The PNS acts as an intermediary between your CNS and the tissues and structures of your body. It does this via the neurons (nerve cells) in these nerves.

The PNS is composed of **efferent** neurons, which transmit information from the CNS to your muscles and glands, and **afferent** neurons, which relay information from your receptors back to the CNS. (Fun mnemonic: **E**fferent info **E**xits, **A**fferent info **A**rrives.) The efferent neurons of your PNS can be divided into two subsystems—the somatic and autonomic nervous systems.

The **somatic nervous system (SNS)** controls muscle movement and relays information from the body's tissues (skin, muscles, joints, etc.) and sensory organs—such as your ears and eyes—to the central nervous system. The **autonomic nervous system (ANS)** regulates involuntary physiologic processes such as your heart rate, blood pressure, respiration, and digestion. Further subgroups of the ANS are the **sympathetic** ("fight or flight") and **parasympathetic** ("rest and digest") **nervous systems** (**A.5**).

Your somatic system controls your hand and wrist to flip the pancakes, as well as your ears to send a message to the CNS that the kettle is whistling. Meanwhile, your autonomic system manages the rumbling of your belly and the salivation in your mouth.

After breakfast, you realize you're running late and start to do three things at once. "I have to get dressed! Load the backpack. Where are my keys?" Neurons are firing.

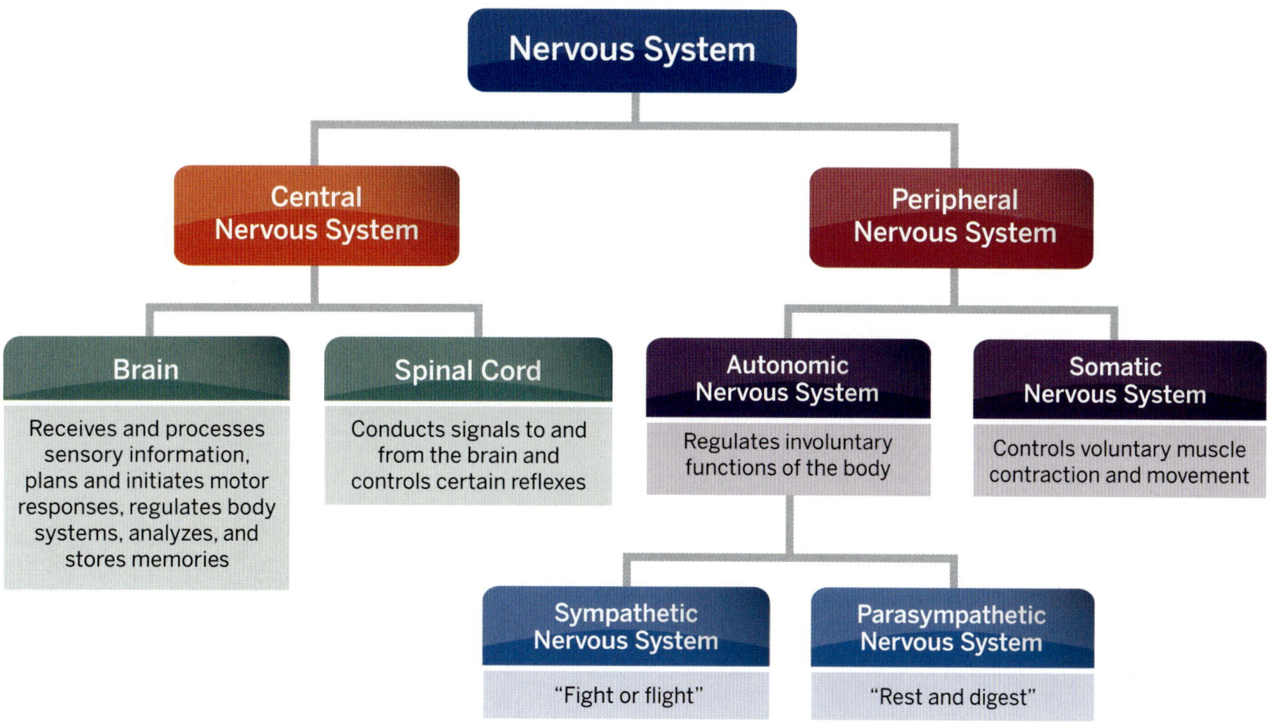

A.5 Organization and functions of the nervous system

A **neuron**, or nerve cell, is the structural and functional unit of the nervous system. Each consists of a **cell body** with two types of extensions—axons and dendrites. **Axons** are typically long and send information away from the cell body. **Dendrites** are generally short and receive information from other cells or the environment (**A.6**).

As we've noted, the neurons of the PNS are designated into two groups—afferent or efferent. **Afferent neurons** (also known as sensory neurons) are the messenger neurons that bring sensory information from other parts of the body to the CNS. The smell of flowers, the pain in your elbow, the feel of sand between your toes are all signals carried by afferent neurons.

Efferent neurons (also called motor neurons) send impulses away from the CNS to muscles, glands, and organs to initiate an action. Considering the staggering quantity of stimuli the body receives every split second, it's not surprising there are far more afferent neurons than efferent neurons located throughout the body.

An interneuron (**A.6**) is a type of nerve cell predominantly found in the CNS. By acting as a "middleman," it integrates information between afferent neurons and efferent neurons. Many interneurons are used in high-functioning activities such as learning, planning, and memory.

Throughout the body, neurons are grouped together to form nerves. There are just a few nerves that contain only afferent fibers or only efferent fibers. Most nerves include both types of transmission and are called **mixed nerves**.

What exactly is a nerve? Located in the peripheral nervous system, a **nerve** is an enclosed, cable-like group of axons (or nerve fibers). A nerve's anatomy begins with a single neuron's axon wrapped in **endoneurium**, a sheath of connective tissue. Then, groups of axons are bundled into **fascicles** and wrapped in **perineurium**, another casing of connective tissue. A final layer of connective tissue, the **epineurium**, bundles the group of fascicles to form a nerve (**A.7**).

*As you step onto the sidewalk, your **afferent** neurons relay messages to your CNS about the air temperature felt on your cheeks, the quantity and sounds of distant traffic, and a small pebble in your right shoe. Your **efferent** neurons send instructions to various muscles to position your body next to a lamppost. While holding yourself steady with one hand and balancing on one foot, you slide off your shoe and shake out the stone. Now let's get to school!*

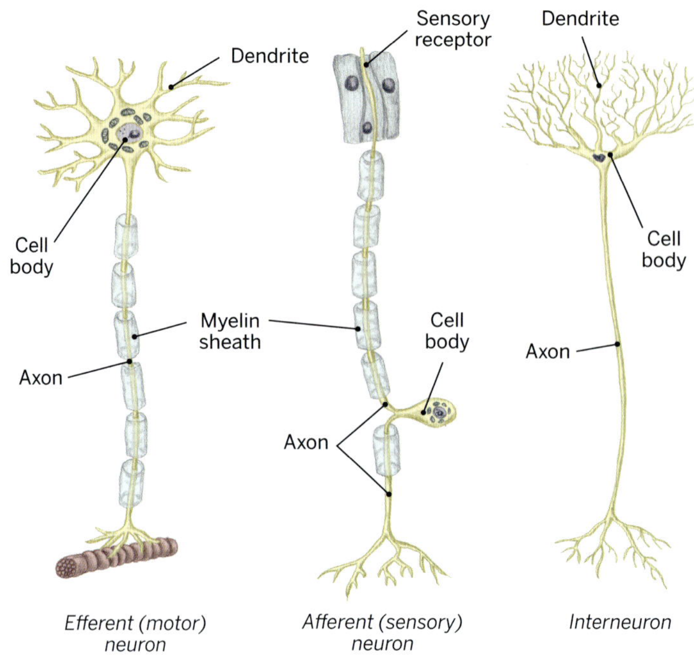

A.6 Types of neurons

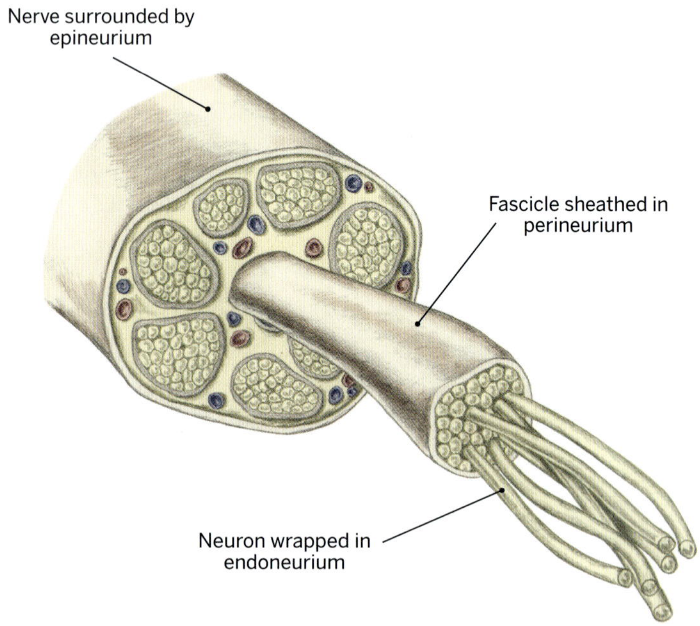

A.7 Parts of a nerve

Cranial Nerves and Spinal Nerves

Cranial Nerves

Sitting in class, soaking up all the images and information, your brain is beginning to feel full. Well, it is, but not in the way you might suspect. There are 12 pairs of cranial nerves that extend from the inferior surface of the brain and brainstem. They primarily innervate (supply) structures of the face and head, but they also innervate some structures of the neck and torso. When you blink your eyes, move your tongue, create a facial expression, smell and taste food, or hear a dog bark, your cranial nerves are chiefly involved (**A.8**).

A pair of cranial nerves is identified by a formal name (such as optic nerve or facial nerve) that relates to its location or function, as well as a Roman numeral (I–XII). Except for the vagus nerve (CN X), each nerve in a pair will exit one side of the brain and function on that corresponding side.

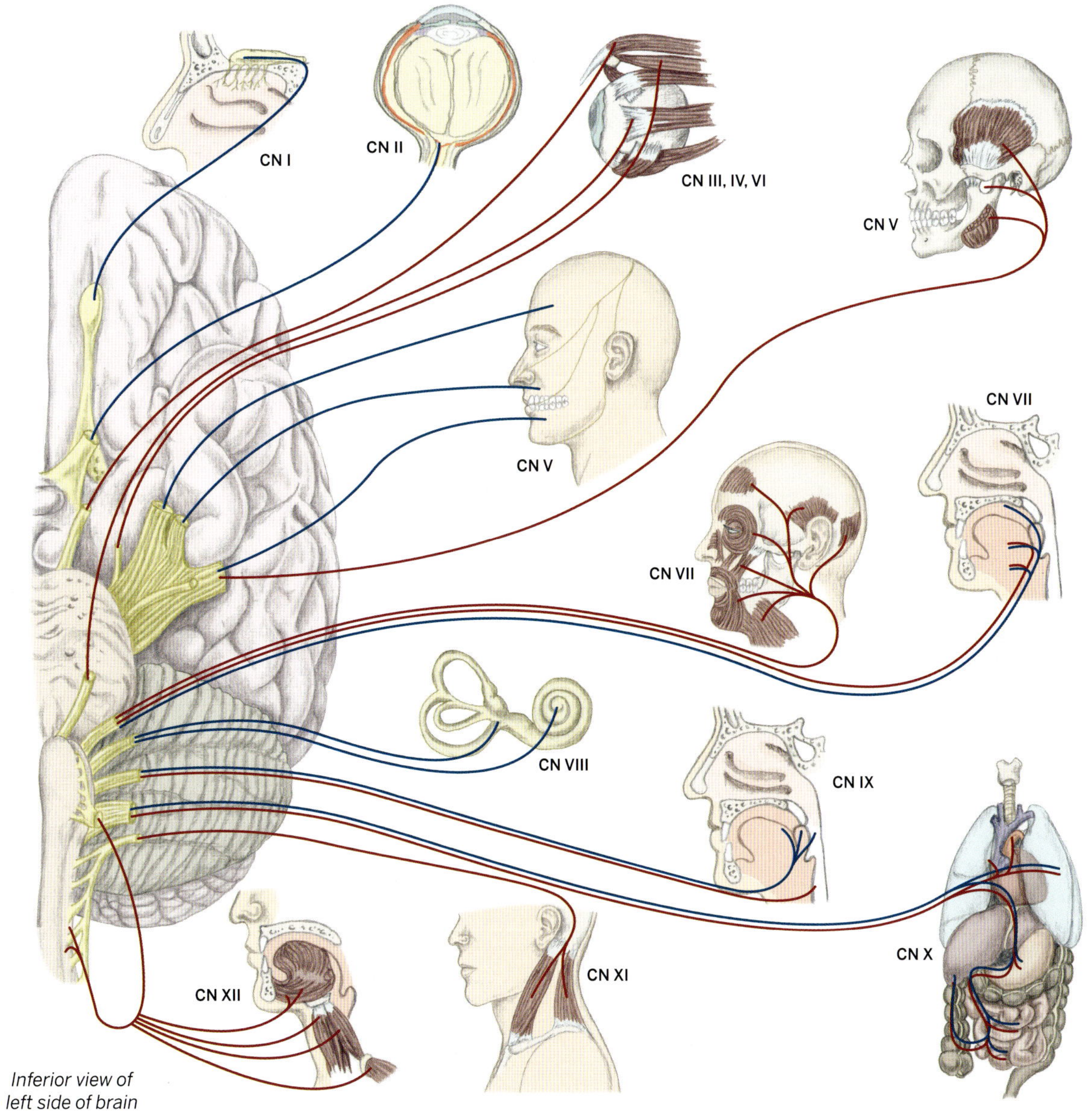

CN I	Olfactory nerve	**CN VII**	Facial nerve
CN II	Optic nerve	**CN VIII**	Vestibulocochlear nerve
CN III	Oculomotor nerve	**CN IX**	Glossopharyngeal nerve
CN IV	Trochlear nerve	**CN X**	Vagus nerve
CN V	Trigeminal nerve	**CN XI**	Spinal accessory nerve
CN VI	Abducens nerve	**CN XII**	Hypoglossal nerve

A.8 Cranial nerves include sensory nerves (**blue**) and motor nerves (**red**).

Spinal Nerves

Thirty-one pairs of spinal nerves emerge from the spinal cord and link the central nervous system to the peripheral nervous system. Based on regions of the vertebral column, these pairs are divided into five groups—cervical (8), thoracic (12), lumbar (5), sacral (5), and coccygeal (1) (**A.9**).

The spinal nerves emerge from the vertebral column through openings (intervertebral foramen) that are situated between adjacent vertebrae. The exception is the first pair of spinal nerves, which exit between the base of the skull and atlas (C-1). The first seven cervical nerves (C1–C7) branch out above their corresponding vertebrae.

The remaining spinal nerves (C8–L5) extend from below their respective vertebrae. For example, spinal nerve T12 exits the foramen located below the twelfth thoracic vertebra and above the first lumbar vertebra.

[Note: "How can there be eight cervical spinal nerves, but only seven cervical vertebrae?" This occurs because spinal nerve C7 exits *above* the seventh cervical vertebra and spinal nerve T1 emerges from *below* the first thoracic vertebra. This gap—between C7 and T1 vertebrae—is filled by spinal nerve C8.]

The arrangement of a spinal nerve is like a tree: Small **rootlets** form into **nerve roots** that combine to form a **spinal nerve** (the tree's trunk) before splitting into **rami** (*ramus* is Latin for "branch") (**A.10**).

More specifically, a spinal nerve begins as tiny **nerve rootlets** that merge to form two **nerve roots**. The **ventral nerve root** comprises efferent axons and runs along the spine's anterior aspect. The **dorsal nerve root** is reserved for afferent axons and is on the posterior side (**A.11**).

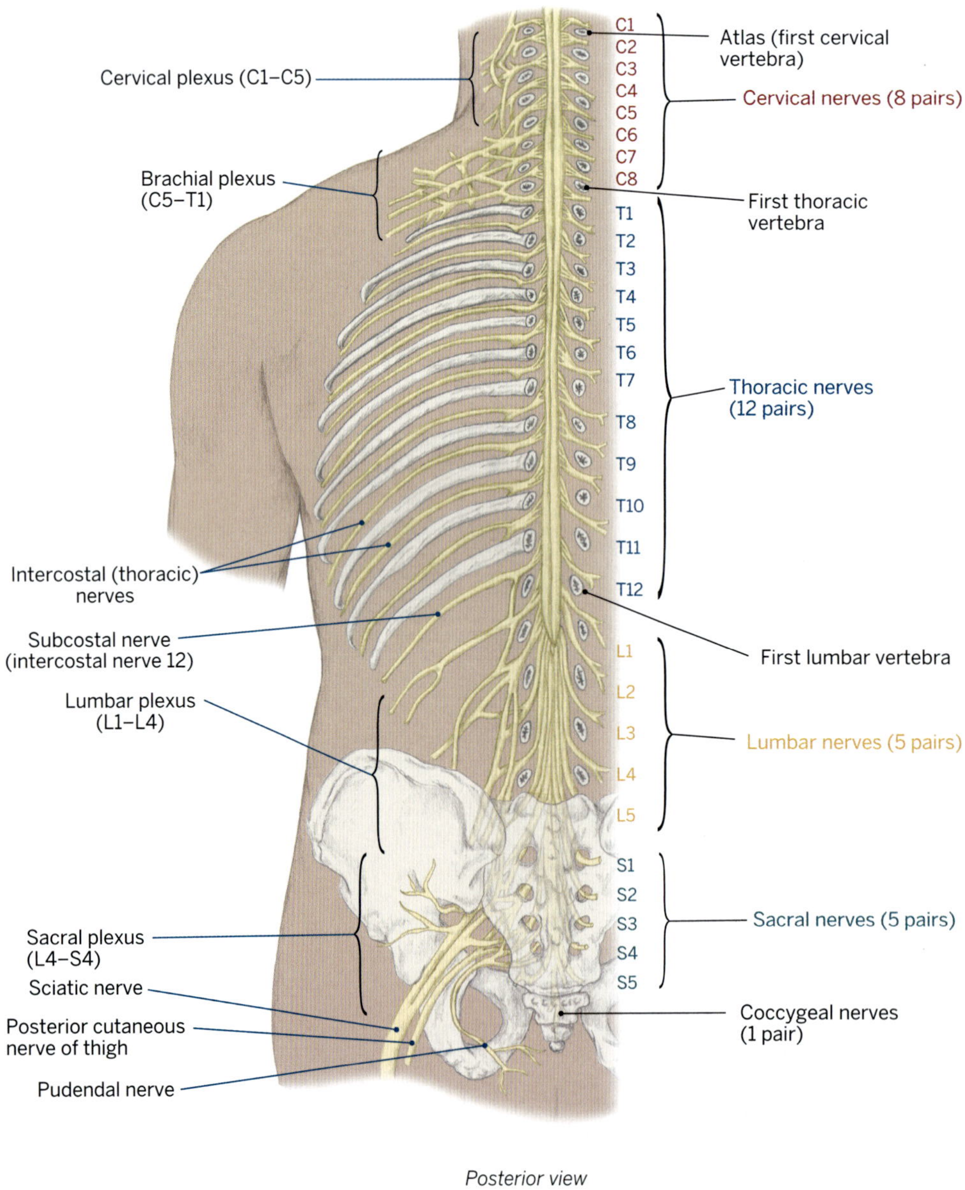

A.9 Posterior view of spine and left side, showing spinal cord and spinal nerves

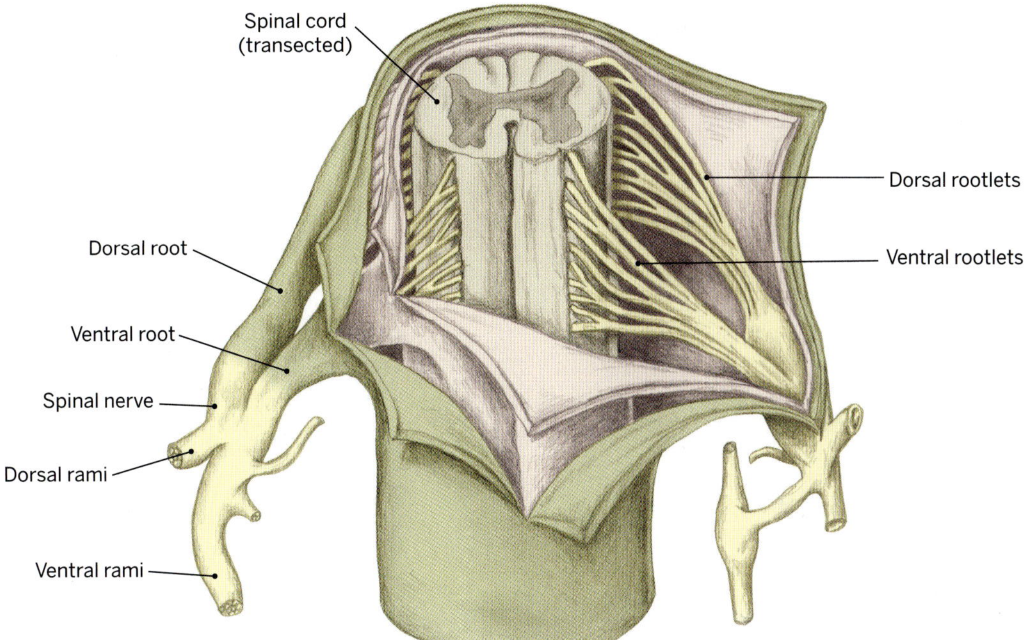

A.10 Anterior view of spinal nerve, showing arrangement of spinal cord, nerve rootlets, and roots

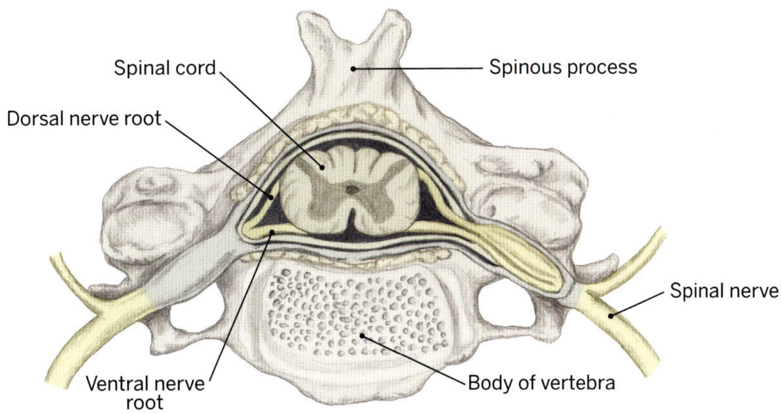

A.11 Cross section of vertebra and spinal cord

Nerve Plexuses and Peripheral Nerve Pathways

Let's continue with our tree metaphor. During a break from class, you step outside and look down at the gnarled, exposed roots of several crowded trees. Initially, you see randomness and disarray. Looking more closely, you detect patterns as roots branch apart but then reconnect elsewhere. Just as a tree interweaves and distributes its roots, so does the body with its nerves.

As we've seen, nerve roots at every level of the spinal cord emerge to form corresponding spinal nerves. A **nerve plexus** is an interconnected group of nerve fiber bundles formed by neurons from the ventral rami of neighboring spinal nerves. This occurs in four areas of the body. Like a house's electrical junction box that distributes specific wires to certain rooms, a plexus sorts nerve fibers from different spinal nerves. Fibers transmitting signals to and from a specific region of the body are combined by the plexus into one nerve.

One result of this mixing process is that a single nerve root might supply more than one peripheral nerve.

For instance, the ulnar and median nerves (which innervate different regions of the upper extremity) both derive from the nerve roots C7, C8, and T1.

The four main spinal nerve plexuses of the body are the **cervical**, **brachial**, **lumbar**, and **sacral**.

Cervical Plexus

Formed by the C1–C4 spinal nerves, the **cervical plexus** is located on the lateral side of the neck and includes numerous branches. Its muscular branches innervate the muscles of the neck, back, and diaphragm. The cutaneous branches of the cervical plexus supply the skin of the neck, upper thorax, scalp, and ear (**A.12**).

Brachial Plexus

Located along the inferior, lateral portion of the neck and axilla, the **brachial plexus** (C5–T1) supplies sensorimotor innervation to the upper extremity (shoulder, arm, and hand). The brachial plexus branches into five major nerves—axillary, musculocutaneous, median, radial, and ulnar (**A.13**).

To reach the upper extremity, the brachial plexus—which begins at the cervical nerve roots—must traverse a narrow pathway through the neck and upper shoulder. Before arriving at the axilla and arm, the plexus passes between the anterior and middle scalenes, over the first rib just under the clavicle, and then under the pectoralis minor against the rib cage. The space is so limited at each of these junctions that the brachial plexus is vulnerable to impingement.

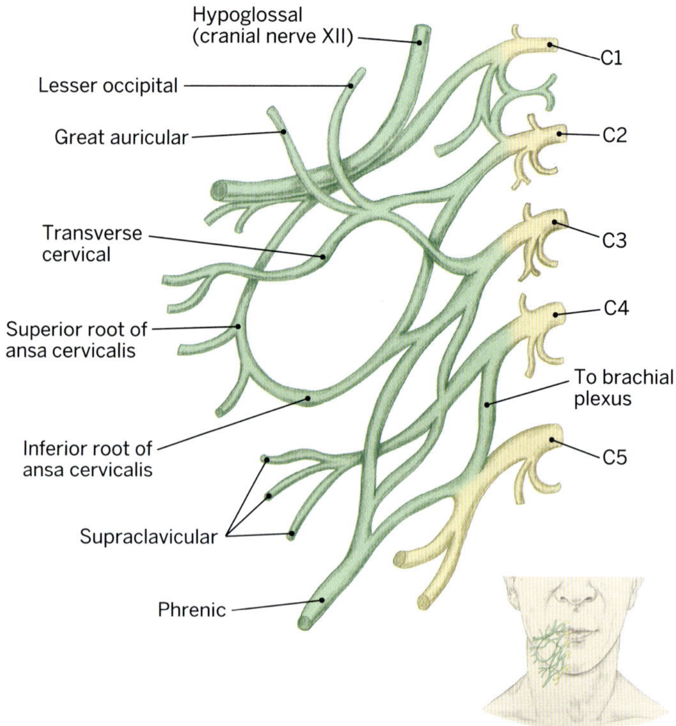

A.12 Anterior view of **cervical plexus**. This bundle of nerves innervates the diaphragm as well as many muscles on both sides of the neck.

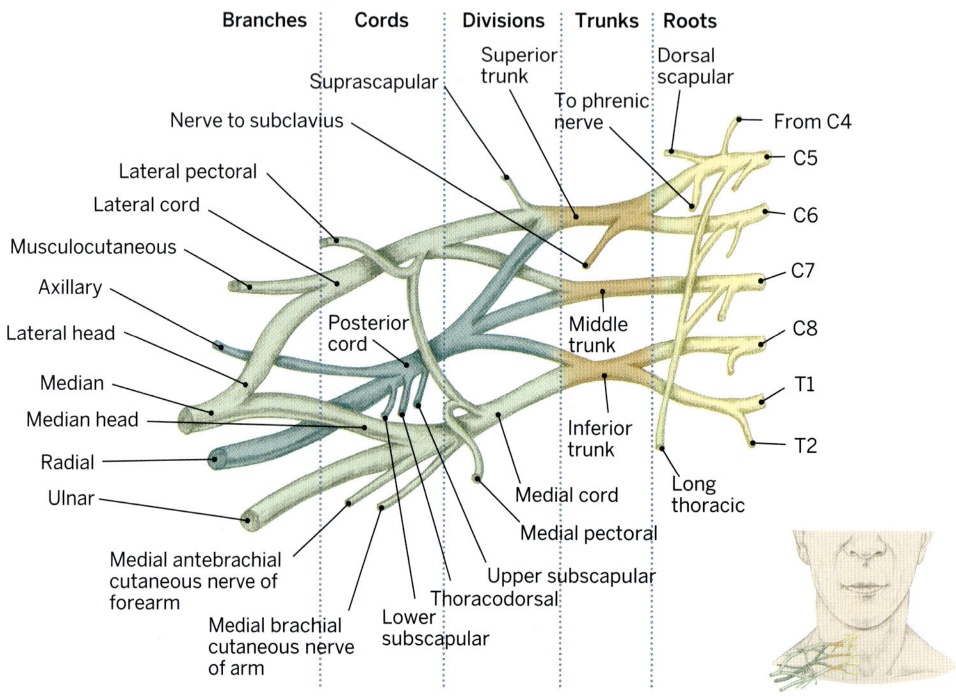

A.13 Anterior view of **brachial plexus**. This plexus contains five branches—axillary, musculocutaneous, median, radial, and ulnar. Together they provide innervation for muscles of the shoulder, arm, and hand.

Lumbar Plexus

The **lumbar plexus** is composed of four spinal nerves (L1–L4). They innervate many muscles of the pelvis and thigh, thus providing mobility, strength, and stability to the hip and knee. Located on the posterior abdominal wall, the plexus lies anterior to the transverse processes of the lumbar vertebrae and along the posterior portion of the psoas major (**A.14**).

[Note: The thoracic spinal nerves do not form a plexus. Instead, each becomes an intercostal nerve that extends laterally along the pathway of its corresponding rib to directly innervate tissues in that region.]

Sacral Plexus

The **sacral plexus** (L4–S4) is located along the posterior side of the sacrum and pelvis, deep to the piriformis. It provides afferent and efferent innervation to portions of the pelvis, posterior thigh, most of the lower leg, and the entire foot. The sciatic nerve, the largest nerve in the body, emerges from the sacral plexus. Roughly the width of a finger, the sciatic nerve divides at the posterior knee into the tibial and common fibular nerves (**A.15**).

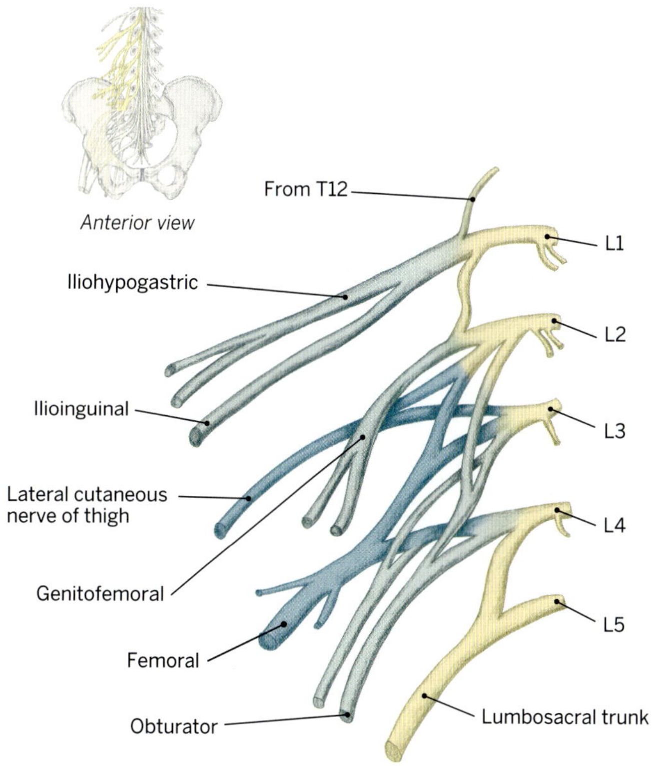

A.14 Anterior view of **lumbar plexus.** This plexus (L1 to L4) innervates much of the pelvis and thigh.

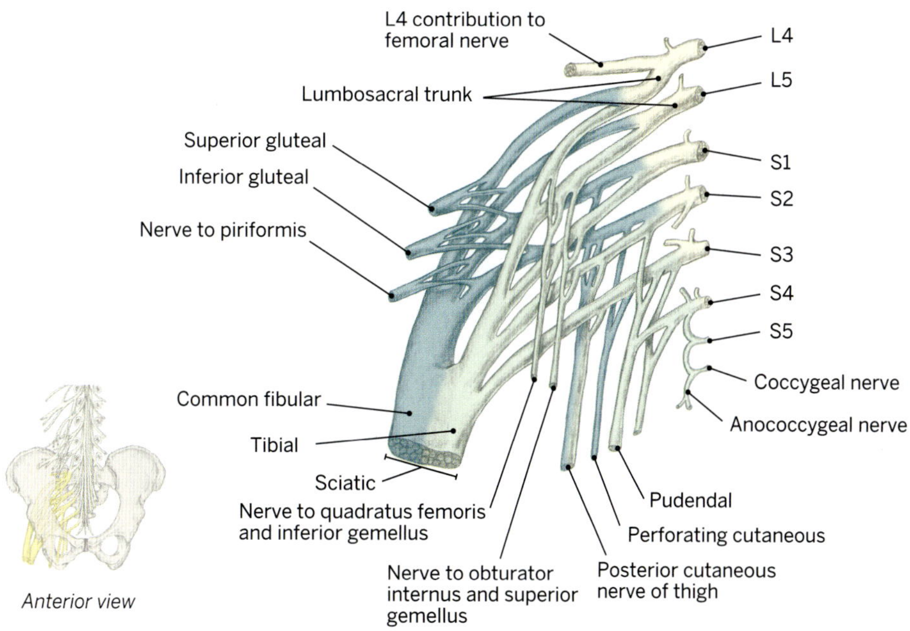

A.15 Anterior view of **sacral plexus**. This plexus innervates the thigh, leg, and foot.

Nerve Distribution in the Upper and Lower Appendages

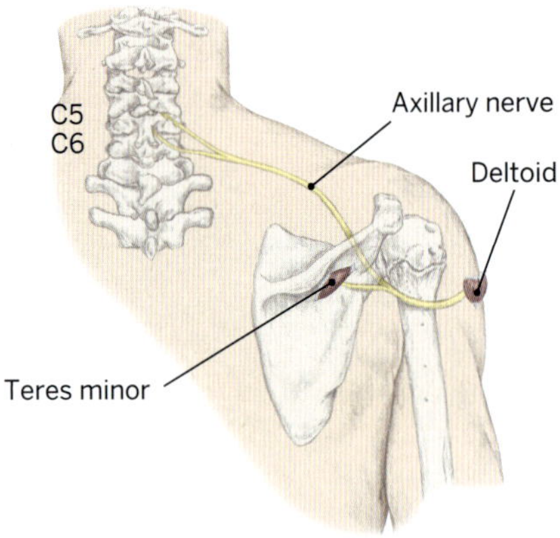

A.16 Posterior view of right shoulder, showing the **axillary nerve**. This short nerve innervates only the deltoid and teres minor.

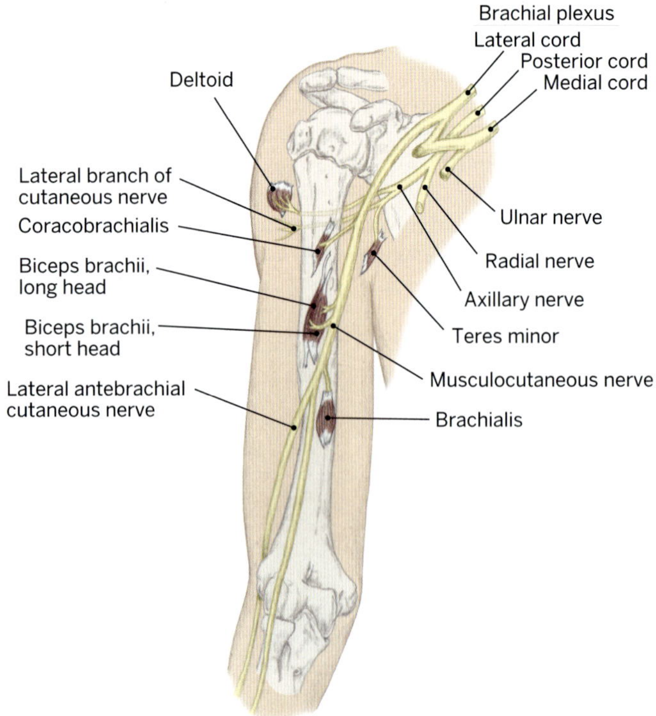

A.17 Anterior view of right arm, showing the **musculocutaneous nerve** (C5–C7). This relatively short nerve supplies innervation to several shoulder and elbow flexors.

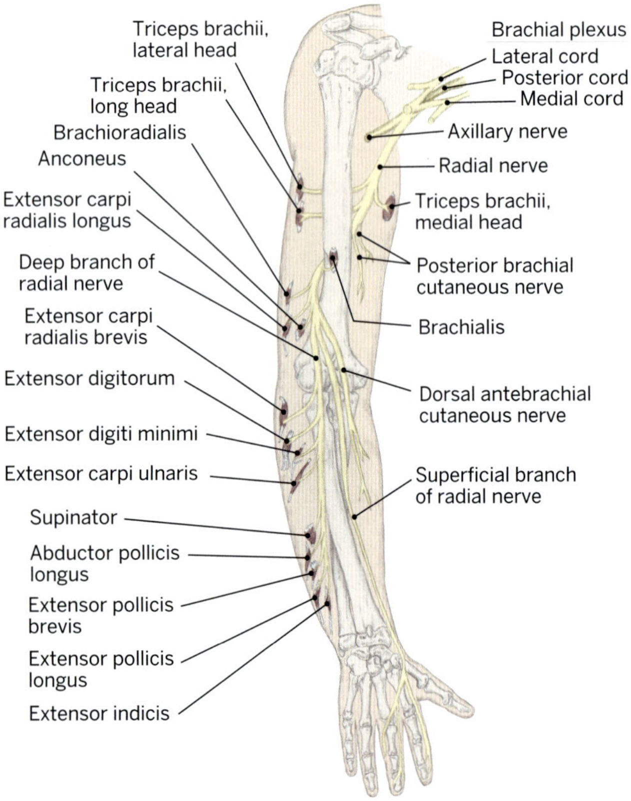

A.18 Anterior view of right upper appendage, forearm pronated, showing the **radial nerve** (C5–T1). The radial nerve innervates all the muscles that extend the elbow, as well as of the extensors of the wrist and fingers.

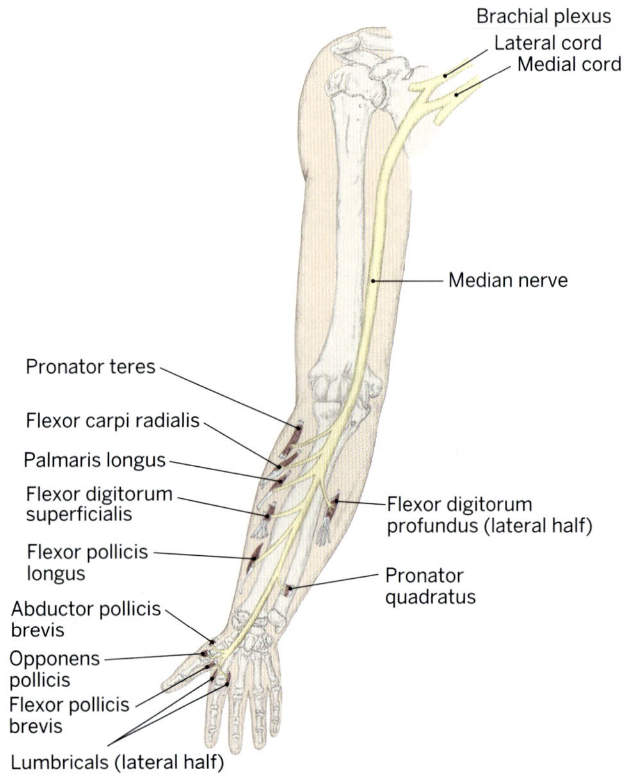

A.19 Anterior view of right upper appendage, showing the **median nerve** (C6–T1). This nerve only begins its motor capacity beyond the elbow. It supplies the pronators of the forearm and some of the flexors of the wrist and fingers, as well as many of the muscles of the thumb. This is the nerve often involved in carpal tunnel syndrome.

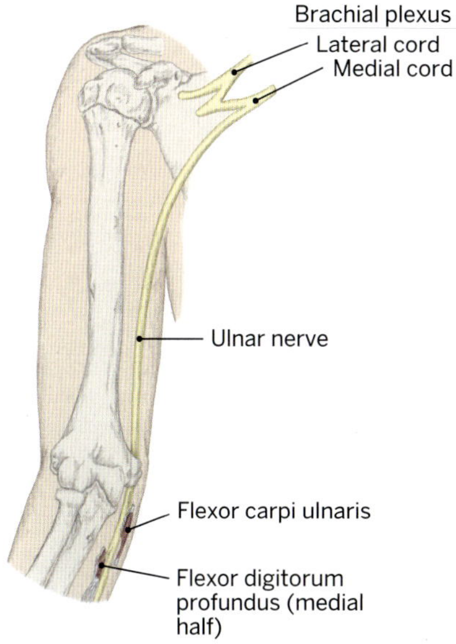

A.20 Anterior view of right arm, showing the **ulnar nerve** (C8, T1). Knocking your "funny bone" is the sensation produced by aggravating the ulnar nerve as it passes between the medial epicondyle and olecranon process.

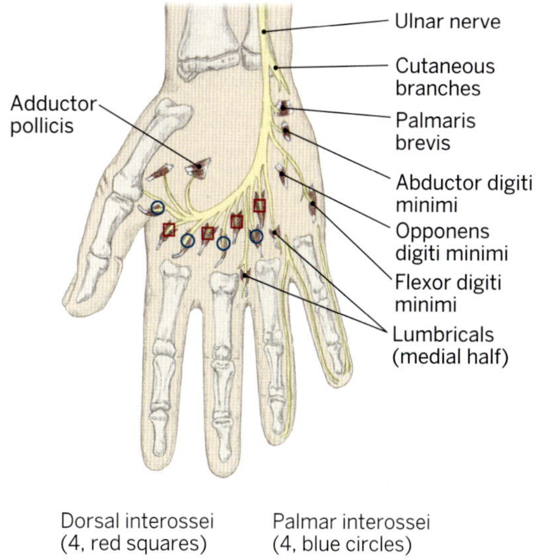

A.21 Palmar surface of right hand, showing the **ulnar nerve** (C8, T1). Aside from a couple of wrist flexors, many of the small muscles of the hand and fingers are supplied by the ulnar nerve.

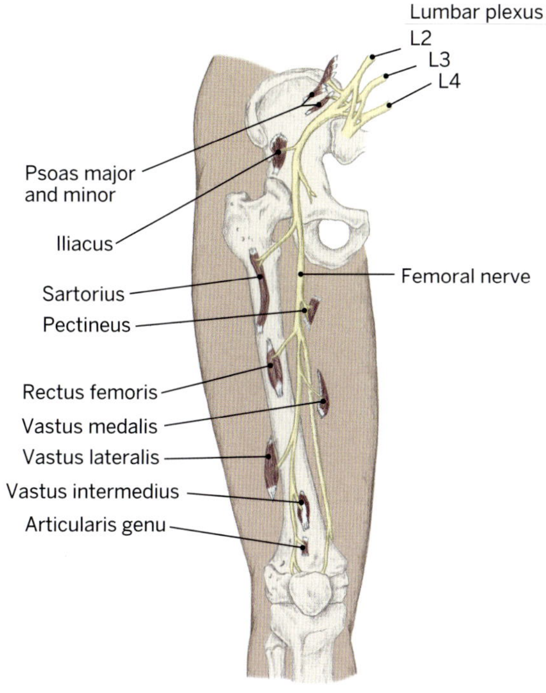

A.22 Anterior view of right hip and thigh, showing the **femoral nerve** (L2–L4). This large nerve innervates the iliacus and quadriceps femoris group, as well as the pectineus and sartorius.

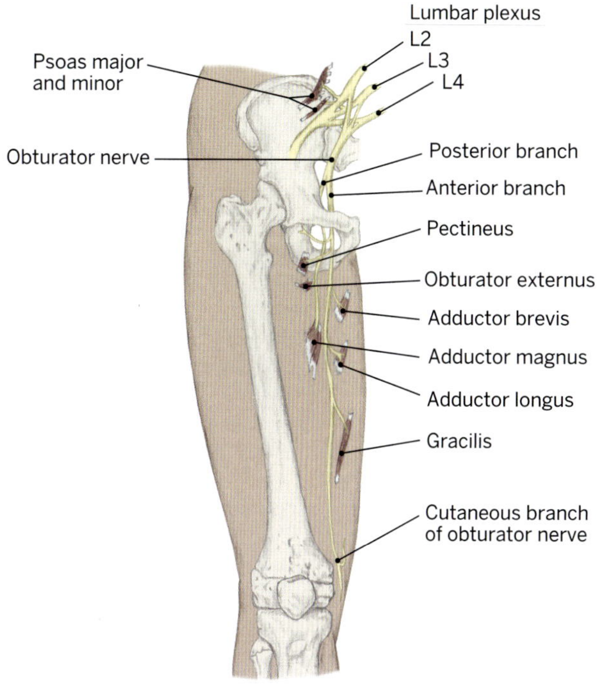

A.23 Anterior view of right hip and thigh, showing the **obturator nerve** (L2–L4). The obturator nerve's pathway is similar to that of the femoral nerve, but it primarily innervates the adductors.

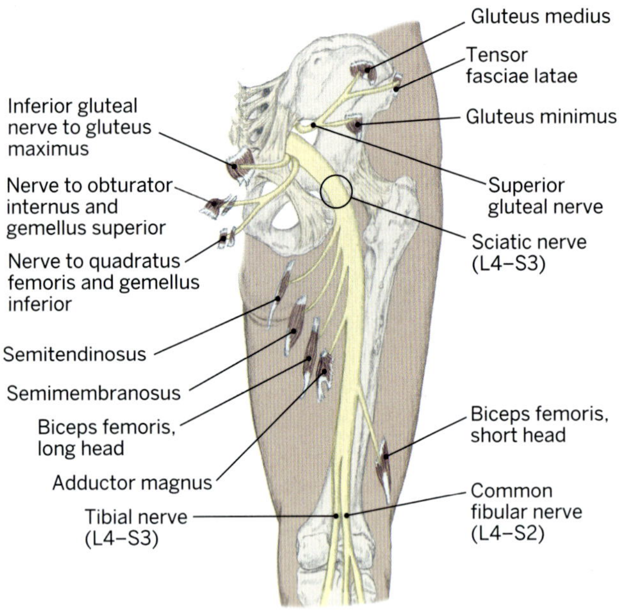

A.24 Posterior view of right hip and thigh, showing the **sciatic nerve** (L4–S3). As the largest nerve in the body, the sciatic nerve is really a bundling of two nerves—the tibial and common fibular. Before it splits off at the knee into those separate branches, it innervates the hamstrings and adductor magnus.

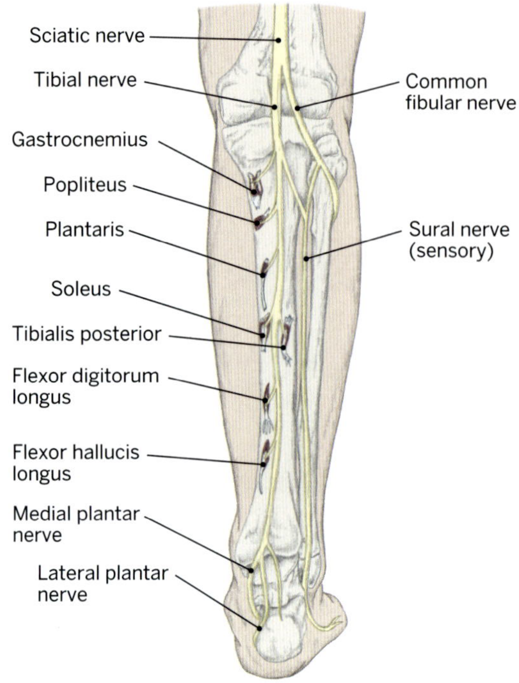

A.25 Posterior view of right leg, showing the **tibial nerve** (L4–S3). Passing straight down the posterior leg, the tibial nerve innervates the gastrocnemius and soleus, as well as the other plantar flexors and more.

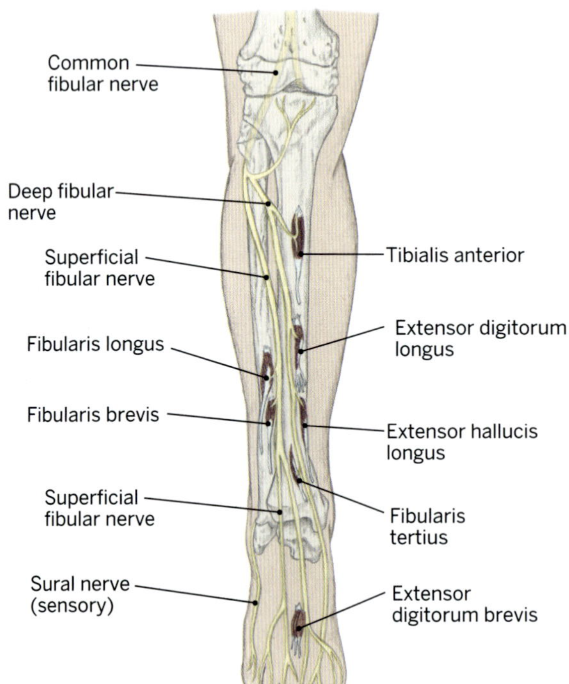

A.26 Anterior view of right leg, showing the **common fibular nerve** (L4–S2). Passing around the front side of the leg, this nerve innervates the fibularis and ankle extensors.

Dermatomes and Myotomes

After school, you walk to your local café and order a cup of tea. In the restroom, you begin to wash your hands and feel the cold water chill your digits. You adjust the knob and sense the water warming. Ouch! It's too hot. You pull your hands away in pain and dry them on a paper towel. To understand how you experienced pressure (touch), temperature, and pain on the surface of your skin, let's take a closer look at dermatomes.

To review, there are thirty-one pairs of spinal nerves that emerge from the spinal cord and link the central nervous system to the peripheral nerves. A **dermatome** is an area of skin primarily supplied by afferent (sensory) nerve fibers of a specific spinal nerve.

Collectively, regional dermatomes form a surface map of the entire body (with exception of the face, which has its own group of neural connections) (**A.27**). Information from a specific dermatome travels through its associated spinal nerve to the brain relaying messages about touch, temperature, and pain.

Although there are thirty-one pairs of spinal nerves, there are only thirty dermatomes because C1 has no corresponding dermatome area. The dermatomes that transmit sensation from a particular region of the skin to the brain include eight cervical nerves, twelve thoracic nerves, five lumbar nerves, and five sacral nerves. Health care providers can use the skin's surface map formed by dermatomes to diagnose or treat certain medical issues. For example, the loss of sensation within a particular dermatome could indicate a compressed nerve root or spinal cord segment.

Along with dermatomes, there are **myotomes**. A myotome is a group of muscles innervated by efferent fibers from a single spinal nerve. Put simply, dermatomes are *skin and sensory*; myotomes are *muscle and motor*.

For example, the C7 myotome includes muscles controlled by the C7 spinal nerve; they produce elbow extension and wrist flexion. Most limb muscles are innervated by more than one spinal nerve root and, therefore, comprise multiple myotomes. For instance, the hamstrings are associated with nerve roots L5, S1, and S2—three nerves intrinsic to actions produced by the hamstrings.

From a clinical standpoint, myotome testing is an important part of a neurological exam when radiculopathy (nerve root compression) is suspected.

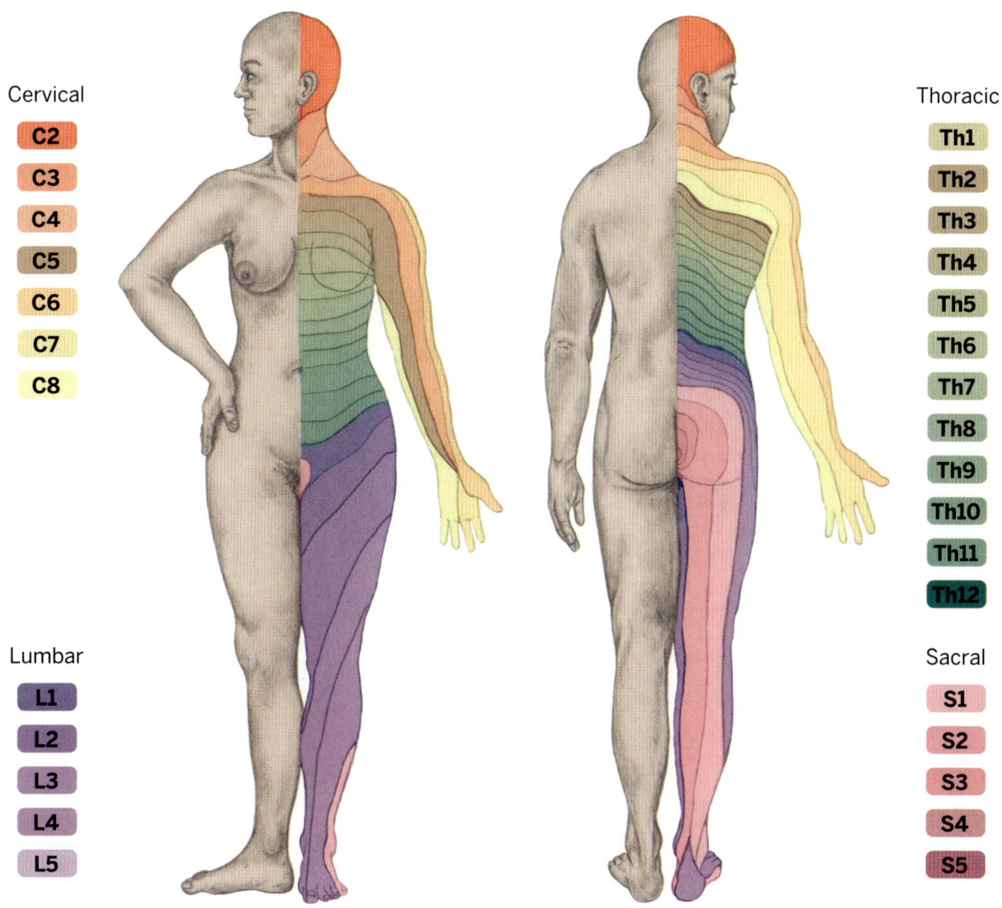

A.27 Dermatomes

derma L. skin
-tome L. *tomus*, section
myo- Grk, muscle

The Autonomic Nervous System

It's been a full day and now you're back at home. After dinner, you relax on the couch. You're nearly falling asleep when the fire alarm goes off. You leap up with your heart pounding and sniff the air for smoke. Then it suddenly stops. You return to the couch feeling agitated and decide to take a few deep breaths. Soon your body begins to settle down and you fall asleep—only to be awoken by the alarm again!

Throughout this entire chaos, many "automatic" unconscious bodily processes were managed, completely unbeknownst to you, by your autonomic nervous system. Let's find out more.

The peripheral nervous system branches into two subsystems—the autonomic and somatic nervous systems. The **autonomic nervous system (ANS)** regulates your unconscious processes such as heart rate, blood pressure, respiration, and digestion (**A.28**).

The ANS affects virtually every function of the body's organ systems, including:

- The rate and force of heartbeats
- The dilation and constriction of blood vessels and, therefore, the control of blood pressure
- The production of sweat and goose bumps on the skin
- A runny nose, a tearing eye, and a watery mouth
- The width of the airways in the lungs
- The digestive process from small intestines to colon

The ANS further divides into the **sympathetic** ("fight or flight") and **parasympathetic** ("rest and digest") **nervous systems**. Although each system produces contrasting functions and effects in the body, they offset each other by helping to maintain homeostasis (physiological equilibrium).

The **sympathetic system** activates during situations of stress, fear, or a perceived threat. Initially, automatic changes occur—the heart rate increases, muscles tense, awareness expands, and sweat glands secrete. By increasing blood flow to areas in need of more oxygen and reducing resources for functions such as digestion and tissue maintenance, this system prepares the body for potential action.

Involuntary stress responses can include a desire to fight, take flight, or freeze. For example, you could brawl with a bear (fight), run from a bear (flight), or stand paralyzed as a bear approaches (freeze). This system also kicks in when sitting down to take a test, striving to score a goal during a game, or having a heated argument.

Conversely, the purpose of the **parasympathetic nervous system** is to conserve energy for later times and focus on rest, digestion, and recovery. Bodily functions stimulated by this system include a decrease in heart and respiratory rates, a lowering of blood pressure, and a shift of blood and resources to the organs for digestion, urination, and defecation. In a *parasympathetic* state, the body can recuperate and rebuild. Therefore, it's not surprising that most of our parasympathetic time happens during sleep. Living in a chronic *sympathetic* state, however, will disrupt sleep and rob the body of its opportunity to recover and restore.

One division of the PNS capable of acting (almost entirely) independently of the sympathetic and parasympathetic nervous systems is the **enteric nervous system (ENS)**. As the PNS's largest and most complex branch—composed of approximately 500 million neurons—the ENS governs gastrointestinal (GI) tract function.

With neurons woven into the lining of the entire GI system, the ENS facilitates efferent (motor), afferent (sensory), secretory, and absorptive functions from the esophagus to the anus. Nicknamed the "second brain," it also releases a host of neurotransmitters, including acetylcholine, dopamine, and serotonin.

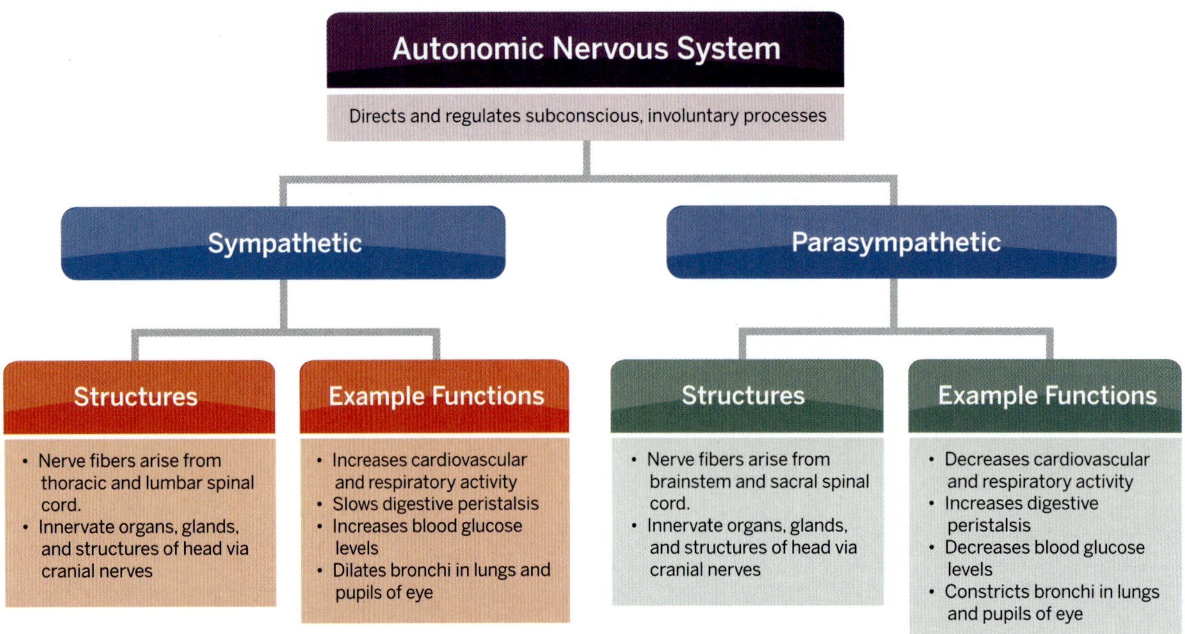

A.28 Organization, structures, and functions of the autonomic nervous system

Proprioception and Muscle Function

Getting ready for bed, you pull out a yoga mat and begin to stretch. Uhh, what a day. You bring yourself into downward-facing dog pose and think, "It's amazing I can even hold this position. The balance, stability, and stretching required—how does the body do it?"

To answer this question, let's finish this appendix by exploring the relationship between muscles and nerves—specifically, **proprioception**, **reflexes**, and **sensory receptors**.

Smooth, coordinated motion (of the arms, legs, and elsewhere) requires **proprioception**—the nervous system's ability to feel the body's position in space. In and around muscles, tendons, and joints are sensors that monitor stimuli involved with movement (**A.29**). These **proprioceptors**—sensory receptors that are sensitive to stimuli pertaining to muscle and joint position—will contribute to the afferent flow of information sent to the CNS for processing. There, the brain will interpret the information and then direct an outgoing efferent response to adjust the balance, posture, and locomotion of the body.

One type of sensory receptor is a **muscle spindle** (**A.30**). As muscle spindles are sensory fibers, their primary role will not be to generate force, but to gauge the stretch of a muscle and its rate of change in length. In doing so, muscle spindles play a key part in setting a muscle's tone.

An entire muscle belly is peppered with these small monitoring units. Muscles that produce fine, accurate movements, such as in the hands and eyes, possess numerous spindle cells. Larger, more coarsely controlled bellies like the hamstrings and quads are invested with fewer spindles.

Like "surveillance devices," muscle spindles provide data from all regions of the muscle to the CNS. Specifically, two pieces of information: the muscle's change in length and the speed at which it happens. Why are these so critical to the body? In a word—protection.

Muscle tissue, for all its amazing properties, is quite vulnerable to damage by tearing when it is stretched beyond its excursion limit or pulled apart too rapidly.

Here's the setup for how muscle spindles participate. The spindles are programmed by the CNS to be a certain length. When a muscle belly is lengthened, so too are its spindle fibers. Thus stimulated, they send an advisory message to the CNS that the muscle is elongated.

If the muscle is experiencing a dangerous amount of stretch, the spinal cord sends a quick reply to the muscle—a reflex—that causes it to contract and thus avoid being pulled apart further and potentially injured. To ensure that the contraction occurs, your nervous system will also engage the muscle's synergists and inhibit its antagonists.

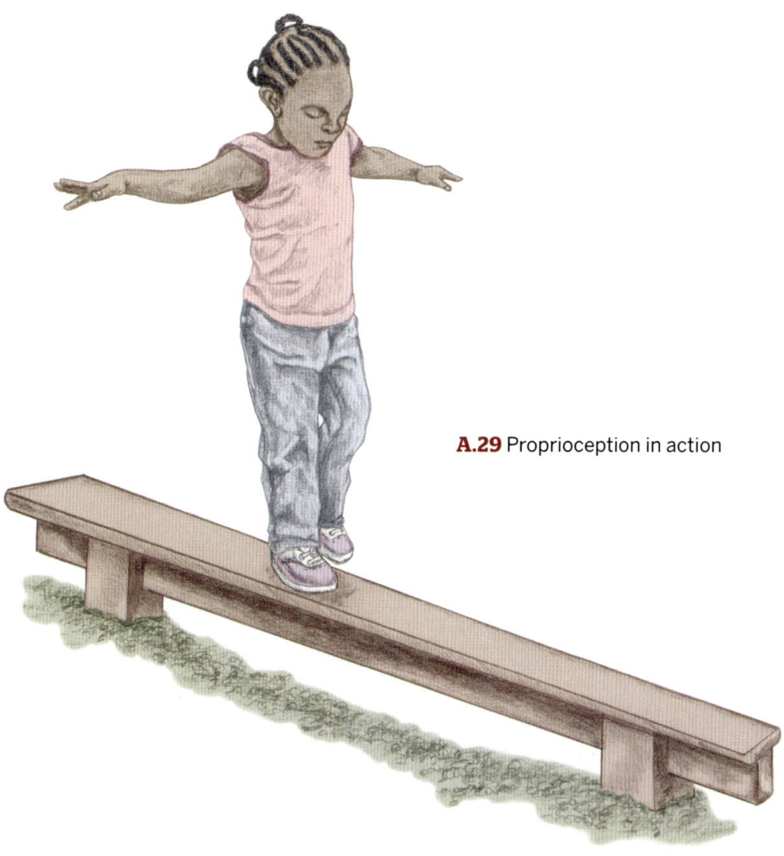

A.29 Proprioception in action

For instance, let's return to your downward-facing dog pose. Your stiff hamstrings are not happy, so you decide to encourage them by quickly pushing back your pelvis and heels into a deeper stretch. This rapid adjustment elongates (and excites) your hamstrings' muscle spindles. As a result, a protective **reflex arc** (which we'll get to in a moment) is activated. This neurological response incites your hamstrings to contract, while another reflex signals your quadriceps to relax. Thus your "rapid stretch" is self-defeating: it counteracts all your lengthening efforts by contracting the very muscles you're hoping to elongate. (This is why it's important to stretch your soft tissues slowly and gently.)

Now let's take a closer look at that reflex arc we witnessed above. A **reflex** is an automatic response to stimuli that involves no conscious thought. A **reflex arc** is the pathway followed by nerve impulses that produce the reflex. When a doctor taps your knee with a reflex hammer, you can watch the reflex—and its corresponding reflex arc—in action as your leg kicks. You didn't think about doing it; it just happened.

One type of reflex is a **stretch reflex**. Activated by the muscle spindles, this reflex affords a muscle to respond to stimuli, such as adjusting its position and tone for balance or movement. As an example, when you did downward-facing dog, a stretch reflex in your hamstrings caused contraction of muscle fibers in response to the lengthening of that same muscle, thereby preventing your hamstrings from being hyper-stretched and potentially injured (**A.31**).

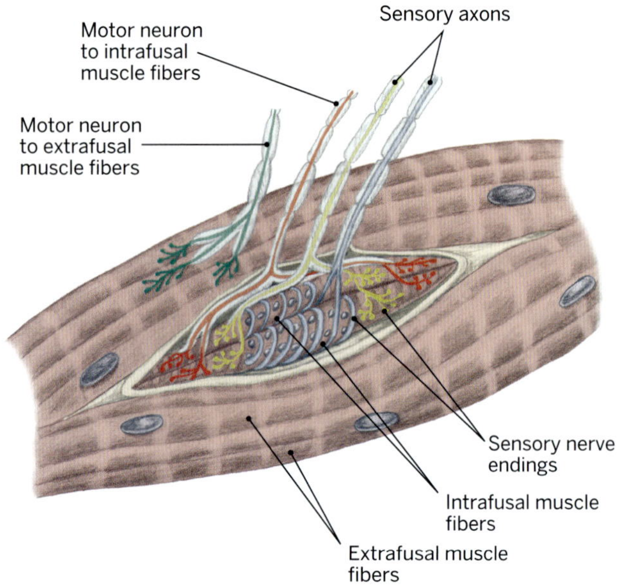

A.30 Muscle spindle cell embedded in muscle fibers

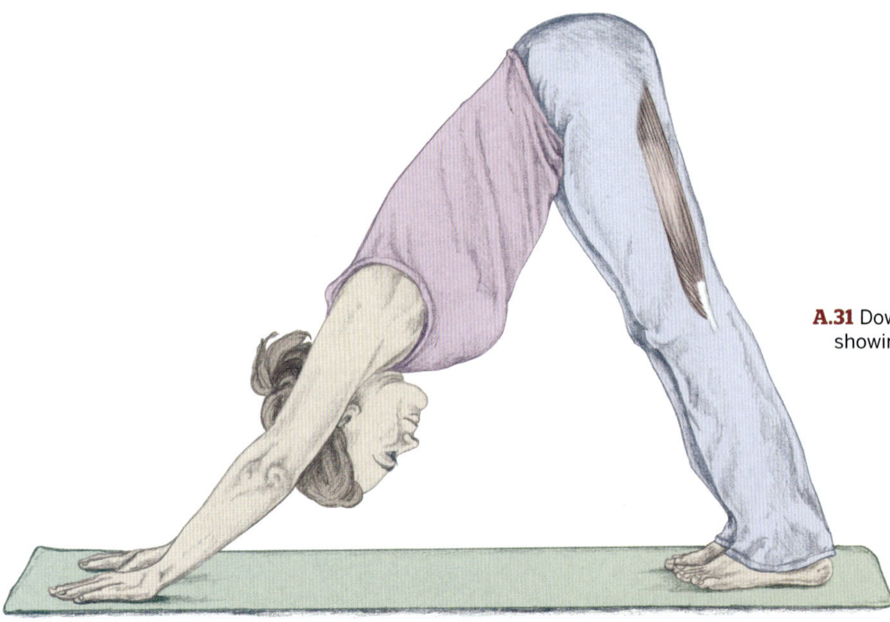

A.31 Downward-facing dog pose, showing hamstring muscles

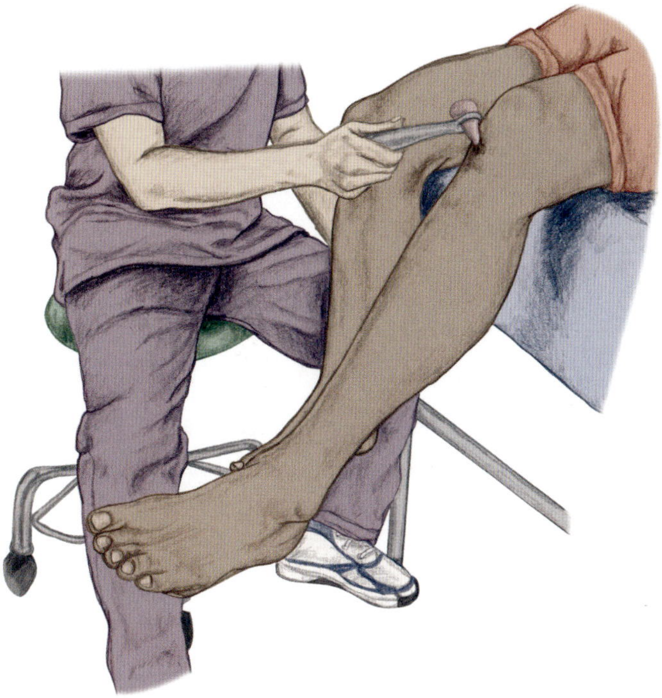

A.32 Eliciting the stretch reflex with a tap on the knee

In the case of the knee-jerk test at your doctor's office, the muscle spindles in your quadriceps were stimulated by a quick stretch induced by a strike of the mallet on your patellar tendon (**A.32**). They sent an afferent message to your spinal cord. There, the reflex arc made a sharp 180° turn and headed directly back to the muscle along efferent neurons stimulating the quadriceps to contract (**A.33**).

In other words, the excitation of your muscle spindles—via the stretch reflex—caused the contraction of your muscle's contractile fibers. This reaction, which causes muscle fibers to contract while they're being stretched, is a fundamental strategy for ensuring that tissue will not be damaged, and that muscle tone is properly maintained. It's so fundamental that you have no conscious control over it.

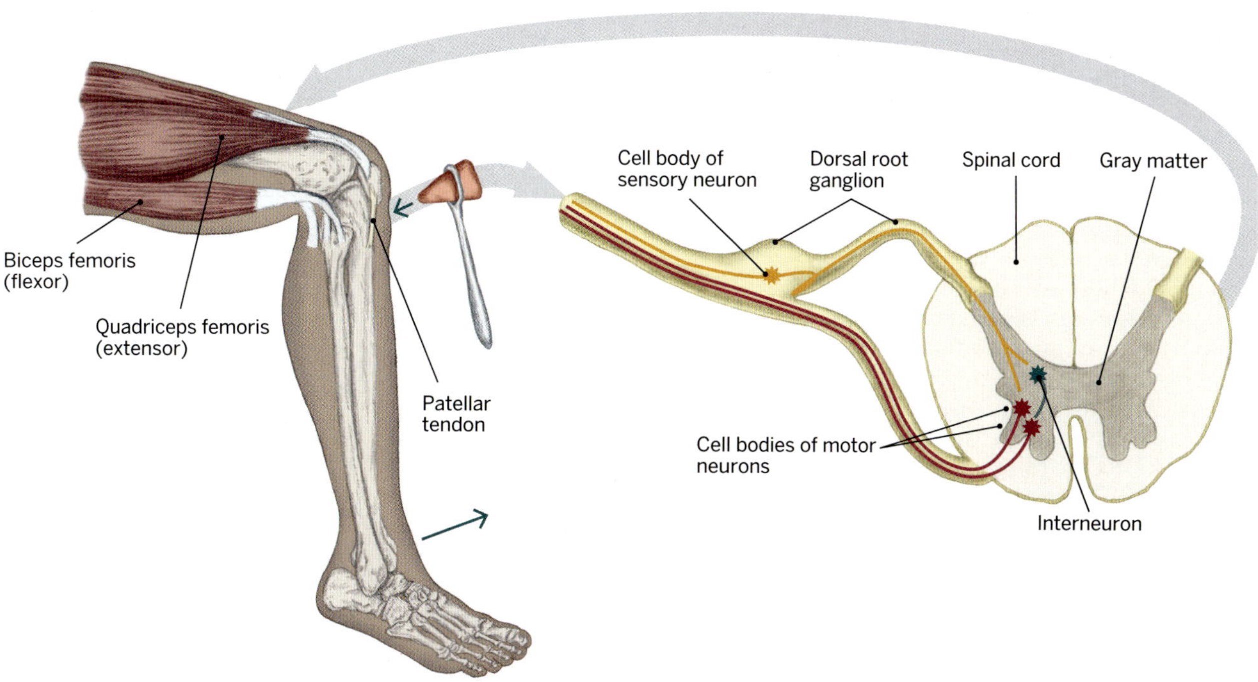

A.33 The knee-jerk reflex is an example of the flow of information in the nervous system. An afferent message is sent from the patellar tendon to the spinal cord, and an efferent message is sent back to the quadriceps.

Working closely with the muscle spindles is another proprioceptor called a Golgi tendon organ (GTO) (**A.34**). Located within the collagen fibers of tendons and joint capsules, these sensory receptors are innervated by afferent nerves that relay information to the CNS. The task of a GTO is to monitor the pulling force placed on a tendon.

While a spindle cell (see **A.30**) gauges the stretch of a muscle and its rate of change in length, a GTO detects a muscle's tension. When combined, the attributes of both receptors increase a muscle's functionality as well as protect its fibers from potentially damaging situations, whether those risks stem from a muscular contraction or a passive stretch. If too much tension is detected at the tendon, the contracting muscle—listening to the inhibitory signals initiated by a GTO—will relax to relieve that tension.

For instance, curl a dumbbell, and a GTO detects the amount of tension generated by the muscle (**A.35**). At the same time, the biceps' spindle cells will keep tabs on the muscle's length and how slow or fast its length changes. If a GTO senses an overload of tension (as you attempt to shorten the muscle), it will inhibit the muscle (via a reflex arc) from creating more force and thus avoid a potential injury.

Conversely, a low-force stretch of your biceps (such as reaching behind you and setting your hand along a wall) will also involve the GTO (**A.36**). If you hold the stretch for more than seven seconds, the increased tension in the muscle—now generated by lengthening the tissue—will trigger the GTO to temporarily impede the spindle cells, thereby reducing the muscle's tension and increase the stretch.

In the dumbbell example, the muscle's tension arose from a concentric (shortening) contraction of the muscle by lifting a weight against gravity. During the low-force stretch, however, the tension resulted not from a contraction, but from a passive lengthening of the muscle. Both of these examples highlight the variety of situations in which muscles and nerves work together to create functional movement and avoid tissue injuries.

You roll into bed, turn out the light, and take a few deep breaths. Thoughts of nerves and dermatomes swim around in your head, soon followed by dreams of connections and plexuses. Sleep well. Tomorrow's another day for the learning to continue.

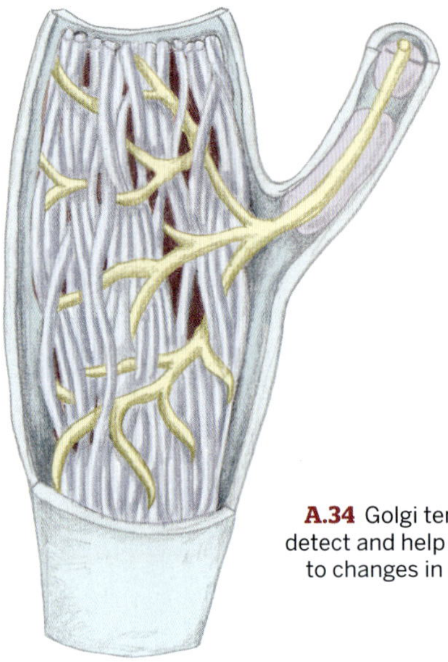

A.34 Golgi tendon organs will detect and help the body respond to changes in muscle tension.

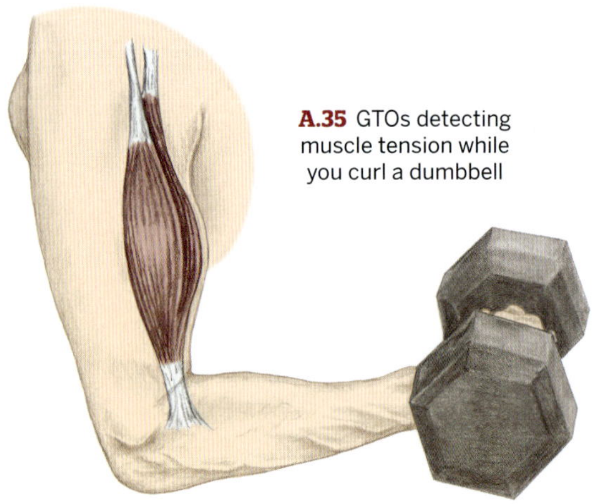

A.35 GTOs detecting muscle tension while you curl a dumbbell

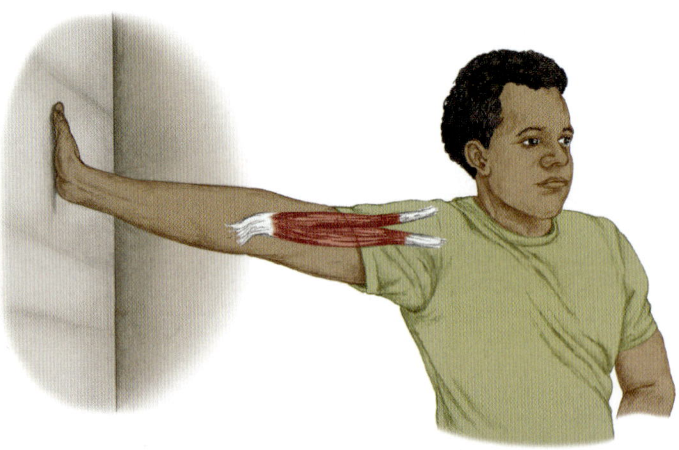

A.36 GTOs detecting muscle tension while you stretch the biceps brachii

Muscles of Facial Expression Attachment Sites

All of these muscles are innervated by the facial nerve (cranial nerve VII).

	Muscle/Nerve (facial)	Action	Origin	Insertion
Mouth	**Buccinator**	Compress the cheeks	Maxilla and mandible	Fascia at the corner of the mouth
	Depressor anguli oris	Draw the corner of the mouth inferiorly and laterally	Mandible	Fascia at the corner of the mouth
	Depressor labii inferioris	Depress the corner of the mouth; Depress, protrude, and draw laterally the lower lip	Mandible	Fascia of the lower lip
	Levator anguli oris	Elevate corner of the mouth	Maxilla	Corner of the mouth
	Levator labii superioris	Elevate and protrude the upper lip	Maxilla	Fascia of the upper lip
	Mentalis	Elevate and protrude the lower lip; Wrinkle the skin of the chin	Mandible	Skin of the chin
	Orbicularis oris	Close the mouth; Shape and protrude the lips	Muscle fibers surrounding opening of mouth	Skin at the corner of the mouth
	Platysma	Depress the mandible; Tighten the fascia of the neck	Fascia covering superior portion of pectoralis major	Lower border of the mandible
	Risorius	Retract the corner of the mouth laterally	Fascia superficial to the masseter	Fascia at the corner of the mouth
	Zygomaticus major	Elevate and draw the corner of the mouth laterally	Zygomatic bone	Fascia at the corner of the mouth
	Zygomaticus minor	Elevate and protrude the upper lip; Deepen the nasolabial fold	Zygomatic bone	Fascia and muscle tissue of the upper lip
Nose	**Levator labii superioris alaeque nasi**	Flare the nostril; Elevate and protrude the upper lip	Maxilla	Fascia of the upper lip and nose
	Nasalis, alar portion	Flare the nostril	Maxilla	Ala of the nose
	Procerus	Draw down the medial eyebrows; Pull the skin of the nose upward	Fascia over the nasal bone	Fascia and skin between the eyes
Eye	**Corrugator supercilii**	Draw the eyebrow medially and inferiorly	Inferior portion of the frontal bone to the fascia	Skin deep to the medial portion of the eyebrow
	Orbicularis oculi	Depress the upper eyelid; Elevate the lower eyelid	Muscle fibers surrounding opening of eye	Skin at the corner of the eye
Scalp	**Frontalis**	Raise the eyebrows; Wrinkle the forehead	Galea aponeurotica	Skin superior to the eyebrows
	Occipitalis	Anchor and retract the galea aponeurotica posteriorly	Galea aponeurotica	Superior nuchal line of the occiput

Synergists—Muscles Working Together

Shoulder (pp. 59-61)
(glenohumeral joint)

Flexion
(antagonists on extension)
Deltoid (anterior fibers)
Pectoralis major (upper fibers)
Biceps brachii
Coracobrachialis

Extension
(antagonists on flexion)
Deltoid (posterior fibers)
Latissimus dorsi
Teres major
Pectoralis major (lower fibers)
Triceps brachii (long head)

Horizontal Abduction
(antagonist on h. adduction)
Deltoid (posterior fibers)

Horizontal Adduction
(antagonists on h. abduction)
Deltoid (anterior fibers)
Pectoralis major (upper fibers)

Abduction
(antagonists on adduction)
Deltoid (all fibers)
Supraspinatus

Adduction
(antagonists on abduction)
Latissimus dorsi
Teres major
Infraspinatus
Teres minor
Pectoralis major (all fibers)
Triceps brachii (long head)
Coracobrachialis

Lateral Rotation (external rotation)
(antagonists on medial rotation)
Deltoid (posterior fibers)
Infraspinatus
Teres minor

Medial Rotation (internal rotation)
(antagonists on lateral rotation)
Deltoid (anterior fibers)
Latissimus dorsi
Teres major
Subscapularis
Pectoralis major (all fibers)

Scapula (pp. 61-62)
(scapulothoracic joint)

Elevation
(antagonists on depression)
Trapezius (upper fibers, unilaterally)
Rhomboid major
Rhomboid minor
Levator scapula (unilaterally)

Depression
(antagonists on elevation)
Trapezius (lower fibers)
Serratus anterior (with the origin fixed)
Pectoralis minor

Adduction (retraction)
(antagonists on abduction)
Trapezius (middle fibers)
Rhomboid major
Rhomboid minor

Abduction (protraction)
(antagonists on adduction)
Serratus anterior (with the origin fixed)
Pectoralis minor

Upward Rotation
(antagonists on downward rotation)
Trapezius (upper and lower fibers, unilaterally)
Serratus anterior (with the origin fixed)

Downward Rotation
(antagonists on upward rotation)
Rhomboid major
Rhomboid minor
Levator scapula (unilaterally)
Pectoralis minor

Elbow (p. 128)
(humeroulnar and humeroradial joints)

Flexion
(antagonists on extension)
Biceps brachii
Brachialis
Brachioradialis
Flexor carpi radialis (assists)
Flexor carpi ulnaris (assists)
Palmaris longus (assists)
Pronator teres (assists)
Extensor carpi radialis longus (assists)
Extensor carpi radialis brevis (assists)

Extension
(antagonists on flexion)
Triceps brachii (all heads)
Anconeus

Forearm (p. 128)
(proximal and distal radioulnar joints)

Supination
(antagonists on pronation)
Biceps brachii
Supinator
Brachioradialis (assists)

Pronation
(antagonists on supination)
Pronator teres
Pronator quadratus
Brachioradialis (assists)

Wrist (pp. 128-129)
(radiocarpal joint)

Extension
(antagonists on flexion)
Extensor carpi radialis longus
Extensor carpi radialis brevis
Extensor carpi ulnaris
Extensor digitorum (assists)
Extensor indicis (assists)

Flexion
(antagonists on extension)
Flexor carpi radialis
Flexor carpi ulnaris
Palmaris longus
Flexor digitorum superficialis
Flexor digitorum profundus (assists)
Flexor pollicis longus (assists)

Abduction (radial deviation)
(antagonists on adduction)
Extensor carpi radialis longus
Extensor carpi radialis brevis
Extensor pollicis longus
Extensor pollicis brevis
Flexor carpi radialis
Abductor pollicis longus

Adduction (ulnar deviation)
(antagonists on abduction)
Extensor carpi ulnaris
Flexor carpi ulnaris

Hand and Fingers (p. 129)

(metacarpophalangeal, proximal and distal interphalangeal joints)

Flexion of the Second through Fifth Fingers

(antagonists on extension of fingers)

Flexor digitorum superficialis
Flexor digitorum profundus
Flexor digiti minimi brevis (5th)
Lumbricals
Dorsal interossei (2nd–4th, assists)
Palmar interossei (2nd, 4th, 5th, assists)

Extension of the Second through Fifth Fingers

(antagonists on flexion of fingers)

Extensor digitorum
Lumbricals
Dorsal interossei (2nd–4th, assists)
Palmar interossei (2nd, 4th, 5th, assists)
Extensor indicis (2nd)

Abduction of the Second through Fifth Fingers

(antagonists on adduction of fingers)

Dorsal interossei (2nd–4th)
Abductor digiti minimi (5th)

Adduction of the Second through Fifth Fingers

(antagonists on abduction of fingers)

Palmar interossei (2nd, 4th, 5th)
Extensor indicis (2nd)

Opposition of the Fifth Finger

Opponens digiti minimi
Abductor digiti minimi (assists)
Flexor digiti minimi brevis (assists)

Thumb (p. 129)

(first carpometacarpal and metacarpophalangeal joints)

Flexion

(antagonists on extension)

Flexor pollicis longus
Flexor pollicis brevis
Adductor pollicis (assists)
Palmar interossei (1st, assists)

Extension

(antagonists on flexion)

Extensor pollicis longus
Extensor pollicis brevis
Abductor pollicis longus
Palmar interossei (1st, assists)

Abduction

(antagonists on adduction)

Abductor pollicis longus
Abductor pollicis brevis

Adduction

(antagonists on abduction)

Adductor pollicis
Palmar interossei (1st)

Opposition

Opponens pollicis
Flexor pollicis brevis (assists)
Abductor pollicis brevis (assists)

Vertebral Column (pp. 194-195)

Flexion

(antagonists on extension)

Rectus abdominis
External oblique (bilaterally)
Internal oblique (bilaterally)
Psoas major (with the insertion fixed)
Iliacus (with the insertion fixed)

Extension

(antagonists on flexion)

Longissimus (bilaterally)
Iliocostalis (bilaterally)
Multifidi (bilaterally)
Rotatores (bilaterally)
Semispinalis capitis
Spinalis (bilaterally)
Quadratus lumborum (assists)
Interspinalis
Intertransversarii (bilaterally)
Latissimus dorsi (assists; see box, p. 67)

Rotation

(all unilaterally)

External oblique (to the opposite side)
Internal oblique (to the same side)
Multifidi (to the opposite side)
Rotatores (to the opposite side)

Lateral Flexion

(unilaterally to the same side)

Iliocostalis
External oblique
Internal oblique
Longissimus
Quadratus lumborum
Psoas major (assists)
Intertransversarii
Spinalis
Latissimus dorsi (assists; see box, p. 67)

Ribs/Thorax (p. 195)

Elevation/Expansion (involved with inhalation)

(antagonists on depression)

Anterior scalene (bilaterally)
Middle scalene (bilaterally)
Posterior scalene (bilaterally)
Sternocleidomastoid (assists)
External intercostals (assists)
Serratus posterior superior
Pectoralis major (all fibers, assists with arm fixed)
Pectoralis minor (with scapula fixed)
Serratus anterior (with scapula fixed)
Subclavius (first rib)

Depression/Collapse (involved with exhalation)

(antagonists on elevation)

Internal intercostals (assists)
Serratus posterior inferior

Muscles of Inhalation

Diaphragm
Anterior scalene (bilaterally)
Middle scalene (bilaterally)
Posterior scalene (bilaterally)
Sternocleidomastoid (assists)
External intercostals (assists)
Serratus posterior superior
Quadratus lumborum
Pectoralis major (assists with arm fixed)
Pectoralis minor (with scapula fixed)
Serratus anterior (with scapula fixed)
Subclavius (first rib)

Muscles of Exhalation

Internal intercostals (assists)
Serratus posterior inferior
External oblique (by compressing abdominal contents)
Internal oblique (by compressing abdominal contents)
Transverse abdominis (by compressing abdominal contents)
Quadratus lumborum

Cervical Spine (pp. 242-243)

Flexion

(antagonists on extension)

Sternocleidomastoid (bilaterally)
Anterior scalene (bilaterally)
Longus capitis (bilaterally)
Longus colli (bilaterally)

Extension

(antagonists on flexion)

Trapezius (upper fibers, bilaterally)
Levator scapula (bilaterally)
Splenius capitis (bilaterally)
Splenius cervicis (bilaterally)
Rectus capitis posterior major
Rectus capitis posterior minor
Oblique capitis superior
Semispinalis capitis
Longissimus capitis (assists; see p. 197)
Longissimus cervicis (assists; see p. 197)
Iliocostalis cervicis (assists; see p. 197)
Multifidi (bilaterally)
Rotatores (bilaterally)
Intertransversarii (bilaterally)
Interspinalis

Rotation

*(unilaterally to the **same** side)*

Levator scapula
Splenius capitis
Splenius cervicis
Rectus capitis posterior major
Oblique capitis inferior
Longus colli
Longus capitis
Longissimus capitis (assists; see p. 197)
Longissimus cervicis (assists; see p. 197)
Iliocostalis cervicis (assists; see p. 197)

Rotation

*(unilaterally to the **opposite** side)*

Trapezius (upper fibers)
Sternocleidomastoid
Anterior scalene
Middle scalene
Posterior scalene
Multifidi
Rotatores

Lateral Flexion

*(unilaterally to the **same** side)*

Trapezius (upper fibers)
Levator scapula
Sternocleidomastoid
Anterior scalene (with ribs fixed)
Middle scalene (with ribs fixed)
Posterior scalene (with ribs fixed)
Splenius capitis
Splenius cervicis
Longus capitis
Longus colli
Longissimus capitis (assists; see p. 197)
Longissimus cervicis (assists; see p. 197)
Iliocostalis cervicis (assists; see p . 197)
Oblique capitis superior
Intertransversarii

Mandible (p. 243)

(temporomandibular joint)

Elevation

(antagonists on depression)

Masseter
Temporalis
Medial pterygoid

Depression

(antagonists on elevation)

Geniohyoid
Mylohyoid
Stylohyoid
Digastric (with hyoid bone fixed)
Platysma (assists)

Protraction

(antagonists on retraction)

Lateral pterygoid (bilaterally)
Medial pterygoid (bilaterally)
Masseter (assists)

Retraction

(antagonists on protraction)

Temporalis
Digastric

Lateral Deviation

(unilaterally)

Lateral pterygoid (to the opposite side)
Medial pterygoid (to the opposite side)

Pelvis

Anterior Tilt (downward rotation)

(antagonists on posterior tilt)

Psoas major
Iliacus
Latissimus dorsi (assists; see box, p. 67)

Posterior Tilt (upward rotation)

(antagonists on anterior tilt)

Biceps femoris
Semitendinosus
Semimembranosus
Rectus abdominis
Psoas minor

Lateral Tilt (elevation)

Quadratus lumborum (unilaterally)
Latissimus dorsi (assists; see box p. 67)

Coxal (pp. 304-306)

(hip joint)

Flexion

(antagonists on extension)

Psoas major
Iliacus
Tensor fasciae latae
Sartorius
Rectus femoris
Gluteus medius (anterior fibers)
Gluteus minimus
Adductor longus (assists)
Pectineus (assists)
Adductor brevis (assists)
Adductor magnus (assists)

Extension

(antagonists on flexion)

Gluteus maximus (all fibers)
Biceps femoris (long head)
Semitendinosus
Semimembranosus
Adductor magnus (posterior fibers)
Gluteus medius (posterior fibers)

Medial Rotation (internal rotation)

(antagonists on lateral rotation)

Gluteus medius (anterior fibers)
Gluteus minimus
Tensor fasciae latae
Adductor magnus
Adductor longus
Adductor brevis
Pectineus
Gracilis
Semitendinosus (assists)
Semimembranosus (assists)

Lateral Rotation (external rotation)

(antagonists on medial rotation)

Gluteus maximus (all fibers)
Piriformis
Quadratus femoris
Obturator internus
Obturator externus
Gemellus superior
Gemellus inferior
Gluteus medius (posterior fibers)
Psoas major
Iliacus
Sartorius
Biceps femoris (assists, long head)

Abduction

(antagonists on adduction)

Gluteus maximus (all fibers)
Gluteus medius (all fibers)
Gluteus minimus
Tensor fasciae latae
Sartorius
Piriformis (when the hip is flexed)

Adduction

(antagonists on abduction)

Adductor magnus
Adductor longus
Adductor brevis
Pectineus
Gracilis
Gluteus maximus (lower fibers)

Knee (p. 307)

(tibiofemoral joint)

Flexion

(antagonists on extension)

Biceps femoris
Semitendinosus
Semimembranosus
Gracilis
Sartorius
Gastrocnemius
Popliteus
Plantaris (weak)

Extension

(antagonists on flexion)

Rectus femoris
Vastus lateralis
Vastus medialis
Vastus intermedius

Medial Rotation of Flexed Knee

(antagonists on lateral rotation)

Semitendinosus
Semimembranosus
Gracilis
Sartorius
Popliteus

Lateral Rotation of Flexed Knee

(antagonist on medial rotation)

Biceps femoris

Ankle (p. 373)

(talocrural joint)

Plantar Flexion

(antagonists on dorsiflexion)

Gastrocnemius
Soleus
Tibialis posterior
Fibularis longus (assists)
Fibularis brevis (assists)
Flexor digitorum longus (weak)
Flexor hallucis longus (weak)
Plantaris (weak)

Dorsiflexion

(antagonists on plantar flexion)

Tibialis anterior
Extensor digitorum longus
Extensor hallucis longus

Foot and Toes (p. 374)

(talotarsal, midtarsal, tarsometatarsal, metatarsophalangeal, proximal and distal interphalangeal joints)

Inversion

(antagonists on eversion)

Tibialis anterior
Tibialis posterior
Flexor digitorum longus
Flexor hallucis longus
Extensor hallucis longus

Eversion

(antagonists on inversion)

Fibularis longus
Fibularis brevis
Extensor digitorum longus

Flexion of Second through Fifth Toes

(antagonists on extension of toes)

Flexor digitorum longus
Flexor digitorum brevis
Lumbricals
Quadratus plantae (assists)
Dorsal interossei (2nd–4th)
Plantar interossei (3rd–5th)
Abductor digiti minimi (5th)
Flexor digiti minimi brevis (5th)

Extension of Second through Fifth Toes

(antagonists on flexion of toes)

Extensor digitorum longus
Extensor digitorum brevis (2nd–4th)
Lumbricals

Adduction of Second through Fifth Toes

(antagonist on abduction of toes)

Plantar interossei (3rd–5th)

Abduction of Second through Fifth Toes

(antagonists on adduction of toes)

Dorsal interossei (2nd–4th)
Abductor digiti minimi (5th, assists)

Flexion of First Toe

(antagonists on extension)

Flexor hallucis longus
Flexor hallucis brevis
Abductor hallucis (assists)
Adductor hallucis (assists)

Extension of First Toe

(antagonists on flexion)

Extensor hallucis longus
Extensor hallucis brevis

Adduction of First Toe

(antagonist on abduction)

Adductor hallucis

Abduction of First Toe

(antagonist on adduction)

Abductor hallucis

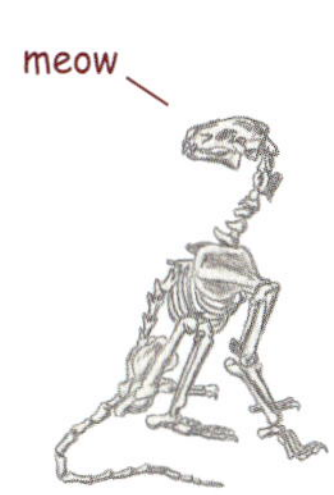

Glossary

abdomen – the region between the diaphragm and the pelvis

acetabulum – the rounded cavity on the external surface of the coxal bone; the head of the femur articulates with the acetabulum to form the coxal joint

adhesion – abnormal adherence of collagen fibers to surrounding structures during immobilization, following trauma or as a complication of surgery, which restricts normal elasticity of the structures involved

afferent – conveying or conducting toward

afferent neuron – neuron transmitting information signals from the body tissues toward the CNS

anatomical position – erect posture with face forward, arms at sides, forearms supinated (so that palms of the hands face forward) and fingers and thumbs in extension

antagonist – a muscle that performs the opposite action of the prime mover and synergist muscles

antecubital – the anterior side of the elbow

anterior – toward the front, or ventral, surface

anterior tilt of pelvis – tilt in which the vertical plane through the anterior superior iliac spines (ASISs) is anterior to the vertical plane through the symphysis pubis

appendage – a structure attached to the body, such as the upper and lower extremities

arm – the portion of the upper limb between the shoulder and elbow joints

arthrology – the study of joints

articular facet – a small articular surface of a bone, especially a vertebra

articular process – a small, flat projection found on the surfaces of the arches of the vertebrae on either side, incorporating the articular surface

articulation – a joint or connection of bones

atlas – first cervical vertebra, articulating with the occipital bone and rotating around the odontoid process of the axis

autonomic – acting or occurring in an involuntary or unconscious mode

autonomic nervous system (ANS) – section of the nervous system that monitors and controls the largely unconscious bodily functions needed for survival (such as respiration, heart action, digestion, sexual response)

axis – the second cervical vertebra

axon – projection, often quite long, that transmits signals from the neuron cell body toward the next neuron in a synaptic chain, or to an effector structure like a muscle fiber or gland tissue

bilateral – pertaining to two sides

brachial plexus – originating from C5–T1 spinal nerves, the plexus that produces nerves that innervate the scapular movers, pectoral actions, and all functions of the upper limb

bursa – a small, fluid-filled sack that reduces friction between two structures

cartilaginous joint – a joint in which two bony surfaces are united by cartilage; the two types of cartilaginous joints are **synchondroses** and **symphyses**

caudal – downward, away from the head (toward the tail)

cell body – command center of a cell that contain its nucleus and other organelles; in the case of neurons, it receives and sends impulses along the synaptic chain; also known as soma

central nervous system (CNS) – composed of the brain and spinal cord, the structures that receive, analyze, and respond to information from the body tissues, as well as initiate directives for body tissue activities

cephalic – toward the head

cervical plexus – a plexus originating from spinal nerves C1–C4 that produces exiting nerves responsible for multiple innervations in the head, neck, and upper torso, including partial innervation of the diaphragm

collagen – the protein of connective tissue fibers

concentric contraction – a shortening of the muscle during a contraction; a type of isotonic exercise

condyle – a rounded articular surface at the extremity of a bone

connective tissue – the supportive tissues of the body, made of ground substance and fibrous tissues, taking a wide variety of forms

contraction – an increase in muscle tension, with or without change in overall length

coronal – a vertical plane perpendicular to the sagittal plane dividing the body into anterior and posterior portions; also called the frontal plane

coronal axis – a horizontal line extending from side to side, around which the movements of flexion and extension take place

cranial – upward, toward the head

crural – pertaining to the leg or thigh; femoral

deep – away from the surface of the body; the opposite of superficial

dendrite – projection of the neuron soma that receives signals from other neurons, converts them from chemical to electrical signals, and communicates them into the cell body

dermatome – an area of skin primarily supplied by afferent (sensory) nerve fibers of a specific spinal nerve

distal – farther from the center or median line or from the thorax

dorsal – relating to the back; posterior

dorsal nerve root – the afferent fibers transmitting along a mixed spinal nerve and separating to reach the sensory reception area in the spinal cord's dorsal horn; also known as posterior root or sensory root

eccentric contraction – an overall lengthening of the muscle while it is contracting or resisting a workload

edema – a local or generalized condition in which body tissues contain an excessive amount of fluid

efferent – conveying or conducting away from

efferent neuron – neuron transmitting directive signals from the CNS toward effector tissues such as muscles, glands, or organs

endoneurium – delicate, fluidy connective tissue sheath enclosing an individual PNS axon, its myelin sheaths, and its capillary network

enteric nervous system (ENS) – division of the ANS responsible for the activities of the digestive tract; semi-autonomous in function, its ancient evolutionary roots lead to its sometimes being called the "little brain"

epineurium – fibrous connective tissue sheath that surrounds the contents of a nerve, serving as a protective outer membrane

facet – a small plane or concave surface

fascia – a general term for a layer or layers of loose or dense fibrous connective tissue

fascicle – bundle of axons inside a peripheral nerve, grouped together because they share a function and/or target tissue

fibrous joint – a joint in which the components are connected by fibrous tissue

flexibility – the ability to readily adapt to changes in position or alignment; may be expressed as normal, limited, or excessive

forearm – the portion of the upper limb between the elbow and wrist joints

frontal plane – a vertical plane perpendicular to the sagittal plane, dividing the body into anterior and posterior portions; also called the coronal plane

genu valgum – "knock-knees," defined as a lateral displacement of the distal end of the distal bone in the joint

genu varum – "bowlegs," defined as a medial displacement of the distal end of the distal bone in the joint

impingement – an encroachment on the space occupied by soft tissue, such as a nerve or muscle

inferior – away from the head

insertion – the more mobile attachment site of a muscle to a bone; the opposite end is the origin

interstitial – the space within an organ or tissue

interstitial fluid – the fluid that surrounds cells

isometric – increase in tension without change in muscle length

isotonic – increase in tension with change in muscle length (in the direction of shortening); concentric contraction

isotonic contraction (dynamic) – a concentric or eccentric contraction of a muscle; a muscle contraction performed with movement

kinesiology – the study of movement

kyphosis – a condition characterized by an abnormally increased convexity in the curvature of the thoracic spine as viewed from the side

lateral – away from the midline

lateral tilt – pelvic tilt in which the crest of the ilium is higher on one side than on the other

leg – the portion of the lower extremity between the knee and ankle joints

ligament – a fibrous connective tissue that connects bone to bone

longitudinal axis – a vertical line extending in a cranial/caudal direction, about which movements of rotation take place

lordosis – an abnormally increased concavity in the curvature of the lumbar spine as viewed from the side

lumbar plexus – originating from T12–L4 spinal nerves, the plexus that produces nerves that innervate parts of the abdominal wall and pelvic contents, and the anterior and medial thigh muscles

lymphatic – pertains to the system of vessels involved with drainage of bodily fluids (lymph)

lymph node – a small oval structure located along lymphatic vessels

medial – toward the midline

mixed nerve – any nerve that contains both motor (efferent) and sensory (afferent) neurons; some also contain autonomic fibers

muscle – an organ composed of one of three types of muscle tissue (skeletal, cardiac, or visceral), specialized for contraction

muscle contracture – an increase of tension in the muscle caused by activation of the contractile mechanism of the muscle

muscle spindle – specialized proprioceptor that senses stretch of skeletal muscle tissue

myofascial – pertains to skeletal muscles ensheathed by fibrous connective tissue

myotome – a group of muscles innervated by efferent fibers from a single spinal nerve

nerve – a grouped set of neurons, usually mixed, existing in the peripheral nervous system as a structure for conveying signals in both directions between specific body tissues and the CNS (grouped neurons in the CNS are called *tracts*)

nerve plexus – networked branching structure in the PNS whose purpose is to infeed neurons from spinal nerves and intermix them to create a group of post-plexus nerves designed to service the motor, sensory, and sometimes autonomic needs of a specific body region

nerve root – the initial neuron grouping at the beginning of a nerve, particularly of those originating from the CNS such as the cranial nerves and spinal nerves; often also known as spinal nerve

nerve rootlet – small cluster of nerve fibers emerging from the spinal cord and coalescing with the anterior and ventral nerve roots of the spinal nerves; also known as nerve filament

neuron – primary (parenchymal) cell of the nervous system, responsible for signal transmission; also known as nerve fiber

occipital condyles – elongated oval facets on the undersurface of the occipital bone on either side of the foramen magnum, which articulate with the atlas vertebra

odontoid process (or dens) – a process projecting upward from the body of the axis vertebra, around which the atlas rotates

origin – the more stationary attachment site of a muscle to a bone; the opposite end is the insertion

palmar – toward the palm

palpable – touchable, accessible

palpate – to examine or explore by touching (an organ or area of the body), usually as a diagnostic aid

parasympathetic nervous system – division of the ANS that predominates during functions of relaxation and body sustenance, growth and repair ("rest and digest")

paravertebrals – alongside or near the vertebral column

pelvic girdle – the two hip bones

pelvic tilt – an anterior (forward), a posterior (backward) or a lateral (vertical) tilt of the pelvis from neutral position

pelvis – composed of the two hip bones, sacrum and coccyx

perineurium – protective connective tissue membrane wrapped around a nerve fascicle

periosteum – the fibrous connective tissue which surrounds the surface of bones

peripheral nervous system (PNS) – composed of the cranial nerves, spinal nerves, and their branches, the structures that carry signal transmission in both directions between the body tissues and the CNS

posterior – toward the back or dorsal surface

posterior tilt of pelvis – tilt in which the vertical plane through the anterior superior iliac spines (ASISs) is posterior to the vertical plane through the symphysis pubis

prime mover – a muscle that carries out an action

proprioception – consisting of elements such as joint position sense and joint motion sense, a component of sensory function that tracks the situation of body parts

proprioceptors – types of receptors that pick up on stimuli specific to sensing body part movement

proximal – nearer to the center or midline of the body

range of motion – the range, usually expressed in degrees, through which a joint can move or be moved

range of motion, active – the free movement across any joint of moving levers that is produced by contracting muscles

range of motion, passive – the free movement that is produced by external forces across any joint or moving levers

reflex – an automatic, involuntary response to a stimulus; reflexes are central to many protective and homeostatic functions

reflex arc – neural loop consisting of an afferent neuron, usually an interneuron, then an efferent neuron; the pathway of reflex response transmission

retinaculum – a network, usually pertaining to a band of connective tissue

sacral plexus – originating from S1–S4 spinal nerves, and collaborating with L4/L5 spinal nerves as the lumbosacral plexus, produces nerves that innervate motor, sensory, and vasomotor functions in the buttocks, posterior thigh, lower leg, and foot

sagittal axis – a horizontal line extending from front to back, about which movements of abduction and adduction take place

sagittal plane – a plane that divides the body into left and right portions

sensory receptor – located at the distal end of a peripheral afferent neuron and activated by stimuli that affect the tissues in which it is embedded, its special property of *transduction* allows it to convert the stimulus energy into electrochemical impulses to be transmitted along its neuron

sesamoid – a bone or fibrocartilage in a tendon playing over a bony surface

soft tissue – usually referring to myofascial tissues, or any tissues which do not contain minerals (such as bone)

somatic nervous system (SNS) – section of the nervous system that oversees the motor and sensory aspects of activities under voluntary control (such as locomotion, body part movements, awareness of body part location)

spinal nerve – mixed nerve that conveys afferent and efferent transmission specifically associated with one spinal cord segment's responsibilities

stretch reflex – reflex response to protect muscle against overstretch damage by causing it to tighten; reflex arc: muscle spindle activates 1a neuron (afferent), which activates alpha motor neuron (efferent to muscle fibers being stretched)

superficial – nearer to the surface of the body; the opposite of deep

superior – toward the head

sural – pertaining to the calf of the leg

surface anatomy – the study of structures that can be identified from the outside of the body

sympathetic nervous system (SNS) – division of the ANS that takes charge in situations of danger and stress, mobilizing the body systems involved in acting effectively ("fight or flight")

symphysis – a union between two bones, formed by fibrocartilage

synchondrosis – a union between two bones, formed by either hyaline cartilage or fibrocartilage

synergist – a muscle that supports the prime mover

synovial joint – a joint containing a lubricating substance (synovial fluid) and lined with a synovial membrane or capsule

tactile – pertaining to touch

tendon – a fibrous tissue connecting skeletal muscle to bone

thigh – the portion of the lower extremity between the coxal and knee joints

thorax – the region between the neck and abdomen

tightness – shortness; denotes a slight to moderate decrease in muscle length; movement in the direction of lengthening the muscle is limited

transverse plane – a plane that divides the body into superior and inferior (or proximal and distal) portions

trunk – the part of the body to which the upper and lower extremities attach

unilateral – pertaining to one side

ventral – a synonym for anterior, usually applied to the torso

ventral nerve root – arising from the anterior horn of the spinal cord, the efferent fibers about to join into a mixed spinal nerve; also known as anterior root or motor root

Pronunciation and Etymology

Grk.	Greek	Fr.	French
L.	Latin	ME.	Middle English
AS.	Anglo-Saxon	NL.	Dutch

etymology **et**-i-**mol**-o-gee the science of the origin and development of a word

ab- (as in *abduct*)		L. away from
abdomen	**ab**-do-men	L. belly
abdominis	ab-**dah**-min-is	
abduct	**ab**-duct	L. to lead away, bring apart
acetabulum	**as**-e-**tab**-u-lum	L. a little saucer for vinegar
acromioclavicular	a-**kro**-me-o-kla-**vik**-u-lar	
acromion	a-**cro**-me-on	Grk. *akron*, top + *omos*, shoulder
ad- (as in *adduct*)		L. toward
adduct	**ad**-duct	L. to bring together
adipose	**a**-di-**pose**	L. fat, copious
alaeque	a-**le**-kwe	L. wing (*ala* of nose)
alar	**ay**-lar	
anconeus	an-**ko**-nee-us	Grk. elbow
annular	**an**-u-ler	L. ringlike
annulus	**an**-u-lus	L. ring
anococcygeal	**a**-no-kok-**si**-je-al	L. *anus*, anus + Grk. *kokkyx*, coccyx
aponeurosis	**ap**-o-nu-**ro**-sis	Grk. *apo*, from + *neuron*, nerve or tendon
appendicular	**ap**-en-**dik**-u-lar	L. to hang to
arrector pili	a-**rek**-tor **pee**-li	L. *arrector*, lifter; *pilus*, hair
artery	**ar**-ter-ee	Grk. windpipe
atlantoaxial	at-**lan**-to-**ak**-se-al	
atlantooccipital	at-**lan**-to-ok-**si**-pi-tal	
auricularis	aw-**rik**-u-**la**-ris	L. little ear
axial	**ak**-see-al	L. axle
axilla	**ak**-sil-a	L. armpit
axillary	**ak**-si-**lar**-ee	
basilic	bah-**sil**-ic	Arabic *basilik*, inner
biceps	**bi**-seps	L. *bis*, twice + *caput*, head
biceps brachii	**bi**-seps **bray**-key-i	L. two-headed (muscle) of the arm
biceps femoris	**bi**-seps fe-**mor**-is	Grk. the two-headed (muscle) of the thigh
brachial	**bray**-key-al	L. relating to the arm
brachialis	**bray**-key-**al**-is	
brachii	**bray**-key-i	L. of the arm
brachioradialis	**bray**-key-o-**ra**-de-**a**-lis	
brevis	**breh**-vis	L. short
buccinator	**buk**-sin-**aye**-tor	L. trumpeter, proclaimer
bulbospongiosus	**bul**-bo-**spon**-je-**o**-sus	L. *bulbus*, bulbous root + Gr. *spongos*, sponge
bursa	**bur**-sah	L. a purse
calcaneocuboid	kal-**ka**-ne-o-**ku**-boyd	
calcaneofibular	kal-**ka**-ne-o-**fib**-u-lar	
calcaneus	kal-**kay**-nee-us	L. heel
capillary	**kap**-i-**lar**-ee	L. hairlike
capitate	**kap**-i-tate	L. head-shaped
capitis	**kap**-i-tis	L. of the head
capitulum	ka-**pit**-u-lum	L. small head
carotid	ka-**rot**-id	Grk. causing deep sleep
carpal	**kar**-pul	Grk. pertaining to the wrist
carpi	**kar**-pi	L. of the wrist
cartilage	**kar**-ti-lij	L. gristle
cephalic	se-**fa**-lic	Grk. pertaining to the head
cervical	**ser**-vi-kal	L. referring to the neck
cervicis	**ser**-vi-sis	L. neck
chest		AS. box
cisterna chyli	sis-**turn**-a **ki**-lee	L. reservoir + Grk. juice
clavicle	**klav**-i-k'l	L. little key
coccyx	**kok**-siks	Grk. cuckoo
collateral	ko-**lat**-er-al	L. of both sides
condyle	**kon**-dial	Grk. knuckle
conoid	**ko**-noyd	Grk. cone-shaped
coracoacromial	**kor**-a-**ko**-a-**kro**-mi-ul	
coracobrachialis	**kor**-a-ko-**bra**-kee-**al**-is	
coracoclavicular	**kor**-a-**ko**-cla-**vic**-u-lar	
coracoid	**kor**-a-koyd	Grk. raven's beak
coronal	ko-**ro**-nal	L. crown-like
coronoid	**kor**-o-noyd	Grk. crown-shaped
corrugator	**kor**-u-**ga**-tor	L. together + to wrinkle
costal	**kos**-tal	L. rib
coxal	**kox**-sal	L. hip
cranio-	**cra**-nee-o	Grk. skull
cranium	**cra**-nium	Grk. skull
cremaster	kre-**mas**-ter	L. to suspend
cricoid	**kri**-koyd	Grk. ring-shaped
cruciate	**kroo**-she-at	L. cross-shaped
crural	**kroo**-ral	
cuboid	**ku**-boyd	Grk. cube-shaped
cuboideonavicular	ku-**boyd**-e-o-na-**vik**-u-lar	
cuneiform	ku-**ne**-i-form	L. *cuneus*, wedge-shaped
deltoid	**del**-toid	Grk. *delta*, capital letter *D* (Δ) in the Greek alphabet
derma	**der**-ma	L. skin
diaphragm	**di**-a-**fram**	Grk. a partition, wall
digastric	di-**gas**-trik	Grk. double-bellied
digit	**di**-jit	L. finger
digitigrade	**di**-ji-tah-grade	L. toe-walking

dorsalis pedis	***dor***-sal-is ***peh***-dis	L. *dorsum*, back; *pedis*, foot
dorsi	***dor***-si	L. of the back
dura mater	***dyoo***-ra ***ma***-ter	L. tough mother
epi-	***eh***-pee	Grk. above, upon
extrinsic		L. without
facet	***fas***-et	Fr. small face
facial	***fa***-shal	L. pertaining to the face
fascia	***fash***-ah	L. a band, bandage
fasciae	***fash***-ay	plural for fascia
fascicle	***fas***-i-kl	L. little bundle
femur	***fee***-mur	L. thigh
fibula	***fib***-u-la	L. pin or buckle
fibularis	***fib***-u-***lar***-is	L. pin or buckle
flavum	***flay***-vum	L. yellow
flex		L. to bend
foot		AS. *fot*
foramen	for-***aye***-men	L. a passage or opening
fossa	***fos***-a	L. a shallow depression
furcula	***fur***-ku-la	L. a little fork
gastrocnemius	***gas***-trok-***ne***-me-us	Grk. *gaster*, stomach + *kneme*, leg
gemellus	jem-***el***-us	L. twin
geniohyoid	***je***-ne-o-***hi***-oyd	Grk. *genion*, chin
genu valgum	***je***-noo ***val***-gum	
genu varum	***je***-noo ***va***-rum	
glabella	gla-***bel***-a	L. *glaber*, smooth
gland		L. acorn
glenoid	***glen***-oyd	Grk. eyeball
glossus	***glah***-sis	Grk. tongue
gluteus	***gloo***-te-us	Grk. *gloutos*, buttocks, which in turn is Anglo-Saxon for *buttuc*, meaning end
gracilis	gra-***cil***-is	L. slender, graceful
hallucis	***hal***-ah-sis	
hallux	***hal***-uks	L. first toe
ham		AS. haunch
hamate	***ham***-ate	L. hooked
hamulus	***ham***-u-lus	L. a small hook
humerus	***hu***-mer-us	L. upper arm
hyoid	***hi***-oyd	Grk. U-shaped
hypothenar	***hi***-po-***thee***-nar	Grk. *hypo*, under or below; *thenar*, palm, flat of the hand
iliacus	i-***lee***-a-cus	L. pertaining to the loin
iliococcygeus	***il***-ee-o-kok-***si***-je-us	
iliocostalis	***il***-ee-o-kos-***ta***-lis	L. from hip to rib
ilium	***il***-ee-um	L. groin, flank
indicis	***in***-di-kis	
inferior	in-***fe***-ree-or	L. below
infraspinatus	***in***-fra-spi-***na***-tus	
inguinal	***ing***-gwi-nal	L. of the groin
integumentary	in-***teg***-u-***ment***-ary	something that covers or encloses
interdigitate	***in***-ter-***dij***-i-tate	L. to interlock, as the fingers of clasped hands
interosseous	***in***-ter-***ah***-see-us	L. between bones
interspinalis	***in***-ter-spi-***na***-lis	
interstitial	***in***-ter-***stish***-al	L. placed between
intertransverserii	***in***-ter-trans-***verse***-er-i	
intertubercular	***in***-tur-tu-***ber***-ku-lar	
intrinsic		L. within
ischiocavernosus	***ish***-she-o-***ka***-ver-***no***-sus	
ischium	***ish***-ee-um	Grk. hip
joint		L. to join
jugular	***jug***-u-lar	L. throat
kyphosis	ki-***fo***-sis	Grk. bent, curved, or stooped
labii	***lay***-bee-eye	L. pert. to the lips
labrum	***lay***-brum	L. lip
lamina	***lam***-i-na	L. thin plate, leaf
latae	***la***-ta	L. broad
lateral	***lat***-er-al	L. to the side
latissimus dorsi	la-***tis***-i-mus ***dor***-si	L. widest of the back
levator	leh-***va***-tor	L. lifter
levator labii superioris alaeque nasi		L. "lifter of the upper lip and of the wing of the nose"
levator scapula	leh-***va***-tor ***skap***-u-la	
ligament	***lig***-a-ment	L. a band
linea aspera	***lin***-e-a ***as***-per-a	L. rough line
longissimus	lon-***jis***-i-mus	L. longest
longus colli	***long***-us ***ko***-li	L. long (muscle) of the neck
lordosis	lor-***doh***-sis	Grk. bent backward
lumbar	***lum***-bar	L. loin
lumborum	lum-***bor***-um	
lumbrical	***lum***-bri-kal	L. earthworm
lunate	***lu***-nate	L. crescent-shaped
lymph	limf	L. pure spring water
magnus	***mag***-nus	L. large
malleolus	***mal***-e-***o***-lus	L. little hammer
mandible	***man***-di-ble	L. lower jawbone
manubrium	ma-***nu***-bree-um	L. handle
masseter	***mas***-se-ter	Grk. chewer
mastoid	***mas***-toyd	Grk. breast-shaped
maxilla	***max***-il-a	L. jawbone
medial	***me***-dee-ul	L. middle
menisci	men-***is***-ki	plural for meniscus
meniscofemoral	men-***is***-ko-fem-***or***-al	
meniscus	men-***is***-kus	Grk. crescent-shaped

mentalis	men-***tal***-is	L. chin
meta-	***met***-a	Grk. after or beyond
metacarpal	***met***-a-***kar***-pul	
metacarpophalangeal	***met***-a-***kar***-po-***fa***-lan-***jee***-al	
metatarsal	***met***-a-***tar***-sal	
metatarsophalangeal	***met***-a-***tar***-so-***fa***-lan-***jee***-al	
mimetic	mi-***me***-tik	relating to, characterized by, or exhibiting mimicry
minimi	***min***-i-mee	L. smallest
multifidi	mul-***tif***-i-di	L. *fidi*, to split
muscle	***mus***-el	L. *musculus*, a little mouse
mylohyoid	***my***-lo-***hi***-oyd	Grk. *myle*, mill
myo-	***my***-o	Grk. muscle
nape		ME. the back of the neck
nasal	***na***-zl	L. nose
nasalis	na-***sa***-lis	
navicular	na-***vik***-u-lar	L. boat-shaped
neck		AS. nape
nerve		L. sinew
nuchae	***nu***-kay	L. nape of neck
nuchal	***nu***-kal	L. the back of the neck
oblique	o-***bleek***	L. diagonal, slanting
obturator	***ob***-tu-***ra***-tor	L. obstructor
occipitofrontalis	ok-***sip***-i-to-fron-***ta***-lis	
occiput	***ok***-si-put	L. the back of the skull
odontoid	o-***don***-toyd	Grk. toothlike
olecranon	o-***lek***-ran-on	Grk. elbow
omohyoid	***o***-mo-***hi***-oyd	Grk. *omos*, shoulder
opponens	o-***po***-nens	L. opposing
orbicularis oris	or-***bik***-u-***la***-ris ***o***-ris	
palpate	***pal***-pate	L. *palpare*, to touch
panniculus carnosus	pan-***ik***-u-lus car-***no***-sis	L. small, fleshy garment
parietal	puh-***ri***-e-tul	L. wall
parotid	pa-***rot***-id	Grk. beside the ear
patella	pa-***tel***-a	L. small pan
pectineus	pek-***tin***-e-us	L. comblike
pectoralis	***pek***-to-***ra***-lis	L. chest
pedicle	***ped***-i-k'l	L. a little foot
pelvis	***pel***-vis	L. basin
penis		L. tail
perineum	***per***-i-***nee***-um	Gr. space between anus and scrotum
peroneus	per-***o***-ne-us	Grk. pin, buckle
pes anserinus	pes ***an***-ser-***i***-nus	L. *pedis*, foot; L. *anserinus*, goose-like
phalanges	fa-***lan***-jeez	Grk. closely knit row, line of battle
phalanx	***fal***-anks	singular for phalanges
philtrum	***fil***-trum	Grk. to love, to kiss
piriformis	***pir***-i-***form***-is	L. pear-shaped
pisiform	***pi***-si-form	L. pea-shaped
plantar	***plan***-tar	L. the sole of the foot
plantaris	plan-***tar***-is	Fr. the sole of the foot
plantigrade	***plant***-i-grad	L. sole-walking
platysma	pla-***tiz***-ma	Grk. plate
plexus	***plek***-sus	L. interwoven
pollex	***pol***-eks	L. thumb
pollicis	***pol***-li-sis	L. thumb
popliteus	pop-***lit***-e-us	L. *poples*, ham of the knee
procerus	pro-***se***-rus	L. slender, elongated
process	***pros***-es	L. going forth
profundus	pro-***fun***-dus	L. deep
pronate	***pro***-nate	L. bent forward
psoas	***so***-as	Grk. muscle of the loin
pterygoid	***ter***-i-***goyd***	Grk. wing-shaped
pubis	***pu***-bis	NL. bone of the groin
pubococcygeus	***pu***-bo-kok-***si***-je-us	
puborectalis	***pu***-bo-rek-***tal***-is	
quadratus	kwod-***rait***-us	L. squared, four-sided
quadratus lumborum	***kwod***-rait-us lum-***bor***-um	L. four-sided muscle of the lumbar region
quadriceps	***kwod***-ri-seps	L. four-headed
quadruped		Grk. four-footed
radiocapitate	***ray***-dee-o-***kap***-i-tate	
radioscapholunate	***ray***-dee-o-***skaf***-o-***loo***-nate	
radiotriquetrum	***ray***-dee-o-tri-***kwe***-trum	
radius	***ray***-dee-us	L. staff, spoke of a wheel
ramus	***ray***-mus	L. branch
rectus	***rek***-tus	L. straight
retinacula	***ret***-i-***nak***-u-la	plural for retinaculum
retinaculum	***ret***-i-***nak***-u-lum	L. halter, band, rope
rhomboid	***rom***-boyd	Grk. in geometry, a parallelogram with oblique angles and only the opposite sides equal
risorius	ri-***so***-re-us	L. to laugh
rotatores	***ro***-ta-***tor***-ays	L. plural for rotator
sacrococcygeal	***sa***-kro-kok-***sij***-e-al	
sacrotuberous	***sa***-kro-***tu***-ber-us	
sacrum	***sa***-krum	L. sacred or holy thing, from the use of the sacrum in Roman animal sacrifice
sagittal	***saj***-i-tal	L. arrow-like
saphenous	***sa***-fe-nus	origin unclear, perhaps Arabic *saphin*, standing; or Greek *saphen*, clearly visible

sartorius	sar-***tor***-ee-us	L. *sartor,* tailor
scalene	***skay***-leen	Grk. uneven
scaphoid	***skaf***-oyd	L. boat-shaped
scapula	***skap***-u-la	L. shoulder blade
scapulae	***skap***-u-lay	plural for scapula
sciatic	si-***at***-ik	Grk. *ischion,* hip joint
sciatica	si-***at***-ika	L. suffering in the hip
semimembranosus	***sem***-eye-***mem***-bra-***no***-sus	L. half membranous
semispinalis	***sem***-eye-spi-***na***-lis	L. half spinal
semitendinosus	***sem***-eye-***ten***-di-***no***-sus	L. half tendinous
septa	***sep***-ta	plural for septum
septum	***sep***-tum	L. enclosure
serratus	ser-***a***-tus	L. notched
sesamoid	***ses***-a-moyd	L. resembling a sesame seed
skeleton	***skel***-et-on	Grk. dried up
skull		ME. bow
soleus	so-***lay***-us	L. *solea,* as in a sole fish
sphenoid	***sfe***-noyd	Grk. wedge-shaped
spinalis capitis	***spi***-na-lis ***kap***-i-tis	
spinalis cervicis	***spi***-na-lis ***ser***-vi-sis	
spine		L. thorn
splenius	***sple***-nee-us	Grk. bandage
splenius capitis	***sple***-nee-us ***kap***-i-tis	L. bandage-like (muscle) of the head
splenius cervicis	***sple***-nee-us ***ser***-vi-sis	
stapedius	sta-***pe***-de-us	L. stirrup
sternoclavicular	***ster***-no-kla-***vik***-u-lar	
sternocleidomastoid	***ster***-no-***kli***-do-***mas***-toyd	
sternohyoid	***ster***-no-***hi***-oyd	
sternothyroid	***ster***-no-***thi***-royd	
sternum	***ster***-num	Grk. chest
stylohyoid	***sti***-lo-***hi***-oyd	
styloid	***sti***-loyd	Grk. a pillar
subclavius	sub-***klay***-vee-us	
subscapularis	sub-***skap***-u-***lar***-is	
supercilii	su-per-***sil***-i-i	L. above eyelid
superficialis	***soo***-per-***fish***-ee-***a***-lis	L. on the surface
supinate	***su***-pi-nate	L. bent backward
supraspinatus	***soo***-pra-spi-***na***-tus	
sural	***soo***-ral	
sustentaculum	***sus***-ten-***tak***-u-lum	L. support
suture	***su***-chur	L. a seam
symphysis	***sim***-fi-sis	Grk. growing together
synchondrosis	***sin***-con-***dro***-sis	
synovial	sin-***o***-ve-al	L. *synovia,* joint fluid
talocalcaneal	***ta***-lo-kal-***ka***-ne-al	
talocrural	***ta***-lo-***kroo***-ral	L. ankle + *crus,* leg
talofibular	***ta***-lo-***fib***-u-lar	
talonavicular	***ta***-lo-na-***vik***-u-lar	
talus	***ta***-lus	L. ankle
tarsal	***tar***-sul	Grk. wicker basket
temporalis	***tem***-po-***ra***-lis	L. time, seen by the graying of hairs in this region
tendon	***ten***-dun	L. to stretch
tensor	***ten***-sor	L. a stretcher
teres	***teh***-reez	L. rounded, finely shaped
tertius	***ter***-she-us	L. third
thenar	***thee***-nar	Grk. palm, flat of the hand
thoracic	tho-***ras***-ik	Grk. chest
thoracolumbar	tho-***rak***-o-***lum***-bar	
thorax	***tho***-raks	Grk. chest
thyrohyoid	***thi***-ro-***hi***-oyd	
thyroid	***thi***-royd	Grk. shield
tibia	***tib***-e-a	L. shinbone
-tome	tohm	L. *tomus,* section
trachea	***tray***-ke-a	Grk. rough
tract		L. extent, drawn out
transverse	***trans***-verse	L. across, turned across
transversospinalis	trans-***ver***-so-spi-***nal***-is	
trapezium	tra-***pee***-ze-um	Grk. little table
trapezius	tra-***pee***-ze-us	Grk. a little table or trapezoid shape
trapezoid	***trap***-e-zoyd	Grk. table-shaped
triceps brachii	***tri***-seps ***bray***-key-i	L. three-headed muscle of the arm
triceps surae	***tri***-seps ***sir***-eye	L. three-headed muscle of the calf
triquetrum	tri-***kwe***-trum	L. three-cornered
trochanter	tro-***kan***-ter	Grk. to run
trochlea	***trok***-lee-ah	Grk. pulley
tubercle	***tu***-ber-kl	L. a little swelling
tuberosity	***tu***-ber-***os***-i-tee	L. a swelling
ulna	***ul***-na	L. elbow, arm
ulnolunate	***ul***-no-***lu***-nate	
ulnotriquetrum	***ul***-no-tri-***kwe***-trum	
umbilicus	um-***bil***-i-kus	L. navel, center
urethral	u-***ree***-thral	relating to the urethra
uvula	***uv***-u-la	L. a little grape
vastus	***vas***-tus	L. vast
vein		L. vessel
vertebra	***ver***-ta-bra	L. joint
xiphoid	***zif***-oyd	Grk. sword-shaped
zona orbicularis	***zo***-na or-***bik***-u-***lar***-is	L. girdle + little circle
zygapophyseal	***zy***-gah-***pof***-i-se-al	
zygomatic	***zy***-go-***mat***-ik	Grk. cheekbone
zygomaticus	***zy***-go-***mat***-i-kus	Grk. cheekbone

Bibliography

Alexander, R. McNeill. *The Human Machine*. New York: Columbia University Press, 1992.

Anson, Barry J. *An Atlas of Human Anatomy*. Philadelphia: W. Saunders, 1963.

Asimov, Isaac. *The Human Body: Its Structure and Operation*. Boston: Houghton Mifflin, 1963.

Backhouse, Kenneth M., and Ralph T. Hutchings. *Color Atlas of Surface Anatomy*. Baltimore: Williams & Wilkins, 1986.

Bates, Barbara. *A Guide to Physical Examination and History Taking*. 4th ed. Philadelphia: J. B. Lippincott, 1987.

Bergman, Ronald A., Sue Ann Thompson, and Adel K. Afifi. *Catalog of Human Variation*. Baltimore: Urban & Schwarzenberg, 1984.

Bodanis, David. *The Body Book: A Fantastic Voyage to the World Within*. Boston: Little, Brown, 1984.

Calais-Germain, Blandine. *Anatomy of Movement*. Seattle: Eastland Press, 2007.

Cartmill, Matt, William L. Hylander, and James Shafland. *Human Structure*. Cambridge, MA: Harvard University Press, 1987.

Chaitow, Leon. *Palpatory Literacy*. London: Thorsons, 1991.

Chaitow, Leon. *Palpatory Skills*. New York: Churchill Livingstone, 1987.

Clay, James H., and David M. Pounds. *Basic Clinical Massage Therapy: Integrating Anatomy and Treatment*. 2nd ed. Baltimore: Lippincott Williams & Wilkins, 2008.

Clemente, Carmine D. *Anatomy: A Regional Atlas of the Human Body*. 3rd ed. Baltimore: Urban & Schwarzenberg, 1987.

Clemente, Carmine D. *Gray's Anatomy*. 30th ed. Philadelphia: Lea & Febiger, 1985.

Craig, Marjorie. *Miss Craig's Face-Saving Exercises*. New York: Random House, 1970.

Cyriax, J. H., and P. J. Cyriax. *Cyriax's Illustrated Manual of Orthopaedic Medicine*. 2nd ed. Oxford: Butterworth-Heinemann, 1992.

Dorland's Illustrated Medical Dictionary. 24th ed. Philadelphia: W. B. Saunders, 1965.

Duin, Nancy, and Jenny Sutcliffe. *A History of Medicine: From Prehistory to the Year 2020*. New York: Barnes & Noble, 1992.

Eaton, Theodore, Jr. *Comparative Anatomy of the Vertebrates*. 2nd ed. New York: Harper & Bros., 1960.

Ekman, Paul. *Darwin and Facial Expression: A Century of Research in Review*. Cambridge, MA: Malor Books, 2006.

Ekman, Paul. *Emotions Revealed: Recognizing Faces and Feelings to Improve Communication and Emotional Life*. 2nd ed. New York: Henry Holt, 2007.

Faigin, Gary. *The Artist's Complete Guide to Facial Expression*. New York: Watson-Guptill, 1990.

Federative Committee on Anatomical Terminology. *Terminologia Anatomica*. Stuttgart: Thieme, 1998.

Feher, Gyorgy, and Andras Szunyoghy. *Cyclopedia Anatomicae*. New York: Black Dog & Leventhal, 1996.

Field, E. J., and R. J. Harrison. *Anatomical Terms: Their Origin and Derivation*. Cambridge, UK: W. Heffer & Sons, 1947.

Gebo, D. L. "Plantigrady and Foot Adaptation in African Apes: Implications for Hominid Origins." *American Journal of Physical Anthropology* 89, no. 1 (September 1992): 29–58.

Gehin, Alain. *Atlas of Manipulative Techniques for the Cranium and Face*. Seattle: Eastland Press, 1985.

Greene, Lauriann. *Save Your Hands! Injury Prevention for Massage Therapists*. Seattle: Infinity Press, 1995.

Gross, Jeffrey, Joseph Fetto, and Elaine Rosen. *Musculoskeletal Examination*. Malden, MA: Blackwell Sciences, 1996.

Guillen, Michael. *Five Equations That Changed the World: The Power and Poetry of Mathematics*. New York: Hyperion, 1995.

Hamrick, M. W., and S. E. Inouye. "Thumbs, Tools, and Early Humans." *Science* 268, no. 5210 (April 1995): 586–87.

Handy, Chester L. "A History of Cranial Osteopathy." *Journal of the American Osteopathic Association* 47, no. 5 (January 1948): 269–72.

Hertling, Darlene, and Randoph M. Kessler. *Management of Common Musculoskeletal Disorders: Physical Therapy Principles and Methods*. 3rd ed. Philadelphia: Lippincott Williams & Wilkins, 1996.

Hildebrand, Milton. *Analysis of Vertebrate Structure*. 4th ed. New York: John Wiley & Sons, 1995.

Hole, John W. *Essentials of Human Anatomy and Physiology*. 4th ed. Dubuque, IA: Wm. C. Brown, 1992.

Hoppenfeld, Stanley. *Physical Examination of the Spine and Extremities*. East Norwalk, CT: Appleton-Century-Crofts, 1976.

Jamieson, E. B. *Illustrations of Regional Anatomy, Sections I–VII*. Edinburgh: E. & S. Livingstone, 1946.

Jenkins, David B. *Hollinshead's Functional Anatomy of the Limbs and Back*. 6th ed. Philadelphia: W. B. Saunders, 1991.

Juhan, Deane. *Job's Body: A Handbook for Bodywork*. Barrytown, NY: Barrytown/Station Hill, 1987.

Kapandji, I. A. *The Physiology of the Joints, Volumes 1, 2, & 3*. 5th ed. Edinburgh: Churchill Livingstone, 1982.

Kapit, Wynn, and Lawrence M. Elson. *The Anatomy Coloring Book*. 2nd ed. New York: HarperCollins, 1993.

Kendall, Florence Peterson, Elizabeth Kendall McCreary, Patricia Geise Provance, Mary McIntyre Rodgers, and William Anthony Romani. *Muscles: Testing and Function with Posture and Pain*. 5th ed. Baltimore: Lippincott Williams & Wilkins, 2005.

Kent, George. *Comparative Anatomy of the Vertebrates*. 6th ed. St. Louis, MO: Mosby, 1987.

Koch, Tankred. *Anatomy of the Chicken and Domestic Birds*. Ames: Iowa State University Press, 1973.

Lumley, John S. P. *Surface Anatomy: The Anatomical Basis of Clinical Examination*. Edinburgh: Churchill Livingstone, 1990.

Luttgens, Kathryn, and Katharine Wells. *Kinesiology: Scientific Basis of Human Motion*. Philadelphia: Saunders, 1982.

MacClintock, Dorcas. *A Natural History of Giraffes*. New York: Charles Scribner's Sons, 1973.

Magee, David J. *Orthopedic Physical Assessment*. 2nd ed. Philadelphia: W. B. Saunders, 1992.

Marzke, M. W. "Evolutionary Development of the Human Thumb." *Hand Clinics* 8, no. 1 (February 1992): 1–8.

McAleer, Neil. *The Body Almanac: Mind-Boggling Facts About Today's Human Body and High-Tech Medicine*. New York: Doubleday, 1985.

McMinn, R. M. H., and R. T. Hutchings. *Color Atlas of Human Anatomy*. Chicago: Year Book Medical Publishers, 1985.

Melloni, John. *Melloni's Illustrated Dictionary of the Musculoskeletal System*. New York: Parthenon, 1998.

Montagna, William. *Comparative Anatomy*. New York: John Wiley & Sons, 1970.

Moore, Keith L. *Clinically Oriented Anatomy*. 3rd ed. Baltimore: Williams & Wilkins, 1992.

Muscolino, Joseph E. *The Muscle and Bone Palpation Manual*. St. Louis, MO: Mosby Elsevier, 2009.

Myers, Thomas W. *Anatomy Trains: Myofascial Meridians for Manual and Movement Therapists*. 2nd ed. Edinburgh: Churchill Livingstone Elsevier, 2009.

Napier, John. *Hands*. Princeton, NJ: Princeton University Press, 1993.

Netter, Frank. *Atlas of Human Anatomy*. Summit, NJ: CIBA-GEIGY, 1989.

Neumann, Donald A. *Kinesiology of the Musculoskeletal System: Foundations for Physical Rehabilitation*. St. Louis, MO: Mosby, 2002.

Norkin, Cynthia C., and Pamela K. Levangie. *Joint Structure and Function: A Comprehensive Analysis*. 2nd ed. Philadelphia: F. A. Davis, 1992.

Oliver, Marcelo V. *Rapid Review: Anatomy Reference Guide*. Skokie, IL: Anatomical Chart Company, 1996.

Olsen, Andrea. *Bodystories: A Guide to Experiential Anatomy*. Barrytown, NY: Station Hill, 1991.

Olsen, Todd. *A.D.A.M: Student Atlas of Anatomy*. Baltimore: Williams & Wilkins, 1996.

Parker, Steve. *Natural World*. London: Dorling Kindersley, 1994.

Peck, Stephen Rogers. *Atlas of Human Anatomy for the Artist*. Oxford: Oxford University Press, 1982.

Platzer, Werner. *Color Atlas of Human Anatomy, Volume 1: Locomotor System*. 5th ed. Stuttgart: Thieme, 2004.

Rohen, Johannes, and Chihiro Yokochi. *Color Atlas of Anatomy*. 3rd ed. New York: Igaku-Shoin Medical Publishers, 1993.

Rolf, Ida. *Rolfing and Physical Reality*. Rochester, VT: Healing Arts Press, 1990.

Rolf, Ida P. *Rolfing: The Integration of Human Structures*. New York: Harper & Row, 1977.

Schider, Fritz. *An Atlas of Anatomy for Artists*. 3rd ed. New York: Dover Publications, 1957.

Schultz, R. Louis, and Rosemary Feitis. *The Endless Web: Fascial Anatomy and Physical Reality*. Berkeley, CA: North Atlantic Books, 1996.

Searfoss, Glenn. *Skulls and Bones: A Guide to Skeletal Structures and Behavior of North American Mammals*. Mechanicsburg, PA: Stackpole Books, 1995.

Seig, Kay W., and Sandra P. Adams. *Illustrated Essentials of Musculoskeletal Anatomy*. 2nd ed. Gainesville, FL: Megabooks, 1993.

Simons, David G., Janet G. Travell, and Lois S. Simons. *Myofascial Pain and Dysfunction: The Trigger Point Manual, Volume 1*. 2nd ed. Baltimore: Lippincott Williams & Wilkins, 1999.

Stern, Jack T. *Core Concepts in Anatomy*. Boston: Little, Brown, 1997.

Stern, Jack T. *Essentials of Gross Anatomy*. Philadelphia: F. A. Davis, 1988.

Stone, Robert J., and Judith A. Stone. *Atlas of Skeletal Muscles*. Dubuque, IA: Wm. C. Brown, 1990.

Taber's Cyclopedic Medical Dictionary. 17th ed. Philadelphia: F. A. Davis, 1993.

Thompson, Clem W. *Manual of Structural Kinesiology*. 11th ed. St. Louis, MO: Times Mirror/Mosby College, 1989.

Todd, Mabel Elsworth. *The Thinking Body*. Brooklyn, NY: Dance Horizons, 1979.

Tortora, Gerard J., and Bryan Derrickson. *Principles of Anatomy and Physiology*. 11th ed. Hoboken, NJ: John Wiley & Sons, 2006.

Traupman, John. *The New College Latin and English Dictionary*. New York: Bantam Books, 1995.

Travell, Janet G., and David G. Simons. *Myofascial Pain and Dysfunction: The Trigger Point Manual, Volume 1*. Baltimore: Williams & Wilkins, 1999.

Travell, Janet G., and David G. Simons. *Myofascial Pain and Dysfunction: The Trigger Point Manual, Volume 2*. Baltimore: Williams & Wilkins, 1992.

Upledger, John E., and Jon D. Vredevoogd. *Craniosacral Therapy*. Seattle: Eastland Press, 1983.

Walker, Judith. *NeuroMuscular Therapy I–IV*. St. Petersburg, FL: International Academy of NMT, 1994.

Walker, Warren F. *Functional Anatomy of the Vertebrates: An Evolutionary Perspective*. Fort Worth, TX: Saunders, 1987.

Walker, Warren F., and Dominique G. Homberger. *A Study of the Cat with Reference to Human Beings*. 5th ed. Fort Worth, TX: Saunders, 1993.

Way, Robert F. *Dog Anatomy—Illustrated*. New York: Dreenan Press, 1974.

Zihlman, Adrienne. *The Human Evolution Coloring Book*. New York: Harper & Row, 1982.

Index

Page numbers in **bold** refer to a principal treatment on a subject.
Page numbers in *italics* refer to illustrations.

D

E

F

K

L

M

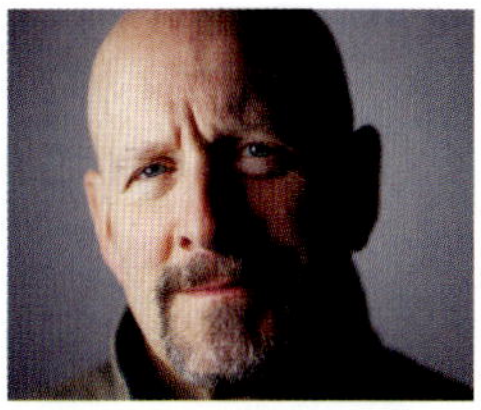

About the Author

Andrew Biel is author of the best-selling textbook *Trail Guide to the Body* and *Trail Guide to Movement*. He has served on the faculties of Boulder College of Massage Therapy and Seattle Massage School and has taught Cadaver Studies for Bodyworkers at Bastyr Naturopathic University. He lives outside of Port Townsend, Washington, with his family—Lyn, Grace, and Elias.

About the Illustrator

Robin Dorn's background as a medical illustrator and licensed massage practitioner gives her the unique ability to create vibrant and detailed anatomical illustrations for *Trail Guide* textbooks. She exhibits her artwork on the West Coast and in France.

Andrew and Robin are also the author and illustrator of two children's books entitled *Lily and Mr. Bones* and *The Tale of Scrawny Billy J.*

Trail Guide to the Body Student Workbook

Great for self-testing, homework, and preparing for national exams.

Improve your memory of anatomical structures by actively working with matching exercises, answering fill-in-the-blank questions, and coloring anatomical drawings. This companion to *Trail Guide to the Body* helps you test your knowledge and retention of information presented in the textbook. It is an outstanding study tool for national exams.

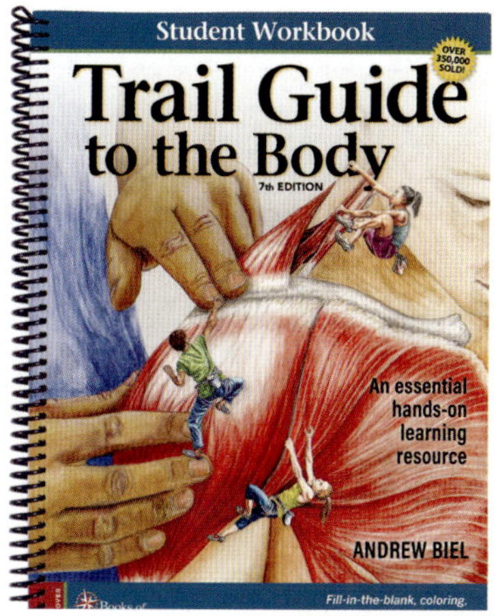

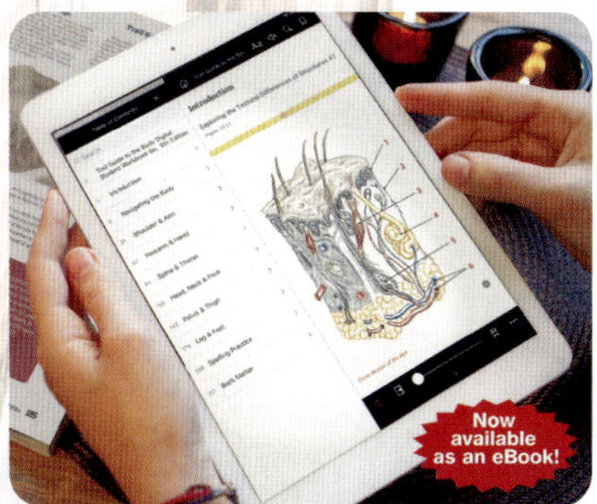

Trail Guide to the Body Digital Student Workbook

The *Digital Student Workbook* is packed with features for students to test their knowledge and increase their retention of information presented in *Trail Guide to the Body*. Convenient and engaging, it includes ways to self-test and re-test: labeling anatomical structures, completing matching exercises, and coloring anatomical drawings.

Trail Guide to the Body eTextbook + Videos

Bring your eTextbook everywhere you go!

Enjoy the same stellar content found in your textbook as an enhanced interactive eTextbook:

- Watch palpation videos directly in your eTextbook
- Bookmark favorite pages
- Enlarge images
- Highlight key information
- Make notes
- Navigate directly to chapters and terms from the Table of Contents
- Search for terms and definitions

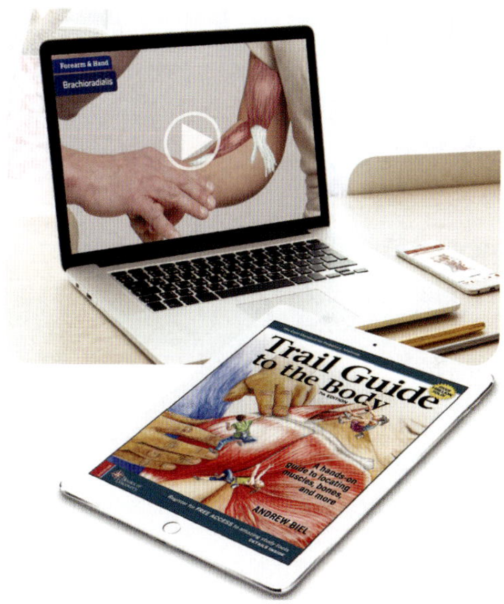

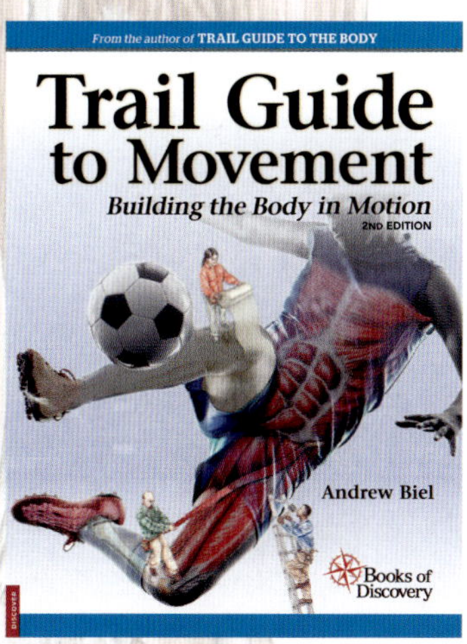

Also available as an eBook!

Trail Guide to Movement

An award-winning textbook revealing the inner workings of the body in motion.

Join author Andrew Biel on a unique and fascinating journey as he helps you build—step by step—a human body in motion! Instead of dissecting the body into smaller, isolated pieces, *Trail Guide to Movement* takes the unique approach of building the body into larger, interconnected components. This award-winning textbook is written with the same encouraging voice and subtle humor as the iconic *Trail Guide to the Body*, making the study of human movement easy to understand, captivating, and memorable. With the purchase of *Trail Guide to Movement*, students gain free access to videos that augment lessons found in the text.

Bones: Quick Reference Index

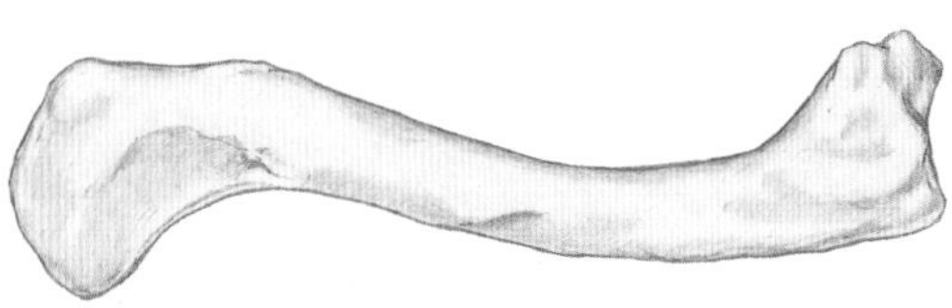